N-MULTISIX®

REAGENT STRIPS FOR URINANALYSIS

DIRECTIONS:
Must be followed exactly.

1. Dip test areas of strip in FRESH, *well-mixed*, uncentrifuged urine. Remove immediately.

2. While removing, run the edge of the strip against the rim of the urine container to remove excess urine. Hold the strip in a horizontal position to prevent possible mixing of chemicals from adjacent reagent areas and/or soiling of hands with urine.

3. Compare test areas closely to corresponding Color Charts at times specified.

PLEASE READ PACKAGE INSERT BEFORE USE.

Ames Division **MILES**

Ames Division, Miles Laboratories, Inc.
P.O. Box 70, Elkhart, Indiana 46515

© 1979 Miles Laboratories, Inc.
3109   R7119   55M

		NORMAL				Ehrlich units/dl urine	
UROBILINOGEN	45 sec.	0.1 / 1		2	4	8	12
NITRITE	40 sec.	NEGATIVE			POSITIVE (any degree of uniform pink color)		
BLOOD	25 sec.	NEGATIVE	NON-HEMOLYZED TRACE / HEMOLYZED TRACE		SMALL +	MODERATE ++	LARGE +++
BILIRUBIN	20 sec.	NEGATIVE			SMALL +	MODERATE ++	LARGE +++
KETONE	15 sec.	NEGATIVE			SMALL +	MODERATE ++	LARGE +++
GLUCOSE	10 sec. qual / 30 sec. quan	g/dl NEGATIVE	1/10 TRACE	1/4 +	1/2 ++	1 +++	2 or more ++++
PROTEIN	TIME NOT CRITICAL MAY BE READ IMMEDIATELY	mg/dl NEGATIVE	TRACE	30 +	100 ++	300 +++	over 2000 ++++
pH	NEAREST HANDLE		5	6	7	8	9

Many simple tests can be done during an office visit to aid the physician in diagnosis. Urine may be analyzed with reagent strips for correct levels of not only glucose, but many other components. (Courtesy of Ames Division of Miles Laboratories, Inc.)

(The color reproductions on these pages are for illustrative purposes only and must not be used to analyze actual test results)

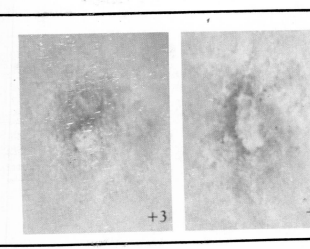

+3   +4

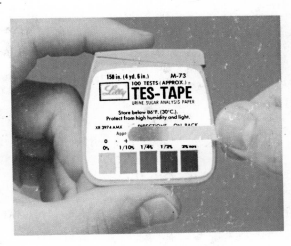

It is important for diabetics to have an immediate, accurate indication of urine sugar level. The patient can be counseled in the use of Tes-Tape®, as shown. (Courtesy of Eli Lilly and Company.)

6TH EDITION

THE MEDICAL ASSISTANT

ADMINISTRATIVE AND CLINICAL

MARY E. KINN, CPS, CMA-A

Assistant Professor, Health Technologies, Retired,
Long Beach City College, Long Beach, California;

Past President, American Association of Medical Assistants;

Former Chairman, American Association of Medical Assistants Certifying Board

ELEANOR F. DERGE, RN, MS, CMA

Formerly Program Director, Medical Assisting Program;
Instructor, Medical Assisting Program,
Madison Area Technical College,
Madison, Wisconsin

with special assistance from

KAREN LANE, CMA-AC

Chairperson, Curriculum Review Board of the
American Association of Medical Assistants Endowment;
Education Consultant, Baltimore, Maryland

1988
W. B. SAUNDERS COMPANY
Harcourt, Brace Jovanovich, Inc.
Philadelphia   London   Toronto   Montreal   Sydney   Tokyo

W. B. SAUNDERS COMPANY
Harcourt Brace Jovanovich, Inc.

The Curtis Center
Independence Square West
Philadelphia, PA 19106

Library of Congress Cataloging-in-Publication Data

Kinn, Mary E.
The medical assistant: administrative and clinical/Mary E.
Kinn, Eleanor F. Derge; with special assistance by
Karen Lane.—6th ed.
   p. cm.

Rev. ed. of: The medical office assistant/Portia M.
Frederick, Mary E. Kinn. 5th ed. 1981.
Bibliography: p.
Includes index.

1. Medical assistants.   I. Derge, Eleanor F.
   II. Lane, Karen, 1946.   III. Frederick, Portia M.
   Medical office assistant.   IV. Title.   [DNLM: 1.
   Allied Health Personnel.   2. Medical
   Secretaries.   W 80 K55m]

R728.8.K493 1988   610.73′7—dc19   88–11445 CIP

ISBN 0–7216–1731–X

DNLM/DLC
for Library of Congress

Editor: Dudley Kay
Developmental Editor: Frances T. Mues
Designer: W. B. Saunders Staff
Production Manager: Frank Polizzano
Manuscript Editor: Gina Scala
Illustrator: Sharon Iwanczuk
Illustration Coordinator: Walt Verbitski
Cover Designer: Charlotte Kay
Indexer: Kathleen Mason

The Medical Assistant: Administrative and Clinical   ISBN 0–7216–1731-X

Last digit is the print number: 9   8   7   6   5   4   3   2   1

PREFACE

In preparing the sixth edition, the authors have kept foremost in their thoughts the standard of excellence established by Portia M. Frederick, one of the original co-authors of this text. Her legacy remains apparent in this revision, and the authors acknowledge with gratitude her contribution to the profession of medical assisting and to this text.

The increasing complexity of providing medical care and the governmental regulations imposed upon medical practice have placed more responsibility on the medical assistant than ever before. The goal of this completely revised edition of *The Medical Assistant* is to continue helping educational institutions and practicing medical assistants meet the challenge of their increased responsibilities. Nearly every chapter has been rewritten and reorganized to include the most up-to-date information. The authors have incorporated the latest principles of competency-based evaluation throughout the text. An entirely new format offers an exciting visual presentation and a writing style that are easier for the reader to follow. **The authors have addressed all the administrative and clinical competencies of the 1984 DACUM Analysis of the Medical Assisting Profession to ensure achievement of the basic entry-level skills of the medical assistant.**

ORGANIZATION AND CONTENT

The text is organized into thirty-nine chapters in three sections that cover the major administrative and clinical responsibilities of the medical assistant. The authors have found the sequence of the chapters, as presented, to be practical in their experience as instructors. However, classroom presentation of chapters can easily be rearranged to meet the needs of students and instructors in any medical assisting program. Content within the chapters progresses from the simple to the complex, enabling the student to build on previously learned skills.

In Section I, Chapters 1 through 5 provide the necessary background information for understanding the significance of being a member of a service profession, a brief history of medicine and the evolution of medical practice, facts about specialty practices, ethics as applied to physicians and medical assistants, and the legal responsibilities of medical practice.

In Section II, Chapters 6 through 20 describe specific administrative skills performed by the medical assistant, directions for performing these skills, ways of streamlining the overall administration of a medical practice, and practical management procedures that may become a part of the medical assistant's responsibilities, including an entirely new chapter, The Computer in Medical Practice. The final chapter in this section explains the externship portion of the training program and the steps for a student to follow in applying for, interviewing for, and performing in a new position.

In Section III, Chapters 21 through 39 cover basic clinical medical assisting principles and procedures. Chapters 21 through 24 present basic concepts and procedures related to nutrition, disease transmission, asepsis, and identification and care of instruments. These chapters prepare the student for more specific clinical duties, such as administration of medications, assisting with examinations and surgery, and performing laboratory procedures, which are covered in Chapters 25 through 38. The final chapter introduces the student to first aid and medical emergencies commonly encountered in medical practices.

SPECIAL FEATURES OF THE SIXTH EDITION

Completely updated in both content and format, this new edition offers numerous features that help make specific information more readily available to both instructors and students:

- A vocabulary list at the beginning of each chapter, with vocabulary words highlighted in boldface type within the chapter and complete definitions in the Glossary at the end of the book.
- Learning objectives for both didactic and practical application at the beginning of each chapter.
- Numerous new illustrations and tables to enhance the reader's understanding of text content.
- Important information highlighted in lists and color.
- Illustrated step-by-step procedures covering all essential entry-level skills of the medical assistant and containing *terminal performance objectives* with conditions and standards of acceptable performance stated in measurable terms.

Highlights of revisions covering *administrative* medical assisting duties include

- Incorporation of instructions on using the telephone and on processing the mail into one chapter, Chapter 9, Oral Communications.
- Combination of The Patient Record and Records Management into Chapter 11, Medical Records Management.
- Additional detailed instructions for operating a pegboard accounting system in Chapter 13, Accounting Systems.
- New material on coding systems, cost containment, prepaid insurance plans, diagnosis-related groups (DRGs), and prospective payment systems in Chapter 16, Health and Accident Insurance.
- Relocation of payroll procedures to Chapter 19, Management Responsibilities, where the reader will also find new material on practice development, patient education, and personnel management.

Highlights of revisions covering *clinical* medical assisting duties include

- Up-to-date information on prevention of disease transmission, especially of hepatitis and AIDS, covered in Chapter 22, Basic Concepts of Asepsis, and Appendix C and incorporated throughout the individual clinical procedures.
- New, easy-to-read approach to clinical pharmacology, with emphasis on drug interactions within the body and procedures for calculating drug dosages for administration to patients, in Chapter 26, Introduction to Clinical Pharmacology.
- Expansion of discussions on laboratory procedures to cover more thoroughly essentials of microbiology, specimen collection, urinalysis, hematology, and electrocardiography, in Chapters 33 through 37. Many medical assisting programs can now eliminate the use of supplemental monographs and textbooks on laboratory procedures.
- Completely updated procedures for first aid and life-threatening emergencies, such as cardiac arrest, based on recommendations of the American Red Cross and the American Heart Association, in Chapter 39, First Aid and Medical Emergencies.
- New quick reference tables that summarize important concepts discussed in the chapters, including clinical and laboratory procedures and testing.

Computers are becoming ever more important in the practice of medicine. To help students and practicing medical assistants who are inexperienced with computers, the authors have added a new chapter, The Computer in Medical Practice. Written simply, the chapter introduces the reader to the elementary language of computers and their various components, provides an overview of the application of computers in the medical facility, and offers brief guidelines on the selection and care of computer systems.

Recognizing that acquired immune deficiency syndrome (AIDS) has become a major health threat, the authors have made every effort to include the most current precautions for prevention of AIDS transmission. Special precautions have been stated in each procedure, where appropriate. Appendix C summarizes the most current recommendations for the prevention of AIDS transmission, providing immediate access to procedures needed to protect medical assistants, other health care workers, and patients alike.

SUPPLEMENTARY MATERIALS

To further aid students and instructors, the authors have also completely revised the *Student Review and Activities Manual*, which includes review questions, forms and instructions for the Procedures presented in the text, and checklists for measuring achievement of the objectives.

The *Instructor's Manual* includes answers to the review questions and suggestions for additional student activities.

ACKNOWLEDGMENTS

Thanks are due the following persons and organizations for providing valuable suggestions, comments, and support during the revision of this text:

Patricia Nelles, CMA, former medical assisting instructor, and owner-operator of Town and Country Personnel Agency, Orange, California, for planning and accessing the photographs by Dan Santucci, and for sharing her expertise in interviewing and hiring for medical facilities.

Marjorie Slaymaker, AAMA Past President, Clinic Manager, Axtell Clinic, Wichita, Kansas, who provided valuable information regarding the group practice of medicine.

Jeanine Verbinski, Medical Insurance Exchange of California, San Francisco, for providing information on professional liability, and for reviewing the chapter on Medicine and the Law.

Don Goethals, Medical Data Management, Glendora, California, for consultations and for illustrations showing the uses of computers in medical practice.

Bibbero Systems, Petaluma, California, and Colwell Systems, Inc., Champaign, Illinois, for their generous support in providing sample forms for illustrating various procedures.

Jack Jackson, owner-operator of Custom Recovery Systems, Santa Ana, California, for his continued interest and review of information on collection practices.

Marilyn Fordney, CMA-AC, CMT, Oxnard, California, author of *Insurance Handbook for the Medical Office*, published by W. B. Saunders Company, for her friendly sharing of information researched for the *Insurance Handbook*.

Regina Masters, CMA, MEd, Instructor, Medical Assisting Program, University of Toledo Community and Technical College, Toledo, Ohio, for reviewing the chapter on Computers in Medical Practice.

Elizabeth Stone, Medical Editor/Writer, and Jeanne Spala, Medical Librarian, Centinela Hospital Medical Center, Inglewood, California, for assistance in preparing the chapter on Editorial Duties.

Janet Parry, RN, President, Medical Management Consultants, Inc., Anaheim, California, for critiquing the discussions of Management Responsibilities and Finding the Right Position.

Teddi Pina, CMA-AC, Medical Assistant Instructor, Fresno, California; Diana Bennett, RN, MA, Program Chairperson, Medical Assisting Program, Indiana Vocational Technical College, Indianapolis, Indiana; and Carol D. Warden, CMA-A, PhD, Coordinator, Medical Assisting, Highline Community College, Midway, Washington, for reviewing the entire administrative portion of the manuscript.

The California Medical Assistants Association, the California Association of Medical Assistant Instructors, and the American Medical Writers Association, for the privilege of membership, from all of whom I have received information on current practices, personal guidance, and, more important, the inspiration to continue this endeavor.

Mary E. Kinn

I wish to thank the following persons and organizations for their valuable comments and support during the revision of this text:

Kathleen Moody, MT(ASCP), Instructor, Medical Assisting and Medical Laboratory Technician Programs, Madison Area Technical College, Madison, Wisconsin, for her original contributions to Chapters 22 and 33 through 37, for her photographs and drawings, and for taking the time to pose for my camera.

Virginia Cascio, MT(ASCP), MS, CMA, former Program Director, Medical Assisting and Medical Laboratory Technician Programs, and current Instructor, Medical Assisting Program, Madison Area Technical College, Madison, Wisconsin, for her reviews, suggestions, and organization of the chapters on medical laboratory procedures for the text, *Student Review Manual,* and *Instructor's Manual.*

Jean Hodge, RN, Supervisor of Central Service, Meriter-Methodist Hospital, Madison, Wisconsin, and President of the Wisconsin Association and Central Service Technicians, for current equipment, supplies, and techniques related to sanitization, disinfection, and sterilization.

Walter Washburn, MD, FACFP, Medical Director, Medical Assisting Program, Madison Area Technical College and Maureen Saunders, CMA, Physician's Plus-Odana Clinic, Madison, Wisconsin, for their suggestions and guidance in all areas of the clinical portion of the text.

David Goodman, MD, Medic-East Urgent Care Clinic, Madison, Wisconsin; Calvin J. Williams, BS, EMT Instructor, and Rich Holmes, MS, EMT Instructor, both at Madison Area Technical College; and Jean Marsch, RN, Emergency Room, Meriter-Madison General Hospital, Madison, Wisconsin, for their suggestions for the chapter on emergencies.

Julie Gilman, CMA, Radiologic Technician, Medic-East Urgent Care Clinic, Madison, Wisconsin, and Becky Elas, Instructor, Medical Assisting, National Education Center, Bryman Campus, Phoenix, Arizona, for their advice on current radiologic techniques.

Graduates of the Madison Area Technical College Medical Assisting Program: Karen Blaska, CMA, Ann Stanisforth, CMA, Mary Beth Arnold, CMA, Judy Barreau, CMA, Mary DeMark, CMA, Becky Lehman, CMA, Julia Brown, CMA, Lynne Funke, CMA, Marsha McCarthy, CMA, Brenda Elgas, CMA, Lisa Heck, CMA, Connie Dennis, CMA, and Kelly Fitzgibbons, who posed for my photographs.

Charlene Mendell, RPT, Director of Physical Therapy, Dean Medical Center, Madison, Wisconsin, who helped with the revision of the medical assisting procedures in Chapter 32.

Carol Gorsuch, RN, Director of Patient Care Services, Dean Medical Center, Madison, Wisconsin, who allowed me unlimited access to all areas of the clinic and personnel.

Beverly Harper, RN, BS, East Madison Clinic, Madison, Wisconsin, who advised me regarding the countless clinic operations and who has nurtured dozens of anxious students through successful externship experiences.

Barbara Hundt, RD, MS, Director of the Dietetic Technician Program, Madison Area Technical College, Madison, Wisconsin, who reviewed and provided suggestions for updating Chapter 21.

Ray Asplund and the Burdick Corporation of Milton, Wisconsin, who provided advice and illustrations from their training manual for electrocardiography techniques.

Walter Klunik and the staff of Badger Medical Supply, Madison, Wisconsin, who directed me to manufacturers of clinical equipment and supplies, and who allowed me to use their instrument catalog for illustrations in Chapter 25.

Special appreciation is expressed to my colleagues Susan Buboltz, BSN, MS, CMA, Program Director, Medical Assisting, Mary Stolen, BSN, CMA, Marge Wimmler, RN, Jean Dueseler, MSN, Pat Bennet, MSN, MSEd, Phyllis Jensen, MSN, RNC, and Judy Monk, BSN, EdS, for their constant help.

I also thank my husband Glen and my daughter Heidi, who posed for countless photographs.

The American Association of Medical Assistants, the Wisconsin Society of Medical Assistants, the American Vocational Association, the Wisconsin Vocational Association, and the American Medical Writers Association have provided direction, teaching techniques, and current professional information for this revision.

Finally, I wish to thank my medical assisting students, past, present, and future, who are the most important persons at Madison Area Technical College and the inspiration for this sixth edition.

Eleanor F. Derge

I wish to express special gratitude to Jeanne Mach, CMA-AC, CLT-ASCP, Education Consultant, Baltimore, Maryland, who has been "transfusing" the rather extensive subject of diagnostic medicine into medical assisting students for the past 20 years with her special ability to draw together the material in a manner that is easily understood by the medical assisting student and is specific to the diagnostic procedures routinely performed in the medical office. She has made a valuable contribution in the revision of several chapters dealing with laboratory medicine, diagnostic testing, nutrition, specialty medicine, and emergency care.

Karen Lane

We wish to acknowledge, with our deepest thanks, the many reviewers whose valuable critiques and suggestions helped shape the manuscript at all stages of development:

Rebecca Jane Ales, CMA, Practical Radiological Technologist, Allied Health, National Education Center, Phoenix, Arizona.

Beverly Badini, RN, EdM, EdD, Vocational Education, School of Technology, Trenton State College, Trenton, New Jersey.

Diana Bennett, RN, BSN, MA, Chairperson, Medical Assistant Program, Indiana Vocational Technical College, Indianapolis, Indiana.

Kathy Bonewit, BS, MEd, CMA-C, Instructor, Medical Assistant Technology, Hocking Technical College, Nelsonville, Ohio.

Alice Covell, CMA-A, Medical Assistant Technology, Kalamazoo Valley Community College, Kalamazoo, Michigan.

Mary Ellen Driver, RN, MEd, Allied Health Division, Community College of Allegheny County, West Mifflin, Pennsylvania.

Patricia U. Fuller, RN, BSAH, Paramedic, Emergency Medical Services, Regional Technical Institute, University of Alabama, Birmingham, Alabama.

Janice D. Hall, BS, Medical Imaging and Therapy–Radiographer Program, University of Alabama, Birmingham, Alabama.

Lois A. Heronemus, RN, BSN, CMA, Health Occupations, Lakeshore Technical College, Cleveland, Wisconsin.

Barbara Madick, MS, RN, Medical Assisting Program/Business Division, College of San Mateo, San Mateo, California.

Regina Masters, CMA, MEd, Instructor, Medical Assisting Program, University of Toledo Community and Technical College, Toledo, Ohio.

Kathy Ann McCall, BS, MA, Allied Health Division, Community College of Allegheny County, Pittsburgh, Pennsylvania.

Lisa McCollum, CMA-AC, Instructor, Health Occupations/Medical Assisting, Olympic Community College, Bremerton, Washington.

Fran Muller, CMA, MT(ASCP), MEd, Department Chair, Medical Assisting, Guilford Technical Community College, Jamestown, North Carolina.

Tom Palko, MT(ASCP), MEd, MCS, Medical Assistant Program Director, Department of Biological Sciences, Arkansas Technical University, Russellville, Arkansas.

Ruth M. Patterson, CMA-AC, EdD, Assistant Professor, Health Occupations, Teacher Education, School of Education, North Carolina State University, Raleigh, North Carolina.

Rosemary Piserchio, CMA-A, MA, MS, Business Division, Medical Assisting, College of San Mateo, San Mateo, California.

Virginia Randolph, MA, Allied Health Department/Clinical Laboratory Sciences Division, University of Alabama, Birmingham, Alabama.

Midge Noel Ray, RN, MSN, MA, CMA-AC, Allied Health Department, Medical Assistant and Multiple Competency Clinical Technician Program, University of Alabama, Birmingham, Alabama.

Janet Stiles, RN, BSN, CMA-C, Medical Assisting/Medical Transcription Program Coordinator, El Centro Community College, Dallas, Texas.

Patricia Suminski, RN, BSN, CMA, Medical Assistant Coordinator-Instructor, Health Occupations, Milwaukee Area Technical College, Milwaukee, Wisconsin.

Carol Warden-Tamparo, CMA-A, PhD, Medical Assistant Coordinator, Highline Community College, Des Moines, Washington.

Mary Ellen Wedding, CMA, MT(ASCP), MEd, Associate Professor, Health and Human Services, University of Toledo Community and Technical College, Toledo, Ohio.

BRIEF CONTENTS

DETAILED CONTENTS

11

Medical Records Management 145

12

Professional Fees and Credit Arrangements 171

16

Health and Accident Insurance 249

17

Editorial Duties and Meeting and Travel Arrangements 273

Section III   The Clinical Assistant

LIST OF PROCEDURES

THE
MEDICAL
ASSISTANT
ADMINISTRATIVE
AND CLINICAL

CHAPTER OUTLINE

VOCABULARY

See Glossary at end of book for definitions.

administrative	freestanding emergency center	regional
allied health professional	group practice	rural
clinical	health maintenance organization	solo private practice
discretion	jargon	technical
empathy	mandatory	therapeutic
externship	protocols	urban

The Medical Assistant Member of the Health Team

1

OBJECTIVES

Upon successful completion of this chapter you should be able to:

1. Define the terms listed in the Vocabulary for this chapter.
2. Identify at least 10 career opportunities that are open to the trained medical assistant.
3. List five characteristics that reflect the type of personality needed by a good medical assistant.
4. Identify at least five skill areas in which the medical assistant should be proficient.
5. Differentiate between administrative and clinical responsibilities of the medical assistant.
6. Describe the programs that are available for training medical assistants and list their required courses.
7. Explain what is meant by an externship for medical assistants.
8. Name three professional organizations that provide certification examinations for medical assistants in addition to supplying members with educational materials.
9. Identify at least 10 allied health occupations and explain the major scope of their functions.

A career as a medical assistant offers variety, excitement, job satisfaction, opportunity for service, opportunity for advancement, and fair financial reward. Both men and women enter into this career.

ADVANTAGES

The advantages of a career in medicine rarely need to be "sold" by enumerating specific benefits. Medicine is of great interest to everyone. It is front page news. Most Americans are better informed on health and medical subjects than ever before, and today more emphasis is placed on prevention and patient education. The continuing struggle of physicians, researchers, and **allied health professionals** to defeat illness and prolong life is a neverending, exciting one.

When you have become trained for medical assisting you will be equipped with a flexible, adaptable career. Acquired skills can be carried all through life, and employment is readily available anywhere in the world that medicine is practiced. While medical assisting holds many opportunities for youth, it is one career that usually does not have **mandatory** retirement. Many medical assistants are still employed beyond the usual retirement age because physicians realize the value of an experienced, mature employee.

CAREER OPPORTUNITIES

Although doctors have employed assistants in their practices for many years, recognition of medical assisting as a profession was slow to develop but is now accelerating rapidly. The delivery of health care has changed dramatically in the last decade, primarily because of the ever-increasing cost. The trend is moving away from hospital-based care, with more procedures and treatments being performed in the physician's office or in outpatient centers. Computerization and high technology have created more opportunities and greater responsibility with an increase in the need for qualified medical assistants.

As the qualifications have become more clearly defined, the quality of training has improved and become more accessible. Medical assisting has become recognized as an important allied health profession. Employment opportunities in allied health are abundant, extremely varied, and increasing every day because of the growing concern for health protection for every individual in the nation. More medical assistants are employed by practicing physicians than any other type of allied health personnel.

As a medical assistant your work can be **administrative, clinical**, or **technical**. You can be a receptionist in a hospital or physician's office, a transcriptionist, insurance specialist, financial secretary, billing and collection specialist, a clinical assistant involved in patient care, or an emergency technician, to name just a few. You may choose to work for a physician in **solo private practice,** for a medical partnership or **group practice,** a **health maintenance organization** (HMO), a hospital, or a **freestanding emergency center.** The physician(s) may be either in general practice or engaged in one of the medical specialties, such as surgery, internal medicine, dermatology, obstetrics, pediatrics, psychiatry, or radiology.

There are career opportunities in public health facilities, hospitals, laboratories, medical schools, research institutions, universities, and with voluntary health agencies and medical firms of all kinds. There are also opportunities for work with such federal agencies as the Veterans Administration, the United States Health Service, and Armed Forces clinics or hospitals.

Although appropriate training will equip you for work in a variety of settings, this text is designed primarily for the person who seeks employment in a medical office or who is already employed as a medical assistant.

Ideally, you should have both administrative and clinical training, even though you may have a personal preference for one or the other. The physician's staff should be able to handle all responsibilities of the office except those requiring the services of a physician or other licensed personnel. Where there are several assistants, each should be able and willing to substitute in an emergency for any of the others. Few physicians in private practice attempt to get along without at least one assistant. The great majority have at least two, and many have five or more.

If there is only one medical assistant, that person reports directly to the physician. With a larger staff, a line of authority must be established. Usually one staff member is designated as supervisor or office manager. This individual should have management skills and the ability to deal with personnel matters. While the career of the medical assistant is more challenging than it ever has been, it also offers more opportunities for advancement today. The recent medical assistant graduate whose first position is as a receptionist may gradually be given more responsibilities and eventually become office manager of a large staff. "The single most critical short supply in health manpower is executive level personnel, specifically individuals competent to develop and operate a health maintenance organization, or prepaid group practice." (Gettys and Zasa, 1977).

EARNINGS

What kind of earnings can the medical assistant expect? As in any other career field, there are **regional** differences. There is usually some difference between earnings in **rural** and in **urban** areas. However, as a medical assistant you will generally get a satisfactory return on your investment in training, experience, and skill. Medical organizations encourage physicians to pay better-than-average salaries to their medical assistants, and most have come to realize that a good medical assistant is worth a good salary. Many have learned through bitter experience that "bargain" help is often the most expensive.

The job turnover among medical assistants is surprisingly low. This fact may indicate that medical assistants derive a high degree of satisfaction from their work. Many cases have been reported of medical assistants who were hired when a physician started practice and remained until the physician's retirement.

PERSONAL ATTRIBUTES

A pleasant, friendly disposition is as necessary to the medical assistant as are administrative or clinical skills. The keys to a good medical office personality are consideration, respect, human kindness, and **empathy.** The services performed by a medical assistant are extremely personal. For this reason the manner in which these services are performed can actually affect the health and welfare of the patient. The effective medical assistant learns to view a situation through the eyes of the patients, and to give attention to their problems, no matter how insignificant they may appear.

As a medical assistant you must be immaculate, dependable, accurate, and have a good head for details. Because you often must assume charge of the office when the doctor is out, you must not hesitate to accept responsibility. If an emergency should arise, you must be able to meet it with composure. **Discretion** and good judgment are also important for the man or woman who works in a doctor's office. The patients' impression of the medical assistant often affects their opinions of the doctor and the care they can expect. More than one patient has been lost because of a seeming lack of concern on the part of a medical assistant.

NECESSARY SKILLS

Every profession or trade has its special vocabulary or **jargon**; the language of medicine must be understood by every allied health professional. The medical assistant must have a basic knowledge of law and ethics as they relate to the medical profession. Additionally, to qualify for secretarial duties, the medical assistant must have good handwriting, be a proficient typist, and have good language, communications, and mathematics skills. Shorthand is helpful, but in most medical facilities electronic dictation and word processing are the current trend. Some training in records management is desirable for both the administrative and clinical assistant, as are skills in human relations and

personal communications. All medical assistants should be trained in cardiopulmonary resuscitation (CPR) and emergency first aid. The clinical medical assistant must be skilled in certain patient care arts and must have the necessary training to perform common medical tests allowed by law. The laws vary from state to state.

DUTIES OF THE MEDICAL ASSISTANT

The duties of the medical assistant will vary from one facility to another, since the schedule must be geared to the type of practice and working habits of the individual physician. In the office with only one employee, the medical assistant's time is divided between administrative and clinical duties. In the multiple-employee office the positions tend to be more specialized.

Administrative Duties

Your administrative duties as a medical assistant will be similar to those of any responsible secretary to a top executive but will have specific medical aspects. They will include answering telephones, scheduling appointments, interviewing and instructing new patients, screening nonpatient visitors and salespersons, explaining the doctor's fees to patients, opening and sorting mail, answering routine correspondence, pulling patient charts for scheduled appointments, and filing reports and correspondence. You may make arrangements for patient admission to a hospital and instruct the patient regarding admission.

You will make financial arrangements with patients, complete insurance claim forms, maintain the financial records and files, prepare and mail statements, prepare checks for the doctor's signature, maintain a file of paid and unpaid invoices, and prepare and maintain employees' payroll records (or submit payroll information to an outside accountant).

Sometimes you may act as an informal editorial assistant to the doctor, helping in the preparation of manuscripts or speeches, or clipping articles from professional journals and assisting with the maintenance of the doctor's personal medical library.

Clinical Duties

Your clinical duties will also be varied. Generally speaking, you will help patients prepare for examinations and other office procedures, take the medical history, stand by to assist the doctor when requested to do so, clean and sterilize instruments and equipment, instruct patients regarding preparation for x-ray and laboratory examinations, and keep the supply cabinets well-stocked. You may collect specimens from patients and either send them to a laboratory or perform certain diagnostic tests for which you have been trained. You may also assist with electrocardiography and radiography, take and record the patient's temperature, pulse, and respiration, prepare treatment trays, and assist with minor surgery. You may occasionally be called upon to administer emergency first aid.

TRAINING

Getting Started

Many community colleges throughout the nation offer vocational courses for medical assistants leading to a certificate and/or associate degree. There are also proprietary schools that offer a certificate in medical assisting. Medical assistants already employed in the field were among the first to recognize the need for more trained personnel for doctors' offices. Through chapters of the American Association of Medical Assistants (AAMA) and aided by medical societies, they have been instrumental in rapidly accelerating the development of such training programs.

The community college programs include course work in medical terminology, anatomy and physiology, biology, psychology, medical law and ethics, human relations, nutrition, first aid, medical laboratory procedures, microbiology, pharmacology, electrocardiography, injections, patient care, accounting practices, medical shorthand, filing and records management, typing and transcription, word processing, business English, and written and oral communications. Some programs have hands-on experience with computers. Most of the college programs include an **externship** in the offices of local physicians as part of the training. Instructors for these courses have been recruited from the ranks of those with practical experience in the field.

Continuing Education

The practicing medical assistant must keep current with the rapid changes within the profession. This can be accomplished by reading, or briefly reviewing, the medical literature that arrives in the daily mail, keeping abreast of medical events publicized in newspapers and news magazines, attending classes and seminars, maintaining an active membership in a professional organization, and having an inquisitive mind. The amount of medical knowledge gained since the beginning of medical history is now said to be doubling every 5 years. Most physicians will appreciate the medical assistant who asks questions about unfamiliar conditions or procedures.

PROFESSIONAL ORGANIZATIONS

American Association of Medical Assistants (AAMA)

The AAMA was formally organized in 1956 as a federation of several state associations that had been functioning independently. In 1986 the AAMA had affiliated societies in 45 states and the District of Columbia, with national headquarters in Chicago, Illinois.

The AAMA has been the force behind establishing a certifying program for medical assistants, the accrediting of medical assisting training programs in community colleges and private schools, and setting minimum standards for the entry-level medical assistant. AAMA members have the opportunity to attend local, state, and regional meetings, where they can participate in workshops, learn of educational advances in their field, hear prominent speakers, and establish a networking system with other medical assistants. The Association publishes a bimonthly journal, *The Professional Medical Assistant* (PMA). Members may wear the AAMA insignia (Fig. 1–1).

Since 1963 the AAMA has offered a certifying examination, with successful completion leading to a certificate and recognition as a Certified Medical Assistant (CMA). The National Board of Medical Examiners participates in the construction and administration of the examination. The examination is given in January and June of each year at designated centers throughout the United States. Certification is available to students or graduates of programs accredited by the Committee on Allied Health Education and Accreditation (CAHEA), medical assisting instructors, and experienced medical assistants. Applicants need not be members of AAMA. Beginning in 1988, revalidation every 5 years will be mandatory, and can be accomplished through continuing education units (CEUs) or reexamination. The Certified Medical Assistant is permitted to wear the CMA pin (Fig. 1–2).

Registered Medical Assistant Program of the American Medical Technologists (RMA/AMT)

In the early 1970s the American Medical Technologists (AMT), the national certifying body for laboratory personnel since 1939, began offering an examination for medical assistants. The examination is given as needed at schools accredited by the Accrediting Bureau of Health Education Schools (ABHES). Applicants must be graduates of a medical assisting course accredited by the ABHES or by a Regional Accrediting Commission, or must meet certain experience requirements. The success of this project brought about the formulation of the Registered Medical Assistant (RMA) Program within AMT in 1976. Since 1976 the RMA Program has

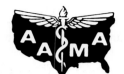

Figure 1–1

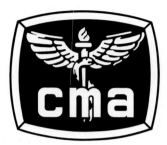

Figure 1–2

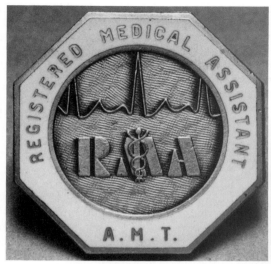

Figure 1–3

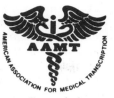

Figure 1–4

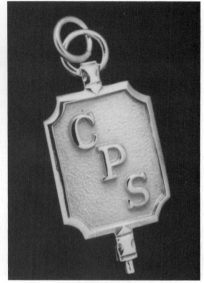

Figure 1–5

Figures 1–1 to 1–5
1–1: Insignia of the American Association of Medical Assistants. (Courtesy of the American Association of Medical Assistants, Chicago, IL.) 1–2: Pin worn by the Certified Medical Assistant. (Courtesy of the American Association of Medical Assistants, Chicago, IL.) 1–3: Pin worn by the Registered Medical Assistant. (Courtesy of RMA/American Medical Technologists, Park Ridge, IL.) 1–4: Insignia of American Association for Medical Transcription. (Courtesy of American Association for Medical Transcription, Modesto, CA.) 1–5: Pin worn by the Certified Professional Secretary. (Courtesy of Professional Secretaries International.)

grown into a respected organization in its own right, with a national RMA Executive Board and state associations. All RMA members are certified medical assistants by examination and are entitled to wear the RMA insignia (Fig. 1–3). Headquarters are in Park Ridge, Illinois.

Benefits from Membership in a Medical Assisting Organization. Both AAMA and RMA/AMT offer opportunities for:

- Participation at local, state, and national levels
- Continuing education events with CEUs being recorded and reported, and a revalidation program
- Group insurance programs
- A professional journal

There are independent unaffiliated medical assistant organizations in some states that offer professional participation at the local and state level.

American Association for Medical Transcription (AAMT)

Many medical offices employ specialists in word processing and machine transcription who will find membership in AAMT valuable. The Association was incorporated in 1978 with headquarters in Modesto, California. Certification by experience was available through December 1983. A certification

examination has been offered since 1981, and since January 1, 1984, the only route to certification has been by successful completion of this examination (Fig. 1–4). Certification is voluntary; once achieved, it must be maintained through continuing education. AAMT publishes a professional journal four times a year and a newsletter six times a year. It offers an outstanding education program and holds an annual national convention.

Professional Secretaries International (PSI)

The administrative medical assistant may profit from membership in the Professional Secretaries International. PSI, formerly known as The National Secretaries Association (International), was founded in 1942, and is headquartered in Kansas City, Missouri. Through its Institute for Certifying Secretaries, PSI sponsors the Certified Professional Secretary (CPS) Examination, covering behavioral science in business, business law, economics and management, accounting, office administration and communication, and office technology. The rating of CPS (Fig. 1–5) is obtained by meeting educational and work experience requirements and passing this six-part, two-day examination. The organization publishes *The Secretary* magazine nine times a year, holds an international convention each July, and sponsors Future Secretaries Association chapters in high schools and colleges.

By joining a professional organization and participating in the activities it affords, you will grow personally and professionally, and will keep abreast of current trends. Participation in a recognized professional organization will indicate to an employer that you are serious about your career and would be an asset to his or her practice. The rewards are limitless.

ALLIED HEALTH OCCUPATIONS

The American Medical Association (AMA) for more than 50 years has been involved in setting standards and the accrediting of allied health education programs. The training of the occupational therapist was the first in allied health education to be accredited by the AMA. This occurred in 1935. By 1967 the AMA Council on Medical Education was accrediting educational programs in eight allied health areas. By 1982, eighteen additional allied health professionals (including the medical assistant in 1969) were being accredited.

The man or woman who seeks employment in a medical office environment must be prepared to function as a member of a team.

> The quantitative and qualitative acceptance of the team approach to health care is reflected in the changing ratio of physicians to other health professionals and in the increasing involvement of organizations representing allied health professionals. In the early 60's, the ratio was eight allied health professionals to one physician; by the late 60's, the ratio was twelve to one; and in the late 70's, the ratio was estimated at twenty to one. (American Medical Association, 1982).

A solo practitioner may practice with only one medical assistant, but the team concept remains. The medical community, unlike competitive commercial enterprise, is very close knit, and the medical assistant is expected to interrelate within this community of physicians and allied health professionals. An understanding of the scope of practice and the training required of other allied health professionals will provide a base for this interaction.

Occupational therapists (OTs) work in hospitals, schools, and mental health and public agencies. A baccalaureate degree is a prerequisite for post-baccalaureate occupational therapy programs. The OT provides services to individuals whose abilities to cope with the tasks of living are threatened or impaired, helping them to attain the highest possible functional level.

Physical therapists (PTs) work in hospitals or nursing homes, rehabilitation centers, or schools for crippled children. They must have a baccalaureate degree. PTs are concerned with the restoration of function and the prevention of disability following disease or injury of the muscles, nerves, joints, or bones, or loss of a bodily part. They treat the patient through application of exercise, heat, cold, water, electricity, ultrasound, and massage.

The *respiratory* (formerly inhalation) *therapist* and the *respiratory therapy technician* are similar in many respects, but differ in length of educational programs and level of responsibility in their jobs. The educational program for the technician is 1 year; the therapist requires a 2-year minimum. Both may be employed in hospitals, nursing care facilities, clinics, doctors' offices, companies providing emergency oxygen services, and municipal organizations. They perform procedures crucial in maintaining the lives of seriously ill patients with respiratory problems, and they assist in the treatment of patients with heart and lung ailments. The therapist, because of higher education, is given more responsibility and discretionary power. The credential initials for a registered therapist are RRT.

The field of radiologic technology includes the *radiation therapy technologist* and the *radiographer*. While most radiographers work in hospitals, some are employed in clinics and private offices. Their educational programs are 2 to 4 years long, with a prerequisite of a high school diploma. The radiographer works under the direct supervision of a physician and must understand the principles of radiation protection for the patient, self, and others, while using imaging modalities. Graduation from a program in radiography is a prerequisite for the more advanced radiation therapy technologist. The RTT training requires another 1 or 2 years, following which the therapist will probably be employed in a hospital to assist radiation oncologists (cancer specialists) in all aspects of the administration of radiation treatment.

Electroencephalography is the scientific field devoted to recording and studying the electrical activity of the brain. *EEG technicians* and *technologists* record this activity with an electroencephalograph, which produces a written tracing of the brain's electrical impulses. They work primarily in the neurology departments of hospitals and in private offices of neurologists and neurosurgeons. The technologist has the more advanced training.

Electrocardiography is the graphic recording from the body surface of the potential of electric currents generated by the heart. The electrocardiogram is a valuable tool used in many routine physical examinations, and most internal medicine specialists and general practitioners will have an *EKG* (ECG) *technician* in their offices. The technique is taught in most medical assistant training programs.

There are several levels of expertise and responsibility in medical laboratory technology. The *histologic technician* prepares sections of body tissue for examination by the physician (pathologist). *Histotechnologists* perform more complex procedures and teach students. *Medical laboratory technicians* perform routine uncomplicated procedures in the areas of hematology, serology, blood banking, urinalysis, microbiology, and clinical chemistry. *Medical tech-*

nologists, in addition to having the skills possessed by the medical laboratory technician, can perform more complex laboratory analyses, fine line discrimination, and correction of errors. Most individuals engaged in medical laboratory technology are employed in hospitals, but they also work in various other settings, including physicians' offices and clinics.

The *EMT-Paramedic* is one of the newest of allied health specialists. Paramedics are usually employed by an ambulance service, fire department, or volunteer emergency care service. They work under the direction of a physician, often through radio communication. Their instruction, which deals specifically with emergency medical care, requires from 500 to 800 hours, including supervised clinical practice experience. The *Basic EMT* has more limited instruction (81 hours), and a narrower scope of practice.

Ophthalmic medical assistants render supportive services to the ophthalmologist, a physician who specializes in the diagnosis and treatment of diseases of the eye. They are qualified by academic and clinical training to carry out diagnostic and therapeutic procedures under the direction and responsibility of the physician. They usually receive their training in a hospital setting.

The management of medical records is of critical importance to patient care, and requires the skill of a specialist. The *registered medical record administrator* (RRA) has a baccalaureate degree and is in charge of medical records and reports in the hospitals. *Accredited medical record technicians* (MRTs) serve as technical assistants to the registered record administrator. In a small institution the MRT may have full responsibility for the records department—compiling, analyzing, and preparing health information needed by the patient and by the health facility.

The *certified medical transcriptionist* (CMT) is a highly skilled and knowledgeable professional who transcribes medical dictation detailing a patient's health care during an illness or after an injury. The CMT is an important member of the health care team in hospitals, clinics, and medical research and teaching centers, as well as in private offices of physicians and surgeons.

A *physician's assistant* (PA) is a medical professional who has graduated from an approved associated medical school program and has been certified by the Physician's Assistant Examining Committee. The *assistant to the primary care physician* and the *surgeon's assistant* perform diagnostic, therapeutic, and preventive activities and services, thus allowing more effective use of the knowledge, skills, and abilities of the primary care physician and the surgeon. This profession originated in the mid-1960s. A study in 1976 indicated that almost half of the physician's assistant graduates were working with physicians in private solo practice or private partnership practice. They may be granted limited hospital staff privileges.

The *surgical technologist* (formerly operating room technician) is frequently employed by a physician as a "private scrub" assisting the physician as a private surgical technologist in the hospital operating room as well as in the physician's private office. The surgical technologist works in patient service settings that call for special knowledge about asepsis, that is, the methods of making or keeping an environment antiseptic. The proliferation of outpatient surgicenters and emergicenters increases the demand for the Certified Surgical Technologist (CST). Education programs for the surgical technologist vary in length from 6 to 20 months and may or may not be designed around an associate degree.

The *licensed practical nurse* (LPN) or *licensed vocational nurse* (LVN) may perform certain clinical procedures under the direction of a physician. The LPN/LVN does not have the extensive training of the registered nurse, and responsibilities are more limited. The scope of practice and **protocols** are determined by the state in which licensure is granted. Many LPNs/LVNs are employed in physicians' offices as well as in hospitals.

The *registered nurse* (RN) may be the product of a 2- or 3-year training program or a 4-year baccalaureate program. All RNs take the same-level licensing examination. The RN is licensed by the state, which also defines the scope of practice.

The *nurse practitioner* is a registered nurse with additional preparation and skills in physical diagnosis, psychosocial assessment, and management of primary health care. The nurse practitioner may work alone, especially in rural areas. The nurse practitioner who is working in collaboration with or under the supervision of a physician may be granted limited hospital staff privileges.

REFERENCES AND READINGS

American Medical Association: *Allied Health Education Directory*, 11th ed. Chicago, The Association, 1982.
Gettys, R. C., and Zasa, R. J.: *Medical Group Practice Management*, Cambridge, MA, Ballinger Publishing Co., 1977.

PROFESSIONAL ORGANIZATIONS

American Association of Medical Assistants, 20 North Wacker, Suite 1575, Chicago, IL 60606.
American Association for Medical Transcription, P.O. Box 6187, Modesto, CA 95355.
Professional Secretaries International, 301 East Armour Boulevard, Kansas City, MO 64111–1299.
Registered Medical Assistant/AMT, 710 Higgins Road, Park Ridge, IL 60068.

CHAPTER OUTLINE

Medical Language and Mythology
Medicine in Ancient Times
Pioneers in Modern Medicine

Women in Medicine
Modern Miracles

VOCABULARY

See Glossary at end of book for definitions.

auscultation	immunology	phagocytosis
bacteria	innovation	protozoa
chemotherapy	microorganism	purulent
contamination	neophyte	stethoscope
dialysis	oviducts	spermatozoa
embryology	pandemic	syphilitic chancre
hemiplegia	pathologic	virulent
histologist	percussion	

A Brief History of Medicine

2

OBJECTIVES

Upon successful completion of this chapter you should be able to:

1. Define the terms listed in the Vocabulary of this chapter.
2. Name the Greek physician who was revered as the God of Medicine.
3. Identify the man who reasoned that blood circulates through the body.
4. Name the first man to observe bacteria and protozoa through a microscopic lens.
5. Identify the physician who pioneered use of the microscope in the study of plants and animals.
6. Identify the 18th century surgeon who was given the title "Founder of Scientific Surgery."
7. Name the physician who discovered the smallpox vaccine and identified the relationship between cowpox and smallpox.
8. Identify the physician who discovered the use of percussion in diagnosis and the physician who developed the stethoscope.
9. Explain what is meant by the term puerperal fever and identify the physician who diagnosed this disorder.
10. List four diseases to which Louis Pasteur devoted many years of study.
11. Identify at least four women who played important roles in the fields of nursing and medicine.
12. Name those individuals who were responsible for the discovery of x-ray therapy, insulin, penicillin, and polio vaccine.

Modern medicine reflects its history in the names given to anatomy, physiology, medications, diseases, instruments, and specialties. Even the latest medical discoveries often have names drawn from the ancients. It is impossible to live in the world of medicine and to talk its language without being constantly touched by this fascinating past. The rich cultural heritage of medicine is interesting to study and to draw upon, but it is also a process filled with hardships and disappointments that were pushed aside by determined men and women who wanted to pursue their dreams and goals. It can be inspiring to think of these pioneers and realize that we too are part of the heritage of caring and discovery that continues to improve health care throughout the world.

MEDICAL LANGUAGE AND MYTHOLOGY

It may seem strange for modern medicine to borrow so liberally from ancient mythology, and to use so actively the classical language that most civilizations abandoned centuries ago. Yet today's medicine uses words whose origins stem from the romance and fantasy of this long "dead" world. Anatomy, especially, seems to reach back to the dawn of history and, although some terms are today erroneous when translated literally, because the ancients did not correctly understand body functions, many early anatomic terms have reached modern times almost unchanged.

Greek and Roman mythology have contributed a major portion of our medical terms, but we have also borrowed liberally from Arabic, Anglo-Saxon, and German sources, with a heavy dash of the Bible added. Here are a few of the many examples from the classical past: the anatomic name for the first cervical vertebra upon which the head rests is aptly named Atlas, for the famous Greek Titan, who, according to mythology, was condemned by Zeus to bear the heavens on his shoulders. The tendon of Achilles reminds us of the story of the youth whose mother held him by the heel and dipped him into the river Styx to make him invulnerable. This particular tendon was not immersed and later a mortal wound was inflicted in Achilles' heel. The dubious honors given in medicine to Venus, the Roman Goddess of Love, are paid to her not so much as the goddess of love but of lust. She has a portion of the female anatomy, the mons veneris, dedicated to her memory. Venereal diseases are also named after her. Aphrodite, the Greek Goddess of Love and Beauty, gave her name to the sex-exciting drugs known as aphrodisiacs.

Aesculapius, the son of Apollo, was revered as the God of Medicine. The early Greeks worshiped the healing powers of Aesculapius and built temples in his honor, where patients were treated by trained priests. His daughters were Hygeia, Goddess of Health, and Panacea, Goddess of All Healing and Restorer of Health. These two names are prominent in our language today.

MEDICINE IN ANCIENT TIMES

Though religion and myth were the basis of care for the sick for millennia, there is evidence of drugs, surgery, and other treatments based on theories about the body from as early as 5000 to 2000 BC. In the well-developed societies of the Egyptians, Babylonians, and Assyrians, certain men acted as physicians, using their scant knowledge to try to treat illness and injury.

Around 1205 BC, Moses incorporated rules of health into the Hebrew religion. He was thus the first advocate of preventive medicine and could even be called the first "public health officer." Moses knew that some animal diseases may be passed on to man and that **contamination** may linger on unclean dishes. Thus, it became a religious law that no one was permitted to eat animals that were not freshly slaughtered or to eat or drink from dirty dishes, lest they become defiled and lose their souls.

Hippocrates (460–377 BC) is the most famous of the ancient Greek physicians and is known as the "Father of Medicine." He did much to separate medicine from mysticism and gave it a scientific basis. He is best remembered for the "Hippocratic Oath" (see Chapter 4) exacted from his pupils. This oath has been administered to physicians for more than 2000 years. Hippocrates' astute clinical descriptions of diseases and his voluminous writings on epidemics, fevers, epilepsy, fractures, and instruments were studied for centuries. He believed that the body tends to heal itself and it is the physician's responsibility to help nature. In his time, very little was known about anatomy, physiology, and pathology, and there was no knowledge of chemistry. Yet, in spite of these handicaps, many of his classifications of diseases and his descriptions of symptoms are being used today.

Many Greek physicians practiced, studied, and taught in Rome in the time after Hippocrates. One was Galen (131–201 AD), who came to Rome in 162 AD and became known as the "Prince of Physicians" (Fig. 2–1). Galen is said to have written 500 treatises on medicine. He wrote an excellent summary of anatomy as it was known at that time, but his work was faulty and inaccurate, for it was based largely on the dissection of apes and swine. He is considered to be the father of experimental physiology, and the first experimental neurologist. He was the first to describe the cranial nerves and the sympathetic system, and he made the first experimental sections of the spinal cord, producing hemiplegia. Galen also produced aphonia by cutting the recurrent laryngeal nerve, and he gave the first valid explanation of the mechanism of respiration.

The profound influence of the writings of Hip-

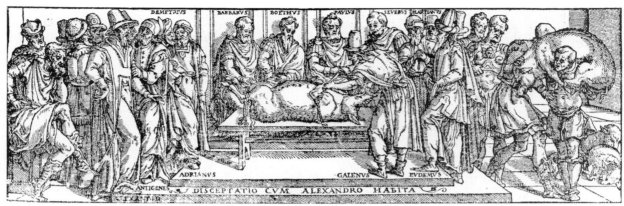

Figure 2–1
Galen. (Courtesy of the National Library of Medicine.)

pocrates and Galen on the course of medicine gives praise to these great thinkers, but their unquestioned authority actually had a negative effect on the progress of science throughout the "Dark Ages." Their theories and descriptions were held to as law, so **innovation** was rarely attempted. Experimenters were scoffed at by their contemporaries. Later, the Christian religion contributed to the learning and teaching of care of the sick because the Christian faith encouraged the establishment of institutions in which the sick could be protected

and cared for. This provided an opportunity for physicians to observe, analyze, and discuss the progress of a variety of patients. The establishment of universities led more to a study of theories of disease rather than to observation of the sick. It was not until the 16th century that Andreas Vesalius (1514–1564) began to correct some of Galen's errors (Fig. 2–2).

Vesalius, a Belgian anatomist, is known as the "Father of Modern Anatomy." At the age of 29 he published his great *De Corporis Humani Fabrica*, in

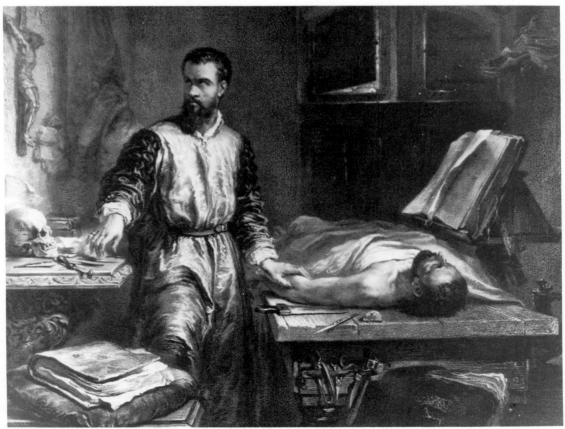

Figure 2–2
Andreas Vesalius. (Courtesy of the National Library of Medicine.)

which he described the structure of the human body. This work marked a turning point in breaking with the past and throwing overboard the Galen tradition. Vesalius introduced many new anatomic terms, but because of his radical approach he was subjected to some persecution from his colleagues, his teachers, and his pupils. Despite his great contributions to the science of anatomy, his name is not used to identify any important anatomic structures. A student of Vesalius, Gabriele Fallopius, was also an accurate and detailed dissector and described and named many parts of the anatomy. He gave his own name to the **oviducts**, known as the **fallopian tubes**. He also gave the vagina and the placenta their present names.

In 1628, William Harvey (1578–1657) made his pronouncement—based on experimental vivisection, ligation, and perfusion, followed by brilliant reasoning—that the heart acts as a muscular force-pump in propelling the blood along, and that the blood's motion is continual, continuous, and in a cycle or circle (Fig. 2–3). The work of this English physician was not fully recognized until 1827, when the full importance of his work was substantiated. Harvey's writings were recognized in Germany before the English permitted their publication at home. Modern England now considers Harvey to be its "medical Shakespeare."

Great advances in medicine were somewhat stilled for a century or so, but the unseen world of microorganisms was opened as Anton van Leeuwenhoek (1632–1723), a Dutch linen draper and haberdasher by trade, pursued his hobby of grinding lenses. He ground over 400 lenses during his lifetime, most of which were very small—some no larger than a pinhead—and usually mounted be-

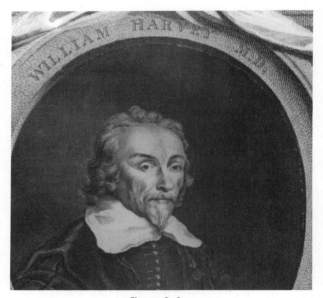

Figure 2–3
William Harvey. (Courtesy of the National Library of Medicine.)

tween two thin brass plates, riveted together. In grinding lenses Leeuwenhoek discovered how to use a simple biconvex lens to magnify the minute world of organisms and structures never seen before. Leeuwenhoek was the first man ever to observe **bacteria** and **protozoa** through a lens. His accurate interpretations of what he saw led to the sciences of bacteriology and protozoology. He described for the first time the **spermatozoa** from insects, dogs, and man. He studied the structure of the optic lens, striations in muscles, and the mouthparts of insects. Leeuwenhoek extended Marcello Malpighi's demonstration in 1660 of the blood capillaries by giving (in 1684) the first accurate description of red blood cells. From 1673 until 1723 he communicated by means of informal letters most of his discoveries to the Royal Society of England, to which he was elected a fellow in 1680.

The greatest of the microscopists was Marcello Malpighi (1628–1694), who was born near Bologna, Italy, entered the University of Bologna in 1646, and in 1653 was granted doctorates in both medicine and philosophy. Malpighi pioneered the use of the microscope in the study of plants and animals, after which microscopic anatomy became a prerequisite for advances in physiology, **embryology**, and practical medicine. He may be regarded as the first **histologist**. In 1661 he identified and described the pulmonary and capillary network connecting the small arteries with small veins, one of the most important discoveries in the history of science. When Malpighi found that the blood passed through the capillaries, it meant that Harvey was right—that blood was not transformed into flesh in the periphery, as the ancients had thought. Malpighi continued to pursue his microscopic studies while teaching and practicing medicine. He identified the taste buds and described the minute structure of the brain and optic nerve. He was the first to see the red blood cells and to attribute the color of blood to them. He discovered the rete mucosum or Malpighian layer of the skin. His work on the structure of the liver, spleen, and kidney is recalled today when we speak of the Malpighian bodies of the kidney and spleen, Malpighi's pyramids (pyramides renales) and Malpighi's vesicles (alveoli pulmonis).

A few years after Leeuwenhoek's death, a famous English surgeon and anatomist, John Hunter (1728–1793), was born (Fig. 2–4). Hunter has been given the title "Founder of Scientific Surgery" because his surgical procedures were soundly based on **pathologic** evidence. He was the first to classify teeth in a scientific manner. In 1778 he introduced artificial feeding by means of a flexible tube passed into the stomach. His description of the **syphilitic chancre** is classic, and the lesion is sometimes called the "Hunterian chancre." In an unsuccessful attempt to differentiate gonorrhea from syphilis, Hunter inoculated himself with what he thought was gonorrhea, but instead acquired syphilis. His

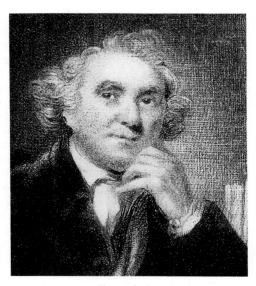

Figure 2–4
John Hunter. (Courtesy of the National Library of Medicine.)

great collection of anatomic and animal specimens formed the basis for the museum of the Royal College of Surgeons. He was also a member of the Royal Society of Medicine and the Royal Academy of Surgery in Paris. Hunter wrote many papers on anatomy and physiology; he was a brilliant lecturer and teacher. Among his many students was one who would become famous and well-loved: Edward Jenner.

PIONEERS IN MODERN MEDICINE

Edward Jenner (1749–1823) was a country physician in Dorsetshire, England (Fig. 2–5). He is listed among the immortals of preventive medicine for his discovery of the smallpox vaccine. The story goes that one day, while Jenner was serving as an apprentice in the office of Daniel Ludlow, a dairy maid was being given treatment. Smallpox was mentioned, and she said, "I cannot take that disease, for I have had cowpox." Smallpox at that time was the deadliest of **pandemics**. Jenner observed that farmers and dairy maids who once had cowpox never contracted smallpox. Later, as a practicing physician, Jenner continued investigating the relationship between cowpox and smallpox, to the extent that other medical society members felt bored and threatened to expel him from their ranks.

On May 14, 1796, Dr. Jenner took some **purulent** matter from a pustule on the hand of Sarah Nelmes, a dairy maid, and inserted it through two small superficial incisions into the arm of James Phipps, a healthy 8-year-old boy. This was the first vaccination. Later, on July 1, a **virulent** dose of smallpox matter was given to young Phipps in the same arm. It had no effect: Phipps had been vaccinated and was safe from the dreaded disease. Edward Jenner's method of vaccination spread throughout the world. The results of his methods and experiments were published in 1798. He called this method of protection "vaccination" because the Latin word *vacca* means cow. Cowpox was called "vaccinia." Pasteur applied the term "vaccine" to suspensions of dead bacteria or attenuated bacteria. This term has come to be used in reference to other immunizing antigens not derived from cows.

Victor Robinson, in *Pathfinders in Medicine*, said of Dr. Jenner, "He died where an intellectual man should die—in his library. The village which gave him birth received his illustrious ashes. When his worn-out body was laid to rest, it would not be surprising if some humble woman, whose child he had saved from smallpox, imagined that Edward Jenner had gone to heaven—to vaccinate the angels."

Percussion and **auscultation** have been the very basics of physical examination for many years. But no physician had a real understanding of what went on inside the body until anatomists had paved the way for an Austrian physician, Leopold Auenbrugger (1722–1809), who developed the use of percussion in diagnosis, and a French physician, René Laënnec (1781–1826), who developed the stethoscope. Auenbrugger became physician-in-chief to the Hospital of the Holy Trinity at Vienna in 1751, and it was there that he tested his discovery, which afterward made him famous but which was generally ignored and scorned by his contemporaries. Laënnec invented the **stethoscope** in 1819, but at first it was only a cylinder of paper in his hands. His book concerning the stethoscope was readily accepted and translated into many languages. It is said to be the most important treatise in diseases of the thoracic organs ever written.

The first American treatise on psychiatry, *Medical Inquiries and Observations upon the Diseases of the*

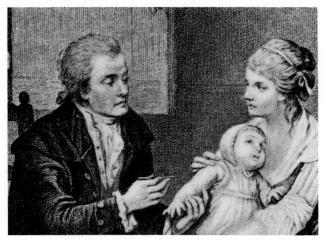

Figure 2–5
Edward Jenner. (Courtesy of the National Library of Medicine.)

Mind, published in 1812, was written by Benjamin Rush (1745–1813), a member of the Continental Congress in 1776 and a signer of the Declaration of Independence.

In the early 1800s there were several men who are remembered for their fight against puerperal fever and for their concern for women's health. Puerperal fever, an infectious disease of childbirth, is also known as puerperal sepsis or childbed fever. This term is from puerpera, denoting a woman in childbed, from the Latin puer, a child, and pario, to bring forth. The word "puerperium" now designates the period from delivery to the time the uterus returns to normal size.

The best known of these men is the Hungarian physician Ignaz Philipp Semmelweis (1818–1865). History has called him the "Savior of Mothers." His fight against puerperal fever is a sad story of hardships and resistance, especially from his instructor in Vienna, Professor Klein. Semmelweis noted the terrible results of puerperal fever in lying-in hospitals and observed that it occurred with special frequency in cases delivered by medical students who came directly from the autopsy or dissecting room. Semmelweis directed that in his wards the students were to wash and disinfect their hands with a solution of chloride of lime after leaving the dissection room and before going to the wards to examine a woman and deliver her child. This brought about a marked reduction of cases of childbed fever on his ward, but violent opposition was given by the hospital's medical men, and especially by Dr. Klein. As his theories were proven correct, Semmelweis began to feel the horror of the deaths that had been caused in the past by doctors themselves.

At the age of 47 Semmelweis died, ironically from the very infection he had fought, brought on by a cut in his finger while he was doing an autopsy. His grave had hardly been closed when Pasteur and Lister began to reveal the secrets that had caused this deadly disease. A monument to Semmelweis in Budapest is given great care and it has been said that if people had been as tender to the man as they are to his statue, his career would have been happier. Surely Semmelweis' death was a matter of tragic timing, for the year of his death was to see the introduction of the great works of Pasteur and a physician in Edinburgh and Glasgow named Joseph Lister.

Louis Pasteur (1822–1895), a Frenchman, did brilliant work as a chemist, but it was his studies in bacteriology that made him one of the most famous men in medical history and earned him the title of "Father of Bacteriology" (Fig. 2–6). He has also sometimes been honored with the name "Father of Preventive Medicine." His skills and studies reached far beyond the outermost boundaries of the knowledge of the time. He pursued everything with the fire of genius. His adventures included

studying the difficulties in the fermentation of wine. He saved the most important industry of France at that time from disaster by a process now called pasteurization. By this process of supplying enough heat to destroy **microorganisms**, wine was prevented from turning into vinegar. This made great improvements in spirit and malt liquors. The French people called on Pasteur again to help the ailing silkworm industry. The silkworm epidemic in the south of France had reached such proportions that whole plantations were ruined. Pasteur devoted five years to the conquest of the two diseases that infected the silkworm. His work was interrupted only when he was stricken with **hemiplegia**. But after a long, difficult recovery time, when his mind was always fully active, he continued his work with a stiff hand and a limping foot.

With the conviction that the "infinitely small" world of bacteria held the key to the secrets of contagious diseases, he again left chemistry, this time to become a medical man. Many renowned scientists denied the germ theory of disease and devoted themselves to degrading Pasteur. In the midst of all this "controversy" he became involved in the prevention of anthrax, which threatened the health of the cattle and sheep of France, as well as of the world. Pasteur's name was also honored for work on many other diseases, such as rabies, chicken cholera, and swine erysipelas.

Pasteur died in 1895, with his family at his bedside. His last words were said to be "There is still a great deal to do."

Joseph Lister (1827–1912) was to revolutionize surgery through the application of Pasteur's discov-

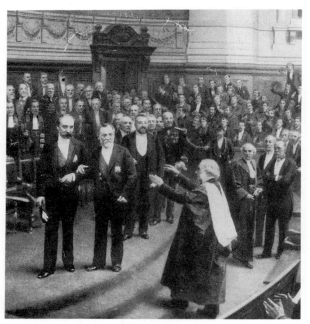

Figure 2–6
Louis Pasteur. (Courtesy of the National Library of Medicine.)

eries. He saw the similarity between the infections that were taking place in postsurgical wounds and the processes of putrefaction which Pasteur had proven were caused by microorganisms. Before this time surgeons accepted infection in surgical wounds as inevitable. Lister reasoned that microorganisms must be the cause of infection and must, therefore, be kept out of wounds. His own colleagues were quite indifferent to Lister's theories since they felt infections were God-given and natural. Lister had once seen pain quelled by the administration of an anesthetic, and pain had been thought to be God-given and inevitable also. He developed antiseptic methods by using carbolic acid for sterilization. By spraying the room with a fine mist of the acid, by soaking the instruments and ligatures, and by washing his hands in carbolic solutions, Lister proved his theory. He is honored with the title of "Father of Sterile Surgery."

Pasteur and Joseph Lister met at the Sorbonne after years of great mutual admiration. The meeting was filled with emotion, and Robinson, in *Pathfinders in Medicine*, has said that "a new star should have appeared in the heavens to commemorate the event. Only a small percentage of the human race entertains any adequate realization of how much we really owe to the combined labors of Louis Pasteur and Joseph Lister."

The name Robert Koch (1843–1910) is familiar to all bacteriologists, for the first law learned as a **neophyte** in this microscopic world is Koch's Postulates, which state rules that must be followed before an organism can be accepted as the causative agent in a given disease.

Robert Koch was a German physician who truly earned great honors in bacteriology and public health. He gave the bacteriology laboratory many of its "tools," such as the culture-plate method for isolation of bacteria. He discovered the cause of cholera and demonstrated its transmission by food and water. This discovery completely transformed health departments and proved the importance of bacteriology. It also established a place of great respect for Koch in the scientific world. A great disappointment in Koch's career was his failure to find a cure for tuberculosis. In this attempt, however, he isolated tuberculin, the substance produced by tubercle bacteria. Its use as a diagnostic aid proved to be of immense value to modern medicine.

Koch's work took him throughout the world. He traveled to America, Africa, Bombay, Italy, and anywhere nations sought his help in ridding themselves of feared diseases. He was investigating anthrax at the same time as Pasteur, but the ill-concealed animosity between the two men prevented any cooperative effort.

In 1885 the University of Berlin created the Chair of Hygiene and Bacteriology in his honor. He became the Nobel Laureate in 1905.

While Robert Koch's brilliant career was nearing

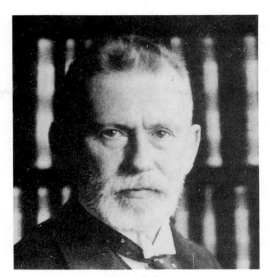

Figure 2–7
Paul Ehrlich. (Courtesy of the National Library of Medicine.)

an end because of age and illnesses, the work of Paul Ehrlich (1854–1915) was reaching its zenith (Fig. 2–7). Ehrlich had been greatly honored when Koch had invited him to work in his laboratory. Koch had known Ehrlich well, since he had been a distinguished student of his and had already made a place for himself in scientific circles.

Ehrlich was a German physician, and one of the pioneers in the fields of bacteriology, **immunology**, and especially **chemotherapy**, a fairly new science. He was only 28 years old when he wrote his first paper on typhoid, but his greatest gift to mankind was to be called his "magic bullet," or "606," and was designed to fight the terrible disease, syphilis. Only three years before, Bordet and Wasserman had identified the organism and devised a test that would smoke it out of hiding. With the offending germ identified, Ehrlich set out to find a chemical that would destroy the organism but not harm the germ's host, the human body. The search was long and tedious, and history tells us it was the 606th drug that Ehrlich tried that finally did the healing. He called the drug salvarsan because he felt it offered mankind salvation from this disease. This also was the beginning of injecting chemicals into the body to destroy a specific organism.

Later, in 1912, Ehrlich discovered a less toxic drug, called neosalvarsan, to replace the original 606. The new drug bore the number 914. In 1908 Ehrlich shared the Nobel prize with Eli Metchnikoff, who is remembered for his theory of **phagocytosis** and immunology.

WOMEN IN MEDICINE

Much time is spent with honoring great men in medical history, but women have also played im-

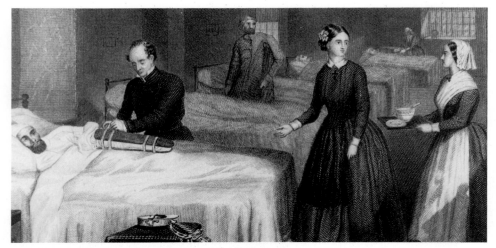

Figure 2–8
Florence Nightingale. (Courtesy of the National Library of Medicine.)

portant roles, which during those times was not an easy thing to do. Two famous women, in particular, are Florence Nightingale (1820–1910) and Clara Barton (1821–1912). You may notice that their careers overlap almost to the year.

Florence Nightingale has been honored and known far and wide as "The Lady with the Lamp" and is immortalized as the founder of nursing (Fig. 2–8). She was of noble birth, and somewhat late in life she sought nurse's training in both England and Europe. By the time of the Crimean War in 1854 she already had a reputation for her work in hospital organization. She was invited by the Secretary of War to visit the Crimea to correct the terrible conditions that existed in caring for the wounded. She created the Women's Nursing Service at Scutari and Balaklava. The doctors at Scutari regarded Florence Nightingale as a troublesome female intruder and treated her and her nurses quite shabbily. Only a crisis that brought thousands of wounded and sick soldiers to army hospitals persuaded the doctors to accept help from her and her nurses.

Miss Nightingale ruled her nurses with an iron hand. Aside from the practical work she did, it was she who insisted the nursing profession get public recognition, and that nursing required special training and experience. From donated funds she organized a school of nursing that bears her name. The modern conception of nursing is based largely on the foundations she laid.

The American counterpart to Florence Nightingale is Clara Barton (Fig. 2–9). She was a nurse and philanthropist whose work during the American Civil War led her to recognize that very poor records, if any at all, were kept in Washington to aid in the search for missing men wounded or killed in combat. This led to the formation of the Bureau of Records. Clara Barton's fame spread as a result of her organization and recruitment of supplies for the wounded. In 1870 she observed the work of the

Red Cross in the Franco-Prussian War, and in 1881 she organized a Red Cross Committee in Washington, forming the American Red Cross, of which she served as the first president from 1881 to 1904.

Elizabeth Blackwell (1821–1910) was the first woman in the United States to receive the Doctor of Medicine degree from a medical school. Blackwell's family immigrated to New York from England in 1832. Young Elizabeth began her medical education by reading medical books and later on had private instruction. Medical schools in New York and Pennsylvania refused her applications for formal study, but finally, in 1847, she was accepted at the Geneva (New York) Medical College. Ten years later when Blackwell was practicing medicine in New York City, she established the New York Infirmary, a hospital staffed by women. In 1869 Dr. Blackwell returned to her native England and became professor of gynecology (1875–1907) at the

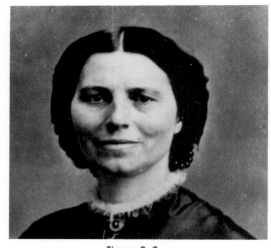

Figure 2–9
Clara Barton. (Courtesy of the National Library of Medicine.)

Table 2–1
Milestones in the History of Medicine

Dates	Person	Achievement	Dates	Person	Achievement
1205 BC	Moses (First "Public Health Officer")	Incorporated rules of health into the Hebrew religion	1781–1826	René Laënnec	Invented the stethoscope
460–377 BC	Hippocrates (Father of Medicine)	Gave scientific basis to medicine Hippocratic Oath	1818–1865	Ignaz Philipp Semmelweis (Savior of Mothers)	Developed theory of childbed (puerperal) fever
131–201 AD	Galen (Father of Experimental Physiology)	First to describe cranial nerves and sympathetic system	1820–1910	Florence Nightingale (Lady with the Lamp)	Founder of nursing
1514–1564	Andreas Vesalius (Belgian anatomist; Father of Modern Anatomy)	Corrected some of Galen's errors Published De Corporis Humani Fabrica describing structure of human body	1821–1912	Clara Barton	Founder of American Red Cross
			1821–1910	Elizabeth Blackwell	First woman in United States to receive Doctor of Medicine degree from a medical school
1578–1657	William Harvey	Described pumping action of heart and circulation of the blood	1822–1895	Louis Pasteur (Father of Bacteriology)	Developed germ theory of disease and destruction of microorganisms through use of heat
1628–1694	Marcello Malpighi (first histologist)	Pioneered microscopic anatomy Identified the taste buds; described minute structures of brain and optic nerve	1827–1912	Joseph Lister	Applied Pasteur's theories and developed sterile techniques in surgery
1632–1723	Anton van Leeuwenhoek	Discovered lens magnification First to observe bacteria and protozoa through a lens Made first accurate description of red blood cells	1843–1910	Robert Koch	Bacteriologist who developed culture-plate method for isolation of bacteria Set down Koch's postulates
			1845–1922	Wilhelm Konrad Roentgen	Discovered x-ray in 1895
1722–1809	Leopold Auenbrugger	Developed the use of percussion in diagnosis	1854–1915	Paul Ehrlich	Began the use of injecting chemicals into the body to destroy a specific organism Developed drug used to fight syphilis
1728–1793	John Hunter (Founder of Scientific Surgery)	Introduced artificial feeding by insertion of flexible tube into stomach Made classic description of syphilitic chancre (Hunterian chancre)	1867–1940	Lillian Wald	New York City nurse who operated a visiting nurse service and helped establish the world's first public school nursing system
1745–1813	Benjamin Rush	Published first American treatise on psychiatry in 1812			
1749–1823	Edward Jenner	Discovered smallpox vaccine			

London School of Medicine for Women, of which she was a founder.

Another great contribution to medical care was made by Lillian Wald (1867–1940), a social worker and nurse who founded the internationally known Henry Street Settlement at 265 Henry Street, New York City. Wald operated a visiting nurse service from this establishment. When one of her nurses was assigned to the city's public schools in 1902, the New York City municipal board of health established the world's first public school nursing system.

MODERN MIRACLES

Anyone who has ever been spared the pain of surgery through the sleep of an anesthetic can give thanks to the memory of two dentists, Dr. Horace Wells and Dr. William T. G. Morton; and a physician, Dr. Crawford Williamson Long. There has been considerable controversy as to whom should be given final credit for the actual discovery of anesthesia, but it now seems to be established that Dr. Long (1815–1878) was the first to employ ether as an anesthetic agent. Early in 1842, after lectures on chemistry, a group of students would have a social gathering and inhale ether as a form of amusement. At one of these so-called "ether frolics," Dr. Long observed that people under the influence of ether did not seem to feel pain. After considerable thought, Dr. Long decided to use ether for a surgical operation. On March 30, 1842, he removed a tumor from the neck of James M. Venable after placing him under the influence of ether. Long did not report this operation or his discovery until 1848. Wells reported his discovery in 1844, and Morton his in 1846, when he extracted a tooth after the patient had been given ether, and he also used it at Massachusetts General Hospital for a surgical procedure.

Surgery undoubtedly owes most to Wilhelm Konrad Roentgen (1845–1922), who discovered the x-ray in 1895. Roentgen was awarded the Nobel prize in physics in 1901. Although he called his ray the x-ray, science has honored him by calling it the roentgen ray.

Walter Reed, U.S. Army pathologist and bacteriologist, in 1900 proved that yellow fever is transmitted by the bite of a mosquito; in 1901 action by U.S. military engineers in Cuba freed Havana from the disease by eliminating the mosquitoes.

Anyone who has had an x-ray or has received radium therapy should know the long struggle of Marie and Pierre Curie leading to the discovery of radium in 1898. Diabetics should be grateful to Frederick Banting, the Canadian physician who discovered insulin in 1922. Children born with cyanosis due to a malformed heart (tetralogy of Fallot) owe thanks to Helen B. Taussig, M.D., of Baltimore,

Maryland, who, together with Alfred Blalock, M.D. (1899–1964), developed the lifesaving operation for so-called "blue babies." While the Blalock-Taussig procedure, first performed in 1944 at Johns Hopkins University Hospital, may seem simple today, 40 years ago it was revolutionary and led to a major change of direction in the treatment of heart disease.

In 1928 Sir Alexander Fleming (1881–1955), a British bacteriologist, discovered penicillin. While working with staphylococcal bacteria, Fleming noticed a bacteria-free circle around a mold growth that was contaminating a culture of the staphylococci. Upon investigation he found a substance in the mold that prevented growth of bacteria even when it was diluted 800 times. He called it penicillin. Fleming shared the 1945 Nobel prize for Physiology or Medicine with Ernst Boris Chain and Howard Walter Florey for further discoveries related to penicillin.

The vaccines developed by Jonas Edward Salk and Albert Sabin in the 1950s almost eradicated polio, once the killer or crippler of thousands, from the United States. The work of Dr. Christiaan Barnard in the 1960s inspired transplantation of hearts and other organs.

William Worrall Mayo, who immigrated to the United States from England in 1845, was the founder, in 1863, of the surgical practice in Rochester, Minnesota, that evolved into today's Mayo Clinic. Mayo's two sons, William James Mayo and Charles Horace Mayo, both became doctors and carried on the work begun by their father. A third-generation Mayo, Charles William Mayo (born in 1899), son of Charles Horace, also became a skilled surgeon and a member of the Mayo Clinic board of governors. The clinic is world renowned and is associated with the University of Minnesota. By the 1980s the staff included more than 800 physicians and over 7000 support staff. Thousands of physicians have received some or all of their residency training at the Mayo Clinic and the Mayo Foundation connected with it.

And history continues. Bypass surgery has made thousands of hearts more functional. Organ transplants are becoming almost commonplace. Great advances have been made in the treatment of cancer—who will find a real breakthrough? Dialysis machines allow people with nonfunctional kidneys, who would have died a few decades ago, to lead relatively normal lives. Countless unnamed people are engaged in research or are implementing new developments. Let us not forget those who are involved in organizing public health services and have thus contributed to bettering the availability and distribution of health care.

It is tremendously exciting simply to be open to such advancements and to be aware of their potential. The supportive role of medical assisting is very important in maintaining the quality of medical service and in making today a strong foundation for the progress of tomorrow.

REFERENCES AND READINGS

Bordley, J., III, and Harvey, A. M.: *Two Centuries of American Medicine*, Philadelphia, W. B. Saunders Co., 1976.

Garrison, F. H.: *History of Medicine*, 4th ed. (reprint). Philadelphia, W. B. Saunders Co., 1929.

Marks, G., and Beatty, W. K.: *The Story of Medicine in America*, New York, Scribners, 1974.

Robinson, V.: *Pathfinders in Medicine*. New York, Medical Life Press, 1929.

Smith, W. D.: *The Hippocratic Tradition*. New York, Cornell University Press, 1979.

Thorwald, J.: *The Century of the Surgeon*. London, Thames & Hudson, 1957.

2

CHAPTER OUTLINE

Early Development of Medical Education

Forms of Medical Practice
    Sole Proprietorship
    Associate Practice
    Group Practice

Types of Medical Care
    General and Family Practice

Prepaid Comprehensive Care through HMOs
Specialty Practice
Preventive Medicine and Public Health

American Board of Medical Specialties
American College of Surgeons
American College of Physicians
Specialties of Medicine

VOCABULARY

See Glossary at end of book for definitions.

accelerating   prudent
dissemination   statutory body
isolation   substantiated

Medical Practice

3

OBJECTIVES

Upon successful completion of this chapter you should be able to:

1. Define the terms listed in the Vocabulary of this chapter.
2. Explain how the printing press affected medicine during the 19th century.
3. Name and briefly describe how a university greatly influenced medical education in the United States.
4. Name a 20th century educator who played a major role in the development of medical education in the United States.
5. State at least two reasons for change in the 20th century delivery of medical care.
6. Name and briefly describe three forms of medical practice.
7. Name and briefly describe three types of available medical care.
8. Match the names of medical specialties with a given set of definitions.

EARLY DEVELOPMENT OF MEDICAL EDUCATION

In our brief review of the history of medicine in Chapter 2, we found that in early times medical knowledge developed slowly, often in **isolation**, and that **dissemination** of knowledge was poor. Before the advent of printing there was very little exchange of scientific knowledge and ideas, and scientists were not well informed about the works of others.

In the middle of the 15th century, Johann Gutenberg's invention of movable type and adaptation of a certain kind of press for printing marked a turning point in history. Gutenberg's invention resulted in a relatively fast way to produce multiple identical copies of any single text. Printing rapidly replaced the laborious method of scribes, who had to copy manuscripts by hand. The greater availability of books enlarged the number of literate people throughout Europe. In turn, ever greater refinements in the printing press were developed to meet the growing demand for books.

Another development of great importance to science, in the 17th century, was the establishment in Europe of academies or societies consisting of small groups of men who met to discuss subjects of mutual interest. The academies provided freedom of expression which, together with the stimulus of exchanging ideas, contributed significantly to the development of scientific thought. One of the earliest of these academies was the Royal Society of London, an organization formed in 1662 by incorporating several smaller groups under one royal charter.

A significant aspect of these societies was their publications, such as the Royal Society of London's *Philosophical Transactions*. Marcello Malpighi and Anton van Leeuwenhoek (mentioned in Chapter 2) both were invited to join the Royal Society, and contributed works to *Philosophical Transactions*.

As the development of communications improved, society also became more complex, and the need for regulation became greater. The passage of the Medical Act of 1858 in Great Britain was considered one of the most important events in British medicine. It established a **statutory body**, the General Medical Council, which controlled admission to the medical register and had great power over medical education and examinations.

In the United States, medical education was greatly influenced by the example set in 1893 by the Johns Hopkins University Medical School in Baltimore. It admitted only college graduates with a year's training in the natural sciences. Its clinical work was superior because the school was supplemented by the Johns Hopkins Hospital, which had been created expressly for teaching and research carried on by members of the medical faculty. The first four professors at Johns Hopkins were Sir William Osler, professor of medicine; William H. Welch, chief of pathology; Howard A. Kelley, chief of gynecology and obstetrics; and William D. Halsted, chief of surgery. Together, these four men transformed the organization and curriculum of clinical teaching and made Johns Hopkins the most famous medical school in the world.

Abraham Flexner (1866–1959), an educator, also played a major role in the development of medical education in the United States. Flexner received a Carnegie Foundation commission to study the quality of medical colleges in the United States and Canada. The Flexner report, published in 1910, rated 155 schools according to the quality of instruction and facilities available to the students. The publication of this report resulted in the closure of many low-ranking schools and the upgrading of many others.

By the mid-20th century, medical practice was experiencing many changes. Rapid developments in medical science encouraged more specialization. The **accelerating** cost of maintaining an office was becoming prohibitive for a solo practitioner, especially the new graduate. Medical insurance for the patient was the rule rather than the exception. More and more government programs, with their accompanying regulations, were developing, and the management of a medical practice required more and better-trained personnel.

All of these developments brought many changes in the delivery of medical care. It is estimated that by the year 2000, 50 percent of the U.S. population will be receiving their medical care in prepaid comprehensive care facilities. Though there are still many solo practitioners in medicine, the trend is toward multiple practitioner practices.

FORMS OF MEDICAL PRACTICE

- *Sole Proprietorship*
- *Associate Practice*
- *Group Practice*
- *Partnership*
- *Professional Corporation*

Sole Proprietorship

Sole proprietorship is commonly referred to as "solo practice." A sole proprietor is an individual who holds exclusive right and title to all aspects of the medical practice. The sole proprietor may employ other physicians to participate in the practice. The employed physician would be entitled to any employee fringe benefits, but the owner would not be so entitled. Additionally, the owner would be potentially liable for all of the acts of his professional employees. Solo practice is steadily declining. In 1984 it was estimated that solo practices were diminishing by 20,000 a year.

Associate Practice

Often two or more physicians will agree to share office space and employees, but conduct their practices as sole proprietors. They will have an agreement among themselves as to the manner in which the practice will be operated.

Group Practice

The governing bodies of the American Medical Association, the American Group Practice Association, and the Medical Group Management Association have formally adopted the following definition of medical group practice:

> Medical Group Practice is the provision of health care services by a group of at least three licensed physician-practitioners, engaged full-time in a formally organized and legally recognized entity; sharing the group's income and expenses in a systematic manner; and sharing facilities, equipment, common records, and personnel, involved in both patient care and business management.

An association of 3 to 7 physicians is considered a small group; 8 to 30 physicians, a medium group; and more than 30 physicians a large group.

A small or medium-sized group might be a single-specialty group with all the physicians engaged in the same specialty. Family practice and anesthesia services are two common examples. A large group would more likely be a multi-specialty practice. Group practice may take the legal form of a partnership or a corporation.

Partnership. When two or more physicians elect to associate in the practice of medicine, they may draw up a partnership agreement. While it is not necessary that the agreement be in writing, no **prudent** person would enter into such an arrangement without a written agreement prepared with the aid of a competent attorney. The agreement should show all the rights, obligations, and responsibilities of each partner. One of the major disadvantages of partnership is the liability of each for the acts and conduct of one another unless otherwise specified in the partnership agreement.

Professional Corporation. A corporation may be defined as an artificial entity having a legal and business status that is independent of its shareholders or employees. Corporations are regulated by state statutes, so their requirements vary but there are many similarities. The physician shareholders are employees of the corporation. Even one physician in solo practice can incorporate. There are income and tax advantages to all employees of the corporation. Usually an attractive fringe benefit package is offered to the employees, which might include pension and profit-sharing plans, medical expense reimbursement, life insurance, disability income insurance and employee death benefit. Fringe benefits to the corporate employee are in addition to salary—tax deductible to the corporation and not taxable to the employee. Professional employees of a corporation are liable only for their own acts. Another advantage of the corporate entity is the continuous life of the corporation.

In an unincorporated solo practice, the practice dies with the owner, and in a partnership practice, the death or discontinuance of practice of a partner necessitates a new agreement. A corporation, however, is an entity unto itself and does not end with a change in shareholders.

TYPES OF MEDICAL CARE

- *General and Family Practice*
- *Prepaid Comprehensive Care*
- *Specialty Practice*
- *Preventive Medicine and Public Health*

General and Family Practice

The physician who does not specialize or limit his or her practice is said to be in general practice. Family or general practice encompasses the care of all members of the family regardless of age or sex, and covers a vast range of medical problems. This allows for continuity of care for the individual, and integration of care for the family as a whole.

Prepaid Comprehensive Care through Health Maintenance Organizations (HMOs)

An HMO is an organization that provides for comprehensive health care to an enrolled group for a fixed periodic payment. HMOs are not an entirely new concept. The Ross-Loos Medical Group of Los Angeles has operated a prepaid group practice since early 1929. For many years, however, organized medicine resisted all arrangements for compensation except on a basis of fee-for-service.

In the early 1970s, the federal government, which bears a great percentage of the costs of medical care, took action to contain the potential abuses of overtreatment and overutilization of health care services. The enactment of Public Law 93-222, the HMO Assistance Act, in December 1973, created Title XIII of the Public Health Service Act. Title XIII is intended to encourage and promote the growth of health maintenance organizations with the intent of cost containment. As the name implies, the HMO concept stresses the maintenance of health and preventive medicine. Members of HMOs are more inclined to see their physician before major and more costly problems arise, because their contract provides for comprehensive care. Employers who provide health care benefits to employees are now required to offer federally qualified HMOs as an option.

Specialty Practice

Many physicians have a special interest in a particular branch of medical practice and eventually direct their efforts to becoming expert in their chosen field. Physicians who decide to limit their practice to a specialized field will have to spend an additional 3 to 6 years in a residency program after completion of internship and will probably seek certification by one of the specialty boards.

Preventive Medicine and Public Health

The practice of medicine does not always involve patient care. The community is the public health physician's patient. All branches of medicine are committed to preventive medicine, and the public health physician complements the efforts of the private physician. The United States Public Health Service and the World Health Organization are both concerned with preventive medicine. The American Board of Preventive Medicine requires completion of 2 years of approved residency, 1 year of study in a School of Public Health, and 3 years of full-time experience in public health work before a candidate is eligible for certification examinations.

General preventive medicine is concerned with the relation of environment to health and with special concern for the health requirements of population groups.

Public Health is a special field of preventive medicine embodying the use of medical and administrative methods to prevent disease and improve general health through community efforts in areas such as sanitation and education.

Occupational medicine, another branch of preventive medicine, is concerned with the medical problems and practices related to occupation and especially to employees in industry.

AMERICAN BOARD OF MEDICAL SPECIALTIES

Presently there are 23 specialty boards under the umbrella of the American Board of Medical Specialties. These specialty boards assist in improving the quality of medical education by elevating the standards of graduate medical education and approving facilities for specialty training. The primary function of each approved specialty board is to evaluate the qualifications of candidates in its field who apply

voluntarily for examination and to certify as diplomates those who are qualified.

To accomplish this function, specialty boards determine if candidates have received adequate preparation in accordance with established educational standards; they provide comprehensive examinations to such candidates; and they issue certificates to those physicians who have satisfied the requirements. Those physicians who are Board-certified are known as diplomates of a specific specialty board—for example, Fredrick B. Mears, M.D., Diplomate of the American Board of Surgery.

A listing of the 23 specialty boards is found in Table 3–1. The American Board of Medical Specialties is located at One American Plaza, Suite 805, Evanston, Illinois, 60201. It regularly publishes a directory listing all physicians certified as diplomates by the specialty boards, including biographic sketches detailing their educational qualifications. Many physicians consult the directory in making referrals.

AMERICAN COLLEGE OF SURGEONS

The American College of Surgeons may also confer a degree on an applicant from a surgical specialty. The applicant is required to have completed a course of postgraduate training equivalent to "Board requirements" and to have submitted 50 detailed, **substantiated** case reports of varied surgical procedures in which the applicant has been the chief surgeon during the last 3 years of practice prior to application. Successful applicants are identified as a Fellow of the American College of Surgeons (FACS).

Table 3–1
Approved Specialty Boards of the United States

American Board of Allergy and Immunology
American Board of Anesthesiology
American Board of Colon and Rectal Surgery
American Board of Dermatology
American Board of Emergency Medicine
American Board of Family Practice
American Board of Internal Medicine
American Board of Neurological Surgery
American Board of Nuclear Medicine
American Board of Obstetrics and Gynecology
American Board of Ophthalmology
American Board of Orthopaedic Surgery
American Board of Otolaryngology
American Board of Pathology
American Board of Pediatrics
American Board of Physical Medicine and Rehabilitation
American Board of Plastic Surgery
American Board of Preventive Medicine
American Board of Psychiatry and Neurology
American Board of Radiology
American Board of Surgery
American Board of Thoracic Surgery
American Board of Urology

AMERICAN COLLEGE OF PHYSICIANS

The American College of Physicians issues a similar fellowship degree (FACP) to applicants who have completed approved postgraduate training and who have exhibited special interest and competence in one of the nonsurgical specialties.

SPECIALTIES OF MEDICINE

Aerospace Medicine. Aerospace medicine is the specialty concerned with the physiologic, pathologic, and psychologic problems encountered by humans in space. At present this field is mostly confined to the space agencies of the federal government.

Allergy & Immunology. An allergy is an abnormal reaction to substances that are harmless to most people. Substances that frequently bother the allergic person include pollens from grass, weeds, and trees, molds, house and other dusts, dog and cat danders, certain foods and medications, and the stings of insects.

There are many kinds of medicines and treatments that can help relieve the allergic symptoms, but it is essential first to identify the cause. The allergist is specially trained to diagnose and treat allergy problems with a high degree of accuracy and success.

The American Board of Allergy and Immunology is a Conjoint Board of the American Board of Internal Medicine and the American Board of Pediatrics. To become an allergist, the pediatrician or internist must take several years of additional specialty training and pass another certifying examination.

Anesthesiology. An anesthesiologist is a physician who administers local and general anesthesia, usually to prepare and maintain a patient for surgery, and in some cases for relief of pain. An anesthesiologist monitors the surgical patient through the surgical process until stable consciousness returns postoperatively.

Dermatology. Dermatologists are medical doctors who have extensive specialized training in the medical and surgical treatment of disorders of the skin, hair, and nails.

Because of specific training, the dermatologist is able to determine the best treatment approach to skin disorders. This approach may involve the use of medicines, both internal and external, or it may involve skin surgery. In addition to common dermatologic procedures such as removal of moles, warts, cysts, benign tumors, and skin cancers, many dermatologists are also trained in certain surgical and cosmetic procedures. These include skin grafts and flaps, hair transplants, dermabrasion, and collagen implants.

Emergency Medicine. The emergency medicine specialist is a physician who specializes in the immediate recognition and treatment of acute illnesses and injuries. These specialists may also be involved in the administration, teaching, and research of systems designed to help patients seeking emergency care. Qualifications for this specialty include a formal emergency medicine residency training or experience and continuing medical education.

Traditionally, specialists in emergency medicine provide 24-hour coverage of emergency departments in acute care hospitals, making emergency care available at all times. These specialists also provide the authority and license under which paramedic pre-hospital care is provided.

Family Practice. Family or general practice encompasses the care of all members of the family regardless of age or sex, and covers a vast range of medical problems. This allows for continuity of care for the individual, and integration of care for the family as a whole.

Internal Medicine. Internal medicine is the specialty concerned with the complete nonsurgical care of the adult. Internists are experts in the medical diagnosis and treatment of adult disorders, as well as in the areas of health maintenance and wellness. General internists are responsible for a broad range of adult medical problems. There are multiple subspecialties within internal medicine, including allergy, cardiology, endocrinology, gastroenterology, gerontology, hematology, infectious disease, nephrology, oncology, pulmonary diseases, and rheumatology.

Neurology. Neurology is concerned with the nonsurgical management of neurologic disease. Generally, the neurologist will manage infectious, metabolic, degenerative, and systemic involvement of the nervous system.

Nuclear Medicine. Nuclear medicine is a specialty field in which radioactive substances are used for the diagnosis and treatment of disease.

Obstetrics & Gynecology. Obstetrics is the specialty involved in the care and management of women during pregnancy, labor, delivery, and the puerperium. Gynecology is the specialty devoted to the medical and surgical treatment of diseases of women, especially those of the reproductive organs and functions.

Ophthalmology. Ophthalmology involves the diagnosis and treatment of eye and vision disorders, utilizing surgery and other corrective techniques.

Otolaryngology. Otolaryngology is professionally known today as Otolaryngology/Head and Neck Surgery. The specialty is broadly based, encompassing medical and surgical treatment of ear, nose, and throat disorders, allergy therapy, facial cosmetic and reconstructive surgery, and tumor problems in the head and neck. Otolaryngology is advancing in the fields of microsurgery and laser surgery.

Pathology. Pathology is the science that deals with the causes, mechanisms of development, and effects of disease. The pathologist seeks to determine the actual nature of disease—not just the physical symptoms or how it feels to the patient, but what the disease is from a biologic standpoint; that is, what visible or measurable changes it produces in the cells, fluids, and life processes of the entire body.

The practice of pathology is divided into two major areas, Anatomic Pathology and Clinical Pathology; and these areas are further subdivided into more numerous subspecialties. The function of the anatomic pathologist is to render a diagnosis on the basis of examination of a tissue specimen, and to determine as precisely as possible the extent of the disease. The clinical pathologist is in charge of the medical laboratory, in which a wide variety of diagnostic studies are performed. Forensic pathology is a subspecialty dealing with various aspects of medicine and the law.

Pediatrics. Caring for the health of children from birth to adolescence is the unique purpose of pediatrics, the medical specialty that continually strives to prevent and treat all aspects of childhood diseases. The extent of the pediatrician's interest and responsibilities spans such areas as infectious diseases, newborn care, hospital care of children, environmental hazards, school health problems, nutrition, accident prevention, children with handicaps, drugs, allergy, cardiology, and pediatric pharmacology. The pediatric specialist is able to handle the problems of acutely ill children, as well as to provide guidance to parents regarding the development and preventive care of children who are well.

The neonatologist deals with the diseases and abnormalities of the newborn.

Physical Medicine and Rehabilitation. Physical Medicine and Rehabilitation is concerned with the diagnosis and treatment of disorders and disabilities of the neuromuscular system. A physician in this specialty is called a physiatrist. He or she uses the physical elements such as heat, cold, water, electricity, and exercise to help restore physical function and independence.

Preventive Medicine. Preventive Medicine is concerned with preventing the occurrence of both men-tal and physical illness and disability. Analysis of present health services and planning for future medical needs are part of Preventive Medicine, as are Occupational Medicine and Public Health.

Psychiatry. A psychiatrist is a physician whose specialty is the diagnosis and treatment of persons with mental, emotional, or behavioral disorders. The psychiatrist is qualified to conduct psychotherapy and to prescribe medications when necessary. This allows the psychiatrist to comprehensively treat complex interactions of biologic, psychologic and social factors that affect patients.

Radiology. Radiology is a specialty in which x-rays (roentgen rays) are used for diagnosis and treatment of disease. A diagnostic radiologist specializes in using x-rays, ultrasound, nuclear medicine, computed tomography (CT), and magnetic resonance imaging (MRI) for detection of abnormalities throughout the body. Therapeutic radiology involves the use of ionizing radiation in the treatment of cancer and other tumors.

Surgery. Surgery is the correction of deformities, defects, diseases, or injured parts of the body by means of operative treatment. By making an incision into body tissue, or by passing instruments through the skin, the diseased or injured tissues or organs can be corrected, modified, removed, or replaced. The various specializations contained within the broad field of surgery are: General Surgery, Colon and Rectal Surgery, Neurosurgery, Orthopedic Surgery, Oral Surgery and Dentistry, Plastic Surgery, Thoracic (Cardiovascular) Surgery, and Urology.

General Surgery. General Surgery may include all aspects of surgery other than those included under special groups. Many general surgeons restrict their practice to surgery of abdominal conditions, traumatic situations, or tumor conditions. However, there is no restriction on the general surgeon's scope of activities, and many take on additional fields as their training, interest, and capabilities dictate.

Colon and Rectal Surgery. Colon and Rectal Surgery is a surgical subspecialty that concentrates on surgical treatment of the lower intestinal tract, which includes the colon and rectum.

Neurosurgery. A neurosurgeon specializes in the diagnosis and surgical treatment of the nervous system (the brain, spinal cord, and nerves) and the surrounding bony structures.

Orthopedic Surgery. Orthopedic Surgery is that branch of medicine that deals with the treatment of maladies of the musculoskeletal system.

It not only involves treatment of musculoskeletal injuries but also deals with congenital deformities and acquired deformities, including spinal curvatures and arthritis. Orthopedic techniques are also used to treat sports injuries, more successfully now than ever with the advent of arthroscopic techniques to maximize rehabilitation.

Although orthopedics is a branch of surgery, many conditions are actually treated without surgery, including most fractures and muscle and tendon infirmities.

Oral Surgery. Oral Surgery is that branch of dentistry dealing with the extraction of teeth, the treatment of fractures of the jaws and adjacent facial bones, and with other surgical procedures on the jaws, oral tissues, and adjacent tissues to treat or correct disease and other abnormal conditions.

Plastic Surgery. Plastic Surgery includes the operative repair of defects by graft, tissue transfer, or cosmetic alteration of tissue. A plastic surgeon specializes in burns, congenital defects, and hand and extremity reconstruction, as well as treating skin wounds and lesions and performing aesthetic surgery of the face and body contouring.

Thoracic (Cardiovascular) Surgery. Thoracic or Cardiovascular Surgery is a surgical subspecialty concerned with the operative treatment of the chest and chest wall, the lungs and respiratory passages. Specialists in this field are involved with heart surgery, including both valvular and coronary heart surgery.

Urology. Urology is a medical specialty concerned with treating diseases and disorders of the urinary tract of men, women, and children, as well as the male genital tract.

As the delivery of medical care has become more fragmented, the close relationship that existed between family physician and patient has declined, and the specialist often enters the picture as a complete stranger. The medical assistant who is skilled in communications can bridge this gap. An understanding of medical ethics and the prevention of malpractice claims is extremely important in communicating with the patient.

REFERENCES AND READINGS

Gerber, P. C., and Petrie, K. J.: What's the Economic Outlook for Medical Practice? *Physician's Management*, August 1984, p. 50.

Manning, F. F.: *Medical Group Practice Management.* Cambridge, MA, Ballinger Publishing Co., 1977.

Stegeman, W.: *Medical Terms Simplified.* St. Paul, West Publishing Co., 1976.

3

CHAPTER OUTLINE

Historical Codes
AMA Principles of Medical Ethics
Judicial Council Opinions
Ethics for the Medical Assistant

VOCABULARY

See Glossary at end of book for definitions.

abet	expulsion	precept
artificial insemination	fee splitting	public domain
censure	genetics	resident
compulsory	ghost surgery	revocation
culminate	in vitro	suspension
dilemma	preamble	technologic
discrepancy		

Medical Ethics

4

OBJECTIVES

Upon successful completion of this chapter you should be able to:

1. *Define the terms listed in the Vocabulary of this chapter.*
2. *Differentiate between the terms ethics and etiquette.*
3. *Identify the earliest written code of ethical conduct for medical practice.*
4. *Name the ancient Greek oath that remains an inspiration to physicians today.*
5. *Identify a code that was an example for the AMA Principles of Medical Ethics.*
6. *Explain the purpose of the 1980 revision of the AMA Principles.*
7. *Identify seven principles of medical ethics found in the present AMA code.*
8. *Name the official body that is charged with interpreting these principles.*
9. *State the prime objective of the medical profession.*
10. *Compare the provisions of the AAMA Code of Ethics with those of the AMA Principles.*

Ethics concerns the thoughts, judgments, and actions on issues that have the greater implications of moral "right" and "wrong." A "morally right" attitude is usually understood to be directed toward an ideal form of human character or action, which should **culminate** in the highest good for humanity. From the desire to achieve this good comes the sense of moral duty and a system of interpersonal moral obligations.

Medical etiquette should not be confused with medical ethics. *Etiquette* deals with courtesy, customs, and manners; *ethics* concerns itself with the underlying philosophies in the ideal relationships of humans. These relationships are often formally set forth in social contracts and codes.

HISTORICAL CODES

Ethics—judgments of right and wrong—have always been a concern of human beings. It is not surprising that for centuries the medical profession has set for itself a rigid standard of ethical conduct toward patients and colleagues. The earliest written code of ethical conduct for medical practice was conceived around 2250 BC by the Babylonians and was called the Code of Hammurabi. It went into much detail regarding the conduct expected of a physician, even prescribing the fees that could be charged. Probably because of its length and detail it did not survive the ages.

About 400 BC Hippocrates, the Greek physician known as the Father of Medicine, developed a brief statement of principles, which has come down through history and remains an inspiration to the physician of today. The Oath of Hippocrates has been administered to medical graduates in many European universities for centuries.

THE OATH OF HIPPOCRATES

I swear by Apollo, the physician, and Aesculapius, and Health, and Allheal, and all the gods and goddesses, that, according to my ability and judgment, I will keep this oath and stipulation, to reckon him who taught me this art equally dear to me as my parents, to share my substance with him and relieve his necessities if required; to regard his offspring as on the same footing with my own brothers, and to teach them this art if they should wish to learn it, without fee or stipulation, and that by precept, lecture, and every other mode of instruction, I will impart a knowledge of the art to my own sons and to those of my teachers, and to disciples bound by a stipulation and oath, according to the law of medicine, but to none other.

I will follow that method of treatment which, according to my ability and judgment, I consider for the benefit of my patients, and abstain from whatever is deleterious and mischievous. I will give no deadly medicine to anyone if asked, nor suggest any such counsel; furthermore, I will not give to a woman an instrument to produce abortion.

With purity and holiness I will pass my life and practice my art. I will not cut a person who is suffering with a stone, but will leave this to be done by practitioners of this work. Into whatever houses I enter I will go into them for the benefit of the sick and will abstain from every voluntary act of mischief and corruption; and further from the seduction of females or males, bond or free.

Whatever, in connection with my professional practice, or not in connection with it, I may see or hear in the lives of men which ought not to be spoken abroad, I will not divulge, as reckoning that all such should be kept secret.

While I continue to keep this oath unviolated, may it be granted to me to enjoy life and the practice of the art, respected by all men at all times, but should I trespass and violate this oath, may the reverse be my lot.

The most significant contribution to ethical history subsequent to Hippocrates was made by Thomas Percival, a physician, philosopher, and writer from Manchester, England. In 1803 he published his Code of Medical Ethics. Percival's personality, his interest in sociologic matters, and his close association with the Manchester Infirmary led to the preparation of a "scheme of professional conduct relative to hospitals and other charities," from which he drafted the code that bears his name.

In 1846, as the American Medical Association was organized in New York City, medical education and medical ethics were being considered from a national point of view. At the first AMA annual meeting in Philadelphia in 1847, a Code of Ethics was formulated and adopted. It specifically acknowledged Percival's Code as its basic example and became a part of the fundamental law of the American Medical Association and of its component parts.

CODES OF MEDICAL ETHICS

2250 BC	*Code of Hammurabi*
400 BC	*Oath of Hippocrates*
1803 AD	*Percival's Code of Medical Ethics*
1980 AD	*AMA Principles of Medical Ethics (latest revision)*

AMA PRINCIPLES OF MEDICAL ETHICS

The AMA Principles of Medical Ethics have been revised on several occasions to keep them consistent with the times, but there has never been a change in their moral intent or overall idealism. Major revisions were made in 1903, 1912, and 1947. In 1957 the AMA Principles of Medical Ethics were condensed to a **preamble** and ten sections, a major change in format from the 1847 code. The 1980 revision of the code (Fig. 4–1), containing a preamble and only seven sections, was done "to clarify and update the language, to eliminate reference to gender, and to seek a proper and reasonable balance between professional standards and contemporary legal standards in our changing society."

As stated in the Preamble, these Principles are

PRINCIPLES OF MEDICAL ETHICS

Preamble

The medical profession has long subscribed to a body of ethical statements developed primarily for the benefit of the patient. As a member of this profession, a physician must recognize responsibility not only to patients, but also to society, to other health professionals, and to self. The following Principles adopted by the American Medical Association are not laws, but standards of conduct which define the essentials of honorable behavior for the physician.

  I. A physician shall be dedicated to providing competent medical service with compassion and respect for human dignity.

 II. A physician shall deal honestly with patients and colleagues, and strive to expose those physicians deficient in character or competence, or who engage in fraud or deception.

III. A physician shall respect the law and also recognize a responsibility to seek changes in those requirements which are contrary to the best interests of the patient.

 IV. A physician shall respect the rights of patients, of colleagues, and of other health professionals, and shall safeguard patient confidences within the constraints of the law.

  V. A physician shall continue to study, apply and advance scientific knowledge, make relevant information available to patients, colleagues and the public, obtain consultation, and use the talents of other health professionals when indicated.

 VI. A physician shall, in the provision of appropriate patient care except in emergencies, be free to choose whom to serve, with whom to associate, and the environment in which to provide medical services.

VII. A physician shall recognize a responsibility to participate in activities contributing to an improved community.

Figure 4–1
AMA Principles of Medical Ethics. (With permission of the American Medical Association, Chicago, IL.)

---

not laws but standards. Laws vary from state to state and from community to community, but ethical standards do not. Ethical standards are never less than the standards required by law; frequently they are greater. Violation of the ethical standards of an association or society may result in **censure, expulsion**, or **suspension** of membership. Violation of a law followed by conviction may result in punishment by fine, imprisonment, or **revocation** of license.

The Judicial Council of the AMA, consisting of five active members of the AMA elected by the House of Delegates, is charged with interpreting the Principles as adopted by the House of Delegates of the American Medical Association. The Council periodically publishes a compilation of its interpretations, opinions, and statements. Some of the interpretations of the Principles set forth in the *Current Opinions of the Judicial Council of the AMA, 1984*, will be discussed in the following pages. While the code and the interpretations are directed specifically toward physicians, the medical assistant, as a member of the medical team, must be familiar with these principles and cooperate with the physician in practicing within their concepts.

JUDICIAL COUNCIL OPINIONS

The opinions of the Judicial Council elaborate and expand the **precepts** in the Principles of Medical Ethics. They are continually updated to encompass developing situations, and they reflect the changing challenges and responsibilities of medicine. In the 1984 issue, a number of situations are dealt with that did not appear in the 1981 issue, such as:

• Abuse of Children, Elderly Persons, and Others at Risk
• Capital Punishment
• **Genetic** Counseling
• Interprofessional Relations with Nurses
• Sports Medicine

For a fuller appreciation of the ethical issues in medicine, the medical assistant should obtain a copy of the *Current Opinions of the Judicial Council* for complete study (Order Department OP-122, American Medical Association, PO Box 10946, Chicago, IL 60610). Only a brief summary will be given here.

Current Opinions, 1984, is presented in nine parts:

1.00 Introduction

The introduction explains the terminology used, and the relation of law and ethics.

2.00 Social Policy Issues

This lengthy section addresses the following issues:
Abortion
Abuse of children, elderly persons, and others at risk

Allocation of health resources
Artificial insemination
Capital punishment
Clinical investigation
Costs
Fetal research guidelines
Genetic counseling
Genetic engineering
In vitro fertilization
Organ transplantation
Quality of life
Terminal illness
Unnecessary and worthless services.

The physician is not prohibited by ethical consid-erations from performing a lawful abortion in ac-cordance with good medical practice.

The discovery that a patient is abusing a child or a parent creates a difficult situation for the doctor's office. The law requires that such abuse be reported.

The physician, being a member of a profession dedicated to preserving life, should not participate in a legally authorized execution.

While participating in the clinical investigation of new drugs and procedures, physicians should show the same concern for the welfare and safety of the person involved as would prevail if the person were a private patient.

Technologic developments add to the ethical **di-lemmas** facing the physician. New expensive treat-ments are available, and the physician must balance the advantages to the patient with the sometimes exorbitant costs. Genetic counseling and organ transplantation may require personal and ethical decisions concerning the quality of the life that is saved. Often in the treatment of deformed new-borns or severely deteriorated victims of injury, illness, or advanced age, the physician must decide what is best for the individual patient.

Patients who live in one of the 35 states having "living will" statutes may have some choice if the patient has made such a will. The living will is a document that states the wishes of that person in the event of a terminal illness. Usually it is done to prohibit heroic measures being taken in a situation in which the patient would be unable or incompe-tent to make such decisions

3.00 Interprofessional Relations

The AMA Principles have always stressed that a physician should not engage in or aid and **abet** in treatment that has no scientific basis. The physician must also be mindful of state laws that prohibit a doctor from aiding and abetting an unlicensed per-son in the practice of medicine, or from aiding or abetting a person with a limited license in providing services beyond the scope of that person's license. The 1984 edition of *Current Opinions* addresses the relationship between nurses and physicians in their mutual ethical concern for patients, and their obli-gations to one another when there is a suspected error or **discrepancy** in the orders to be carried out by the nurse.

The physician who serves in a medical capacity at an athletic contest or sporting event is reminded that her or his professional responsibility is to protect the health and safety of the contestants, and that the physician's judgment should be gov-erned by medical considerations only.

4.00 Hospital Relations

Most practicing physicians have staff privileges at one or more hospitals. Guidelines for the physi-cian-hospital relationship are developed in this sec-tion and include the following:

- Charging a separate and distinct fee for the incidental, administrative, non-medical service the physician performs in securing the admis-sion of a patient to a hospital is considered unethical.
- **Compulsory** assessments should not be a con-dition of granting medical staff membership or privileges.
- The physician may ethically bill a patient for services rendered the patient by a **resident** un-der the physician's personal observation, direc-tion and supervision, if the physician assumes responsibility for the services.
- A physician may ethically own or have a finan-cial interest in a health facility, but must disclose this information to a patient prior to admission or utilization.
- Decisions regarding hospital privileges should be based upon the training, experience, and demonstrated competence of candidates.

5.00 Confidentiality, Advertising and Communications Media Relations

A great deal of emphasis is placed on the confi-dentiality of patient information, and the limits placed on access to this information. The expanding use of computer technology permits the accumula-tion and storage of an unlimited amount of medical information, and the possibility of access to this information is greater than with the traditional written form in a physician's office. Detailed guide-lines are set forth for the care of computerized information.

Standards regarding advertising and publicity have been somewhat liberalized over the years, but any advertisement or publicity must be true and not misleading. Testimonials of patients, for in-stance, should not be used in advertising, as they are difficult, if not impossible, to verify or measure by objective standards. Physicians practicing in pre-paid plans or HMOs are subject to the same ethical principles as are other physicians.

Although information regarding some patients, such as celebrities and politicians, may be considered "news," the physician may not discuss a patient's condition with the press without authorization from the patient or a lawful representative. The physician may release only authorized information or that which is public knowledge. Certain news is a part of the public record. News in this category is known as news in the **public domain**, and includes births, deaths, accidents, and police cases. Explicit guidelines are given to assist physicians in their ethical and legal obligation to protect the personal privacy and other legal rights of patients.

One item of particular interest to the medical assistant is what information may be disclosed by the physician's office to insurance company representatives. It is important to remember at all times that the history, diagnosis, prognosis, and other information acquired during the physician-patient relationship may be disclosed to an insurance company representative *only* if the patient or the patient's lawful representative has consented to the disclosure.

In the case of a pre-employment physical examination, although no physician-patient relationship exists, the physician is still bound to the rule of confidentiality.

6.00 FEES AND CHARGES

A physician should not charge or collect an illegal or excessive fee, and *Current Opinions* lists factors to be considered as guides in determining the reasonableness of a fee.

Fee splitting, whether with another physician, a clinic or laboratory, or a drug company, is unethical. All referrals and prescriptions must be based on the skill and quality of the physician to whom the patient has been referred or the quality and efficacy of the drug or product prescribed.

The medical assistant whose duties include the collection of fees should note the opinion that the attending physician should complete without charge the appropriate "simplified" insurance claim forms as a part of the service to the patient, but that a charge for more complex forms may be made in conformity with local custom.

Traditionally, the use of harsh or commercial practices in the collection of fees has been discouraged. However, it is proper to request that payment be made at the time of treatment or to add interest or other reasonable charges to delinquent accounts. It is important that the patient be notified in advance of such charges. This can be accomplished by posting a notice in the physician's reception room or by appropriate notations on the billing statement. A patient information folder that includes billing information may be given to patients on their initial visit. Federal laws and regulations applicable to the imposition of interest charges will be discussed in Chapter 12, Professional Fees and

Credit Arrangements. If there are outside laboratory charges, these may be included on the physician's bill by showing the actual charges for laboratory services and the name of the laboratory.

When services are provided by more than one physician—for example, a surgeon and an assisting surgeon or surgeons—each physician should submit a separate bill to the patient and be compensated separately, if possible. In some instances the surgeon and the assisting surgeon may be partners or associates in the same office, in which case one statement with itemized services would be appropriate.

7.00 PHYSICIAN'S RECORDS

Information regarding the patient's medical history must be made available to other physicians upon request of the patient. A physician who formerly treated a patient should not refuse for any reason, including nonpayment for services, to make the records of that patient promptly available on request to another physician presently treating the patient. Proper authorization for the use of records must have been granted by the patient.

Sometimes a question arises regarding ownership of the record. Notes made in treating a patient are primarily for the physician's own use and are considered the physician's personal property. Original records should never be released except on the physician's retirement or sale of a medical practice. However, on request of the patient, a physician should provide a copy or a summary of the record to the patient or to another physician.

Several states have statutes that authorize patient access to medical records. The statutes vary in scope, and some limit access to mental health records. Health care professionals should familiarize themselves with the laws in their own state. Of primary concern regarding all records is the authorization of the patient before releasing any information, unless it is required by law.

8.00 PRACTICE MATTERS

Section 8.00 of *Current Opinions* deals with many practice matters, including:

a. *Appointment Charges.* A physician may charge a patient for a missed appointment or for one not cancelled 24 hours in advance if the patient is fully advised that the physician will make such a charge.

b. *Consultation.* Physicians should obtain a consultation whenever they believe that it would be helpful in the care of the patient or when requested by the patient or the patient's representative.

c. *Contingent Physician Fees.* A physician's fee for medical services should be based on the value of the service provided by the physician to the patient and not on the uncertain outcome of a contingency unrelated to the value of the medical service.

d. *Contractual Relationships.* The contractual relationships that physicians assume when they enter prepaid group practice plans are varied. Physicians should not be subjected to lay interference in professional medical matters, and their primary responsibility should be to the patients they serve.

e. *Drugs and Devices: Prescribing.* A physician should not be influenced in the prescribing of drugs, devices, or appliances by a direct or indirect financial interest in a pharmaceutical firm or other supplier.

f. *Informed Consent.* The patient's right of self-decision can be effectively exercised only if the patient possesses enough information to enable an intelligent choice. (Informed consent is discussed in more detail in Chapter 5.)

g. *Laboratory Services.* The physician's ethical responsibility is to provide the patients with high quality services. This includes services which are personally performed by the physician and those which are delegated to others.

h. *Lien Laws and Neglect of Patients.* These are discussed in Chapter 5.

i. *"Ghost Surgery."* The last subparagraph in 8.00 addresses the practice of **"ghost surgery,"** that is, substitution of surgeon without the patient's knowledge or consent. To have another physician operate on one's patient without the patient's knowledge and consent is a deceit. The patient is entitled to choose his own physician, and he should be permitted to either agree or refuse to accept the substitution.

9.00 PROFESSIONAL RIGHTS AND RESPONSIBILITIES

The final part of *Current Opinions* stresses the professional rights and responsibilities of physicians regarding such matters as their involvement in accreditation programs; agreements restricting the practice of medicine; civil rights; and professional responsibility in exposing incompetent, corrupt, or unethical conduct of professional colleagues; free choice of physician; and peer review.

ETHICS FOR THE MEDICAL ASSISTANT

The Code of Ethics of the American Association of Medical Assistants (Fig. 4–2) is a standard for all medical assistants to honor. The Code is patterned after the AMA Principles and is adapted to the professional medical assistant who accepts this discipline as a responsibility of trust.

The prime objective of the medical profession is to render service to humanity, and this must be the medical assistant's first concern also. The importance of respecting the confidentiality of information learned from or about patients in the course of employment cannot be overemphasized. It is not right to reveal patient confidences to *anyone*—this

CODE OF ETHICS

The Code of Ethics of this Association shall set forth principles of ethical and moral conduct as they relate to the medical profession and the particular practice of medical assisting.

Members of this Association dedicated to the conscientious pursuit of their profession, and thus desiring to merit the high regard of the entire medical profession and the respect of the general public which they serve, do pledge themselves to strive always to:

(a) Render service to humanity with full respect for the dignity of person.

(b) Respect confidential information gained through employment unless legally authorized or required by responsible performance of duty to divulge such information.

(c) Uphold the honor and high principles of the profession and accept its disciplines.

(d) Seek to continually improve our knowledge and skills of medical assisting for the benefit of patients and professional colleagues.

(e) Participate in additional service activities which aim toward improving the health and well-being of the community.

Figure 4–2
AAMA Code of Ethics. (With permission of the American Association of Medical Assistants, Chicago, IL.)

includes your family, your spouse, your best friend, your beautician, other medical assistants—in short, anyone at all! The medical assistant must avoid even mentioning the names of patients, for sometimes the doctor's specialty reveals the patient's reason for consulting that doctor.

Never discuss one patient's case with another patient; if you are asked questions by a curious patient, change the subject. When patients ask questions of a medical nature about their own case, they should be referred to the doctor for information. Patients may also ask for your advice on personal matters, and you should avoid such involvements. Patients tend to identify your remarks as being those of the doctor. By staying mum in all instances, you will be protecting the physician, yourself, and the patient. Confidential papers, case histories, and even the appointment book should be kept out of reach of curious eyes, to protect the patient as well as the doctor and office staff.

It is also the obligation of the medical assistant to keep abreast of developments that affect the practice of medicine and care of the patients. Membership in a professional organization provides access to continuing education that will improve your knowledge and skills.

On rare occasions a medical assistant is faced with a situation in which the physician employer's conduct appears to violate established ethical standards. Before making any judgments, the medical assistant must be absolutely sure of all the facts and circumstances. If there has in fact been a history of unethical conduct, the medical assistant must then make some decisions. Is it wise to remain under these circumstances or would it be better to seek other employment? This is a difficult decision, particularly if the relationship and employment conditions have been satisfactory and congenial. Will a decision to remain adversely affect future opportunities for employment with another physician?

A medical assistant is not obligated to report questionable actions of the physician, or to attempt to change the practice. However, an ethical medical assistant will not wish to participate in the continuance of known substandard practices that may be harmful to the patients, or that are unlawful.

REFERENCES AND READINGS

American Medical Association: *Current Opinions of the Judicial Council.* Chicago, The Association, 1984.
Lewis, M. A., and Warden, C. D.: *Law and Ethics in the Medical Office,* Philadelphia, F. A. Davis Co., 1983.

4

CHAPTER OUTLINE

Licensure and Registration
Classifications of Law
Law of Contracts

Professional Liability
   Negligence

Arbitration
Securing Patient's Informed Consent or Informed
   Refusal

Who May Give Consent?
Good Samaritan Acts
Uniform Anatomical Gift Act
Legal Disclosures
Legal Responsibilities of the Medical Assistant
Claims Prevention
Glossary of Legal Terms

VOCABULARY

See Glossary at end of book for definitions.

arbitration	informed consent	prudent
arbitrator	liability	quackery
assault	litigation	reciprocity
battery	malfeasance	revocation
communicable	malpractice	substantive law
contagious	misfeasance	suspension
continuing education units	nonfeasance	tort
emancipated minor	perjured testimony	trespass
endorsement	probate	venereal

Medicine and the Law

5

OBJECTIVES

Upon successful completion of this chapter you should be able to:

1. Define the terms listed in the Vocabulary of this chapter.
2. State the purpose of medical practice acts and how they are established.
3. List the three methods by which licensure may be granted.
4. List three general categories of cause for revocation or suspension of license.
5. Briefly explain the difference between a crime and a tort.
6. Explain what steps a physician must take for legal protection when terminating an established doctor-patient relationship.
7. List the four D's of Negligence as published by the AMA.
8. Describe briefly what is meant by an arbitration procedure, and identify at least three advantages from using this process.
9. List at least five points that must be included in an informed consent.
10. State five conditions under which a minor may give consent for treatment.
11. Explain the purpose of Good Samaritan Acts.
12. State two restrictions imposed on physicians by the Uniform Anatomical Gift Act.

Closely allied with medical ethics are certain medicolegal principles that must be considered in the daily operation of the doctor's office.

LICENSURE AND REGISTRATION

Medical Practice Acts. Medical practice acts are established by **statute** in each of the 50 states. They define what is included in the practice of medicine within that state and govern the methods and requirements of licensure and the grounds for suspension or revocation of license.

Although medical practice acts existed as early as colonial days, these were later repealed, and in the mid-19th century practically none of the states had laws governing the practice of medicine. As might be expected, there was rapid decline in professional standards. The general welfare of the people was endangered by medical **quackery** and inadequate care; by the beginning of the 20th century, medical practice acts were again in effect in every state.

Licensure. A Doctor of Medicine degree (MD) is conferred upon the graduate from medical school. Some graduates may not wish to actually engage in the practice of medicine; their interests may lie in research or administration, or even in the practice of law with a special interest in medical **liability**. In such cases it is not necessary for them to be licensed. However, before an MD can engage in the practice of medicine, he or she must be licensed.

Physicians in the Armed Forces, Public Health Service, or Veterans Administration facilities need not be licensed in the state where they are employed.

The license to practice medicine is granted by a state board, frequently known as the Board of Medical Examiners, or Board of Registration.

Licensure may be by any one of the following:

• Examination
• Reciprocity
• Endorsement

All states require a written exam for initial licensure. All U.S. licensing jurisdictions except Puerto Rico use the Federation Licensing Examination (FLEX) as the official medical licensing examination. Puerto Rico endorses scores from both the National Board of Medical Examiners (NBME) and FLEX for licensing purposes.

To be eligible for NBME certification, an individual must fulfill all of the following prerequisites:

• Have received the MD degree from a medical school in the United States or Canada which was accredited by the Liaison Committee on Medical Education (LCME) at the time the MD degree was granted.
• Have passed Parts I, II and III of the NBME examination.

• Have completed, with a satisfactory record, one full year of an accredited residency.

Most graduates of U.S. medical schools are now licensed by endorsement of their National Board certificate. Those graduates who are not licensed by endorsement must pass a state board examination, usually FLEX.

Some states grant a license to practice medicine by reciprocity; that is, they endorse a license held in another state or jurisdiction. If an applicant is certificated by the National Board of Medical Examiners, he or she may be granted a license by endorsement in all licensing jurisdictions except Louisiana, Texas, and the Virgin Islands.

In all states, graduates of foreign medical schools seeking licensure by endorsement must meet the same requirements as U.S. graduates, in addition to various other qualifying factors.

Registration. After a license is granted, periodic re-registration is necessary. A physician can be concurrently registered in more than one state. The issuing body will notify the physician when re-registration is due; however, not all states do this at the same time of the year.

Periodic re-registration is necessary annually or biennially

The medical assistant can aid the physician by being aware of when the registration fees are due and thereby prevent a possible lapsing of the registration. Pennsylvania is the only jurisdiction that does not require a re-registration fee. The other states charge fees ranging from $15 to $200. Many states require proof of continuing education in addition to payment of a registration fee.

Continuing education units (CEUs) are granted for attending approved seminars, lectures, and scientific meetings, as well as formal courses in accredited colleges and universities. Fifty hours a year is the average requirement. The medical assistant may be expected to remind the physician and help make arrangements for completing the required units for license renewal.

Revocation or Suspension. Under certain conditions the license to practice medicine may be revoked or suspended.

Grounds for revocation or suspension of medical license generally fall within three categories:
(1) Conviction of a crime
(2) Unprofessional conduct
(3) Personal or professional incapacity

Conviction of a crime may include felonies such as murder, rape, larceny, narcotics violations, and others.

Unprofessional conduct is a failure to uphold the ethical standards of the profession. Betrayal of patient confidences, giving or receiving rebates, and excessive use of narcotics or alcohol are examples.

Personal or professional incapacity is more difficult to label or prove. For instance, advanced age or an injury may reduce the apparent capacity of some physicians. Certain illnesses can affect the memory or judgment necessary to practice medicine.

CLASSIFICATIONS OF LAW

Law is the system by which society gives order to our lives. For our purposes, the law may be divided into two general categories: criminal law and civil law.

Criminal law governs violations of the law that are punished as offenses against the state or government. Such offenses involve the welfare and safety of the public as a whole rather than one individual. Criminal offenses are classified as:

- Treason
- Felony
- Misdemeanor

Treason is defined by the Constitution of the United States and is a crime against the United States. Felonies affecting business include robbery, arson, using bad checks, forgery, using the mail to defraud, and so forth. Misdemeanors are lesser offenses such as reckless driving or disturbing the peace.

Civil law is concerned with relations between individuals.

- Contract law governs enforceable promises.
- Tort law governs acts that bring harm to a person or damage to property caused negligently or intentionally.

The physician-patient relationship is governed by the law of contracts. Professional liability is governed by the law of torts.

LAW OF CONTRACTS

Although we do not give it much thought, the law of contracts touches us in many ways, practically every day of our lives. For instance, when you order medications or supplies for the office, you have entered into a contract. In fact, your employment is in itself a contract, though not necessarily in writing.

A contract is an agreement creating an obligation. To be valid or enforceable, a contract must have the following four basic elements:

1. *Manifestation of assent* (an offer and an acceptance). The parties to the contract must understand and agree on the intent of the contract.

2. *Legal subject matter.* An obligation that requires an illegal action is not an enforceable contract.

3. *Legal capacity to contract.* Both parties to the contract must be adults of sound mind.

4. *Consideration.* There must be an exchange of something of value.

If any of these four elements is missing, there is no contract.

A contract may be written or oral, express or implied. The party making the offer is known as the offeror and the party to whom the offer is made is the offeree. The physician-patient relationship is generally held by the courts to be a contractual relationship that is the result of three steps:

1. The physician invites an offer by establishing availability.

2. The patient makes an offer by arriving for treatment.

3. The physician accepts the offer by undertaking treatment of the patient.

Prior to accepting the offer, the physician is under no obligation, and no contract exists. Once the physician has accepted the patient, however, an implied contract does exist that the physician (1) will treat the patient, using reasonable care, and (2) possesses the degree of knowledge, skill, and judgment that might be expected of another physician in the same locality and under similar circumstances. It is extremely important that no express promise of a cure be made, for this then becomes a part of the contract.

The patient's part of the agreement includes the liability for payment for services and a willingness to follow the advice of the doctor. Most physician-patient relationships are implied contracts.

Termination of Contract. After the physician-patient relationship has been established, the physician is obligated to attend the patient as long as attention is required, unless a special arrangement is made.

The physician-patient relationship may be terminated by the physician or the patient.

When the physician terminates the relationship, the patient must be given notice of the physician's intention to withdraw in order that the patient may secure another physician. The physician may write a letter of withdrawal from the case to the patient, similar to the one shown in Fig. 5–1. The letter should state that professional care is being discontinued, that the physician will turn over the patient's records to another physician, and that the patient should seek the attention of another physician as soon as possible. The letter should be sent by certified or registered mail with a return receipt requested. The returned receipt should be attached to a copy of the letter and retained permanently. The patient's medical record should include details of the circumstances under which the physician is withdrawing from the case, to protect the physician against a suit for abandonment. Before withdrawing, the physician may want to take into consider-

Dear (patient):

I find it necessary to inform you that I am withdrawing from providing you medical care for the reason that _____
_____ .

As your condition requires medical attention, I suggest that you promptly place yourself under the care of another physician. If you do not know of other physicians, you may wish to contact the county medical society for a referral.

If you so desire, I shall be available to attend you for a reasonable time after you have received this letter, but in no event for more than fifteen days.

When you have selected a new physician, I would be pleased to make available to him or her a copy of your medical chart or a summary of your treatment.

Very truly yours,

Figure 5–1
Letter of withdrawal from case.

ation the condition of the patient, the size of the community, and the availability of other physicians.

In the event that the patient terminates the relationship, the termination of the contract and the circumstances surrounding it should be carefully documented in the physician's records. This may be accomplished by the physician's confirming the discharge by a certified mail letter similar to the one shown in Fig. 5–2.

Statute of Frauds. In 1677, a statute was adopted in England aimed at reducing the evil of **perjured testimony** by providing that certain contracts could not be enforced if they depended upon the testimony of witnesses alone and were not evidenced in writing. The provisions of this English statute have been closely followed by statutes adopted in all the states of this country. Under the Statute of Frauds some contracts, in order to be enforceable, must be in writing. One of these is the promise to pay the debts of another. Thus, if a third party, not otherwise legally responsible for the person's debts, agrees to pay a patient's medical bills, the agreement cannot be enforced unless it is in writing. Another contract that falls within the Statute of

Dear (patient):

This will confirm our telephone conversation of today in which you discharged me from attending you as your physician in your present illness.

In my opinion your condition requires continued medical treatment by a physician. If you have not already done so, I suggest that you employ another physician without delay.

At your request, I would be pleased to make available to him or her a summary of the diagnosis and the treatment you have received from me.

Very truly yours,

Figure 5–2
Letter to confirm discharge by patient.

Frauds is one that cannot be completed within a year. If the physician entered into an agreement to perform a series of treatments for a given sum, and this series covered a time span of more than 1 year, it would have to be in writing to be enforceable.

PROFESSIONAL LIABILITY

The term "medical professional **liability**" encompasses all possible civil liability that a physician can incur as a result of professional acts. It is preferred over the term "medical **malpractice**" because the latter carries some negative overtones. Medical professional liability is more easily prevented than defended.

Negligence

Negligence is a tort liability. When applied to the medical profession, negligence is called malpractice.

*Negligence is generally defined as the doing of some act which a reasonable and **prudent** physician would not do, or the failure to do some act which such a person should or would do.*

The standard of prudent conduct is not defined by law but is left to the determination of a judge or jury.

All medical professional liability claims fall into one of three classifications: **malfeasance, misfeasance,** or **nonfeasance.** Feasance simply means "performance" or the doing of an act. Add the prefix "mal" and you have malfeasance—the performing of an act that is wholly wrong and unlawful. Misfeasance is the improper performance of some lawful act, and nonfeasance is the failure to do something that should have been done.

CLASSIFICATIONS OF MEDICAL PROFESSIONAL LIABILITY

- *Malfeasance*
- *Misfeasance*
- *Nonfeasance*

A physician who performs an operation carelessly or contrary to accepted standards, who performs an unnecessary operation, or who fails to render care that should have been given may be found guilty of negligence or malpractice.

A medical assistant whose responsibilities are clearly set forth in a policy and procedure manual may be guilty of negligence through failure to carry out these responsibilities or to exercise reasonable and ordinary care in so doing. The medical assistant must also avoid rendering any care to a patient that might be construed as the practice of medicine.

If a physician were held legally responsible for every unsuccessful result occurring in treatment, no person would undertake the responsibility of practicing medicine. The courts hold that a physician must use reasonable care, attention, and diligence in the performance of professional services, follow his or her best judgment in treating patients, and possess and exercise the skill and care that are commonly possessed and exercised by other reputable physicians in the same or a similar locality. Physicians who represent themselves as specialists must meet the standards of practice of their specialty. Whether or not they have met these requirements in treating a particular patient is generally a matter for the court to decide upon the basis of expert testimony provided by another physician. Negligence is not presumed; it must be proved.

Physicians are not required to possess extraordinary learning and skill, but they must keep abreast with medical developments and techniques, and they cannot experiment. They are also bound to advise their patients if they discover that the condition to be treated is one beyond their knowledge or technical skill.

When injury results to a patient through a physician's negligence, the patient can legally initiate a malpractice suit to recover financial damages. Experience has shown, however, that the incidence of malpractice claims is directly related to the personal relationship existing between the physician and the patient. Deterioration of the physician-patient relationship is a frequently demonstrated reason for a patient's going to a lawyer to initiate a malpractice suit, even though there was no real injury to the patient.

> *The incidence of malpractice claims is directly related to the personal relationship existing between the physician and the patient.*

The medical assistant also has an important role in claims prevention. For instance, a patient who is kept waiting for an inexcusably long time without explanation or reassurance has developed some feeling of hostility before ever seeing the physician. A few words from the medical assistant at the proper time may forestall hostility and promote understanding.

Any time a medical assistant has reason to believe that a patient is dissatisfied, it is the medical assistant's duty to pass along such information to the physician. The medical assistant must be very careful in the choice of words while reassuring an apprehensive patient. Rather than saying, "I'm sure you will soon be entirely well," a gentle touch or a friendly smile will comfort the patient but be noncommital.

WHEN THE PHYSICIAN IS SUED

Malpractice suits are far from rare, and it is estimated today that one out of four physicians will be sued at least once during his or her career. When a suit is filed, the medical assistant sometimes becomes involved in scheduling depositions or court appearances, and preparing materials for court.

Interrogatory. Before the trial, the physician may be requested to complete an interrogatory. An interrogatory is a list of general questions from another party to the lawsuit. Answers to the interrogatory must be provided within a specified time and must be answered under oath. Interrogatories are limited to parties named in the lawsuit.

Deposition. There may be a request for a deposition. A deposition is oral testimony taken from a party or witness to the litigation and is not limited to parties named in the lawsuit. A witness who is not a party to the lawsuit will be summoned by subpoena for the deposition. The deposition is usually taken in the attorney's office in the presence of a court reporter, and must be taken under oath to tell the truth, just as in a court of law. The person giving the deposition is called the deponent. The transcribed deposition is sent to the deponent for review, and the deponent is at liberty to make any necessary changes or corrections. Only deponents who are not parties to the suit are compensated for their time.

Subpoena. A subpoena is a document issued by the court requiring the person to whom it is directed to be in court at a given time and place to testify as a witness in a lawsuit.

Subpoena duces tecum. A subpoena duces tecum is an order to provide records or documents of some sort and is usually addressed to the custodian of the records. This may be the medical assistant. The custodian of the records may expect to be compensated for the time spent in compiling the records and for photocopying charges. The fee must be demanded at the time the subpoena is served, or it is considered to be waived.

Some states have laws that permit patients to obtain a copy of their records upon request, although a photocopying charge may be made. It is never wise to release the original records.

THE FOUR D'S OF NEGLIGENCE

In a report by the Committee on Medicolegal Problems of the American Medical Association it was stated that:

> To obtain a judgment against a physician for negligence, the patient must present evidence of what have been referred to as the "four D's." He must show: (1) that the physician owed a *duty* to the patient, (2) that the physician was *derelict* and breached that duty by failing to act as the ordinary,

competent physician in the same community would have acted under the same or similar circumstances, (3) that such failure or breach was the *direct cause* of the patient's injuries, and (4) that *damages* to the patient resulted therefrom.

The four D's of negligence are:
- *Duty*
- *Derelict*
- *Direct cause*
- *Damages*

Duty. Duty exists when the physician-patient relationship has been established. That is, the patient has sought the assistance of the physician and the physician has knowingly undertaken to provide the needed medical service.

Derelict (Neglectful of Obligation). Proof of dereliction, or proof of negligence of an obligation, must be shown in obtaining a judgment for malpractice.

Direct Cause. There must be proof that the injury or death was directly caused by the physician's actions or failure to act, and that it would not otherwise have occurred.

Damages. There are three kinds of damages recognized by the law: (1) nominal, (2) punitive or exemplary, and (3) compensatory or actual. Nominal (existing in name only) damages are a token compensation for the invasion of a legal right in which no actual injury was suffered. Punitive (inflicting punishment) or exemplary (serving as a warning) damages require allegations and proof of willful misconduct and are unusual in suits against physicians. It is the compensatory or actual damages that are most frequently involved in professional liability cases. Compensatory damages may be general or special.

Compensatory or actual damages for injuries or losses that are the natural and necessary consequences of the physician's negligent act or omission are referred to as "general damages." General damages include compensation for pain and suffering, for loss of a bodily member or faculty, for disfigurement, or for other similar direct losses or injuries. The fact of the losses must be proved—the monetary value need not be proved.

Special damages are those injuries or losses that are not a necessary consequence of the physician's negligent act or omission. These may include the costs of medical and hospital care, loss of earnings, cost of travel, and so forth. Both the fact of these injuries or losses and the monetary value must be proved.

The Committee on Professional Liability of the California Medical Association in 1971 called these same four elements the "ABCD's" of negligence in medical practice:

A Acceptance of a person as a patient
B Breach of the physician's duty of skill or care
C Causal connection between the breach by the physician and the damage to the patient
D Damage of a foreseeable nature—that is, injury, pain, loss of earnings, and so on, which could reasonably have been foreseen to result

ARBITRATION

Arbitration, the settlement of a dispute by a third party or parties, selected because of their familiarity with the practices involved, is common in modern business life. It has only recently been implemented in the medical profession. Arbitration is an alternative method of resolving legal disputes between doctor and patient. Many physicians and lawyers see it as one way to help solve the malpractice crisis. Instead of taking the disagreement through the long and expensive process of court **litigation**, which may take as long as 7 or 8 years, the patient and the physician (or hospital) agree in advance to submit the dispute informally to a neutral person or persons.

An arbitration agreement is a contract and is subject to the judgment of the courts only as to the fairness of the agreement. The agreement is precisely worded by an attorney and should not be paraphrased in explaining it to a patient (Fig. 5–3). Signing the agreement is a voluntary act on the part of the patient, who has a period of grace in which to revoke the agreement if he or she later decides against it. Both the patient and the physician have the opportunity to agree on who will arbitrate the case, so that it does not favor one side over the other. By prior agreement, the **arbitrator**(s) may be appointed by or from the American Arbitration Association, which is a neutral, private, nonprofit association dedicated solely to the advancement of out-of-court remedies. Its panels of arbitrators are made up of persons from business, the professions, and public interest groups.

Advantages of Arbitration:
- *Less expensive*
- *Faster*
- *More confidential*

After an informal hearing the arbitrator(s) then renders a binding decision, based on very specific rules of arbitration, as to any award. Arbitration is established by statute and applies essentially the same **substantive law** and the same measure of damages as a court. Arbitration is fair, it is less expensive, it is faster, and it is more confidential than court litigation.

If an arbitration statute exists in your state, you

Physician's Copy

PATIENT-PHYSICIAN ARBITRATION AGREEMENT

1.   It is understood that any dispute as to medical malpractice, that is as to whether any medical services rendered under this contract were unnecessary or unauthorized or were improperly, negligently or incompetently rendered, will be determined by submission to arbitration as provided by California Law and not by a lawsuit or resort to court process except as California Law provides for judicial review of arbitration proceedings. Both parties to this contract, by entering into it, are giving up their constitutional right to have any such dispute decided in a court of law before a jury, and instead are accepting the use of arbitration.

2.   I have read and understood Article 1 above and I voluntarily agree, for myself and all persons identified in Article 3 below, to submit to arbitration any and all claims involving persons bound by this Agreement whether those claims are brought in tort, contract or otherwise. This includes, but is not limited to, suits for personal injury, actions to collect debts, or any other kind of civil action.

3.   I understand and agree that this Arbitration Agreement binds me and anyone else who may have a right to assert a claim on my behalf. I further understand and agree that if I sign this Agreement on behalf of some other person for whom I have responsibility (including my spouse or children, living or yet unborn) then, in addition to myself, such person(s) will also be bound, along with anyone else who may have a right to assert a claim on their behalf. I also understand and agree that this Agreement relates to claims against the physician and any consenting substitute physician, as well as his/her partnership, professional corporation, employees, partners, heirs, assigns or personal representatives. I also hereby consent to the intervention or joinder in the arbitration proceeding of all parties relevant to a full and complete settlement of any dispute arbitrated under this Agreement, as set forth in the Medical Arbitration Rules and/or CHA-CMA Rules for the Arbitration of Hospital and Medical Fee Disputes.

4.   I agree to accept medical services from the undersigned physician and to pay therefor. I UNDERSTAND THAT I DO **NOT** HAVE TO SIGN THIS AGREEMENT TO RECEIVE THE PHYSICIAN'S SERVICES, AND THAT IF I DO SIGN THE AGREEMENT AND CHANGE MY MIND WITHIN 30 DAYS OF TODAY, THEN I MAY REVOKE THIS AGREEMENT BY GIVING WRITTEN NOTICE TO THE UNDERSIGNED PHYSICIAN WITHIN THAT TIME STATING THAT I WANT TO WITHDRAW FROM THIS ARBITRATION AGREEMENT. I further understand that after those 30 days, this Agreement may be changed or revoked only by a written revocation signed by both parties.

5.   On behalf of myself and all others bound by this Agreement as set forth in Article 3, agreement is hereby given to be bound by the Medical Arbitration Rules of the California Hospital Association and California Medical Association and the CHA-CMA Rules for the Arbitration of Hospital and Medical Fee Disputes, as they may be amended from time to time, which are hereby incorporated into this Agreement.

6.   I have read and understood the attached explanation of the Patient-Physician Arbitration Agreement and I have read and understood this Agreement, including the Rules. I understand and agree that this writing makes up the entire arbitration agreement between me and/or the person(s) on whose behalf I am signing and the undersigned physician and/or consenting substitute physicians.

   NOTICE: BY SIGNING THIS CONTRACT YOU ARE AGREEING TO HAVE ANY ISSUE OF MEDICAL MALPRACTICE DECIDED BY NEUTRAL ARBITRATION AND YOU ARE GIVING UP YOUR RIGHT TO A JURY OR COURT TRIAL. SEE ARTICLE 1 OF THIS CONTRACT.

Dated: _____, 19___ _____
                                                                   (Patient)

Physician's Agreement to Arbitrate

   In consideration of the foregoing execution of this Patient-Physician Arbitration Agreement, I likewise agree to be bound by the terms set forth in this Agreement and in the Rules specified in Article 5 above.

Dated: _____, 19___ _____
                                                                   (Physician)

_____   _____
      (Name of partnership or   (Title — e.g., Partner, President, etc.)
      professional corporation)

©California Medical Association, 1977, 1981

Figure 5–3
Arbitration agreement used in the state of California.

should get details of the procedure from your state or local medical society. If a physician elects to implement the procedure, every member of the physician's staff should know the details of the agreement, how to sign patients up, and how to answer the patient's questions. The fairness with which the physician's personnel present the program to the patient and the willingness with which the personnel answer the patient's questions will largely determine whether or not the court will uphold the arbitration agreement. Furthermore, when the physician's personnel "speak for the physician," any representations made by the personnel could be held against the physician.

SECURING PATIENT'S INFORMED CONSENT OR INFORMED REFUSAL

A physician must have consent to treat a patient even though this consent is usually implied by virtue of the patient's having come to that physician for treatment. Consent may be express or implied, and, if express, may be either written or oral.

In *Medicolegal Forms with Legal Analysis*, the American Medical Association explains some of the implications of consent in this way:

> Usually authority to treat or operate arises from the valid consent of the patient or someone authorized to act in his behalf. A statute in Georgia (Georgia Code, Chapter 88-29) enumerates those who may consent to treatment for themselves or for others. The consent given may be either express or implied and, if express, it may either be written or oral. The consent given must be an **informed consent** with an understanding of what is to be done and of the risks involved. The procedure involved and its attendant risks should be explained to the patient in understandable nontechnical terms. The consent given may be invalid (a) because the act consented to is unlawful, (b) because the consent was given by one who had no legal right to give it, or (c) because it was obtained by misrepresentation or fraud.

An informed consent implies an understanding of:
- *What is to be done*
- *Why it should be done*
- *The risks involved*
- *Alternative treatments, including the failure to treat*
- *The attendant risks of alternative treatment*

Even in cases in which the treatment was not negligent, the physician can be sued for failing to obtain an informed consent. Under such circumstances, the physician must be prepared to prove in court that a full explanation was given to the patient before obtaining the patient's consent.

To be legally binding, the consent given must be an informed consent with an understanding of what is to be done and of the risks involved, why it

should be done, and alternative methods of treatment available and their attendant risks. The alternatives include the failure to treat and the attendant risk.

To obtain informed consent, a discussion must occur during which the physician provides the patient with enough information to decide whether or not to undergo the proposed therapy. After such a discussion the patient either consents or refuses to consent to the proposed therapy. There should be a note placed on the medical record that such a discussion took place and the patient's decision. Treatment may not exceed the scope of the consent. Remember that a discussion must take place. Having the patient sign a form is not informed consent.

Sometimes, if a physician fails to secure some formal expression of consent, he can be charged with **trespass** or **assault** and **battery**. The American

---

CONSENT TO OPERATION, ANESTHETICS, AND OTHER MEDICAL SERVICES

Date_____ Time_____ A.M. P.M.

1. I authorize the performance upon _____
(myself or name of patient)

of the following operation _____
(state nature and extent of operation)

to be performed by or under the direction of Dr._____.

2. I consent to the performance of operations and procedures in addition to or different from those now contemplated, whether or not arising from presently unforeseen conditions, which the above-named doctor or his associates or assistants may consider necessary or advisable in the course of the operation.

3. I consent to the administration of such anesthetics as may be considered necessary or advisable by the physician responsible for this service, with the exception of _____
(state "none," "spinal anesthesia," etc.)

4. The nature and purpose of the operation, possible alternative methods of treatment, the risks involved, the possible consequences, and the possibility of complications have been explained to me by Dr._____ and by_____.

5. I acknowledge that no guarantee or assurance has been given by anyone as to the results that may be obtained.

6. I consent to the photographing or televising of the operations or procedures to be performed, including appropriate portions of my body, for medical, scientific or educational purposes, provided my identity is not revealed by the pictures or by descriptive texts accompanying them.

7. For the purpose of advancing medical education, I consent to the admittance of observers to the operating room.

8. I consent to the disposal by hospital authorities of any tissues or body parts which may be removed.

9. I am aware that sterility may result from this operation. I know that a sterile person is incapable of becoming a parent.

10. I acknowledge that all blank spaces on this document have been either completed or crossed off prior to my signing.

(CROSS OUT ANY PARAGRAPHS ABOVE
WHICH DO NOT APPLY)

Signed _____
(Patient or person authorized
to consent for patient)

Witness_____

Figure 5–4

Patient consent form. (From Medicolegal Forms with Legal Analysis, *3rd ed. Office of the General Counsel, 1973, p. 57. Copyright © 1973. American Medical Association.)*

Medical Association's Law Division states that "a prudent physician will demand a written consent or authorization with respect to any operation which involves an element of recognized danger to the patient or which requires hospitalization." This is desirable in order to avoid misunderstandings that can lead to lawsuits; it also facilitates proof when necessary.

Forms on which a patient can grant written consent for operations or other procedures are kept in most physicians' offices. Figures 5–4 and 5–5 illustrate a general form of consent to operation.

CONSENT TO OPERATION, ANESTHETICS, AND OTHER MEDICAL SERVICES (ALTERNATE FORM)

Date_____Time_____ A.M. / P.M.

1. I authorize the performance upon _____
   (myself or name of patient)

of the following operation _____
   (state name of operation)

to be performed under the direction of Dr. _____.

2. The following have been explained to me by Dr._____:

   A. The nature of the operation _____
      (describe the operation)

      _____

      _____

   B. The purpose of the operation_____
      (describe the purpose)

      _____

   C. The possible alternative methods of treatment _____

      _____
      (describe the alternative methods)

   D. The possible consequences of the operation _____

      _____
      (describe the possible consequences)

   E. The risks involved _____
      (describe the risks involved)

      _____

   F. The possibility of complications _____

      _____
      (describe the possible complications)

   3. I have been advised of the serious nature of the operation and have been advised that if I desire a further and more detailed explanation of any of the foregoing or further information about the possible risks or complications of the above listed operation it will be given to me.

   4. I do not request a further and more detailed listing and explanation of any of the items listed in paragraph 2.

Signed _____
   (Patient or person authorized to consent for patient)

Witness_____

Figure 5–5

Alternate patient consent form. (From Medicolegal Forms with Legal Analysis, *3rd ed. Office of the General Counsel, 1973, p. 59. Copyright © 1973. American Medical Association.)*

Birth control through voluntary surgical sterilization procedures such as vasectomy or tubal ligation is lawful in some states. It is recommended that for every such procedure the physician should obtain from the patient and the spouse, if any, a signed, written informed consent (see Fig. 5–6).

WHO MAY GIVE CONSENT?

If a mentally competent adult expressly indicates assent to a particular form of treatment, then consent has been obtained.

Emergencies. In an emergency one may render aid or care to prevent loss of life or serious illness or injury. However, implied consent in this circumstance lasts only as long as the emergency, and formal consent must be obtained for follow-up procedures done after the emergency has passed.

Incompetent Adults. Adults who have been found by a court to be insane or incompetent usually cannot consent to medical treatment. Consent must be obtained from the guardian.

Minors. Except for emergency circumstances, minors as a general rule cannot consent to medical treatment. However, there are many statutory exceptions. These statutes will vary from state to state but may include the following exceptions:
1. Married minors, and minors in the armed forces.
2. Emancipated minors—those minors who are 15 years of age or older, living separate and apart from their parents or legal guardians (with or without their consent), and who are managing their own financial affairs regardless of the source of income.
3. A pregnant minor may consent to care related to the prevention or treatment of pregnancy (including abortion and birth control).
4. Minors 12 years old or older may consent to:
   a. Treatment for any reportable infectious or communicable disease.
   b. Treatment for sexual assault.
   c. Medical care and counseling relating to the diagnosis and treatment of a drug- or alcohol-related problem.

Unless a statute declares otherwise, a minor who has the right to consent to treatment is entitled to the protection of his or her confidences, even from parents.

GOOD SAMARITAN ACTS

The purpose of a Good Samaritan Act is to protect the physician from liability for any civil damages as a result of rendering emergency care.

Physicians are sometimes reluctant to fulfill an ethical obligation to render aid in an emergency to

REQUEST FOR STERILIZATION

A.M.
Date_____ Time_____P.M.

We, the undersigned husband and wife, each being more than twenty-one years of age and of sound mind, request Dr.

_____, and assistants of his choice, to perform upon

_____, the following operation: _____.
(name of patient)　　　　(state nature and extent of operation)

It has been explained to us that this operation is intended to result in sterility although this result has not been guaranteed. We understand that a sterile person is NOT capable of becoming a parent.

We voluntarily request the operation and understand that if it proves successful the results will be permanent and it will there-after be physically impossible for the patient to inseminate, or to conceive or bear children.

Signed_____
(Husband)

Signed_____
(Wife)

Witness_____

Figure 5–6

Sterilization request. (From Medicolegal Forms with Legal Analysis, 3rd ed., Office of the General Counsel, 1973, p. 69, Copyright © 1973. American Medical Association.)

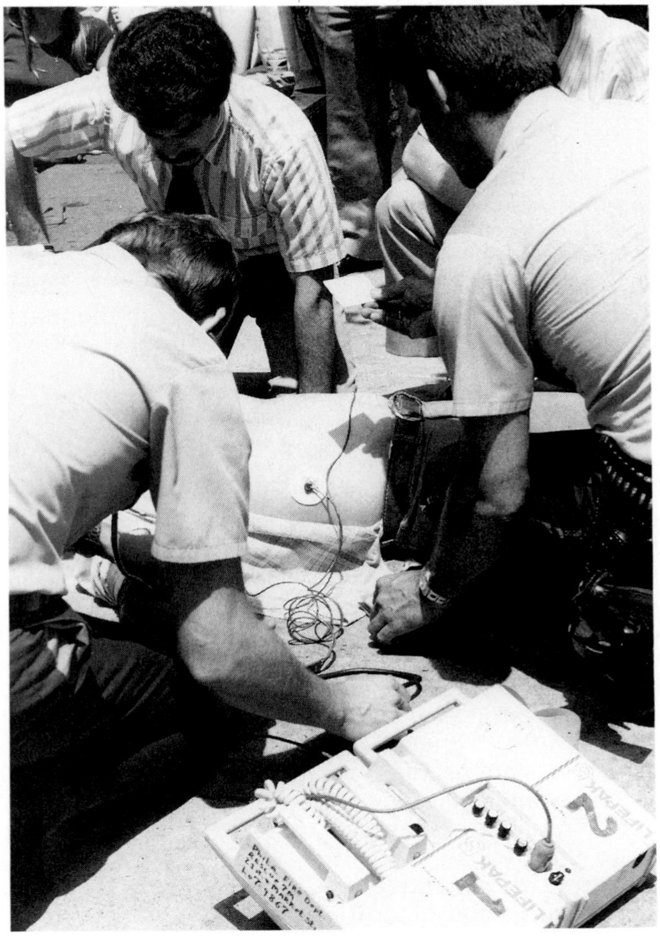

5

Figure 5–7

Physician treating at the scene of an accident. The Good Samaritan Act protects the physician from liability for any civil damages as a result of rendering emergency care. (Courtesy of H. Armstrong Roberts.)

UNIFORM DONOR CARD

OF _____

Print or type name of donor

In the hope that I may help others, I hereby make this anatomical gift, if medically acceptable, to take effect upon my death. The words and marks below indicate my desires.

I give: (a) _____ any needed organs or parts

(b) _____ only the following organs or parts

_____

Specify the organ(s) or part(s)

for the purposes of transplantation, therapy, medical research or education;

(c) _____ my body for anatomical study if needed.

Limitations or
special wishes, if any :_____

Signed by the donor and the following two witnesses in the presence of each other:

_____   _____
Signature of Donor   Date of Birth of Donor

_____   _____
Date Signed   City & State

_____   _____
Witness   Witness

This is a legal document under the Uniform Anatomical Gift Act or similar laws.

Figure 5–8
Uniform donor card.

someone who is not their patient, for fear they may later be charged with negligence or abandonment by a total stranger (Fig. 5–7). In 1959 California passed the first **Good Samaritan Act**, and today all 50 states have Good Samaritan statutes. Although there are minor variations in the state statutes, their purpose is to protect the physician from liability for any civil damages as a result of rendering emergency care, provided such care is given in good faith and with due care under the circumstances. In some states the law applies to nurses and other health professionals as well as to physicians. There is no creation of a contract in giving emergency care.

UNIFORM ANATOMICAL GIFT ACT

The Uniform Anatomical Gift Act was approved by the National Conference of Commissioners on Uniform State Laws in 1968. Although many states had passed laws prior to this time that permitted living persons to make a gift of their body or portions of it after death, the laws were so different from state to state that arrangements for a donation in one state might not be recognized in another. All states have adopted the Uniform Anatomical Gift Act or similar legislation.

Essentially, the model law for donation states that:

- Any person of sound mind and 18 years of age or over may give all or any part of his body after death for research, transplantation, or placement in a tissue bank.
- A donor's valid statement of gift is paramount to the rights of others except where a state autopsy law may prevail.
- If a donor has not acted during his lifetime, his survivors, in a specified order of priority, may do so.
- Physicians who accept organs or tissues, relying in good faith on the documents, are protected from lawsuits. The physician attending at the time of death, if acquainted with the donor's wishes, may dispose of the body under the Uniform Anatomical Gift Act.
- The time of death must be determined by a physician who is not involved in the transplantation, and the attending physician cannot be a member of the transplant team.
- The donor may revoke the gift, or the gift may be rejected.

The most important clause permits the donation to be made by a will (without waiting for probate) or by other written or witnessed documents, such as a card designed to be carried on the person (Fig. 5–8). The Uniform Donor Card is considered a legal document in all 50 states.

The provisions of the Uniform Anatomical Gift Act are so designed that the offer is exercised only after death. Therefore, the donors should reveal their intentions to as many of their relatives and friends as possible, and to their physician. Since the human body or its parts are not commodities in commerce, no money can be exchanged in making an anatomical donation.

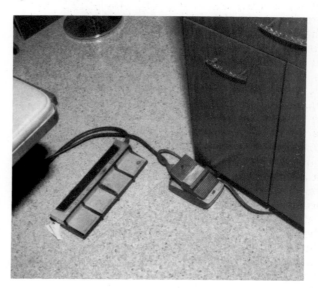

Figure 5–9
Example of a possible safety hazard.

LEGAL DISCLOSURES

The physician is charged with safeguarding patient confidences within the constraints of the law, but according to state laws, which vary somewhat throughout the nation, certain disclosures must be made. Births and deaths must be reported. Births out of wedlock must be reported on special forms in some states; some require detailed information about stillbirths. Physicians are required to report cases that may have been a result of violence, such as gunshot wounds, knifings, or poisonings. They also must report deaths from accidental or unexplained causes. In some states occupational diseases must be reported within 10 days or 2 weeks. Venereal diseases are reportable in every state. Child abuse is now a leading cause of death in children under 5 years of age, and health professionals are required by law to report any suspected cases of child abuse. This should be done as soon as evidence is discovered. The physician must report any cases of contagious, infectious, or communicable diseases. Local health departments publish lists of diseases that are reportable, and the method of reporting. Often the report may be made by telephone. When reporting by mail, the appropriate forms, supplied by the Health Department, must be used. In many areas the County Health Department issues regular bulletins that are sent to all physicians in the county. Check with the local authorities for specific procedures in your area.

LEGAL RESPONSIBILITIES OF THE MEDICAL ASSISTANT

Generally, the law holds that every person is liable for the consequences of his or her own negligence when another person is injured as a result. In some situations this liability also extends to the employer. Physicians may be held responsible for the mistakes of those who work in their offices and sometimes must pay damages for the negligent acts of their employees.

Physicians are legally responsible for the acts of their employees when the employees are acting within the scope of their duties or employment. Physicians are also responsible for the acts of assistants who are not their own employees if they commit acts of negligence in the presence of the physician while under the physician's immediate supervision. For example, a nurse who is a hospital employee makes an error in a procedure while acting under a physician's direction. The court may determine that the nurse came so completely under the direction and supervision of the physician that the physician is liable for the nurse's negligence. This is known as the doctrine of *respondeat superior* (let the master answer). On the other hand, if a special nurse is employed by the patient, the physician is not usually held liable for negligent acts of the special nurse. When physicians practice as partners, they are liable not only for their own acts and those of their partner but also for the negligent acts of any agent or employee of the partnership. The medical assistant, while acting within the scope of the employment contract, is considered an agent of the employer.

A physician who properly writes a prescription is not liable for a pharmacist's negligence in compounding it, but may be liable in cases in which there is misunderstanding as to the ingredients when the prescription is ordered over the telephone.

Need for Extreme Care. Medical assistants who are guilty of negligence are liable for their own actions, but the injured party generally sues the physician because there is a better chance of collecting. However, even an assistant who has no money can still be liable for any negligent actions. This fact illustrates the continuing importance of exercising extreme care in performing all duties in the professional office. While working under pressure there is always the danger of interchanging blood, serum, or medications, or of mixing names or improperly preparing labels. Medication and treatment solutions should be labeled clearly and their expiration dates checked. Never proceed with administration of a medication or treatment without checking all details at least three times. It is an accepted rule that the medication label should be read three times: (1) when removing the container from its storage place; (2) when you are preparing the medication and (3) when you return the medication to the storage place.

Rechecking Equipment. One person in the office should be designated to make periodic safety checks of reception room and treatment room furniture, and the condition of instruments and supplies. Every person on the staff should be alert for potential hazards, such as slipping rugs, exposed telephone and light cords, highly waxed floors, and protruding objects, since patients who are harmed as a result of these conditions can sue for damages (Fig. 5–9).

Illegal Practice of Medicine. A physician studies many years to learn the profession before becoming licensed by the state to practice medicine. The medical assistant is not licensed to practice medicine and must never prescribe or try to diagnose a patient's ailment. This is the illegal practice of medicine. For this reason, it is not good policy for the medical assistant to discuss patients' complaints with them, because patients tend to identify the medical assistant's remarks as being the opinion of the physician.

Instructions to Patients. Both the physician and the medical assistant must be thorough when giving instructions to patients. Written instructions should be provided whenever possible. A patient might forget oral instructions, resulting in drug-related injuries stemming from poor understanding of the proper use of the medications, their limitations, and their contraindications. The American Medical Association has developed a Patient Medication Instruction program consisting of printed 5½″ × 8½″ sheets with information on over 80 common drug types (Fig. 5–10).

Assisting at Patient Examinations. Except in an actual emergency, the physician should not examine a patient unless a third person is present. Allegations of sexual misconduct are increasing against physicians of all specialties. The charge of undue familiarity against a physician is very damaging. For this reason, the assistant generally stands by during examinations.

Emergency Aid. The question sometimes arises: Should the medical assistant give emergency care to a patient brought into the office during the physician's absence? In a medical emergency, the medical assistant, like any other layperson, may do whatever is reasonably necessary, provided the action taken is within that person's skill and competence. The physician should instruct the medical assistant regarding what course of action to take in such instances. The medical assistant must immediately get in touch with a physician to care for the patient, once any emergency measures have been performed.

CLAIMS PREVENTION

The majority of patients never entertain the thought of taking legal action against their physicians, and the medical assistant should not develop an attitude of skepticism. The medical assistant can, however, play a role in claims prevention by following these suggestions:

- Give scrupulous attention to the needs of each patient.
- Avoid leaving patients alone (especially children and elderly patients).
- Avoid destructive and unethical criticism of the work of other physicians.
- Do not give out information either orally or in writing without the patient's consent.
- Verify the identity of anyone requesting information.
- Use discretion in telephone and office conversations.
- Keep records that clearly show what was done and when it was done.
- Make no promises as to outcome of treatment.
- Record the facts if a patient discontinues treatment or fails to follow instructions.

- Avoid making any statement that might be construed as an admission of fault.
- Check the office equipment regularly to see that it is operating properly and safely.
- Make periodic safety inspections of furniture.
- Keep toxic substances out of reach of patients and clearly labeled.
- Keep drug samples and prescription pads out of sight.
- Never diagnose, prescribe, or offer a prognosis.

GLOSSARY OF LEGAL TERMS

burden of proof The necessity or duty of affirmatively proving a fact or facts in dispute on an issue raised between the parties in a cause.

civil law That division of municipal law occupied with the exposition and enforcement of civil rights as distinguished from criminal law.

common law Law derived from court decisions, judge-made law.

contributory negligence The act or omission amounting to want of ordinary care on the part of the patient, which, concurring with defendant's negligence, is proximate cause of injury.

criminal case An action, suit, or cause instituted to punish an infraction of the criminal laws.

criminal law Law that deals with conduct offensive to society as a whole, or the state.

defamation Offense of injuring another's reputation by false and malicious statements.

defendant The person defending or denying; the party against whom relief or recovery is sought in an action or suit.

feasance The doing of an act; a performing or performance.

>*Malfeasance.* The doing of an act which is wholly wrongful and unlawful.

>*Misfeasance.* The improper performance of some act which a man may lawfully do.

>*Nonfeasance.* The omission of an act which a person ought to do.

felony A crime of a graver or more atrocious nature than those designated as misdemeanors; generally, an offense punishable by imprisonment in a penitentiary.

grievance committee A committee established by a local medical society to hear and investigate the complaints of patients respecting professional care rendered by an attending physician or allegedly excessive fees charged by the physician.

invasion of privacy An encroachment on the right of privacy, the right to be "left alone" or to live in seclusion without being subjected to unwarranted or undesired publicity. Thus, without the knowledge and authorization of the patient, there should be no publication of his medical case record and no showing of a photograph or motion picture from which the identity of the patient is determinable.

PMI 008   **Tetracyclines**

Patient Medication Instruction Sheet

For: _____

Drug Prescribed: _____

Directions for Use: _____

_____

Special Instructions: _____

Please Read This Information Carefully

This sheet tells you about the medicine your doctor has just prescribed for you. If any of this information causes you special concern, check with your doctor. **Keep this and all other medicines out of the reach of children.**

Uses of This Medicine

Tetracyclines are used to help the body overcome bacterial infections. However, they will not work for colds, flu, or other virus infections. Some tetracyclines may help control acne and also may be used for other conditions as determined by your doctor. Take this medicine only as directed by your doctor.

Before Using This Medicine

BE SURE TO TELL YOUR DOCTOR IF YOU . . .
- are allergic to any medicine;
- are pregnant or intend to become pregnant while using this medicine;
- are breast-feeding;
- are taking any other prescription or nonprescription medications, or if you have any other medical problems.

Proper Use of This Medicine

DOSAGE
Tetracyclines should be taken with a full glass (8 ounces) of water to prevent irritation of the esophagus or stomach. In addition, most tetracyclines (except doxycycline or minocycline) are best taken on an empty stomach (either 1 hour before or 2 hours after meals). However, if this medicine upsets your stomach, your doctor may want you to take it with food. **You should not, however, take milk, milk formulas, or other dairy products within 1 or 2 hours of the time you take tetracyclines.** Also, you should not take antacids, iron pills, or vitamins with minerals within 2 hours after you take tetracyclines. Consult with your doctor if you have any questions.

To help clear up your infection completely, **keep taking this medicine for the full time of treatment** even if you begin to feel better after a few days; **do not miss any doses.**

(continued on reverse side)

Figure 5–10
Example of a patient instruction sheet for taking medications. (Copyright © 1982, American Medical Association. Portions of this text have been taken from USP DI © 1982, USP Convention. Permission granted.)

If you do miss a dose of this medicine, take it as soon as possible. However, if it is almost time for your next dose and your dosing schedule is:

- 1 dose a day (for example, for acne)—Space the missed dose and the next dose 10 to 12 hours apart.
- 2 doses a day—Space the missed dose and the next dose 5 to 6 hours apart.
- 3 or more doses a day—Space the missed dose and the next dose 2 to 4 hours apart or double your next dose.

Then go back to your regular dosing schedule. Consult with your doctor if you have any questions.

Precautions While Using This Medicine

If your symptoms do not improve within a few days (or a few weeks or months for acne patients) or if they become worse, check with your doctor.

If this medicine has become outdated, do not use it.

Do not give tetracyclines to infants or children under 8 years of age unless directed by your doctor. Tetracyclines may cause permanently discolored teeth and other problems in this age group. Also, tetracyclines should generally not be taken by pregnant or breast-feeding women.

This medicine has been prescribed for your present infection only. Another infection later on may require a different medicine. Also, even though other people may have the same symptoms you do, they may have a different kind of infection. Your medicine may not work at all for them and may even cause them harm. Therefore, **your medicine must not be given to other people or used for other infections** unless otherwise directed by your doctor.

Side Effects of This Medicine

SIDE EFFECTS THAT SHOULD BE REPORTED TO YOUR DOCTOR

- Severe cramps or burning of the stomach; vomiting; severe or watery diarrhea
- Increased sensitivity of skin to sunlight resulting in sunburn (rare with minocycline)
- Skin rash, itching, fever, wheezing
- Excessive thirst, greatly increased frequency of urination or amount of urine, or unusual tiredness (most likely to occur with demeclocycline)
- Itching of the rectal or genital areas

SIDE EFFECTS THAT MAY NOT REQUIRE MEDICAL ATTENTION
These possible side effects may go away during treatment; however, if they persist, contact your doctor.

- Mild cramps or burning of the stomach; mild nausea, mild diarrhea
- Dizziness, lightheadedness, or unsteadiness (most likely to occur with minocycline)
- Sore mouth or tongue

The information in this PMI is selective and does not cover all the possible uses, actions, precautions, side effects, or interactions of this medicine.

This PMI is produced by the AMA, which assumes sole responsibility for its content. Appreciation is acknowledged to the other organizations that provided assistance and information to the AMA and, in particular, the U.S. Pharmacopeia.

© 1982, American Medical Association. Portions of this text have been taken from USP DI © 1982, USP Convention. Permission granted.

PMI 008

HDA: 82-455: 10/82: 30M

Figure 5–10 Continued

judicial Relating to or connected with the administration of justice.

jurisprudence The philosophy of law, or the science which treats of the principles of positive law and legal relations.

libel Defamatory words that are printed, written or published which injure the character or reputation of another by holding him up to ridicule, contempt, shame, disgrace or degrade him in the estimation of the community. (See **slander**.)

locum tenens "Holding the place." A deputy, substitute, lieutenant, or representative.

medical audit A study of the patient's medical record for the purpose of determining the quality of medical care the patient received.

non compos mentis Not sound of mind; insane. This is a very general term, embracing all varieties of mental derangement.

plaintiff The person who brings an action; the party who complains or sues in a personal action and is so named in the record.

proximate cause That which, in a natural and continuous sequence, unbroken by any efficient intervening cause, produces the injury, and without which the result would not have occurred.

qui facit per alium facit per se "He who acts through another acts himself."

quid pro quo Something for something.

res gestae "Things done." Res gestae is considered as an exception to the hearsay rule. In its operation it renders acts and declarations which constitute a part of the things done and said admissible in evidence, even though they would otherwise come within the rule excluding hearsay evidence or self-serving declarations.

res ipsa loquitur "The thing speaks for itself."

res judicata A matter adjudged; a thing judicially acted upon or decided; a thing or matter settled by judgment.

rule of discovery Statute of limitations does not begin to run until the patient knew or should have known of the injury.

slander Oral defamation; speaking falsely about another with resulting injury to his reputation. (See **libel**.)

statute of limitations A legal limit on the time one has to file suit in civil matters, usually measured from the time of the wrong or from the time a reasonable person would have discovered the wrong.

tort A private or civil wrong or injury.

REFERENCES AND READINGS

American Medical Association: *Medicolegal Forms with Legal Analysis*, Chicago, The Association, 1973.

California Medical Association: *Arbitration for Physicians in Private Practice*, San Francisco, The Association, 1975.

California Medical Association: *Professional Liability*, San Francisco, The Association, 1971.

Cowdrey, M. L.: *Basic Law for the Allied Health Profession*. Monterey, CA, Wadsworth Health Sciences Division, 1984.

Hemelt, M. D., and Mackert, M. E.: *Dynamics of Law in Nursing and Health Care*. Reston, VA, Reston Publishing Co., 1979.

Hirsch, C. S., Morris, R. C., and Moritz, A. R.: *Handbook of Legal Medicine*, 5th ed. St. Louis, C. V. Mosby Co., 1979.

Lewis, M. A., and Warden, C. D.: *Law and Ethics in the Medical Office*. Philadelphia, F. A. Davis Co., 1983.

Medical Insurance Exchange of California: *Malpractice Prevention Guide for California Medical Practices*. San Francisco, The Exchange, 1983.

5

SECTION II THE ADMINISTRATIVE ASSISTANT

CHAPTER OUTLINE

Elementary Language of Computers
    Hardware
    Software

Types of Computers
Outside Computer Services
Software Capabilities
    Collections, Billing, and Insurance
    Accounting
    Medical Records
    Appointment Scheduling

Telecommunications
Text or Word Processing

Applying Your Knowledge
Helping the Physician Select a Computer System
    Choosing a Vendor
    Desirable Hardware Features
    Choosing Software
    Training

Computer Vocabulary

VOCABULARY

See Glossary at end of book for definitions. Also see Computer Vocabulary at end of chapter.

batch	floppy disk (diskette)	monitor
central processing unit (CPU)	hard copy	peripheral
computer	hardware	random access memory (RAM)
daisy wheel printer	I/O (input/output)	read only memory (ROM)
disk drive	main memory	software
dot matrix printer	microcomputer	telecommunications
electronic mail	minicomputer	tutorial
file	modem	word processing (WP)

6

The Computer in Medical Practice

OBJECTIVES

Upon successful completion of this chapter you should be able to:

1. *Define the terms listed in the Vocabulary of this chapter.*
2. *Demonstrate the ability to use elementary language of computers effectively.*
3. *Discuss the advantages and disadvantages of the four kinds of printers.*
4. *Distinguish between the two kinds of outside computer services.*
5. *Cite at least 10 general office functions that can be performed by a computer.*
6. *Identify at least eight specific functions that a well-designed computer system can perform in the areas of collections, billing, and insurance.*
7. *Explain why the patients' clinical records are seldom fully computerized in a doctor's office.*
8. *List at least eight demographic entries that are usually found on a patient's profile.*
9. *List three available functions of computer appointment scheduling programs.*
10. *Explain what telecommunication equipment and software allows the computer to do.*
11. *List three types of equipment used in word processing.*
12. *Describe the advantages of using a word processing software package in a physician's office.*

Optional Objectives: The student with hands-on computer experience, given the necessary information and equipment, should be able to perform the following activities:

1. *Generate a patient record.*
2. *Prepare a billing statement.*
3. *Complete a patient insurance form.*
4. *Personalize a computerized form letter.*
5. *Access, add, correct, and delete information on the computer.*

Only 40 years ago, in 1946, the first electronic computer (ENIAC) was completed, after 2½ years in the making. It weighed 30 tons, required a space of 15,000 square feet, and cost over a million dollars. In those 40 years a computer explosion has taken place, brought about by, first, the transistor, then integrated circuits, and now silicon chips. A compact personal computer in the home, and a desktop monitor on the office desk, are now commonplace.

The age of the computer has also arrived in the physician's office. For many years the computer has been used in hospitals and large group practices, but the proliferation of software, the drop in cost of hardware, and the sharp increase in paperwork that must be done in the medical marketplace have brought computerization into private medical practices. A computer in the physician's office is no longer a question of "if" but "when."

The development of computers, their programming, and internal operation is extremely complicated. Entire volumes are written on the minute technical details of the computer. Fortunately this technical knowledge is not necessary in order to use the computer, just as it is not necessary to be a mechanic in order to drive an automobile or an electrician in order to operate a light switch. But a knowledge of the functions that a computer can perform, how it influences our daily lives, and how it is used to perform tasks in the workplace has become a necessary part of the general education of all students. This chapter is intended to deal only with the use of the computer by the medical assistant as a tool in a medical facility.

ELEMENTARY LANGUAGE OF COMPUTERS

The physical equipment is called **hardware. Software** is the programming necessary to direct the hardware of a computer system. **Peripherals** are devices connected to the computer but which are not part of the computer itself, for example, **disk drives** and **printers. Input** to the computer is accomplished via a keyboard, which looks very much like an ordinary typewriter keyboard with a few extra keys, called special function keys. These are used to perform particular word processing or computer-related operations. **Output** is information processed by the **central processing unit (CPU)** and displayed on the **monitor** of the terminal, which resembles a television screen (Fig. 6–1).

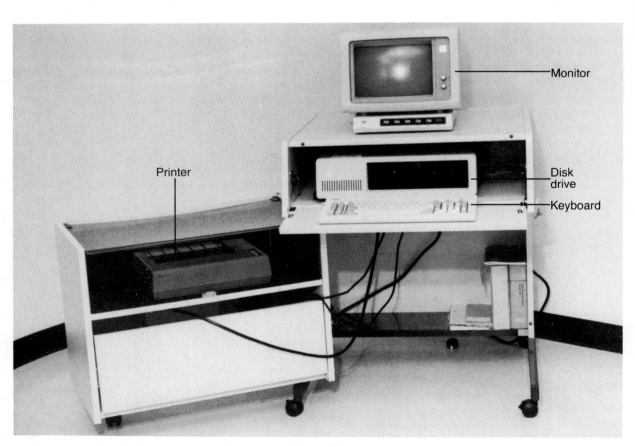

Figure 6–1
Basic components of computer hardware: monitor, disk drive, keyboard, and printer.

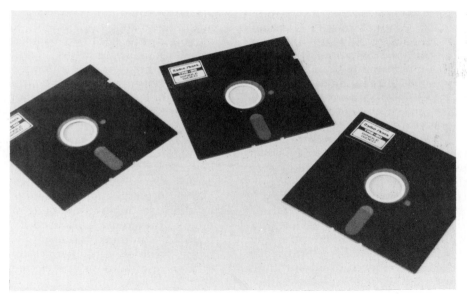

Figure 6–2
Floppy disks.

6

SYSTEM COMPONENTS

Hardware: the electrical, electronic, and mechanical equipment (the computer and various peripherals, such as disk drives and printer)

Software: the programming (instructions) that instructs the hardware how to complete the desired task

Input and Output Devices: the components that allow the computer to communicate with the operator or other computers

Hardware

The CPU is the most important piece of hardware. It is the "brain" of the computer. Although you cannot see it, within the CPU is the memory, consisting of electronic or magnetic cells, each of which contains information.

Memory. There are two kinds of **memory: ROM,** or read-only memory, and **RAM,** or random access memory. ROM is internal memory that contains the entire operating system and a computer language. With this permanent memory, much less information has to be transferred from a disk to start the computing process. The ROM cannot be overwritten and is not erased when the power is shut off. RAM can be thought of as the internal scratch pad of the computer. It contains the program instructions and the data it is currently processing. This memory is normally erased automatically when the power is turned off.

Information may be saved on a **disk** for future reference or printing. The amount of information that can be stored depends on the type of disk the system uses. Storage is achieved on either "hard" disks or **"floppy" disks (diskettes),** or both (Fig. 6–2). Floppy disks may be 8", 5¼", or 3" in diameter. Floppy disks are more often found on personal and small-business computer systems, and the size of the disk will depend upon the type of computer you have. Rigid or hard disks will store much more information than floppy disks and allow for faster access. They may be fixed or removable. Hard disks come in different sizes (from 10 to 80 or more megabytes of storage). The hard disk is usually necessary in a medical practice. A collection of

Table 6–1
Care of Diskettes

1. Avoid exposing the diskette to extremes of temperature.
2. When the diskette is not in use, always return it to its storage envelope, where it will not collect dust.
3. Avoid laying a diskette on top of the monitor, because that could scramble information on the diskette.
4. Keep your fingers off the surface of the diskette, especially around the window in the jacket. Body oils can permanently destroy data.
5. Do hold the diskette with your thumb on the label.
6. Write or type on the label before attaching it to the diskette if possible, or write with a soft felt tip pen. Never write with a ballpoint pen or pencil on a label that is on a diskette, and do not erase. All of these can cause impressions in the diskette, and the ink can run.
7. Don't force a diskette into a disk drive or its storage envelope. If there is resistance, pull it out and try again. Bending or folding a diskette will render it useless.
8. Store the diskettes vertically in dust-tight containers.
9. Keep smoke, food, and drink away from the area of use.

related records organized and stored on the disk is called a **file.**

Printers. In word processing, the material on the screen is directed to a printer for what is called a **hard** (paper) **copy.** Some printers have built-in paperfeeders, while others require accessory feeders. The single-sheet or cut-sheet feeder is used for feeding single sheets of letterhead into the printer. Continuous forms such as bills, insurance forms, reports, and so forth require a tractor feeder, which feeds in the continuous sheets, aligns the paper, and automatically advances it as necessary.

Four methods of printing are commonly used in connection with data processing: (1) thermal, (2) **dot matrix,** (3) letter-quality or print wheels, and (4) laser printers. Many are bidirectional (print from both left to right and right to left). Some are capable of both draft- and correspondence-quality printing. Other desirable first class word processing features are text centering, bold face, shadow printing, underscoring, and superscript and subscript.

Thermal printers, which require a chemically treated paper, are the least expensive, but the operating costs are higher and the printing quality is the poorest. A thermal printer would not be used in a medical office.

Dot matrix printers cost more than thermal printers, but are generally less expensive and operate faster than letter-quality machines. The printing is readable but lacks the clarity generally desired for a professional look. They are steadily being improved, however.

Letter-quality printers may be either mechanical or electronic. The electronic letter-quality printer generally uses a print wheel or "**daisy wheel**," which is interchangeable for variations in print style or size. Many printers have 10-, 12-, and 15-pitch typing capability as well as proportional spacing.

Laser printers are the latest generation of quality printers. They are very fast and the quality is comparable to typeset. They are also expensive.

Software

Software is the most important component of a computer system. The software, or program, is the "roadmap" for the computer. It contains the instructions on what the computer is to do with the data you input. It can be a major portion of the cost of a system.

TYPES OF COMPUTERS

Computers may be roughly divided into:

- Microcomputers
- Minicomputers
- Main frames

The **microcomputer** is a desk-top computer. Originally designed as a personal computer, today's microcomputer has many business applications and may be suitable for the small medical practice. The **minicomputer,** more commonly found in health agencies, historically has had larger storage capacity and multi-location terminals. Both the micro- and the minicomputer can be installed in an average environment without the necessity of special rooms or air conditioning.

Main-frame computers are capable of manipulating and storing great amounts of information and are found in large facilities such as hospitals, clinics, and service bureaus. Because main-frame computers are susceptible to changing environmental conditions, they must be housed in temperature- and humidity-controlled rooms.

Any complete computer system located within an office is known as a stand-alone system.

OUTSIDE COMPUTER SERVICES

Computer services are also available through service bureaus. This is not a new concept in medical facilities. Service bureaus have been providing computer services for 20 years or more in batch mode or on-line mode. It is estimated that about 10% of the medical practices in the United States use a computer service bureau.

Batch System. The physician who uses a **batch** system sends financial information daily by mail or messenger to a central location where the data is entered into a main-frame computer. The service bureau then prepares statements, insurance forms, and reports for the physician. One of the major problems with this system is the time lag in sending and receiving information.

On-Line System. With the on-line system, the office is supplied with a terminal and the practice is "on-line" to the computer, using telephone lines. There may also be a printer at the user site for the preparation of reports.

SOFTWARE CAPABILITIES

A partial list of functions in the physician's office for which computer software has been designed includes:

- Processing insurance claims (Fig. 6–3)
- Billing and collections
- Accounting processes
- Storing medical records
- Generating reports for clinical research
- Scheduling appointments
- Accessing medically oriented data bases
- Accessing business and financial information

PLEASE DO NOT
STAPLE IN
THIS AREA

→

COLONIAL PENN LIFE INS. CO.
CLAIMS OFFICE
P.O. BOX 797
ROCHESTER   MI 48308

FORM APPROVED
OMB NO. 0938-0008

HEALTH INSURANCE CLAIM FORM

(CHECK APPLICABLE PROGRAM BLOCK BELOW)

| ☐ MEDICARE (MEDICARE NO.) | ☐ MEDICAID (MEDICAID NO.) | ☐ CHAMPUS (SPONSOR'S SSN) | ☐ CHAMPVA (VA FILE NO.) | ☐ FECA BLACK LUNG (SSN) | ☒ OTHER (CERTIFICATE SSN) |

PATIENT AND INSURED (SUBSCRIBER) INFORMATION

1. PATIENT'S NAME (LAST NAME, FIRST NAME, MIDDLE INITIAL)
STEPHEN   C

2. PATIENT'S DATE OF BIRTH
1 | 28 | 53

3. INSURED'S NAME (LAST NAME, FIRST NAME, MIDDLE INITIAL)
STEPHEN   C

4. PATIENT'S ADDRESS (STREET, CITY, STATE, ZIP CODE)
FULLERTON   CA 92635

TELEPHONE NO.   871-6278

5. PATIENT'S SEX
MALE ☒   FEMALE ☐

7. PATIENT'S RELATIONSHIP TO INSURED
SELF ☒   SPOUSE ☐   CHILD ☐   OTHER ☐

6. INSURED'S I.D. NO. (FOR PROGRAM CHECKED ABOVE, INCLUDE ALL LETTERS)
162-44-0273

8. INSURED'S GROUP NO. (OR GROUP NAME OR FECA CLAIM NO.)
SHU032
INSURED IS EMPLOYED AND COVERED BY EMPLOYER HEALTH PLAN

9. OTHER HEALTH INSURANCE COVERAGE (ENTER NAME OF POLICYHOLDER AND PLAN NAME AND ADDRESS AND POLICY OR MEDICAL ASSISTANCE NUMBER)

10. WAS CONDITION RELATED TO:

A. PATIENT'S EMPLOYMENT
YES ☐   NO ☒

B. ACCIDENT
AUTO ☐   OTHER ☒

11. INSURED'S ADDRESS (STREET, CITY, STATE, ZIP CODE)
FULLERTON   CA 92635
TELEPHONE NO.

11.a. CHAMPUS SPONSOR'S:
STATUS: ACTIVE DUTY ☐   DECEASED ☐   RETIRED ☐   BRANCH OF SERVICE

12. PATIENT'S OR AUTHORIZED PERSON'S SIGNATURE (READ BACK BEFORE SIGNING) I AUTHORIZE THE RELEASE OF ANY MEDICAL INFORMATION NECESSARY TO PROCESS THIS CLAIM. I ALSO REQUEST PAYMENT OF GOVERNMENT BENEFITS EITHER TO MYSELF OR TO THE PARTY WHO ACCEPTS ASSIGNMENT BELOW.

SIGNED _____ DATE _____

13. I AUTHORIZE PAYMENT OF MEDICAL BENEFITS TO UNDERSIGNED PHYSICIAN OR SUPPLIER FOR SERVICE DESCRIBED BELOW.

SIGNED (INSURED OR AUTHORIZED PERSON) _____

PHYSICIAN OR SUPPLIER INFORMATION

14. DATE OF: ILLNESS (FIRST SYMPTOM) OR INJURY (ACCIDENT) OR PREGNANCY (LMP)
2/14/86 ◄

15. DATE FIRST CONSULTED YOU FOR THIS CONDITION
2/15/86

16. IF PATIENT HAS HAD SAME OR SIMILAR ILLNESS OR INJURY, GIVE DATES

16.a. IF EMERGENCY CHECK HERE ☐

17. DATE PATIENT ABLE TO RETURN TO WORK

18. DATES OF TOTAL DISABILITY
FROM _____ THROUGH _____

DATES OF PARTIAL DISABILITY
FROM _____ THROUGH _____

19. NAME OF REFERRING PHYSICIAN OR OTHER SOURCE (e.g. PUBLIC HEALTH AGENCY)

20. FOR SERVICES RELATED TO HOSPITALIZATION GIVE HOSPITALIZATION DATES
ADMITTED _____ DISCHARGED _____

21. NAME AND ADDRESS OF FACILITY WHERE SERVICES RENDERED (IF OTHER THAN HOME OR OFFICE)

22. WAS LABORATORY WORK PERFORMED OUTSIDE YOUR OFFICE?
YES ☐   NO ☒   CHARGES: .00

23. A. DIAGNOSIS OR NATURE OF ILLNESS OR INJURY. RELATE DIAGNOSIS TO PROCEDURE IN COLUMN D BY REFERENCE NUMBERS 1, 2, 3. ETC. OR DX CODE
1.
2. 727 67 RUPTURE ACHILLES TENDON - BILATERAL
3.
4.

B.
EPSDT   YES ☐   NO ☒
FAMILY PLANNING   YES ☐   NO ☒
PRIOR AUTHORIZATION NO.

24. DATE OF SERVICE FROM	TO	B. PLACE OF SERVICE	C. PROCEDURE CODE (IDENTIFY)	(EXPLAIN UNUSUAL SERVICES OR CIRCUMSTANCES)	D. DIAGNOSIS CODE	E. CHARGES	F. DAYS OR UNITS	G. T.O.S.	H. LEAVE BLANK
2 15 86		3	90020	INITIAL VISIT	^	50.00			
2 15 86		3	29405	CAST-SHORT LEG, 10+	^	85.00			
2 15 86		3	29405	CAST-SHORT LEG, 10+	^	85.00			
2 28 86		3	90050	REVISIT OFFICE	^	30.00			
2 28 86		3	29425	CAST,WALK/AMBL,10+SL	^	95.00			
2 28 86		3	29425	CAST,WALK/AMBL,10+SL	^	95.00			

25. SIGNATURE OF PHYSICIAN OR SUPPLIER (INCLUDING DEGREE(S) OR CREDENTIALS (I CERTIFY THAT THE STATEMENTS ON THE REVERSE APPLY TO THIS BILL AND ARE MADE A PART THEREOF)
JOSEPH K. CUMMINGS M.D.
DATE: 3/19/86

26. ACCEPT ASSIGNMENT (GOVERNMENT CLAIMS ONLY) (SEE BACK)
YES ☐   NO ☒

30. YOUR SOCIAL SECURITY NO.

27. TOTAL CHARGE
440.00

28. AMOUNT PAID

29. BALANCE DUE
440.00

31. PHYSICIAN'S, SUPPLIER'S, AND/OR GROUP NAME, ADDRESS, ZIP CODE AND TELEPHONE NO.
JOSEPH K. CUMMINGS,M.D.,INC.
1201 W. LA VETA AVE.
ORANGE   CA 92668
714-558-9182   00C285170
I.D. NO. C28517   00C285170

32. YOUR PATIENT'S ACCOUNT NO.
500181

33. YOUR EMPLOYER I.D. NO
95-2791122

★PLACE OF SERVICE AND TYPE OF SERVICE (T.O.S.) CODES ON THE BACK
REMARKS:

APPROVED BY AMA COUNCIL ON MEDICAL SERVICE 6/83

Form HCFA-1500-C2-SC(1-84)   Form OWCP-1500
Form CHAMPUS-501   Form RRB-1500

Figure 6–3
Patient's insurance billing generated through on-line computer system.

```
DONALD      GOETHALS              51049    FC 1, U 2, X  8/29/86 10:00        8608290001
Apt Dr JULIAN MONTES, M.D.
Asn Dr JULIAN MONTES, M.D.
Ref Dr BEN GOODMAN M.D.




Dx1    250        250      DIABETES MELLITUS&&
Dx2
Dx3
Dx4

**** Last Payment ****
* Date    Code    Amount*   Bal      8/86     7/86     6/86     5/86     4/86
 8/28/86 00999   25.00CR 3663.00   429.00   220.00   825.00  1878.00   311.00
```

Figure 6–4

Age analysis of one patient's account. (Courtesy of Medical Data Management, Glendora, CA.)

- Receiving and sending electronic mail
- Information or data processing (correspondence, reports, form letters, practice-building mailers, manuscripts)

In most practices the list is headed by processing insurance claims, billing, and collections. These are the most repetitive daily tasks in the average office. Having them computerized can free the staff for more creative and productive activities.

Collections, Billing, and Insurance

A well-designed system will:

- Store patient demographic and financial data
- Post and store financial transactions

- Store CPT and other codes most commonly used
- Total transactions daily and monthly
- Produce patient bills
- Identify delinquent accounts
- Keep a running age-analysis of patient accounts (Fig. 6–4)
- Produce insurance claims
- Analyze activity in the practice

Other capabilities to consider include personalized collection letters, custom design of insurance forms, recall and reminder notices, and production of a superbill at the time of service. The computer can prepare trial balances, balance sheets, and income statements. With the appropriate software, patient bills and insurance claims may be instantly produced in a variety of formats (Fig. 6–5).

```
   1      Pt nm           Uniform Claim form top section                  899 01
CHET       SOUTHLAND                            Rp nm CHET        SOUTHLAND
1422 E WICKER                    DOB 12/04/10
                                 Sex M          MCE# 227104525A
PASADENA            CA 92430     Rl to Rp I     Rp addr.
Other health ins.                               1422 E WICKER

                                 Emp  N         PASADENA               CA 92430
                                 Accd N
                                                Champus Status   Branch
   Onset              1st consult              Prior symptoms  0/00/00
   0/00/00            0/00/00                  Emergency N
Rt work    TDsp fm  to                         Pdsp fm     to
   0/00/00     0/00/00   0/00/00                  0/00/00     0/00/00
Rf Dr. or other source                         Admit     Disc
                                                  0/00/00   0/00/00

   Facility Name                               EPSDT N
                                               Family planning srv
      Dx        Dx9      Desc                  Prior Auth.
      D 115     521      AORTIC INSUFF.
A
```

Figure 6–5

*Computer-generated Uniform Insurance Claim Form. **A**, Top section. **B**, Bottom section. (Courtesy of Medical Data Management, Glendora, CA.)*

Illustration continued on opposite page

```
   i RU RD 13 14 15      Uniform Claim Form bottom section              899 01
      Dx          Dx9     Desc
   D 115         521      AORTIC INSUFF.


St Dr Fac   Sv Dt    Sv Cd Desc              HCPCS Mi    Dx      Fq       Amt
   AB 84    8/22/86  00072 NP-INTMED.HIST/EXAM 90015    D 115    i      95.00
   AB 84    8/22/86  00544 CHEMFILE 25                  D 115    i      25.00
   AB 84    8/22/86  00550 CBC/GLUCOSE/POTASSIU         D 115    i       .00
   AB 84    8/22/86  00551 SGPT/GGTP/TOT. PROTE         D 115    i       .00
   AB 84    8/22/86  00552 ALBUMIN/GLOBULIN             D 115    i       .00
   AB 84    8/22/86  00553 A/G RATIO/ALK PTASE          D 115    i       .00
   AB 84    8/22/86  00554 PHOSPHORUS/URIC ACID         D 115    i       .00
   AB 84    8/22/86  00555 BUN/CREATININE/CHLOR         D 115    i       .00  +
                                                              Tot     132.00

ANNE MARIE BURROS, M.D.        Accept assgn Y
                               00000000000            ANNE MARIE BURROS, M.D.
                               95-638541

000048923 SOUTHLAND       CHET                        541 WEST LIGHTHOUSE DR.
                                                      SUITE 501
                                                      GLENDORA        CA 91740
B                                                     818-963-6070
```

Figure 6–5 Continued

Because some third-party insurance carriers are now accepting claims on magnetic media or directly through **telecommunications**, consideration should be given to equipping the system with a **modem** and a special telephone line if the volume warrants this. When insurance information is delivered electronically, a great deal of time is saved and the cash flow is improved. One of the big advantages is that errors in coding or procedure can be corrected immediately.

Accounting

With the appropriate software, the computer can easily handle all of the accounting processes, such as:

• Recording payables and receivables (Fig. 6–6)
• Computing the payroll
• Keeping track of bills to be paid
• Generating checks
• Reconciling bank statements
• Preparing daily, monthly, and annual financial and statistical reports (Fig. 6–7).

Patient account information is kept current and available for review at any time.

Medical Records

Computer systems can store clinical information about the patients. Although it is possible to fully computerize the patient's clinical record—with no paper records and no filing cabinets—relatively few practices have gone this far, because of the high cost and because most doctors are more comfortable working with manual records. However, many have found it practical to store an abbreviated record or patient profile in the computer. *It must be kept in mind that medical information in the computer is subject to the same confidentiality as any other medical information.*

The content of the patient profile depends upon what the individual physician considers important and its intended use. It would certainly include demographic information—date of birth, sex, address, telephone number, and so forth; the current primary diagnosis and any ongoing problems; current medications; any known allergies; treatment plan; and date last seen (Fig. 6–8).

Appointment Scheduling

The computer can replace the appointment book, but this is practical only with large practices and clinics (Fig. 6–9). The computer programs for appointment scheduling range from relatively simple ones that merely display available and scheduled times, to sophisticated systems in which the operator may enter information such as the length of appointment required, type of appointment, and day and time preferences, with the computer selecting the best appointment time based on this information.

The computer can keep track of future appointments so that when a patient calls and inquires about an appointment, the system can search by name to find the time and date. The computer can print copies of the daily schedule, including the patient name, the reason for the visit, and the

```
CORONA MEDICAL GROUP                                    SERVICE DATE
A PROFESSIONAL CORP.                                       8/29/86
245 WEST MERCED AVENUE
C5524842485
CORONA DEL MAR        CA 91740                          INT.860829
714-569-8234  FED ID 95-4523689


PATIENT:  DONALD    GOETHALS      SEX M  DOB 5/10/49  ACCOUNT#    51049

PHYSICIAN: JULIAN MONTES, M.D.           REF PHY BEN GOODMAN M.D.

DIAGNOSIS: OFFICE CODE ICD-9-CM DESCRIPTION
             250      250.      DIABETES MELLITUS&&

PROCEDURE: DESCRIPTION            CPT4 M1 M2 FRQ   AMOUNT   DR  CODE Dx CODE
           OFFICE VISIT           90030       1    35.00   JM 00074  250.
           CK PAYMENT-THANK YOU                1    25.00CR JM 00999

                        TODAYS CHARGES       35.00
                            ADJUSTMENTS        .00
                            PAYMENTS        25.00CR
                                          -------------
                        CHARGE TICKET NET    10.00
                        PREVIOUS BALANCE   3,663.00
                        ACCOUNT BALANCE    3,673.00
```

Figure 6–6

Printout of patient's account serves as receipt. (Courtesy of Medical Data Management, Glendora, CA.)

```
PRACTICE # 123-1                 ANALYSIS OF CHARGES
                                 DOCTOR AT GROUP LEVEL

         DESC                 ------SEPTEMBER 85-------    -------FISCAL Y T D------
         CODE   RVS  MOD  DESCRIPTION    AMOUNT      FREQ    NET AMOUNT       FREQ
 DR 1   0001 90620 01  INITIAL OFFICE VISIT   942.50    65    4,511.50      303
 DR 1   0002 90621     OFFICE VISIT         4,590.00   370   28,460.00    2,315
 DR 1   0003 62270 52  COMPLETE H&P            40.00     2      297.68       19
 DR 1   0004 98721     PHY.EXAM.SCH/INS/EMP    58.00     3      772.57       42
 DR 1   0009 56841     CAST CHECK              8.00      1        8.00        1
 DR 1   0010 86482     CONSULTATIVE VISIT     45.00     12      105.00       50
 DR 1   0013 75612     ANOSCOPIC EXAM                            20.00        3
 DR 1   0018 56184 90  XRAY CHEST IV W/INT    277.50    18    2,293.50      125
 DR 1   0157 89103     PENC.TABS. 250MG.#40    80.50    23      437.50      124
 DR 1   0161 53156     ORNADE SPANSULES #20     3.00     1       50.00       17
 DR 1   0182 52144 02  HOT PACKS              282.50    38    2,835.00      379
 DR 1   0185 69548     ULTRASOUND             15.00      2      172.50       23
 DR 1   0189 86123     SPECIAL REPORTS        17.00      3      495.00       23
 DR 1   0238 75692     PENICILLIN 600,000     90.00     13      555.00       76
 DR 1   0351 63534     INIT. HOSP. HX & PHY  525.00     10    6,950.00      140
 DR 1   0358 12358     ASSISTANT SURGEON     420.00     10    4,563.20       42
 DR 1   0650 45626 50  E.R. VISIT              .00       0       89.50        4

                        IN-OFFICE TOTAL    5,504.00   536  85%  41,013.25   3500  78%
                       OTHER    TOTAL        945.00    33  15%  11,602.70    186  22%
                    ÷ COMBINED  TOTAL      6,446.00   569 100%  52,615.95   3686 100%

             THIS LISTING IS ONLY A SAMPLE. YOUR OFFICE
            COULD HAVE AS MANY AS 700 OR MORE DESCRIPTIONS
                 TAILORED TO YOUR PRACTICE NEEDS.


                 XXXXXXXXXXXXXXXXXXX
                 X                 X
                 X                 X
                 X   S A M P L E   X
                 X                 X
                 X                 X
                 XXXXXXXXXXXXXXXXXXX
                   SERVICE ANALYSIS

         THIS REPORT IS A COMPLETE ANALYSIS OF SERVICE FOR THE CURRENT MONTH
         AND YEAR-TO-DATE, PROVIDING ESSENTIAL INFORMATION TO BE USED FOR MORE
         EFFECTIVE PRACTICE MANAGEMENT. IT IS DELIVERED MONTHLY.
```

Figure 6–7

Computer-generated analysis of charges for month and year to date by practice management system. (Courtesy of Medical Data Management, Glendora, CA.)

patient's telephone number. Multiple copies can be made according to the needs of the practice.

A big advantage of computer scheduling is that more than one person can access the system at one time, and the information will be available to all operators. In most facilities one employee still keeps an appointment book as a back-up to computer scheduling.

Telecommunications

Telecommunications software allows one computer to communicate with another computer. The system must include a modem linking the computer and the telephone line. There are two basic types of modems, acoustically-coupled and wire-connect. Acoustical devices require the user to use a telephone handset and tend to be less reliable than wire-connect devices, which go from the computer directly to the telephone jack. Advantages of the wire-connect modem are faster data transfer and the ability to automatically answer an incoming call from another computer without your being there.

Since modems allow the user to access other users, data bases, electronic bulletin boards, and so forth, they can be quite useful. Modems make communication to satellite offices possible. The phy-

```
Account No.:          1645
Name:                 MARY G JONES
Street:               1234 MAIN ST
City:                 PODUNK
State:                WY
Zip:                  80680
Home Phone:           333 154 3678
Work Phone:
Insurance Cd.:        4
Charge Type:          4    PRIVATE INS CHARGE
Statement Code:       Y
Sex:                  F
Birthdate:            05-05-73
Soc Sec No.:          555-55-5555
State I.D.#:
Driv. Lic.#:
CPT Code:             1
Fee Code:             1
Diagnosis 1:          7    ABDOMINAL PAIN                      789.0
Diagnosis 2:
Referring Dr.:        4    JOHN          M D
Normal Dr.:           2    BHARAT K            M D
Recall Date:
Recall Message:
Relationship 1:
Relationship 2:
Date of Injury:
1st Consult Date:     05-05-86
Cond. Employment:     N
Cond. Automobile:     N
Prev. Symptoms:       Y
Accept Assign.:       N
Medicare Status:      0
Sig. on File:         Y

Insured's Name:       MARY G JONES
Insur. Co. Name:      HEALTH PLAN OF AM
Insur. Co. Street:    2200 POWELL ST., #760
Insur. Co. City:      EMERYVILLE CA
Insur. Co. Zip        94608
Group Name/No.:       NORTHROP
Alt Insured's Name:   JOHN G JONES
Alt Insured's I.D.:   444 44 4444
Alt Ins Co. Name:     BLUE CROSS
Alt Ins Co. Street:   P O BOX 70000
Alt Ins Co. City:     VAN NUYS CA
Alt Ins Co. Zip:      91470
Alt Group Name/No.:   16005 A

Responsible For:      SELF
```

Figure 6–8
Example of patient information generated on in-house personal computer.

```
Report # MB03010              Appointments for  8/29/86              Page    1
Practice 899-01               By time then doctor                    8/29/86

Time    Dr Last name    First        Account    Phone Note1  Note2

10:00   JM GOETHALS     DONALD         51049  818-125-6895         COMPLETE PHYSICAL

10:15   AL COTA         SUSAN          27851  714-599-6587         CONSULT

10:30   JM PETERSON     BARBARA        65432  818-745-2364         FLU SHOT

10:45   JM FULLER·      NINA           12386  714-599-6587         POS WHIPLASH

11:00   RG ZALTA        NOURI             26  818-785-6985         BP CK

11:10      PACMAN       LOUIS           8965  213-963-6070         EKG

11:30      SYSTEM       JOE           100000  714-983-4563         POS SINUS INFECTION

11:45      KIM          MARY                  714-555-4569  NEW    PHYSICAL
```

Figure 6–9

Computer appointment schedule showing time, patient's name, account number, telephone number, and reason for visit. (Courtesy of Medical Data Management, Glendora, CA.)

sician may have a computer at home and wish to access information that is stored in the office computer files. This is possible with a modem. (Accessing data bases is discussed in Chapter 17, Editorial Duties and Meeting and Travel Arrangements).

Electronic transmission of insurance claims is mentioned earlier in this chapter. It is possible for computer users to subscribe to a service that allows users to communicate with each other using "**electronic mail**." (See Chapter 10, Written Communication.)

Text or Word Processing

In offices in which a great deal of typing is done, electronic **word processing** can ease the burden of the typist and improve efficiency (Fig. 6–10). The term "word processing" was coined by IBM in the 1960s to describe its innovative Magnetic Tape Selectric Typewriter (MT/ST). The MT/ST was costly and met with some resistance because it required special training. A few years ago electronic typewriters made their appearance. They have been termed "intelligent typewriters" and are beginning to challenge the electric typewriter.

There are three ways to go with word processing: the intelligent typewriter, the dedicated word processor, and the small computer that can also perform other functions. All are an improvement over even a very good electric typewriter.

The electronic typewriter has many automatic features, such as number alignment, automatic centering, underlining, indenting, caps lock, carrier return, and so forth, depending on the make and model. One drawback is the inability to store information.

Dedicated word processors are computers that are especially designed to perform one function—word processing. They are expensive, and the financial outlay may not be feasible for the smaller practice.

Word processing software is available for use on all small computers that can also perform other

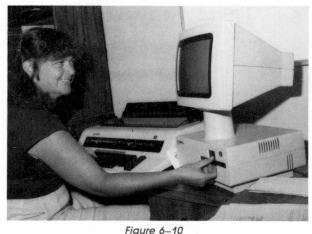

Figure 6–10

Word processing. (Courtesy of Vista Medical Group, El Toro, CA. Photo by Dan Santucci.)

functions in the medical office. The person who uses a word processor can throw away the eraser and correcting fluid, for the entire text can be edited on the monitor, any necessary corrections or changes made, and a perfect copy obtained before any printing is done. Revisions can be made easily without retyping a whole document. Blocks of text can be moved from one section of the document to another with just a few keystrokes. Even whole sections of text can be inserted in a document easily and quickly. With the text stored in memory, additional editing can be done and a corrected copy printed out almost effortlessly at any future time.

Many word processors can instruct the printer to print in boldface or in alternate type fonts. Some can create subscripts and superscripts. The software may include a spelling checker that can proofread a lengthy document in minutes with complete accuracy. One disadvantage is that the checker can determine only whether the word is spelled correctly. If an incorrect word, correctly spelled, is typed, the checker will not pick it up (for example, the use of "ilium" in place of "ileum").

The office that regularly sends out identical letters, such as recall notices or collection letters, will find word processing very helpful.

The physician who does academic writing will want a program that can create footnotes, bibliographies, indexes, and so forth.

The most difficult part of using a word processor is learning the commands. These are usually printed on cards for quick reference. Some software packages have built-in HELP screens that can be called up on the monitor for immediate assistance.

APPLYING YOUR KNOWLEDGE

Even with some basic knowledge of computer components and of what computers can do, if you have had no "hands on" experience with a computer, you may feel some initial fear—fear of the unknown, fear of machines, or fear of not being able to master the computer. You will soon overcome any such fears if you will remember that you really are smarter than the computer. All it can do is perform the tasks that you tell it to do. It cannot think. It cannot make decisions, and it will wait for your commands. What it can do is relieve you of repetitive clerical tasks, reduce errors, speed up production, recall information on command, save time, reduce paperwork, and allow more creative use of your time.

As you begin your familiarization with the computer, you may key in some wrong information. As a result, the computer will become confused and will respond with a question mark or a comment. It will give you the opportunity and time to figure out the correct information and input it. If you are in doubt about what to do next, take a look at the

screen. Most of the time it will indicate what to do next. If the answer is not readily available on the screen, check the list of commands and instructions in your manual. The answer should be there. Most programs have a **tutorial**. Refer to it frequently until you are thoroughly familiar with operation of the program.

You cannot break the computer simply by hitting the wrong keys. It is even unlikely that you will destroy records accidentally; a specific command is necessary. However, if you shut off the computer without saving the information on disk or tape you will lose what you have put in. By using a computer in the classroom you will gain familiarity with computer operation, and confidence that you can master it. But mastery can be accomplished only through practice.

The computer that you will actually encounter on the job is likely to be different from the one on which you will learn in the classroom. The programs and tasks performed may also be different, but you will be given training with that specific system, either by the vendor or by a member of the staff. It is important to keep an open mind while learning to operate any system. With a knowledge of computer terms, the ability to follow step-by-step instructions, and a reasonable facility with a typewriter keyboard, you should have no problem with learning and using any computer system. In fact, many computer users consider them their best friend. You probably will, too.

HELPING THE PHYSICIAN SELECT A COMPUTER SYSTEM

The medical assistant who is already in the employ of a physician when the decision is made to invest in a computer system may be asked to participate in the selection of the system. The first step is to determine just what the computer can do for the practice and whether the practice really needs a computer. Types of computers, system components, and software capabilities have already been discussed in this chapter.

Choosing a Vendor

After determining what you want the computer to do, the next important step is choosing a vendor. It is best to deal with an established vendor who has a reputation for reliability and who can be expected to remain in business. Ask how many medical systems they have installed and the name of users who can be contacted for references. The success of the computer application may depend a great deal upon the selection of the vendor, who will advise on the environmental requirements for temperature control, ventilation, power source, and so forth. The vendor's representative should be knowledgeable about medical practice and be able to advise what software can best perform the functions that you need and help you select compatible hardware. He or she will understand your need for adequate instruction and continuing support after the system is installed. Ask how this support will be provided and what it will cost. How many experienced support personnel are available or on call? Satisfaction is usually greatest when the complete system is purchased from one vendor.

Desirable Hardware Features

There are certain physical features to look for that will assure the user's comfort:

1. A tilt and swivel screen that can be adjusted to individual comfort when several persons will be using the terminal.

2. Adjustable screen brightness/contrast.

3. Easy-access disk drives.

4. A keyboard that is separate from the unit.

5. A separate numerical keypad for accounting entries.

6. Keys that are not over- or under-responsive.

Choosing Software

Available software has a wide range of capabilities. Programs also require various degrees of training to attain proficiency. Software is sometimes referred to as being user-friendly, meaning that it is relatively easy to learn and use. User-friendly may also mean that the performable functions are limited, possibly too limited for a medical practice. In choosing software it is important to consider the requirements of the practice first, and to make arrangements for whatever training is necessary to operate the system.

Training

After a well-chosen system is in operation, its ultimate success will depend largely on the people who operate it. Formal training sessions are the best way to introduce new users to the system, and each person on the staff who will be operating the computer should receive this formal training. In the learning sessions, the new operators should practice their skills, using data similar in form and content to the actual data that will be processed by the system. Along with the formal training, the vendor should supply good operating manuals, and a telephone number to call when difficulties arise that the operator cannot solve.

Computers are here to stay. Let's use and enjoy them.

COMPUTER VOCABULARY

backup: duplicate of file made to protect information

batch: a collection of similar work that can be processed in one operation

bit: a binary digit, the smallest unit of data in a computer

boot: starting up a computer

buffer: temporary storage for data in a computer's memory

bug: an error in a computer or program that keeps it from working properly

byte: eight bits or units of memory; a byte is roughly equal to one letter or digit

CAI: an acronym for Computer-Assisted Instruction

catalog: a list of files on the storage media

central processing unit (CPU): the heart of a computer system

characters per second (CPS): term used to measure printer output

command: an instruction

computer: a device that manipulates data according to a series of instructions stored in its memory

crash: a breakdown resulting from software or hardware malfunction

cursor: the display screen's indicator where the next character will be typed

daisy wheel printer: a printer that uses a changeable printwheel, named for its shape

debugging: finding errors and correcting them in computer programs

disk drive: manual device that operates the disk

DOS (disk operating system): a program that tells the computer how to use the disk drive

dot matrix printer: printer that uses dots to form letters and numbers

electronic mail: the transmission of letters, messages, and memos from one computer to another over telephone lines

file: an orderly, self-contained collection of data that is usually stored on a permanent storage device such as a disk

floppy disk (diskette): a thin disk of magnetic material capable of storing a large amount of information; it was developed to give small computer systems an inexpensive and convenient way of storing information

hard copy: the readable paper copy or printout of information

hardware: the electronic, magnetic, and electromechanical equipment of a computer system (the physical equipment)

I/O (input/output): *Input* is any information that goes into and is used by the computer; *output* is any information that is processed by the computer and displayed to the terminal, printer, or other device

initialize: to prepare a diskette to receive data

kilobyte (abbreviated "K"): in electronics, K is short for kilo, a prefix meaning one thousand; for example, 64 K = 64,000 bytes

main memory: the internal memory of the computer

memory: data held in storage

menu: the list of commands in a program available to the user

microcomputer: a small computer system that uses a microprocessor as its central processing unit

microprocessor: a single chip where the computer computes

minicomputer: a computer significantly smaller in size, capacity, and software capability than its larger main-frame counterparts

modem: an abbreviation for MOdulator DEModulator; a device that enables data to be transmitted over telephone lines

monitor: a device used to display computer generated information

peripheral: a device, such as a printer, disk drive, or game paddles, that can be attached to a computer for input, output, or storage purposes

program: a sequence of instructions written in a computer language designed to make the computer carry out a given task

RAM (random access memory): the working area of a computer that stores instructions and data during execution of a program. The information need not be retrieved in the order in which it was written. Information stored in RAM may be lost when the computer is turned off

ROM (Read-Only Memory): Memory that can be altered only by changing the physical structure of the chip. ROM chips are usually used to store information that is essential to the operation of the computer

scrolling: moving through information on a computer display, either vertically or horizontally, to view information otherwise excluded

software: The programming necessary to direct the hardware of a computer system (computer programs)

syntax error: a system response to a mistake in instruction, such as a transposition of characters or an omission of a character or word

telecommunications: The use of telephone lines to transmit data between computers or terminals

WP (word processing): The transformation of ideas and information into a readable form of communication through the management of procedures, equipment, and personnel

write-protect: process or code that prevents overwriting of data or programs on a disk

REFERENCES AND READINGS

Ehrlich, A.: *Computers: The Key to Medical Practice Management,* Champaign, IL, Colwell Systems, 1985.

Neiburger, E. J.: *Computers for Professional Practice,* Waukegan, IL, Andent, Inc., 1984.

Sellars, D.: *Computerizing Your Medical Office,* Oradell, NJ, Medical Economics Co., 1983.

Superintendent of Documents, U.S. Government Printing Office: *Computers, Health Records, and Citizen Rights,* 1976.

Stwertka, E., and Stwertka, A.: *Computers in Medicine,* New York, F. Watts, 1984.

Tolos, P. C., and Moody, D.: *How to Choose the Right Computer for Your Medical Practice,* Santa Rosa, CA, Burgess Communications, 1986.

6

CHAPTER OUTLINE

VOCABULARY

See Glossary at end of book for definitions.

allergic reaction	intercom	prevail
controversial	oral hygiene	propriety
haughty	phonetic	psychologic

Patient Reception

OBJECTIVES

Upon successful completion of this chapter you should be able to:

1. *Define the words listed in the Vocabulary of this chapter.*
2. *Discuss the three essentials of an attractive professional appearance.*
3. *List six considerations in planning a comfortable reception room.*
4. *Briefly discuss seven steps in collating patient charts for a day's appointments.*
5. *State two reasons for checking supplies at the beginning of each day.*
6. *Identify and discuss the importance of the three components of greeting an arriving patient.*
7. *Instruct a new patient about providing personal data for the records and completing a registration form.*
8. *List three actions a medical assistant might take to reduce stress caused by a delayed schedule.*
9. *Discuss ways a medical assistant might help a handicapped, uncomfortable, or ill patient.*
10. *Cite at least four measures a medical assistant might take in effecting a friendly farewell to a departing patient.*

Upon successful completion of this chapter you should be able to perform the following activities:

1. *Demonstrate how the medical assistant maintains a professional appearance.*
2. *Collate patient charts for one day.*
3. *Through role play and under the observation of the instructor:*
   a. *Greet an arriving patient.*
   b. *Respond to a patient's complaint.*
   c. *Escort a patient to an examination room and give the patient appropriate instructions.*

Appearances and first impressions mean a great deal in any situation. This is especially true in the physician's office, where an atmosphere of cleanliness and order must **prevail**. The impression that the medical assistant makes upon the patients often colors their impressions about the doctor and the care they can expect. The patient who feels comfortable with the assistant will probably feel comfortable with the doctor.

FIRST IMPRESSIONS

The Assistant

A well-groomed assistant in professional attire has a good **psychologic** effect upon patients. The essentials of a professional appearance are good health, good grooming, and appropriate dress.

Good health means getting plenty of sleep, eating balanced meals, and getting sufficient exercise to keep fit. Medical assistants need a sensible regimen of healthful living and regular checkups of their own physical condition. A radiantly healthy office staff is the best possible public relations for the physician.

Medical assistants usually wear a uniform. The uniform not only gives a professional look but identifies the assistant as a member of the team. Uniforms are no longer limited to the traditional white. Modern fabrics and styling have made it possible for the medical assistant's uniform to be attractive as well as practical. Women have a choice of a pantsuit, in white or color, or perhaps with contrasting top; a two-piece dress uniform in white or color (Fig. 7–1); or an attractive design in the traditional white dress uniform. Men usually wear white slacks with a white or light-color shirt, jacket, or pullover top. A laboratory coat over street clothes may be worn by men or women if this is within the facility's dress code.

Whatever style of uniform the assistant chooses, it should be one that is personally becoming, worn over appropriate undergarments and without ornamentation. Jewelry should be limited to an engagement ring, wedding band, and professional pin. If there is more than one assistant in the office, name pins worn by everyone in the office will help the patient to identify each assistant by name.

Because today's fabrics are so easy to care for, there should be no temptation to wear a uniform a second day without laundering. Even spills and spots that occur during the course of the working day can usually be rinsed out immediately.

The shoes the assistant wears should be appropriate for a uniform, spotless, and comfortable. White shoes must be kept white by daily cleaning. A damp sponge and Ivory soap will take care of quick cleanups during the working day; when you

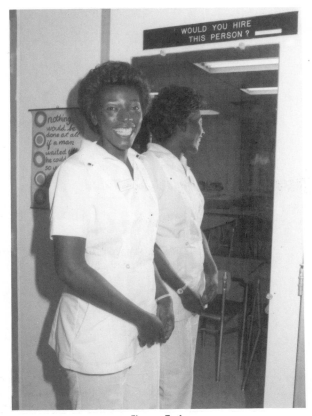

Figure 7–1
Medical assisting student checking her appearance. (Courtesy of Southern California College of Medical and Dental Careers, Anaheim, CA. Photo by Dan Santucci.)

give them a thorough cleaning at night, don't forget that shoestrings need cleaning, too, if you wear a tie shoe.

In some offices the physician prefers that the assistant not wear a uniform. Some psychiatrists, for example, feel that the clinical appearance of a uniform may have an adverse effect upon patients. The medical assistant who does not wear a uniform should still follow the dictates of good taste and **propriety** in choosing an office wardrobe. The garments worn on the job must be comfortable, becoming, allow easy movement, and still look fresh at the end of a busy day.

Good grooming is little more than attention to the details of personal appearance. Personal cleanliness, which includes taking a daily bath or shower, using a good deodorant, and practicing good **oral hygiene**, is vital. The female medical assistant's makeup should be carefully selected and applied. Harsh or exaggerated makeup is out of place in the professional office. Subtle eye makeup and clear or natural shades of nail polish may enhance the assistant's appearance. Both the male and the female medical assistant should have hair that is clean, neatly styled, and off the collar.

Procedure 7–1

PRESENTING A PROFESSIONAL IMAGE

PROCEDURAL GOAL

To present an appropriate professional image to the physician, your co-workers, the patients, and visitors in your medical setting.

PROCEDURE

1. Appear ready to work in fresh, clean, pressed professional clothing in accordance with your facility's dress code.
2. Clean and polish your shoes daily.
3. Wear your name pin and professional pin proudly.
   Purpose: Name pins are required by law in some states.
4. Use a non-scented deodorant daily and pay particular attention to oral hygiene.
   Purpose: Body odors offend your patients and your co-workers.
5. Style your hair so that it is up and off your collar (female assistants may wear an appropriate hairnet).
   Purpose: Hair harbors numerous germs, which may fall from the hair onto medically and surgically aseptic areas. Hair can also get caught in equipment or be pulled by children.
6. Trim your nails and polish them as appropriate.
   Purpose: Long nails harbor bacteria, or you may scratch your patient's skin.
   Female Assistants:
7. Wear full-length, neutral shade, run-free hosiery.
8. Keep makeup conservative and use no cologne or perfume.
   Purpose: Strong odors may make an already ill patient feel more uncomfortable. Some patients are allergic to colognes and perfumes.
   Male Assistants:
7. Wear hosiery compatible with your shoes and uniform.
8. The face should be clean-shaven, or if a mustache or beard is worn it should be neatly trimmed and clean.

TERMINAL PERFORMANCE OBJECTIVE

Given your agency's dress code, present an appropriate professional image at all times to a performance level of 95%.

The Reception Room

Take an objective look around the reception room periodically. Could it use a little brightening or freshening up? Try to look at it as if you were seeing it for the first time. The reception room is just that—a place to receive patients. It should be planned for the patient's comfort, made as attractive and cheerful as possible, and kept clean and uncluttered.

Fresh harmonious colors and cleanliness are the basis of an attractive room. Add comfortable furniture, adequate to accommodate the peak load of patients seen each day, and arrange it in conversational groups. Individual chairs are usually best. People will sometimes stand rather than sit next to a stranger on a sofa. Provide good lighting, ventilation, and a regulated temperature for additional comfort, and you have the essentials of an attractive reception room that tells the patient you care. A place to hang coats, rainwear, and umbrellas will help reduce reception room clutter (Fig. 7–2).

Plants, pictures, travel posters, and bulletin board displays can add charm and individuality to a reception room. Indoor plants are suitable, but fresh flowers may cause **allergic reactions.** Artificial flower arrangements and plants can be just as attractive, but one word of caution is in order—don't allow those artificial arrangements to collect dust. Either wipe them off regularly or take time to "dunk" them in water occasionally.

Most physicians' offices are well-supplied with recent magazines in washable plastic covers. Patients seem to enjoy looking at pictures rather than something that requires concentrated reading. Pictorial travel books and magazines with short items of popular interest are favorites. The reception room, incidentally, is not the place for the physician's professional journals.

ADDED ATTRACTIONS FOR RECEPTION AREA

- *Plants (fresh or artificial)*
- *Pictures*
- *Travel posters*
- *Bulletin board displays*
- *Recent general interest magazines*
- *Pictorial travel books*
- *Aquarium (built-in for safety)*
- *Safe toys for children's corner*

Some doctors place a writing desk and writing paper in the room for the convenience of patients; some play restful music over a concealed speaker. Even such additions as a television set, a lighted

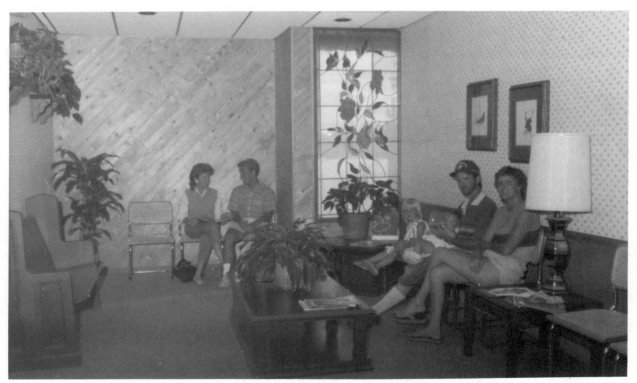

Figure 7–2
A comfortable, tasteful reception room. (Courtesy of Vista Medical Group, El Toro, CA. Photo by Dan Santucci.)

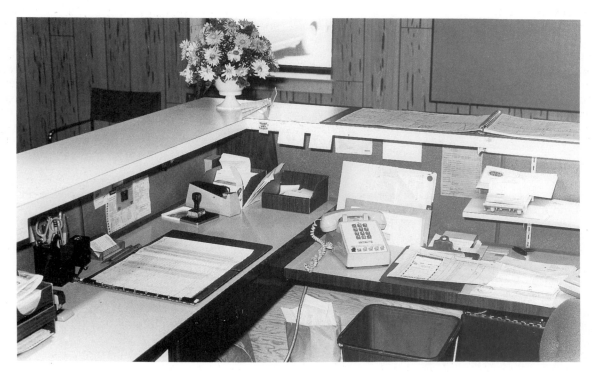

Figure 7–3
Desk with shoulder-high shield for privacy.

aquarium, or an educational display of some sort will enhance the attractiveness and individuality of the front door to the doctor's practice.

In pediatric practices, a children's corner, equipped with small-scale furniture and some playthings, is a good idea. It helps keep youngsters occupied who might otherwise get into mischief. Toys should be easily cleanable; plastic washable ones are especially good. Be scrupulously careful that the toy has no sharp corners that could injure a child, or small parts that could be swallowed. Also, in selecting toys, make sure that they will not stimulate the child toward noisy activity. And no rubber balls, for obvious reasons.

It may be necessary to engage a professional designer to suggest reception room improvements that will add to the patient's comfort and enjoyment. The medical assistant is at least partly responsible for the appearance of the reception room by making sure that the room remains neat and orderly throughout the day. A quick check at intervals during the day and a minute or two devoted to putting the room in order help keep it looking its best.

If the medical assistant's desk is in the reception room or in open view of the patients, it should be free of clutter. In particular, patients' charts or financial cards should not be in sight. Personal articles, coffee cups, and ashtrays should not be on the receptionist's desk (Fig. 7–3).

PREPARING FOR PATIENT ARRIVAL

Advance preparation will make your day smoother and will contribute toward a more relaxed atmosphere for all concerned.

Appointment List

If the appointment list was typed (or a printout made from the computer) before you left the previous evening, refresh your memory of the patients' names by going over the list at the start of the day, and place a duplicate copy on the physician's desk. On this schedule, special notations should be made concerning new patients, special examinations, and so forth. Pull the charts for the patients to be seen that day, noting any special instructions, and place them in the order they are expected to be seen. You should check each history before the physician sees it, to make certain that any recently received information, such as laboratory reports and x-ray readings, has been correctly entered and that the chart is up-to-date. You may be expected to place the charts on the physician's desk for all the patients to be seen that day, but more than likely the physician will prefer to receive each chart just prior to seeing the patient.

7—2

EQUIPMENT AND SUPPLIES

Appointment schedule for current date
Clerical supplies (pen, tape, stapler, etc.)
Access to patient files

PROCEDURAL GOAL

To collate patient charts for daily appointment schedule and have them ready for the physician before patients' arrival.

PROCEDURE

1. Review the appointment schedule.
2. Identify full name of each scheduled patient.
3. Pull patients' charts from files, checking each patient's name on your list as each chart is pulled.
   Purpose: To determine that the correct charts have been pulled and that none have been omitted.
4. Review each chart.
   Purpose: To reaffirm that:
   a. All information has been correctly entered
   b. Any previously ordered tests have been performed
   c. The results have been entered on the chart
5. Annotate the appointment list with any special concerns.
   Purpose: To alert the physician regarding matters that should be checked or discussed with the patient.
6. Arrange all charts sequentially according to each patient's appointment.
7. Place the charts in the appropriate examination room or other specified location.

TERMINAL PERFORMANCE OBJECTIVE

Given the listed equipment and supplies, collate and arrange the patient charts sequentially, and annotate the appointment schedule as necessary to a performance level of 100% within 30 minutes (time will vary based on the number of patients).

Clinical Supplies

When the patients start arriving, you will want to have everything ready for the day so that you and the doctor can give undivided attention to the patients' needs. If the previous day was a busy one, the supplies in the treatment rooms may be low, and instruments may need sterilizing. The doctor may have had to return to the office to care for a patient during the previous evening.

> *Check the rooms to make certain that everything is clean, the cabinets are well-stocked, and everything is ready for the first patient of the day.*

If reserve supplies are kept in another room, you may wish to use a hand basket or a cart on wheels so that everything can be carried at one time rather than requiring several trips to the stock room.

Administrative Supplies

Supplies at the medical assistant's desk should also be checked periodically. Stationery, appointment cards, charge slips, sharpened pencils, and any items you are likely to use during the day should be on hand, to avoid needless trips to the supply closet.

GREETING THE PATIENT

1. *Greet each patient immediately upon arrival.*
2. *Introduce yourself to a new patient.*
3. *Greet the established patient by name.*
4. *Pronounce the patient's name correctly.*

Every patient has the right to expect courteous treatment in the physician's office. No matter what the patient's economic or social status, each individual who enters the reception room should receive a cordial, friendly greeting.

The medical assistant can do a great deal to give each patient reassurance and a feeling of importance by the manner in which the patient is greeted. Contrast the closed opaque window over a sign that reads "Ring Bell and Be Seated" with the friendly greeting of the medical assistant: "Good morning, Mr. Barker. I see you are right on time! The doctor will see you in just a few minutes."

Ideally, the medical assistant's desk is placed for a clear view of all visitors who come into the office. If there is only one medical assistant, it is sometimes impossible for each new caller to be welcomed personally. In this situation some announcement system must be worked out. The patient who enters an empty reception room does not know whether to sit down or to try to announce his presence in some way. Sometimes a register is placed in the reception room with a sign above it reading: "Please sign the register when you arrive. Doctor will see you shortly." This is a makeshift arrangement, as is the bell advising the patient to ring and be seated. Either of these arrangements is better than no reception at all, but cannot compare with the personal greeting of the medical assistant.

The importance of the personal touch in receiving patients should not be overlooked. A good medical assistant cultivates the habit of greeting each patient immediately in a friendly, self-assured manner, without being overly familiar. If the patient is new, introduce yourself. Greet the established patient by name. Learn how to pronounce each patient's name correctly, since incorrect pronunciations may offend and irritate some people. If the name is unusual, write the **phonetic** spelling on the history for reference. This may save embarrassment at future visits.

Try to learn each patient's name and to remember something personal about each one so that on return visits you can inquire about their hobbies or the activities of their children. It is unwise to appear overcurious about patients' personal lives, but most patients appreciate the interest of the doctor and the staff in their family, hobbies, or work. Sometimes the medical assistant can jot down key words on the patient's history that provide subjects for future conversations.

REGISTRATION FORMS: PERSONAL HISTORY

A patient coming in for a first visit will require certain introductory procedures. Most physicians use a patient information form of some kind to gather subjective information about the patient. The medical assistant may complete the form while interviewing the new patient or have the patient complete the form upon arrival for the first appointment. The form may be attached to a clipboard and handed to the patient with instructions to complete all parts of the form, with assurance that the assistant is ready and willing to answer any questions (Fig. 7–4). The form will include space for personal data about the patient, such as:

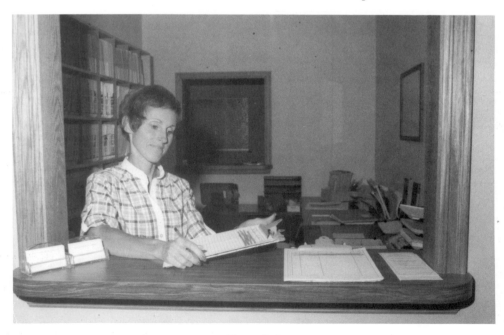

Figure 7–4
The new patient is given a patient information form on a clipboard. (Courtesy of Vista Medical Group, El Toro, CA. Photo by Dan Santucci.)

- Full name
- Address
- Telephone number
- Social Security number
- Date of birth
- Occupation
- Name and address of employer
- Name of spouse
- Referring physician, if any
- Medical insurance information

When the completed form is returned to the medical assistant, it should be checked carefully to be certain that all the necessary information has been included (Fig. 7–5).

The personal and medical history, and the patient's family history, may be secured by asking the patient to complete a questionnaire, with the physician augmenting this during the patient interview. The more experienced medical assistant may be expected to interview the patient for the patient's personal and medical history, family history, and chief complaint. This is a very specialized procedure, and the interviewer will most likely be specifically trained for the individual practice.

CONSIDERATION FOR PATIENTS' TIME

The patient's first question, once he or she has been received, frequently is, "When can I see the

PATIENT INFORMATION FOR MEDICAL RECORDS *(Please Print)* DATE: 04-20-88

PATIENT — MR.✓ MRS. MISS — LAST NAME: MORRIS — FIRST NAME: SAMUEL — MIDDLE: ALBERT

PATIENT ADDRESS — STREET CITY STATE ZIP HOME PHONE: 3810 Commonwealth Avenue, Los Angeles, CA 90056 213 862 9917

SOCIAL SECURITY NUMBER: 012 34 5678 — DATE OF BIRTH: 04-05-40 — AGE: 48 — DRIVER'S LICENSE NO.: Z80037

PATIENT EMPLOYER: Morris Appliances — OCCUPATION: Merchant

EMPLOYER'S ADDRESS — STREET CITY STATE ZIP BUS PHONE: 5400 Hollywood Blvd., Los Angeles 90036 213 462 8122

SPOUSE'S NAME: Louise Marie — MARITAL STATUS: M✓ S D W SEP. — REFERRED BY: Frank Gentry, M.D. 714 635 4300

SPOUSE'S EMPLOYER — STREET CITY STATE ZIP BUS. PHONE: Morris Appliances (see above)

IN CASE OF EMERGENCY CONTACT: NAME ADDRESS CITY STATE ZIP TELEPHONE: (Daughter) Ellen Spivak, 486 Vine Street, Los Angeles 90036 213 536 4142

MEDICAL INSURANCE INFORMATION

COMPANY: Occidental Insurance Company — POLICY NUMBER: WD 4305

COMPANY — POLICY NUMBER

COMPANY — POLICY NUMBER

IF SOMEONE OTHER THAN PATIENT IS RESPONSIBLE FOR PAYMENT PLEASE COMPLETE THIS SECTION

RESPONSIBLE PARTY — MR. MRS. MISS — LAST NAME — FIRST NAME — MIDDLE — RELATION

ADDRESS — STREET — CITY — STATE — ZIP — TELEPHONE

OCCUPATION — EMPLOYED BY

EMPLOYER'S ADDRESS — STREET — CITY — STATE — ZIP — BUS. PHONE

I hereby authorize Dr. Theodore Wilson to release any and all medical (including dental) information to the above-named insurance carrier (or to a designated attorney) for purposes of claims administration and evaluation, utilization review and financial audit. This authorization remains valid and effective from the date of signing until revoked in writing. I understand that I may request a copy of this authorization. I have read this authorization and understand it. I hereby assign to Dr. Theodore Wilson all money to which I am entitled for medical and/or surgical expense relative to the service rendered by him, but not to exceed my indebtedness to said physician and/or surgeon. It is understood that any money received from the above named insurance company, over and above my indebtedness will be refunded to me when my bill is paid in full. I understand I am financially responsible to said doctor(s) for charges not covered by this assignment. I further agree in the event of non-payment, to bear the cost of collection, and/or Court cost and reasonable legal fees should this be required.

INSURED OR GUARDIAN'S SIGNATURE ________ PATIENT'S SIGNATURE Samuel A. Morris

58-8409 © 1976 BIBBERO SYSTEMS, INC. PETALUMA, CA

Figure 7–5
Patient registration form. (Courtesy of Bibbero Systems, Inc., Petaluma, CA.)

Procedure 7–3

EQUIPMENT AND SUPPLIES

Registration form
Clerical supplies (pen, clipboard)
Private conference area

PROCEDURAL GOAL

To complete registration form for a new patient, obtaining adequate information for credit and insurance claims.

PROCEDURE

1. Determine that the patient is new.
2. Obtain and record the necessary information:
   a. Full name, birth date, name of spouse (if married)
   b. Home address, telephone number (include ZIP code and area code)
   c. Occupation, name of employer, business address, telephone number
   d. Social Security number
   e. Name of referring physician if any
   f. Name and address of person responsible for payment
   g. Method of payment
   h. Health insurance information
      (1) Name of primary carrier
      (2) Type of coverage
      (3) Group policy number
      (4) Subscriber number
      (5) Assignment of benefits, if required
   Purpose: This information is necessary for credit and insurance claims.
3. Review the entire form.
   Purpose: To be certain that information is complete and legible.

TERMINAL PERFORMANCE OBJECTIVE

Given the listed equipment and supplies, complete the registration form for a new patient, including all the required information, to 100% accuracy, within 10 minutes.

---

doctor?" The medical assistant should get the patient in to see the doctor as near the appointment time as possible or explain why the patient must wait. It is your responsibility as the medical assistant to convey both your own and the doctor's concern if there will be a delay. Consideration for the patient's time is extremely important.

Most experts agree that in a well-managed, busy office there are seldom more than three to five patients in the reception room. "Too long a wait in the doctor's office" is one of the most frequently heard criticisms of the medical profession. The patient who complains about medical fees or care may in actuality be complaining about the long wait or discourteous service.

A crowded waiting room is not always an indication of a doctor's popularity. It may reveal, instead, that the doctor or the assistant is inefficient in scheduling patients. In some rare instances it can be a **haughty** disregard for the patient. Patients do not seem to mind waiting 15 to 20 minutes to see the doctor, but they do consider a wait of more than this excessive.

Business people, for example, who are in the habit of making the most of their time, are particularly displeased at what may appear to them to be inefficient scheduling of appointments. Any delay of longer than 15 minutes should be explained to the person waiting.

When a prolonged wait is unavoidable, the medical assistant may be able to help the patients pass the time by suggesting a particularly good story or article in a magazine to a patient who wants to read, or by chatting briefly with a restless patient. It should, however, be the patient's decision as to whether or not to talk. Select conversation subjects that interest the patient—hobbies, family, business, profession, or recreational interests—and steer clear of **controversial** subjects such as religion and politics.

The medical assistant can sometimes increase a patient's esteem for the physician by mentioning the physician's hobby or telling about a forthcoming trip to a medical meeting to present a scientific paper. A patient is favorably impressed with an assistant who is well versed on such subjects as health insurance, new medical discoveries, local health agencies, and other topics pertaining to medical care that patients may raise during conversation. Printed literature to answer patients' questions on these subjects is usually available from medical organizations. Active members of medical assistants' groups keep well informed on such subjects by attending local meetings regularly.

Some personal attention, such as offering a drink of water, a cup of coffee, or a new magazine, sometimes will quiet a patient who is becoming visibly irritated at waiting.

Many patients are fearful and tense, but the medical assistant can often put them in a better frame of mind merely by a friendly smile and show of concern.

The experienced medical assistant keeps the appointment schedule operating smoothly by tidying each examination room immediately and moving the next patient in so that the doctor need have no idle moments waiting for a patient to be prepared. It is inconsiderate, however, to place a patient in an examining room just to get him out of the reception area, and then keep him waiting a long time, particularly if he has been gowned, draped, and left in an uncomfortable position on the examining table. If you think there might be some delay, suggest that the patient take along a magazine or something to occupy his time during the additional wait. Avoid the assembly line atmosphere.

ESCORTING AND INSTRUCTING THE PATIENT

Sometimes we become so accustomed to our own surroundings that we forget that the stranger may be confused or disoriented by all the hallways, doors, and rooms. Do take time to personally escort the patient to the appropriate examination or treatment room. If the patient is to disrobe, explain what garments, if any, can be left on, whether shoes are to be removed, the removal of jewelry if an x-ray is to be taken, and so forth. If a gown is to be worn, specify whether the opening should be in front or

back, and tell the patients where they can hang their clothes if this is not obvious. All instructions must be clear. Do not assume that patients will know what you want if you have not told them.

Be equally clear when the examination has been completed: "You can get dressed now and return to the consultation room," or "After you are dressed please stop by the desk to make your next appointment."

ASSISTING THE DISABLED PATIENT

Some patients will have a physical handicap, some will be very ill, and some will be severely uncomfortable.

Observe the patient's appearance and behavior. Is the patient pale or drawn looking? Do the eyes or voice reflect pain or discomfort? Find out how the patient is feeling before you suggest that he or she be seated to wait for the doctor. The patient may need to lie down in a cool room, or perhaps should be seen as an emergency. The patient in a wheelchair or walker, or using crutches, may need a bit of personal attention. Some patients may need help in disrobing even when a disability is not obvious. Ask if you can be of assistance. The medical assistant must use good judgment in helping disabled patients, perhaps even bypassing some of the usual routines (Fig. 7–6).

HANDLING PATIENTS' COMPLAINTS

Even under the best of conditions, there will at times be complaints from patients. Remember that the practice of medicine is a personal service for

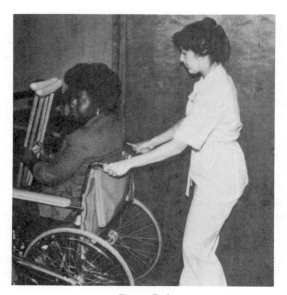

Figure 7–6
The medical assistant helps a disabled patient. (Courtesy of Ferris State College, Big Rapids, MI.)

individual personalities, and the medical assistant must cultivate the skill of listening. Each patient is a very important person, and any complaint should be taken seriously. Try to resolve the matter if it is within your realm of responsibility. Otherwise, assure the patient of your concern and explain that you will try to find a solution. Then be sure to carry through.

PROBLEM SITUATIONS

The Talker. There are certain problem patients in any professional office. The talker, for example, takes up far more of the doctor's time than is justified. An alert medical assistant can usually spot these individuals during the initial interview. The patient's history can be checked with a symbol to alert the doctor. A prearranged agreement to contact the doctor on the **intercom** at the end of the appointment time, with the message that the next patient has arrived, gives the doctor an opportunity to conclude the interview. Once you have learned which patients take extra time, you can book them for the end of the day or simply allow more time for them.

Children. Children sometimes present special management problems. It is often advisable for young patients to go into the treatment room without the parent. This, of course, should be at the discretion of the physician.

While this practice of separating children from their parents to treat their needs is not always feasible, it sometimes can be applied with great success. In some offices a token of the doctor's friendship, such as a trinket or toy, is given the child at the completion of the visit.

The Angry Patient. Every medical assistant at some time is confronted with an angry patient. The anger may be simply a reflection of the patient's pain or fear of what the doctor may discover on the examination. It is usually best to let such patients talk out their anger. A calm attitude on the part of the medical assistant, with a few remarks interjected in a low voice, will often quiet the patient. Under no circumstances should the assistant return the anger or become argumentative.

The Patient's Relatives. A patient will sometimes be accompanied by a relative or well-meaning friend who may become restless while waiting for the patient and attempt to discuss the patient's illness. The medical assistant should sidestep any discussion of a patient's medical care, except by direction of the physician. Also avoid a too casual attitude, such as, "I'm sure there's nothing to worry about." A show of moderate concern, offering reassurance

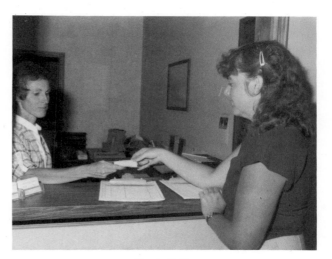

Figure 7–7
Handing appointment card to patient for next visit. (Courtesy of Vista Medical Group, El Toro, CA. Photo by Dan Santucci.)

that "the patient is in good hands" will usually take care of the situation.

FRIENDLY FAREWELLS

The medical assistant should be ready to take charge of the patient as soon as the visit with the physician has been completed by assisting the patient in dressing, if necessary, and making sure that any questions are answered. Ask the patient whether another appointment is necessary and, if so, be sure the appointment time is arranged before the patient leaves the office (Fig. 7–7).

If a patient seems hesitant to leave, there may be some unanswered question still on his mind. A friendly offer on the part of the medical assistant to help or explain a problem will often relieve anxiety and save a telephone call later. The assistant can help convey the impression of friendliness by terminating the patient's visit cordially. If there is time, walk to the door with the patient. If the patient is returning for another visit, the medical assistant can say something like "We'll see you next week." If it is the patient's last visit, a pleasant "I certainly hope you'll be feeling fine from now on" is appropriate. The assistant may want to tell a patient on his last visit that he has been a fine patient and that it has been a pleasure to serve him. Whatever words of goodbye are chosen, all patients should leave the doctor's office feeling that they have received top quality care and were treated with friendliness and courtesy.

REFERENCES AND READINGS

American Medical Association: Winning Ways with Patients. Chicago, The Association, 1979.

7

CHAPTER OUTLINE

VOCABULARY

See Glossary at end of book for definitions.

deviation	intermittent	stat report
disruption	matrix	tickler (file)
integral	prerogative	

Appointment Scheduling

OBJECTIVES

Upon successful completion of this chapter you should be able to:
1. Define the terms listed in the Vocabulary of this chapter.
2. Discuss the advantages and disadvantages of open office hours vs. scheduled appointments.
3. Describe four important features of an appointment book.
4. List and explain the three basic guidelines to follow in scheduling appointments.
5. Identify and discuss the advantages of wave scheduling.
6. Cite three common situations that would require adjusting the appointment schedule.
7. Describe how you will determine when a request for an appointment is an emergency.
8. State the reason for recording a failed appointment on the patient's chart.
9. Discuss the handling of cancellations and delays brought about by office situations.
10. State one question that should be avoided in arranging a patient appointment.
11. List at least six points of information that will be necessary in scheduling surgery with a hospital.
12. State four items of information that must be available before arranging an outside laboratory appointment for a patient.

Upon successful completion of this chapter you should be able to perform the following activities:
1. Select an appropriate appointment book to suit a given type of practice.
2. Demonstrate the advance preparation that must be done before using a new appointment book.
3. Schedule patients according to the urgency of the appointment and the anticipated treatment time.
4. Rearrange the schedule in the event the physician's arrival is delayed.
5. Explain the physician's unavailability to patients in the reception room.
6. Arrange a referral appointment for a patient.
7. Schedule a patient for a diagnostic test as indicated by the physician.
8. Schedule a surgery with the hospital, notifying all the persons and departments concerned.
9. Instruct a patient regarding pre-admission requirements, hospital stay, and insurance information needed.
10. Arrange for a patient's admission to a hospital as ordered by the physician.

IMPORTANCE OF TIME MANAGEMENT

Open Office Hours. With open office hours the facility is open at given hours of the day or evening, and the patients are probably "scheduled" by saying something such as, "Come back in a couple of weeks." At a convenient time the patients come in to see the doctor, knowing in advance that they will be seen in their order of arrival. Physicians who use this method say that it eliminates the annoyance of broken appointments and "running late."

Few doctors' offices in metropolitan areas have open office hours—no scheduled appointments—but this system is common in some rural areas, where the way of life is governed not so much by the clock as by the sun and the seasons. Another type of practice that has open hours is the growing number of emergency centers, many of which are open on a 24-hour basis. Although they are frequently called "emergicenters," they may in reality deal with many general practice types of cases.

There can be many disadvantages to open office hours:

- The office may be crowded when the doctor arrives, resulting in extremely long waits for some patients.
- There is the danger of rushing some patients through without giving them full attention.
- It is also possible that few or none will arrive before afternoon, and both doctor and staff will have to stay late to see everyone.
- Without planning, the facilities as well as the staff can be overburdened.

Scheduled Appointments. Studies have shown that physicians are able to see more patients with less pressure when they schedule appointments. Most providers of medical care find that efficient scheduling of appointments is one of the most important factors in the success of a practice.

If appointments are made by telephone, that first telephone interaction creates the patient's impression of the medical facilities. Unfortunately, the skill required for the scheduling of appointments is often not fully appreciated by the physician, and this responsibility may be delegated to the least qualified medical assistant. But while the skill and attitude of the assistant who manages the appointment schedule is very important, the ultimate success of the system lies in the cooperation of the physician(s).

Efficient scheduling requires an understanding

- of the practice,
- of the personality and habits of the physician, and
- a close estimate of the time needed for each patient.

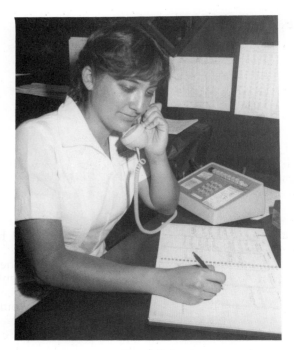

Figure 8–1
Medical assistant at appointment desk. (Courtesy of Southern California College of Medical and Dental Careers. Photo by Dan Santucci.)

Planning appointments realistically and seeing that the physician starts on time and sticks to the schedule will please the patients, bring economic gain to the physician, and assure a more regular schedule for both the medical assistant and the physician (Fig. 8–1).

THE APPOINTMENT BOOK

Selection. Office suppliers and stationers carry a variety of appointment book styles. One of the standard preprinted styles will be satisfactory for a physician who is just starting a practice, but as the practice develops, the physician may find the preprinted books too restrictive. When this happens, it is time to look for an appointment book that more closely suits the practice, or, failing this, to personally design one. In either case, there are certain basic features to consider.

Basic Features of Appointment Book:

- *Size conforms to the desk space available*
- *Large enough to accommodate the practice*
- *Opens flat for easy writing and reference*
- *Allows space for when, who, and why*

Additional Considerations:

- *Pages that show an entire week at a glance*
- *Color coding with a special color for each day of the week*
- *Multiple columns corresponding with the number of doctors in a group practice*
- *Division into time units suitable to the practice*

Many professional stationers will furnish planning kits and work with you to develop what is best for the practice. Some of these resources are listed at the end of the chapter.

Advance Preparation. Having chosen an appropriate book, some advance preparation should be done. This is sometimes called "establishing the matrix." Block off, in pencil, those periods when the doctor is routinely not available to see patients (days off, holidays, hospital rounds, lunch, meetings, and so forth). In the space where you would ordinarily write the patient's name, write a memo showing the reason for blocking off these spaces. Always try to account for every time period in each day.

If the physician keeps you informed of social or family engagements, make a note of these also as a reminder.

GUIDELINES FOR SCHEDULING

The scheduling system must be individualized to each specific practice. There are, however, certain general guidelines to be followed in each practice:

- Patient need
- Doctor's preferences and habits
- Available facilities

Patient Need. A major general consideration in determining office hours and appointment times is the socioeconomic status of the area—Is it agricultural? a retirement community? industrial? Who are the patients? Are evening and Saturday appointments essential for some?

More specifically, time must be allotted to patients on the basis of each one's particular needs, which can be assessed by asking such questions as:

- What is the purpose of the visit?
- What is the age of the patient? (A teenager will probably not require as much time as an older patient.)
- Will the patient require the doctor's time for the entire visit, or will another member of the staff be performing part or all of the service?
- Is the patient a young mother who prefers to schedule her appointments during the school hours?

Whenever possible, attempt to make the appointment suit the needs of the patient.

Doctor's Preferences and Habits. Is the doctor methodical and careful about being in the office when patient appointments are scheduled to begin? Some doctors are habitually late.

Does the doctor move easily from one patient to the next? Some require a "break" time between patients.

Would the physician rather see fewer patients and spend more time with each one? If so, this must be taken into account in the scheduling process.

Some doctors become restless if the reception room is not packed with waiting patients; others worry if one patient is kept waiting. All these personal preferences and habits become an integral part of the scheduling process.

Available Facilities. There's no point in getting a patient into the office at a time when no facilities are available for the services needed. For instance, suppose that in a two-physician office there is only one room that can be used for minor surgery. You wouldn't schedule two patients requiring minor surgery for the same time block even though both doctors could be available. If there is only one electrocardiograph, you would not book two EKGs at the same time. As you become proficient in scheduling, you should be able to pair patients' needs with the available facilities.

Appointment Time Pattern. The physician who has been practicing for years knows how much time is needed for the various kinds of office visits: complete physical, presurgery workup, well-child visit, eye examination, and so forth. The physician is the one who should decide how long a visit should be, and an estimated time schedule should be at the appointment desk. Since the doctor's timing does change through the years, an annual review of the time schedule should be made to accommodate these changes as well as changes in the patient profile.

It may be, however, that a time pattern has never been determined. The medical assistant can do the preliminary work on this through an informal practice analysis, noting the arrival time, treatment or conference time, departure time, and service performed (Fig. 8–2). After a few weeks a definite time pattern should be distinguishable for each type of service. When possible, smooth out the schedule by having some long and some short appointments, and go over the schedule with the doctor at the beginning of each day.

Same-Day Service. Ideally, the scheduling system should provide for same-day service for acutely

APPOINTMENT TIME ANALYSIS

NAME	ARRIVED	BEGIN TREATMENT	END TREATMENT	SERVICE CODE

SUMMARY

SERVICE	AVERAGE WAITING TIME	AVERAGE TREATMENT TIME

Figure 8–2
Sample form for determining appointment pattern.

ill patients, for emergencies, and for seeing all scheduled patients on time. New patients are sometimes treated as emergencies.

Every doctor's schedule should have at least one, or preferably two, appointment slots open each day. Family practitioners may want to leave as much as 25 per cent of their time open for emergencies and work-in patients. Many doctors find that reserving one time slot at the end of the morning and one at the end of the afternoon works well and causes the least disruption of schedule.

TIME MANAGEMENT

Wave Scheduling

Many scheduling systems lack flexibility. Wave scheduling is an attempt to correlate a time schedule with the variables brought about by patients who need more time or less time than planned for, by a patient who arrives late, and by other unavoidable deviations from the schedule, such as the patient who fails to keep an appointment (no-show) and unscheduled (work-in) patients. In wave scheduling an attempt is made to start and finish each hour on time.

What happens when all patients are assigned the same length of time? With a patient scheduled every 20 minutes the schedule might look like this:

10:00 Alicia Barker
10:20 Colleen Davies
10:40 Edna Farber

11:00 Gertrude Havens
11:20 Irene Jackson
11:40 Katherine Lambert

Mrs. Barker, the first patient, arrives at 10:15. The physician has already lost 15 minutes. The patient needs 25 minutes instead of the allotted 20 minutes. Mrs. Davis, the second patient, also arrived at 10:15, 5 minutes early for her appointment, but is kept waiting until 10:40, the time that Mrs. Farber, the third patient, was to have been seen. Mrs. Farber is on time but will also be kept waiting. Fortunately, Mrs. Davis actually needs only 10 minutes, so Mrs. Farber can be seen at 10:50, but if she requires the allotted 20 minutes, Mrs. Havens, the fourth patient, will also have to wait, and so on throughout the day.

Wave scheduling assumes that the actual time needed will average out. If the average time is 20 minutes per patient, three patients will be scheduled for each hour and be seen in order of arrival. Thus, one person's late arrival will not disrupt the entire schedule. The appointment schedule would then look like this:

10:00 Alicia Barker
Colleen Davis
Edna Farber

Procedure 8–1

EQUIPMENT AND SUPPLIES

Page from appointment book
Office policy for office hours, and doctor's availability
Clerical supplies
Calendar
Description of patients to be scheduled

PROCEDURAL GOAL

To establish the matrix of the appointment page, arrange appointments for one day, and enter information according to office policy.

PROCEDURE

1. Determine the hours that the physician will not be available.
   Purpose: So that those hours can be blocked out on the appointment page.
2. Establish the matrix of the appointment page for the day.
   Purpose: To leave available only those time slots that can be used for patient appointments.
3. Identify each patient's complaint.
   Purpose: You must have this information in order to allot time and space for the appointment.
4. Consult guidelines to determine the length of time necessary for each patient.
5. Allot appointment time according to complaint and facilities available.
6. Enter information in appointment book.
   Note: Telephone number must follow patient's name. If patient is new, add the letters NP (new patient) after name.
7. Allow buffer time in morning and afternoon.
   Purpose: To allow the physician and staff a short breather and catch-up time.

TERMINAL PERFORMANCE OBJECTIVE

Given the listed equipment and supplies, prepare the appointment page and schedule all appointments requested for one day within 30 minutes to 100% accuracy. Upon completion, the book must show names of patients, reasons for appointments, and telephone numbers (including notation of new patients and source of referral), with the estimated time needed for each patient marked off.

11:00 Gertrude Havens
Irene Jackson
Katherine Lambert

Given the circumstances illustrated above, Mrs. Davis would have arrived first (5 minutes early), Mrs. Farber would be next (on time), and Mrs. Barker would be third (15 minutes late). All could have been seen within the hour, with no delay affecting the patients scheduled for the next hour.

Modified Wave Scheduling. There are several ways of modifying the wave schedule. One method is to have two patients scheduled to come in at 10:00 and the third at 10:30, with this hourly cycle repeated throughout the day. Another application is to have patients scheduled to arrive at given intervals during the first half of the hour, and none scheduled to arrive during the second half of the hour.

Double Booking

Booking two patients to come in at the same time, both of whom are to be seen by the doctor, is poor practice. Of course, if each is expected to take only 5 minutes or so, there is no harm in telling both to come at 2:00 and reserving a 15-minute period for the two. This is an application of wave scheduling.

But if each one will require 15 minutes, two will require 30 minutes no matter how their names are written in the book. It is not double booking if a patient comes to the office for a treatment or injection from the medical assistant.

Grouping Procedures

Another method of time management that appeals to some practitioners is grouping of procedures; for example:

- An internist might reserve all morning appointments for complete physicals.
- A surgeon whose practice depends upon referrals might reserve one day a week or specific hours on each day for referrals.
- A pediatrician might have well-baby hours.

Experimenting with different groupings may help in arriving at the best arrangements. In applying a grouping system of appointments, the medical assistant may find it helpful to lightly color-code those sections of the appointment book being reserved for special procedures.

Advance Booking

When booking appointments weeks or months ahead, make it a policy to leave some open time during each day's schedule. Then, if a patient calls with a special problem that is not an immediate emergency, you will be able to book the patient for at least a brief visit. The busy doctor will always be able to fill these open slots, and the patients will appreciate being able to see their doctor within a reasonable time when the circumstances warrant it. Some authorities say that appointments should not be scheduled more than 3 months in advance.

If possible, set time aside in the morning and afternoon for a breather, or work break. Even 15 or 20 minutes will give the doctor an opportunity to return calls from patients, verify prescription calls, or answer questions you may have that were not an emergency.

DETAILS OF ARRANGING APPOINTMENTS

Many return appointments are arranged while a patient is in the office. The patient's first appointment, though, will probably be made by telephone. Pleasantness on the part of the medical assistant who sets up the appointment is extremely important, whether the encounter is in person or by telephone.

In Person

The physician will probably ask the patient to stop at the desk and make another appointment before leaving the office. While you reach for your pencil and the appointment book, look at the patient and say something like this: "Will next Thursday, the 8th, at 10:00 AM be satisfactory?" Avoid asking the question, "When would you like to come in?" Chances are this will only open up a debate and the patient may finally decide on a time that you don't have available. Write the patient's name and telephone number in the book and give the patient a completed appointment card (after you have double-checked the date and time with your book), along with your best smile. Give the patient any necessary instructions.

Appointment Cards and Reminders

Most offices use cards to remind patients of appointments, as well as to eliminate misunderstandings about dates and times.

Make a habit of reaching for an appointment card while making an entry in the appointment book. After you have written the date and time on the appointment card, double-check with the book to see that the entries agree. Some practices mail reminder cards to patients who have made appointments several weeks in advance. Patients who telephone for appointments may also be sent reminder cards.

Some patients like to be sent recall reminders of when they are to return to see the doctor. A simple way of handling this is to have a supply of postal cards on hand and while the patients are still in the office have them write their name and address on a card. Then place it in a file box under the date it is to be mailed.

Appointments by Telephone

It is as important for the medical assistant to express pleasantness and a desire to be helpful when using the telephone as it is when meeting patients face to face. This is particularly essential in the arranging of appointments, since it is often the manner in which the booking is made rather than the actual time of appointment that is important to the patient.

Study the principles of telephone technique as set forth in the next chapter, Oral Communications. Be especially considerate if you must refuse an appointment for the time requested. Explain why and offer a substitute time and date. It should also be determined whether the patient has been in before and whether any necessary insurance information has been obtained. Comply with the patient's desires as much as possible and do not show impatience if a few patients are not understanding of the problems involved in scheduling appointments. Most people do appreciate the need for a well-managed office and are willing to cooperate. End the conversation pleasantly with something like this: "Thank you for calling, Mrs. Albright. Dr. Wright will see you next Wednesday, the 28th, at 2:30. Goodbye." This little courtesy adds to the patient's feeling of esteem, along with reinforcing the time of the appointment. While you are saying this, you should be rechecking your appointment page to be certain you have written it in the right time slot on the right day.

Appointments for New Patients

Arranging the first appointment for a new patient requires a bit more time and attention to detail. Carefully check the correct spelling of the name by repeating it or spelling it back. Obtain the address,

Procedure 8-2

SCHEDULING A NEW PATIENT

EQUIPMENT AND SUPPLIES

Appointment book
Scheduling guidelines
Appointment card
Telephone

8

PROCEDURAL GOAL

To schedule a new patient for a first office visit.

PROCEDURE

1. Obtain patient's full name, birthdate, address, and telephone number.
   Note: Verify spelling of name.
2. Determine whether the patient was referred by another physician.
   Purpose: You may need to request additional information from the referring physician, and your physician will want to send a consultation report.
3. Determine the patient's chief complaint and when the first symptoms occurred.
   Purpose: To assist in determining the length of time needed for the appointment and the degree of urgency.
4. Search the appointment book for the first suitable appointment time and an alternate time.
5. Offer the patient a choice of these dates and times.
   Purpose: Patients are better satisfied if they are given a choice.
6. Enter the mutually agreeable time in the appointment book followed by patient's telephone number.
   Note: Indicate that the patient is new by adding the letters N.P.
7. If new patients are expected to pay at the time of the visit, explain this financial arrangement when the appointment is made.
   Purpose: Patient will be aware of payment policy and can come prepared to pay at time of visit.
8. Offer travel directions for reaching office and parking instructions.
   Purpose: To relieve any anxiety about being able to find medical facility.
9. Repeat the day, date, and time of the appointment before telling the patient goodbye.
   Purpose: To verify that the patient understands the date and time of the appointment.

TERMINAL PERFORMANCE OBJECTIVE

Given the listed equipment and supplies, schedule a new patient at an appropriate time, obtaining all the necessary information and entering it in the agreed-upon slot in the appointment book within 10 minutes to a performance level of 100%.

the telephone number where the patient can be reached, the patient's age, and the name of the referring doctor or individual. If possible, determine the nature of the visit so that the proper amount of time can be allotted on the appointment book. Financial arrangements should be made at the time of the first visit.

If another physician has referred the patient, the medical assistant may need to call the referring physician's office and obtain additional information before the patient's appointment. This information should be typed and given to the doctor in advance of the patient's arrival.

Special Problems

Probably every doctor has a few patients who are habitually late for appointments. This seems to be a problem for which no cure has yet been found; consequently, you must find a way of booking this patient as the last appointment of the day. Then, if closing time arrives before the patient does, you need feel no obligation to wait. Some medical assistants simply tell the patient to come in a half hour earlier than the time they actually write in the book. The point to remember is that you must learn to work around this patient, with the realization that in all likelihood he or she is not going to change.

When a former patient returns after a lengthy absence, the medical assistant should recheck the address, telephone number, insurance, and employment information. If the appointment is made by telephone, be sure to ask for the patient's telephone number. You may need to place a call to the patient, and you cannot safely assume that the number has not changed. You should also inquire into the nature of the current complaint.

Use a pencil for making entries in the appointment book. Trying to change an entry made in ink is difficult and messy. At the end of the day the names may be written over in ink for a permanent record, if desired.

Always write the patient's name in full, last name first, together with the reason for the appointment, immediately. DO NOT TRUST TO MEMORY! Be sure to cross off sufficient time for the appointment. It's a good idea to write the patient's telephone number after every entry in the appointment book. You may have to cancel or rearrange that day's schedule in a hurry, and many precious minutes can be saved if you don't have to look up each patient's telephone number.

Rescheduling an Appointment

Sometimes changes must be made in the appointment schedule. For instance, the patient who has a 3:00 PM appointment next Monday calls and asks to have this changed to 1 week later. You find an opening at 3:00 PM on the following Monday and write in the patient's name, but in your haste you fail to cross out the first appointment. Someone else looking at the appointment book (or possibly even yourself a couple of days later) will either expect the patient on both days or be unable to determine which day is correct. Avoid this embarrassing situation by making it a habit to cross out the first appointment before writing in the new one.

You may have a patient who requires a series of appointments, say at weekly intervals. Try to set up the appointments on the same day of each week at the same time of day if possible. This considerably reduces the risk of a forgotten appointment. A calendar that shows the dates several months in advance at a glance is useful to have on or near the appointment desk.

At the end of each day, prepare a daily schedule on the typewriter or computer listing the appointments for the following day, showing each patient's name and reason for visit. This should be made available to the physician and any other members of the staff who have patient contact. If changes occur during the day, be sure to correct the daily schedule sheet as well as your appointment book.

EXCEPTIONS TO APPOINTMENT SYSTEM

With even the best of appointment systems, certain situations will require an immediate adjustment in the schedule. Some examples are discussed in the following paragraphs.

Emergency Patients. If someone telephones to report an emergency that can be taken care of in the office, the medical assistant will have no hesitancy in having the patient come immediately. In making such determinations, however, there must be some previous understanding with the doctor on what kinds of emergencies will be seen in the office, the criteria for determining whether a particular case *is* an emergency, and what procedures the medical assistant should follow. Try to have a list of questions to ask the caller appropriate to the situation. For instance:

- Is there bleeding?
- Where is the blood coming from?
- What is the patient's temperature?
- Are there chills?
- Is there nausea or vomiting?
- If there is pain, is it steady or intermittent?
- Is the pain severe? sharp? dull?
- How long have the symptoms been present?

Acutely Ill Patients. Patients cannot always give advance notice of when they will need a doctor. There is sometimes a very fine line between an

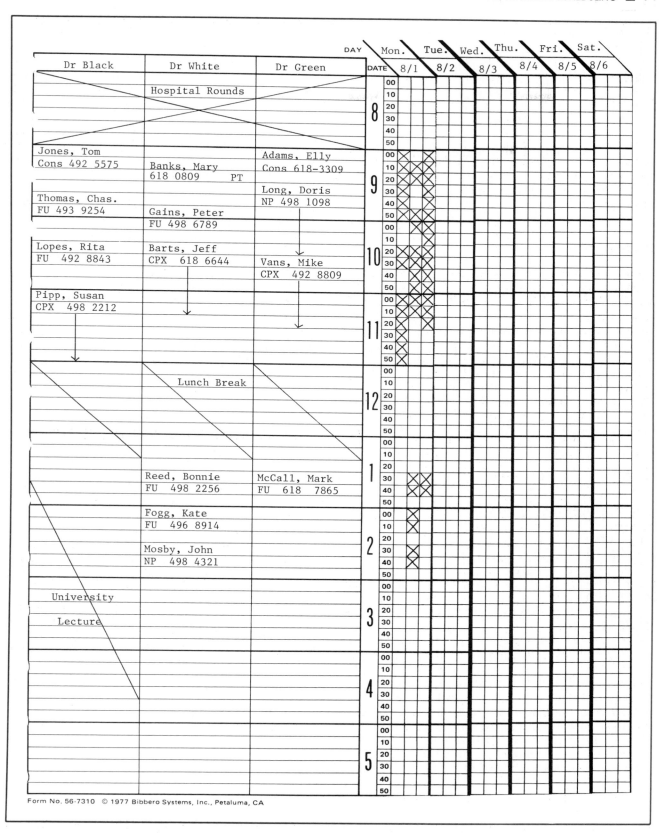

Figure 8–3
Sample appointment book page for three physicians.

emergency patient and the acutely ill patient, but the latter should be seen as soon as possible. At the very least, let the physician decide whether the patient should be seen immediately or whether an appointment should be made for another day. The 15- to 20-minute breather time you saved in the middle of the morning and the afternoon may rescue your schedule.

Physician Referrals. If another physician telephones and requests that a patient be seen by your doctor today, this is another exception you will have to make. Most physicians recognize the importance of keeping a schedule and will not be inconsiderate in this respect.

FAILED APPOINTMENTS

Reasons for Failed Appointments. Why do patients fail to keep appointments? Some patients are simply forgetful. If you detect this tendency in a patient, form the habit of telephoning a reminder the day before the appointment, or send a postcard timed to arrive a day or two in advance of the appointment. If your office consistently runs behind schedule, with patients being kept waiting for more than 20 to 30 minutes, the patient whose own time is well-planned may simply elect not to run the risk of losing so much valuable time. Perhaps you gave a patient an appointment at a time that really was not agreeable to him. Or a patient who has been pressed for payment may stay away because of being unable to pay on that day. Try to determine the reason for failed appointments and do what you can to remedy the situation.

No-Show Policy. Some patients may not realize the importance of keeping their appointments. A busy practice must have a very specific policy on appointment "no-shows" and enforce it effectively. Michael Silver, Practice Management Consultant of Williamsville, New York, makes these suggestions in *Physician's Management*, October 1978:

> The first time a patient fails to show, note the fact on the medical record or ledger card. The second time this happens, you'll have a warning, and if the patient is more than a half-hour late, call his or her home. The third time a patient fails to show without good reason, I suggest dropping the patient by using the customary methods that avoid legal problems.
> Incidentally, a patient with a major appointment—physical exams, counseling or the like—should be reminded by phone 24 to 48 hours before the appointment.

Charging for Failed Appointments. Legally a patient may be charged for failing to keep an uncanceled appointment, if the patient was informed in advance about this policy and if it can be shown that this time was not used for another patient. However, few doctors attempt to collect for such occasions. The risk of poor public relations is too great; it generally results in a lost patient. Some other way must be found to handle failed appointments if they become a problem.

Recording the Failed Appointment. Whenever a patient fails to keep an appointment, a notation should be made in the patient's chart. If the patient is seriously ill, the doctor should also be told about the failure. This may be a legal consideration at some later date. In some cases it may be necessary for the doctor or the medical assistant to call and remind the patient that an unkept appointment may have serious effects on the patient's health.

HANDLING CANCELATIONS AND DELAYS

When the Patient Cancels. It is inevitable that some cancelations will occur. If you keep a list of patients with advance appointments who would like to come in sooner, get busy on the telephone and try to get one of them in to fill the available time.

When the Doctor is Delayed. There are days when the doctor is delayed in reaching the office. If you have advance notice of the delay you can start calling those patients with early appointments and suggest they come later. If some have already arrived before you learn of the delay, you will have to explain that an emergency has prevented the doctor from getting in. Show concern for the patient, but avoid being overly apologetic, which might imply some degree of guilt. Most patients realize that a doctor has certain priorities, and that the patient who is able to be in the office may be inconvenienced but it is not a life-or-death matter. If this kind of situation occurs frequently, though, you may have to devise a different scheduling system.

When the Doctor Is Called Out on Emergencies. Physicians are conscious of their responsibilities for responding to medical emergencies, and most patients will be sympathetic to such occurrences if the medical assistant takes the time to explain what has happened. You may say something like this: "Dr. Wright has been called away to answer an emergency. She asked me to tell you she is very sorry to keep you waiting. There will be at least an hour delay."

Ask the patient, "Do you wish to wait? If it is inconvenient, I'll be glad to give you an appointment on another day. Or perhaps you'd like to have some coffee or do some shopping and return in an hour.''

As quickly as possible, call the patients who are scheduled for a later hour. In many offices, especially those of obstetricians, surgeons, and general practitioners, it is sometimes necessary to cancel a whole day's appointments. For this reason it is particularly important that you have the telephone number of each patient available so that you can cancel the appointment and make a new one without delay. If it is at all possible, cancel appointments *before* the patient arrives in the office to find that the doctor is not in.

When the Doctor Is Ill or Is Called Out of Town. Physicians do get ill, too, and the patients who are scheduled to be seen during the course of the doctor's expected recovery period must be informed of this. They need not be told the nature of the illness. When the physician is called out of town for personal or professional reasons, the appointments will have to be canceled or rescheduled. It is customary to provide the patient with the name of another physician, or possibly a choice of several, who will take care of the doctor's patients during such absences.

SCHEDULING OUTSIDE APPOINTMENTS

There are other appointments that the medical assistant will make and that will appear on the appointment book, such as scheduled surgery at a hospital, consultations at a hospital or at another physician's office, and house calls at extended care facilities or in the home. The doctor must have time to get from one place to another, so allowance must be made for traveling time when arranging these appointments.

Surgeries

You may be responsible for scheduling surgeries. In scheduling with most hospitals you should call the secretary in surgery first when your doctor plans an operation. Give the surgical secretary:

- The preferred date and time
- The type of surgery to be performed
- The approximate time required

After the date and hour have been established, give:

- The patient's full name
- Sex
- Age
- Telephone number

Then explain any special requests the doctor may have, such as the amount of blood to have available.

Be sure you have all this information at hand before placing the call.

It may also be your responsibility to arrange for an assistant surgeon, the anesthesiologist, and the bed reservation.

Some hospitals request that the patient complete a preadmittance form so that all records can be processed before the patient is admitted. In such cases it may be the medical assistant's responsibility to see that this is done. These are general guidelines only, as procedures will vary in different areas and different hospitals.

House Calls

If the physician regularly makes house calls or sees patients in convalescent homes, you will probably set aside a special block of time for this on your appointment schedule. In arranging such appointments be sure to get all the pertinent details:

- Name and address of patient
- Telephone number
- Best way to reach the home
- Nearest cross street
- Name of person making the request

Again, traveling time must be allowed for. Many physicians never make house calls, believing that the patient can best be examined and treated in the medical facility or in a hospital.

Outside Appointments for Patients

The medical assistant is often requested to arrange laboratory or x-ray appointments for patients. Before calling the laboratory or x-ray facility, you need to know:

- The exact procedure required
- Whether expediency is a factor
- Whether a **stat report** is necessary
- The patient's availability

With this information before you, you can set up the appointment with confidence. When you inform the patient of the time and place for the appointment, you can also relay any special instructions that may be necessary. Then note these arrangements on the patient's chart, and place a follow-up reminder on your **tickler** or desk calendar.

PATIENTS WITHOUT APPOINTMENTS

What will you do about patients who arrive without an appointment? There must be a policy agreed upon by the doctor and then carried out by the medical assistant.

The patient who requires immediate attention will

8

Procedure 8–3

SCHEDULING OUTPATIENT DIAGNOSTIC TESTS

EQUIPMENT AND SUPPLIES

Diagnostic test order from physician
Name, address, and telephone number of diagnostic facility
Patient chart
Test preparation instructions
Telephone

PROCEDURAL GOAL

To schedule patient for outpatient diagnostic test ordered by physician within the time frame needed by physician, confirm with patient, and issue all required instructions.

PROCEDURE

1. Obtain oral or written order from physician for exact procedure to be performed and time frame for results.
   Purpose: The urgency of the test results will affect the time and date of appointment needed.
2. Determine the patient's availability.
   Purpose: To be sure that the patient will be able to comply with arrangements for test.
3. Telephone diagnostic facility:
   a. Order specific test needed.
   b. Establish date and time.
   c. Give name, age, address and telephone number of patient.
   d. Determine any special instructions for patient.
   e. Notify facility of any urgency for test results.
4. Notify patient of arrangements, including:
   a. Name, address and telephone number of diagnostic facility.
   b. Date and time to report for test.
   c. Instructions concerning preparation for test (eating restrictions, fluids, medications, enemas, and so forth).
   d. Ask patient to repeat instructions.
   Purpose: To be certain that patient understands preparation necessary and importance of keeping appointment. If time permits issue written instructions to patient.
5. Note arrangements on patient chart.
   Purpose: To ensure follow-up on diagnosis and/or treatment.
6. Place reminder on tickler or desk calendar.
   Purpose: To check on whether appointment was kept and report received from testing facility.

TERMINAL PERFORMANCE OBJECTIVE

Given the listed equipment, information, and supplies, schedule a patient for a diagnostic test in an outpatient facility, all steps to be completed in 15 minutes with 100% accuracy.

most likely be fitted into the schedule somehow. If the patient does not need immediate care, a brief visit with the doctor and a scheduled appointment at a later time may be the answer. Or you may simply have to turn down the request.

The medical assistant should always make it clear, even when sending patients without appointments in to see the doctor, that the office runs on an appointment basis. You might say, for example:

"The doctor will be able to see you today, but we would appreciate it very much if you would make an appointment for your next visit." Or, "The doctor can see you now and I'm sorry you had to wait so long. Perhaps it would be possible for you to make an appointment the next time."

Try to convey the message that appointments save not only the doctor's time but the patient's as well. Emphasize that the doctor will be able to give them full attention and more time if an advance appointment is made.

OTHER CALLERS

Physicians. Another physician calling at your doctor's office should be ushered in to see the doctor as soon as possible regardless of the appointment schedule. If the doctor is seeing a patient, explain the situation and, if possible, take the visiting physician into a private room to wait. Then notify your doctor as soon as possible. The visits of other physicians are usually brief and will not appreciably affect your schedule.

Pharmaceutical Representatives. Also known as "detail persons," representatives from leading pharmaceutical houses are frequent visitors to physicians' offices and are generally welcomed when the schedule permits. They are well-trained and bring valuable information on new drugs to the physician. The medical assistant is often expected to screen such visitors and turn away those whose products would not be used in that practice. If you do not know the representative or the pharmaceutical company, ask for a business card, then check with the doctor, who will then decide whether or not to see the caller.

If the doctor is in a specialty practice or wishes to confer with only selected pharmaceutical company representatives, the medical assistant and the doctor can prepare a list of the representatives who will be seen by the doctor. Then, when a detail person calls, the medical assistant can deal with the caller confidently.

The medical assistant can say whether or not the doctor will be available that day and give an estimate of the waiting time, or suggest a later time at which to return. The caller can then make a decision regarding whether to wait or return later. The pharmaceutical representative is usually quite understanding and cooperative and is willing to wait patiently a long while for just a brief visit with the doctor. The medical assistant should in turn treat the representative with courtesy, showing as much cooperation as possible. In some cases, the representative will just leave literature or materials for the doctor with the medical assistant. The detail person who is not on the calling list for a particular doctor will also appreciate the saving in time by knowing this. Most representatives say they would rather be told outright if the doctor does not wish to see them than to be given some evasive reply.

Salespersons. Salespersons from medical, surgical, and office supply houses call regularly at physicians' offices. Sometimes they want to see the doctor, but the medical assistant who is in charge of ordering supplies usually is able to handle these calls personally.

Unsolicited salespersons sometimes present a problem in the professional office. If the physician does not wish to see such callers, the medical assistant must firmly but tactfully send them away. You can suggest that they leave their literature and cards for the doctors to study, and say that the doctor will contact them if further information is desired. Persistent callers who ignore a polite "No" can be discouraged by the suggestion that perhaps they would like to schedule an appointment, at the doctor's customary fee.

Miscellaneous. From time to time, other callers appear in the doctor's office. Some are civic leaders seeking the doctor's aid in community projects. Others may be church leaders, insurance representatives, solicitors for fund drives, and so forth. Most physicians inform their medical assistants of their general policy in regard to seeing such callers. Civic leaders should be treated with courtesy and consideration when they telephone or come into the office. Most doctors feel a responsibility to take an active part in community affairs, but no one can participate in all activities. Sometimes the responsibility for accepting or refusing such community appointments is delegated to the medical assistant. In this event, you must use discretion and exercise great tact and courtesy. Turning away community leaders with a blunt refusal does not create good medical public relations. If it is necessary to refuse such requests, be sure to explain that the doctor is already participating in such community projects as, for example, the Boy Scouts, Girl Scouts, Kiwanis, and the Health Council (naming specific activities or organizations), and cannot accept additional responsibilities at this time. The rules regarding tact, courtesy, and consideration apply to every caller in a physician's office.

REFERENCES AND READINGS

American Medical Association: *Winning Ways with Patients.* Chicago, The Association, 1979.
Beck, L. C.: *The Physician's Office.* Princeton, NJ, Excerpta Medica, 1977.
Manning, F. F. (ed.): *Medical Group Practice Management.* Cambridge, MA, Ballinger Publishing Co., 1977.

RESOURCES

Colwell Company, 275 Kenyon Road, Champaign, IL 61820.
Patient Care Systems, 16 Thorndal Circle, Darien, CT 06820.
VISIrecord Systems, 160 Gold Star Boulevard, Worcester, MA 01606.

8

CHAPTER OUTLINE

VOCABULARY

See Glossary at end of book for definitions.

clarity	monitor	pronunciation
diction	pitch	transmitter
enunciation		

Oral Communications

9

OBJECTIVES

Upon successful completion of this chapter you should be able to:

1. Define the terms listed in the Vocabulary of this chapter.
2. Discuss the importance of oral communication and effective listening.
3. List ways by which the medical assistant can develop a pleasing telephone personality.
4. Cite seven items to be included in taking a complete telephone message.
5. Identify ten kinds of telephone calls that the medical assistant should be able to handle successfully.
6. Identify six kinds of telephone calls that will need to be referred to the physician for response.
7. Explain what is involved in monitoring telephone calls.
8. Discuss the useful information that may be found in a telephone directory in addition to telephone numbers.
9. Discuss ways of controlling telephone expenses by using optional services.
10. Explain the ways in which an operator-answered telephone answering service can benefit a medical practice.

Upon successful completion of this chapter you should be able to perform the following role-play activities:

1. Demonstrate the appropriate method of placing and receiving telephone calls.
2. Using a multiple-line telephone, demonstrate the correct handling of two incoming calls, one of which must be transferred to another party.
3. Correctly record a telephone message from a laboratory facility reporting test results on a patient.
4. Respond to a call from a pharmacist regarding a request for a prescription refill, demonstrating appropriate precautions and completing necessary documentation.
5. Using a list of local social service agencies, respond to telephone calls for emergency treatment (poison or burn center) and for non-emergency services (such as crippled children or cancer-screening center).
6. Check a telephone answering device for recorded messages; prepare and distribute message slips.
7. Call an operator-answered exchange to report on-call information for out-of-office messages.

EFFECTIVE COMMUNICATIONS

Effective communication is a major requirement for success in any endeavor. Effective communication is necessary to establish and maintain rapport between staff members, between staff and physician, between physician and physician, and between all of these individuals and the patient.

Oral Communication. Oral communication will be addressed in this chapter, and written communications in the following chapter. Oral communication includes not only what you say but also how you look when you say it—your body stance; whether you are smiling, frowning, or expressionless; and whether you appear agitated or calm and relaxed. Communication is never one-way. There must be a receiver as well as a sender. Remember that it is as important to listen as it is to speak. The listener who maintains eye contact with the person speaking will be communicating interest in what is being said.

Non-listeners. True communication can exist only when there is understanding among all parties. The communicator must be aware of possible language barriers. The worried patient may be a "non-listener" because of a high anxiety factor. When giving instructions to a patient it may be necessary to have the patient repeat what you have said, to verify understanding of the message. At other times it may be wise to repeat to the patient what he or she has said, or to rephrase the message if you think that the person speaking is failing to state clearly the intended remark or question. Patience and courtesy are extremely important.

Staff Harmony. Patients are usually quite sensitive to the degree of harmony that exists in the medical facility, and it is important to their well-being that they be treated in a harmonious atmosphere. If there are personality problems, the persons involved should deal with them in open discussion so that the problems can be resolved. Where there are several staff members, care must be taken to avoid chronic criticism of others and office gossip.

Staff interaction with patients occurs in the making of appointments, in greeting patients, and especially in telephone conversations. Since 90% of the patients make their initial contact with the medical facility by telephone, it is obvious that the telephone is a powerful public relations instrument. Its proper use can build a beginning medical practice; its improper use can do much to destroy a flourishing one. The physician's office without one or more telephones is difficult to imagine, and the medical assistant who regards the telephone as a nuisance has no place in the medical office.

The telephone is the lifeline of the office. The majority of telephone contacts will be incoming calls. They may be coming from:

- A former patient calling for an appointment or to seek advice
- Someone reporting an emergency
- A physician calling to make a referral
- The laboratory reporting vital information regarding a patient
- A new patient making a first contact

YOUR TELEPHONE PERSONALITY

To a telephone caller, your voice is your entire personality. The caller cannot see you, your smile, or your facial expression. The total impression of you and the office will be formed from your voice. What image will you create with your telephone personality?

- Is your voice warm and friendly?
- Does it sound confident?
- Is your conversation courteous and tactful?

All of these qualities create a favorable impression and promote good public relations. Try to visualize the person with whom you are speaking. A small mirror, placed near the telephone, will remind you to smile. Now pretend that each caller is a new patient meeting you for the first time.

Every caller should be made to feel that you have time to attend to his or her wishes. If you are rushed when you pick up the telephone, wait a few seconds until you are able to answer graciously without seeming breathless or impatient.

Because the telephone is the lifeline of the medical office, personal calls should be kept to a bare minimum. Physicians usually are understanding about occasional urgent calls from the medical assistant's family. The medical assistant who is active in a professional organization will sometimes find it necessary to take calls from colleagues or others involved in the profession. While these communications are not considered entirely personal, they should also be kept to a minimum. The doctor's telephone lines should be clear to receive the doctor's professional calls.

INCOMING CALLS

You will be receiving many calls during the course of a single day. Each one deserves your most competent attention. Here are a few guidelines to follow in answering all telephone calls.

Receiving Calls

Answer Promptly. Whenever possible, answer the telephone on the first ring. If you are unable to complete the conversation when you first answer the telephone, you might say, "Will you please hold the line for one moment and I will be with you." Then wait for the caller to respond. Avoid such responses as "Just a minute" or "Doctor's office, hold please." When you return to the telephone, thank the caller for waiting.

Hold the Instrument Correctly. Hold the handset around the middle, with the mouthpiece about one inch from the lips and directly in front of the teeth. Never hold it under the chin. You can check the proper distance by taking your first two fingers and passing them through sideways in the space between your lips and the mouthpiece. If your fingers just squeeze through, your lips are the correct distance from the telephone and your voice will go over the line as close to its natural tone as possible. Speak directly into the telephone immediately after removing it from the cradle. If you turn to face a window or another part of the room, make sure the telephone **transmitter** moves too, or your voice will be lost.

Develop a Pleasing Telephone Voice. What are the qualities of a good telephone voice? And how do your cultivate good voice quality? Here are some tips from the Bell Telephone system:

- *Stay Alert.* Give the impression you are wide-awake and alert, and interested in the calling person. Let the caller know he or she has your full attention.
- *Be Pleasant.* Build a pleasant, friendly image for you and your office. Be the "voice with a smile."
- *Talk Naturally, Be Yourself.* Use your own words and expressions. Avoid repetition of mechanical words or phrases. Do not use slang. Avoid the use of professional jargon.
- *Speak Distinctly.* Clear, distinct **pronunciation** and **enunciation** are vital. Move the lips, tongue, and jaw freely. Talk directly into the transmitter. Never answer the telephone when you are eating or chewing gum.
- *Be Expressive.* A well-modulated voice carries best. Use a normal tone of voice, neither too loud nor too soft. Talk at a moderate rate, neither too fast nor too slow. Vary your tone. It will bring out the meaning of sentences and add color and vitality to what you say.

Everyone should have the experience of hearing his or her own voice; it reveals immediately the importance of careful **diction.** Try putting your voice on tape and listening to a playback. Each word and each sound must be given individual attention in order to achieve clarity. Slurring your words or dropping your voice too much at the end of a sentence can place a strain on your listener.

Try to avoid the habit of dropping "ers," "uhs," and long pauses into your conversation. Remember,

too, that it is seldom necessary to raise the **pitch** of your voice in order to be heard. The person who has trouble being heard is generally speaking too fast, enunciating poorly, or not speaking into the transmitter.

Guides to Good Diction

NUMERAL OR LETTER	SOUNDED AS	PRINCIPAL SOUNDS
0	oh	Round and long O
1	wun	Strong W and N
2	too	Strong T and long OO
3	th-r-ee	A single roll of the R and long EE
4	fo-er	Strong F, long O, and strong final R
5	fi-iv	I changing from long to short, strong V
6	siks	Strong S and KS
7	sev-en	Strong S and V, well-sounded EN
8	ate	Long A and strong T
9	ni-en	Strong N, long I, well-sounded EN
10	ten	Strong T and N
J	jay	Strong J and long AY
R	ahr	Strong R
M	em	Short E and strong M
W	dubble-yoo	Full value given to every syllable
F	ef	Short E and strong F

Do not over-accentuate; it causes you to sound artificial. Use a friendly natural style. Few words need to be spelled over the telephone if a person speaks slowly and clearly. Below are key words you can use when it is necessary to verify letters in spelling back over the telephone:

A as in Adams	J as in John	S as in Samuel
B as in Boston	K as in Katie	T as in Thomas
C as in Charles	L as in Lewis	U as in Utah
D as in David	M as in Mary	V as in Victor
E as in Edward	N as in Nellie	W as in William
F as in Frank	O as in Oliver	X as in X-ray
G as in George	P as in Peter	Y as in Young
H as in Henry	Q as in Queen	Z as in Zebra
I as in Ida	R as in Robert	

Any conversation necessarily involves two or more persons, and while we put a great deal of emphasis upon rules for speaking, we often neglect the importance of good listening. The same attention should be given a telephone conversation that would be given a face-to-face conversation. Concentration is not always easy; it must be practiced. Effective listening is vital to the medical assistant.

Identify Yourself. Your response to an incoming call should identify first the office and then yourself. There are numerous telephone greetings that can be used, which you will probably wish to discuss with the doctor. Your response might be something like this: "Dr. Black's office—Miss Anderson." If the doctor's surname is fairly common to your area, you may wish to use the given name also, to provide further identification, saying, "Dr. Sherman Black's office—Miss Anderson."

The use of salutations in telephone identifications is optional. Sometimes the addition of "Good morning" or "Good afternoon" to the identification is awkward. A rising inflection or a questioning tone in your voice will indicate interest and a willingness to assist, eliminating the need for an additional greeting.

If there are two doctors in the office, both names should be included in the identification. Say "Drs. Smith and Taylor," or "Drs. Taylor and Smith's office." Some names will not blend smoothly; then you must modify the identification so that it will be easy to say and easy to understand. Keep in mind the reason for using the doctor's name. You are telling the caller that the correct number has been reached. If callers frequently ask you to repeat, you must analyze the failure to communicate and modify your response in some way. Some authorities suggest preceding the identification with the words, "This is. . ." by saying "This is Dr. Black's office," theorizing that the first two words are probably lost on the listener, who only begins to hear you when you have reached ". . . Dr. Black's office."

Answering an office telephone merely by repeating the telephone number or saying "Hello" is undesirable. The caller will invariably ask, "Is this Dr. Black's office?" Rarely can a person immediately recall the number he has just dialed. Time is wasted, the caller is psychologically rebuffed, and you have lost another opportunity to create a favorable impression of your office.

When you have decided upon the greeting to be used, practice it until you can say it easily and smoothly without having to think about what you are saying.

Identify the Caller. If the caller does not identify himself, you should ask to whom you are speaking. It is a good idea to repeat the name by using it in the conversation as soon as possible, unless there are other patients within the range of your voice and the caller's privacy should be respected.

Offer Assistance. You can offer assistance both by the tone of your voice and by what you say. The phrase "May I help you?" or "How may I help you?" will open the conversation and assure the caller that you are both willing and capable of being of service.

Screen Incoming Calls. Most doctors expect the medical assistant to **screen** all telephone calls. Good judgment in deciding whether or not to put calls through to the doctor comes with experience.

Do put through calls from other physicians at once. If your doctor is busy and cannot possibly come to the telephone, explain this briefly and politely, then say that you will ask the doctor to return the call as soon as possible.

Many callers will ask, "Is the doctor in?" Avoid answering this question with a simple "Yes" or "No" or responding with the question, "Who is calling, please?" If the doctor is not in, say so *before* asking the identity of the caller. Otherwise the impression is created that the doctor is simply not willing to talk with this person.

If the doctor is away from the office, the rule of offering assistance still holds. You can say, "No, I am sorry, Dr. Black is not in. May I take a message?" or "No, I am sorry, but Dr. Black will be at the hospital most of the morning. May I ask the doctor to return your call after 12 o'clock?"

If the doctor is in and is available to speak on the telephone, a typical response would be, "Yes, Dr. Black is in; may I say who is calling, please?" If your doctor prefers to keep telephone calls to a minimum, you might say, "Yes, Dr. Black is here, but I'm not sure she is free to come to the phone. May I say who is calling, please?" That way, the doctor is not committed to taking the call.

The doctor who is with a patient probably will not wish to be disturbed for a routine call. In this case, you might say, "Yes, Dr. Black is in, but with a patient right now. May I help you?" or "Yes, Dr. Black is in but is with a patient right now. Is there anything you want me to ask?"

You must guard against being overprotective. A patient has a right to talk with the doctor; however, unless it is an emergency, the patient is probably willing to do so at the doctor's convenience. Don't let it be said of your doctor, "He's a good doctor, but you can never talk to him." The medical assistant who answers the telephone should act as a screen, not a block.

Find out exactly how calls are to be handled when the doctor is out of the office, and under what circumstances you can interrupt when the doctor is in the office. Be firm in your commitment to those preferences, and cultivate a reputation for being helpful and reliable. You will save the doctor many trips to the telephone if patients develop confidence in your ability to help them, and have faith in your promise to take their messages and deliver them properly.

Minimize Waiting Time. When a call cannot be put through immediately, ask "Will you wait, or shall I call you back when the doctor is free?"

If the caller elects to wait, remember that waiting with a silent telephone can be irritating. The waiting time, no matter how brief, always seems long. Let no more than one minute pass without breaking in with some reassuring comment, for instance, "I'm sorry, Dr. Black is still busy."

If the wait is longer than expected, the caller may

wish to reconsider and call back another time or have the call returned, but he or she needs to communicate this to you. By going back on the line at frequent intervals, you give the caller an opportunity to express such concerns. In fact, you may ask the caller if he wishes to continue waiting. Say something like, "I'm sorry to keep you waiting so long, Mr. Hughes. Would you prefer to have me return your call when Dr. Black is free?" Try to give the caller some estimate of when he may expect the return call. In any event, irritation can be lessened by your consideration in saying, "Thank you for waiting, Mr. Hughes."

When it is necessary for you to leave the telephone to obtain information, ask the caller, "Will you please wait while I get the information?" and then wait for a reply. When you return to the telephone, thank the caller for waiting. If it will take longer than a few seconds to get the information, give some estimate of the time required and offer to call back. When a patient calls and asks a question that requires the chart, it may be best to take a message and call back.

Transferring a Call. Always identify the caller when transferring a call to the doctor. Any person who refuses to give a name should not be put through unless your doctor instructs you otherwise.

If it is a patient calling, the doctor will presumably want the patient's history at hand during the conversation. If there is no concern about others hearing your conversation, you can announce the caller's name on the intercom and tell the doctor you will bring the history. If there are others within hearing, you might simply take the history to the doctor and say, "Dr. Black, this party is waiting on the telephone to speak with you." In this way, the patient's right to privacy is protected.

Answering a Second Call. If your office has several incoming lines, or more than one telephone, it will sometimes be necessary for you to interrupt a conversation to answer another ring. Excuse yourself by saying, "Pardon me just a moment, the other line is ringing." Answer the second call, determine who is calling, and ask that person to hold while you complete the first call. Return to your first call as soon as possible, and apologize briefly for the interruption.

Do not make the mistake of continuing with the second call while the first one waits. Think what you would do if there were a face-to-face conversation. You would not allow a second person to just interrupt a conversation and then ignore the one you were speaking with first.

If the second call is an emergency, you can still take a moment to return to the first line and alert the caller that you will have to keep him or her waiting or call back. *Never* answer a call by saying, "Hold the line, please," without first finding out who is calling. It could be an emergency. It takes only a moment to be courteous—this courtesy could save a life.

Ending a Call. When a caller's requests have been satisfied, do not encourage needless chatting or permit the call to monopolize your time unnecessarily. The telephone lines should be cleared for other calls.

End the call pleasantly. It is considered good telephone etiquette to allow the person who placed the call to hang up first. It is a gracious gesture to thank a person for calling. Always close the conversation with some form of goodbye; do not just hang up abruptly. Replace the telephone on the cradle as gently as if you were closing a door in the office.

SUMMARY OF OFFICE TELEPHONE RULES

- *Answer promptly*
- *Visualize the person to whom you are talking*
- *Hold the instrument correctly*
- *Develop a pleasing telephone voice*
- *Identify your office and yourself*
- *Identify the caller*
- *Offer assistance*
- *Screen incoming calls*
- *Minimize waiting time*
- *Identify the caller when transferring a call*
- *When answering a second call, identify the caller, then return to first call*
- *End each call pleasantly and graciously*

The Telephone Message

Be Prepared. Always have a pen or pencil in your hand and a message pad nearby when you answer the telephone. You may be answering several calls before you have an opportunity to relay a message or carry out a promise of action. Therefore, the *written* message is vital.

What kind of message pad will you use? Probably the most satisfactory is an ordinary spiral-bound stenographer's notebook. It is inexpensive, sturdy, well-proportioned, will lie flat on your desk, and can be filed for future reference if desired. Do not be guilty of using small scraps of paper for messages. They are too easily lost. Date the bottom of the first blank page in your notebook at the beginning of each day. You will then have a permanent record that can be referred to later if the need arises. If you will draw a half-inch column down one side of each page, you can use this area to check off each message as it is delivered or taken care of. This is a good reminder system for yourself.

Minimum Information Required. The minimum information you will need from each call includes:

- Name of person called
- Name of caller
- Caller's telephone number
- Reason for the call
- Action to be taken
- Date and time of the call
- Your initials

Transmitting and Recording the Message. Messages that are to be transmitted to another person may be rewritten on individual slips and delivered or posted on a message board later. Message pads that provide for a carbon copy of each page are good insurance that no message will be forgotten. The nature of the message will determine whether you must report it immediately or not. Figure 9–1 illustrates a model message form that can be adapted to the practice by inserting the patient symptoms and requests you hear most often. The person who completes the call must sign and date it. It is also possible to get message forms with a self-adhesive back that can be placed permanently in the patient's case history (Fig. 9–2). If the call is from a patient and relates in any way to the medical history, or if any instructions were given, or queries answered, this information should be placed in the patient's chart.

Taking Action. The message procedure is not complete until the necessary action has been taken. Notations on the memo pad should be carried over to the following day if they have not been attended to. Just place an X in front of the item and move it onto the next page. Sometimes a notation will be carried over for several days until action can be completed. Do not trust to memory in regard to messages unattended to from previous days; always carry them forward in writing.

Make brief notations of patients' reactions while you are talking to them on the telephone. The doctor does not require a character study, but it is helpful to know when a patient appears fearful, apprehensive, or nervous. If a patient shows such symptoms, it may be wise to transfer the call to the doctor.

When your employer is talking to another physician in regard to a referral, you may sometimes be requested to take down a brief outline of the patient's case history by listening on the extension telephone. This information can be typed and placed on the doctor's desk just before the patient arrives in the office.

PITFALLS TO AVOID

Having too few telephone lines. On request the telephone company will do a traffic survey to determine how many busy signals are occurring and advise you as to whether you need additional lines. If collections and insurance processing require extensive use

TELEPHONE MESSAGE LOG

Date 1/26/88 Time Of Call 9:35 a

Caller Ernest Dinero Patient Stella (wife)

Address 420 Baker Street, S.C. Age 58

Complaint sore throat, congestion

Medication Taken aspirin How Long Sick 2 days

Cough ✓ Productive Temp 101°

Vomiting — Diarrhea —

Pain — Location —

Bleeding — How Long From How Much

Nurse Return Call Doctor Return Call ✓ Phone No. 643-2319

Appointment Made and Response or/Prescription given

MK

Figure 9–1
Telephone message log. (Courtesy of Colwell Systems, Inc., Champaign, IL.)

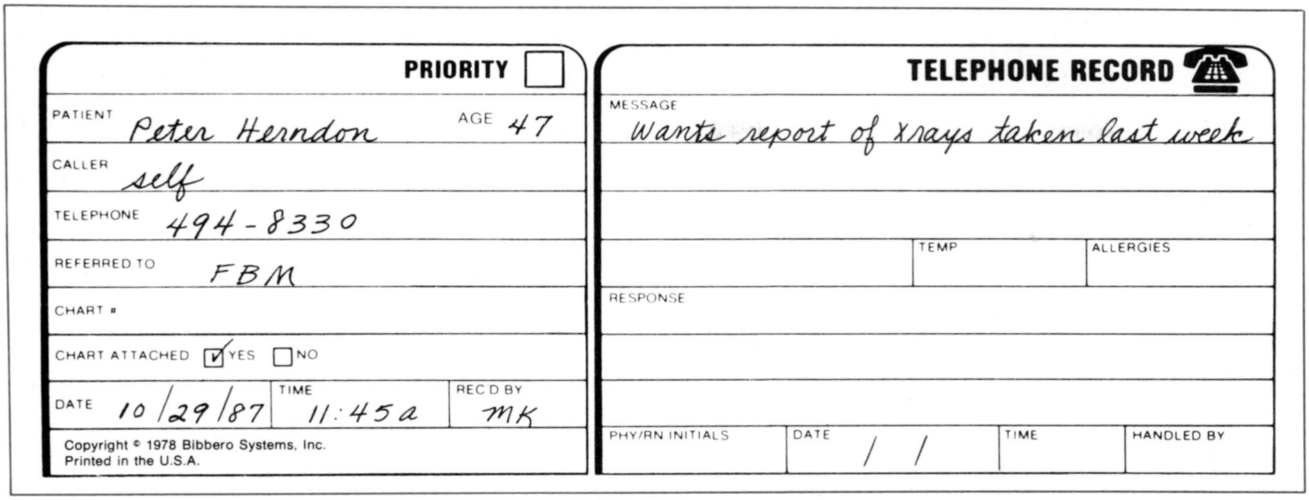

PRIORITY ☐		TELEPHONE RECORD ☎

PATIENT *Peter Herndon*   AGE *47*

CALLER *self*

TELEPHONE *494-8330*

REFERRED TO *FBM*

CHART #

CHART ATTACHED ☑ YES ☐ NO

DATE *10/29/87*   **TIME** *11:45a*   **REC'D BY** *MK*

Copyright © 1978 Bibbero Systems, Inc.
Printed in the U.S.A.

MESSAGE *Wants report of xrays taken last week*

TEMP   ALLERGIES

RESPONSE

PHY/RN INITIALS   DATE / /   TIME   HANDLED BY

Figure 9–2
Message form with self-adhesive backing. (Courtesy of Bibbero Systems, Inc., Petaluma, CA.)

of the telephone, a special line just for this purpose may be advisable.

- Having too few assistants to handle the existing lines. One assistant can handle two incoming lines, but three lines are probably too many for one person. Another assistant should be assigned to pick up the phone after a specified number of rings.
- Wasting time looking up frequently called numbers. Keep these in a personal directory where they can be quickly and easily located.
- Incoming or outgoing personal calls by employees, except in emergencies. Most doctors have an unlisted private line to take care of their own personal and priority calls.
- Using the telephone to give travel directions to new patients (except for short notice appointments). This information should be included in a Patient Information Sheet or Folder sent to every new patient.
- Taking extensive patient histories over the telephone when this can be done more efficiently at the time of the patient visit.
- Diagnosing or giving medical advice without authorization from the physician.
- Releasing patient information without authorization.

Incoming Calls the Medical Assistant Can Handle

One reason for having a medical assistant answer the incoming calls is to spare the physician unnecessary interruptions during visits with patients. Additionally, many calls relate to the administrative aspects of the office and can actually be better handled by the medical assistant. The doctor's pol-

icy regarding how calls are to be handled should be set forth in the office procedure manual. Figure 9–3 shows how the instruction page might be arranged in the manual. Listed below are some kinds of calls that can be handled by the medical assistant in most offices.

Appointments for New Patients. As mentioned in the chapter on scheduling appointments, the first appointment for a new patient requires more time and attention to detail. The medical assistant who is in charge of scheduling appointments should handle these calls. It is well to remember that you are in a sense "opening the door." The patient will form a first impression of the office, of you, and of the doctor from that first telephone contact. Follow all the prescribed rules of telephone courtesy in offering your friendly assistance.

Take the patient's full name, age, complete address and telephone number, name of person who referred him, and the general type of examination required. This helps decide how much time to allot the patient on the appointment schedule. Your doctor also may ask you to give general instructions to patients seeking care for specific complaints; for example, to request the patient to bring in a urine specimen.

When you have recorded the necessary data, you may ask the patient, "Do you prefer morning or afternoon?" and then offer the first available date. Make certain the patient knows where the office is located and, if necessary, how to get there. If there are special parking conveniences, tell the patient. Ideally, transportation and parking instructions would be described in a Patient Information Folder to be mailed to the patient prior to a first visit if time permits. Before hanging up, repeat the appointment date and time agreed upon and thank the person for calling.

STANDARD PROCEDURE FOR TELEPHONE CALLS IN THE OFFICE OF

_____ :

CALLS THE ASSISTANT CAN HANDLE:

    Appointments for New Patients _____

    Office Administration Problems _____

    _____

    _____

    _____

    _____

    _____

    _____

    _____

CALLS TO BE PUT THROUGH IMMEDIATELY:

    Calls from Other Physicians _____

    Emergency Calls _____

    _____

    _____

CALLS TO BE REFERRED TO PHYSICIAN:

    Unsatisfactory Progress Reports _____

    Third Party Requests for Information _____

    _____

    _____

    _____

    _____

Figure 9–3
Page from procedure manual.

Return Appointments. Usually it is necessary only to determine when the patient is expected to return, and then to find a suitable time on the schedule. It is not necessary to give extensive explanations about the location of the office and parking facilities. However, if it has been some time since the last visit, it is advisable to ask whether the patient's address and telephone number remain the same. You may also wish to inquire whether the patient wants to see the doctor about a condition similar to the former one. A different complaint may require a longer or shorter visit than usual.

Inquiries About Bills. A patient may request to speak with the doctor about a recent bill. Ask the caller to "Hold" for a moment while you pull the ledger. If you find nothing irregular on the ledger, you can return to the telephone and say, "I have your account in front of me now. Perhaps I can answer your question." The chances are that the patient will have some simple inquiry such as "Is that my total bill?" "Has my insurance paid anything?" or "May I wait until next month to make a payment?" Not all patients realize that it is the medical assistant who usually takes charge of these matters.

Inquiries About Fees. In some offices the medical assistant is instructed *not to quote fees.* However, a caller who inquires, "How much does Dr. Arnold charge for an examination?" may not be pleased to hear "That's impossible to say—it depends entirely on how extensive an examination is necessary." The following response is equally noncommittal but far more satisfying to the caller: "Mr. Barker, that naturally varies with the nature of the problem. An uncomplicated physical examination without any laboratory tests or x-rays might run as little as $. . . . On the other hand, it could run considerably more if special tests are required." If fees are regularly discussed on the telephone, write a suggested script in the policy manual. Don't be evasive. Have a schedule of fees available.

Requests for Insurance Assistance. Again, it is the medial assistant who is in a better position to answer inquiries about insurance. Often patients find insurance claims very confusing and think they must answer questions with precise medical terminology. A simple statement to "just put it in your own words" may take care of this kind of inquiry. It is best to avoid interpreting insurance coverage by telephone. If the patient has a complicated problem, the medical assistant can ask that the policy form be mailed or brought into the office.

Receiving X-ray and Laboratory Reports. Many physicians have x-ray and laboratory reports telephoned to their offices on the day the test is completed. The medical assistant can take these reports. Your task will be greatly simplified if you have blank forms on which you can just fill in the results rather than having to write the names of all the tests, particularly on laboratory reports. If it is impossible to get blank forms from the laboratory, you can type up your own and run it through the copy machine. By typing four or six to a page, the expense of duplication will be cut considerably. They can then be cut to size. Save the original for future duplicating.

Satisfactory Progress Reports from Patients. Doctors sometimes ask a patient to "phone and let me known how you're feeling in a few days." The medical assistant can take such a call and relay the information to the doctor if it is a satisfactory report.

Assure the patient that you will inform the doctor about the call by saying, for example, "I'll relay this information as soon as the doctor arrives."

Routine Reports from Hospitals and Other Sources. There may be routine calls from the hospital and other sources reporting a patient's progress. If it is only a reporting procedure, take the message carefully, make sure that the doctor sees it, and then place it in the patient's history.

Office Administration Matters. Not all calls concern patients. There may be calls from the accountant or auditor, or calls regarding banking procedures, office supplies, office maintenance, and so forth, all of which the medical assistant can either handle immediately or get the necessary information on and call back.

Requests for Referrals. Doctors who are liked and respected by their patients are frequently asked for referrals to other specialists, for themselves or for friends. If the physician has furnished the medical assistant with a list of doctors for this purpose, these inquiries can usually be handled without referring them to the physician. The physician should, however, be told of such requests.

Prescription Refills. If the physician has placed a note on the patient's chart indicating that a prescription may be filled a certain number of times, the medical assistant can give an okay to the pharmacist after determining the number of times it has already been filled. This information should appear on the patient's chart, but it is always best to double-check. If there is any question, tell the pharmacist you will have to check with the doctor and call back.

Calls that Require Transfer to the Doctor or Call Back

Calls from Other Physicians. As stated earlier, calls from other physicians should be put through immediately. If it is impossible for the doctor to take the call at once, be sure to offer to call back as soon as possible.

Patients Who Will Not Reveal Symptoms. Occasionally patients will call and wish to talk with the doctor about symptoms that they are reluctant to discuss with a medical assistant. Do not make the mistake of pressing for details. Even though you may not be embarrassed, patients have the right to privacy. Put these calls through or offer to have the doctor call back.

Unsatisfactory Progress Reports. If the patient reports that he or she "still is not feeling well," or the "prescription the doctor gave me makes me feel sick," do not try to practice medicine by telling the patient "this is to be expected." Even if you think the doctor will say the same thing, the patient should hear it directly from the doctor for reassurance.

Requests for Test Results. When the physician orders special tests for the patient, the patient may be told to call the office in a couple of days for the results. Be sure the physician has seen the results and has given you permission to tell the patient before giving out any information. Particularly if the result is unfavorable, the physician should be the one to inform the patient and give further instructions. This call must be handled tactfully; otherwise, the patient may get the feeling that you are hiding something. Some patients do not understand that the medical assistant does not have the privilege of giving out information without the permission of the physician. You might answer the inquiry like this: "The doctor has not seen the report yet; will you please call back after 2 o'clock? I will try to have the information for you then." Or offer to call the patient as soon as you have the necessary information.

Third-Party Requests for Information. If there is no legal requirement for disclosure of information, you must have the written permission of the patient before giving information to third-party callers. This includes insurance companies, attorneys, relatives, neighbors, employers, or any other third party.

Complaints About Care or Fees. You may be able to offer a satisfactory explanation to a patient who complains about the care he received or the fee charged. If a patient seems angry, you may say that it will take a few moments to pull the chart, and offer to call back. This reassures the patient that someone is willing to talk about the problem, and also gives the patient a chance to "cool off." If you are unable to appease the patient easily, though, the doctor would probably prefer to talk directly to the patient.

Call-Back System. The transfer of nonemergency calls as they occur may cause needless interruption in the physician's daily schedule. Some offices set aside a special time once or twice a day when the physician will accept or return calls—for instance, at the end of the morning office hours and again at the end of the afternoon. The person answering the telephone logs each caller's name, telephone number, and reason for calling. Patients' charts are pulled and given to the physician along with the log. When calls are handled in this manner, the physician is better prepared to answer questions and the caller is better assured of undivided attention to the call.

Special Telephone Problems

Emergency Call Procedures. The handling of telephone calls involving a possible emergency situations was briefly discussed in Chapter 8. According to the American Medical Association's *The Business Side of Medical Practice*:

> Many emergency calls are judgment calls on the part of the person answering in the physician's office. Good judgment only comes from proper training by the physician as to what constitutes a real emergency in his/her type of practice and how such calls should be handled. If you are not immediately available, what should your assistant do?

The person answering the telephone should first determine, "Is it urgent?" If the physician is in, the call should probably be transferred immediately. Some plan for the action to be taken when the physician is not present should be agreed upon (Fig. 9–4). It is estimated that fewer than 10% of medical assistants have such guidance.

The physician and medical assistant may also jointly develop typical questions to ask the caller, to determine the validity and disposition of an emergency. For example:

- What are the chief symptoms?
- When did they start?
- Has this happened before?
- Are you alone?
- Do you have transportation?
- What is the telephone number where you can be reached?

Unidentified Callers. Although it will happen rarely, you will sometimes encounter individuals who refuse to give you their name or business but are insistent upon speaking to the doctor. Such callers frequently are salespersons who are fully aware that if their identity is revealed they will never get the opportunity to speak to the doctor. Your own course in such instances is to say firmly, "Dr. Jones is very busy with a patient and has asked me to take all messages. If you will not give me a message, I suggest you write the doctor a letter."

Calls from Family and Friends. Every doctor receives a certain number of personal calls at the office from family and friends. As you become acquainted with the doctor's practice, you will soon know how to handle these calls. However, some persons abuse the telephone privilege. If a friend of the doctor calls too often and the doctor does not wish to take the calls, the medical assistant must deal with it. You can say, "Dr. Wilson is with a patient now and cannot be disturbed. We are booked rather heavily this afternoon, and you may have more time to talk with the doctor if you call

EMERGENCY CALL PROCEDURES

When the physician is not in the office, follow these emergency procedures:

Patient Complaint	Refer to Physician Below	Call RN	Call Paramedics	Have Patient	
				Go to Hospital	Come to Office
Severe bleeding					
Head injury					
Severe chest pain					
Broken bone					
Severe laceration					
Unconscious					
High fever					
Difficulty in breathing					

Figure 9–4
Form for instructions on emergency call procedures (when physician is not in office).

at home this evening. The home telephone number is . . .

Angry Callers. No matter how efficient you are at the telephone or how well-liked your employer may be, sooner or later you will have an angry caller on the line. There may be a legitimate reason for the anger, or it may have resulted from a misunderstanding. It is a real challenge to handle such a call. You must:

- Avoid getting angry yourself
- Try to find out what the real problem is
- Provide the answers, if possible

If answers are not readily available, a friendly assurance that you will find the answer and call back will usually calm the angry feelings. Be sure to:

- Really listen while you let the caller talk
- Express interest and understanding
- Do not "pass the buck"
- Take careful notes
- Maintain your own poise
- Take the required action—even is it is to say that you will take the matter up with your employer as soon as possible and call back later.

Monitoring Calls. Occasionally you may be asked by your employer to **monitor** a telephone call. You will be expected to listen from an extension phone and take notes on the conversation. It is possible to record both sides of a telephone call by placing a dictating machine close to the telephone receiver. However, you should be aware that this is illegal unless the other person is told that the conversation is being recorded.

Requests for House Calls. Scheduling house calls was discussed briefly in Chapter 8. In response to a telephone request for a home visit, be sure to inquire as to the nature of the illness. There are certain conditions that are impossible to treat at home, and time will be saved if the patient is sent directly to the hospital, where the doctor can meet him. Or urge the patient to come to the office. You can point out that facilities for giving the best medical treatment are available there and that office calls are more economical. This also conserves the doctor's time.

Consult the doctor, if possible, before scheduling a house call. In most cases you can explain to the patient that you will check with the doctor and call back immediately. If your doctor cannot make the house call, you should attempt to find other assistance for the patient. It is easier for you to call another physician than it is for the distraught patient. One of the most common complaints about the medical profession is being unable to get a doctor in an emergency. In communities that have paramedic teams, this is not such a problem.

Routine But Troublesome Calls

Many of the so-called "routine" calls coming into the physician's office will be difficult for a new medical assistant to handle (Fig. 9–5). Though no stock answer can be phrased for these calls, a gracious and prompt reply paves the way for a quicker handling of the call, since it tells the patient that you are capable, pleasant, and willing to offer assistance.

Here are a few typical calls that any medical assistant may receive:

1. The Call   "I have an appointment with the doctor this morning and cannot keep it. May I come in this afternoon instead?"

    The Answer   Even though this type of call throws the appointment book into confusion, showing irrita-

ASSISTANT'S GUIDE FOR HANDLING ROUTINE TELEPHONE CALLS	Refer immediately to physician	Physician will call back	Refer to clinical personnel: RN, CMA, PA	Other
New patient—ill and wants to talk to physician				
Established patient—wants to talk to physician				
Patient—request for lab results				
Family requesting patient information				
Patient or pharmacy—regarding Rx refill				
Another physician—wants to talk to physician				
Hospital—regarding a patient				
Insurance carrier or attorney requesting patient information				
Business calls for physician (attorney, accountant, broker)				
Professional society calls for physician				
Personal calls for physician (family, friends)				

Figure 9–5
The new assistant needs a guide for handling even routine calls.

tion with the patient won't help the situation. Make a sincere effort to help the caller make a new appointment. Explain that appointments are made in order that the doctor can give the very best care without rushing the patients and that consequently keeping appointments is to each patient's personal benefit.

2. The Call "I received my statement this morning and I don't understand why it is so high."

The Answer When this type of call comes in, politely ask the patient to hold the line while you pull the financial card. When you return to the line, thank the patient for waiting and explain the charges carefully. If there is an error, apologize and say a corrected statement will be sent out at once. Thank the patient for calling. If patients are properly advised about charges at the time

services are rendered, the number of these calls will be considerably reduced.

3. The Call "Last time I had an office call, Doctor gave me a prescription for some sleeping tablets. I want you to call the druggist and okay a refill."

The Answer Remember that the medical assistant is not licensed to practice medicine. Ask the patient for the prescription number, the date, the name, address and telephone number of the druggist, and obtain the patient's phone number. Explain that you will give the message to the doctor as soon as possible. At this point it may be advisable to pull the patient's chart and have it ready with the message when the doctor comes in. If the doctor okays the refill, you may be asked to phone the pharmacy and the patient with the information.

4. The Call   "Does the doctor treat stomach trouble?"

The Answer   It depends upon the doctor's field of practice. Many people don't understand the various medical specialties, and this call may come from a person referred to the doctor by a friend who didn't explain that the doctor is a specialist. If your doctor is unable to handle the case, you may have to refer the patient to another doctor. Give the patient the names of at least three physicians when possible; these should be only names that your employer has had you place on the referral list. Do not presume to make a diagnosis when a patient calls in with bizarre complaints; transfer the call to the doctor, or take the caller's name and number and have the doctor return the call later.

Procedure 9–1

ANSWERING THE TELEPHONE

PROCEDURAL GOAL

To answer the telephone in a physician's office in a professional manner, respond to request for action, and accurately record message.

EQUIPMENT AND SUPPLIES

Trainer telephone
Role-play partner
Message pad
Pen or pencil
Appointment book

PROCEDURE

1. Answer telephone on first ring, speaking directly into mouthpiece positioned one inch from mouth.
 Purpose: Answering promptly conveys interest in the caller. Proper positioning of handset carries voice best.
2. Speak distinctly with a pleasant tone and expression, at a moderate rate, and with sufficient volume for calling party to understand every word.
 Purpose: Conveys interest in caller and prevents stressful response.
3. Identify office and self.
 Purpose: Caller will know correct number has been reached and identity of staff member.
4. Verify identity of caller.
 Purpose: To confirm origin of call.
5. Provide caller with the requested information or service if possible.
 Purpose: Medical assistant can handle many calls and conserve time and energy of physician or other staff members.
6. Take message for further action if required.
 Purpose: Not all calls can be responded to immediately.
7. Terminate call in a pleasant manner and replace receiver gently.
 Purpose: Promotes good public relations.

TERMINAL PERFORMANCE OBJECTIVE

Given the listed equipment and supplies, take a variety of telephone calls in a physician's office, follow the agency's accepted procedures, and complete each call within 5 minutes with no errors in message, to a performance level of 90%.

5. The Call   "My next-door neighbor is a patient of the doctor's and I am quite concerned about her. Could you tell me what is wrong with her?"

The Answer   Professional ethics is involved here. It is not the role of the medical assistant to give out any information about a patient's condition, except information that the physician has specifically okayed for "release." The caller in this case may be merely curious, or may actually be a kindly neighbor who wishes to help a friend. Generally, refer such calls to the doctor.

Telephone Answering Services

Because a physician's telephone is an all-important tool of the practice, it must be constantly "covered"—that is, there must be someone to answer it at all times—day and night, weekends and holidays. This presents no problem during weekdays, but nights and weekends require special attention. Most doctors subscribe to telephone answering services that provide around-the-clock coverage. Some telephone answering services are privately owned; others are owned and operated by the local medical society. Alternatively, the doctor may use an automatic answering device.

Operator-Answered Services. There are two types of operator-answered services:

1. Doctor-subscribers leave messages with, or obtain patients' messages from, a service whose number appears in the local telephone directory in this way, "After _____ PM, call _____ [number]," or "If no answer, call _____ [number]." Such listings are placed immediately below the doctor's own telephone number in the directory. This form of service is somewhat inconvenient for the patient but is far better than no coverage at all.

2. The answering service has a direct connection with the office telephone. When the telephone rings in the physician's office or at home, it also signals on the switchboard of the answering service. As long as the telephone is ringing, it will continue to signal at the answering service. If no one answers within a certain agreed-upon number of rings, the answering service operator takes the call. This method provides continuous telephone coverage.

Even during the day, such an answering service can function effectively. There may be times when you are assisting the doctor and it is impossible for you or anyone else to answer the telephone. An unanswered telephone is extremely poor policy, but if you have an agreement with the answering service (sometimes referred to as the exchange), its operators will accept calls for you in such situations. With this direct-wire answering method, the operator answers the telephone in your employer's name, as you would in the office, explaining. "This is Dr. Wilson's exchange. May I take a message?" The operators on the exchange switchboards are usually exceptionally well trained, especially if the service is owned by the local medical society.

The answering service will greatly appreciate your cooperation if you call them every day before leaving the office, telling them where the doctor will be during the evening or giving them other special messages. Then, in the morning when you return to the office, call the exchange and ask for any messages they may have. Usually there will be messages from patients who called during the evening but whose calls were not urgent enough to merit an emergency call to the doctor. An exchange can act as a buffer for the physician and help eliminate too frequent, unnecessary calls during the night.

Here is how the system works: During the hours that the office is closed, the exchange will answer the doctor's office telephone, take a message, and immediately relay it to the doctor. If it is urgent, the doctor will then return the call to the patient; if not, the exchange will call the patient and explain that the doctor will call first thing in the morning. Emergency calls, of course, are immediately put through by the exchange to the doctor.

Occasionally it is a good idea to check up on your answering service by placing a few random calls at various hours. It may be that now and then the service does not answer the call or the response may not meet your standards. The service may be enhanced by inviting the manager of the answering service in to see the office, or by having the medical assistant go to the exchange facility to meet with the manager and staff. This personal contact frequently improves the rapport and quality of service you may expect.

Automatic Answering Devices. Some doctors use an automatic answering device after office hours. Callers who dial the office hear a recorded message either telling them how to reach the doctor (or a colleague who may be covering the practice) or inviting the caller to leave a message. The caller's message is recorded for later checking by the doctor or a staff member.

Some telephone answering devices are equipped with a remote control with which the doctor can call the office from any telephone and, by simply holding the remote control near the mouthpiece of the telephone, receive the messages that have been recorded. Some machines have a code access that may be set in the machine, and the messages may be picked up by dialing the number and then punching in the code access during the outgoing message.

The automatic telephone answering devices are particularly useful in areas where no competent answering service is available.

Optional Services

Call Forwarding. Though not yet available in all areas, call forwarding is something the physician may want to investigate. This is a particularly attractive feature for the physician who has two offices and does not want to confuse patients with different numbers for different days of the week. With the call forwarding feature, all you do is dial a special code followed by the number of the other office (or the number at which the doctor can be reached). Then all phone calls will be automatically transferred to the new location. Calls may also be forwarded to the doctor's home or to any other number that can be dialed directly, without operator assistance.

Call Waiting. Call waiting service lets you know someone else is calling when you're using the telephone. You hear a beep tone, but the calling party hears only the normal ringing. If you wish, you can answer the second call while keeping the first call on "hold." You can even switch back and forth between the two calls as often as you want.

Mobile Service and Radio Paging. In order to guarantee continual availability to patients, some physicians have telephones in their automobiles and/or have pocket radio paging equipment. There are several types of radio receivers. One is tone only, and one is tone and voice. Another has a visual display of messages. The doctor carries the radio receiver, sometimes called a "beeper," and access is effected by dialing the paging equipment by telephone. The physician is alerted by the beeper and then calls the office or answering service. The Bell System's unit is called Bell Boy.

Telephone Dictation. In hospitals, dial dictation and recording services are quite common. A physician can dictate a case history or report by telephone into a centrally located recording machine. The report will then be transcribed by word processors at the central location. In a group practice, the recording machine may be in the doctor's office, where the office staff will do the typing.

New concepts in telecommunications are being developed continually. A call to the marketing division of your local telephone company will help keep you formed of what is available in your locality.

USING THE TELEPHONE DIRECTORY

The primary purpose of the telephone directory, of course, is to provide lists of those who have telephones, with their numbers and in most cases their addresses. In addition, the directory is an aid in checking the spelling of names and in locating certain types of businesses through the yellow pages. Directories are usually organized in three sections:

1. Introductory pages
2. Alphabetical pages (white pages)
3. Yellow pages

In metropolitan areas the yellow pages appear in a separate volume.

The introductory pages are sometimes entirely overlooked by the subscribers. This section precedes the white alphabetical pages and provides basic information concerning the telephone services in the area, including:

- Emergency services (fire, police, ambulance, highway patrol)
- Service calls
- Dialing instructions for local and out-of-town calls
- Area codes for some cities

The introductory pages may also include:

- A survival guide
- Community service numbers
- Prefix locations
- Rates
- Long distance calling information
- International calling information
- Time zones
- Government listing

Some directories include zip code maps for the local area. Take a few moments to familiarize yourself with your local directory; then use it frequently for getting information fast.

The white pages are an alphabetical listing of telephone subscribers with their telephone numbers, and in most cases their addresses.

The yellow pages directory, sometimes published separately, contains listings for businesses arranged by the product or services they sell. Physicians are listed alphabetically, usually under the heading Physicians and Surgeons, and have the option of another listing by type of practice.

In some areas a Street Address Telephone Directory is published that lists street addresses, with the name and telephone number of the person or business at that address.

9

ORGANIZING A PERSONAL TELEPHONE DIRECTORY

Organize your telephone numbers in an indexed 3 × 5 inch desktop file or a rotary file. Emergency numbers might be typed on a colored card or flagged with a color tab. Your personal directory of telephone numbers should include all the numbers that you call frequently, including:

- Specialists to whom your employer sometimes refers patients
- Professional facilities, such as hospitals, the Poison Control Center, pharmacies, ambulance companies, laboratories
- Special duty nurses, along with their specialties and other pertinent information
- Administrative contacts, such as stationers, equipment dealers and repair services, laundry and maintenance services, surgical supply houses
- Personal numbers, such as the doctor's family, special friends, insurance agent, stockbroker, accountant, lawyer.

OUTGOING CALLS

Pre-Planning the Call. Before placing a call, make certain you have the correct telephone number and the information you will need during the call at your fingertips.

If you are reporting a patient's history, have the complete record before you, including all the latest laboratory and x-ray reports.

If you are placing a call to order supplies, have the catalog in front of you, along with any previous order sheets or invoices. Also have a list of the items desired, the specifications for them, and any questions you may have regarding them.

Apply this rule to every call you make. The called party will be impressed with your competent organization, and you will save a great deal of time and prevent errors.

Placing the Call. Lift the receiver, listen for the dial tone, then start dialing your number. It sometimes happens that just as you pick up the telephone to place a call, an incoming call has reached your line but you lifted the receiver before the telephone had a chance to ring. If you start dialing without listening for the dial tone, you will not only fail to reach your number, you will have offended the ear of the party trying to reach you.

If your telephone has a rotary dial, use the index finger or a special dialing instrument for dialing your call. Do not use the eraser end of a pencil and do not let finger remain in the dial openings on the return of the dial. It is the return of the dial that

determines the number you reach, and if it is not allowed to return freely you may reach a wrong number.

Calling Etiquette. When placing a call to another doctor or to a patient at the doctor's request, your doctor should be ready to receive the call. Doctors, because of their busy schedules, sometimes are negligent in this respect. The telephone company's courtesy rule is that the person placing the call should be on the line and ready to speak when the called party answers.

If you are calling a patient to change an appointment, be ready to offer a new appointment time. Also, give the patient a logical reason for the inconvenience of having to change the original appointment. This change may cause considerable disruption of plans, and the patient is fully entitled to an explanation.

Remember that if your telephone is within hearing range of office patients, you should be careful in mentioning names or diagnoses.

By following these suggested techniques you will be able to use the telephone wisely and efficiently. Correct use of the telephone is a skill and an art that can be developed only through actual practice. It is one of the most important skills the medical assistant can possess.

Long Distance Service. Long distance calls are no longer reserved for special occasions. The calls are simple to place, inexpensive, and efficient. When information is needed in a hurry, it is much more expedient to telephone rather than wait for an exchange of letters.

Before placing a long distance call, have the correct number ready. This number often may be obtained from a letterhead or from other records. The telephone company also has a collection of major city telephone directories in every town. If you do not have the number, you may obtain directory assistance by dialing the area code of the party you are calling, then 555–1212. In some areas you must dial "1" before the area code.

It is important to keep in mind the different time zones when you are calling long distance (Fig. 9–6). The continental United States is divided into four standard time zones: Pacific, Mountain, Central, and Eastern. When it is 12:00 noon Pacific time, it is 3:00 PM Eastern time. If you are calling from San Francisco to New York, you will probably want to make the call no later than 2:00 PM if you are calling a business or professional office, because it will already be 5:00 PM on the East Coast.

Dialing Direct. By dialing your own long distance calls, you will pay the lowest rate and pay for only the minutes you talk (minimum 1 minute). Use direct dialing when you are willing to talk with anyone who answers the phone and you want the

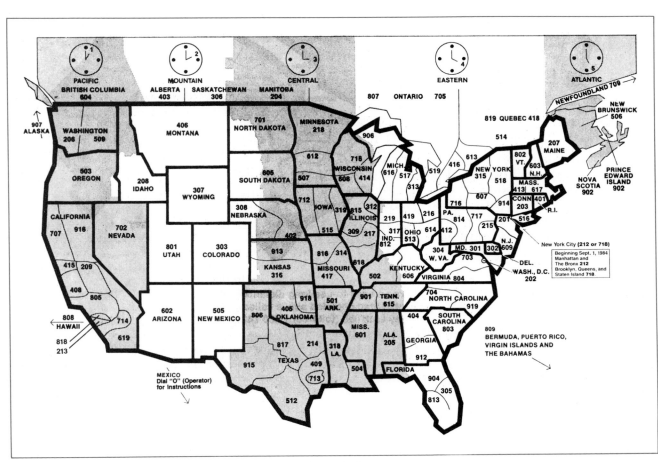

Figure 9–6
Time zones across the United States. (Courtesy of Bell Telephone.)

call charged to the number from which you are calling.

"800" WATS (Wide Area Telephone Service) Numbers. Many businesses and professional people have "800" WATS numbers, to which long distance calls can be made without charge to the caller. To call an "800" number, dial 1 + 800 + the 7-digit telephone number. You can get the telephone numbers of those businesses and people who have 800 numbers by dialing 1 + 800 + 555–1212.

Operator-Assisted Calls. Operator-assisted calls include calls such as:

- Person-to-person
- Bill to a third number
- Collect
- Requests for time and charges
- Certain calls placed from hotels

There is a 1-minute initial period charge, and the rates are the dial-direct rates plus a service charge.

International Service. International Direct Distance Dialing (IDDD) is available in many areas. International dialing codes are the same for all companies offering IDDD. Depending on your long distance company, additional numbers or codes may preface the international access, country, and city codes. IDDD is still not available in all areas. If it is available, you may place international station-to-station calls by dialing in sequence the:

- International code 011
- Country code
- City code
- Local telephone number
- "#" button if your telephone is touch-tone

For example, to place a call to London you would dial:

International Access Code		Country Code		City Code
011	+	44	+	1

plus the local telephone number and "#" if touch-tone dialing. After dialing any international code, allow at least 45 seconds for the ringing to start.

Wrong Numbers. One slip in direct distance dialing can give you Los Angeles or New York instead of Dallas. If you reach a wrong number when dialing long distance, be sure to obtain the name of the city and state you have reached. By reporting this information promptly to the operator in your own city, you will not be charged for the call. If you are cut off before terminating your call, this too should be reported to the operator, who will either reconnect your call or make an adjustment of the charge.

Conference Calls. Conference telephone service is of great value to the medical profession in notifying and explaining to a family how a patient is progressing. It has exceptional value in family conferences requiring a quick decision by the entire family in regard to a patient's condition.

This service can connect from 3 to 14 points for a two-way conference in which each person can hear or talk to all others participating. Conference calls may be local or long distance calls. Charges are added for the number of places connected, mileage, and the length of the conversation.

To place a call, dial the operator and say you wish to make a conference call. Give the operator the names and telephone numbers of the people you want to connect. If prior arrangements are made with all parties, there is a better chance of reaching everyone at a given time.

TELEPHONE EQUIPMENT

Number and Placement of Telephones

Few health care facilities can get along with just one telephone line. A busy signal can be very irritating to a caller, especially when it is a new patient attempting to reach the physician for the first time. One medical assistant can handle no more than two incoming lines, so the addition of more lines may also involve additional staffing.

If there is a staff member assigned solely to dealing with insurance and billing, a separate line and listing in the telephone directory for this service may considerably lessen the load on the main incoming lines.

Where should the phones be located?— Everywhere you need them, except in the examining rooms, according to Conomikes Associates, Inc., a nationally recognized practice management consulting firm.

Obtaining Equipment and Services

There are many options today in acquiring telephone equipment and services. In the past the source of equipment was by lease from the Bell System. The Bell System is still the major source, but the equipment may be either leased or purchased. Equipment may also be purchased from private sources.

Long distance service is available from sources outside the Bell System. The use of a private long distance provider may require dialing an access number in addition to the usual area code plus telephone number. Equipment leasing fees, monthly service charges, and long distance charges are each billed separately.

Multiple-Line Telephones

Familiarity with a multiple-line telephone is a must for the medical assistant. The multiple-line instrument allows holding one or more calls while answering another, or while speaking with another person within the office on an intercom line.

Six-Button Key Set. The most common telephone instrument in the doctor's office is the six-button key set. It can have several outside lines, can hold calls, and can be used as an intercom or for signaling. Lights within the buttons flash for incoming calls and wink rapidly to remind of calls being held. A steady light indicates that the line is in use. Although many rotary dial telephones are still in use, they are gradually being phased out and replaced with the speedier touch-tone instrument (Fig. 9–7).

Speakerphone. Some doctors like the Speakerphone, a small receiver-transmitter which sits on the desk and picks up and amplifies normal conversation, freeing the hands for note-taking. This same device can be very useful to the medical assistant who may receive frequent calls that require going to another location to refer to charts or financial records. With the Speakerphone there is no break in communication. The Speakerphone is convertible; at the touch of a button it changes from a regular telephone to a hands-free communications system.

10-Button Phone. As the practice grows, it may become necessary to add additional telephone lines. The 10-button phone handles as many as nine lines, with the subscriber choosing the appropriate number and "mix" of outside and inside lines serving each phone.

Com Key. Ideal for the larger office is the flexible Com Key, which utilizes 10-button phones. It provides up to seven incoming lines, plus built-in equipment for multi-line intercom conferencing as well as one-way voice signaling on the intercom. A built-in loudspeaker system is an added convenience. A simple control switch at each phone allows the selection of which phones will ring on any combination of outside lines—ideal for "after hours" assignments or reduced staff situations.

11- and 20-Button Desk Telephone Sets. The office that has frequent need for outside conferencing will find this instrument convenient. Up to 7 lines of the 11-button set and up to 15 lines of the 20-button set may be used as conferencing lines by simultaneously pressing the line buttons on the lines to be used without going through an operator. These instruments also have a special recall button that lets you flash your operator without losing a call or breaking a conference connection.

Call Director or Call Commander Telephone. This piece of equipment may have 18 or 30 buttons. One button is reserved for "Hold," and the remainder may be a mix of outside and inside lines. It is a compact desktop instrument and may be thought of as a desk-sized switchboard offering many optional features (Fig. 9–8).

Touch-a-Matic. The Bell System refers to its Touch-a-Matic telephone as "the telephone that remembers." It has the ability to store up to 31 telephone numbers electronically and can dial any one of them for you at the touch of a single button. The names of the people or places you call most frequently are displayed on the face of the instrument, eliminating the need for an index or cards to insert. A very attractive feature of this instrument is its *last number dialed* button. If you want to call back someone you've just spoken to, or try a number that was busy a few minutes ago, the number is re-dialed for you electronically by simply touching the *last numbered dialed* button. By following simple recording instructions you can add to, delete, or change the numbers assigned to the memory system.

TeleDialer 32. The same features that are found in the Touch-a-Matic may be added to your present phone by installing the auxiliary TeleDialer 32.

Headsets. A popular headset is a very light plastic earphone and microphone combination that allows the medical assistant or the doctor to move about the room and to have the hands free. One brand name is StarSet (Fig. 9–9). It was originally designed for the astronauts and weighs less than 1 ounce. Instead of being worn over the head, it is worn behind the ear or clipped to your glasses. It can be equipped with a cord up to ten feet long for easy movement about the room. There is also an optional quick-disconnect feature that allows the user to separate the headset even during a call without breaking the connection.

TELEGRAPH SERVICES

Although most long distance communications from the physician's office will be via the telephone, there are instances in which the telegraph message is the one of choice. The preferred delivery time and the urgency of the message would determine the type of service to be used. There are two basic classes of domestic telegraph service: the *regular telegram* and the more economical *overnight telegram*.

9

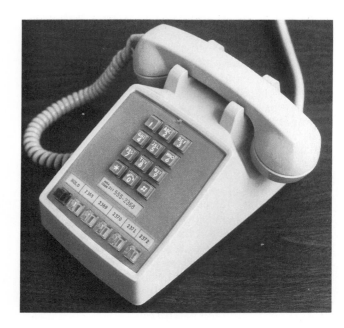

Figure 9–7
Key Set Touch-Tone. The Key Set features one "hold" button and five others for calling, signaling, or access to other extensions. (Courtesy of American Telephone and Telegraph.)

Figure 9–8
Call Director Touch-Tone. Thirty-button Call Director with self-designating keys. (Courtesy of American Telephone and Telegraph.)

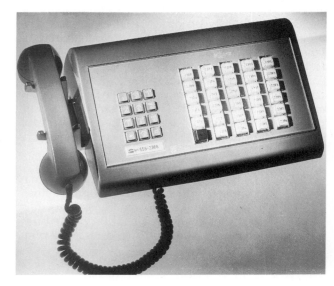

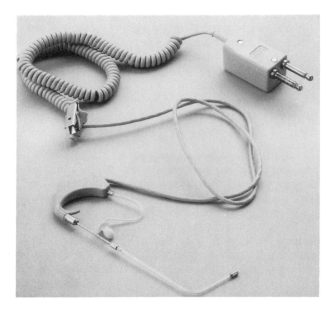

Figure 9–9
StarSet telephone. (Courtesy of American Telephone and Telegraph.)

Regular Telegram. The regular telegram is accepted at any time and transmitted immediately. Usually delivery may be expected within two hours. The minimum charge is based on 15 words, and an extra charge is made for each additional word.

Overnight Telegram. The overnight telegram may be sent up until midnight for delivery the next morning. The minimum charge is based on 100 words, and an extra charge is made for each additional word.

Mailgram. The mailgram is a variation of the overnight telegram. It is wired to the office of the US Postal Service nearest the recipient, where it is placed in a special Mailgram envelope and delivered by the regular letter carrier.

You should be familiar with the methods used in counting the chargeable words and characters. One address and one signature are free. Punctuation marks are not charged for: however, if such words as *stop, period,* or *quote* are used, they are considered chargeable words. Three of the characters on your typewriter cannot be transmitted and must be written as words in a telegram: these are &, @, and ° (for degree).

Telegrams may be telephoned to the telegraph company and charged on your telephone bill. However, before telephoning, the message should be carefully composed and a copy typed for the office files, including the date and time sent. Telegrams may be addressed to airports, to sailing or arriving ships, to ships at sea, and even to isolated places if there is a telephone there.

Other Services from Western Union. Your Western Union office will make and confirm hotel or motel reservations. They will sometimes call as many as eight hotels or motels in the same city in order to get the accommodations you wish.

It is possible to send money by telegraph and cable to all parts of the world. Payments in foreign countries are made in the currency of that country. In addition to the amount of money being wired, you must pay for the cost of a 15-word telegram or a 100-word overnight telegram, plus a service charge based on the amount of money to be sent.

Western Union offers many additional services, although there would be little need for most of them in the average doctor's office.

REFERENCES AND READINGS

What Every Telephone User Should Know, General Telephone System.
Your Telephone Personality, Bell Telephone System.
Your Voice is You, Bell Telephone System.
The Business Side of Medical Practice, American Medical Association, 1979.

9

CHAPTER OUTLINE

Equipment
Stationery
Language Skills
    Procedure 10–1: Transcribing Machine-
      Dictated Letters

Composing Responsibilities
Letter Styles
Punctuation
Parts of Letters
Signature
    Procedure 10–2: Composing Business
      Correspondence
    Procedure 10–3: Writing Instructions

Addressing the Envelope
Folding and Inserting Letters
Preparing the Outgoing Mail
Postage Meters
Mailing Costs
Classifications of Mail
Size Standards for Domestic Mail
Private Mail Services
Electronic Mail
Postal Services
Handling Special Problems
Incoming Mail
Mail the Assistant Can Handle
Vacation Mail

VOCABULARY

See Glossary at end of book for definitions.

annotate	dual-pitch	proofread
concise	edit	tabulation
continuation page	elite	transcription
daisy wheel	pica	

10

Written Communications

OBJECTIVES

Upon successful completion of this chapter you should be able to:

1. *Define the terms listed in the Vocabulary of this chapter.*
2. *Select equipment and stationery suitable for producing professional correspondence.*
3. *Discuss the importance of correct grammar, spelling, and punctuation.*
4. *Name three types of essential references for the medical assistant's library.*
5. *List three kinds of possible corrections to look for in transcription editing and proofreading.*
6. *Discuss the five steps in composing a reply to a business letter.*
7. *Name and describe the two most commonly used letter styles and punctuation patterns.*
8. *List and describe the seven essential parts of every standard business letter.*
9. *Discuss and compare the uses of certified mail and registered mail.*
10. *Cite the advantages of using a postage meter and the procedure for replenishing the supply of postage.*
11. *Discuss the importance of having a return address on every piece of mail, and how you would obtain a change of address of an addressee.*
12. *Outline the procedure for processing mail during vacation periods.*

Upon successful completion of this chapter you should be able to perform the following activities:

1. *Open, sort, and annotate incoming mail.*
2. *Prepare a response to an inquiry letter.*
3. *Compose original letters.*
4. *Produce mailable letters and reports from transcription.*
5. *Address envelopes for optical scanning.*
6. *Fold outgoing mail for insertion into three styles of envelopes.*

Written communications offer a perfect opportunity for making a good impression on others—but they don't just happen. They require thought, preparation, skill, and a caring attitude. Written communications take many forms in the medical office. The medical assistant may be required to:

- Transcribe from machine or shorthand dictation
- Compose original letters
- Reply to inquiries
- Respond to requests for information
- Write collection letters
- Order supplies
- Write instructions for patients
- Type consultation and surgical reports
- Process a variety of other communications

Written communications should be courteous to the reader, correct in content, and concise without being curt. In order to create a good impression, one begins with good equipment and quality stationery.

EQUIPMENT

The typewriter should be one that will produce good copy; the typewriter ribbon should be dark enough that the letters will be easily read but not so heavily inked as to result in smudged copy. If the typewriter has keys, they must be kept clean. This is easily accomplished by the regular use of a commercial cushion sheet made especially for this purpose that cleans the keys as you type on it. If the typewriter is equipped with a carbon ribbon, the print will be uniform, never lighter or darker, and the keys will not fill with ink from the ribbon.

Most typewriters purchased today do not have keys but are equipped with either a printing ball, called a single element, or a **daisy wheel**. The daisy wheel is a thin wheel with the letters and symbols at the end of each "spoke." Both the ball and the daisy wheel are very durable, easily changed, and available in many type styles. Such typewriters have an immovable carriage, and consequently are quieter and require less desk space. The newer typewriters are usually **dual pitch** and can be changed by the flip of a switch from pica type, with 10 characters to the linear inch, to elite type, with 12 characters to the linear inch. Many models also have 15-pitch and proportional spacing. The single element or daisy wheel typewriter with dual-pitch allows great versatility in the appearance of written communications. Professional correspondence usually looks best when done with the smaller **elite** type; reports may preferably be done with the larger **pica** type. Both elite and pica produce the standard six lines to the vertical inch.

The typewriter may also have a correcting device that lifts an incorrect character or even a full line off the paper, allowing the typist to put in the correct character with no visible evidence of an error having occurred.

In Chapter 6 we discussed the electronic typewriter and the dedicated word processor. These are definitely the wave of the future.

STATIONERY

The quality of paper unquestionably affects the total impression on the reader. Your stationer or printer is qualified to advise on the selection of paper, which can range from all-sulfite (a wood pulp) to all-cotton fiber (sometimes called rag). Letterhead paper is usually made of 25% (or more) cotton fiber bond. The weight of paper is described by a substance number. This number is based on the weight of a ream consisting of 500 sheets of 17 × 22 inch paper. The larger the number, the heavier the paper. If the ream weighs 24 pounds, the paper will be referred to as Sub 24 or 24-pound weight. Letterhead stationery and matching envelopes are usually 16-, 20-, or 24-pound weight.

There are three basic sizes of letterhead: Standard; Monarch or Executive; and Baronial. Standard letterhead, 8½ × 11 inches, is used for general business and professional correspondence. Some executives and professional persons also have letterheads in Monarch (Executive) size, 7¼ × 10½ inches, for informal business and social correspondence. The third size, which is a half-sheet called Baronial, 5½ × 8½ inches, is used for very short letters or memoranda. Each size letterhead should have its matching envelope (Table 10–1).

Continuation pages of a letter or report are typed on plain bond that matches the letterhead in weight and fiber content. Bond paper has a "felt" side and a "wire" side. Printing and typing is done on the felt side. Pick up a sheet of letterhead, hold it to the light, and you will see a design or letters that can be read from the printed side. This design is called a watermark and is an indication of quality. The side from which you can read the watermark is the "felt" side of the paper and is the side on which typing should be done. Always have the watermark read across the page in the same direction as the typing.

Table 10–1
Letterhead

Type	Size	Uses
Standard	8½ × 11	General correspondence
Monarch or Executive	7¼ × 10½	Information, business, and social correspondence
Baronial	5½ × 8½	Very short letters or memoranda

LANGUAGE SKILLS

Most persons, before they reach adulthood, have been exposed to considerable instruction in language skills. Unfortunately, through lack of use, much of the basic information is forgotten. A little book published by The Macmillan Company, *The Elements of Style*, by William Strunk, Jr., and E. B. White, is probably the most interesting and best refresher manual available. In its 85 pages, one can find practical information regarding punctuation, elementary principles of composition, explanations of many words and expressions commonly misused, and some very pointed hints on developing style in writing.

Table 10–2
150 English Words Frequently Misspelled or Misused

absence	exceed	prevalent
accede	exhilaration	principal
accessible	existence	principle
accommodate	February	privilege
achieve	forty	procedure
affect	grammar	proceed
agglutinate	grievous	professor
all right	height	pronunciation
altogether	incidentally	psychiatry
analyze	indispensable	psychology
analyses (pl.)	inimitable	pursue
analysis (s.)	inoculate	questionnaire
anoint	insistent	rearrange
argument	irrelevant	recede
assistant	irresistible	receive
auxiliary	irritable	recommend
balloon	judgment	referring
believe	labeled	repetition
benefited	led	rheumatism
brochure	leisure	rhythmical
bulletin	license	ridiculous
category	liquefy	sacrilegious
changeable	maintenance	seize
clientele	maneuver	separate
committee	miscellaneous	siege
comparative	mischievous	similar
concede	misspell	sizable
conscientious	necessary	stationary
conscious	newsstand	stationery
coolly	noticeable	subpoena
corroborate	occasion	succeed
definitely	occurrence	suddenness
description	oscillate	superintendent
desirable	paid	supersede
despair	pamphlet	surprise
development	panicky	tariff
dilemma	parallel	technique
disappear	paralyze	thorough
disappoint	pastime	tranquility
disastrous	perseverance	transferred
discreet	persistent	truly
discrete	personal	tyrannize
discriminate	personnel	unnecessary
dissatisfaction	possession	until
dissipate	precede	vacillate
drunkenness	precedent	vacuum
ecstasy	predictable	vicious
effect	predominant	warrant
eligible	predominate	Wednesday
embarrass	prerogative	weird

Table 10–3
Medical Words Frequently Misspelled

abscess	homeostasis	peritoneum
additive	humerus	petit mal
aerosol	idiosyncrasy	pharynx
agglutination	ileum	pituitary
albumin	ilium	plantar
anastomosis	infarction	pleura
aneurysm	intussusception	pleurisy
anteflexion	ischemia	pneumonia
arrhythmia	ischium	polyp
bilirubin	larynx	prophylaxis
bronchial	leukemia	prostate
cachexia	malaise	prosthesis
calcaneus	malleus	pruritus
capillary	melena	psoriasis
cervical	mellitus	pyrexia
chromosome	menstruation	respiratory
cirrhosis	metastasis	rheumatic
clavicle	neurilemma	roentgenology
curettage	neuron	sagittal
cyanosis	occlusion	sciatica
defibrillator	optic chiasm	scirrhous
desiccate	oscilloscope	serous
ecchymosis	osseous	sessile
effusion	palliative	sphincter
epididymis	parasite	sphygmomanometer
epistaxis	parenteral	squamous
eustachian	parietal	staphylococcus
fissure	paroxysmal	suppuration
flexure	pemphigus	trochanter
glaucoma	percussion	venous
gonorrhea	perforation	wheal
graafian	pericardium	xiphoid
hemorrhage	perineum	
hemorrhoids	peristalsis	

10

The medical assistant needs a basic knowledge of composition, including sentence structure, spelling, and punctuation. A personal reference library should include an up-to-date standard dictionary, a medical dictionary, and a secretary's reference manual.

Spelling. The medical assistant who has difficulty with spelling may wish to keep a small looseleaf, indexed notebook or card index of words that are troublesome. Whenever it is necessary to look up a word in the dictionary for spelling, record it in the notebook or card index where it will be easy to refer to next time. The doctor or a medical assistant who is familiar with the doctor's specialty might compile a basic list of medical terms and abbreviations used in the practice, as a reference for the trainee. Table 10–2 lists 150 frequently misspelled or misused English words. Table 10–3 lists 100 frequently misspelled medical terms. Your list may be entirely different, depending upon your capabilities and the branch of medicine involved.

The medical assistant who uses a word processor or a computer with word processing software may have a spelling checker within the program that can **proofread** an entire document in seconds. (See Chapter 6.)

Transcription. Much of the doctor's correspondence is dictated either to a machine for later **transcription** (Fig. 10–1) or directly to the medical assistant who writes shorthand. The medical assistant who is responsible for transcribing the dictation should be able to check for errors in sentence structure, punctuate sentences correctly, and spell every word correctly. As a final step, the finished typewritten page should be checked twice—once for typing accuracy and once to be sure it makes sense. Never present material for signature unless it makes sense to you and is free of errors.

Editing and Proofreading. Whether you are transcribing from shorthand or from machine dictation, the material will probably need some **editing.** This involves proper placing of insertions, verifying dates and spelling of names, checking sentence structure, and making all dictated changes. Many machine transcriptionists first type a rough draft on which they make corrections, and then retype for the final copy. Proofreader's marks are simple to learn and are very useful in such editing (see Fig. 17–5). Shorthand transcriptionists usually read over their notes for editing before typing the finished

Procedure 10–1

TRANSCRIBING MACHINE-DICTATED LETTERS

EQUIPMENT AND SUPPLIES

Machine-dictated letter
Typewriter or word processor
Draft paper
Pen or pencil for use in editing
Letterhead paper
Dictionary
Correcting tape, liquid, or eraser (optional)

PROCEDURAL GOAL

To transcribe a mailable letter from machine dictation, following the guidelines of a commonly used business letter style, with no errors in grammar, spelling, or punctuation.

PROCEDURE

1. Turn on equipment for machine dictation.
2. Insert draft paper into typewriter.
   Purpose: To produce a rough copy for editing.
3. Set line for double spacing, and keyboard draft of letter.
4. Remove draft copy and edit for spelling, insertions, and sentence structure.
   Explanation: Some dictators make insertions and changes without alerting the transcriptionist by appropriate signals. Use the dictionary to check any doubtful spelling.
5. Insert letterhead paper into machine.
6. Set the line and margins for attractive centering of letter.
7. Keyboard the edited draft, using standard placement of letter parts according to chosen letter style.
8. Type your identification initials.
9. Proofread letter for content and errors,
   Purpose: Any necessary corrections are more easily accomplished while paper is still in typewriter.
10. Remove completed letter for signature.

TERMINAL PERFORMANCE OBJECTIVE

Given the listed equipment and supplies, transcribe a machine-dictated letter into a mailable document without error or detectable corrections, within 15 minutes, to a performance level of 95%.

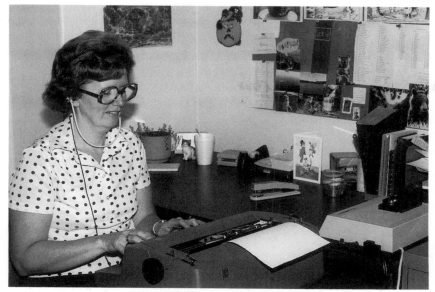

Figure 10–1
The medical assistant using transcribing equipment. (Courtesy of Vista Medical Group, El Toro, CA.)

product. In making corrections, be careful not to change the meaning. When in doubt, ask! Before taking the final copy from the machine, check for any typographical errors. Corrections are more easily made before the paper is removed from the typewriter.

COMPOSING RESPONSIBILITIES

Many doctors, when queried about the skills they most desire in an administrative medical assistant, have said, "Send me someone who can write a good letter." When the physician delegates to the medical assistant the responsibility for composing letters (which will certainly reflect positively or negatively on the practice), this is a mark of confidence, a "plus" that increases the medical assistant's value to an employer.

Letter composition can be speeded up by developing a portfolio of sample letters to suit the various situations that arise frequently. Suppose, for instance, you need to write to a patient to change an appointment. Compose the very best letter you can—clear, **concise,** and courteous—and make an extra copy to place in your portfolio of letters. Do this each time you write a new kind of letter and soon you will be able to select a letter from your samples, change it slightly to suit the current situation, and have your letters written in no time. Watch for sample letters that appear from time to time in the doctor's business journals, and clip them for your portfolio. Scan the textbooks and office manuals on the market or in your public library for additional help. Word processing by computer allows storage of model letters on the disk.

Written communications include more than letter writing. Consider, for instance, those telephone messages you take. Are you sure they are clearly stated and convey to the reader what you intended? You may need to mail a prescription to a patient, with instructions from the doctor. Will the patient "read" what you intended to say? Communication is an art, as well as a skill. The ability to communicate effectively is extremely important to the medical assistant on the way "up the ladder."

Composing Tips. If your only experience in letter writing has been social correspondence, you will have a new set of rules to learn. Social letters tend to be long and chatty, "I" oriented, and do not necessarily follow any organized plan. Most business letters should be less than one page long, "you" oriented, and carefully organized. This takes practice and preparation.

Getting Ready to Write. If you are asked to answer a letter, first organize your facts.
1. Read carefully the letter you are to answer.
2. Make note of or underline any questions asked or materials requested.
3. Decide on the answers to the questions and verify your information.
4. Draft a reply, using the tools you are most comfortable with—typewriter, longhand, or shorthand.
5. Rewrite for clarity.

Keep most of your sentences short. Put only one idea in each sentence. Eliminate the superfluous words. Be careful about using medical terms in correspondence with patients; use only language that the reader will understand.

Every person who writes letters develops his or

her own personal style. Most physicians conform to a highly professional, formal style in their dictation. The medical assistant who is given the responsibility of composing correspondence for the medical office should strive for the same degree of formality that the physician has. It would be inappropriate for the assistant to write in a breezy, informal style when acting as the representative of an employer who is strictly formal in approach. The main thing to remember is that every letter produced in your office should project the image of the physician, irrespective of who composes or signs it.

LETTER STYLES

A business letter is usually arranged in one of three styles: block, semiblock, or full block. A fourth style, called simplified, is occasionally used. The blocked and semiblocked are most commonly used in the physician's office.

Blocked Style. The date line, the complimentary closing, and the typewritten signature all begin at the center. All other lines begin at the left margin (Fig. 10–2).

Semiblocked Style. This is identical to the blocked style except that the first line of each paragraph is indented five spaces (Fig. 10–3).

Full Blocked Style. All lines start flush with the left margin. This is considered more efficient but is less attractive on the page (Fig. 10–4).

Simplified Style. All lines begin flush with the left margin. The salutation is replaced with an all-capital subject line on the third line below the inside address. The body of the letter begins on the third line below the subject line. The complimentary closing is omitted. An all-capital typewritten signature is typed on the fifth line below the body of the letter (Fig. 10–5).

PUNCTUATION

Traditionally, the punctuation pattern is selected on the basis of letter style. The message within the body of a business letter is always punctuated with normal punctuation. The other parts follow one of the following patterns.

Standard (Mixed) Punctuation. A colon is placed after the salutation and a comma after the complimentary closing. This is the punctuation pattern most commonly used and is appropriate with the blocked, semiblocked, and full blocked letter.

Open Punctuation. No punctuation is used at the end of any line outside the body of the letter unless that line ends with an abbreviation. This pattern is often used with the full block and always with the simplified letter styles.

PARTS OF LETTERS

The parts of letters and their placement are fairly standard, but there is some degree of flexibility and some variation in published guidelines. Just remember the objective—an attractively arranged communication that reflects dignity and clarity and says to the reader what you want to say.

Letterhead. The printed letterhead is usually centered at the top of the page and includes the name of the physician or group and the address. It may include the telephone number and the medical specialty (or specialties). In a group or corporate practice, the names of the physicians may also be listed.

Date Line. On standard stationery, the date line is typed two to three lines below the last line of the letterhead or on line 15, whichever is lower. The name of the month is written in full, followed by the day and year. The date should not be abbreviated, nor should ordinal numbers such as 1st, 2nd, and 3rd be used following the name of the month.

Inside Address. The inside address has two or more lines, starts flush with the left margin, and contains at least the name of the individual or firm to whom the letter is addressed, and the mailing address. When the letter is addressed to an individual, the name is preceded by a courtesy title, such as Dr., Mr., Mrs., Miss, or Ms. When addressing a letter to a physician, omit the courtesy title and type the physician's name followed by academic degree. Do not use both a courtesy title and a degree that mean the same thing, such as Dr. Herbert H. Long, M.D.

Attention Line. The attention line, if used, is placed on the second line below the inside address. The current trend, however, is to avoid using an attention line. If you know the name of the person for whom the letter is intended, use that person's name in the inside address, and address him/her personally. Use the same procedure if the letter is being directed to a division or department within a company.

Salutation. The salutation is the letter writer's introductory greeting to the person being addressed. It is typed flush with the left margin on the second line below the last line of the inside address. It is followed by a colon unless open

Text continued on page 129

```
        MEDICAL ARTS PROFESSIONAL ANNEX
            3578 North Willow Avenue
             Palm Beach, FL 33480



                            January 29, 1987



Elizabeth Blackwell, M.D.
223 Orange Avenue, N.W.
Cottonwood, UT 84121

Dear Doctor Blackwell:

We have two remaining street-level suites available
for occupancy about July 1.  These are marked on
pages 3 and 4 of the enclosed descriptive brochure.
If either of these suites appeals to you, we will be
pleased to customize it for your practice.

Please feel free to call me collect at the number on
the brochure for further discussion of your needs.

                        Sincerely yours,


                        Richard Fluege
                        Business Manager

RF:mk

Enc.
```

10

Figure 10–2
Blocked letter style.

WILLIAM OSLER, M.D.
1000 South West Street
Park Ridge, NJ 07656

January 26, 1987

Robert Koch, M.D.
398 Main Street
Park Ridge, NJ 07656

Dear Doctor Koch:

<u>Mrs. Elaine Norris</u>

Thank you for referring your patient, Mrs. Elaine Norris, for consultation and care. She was examined in the office today.

FINDINGS: The patient complained of pain in the left lower quadrant and some abdominal tenderness. She had a temperature of 100.2 degrees.

RECOMMENDATIONS: The patient was placed on a soft, low-residue, bland diet, antibiotics, and bedrest for a few days. Upper and lower gastrointestinal X-rays will be performed next week.

TENTATIVE DIAGNOSIS: Diverticulitis of large bowel.

Mrs. Norris has been asked to return here for re-evaluation in about ten days.

Sincerely yours,

William Osler, M.D.

WO:mk

Figure 10–3
Semiblocked letter style.

ELIZABETH BLACKWELL, M.D.
223 Orange Avenue, N.W.
Cottonwood, UT 84121

January 26, 1987

Mr. Richard Fluege
3578 North Willow Avenue
Palm Beach, FL 33480

Dear Mr. Fluege:

Please send me full particulars on the professional
suites you expect to offer for sale or rent in the
Medical Arts Professional Annex.

In about six months I will be ready to open my
practice, and I am interested in locating in Florida.
My preference is a street-level suite of approximately
2,000 square feet.

After I have had an opportunity to study the information
you send me, I will write or telephone you if I have
further questions.

Very truly yours,

Elizabeth Blackwell, M.D.

EB:mk

10

Figure 10–4
Full blocked letter style.

ROBERT KOCH, M.D.
398 Main Street
Park Ridge, NJ 07656

January 30, 1987

William Osler, M.D.
1000 South West Street
Park Ridge, NJ 07656

ANNABELLE ANDERSON

You'll be glad to know, Bill, that Mrs. Anderson is
progressing nicely. Her wound is healing. Her
temperature has returned to normal, and she is
beginning to resume her usual activities.

Mrs. Anderson has an appointment to return here
for one more visit next week. At that time, I will
ask her to return to you for any further care.

ROBERT KOCH, M.D.

mk

Figure 10–5
Simplified letter style.

punctuation is used. The words used in the salutation will vary depending upon the degree of formality of the letter. In addressing a physician, spell out the word "Doctor" (Dear Doctor Long).

Subject Line. Often in medical office correspondence, the subject of a letter is the patient. The patient's name is used as the subject line. Because the subject line is considered a part of the body of the letter, it is typed on the second line below the salutation. It may start flush with the left margin, at the point of indentation of indented paragraphs, or be centered. The word Subject, followed by a colon, may be used or may be omitted entirely.

Body of Letter. Begin typing the body of the letter (the message) on the second line below the subject line or the second line below the salutation if there is no subject line. The first line of each paragraph may be indented 5 spaces or may start flush with the left margin, depending upon the letter style being used.

Complimentary Close. The complimentary close is the writer's way of saying goodbye. The words used are determined by the degree of formality in the salutation. For instance, if the salutation is "Dear Herb:" the close might be "Cordially" or "Sincerely." If the letter is addressed to a business firm, the complimentary close generally used is "Very truly yours." The complimentary close is typed on the second line below the last line of the body of the letter, and followed by a comma unless open punctuation is used. Only the first word is capitalized.

Typewritten Signature. Typing the name of the signer of the letter is a courtesy to the reader, especially if the name does not appear on the printed letterhead. Type the signature on the fourth line directly below the complimentary close.

Reference Initials. The reference initials identify the dictator and the transcriptionist, and are typed flush with the left margin on the second line below the typed signature. If the medical assistant composes the letter, only the medical assistant's initials are used. There are variations in typing the reference initials, but the form most generally used has the dictator's initials in caps followed by a colon and the typist's initials in lower case (PF:mk).

Enclosure and Carbon Copy Notations. If the letter indicates an enclosure, type the word Enclosure or Enc. on the first or second line (authorities differ) below the reference initials. If there is more than one enclosure specify the number (Enclosures 3). If carbon copies are to be sent to others, type this notation in the same manner as the enclosure notation, or following it if both notations are

needed. The carbon copy notation is usually written cc:E.F. Duggan, M.D. If more than one carbon copy is to be distributed, list the names of the individuals either alphabetically or according to rank.

Second Page Heading. If the letter requires one or more continuation pages, the heading of the second and subsequent pages must contain three bits of information: (1) the name of the addressee, (2) the page number, and (3) the date. Three accepted forms for the heading are illustrated:

Elizabeth Blackwell, M.D.   -2-   March 14, 19xx

William Osler, M.D.
Page 2
March 14, 19xx

William S. Halsted, M.D.
Page 2
March 14, 19xx
Subject: Susan Barstow

The heading should be typed on the seventh line from the top of the page; continuation of the body of the letter begins on the tenth line or the third line below the heading.

Always carry at least two lines of the body of the letter over to the second page. Do not use a continuation page just to type the closing section of a business letter.

SIGNATURE

Some physicians prefer to sign all letters that leave their offices, but the majority do delegate to the medical assistant the responsibility of composing and signing some letters. Although not all authorities agree on the form to be followed, most recommend that a woman's typewritten signature include a title, Miss, Mrs., or Ms., and that the title not be enclosed in parentheses. It is not necessary to include the title in the handwritten signature.

How will you know which letters to sign? In general, the physician will sign all of the following:

- Letters that deal with medical advice to patients
- Letters to officers or committees of the medical society
- Referral and consultation reports to colleagues
- Medical reports to insurance companies
- Personal letters
- Any letters of a personal nature

The medical assistant usually signs letters concerning the following:

- Strictly routine or business matters, such as arranging or rescheduling appointments
- Ordering office supplies

Procedure 10-2

EQUIPMENT AND SUPPLIES

Typewriter or word processor
Draft paper
Letterhead paper
Pen or pencil
Want List of supplies needed
Medical and Office Supply Catalog
Correcting tape, liquid, or eraser (optional)

PROCEDURAL GOAL

To compose and type a letter ordering medical and office supplies, using tabular placement of items, and following the guidelines of a commonly used business letter style.

PROCEDURE

1. Locate items from Want List in catalog.
2. Note catalog number of each item, unit price, size and color, and any special information requirements.
   Explanation: Compare this information with Want List to confirm correctness of order.
3. Prepare a draft of letter by hand or typewriter, tabulating the items ordered.
   Purpose: To provide practice in composing a letter and the use of tabulation. (With sufficient experience this step can be eliminated.)
4. Edit draft carefully for correct information, grammar, spelling, and punctuation.
5. Insert letterhead in typewriter.
6. Set line and margins for attractive placement of letter.
7. Type letter from corrected draft.
8. Type your signature and identification initials.
   Explanation: The medical assistant signs letters ordering supplies.
9. Proofread letter for composition errors and accuracy of order.
   Purpose: Any necessary corrections are more easily accomplished while paper is still in typewriter.
10. Remove completed letter and sign.

TERMINAL PERFORMANCE OBJECTIVE

Given the listed equipment and supplies, compose a mailable letter without error or detectable corrections, within 20 minutes, to a performance level of 95%.

- Reserving hotel accommodations
- Notifying patients of surgery or hospital arrangements
- Collecting delinquent accounts
- Ordering subscriptions

ADDRESSING THE ENVELOPE

The Postal Service expects to soon have all mail (in No. 10 and No. 6¾ envelopes) read, coded, sorted, and cancelled automatically at regional sorting stations where mail can be processed at a rate of 30,000 letters per hour. The success of automatic sorting depends upon the cooperation of mailers in preparing envelopes in the format that can be read by automatic equipment. Key points are as follows:

- Use dark type on a light background. Black on white is best.
- Do not use script or italic type, because these cannot be read by the electronic scanner.
- Type all envelope addresses in the blocked format and in the area on the envelope that the scanner is programmed to read:
  No. 10 envelope—Type the address 12 lines from the top of the envelope and 4 inches from the left edge of the envelope.

No. 6¾ envelope—Type the address 12 lines from the top of the envelope and 2½ inches from the left edge of the envelope.
- Capitalize everything in the address.
- Eliminate all punctuation in the address.
- Use the standard two-letter state code instead of the spelled out name of the state (Fig. 10–6).
- The last line of the address must contain the city, state code, and ZIP code, and it must not exceed 22 digits. The digits should be distributed so they will not exceed the following limits:

Allowance for city name	13
Space between city name and state code	1
Allowance for state code	2
Space between state code and ZIP code	1
Allowance for ZIP code	5
	22

If a city name contains more than 13 digits

Procedure 10–3

WRITING INSTRUCTIONS

EQUIPMENT AND SUPPLIES

Local map
Name and address of patient
Typewriter or word processor
Draft paper
Pen or pencil
Bond paper
Envelope
Dictionary
Correcting tape, liquid, or eraser (optional)

10

PROCEDURAL GOAL

To inform new patient of most desirable automobile route to doctor's office, including any known landmarks, and description of parking facilities at destination.

PROCEDURE

1. Locate doctor's office on map.
2. Locate the patient's address on map.
   Purpose: To determine most desirable route between these two points.
3. On draft paper, using pencil or typewriter, compose directions, using street names and including any prominent intersections, right or left turns, landmarks just preceding destination, and means of identifying destination.
   Purpose: To create a mental picture of route and directions that can be easily followed.
4. Read your copy for clarity and recheck with map for accuracy.
   Purpose: Note spelling of street names and check for accuracy of direction turns.
5. Describe parking facilities and their utilization.
   Explanation: Include information about meters, validation, time limit, and so forth.
6. Describe route to doctor's office entrance from parking facility.
   Purpose: To provide peace of mind to patients who feel apprehensive about traveling to an unfamiliar location.
7. Check complete draft for clarity and detail.
   Purpose: It is very important that directions be accurate, clear, and complete.
8. Typewrite directions in narrative form on bond paper.
9. Proofread and correct any typographical errors.
10. Typewrite patient's mailing address on envelope using format for optical scanning.

TERMINAL PERFORMANCE OBJECTIVE

Given the listed equipment and supplies, write instructions that are clear, concise, and accurate, within 20 minutes, to a performance level of 100%.

<u>TWO-LETTER ABBREVIATIONS</u>

UNITED STATES AND TERRITORIES

Alabama	AL	Montana	MT
Alaska	AK	Nebraska	NE
Arizona	AZ	Nevada	NV
Arkansas	AR	New Hampshire	NH
California	CA	New Jersey	NJ
Canal Zone	CZ	New Mexico	NM
Colorado	CO	New York	NY
Connecticut	CT	North Carolina	NC
Delaware	DE	North Dakota	ND
District of Columbia	DC	Ohio	OH
Florida	FL	Oklahoma	OK
Georgia	GA	Oregon	OR
Guam	GU	Pennsylvania	PA
Hawaii	HI	Puerto Rico	PR
Idaho	ID	Rhode Island	RI
Illinois	IL	South Carolina	SC
Indiana	IN	South Dakota	SD
Iowa	IA	Tennessee	TN
Kansas	KS	Texas	TX
Kentucky	KY	Utah	UT
Louisiana	LA	Vermont	VT
Maine	ME	Virgin Islands	VI
Maryland	MD	Virginia	VA
Massachusetts	MA	Washington	WA
Michigan	MI	West Virginia	WV
Minnesota	MN	Wisconsin	WI
Mississippi	MS	Wyoming	WY
Missouri	MO		

CANADIAN PROVINCES AND TERRITORIES

Alberta	AB	Nova Scotia	NS
British Columbia	BC	Ontario	ON
Manitoba	MB	Prince Edward Island	PE
New Brunswick	NB	Quebec	PQ
Newfoundland	NF	Saskatchewan	SK
Northwest Territories	NT	Yukon Territory	YT

Figure 10–6
Two-letter abbreviations for states and territories should be used only with ZIP Codes in addresses.

you must use the approved code for that city as shown in the Abbreviations Section of the National Zip Code Directory.

The Postal Service provides three special sets of abbreviations: (1) state names; (2) long names of cities, towns, and places; and (3) names of streets and roads and general terms like University or Institute. By using these abbreviations it is possible to limit the last line of any domestic address to 22 strokes (see Postal Service Publication 59). The next-to-last line in the address block should contain a street address or post office box number, as in the following examples:

MEDICAL ASSOCIATES INCORPORATED
4444 WILSHIRE BOULEVARD
LOS ANGELES CA 90013

HENRY B TURNER MD
PO BOX 845
ALBANY NY 12210

Leave a bottom margin of at least ⅝ inch and a left margin of at least 1 inch. Nothing should be written or printed below the address block or to the right of it.

Any notations on the envelope directed toward the addressee, such as "personal" or "confidential," should be typed two lines below the return address and three spaces from the left edge of the envelope in all capitals. Any notations directed toward the post office, such as "special delivery" or "certified mail," should be typed in all capital letters in the upper right corner of the envelope immediately below the area where the stamp will be placed. If an address contains an attention line, it should be typed as the second line of the address. One visit to a regional postal center where automated letter-sorting machines are operating will convince anyone of the value of preparing machine-readable envelopes.

Return Address. Always place a complete return address on your envelope. The Postal Service will not deliver mail without postage, and if you should forget to stamp the envelope or if your stamp should fall off and there is no return address, it will go to the dead letter office. There the postal employees will open the mail in an attempt to identify the sender. If they find an address for the sender they will return the mail in a brown envelope with a notice of postage due. If they do not find an address for the sender, the mail is destroyed and you may never know what happened to it. At best it causes a great delay. If there is inadequate postage on your envelope it will be delivered to the addressee marked "postage due."

ZIP Codes. The Postal Service is continually striving to improve the mail service and keep costs down. The ZIP code is a very important part of the address, just as the area code is necessary for telephone numbers. When the USPS introduced its 5-digit ZIP Code in 1961, most people said it would never catch on. Today, they're saying the same thing about the ZIP-plus-4 program. In the ZIP-plus-4 system, the first five numbers of the ZIP code signify the delivery office, and the next four numbers signify street information, including what side of the street the addressee is on. The USPS says that ZIP-plus-4, used with the new automated letter-sorting machinery, can eliminate 20 mail handling steps and result in considerable cost savings. Mailers who use 9-digit ZIP codes on machine-readable mail first-class letter-size envelopes with typewritten addresses can save 0.9 of a cent per letter on mailings of at least 250 pieces. ZIP-plus-4 mailings of at least 500 pieces of presorted mail receive a discount of 0.5 cent per piece in addition to the basic presort rate.

Pre-Sorting. Large mailers can get a discount on postage for pre-sorting their mail. A discounted pre-sort rate is charged on each piece that is part of a group of 10 or more sorted to the same 5-digit code or a group of 50 or more pieces sorted to the same first 3-digit ZIP code (Information Guide on Pre-Sorted First Class Mail, Publication 61).

FOLDING AND INSERTING LETTERS

Standard ways of folding and inserting letters are used so that the letter will fit properly into the envelope and so that it can be removed easily without damage. The following three methods may be useful (Fig. 10–7):

1. To fold a standard-size letter for a No. 10 envelope, bring the bottom third of the letter up and make a crease. Fold the top of the letter down to within about ⅜ inch of the creased edge and make a second crease. The second crease goes into the envelope first.

2. To fold a standard-size letter for a 6¾ envelope, bring the bottom edge to within about ⅜ inch of the top edge and make a crease. Then, folding from the right edge, make a fold a little less than one-third the width of the sheet and crease it. Folding from the left edge, bring the edge to within about ⅜ inch of the previous crease. Insert the left creased edge into the envelope first.

3. To fold a letter for insertion into a window envelope, bring the bottom third of the letter up and make a crease, then fold the top of the letter back to the crease you made before. (The inside address should now be facing you.) This method is often followed for mailing statements.

PREPARING THE OUTGOING MAIL

Sealing and Stamping Hints. Here's a suggestion for speeding up the sealing of a number of envelopes. At statement time, for example, many envelopes will be going into the mail at once. Fan out unsealed envelopes, address side down, in groups of six to ten. Then draw a damp sponge over the flaps and, starting with the lower piece, turn down the flaps and seal each one. Do not use too much moisture, as this will cause the glue to spread and several letters will stick together.

A similar process simplifies stamping several letters at a time. If possible, purchase your stamps by the roll. Tear off about ten stamps. Fanfold them on the perforations so that they will separate easily. Again fan the envelopes, this time address side up. Wet a strip of stamps with the sponge and, starting at one end of the fanned envelopes, attach the stamp at the end of the strip, tear it off, and proceed to the next envelope.

Getting Faster Mail Service. Post offices that handle a large volume of mail will appreciate your mailing early in the day whenever possible. Place a letter tray on your desk or some other convenient place so that you can keep all outgoing mail together until you are able to send it on its way. For large mailings, local letters should be separated from out-of-town letters. Letters or packages that need to be rushed should be taken directly to the post office for mailing. Others can be placed in street boxes or your own building mail chute for pickup. Never leave packages on top of public mail boxes; these should always go to the post office.

10

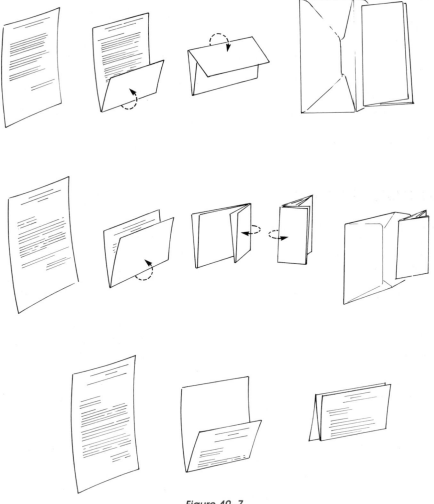

Figure 10–7
Correct methods for folding letters.

POSTAGE METERS

Metered mail does not have to be canceled or postmarked when it reaches the post office. This means that it can move on to its destination faster. The postage meter is the most efficient way of stamping the mail in a business office (Fig. 10–8). It can print postage onto adhesive strips that are then placed onto the envelopes or packages, or it can print the postage directly onto the envelope. Meters vary in size and capabilities. Consult your office equipment dealer for your own needs.

In order to use a postage meter, the user applies to the post office for a license, indicating the make and model of the meter desired. The postage meter machine is purchased, but the meter itself is leased from the manufacturer. The meter must be taken to the post office, where the user pays in advance for a specified amount of postage. This is recorded by the post office on the dials of the postage meter. When the meter is in operation, it records the amount of postage used and the amount remaining. Before the postage is exhausted, the meter should be taken to the office and more purchased. If the postage is entirely used up, the meter locks until it is again taken to the post office and more postage purchased. Planning can avoid this inconvenience.

Some of the newer models have an electronically controlled meter that can be reset without taking it to the post office.

MAILING COSTS

Although mailing fees are still one of our better bargains, the mailing costs for even a small office are a sizable item in the annual budget, and carelessness can cause them to soar. If your office does not have a postage meter that dispenses postage exactly, then be sure that you are not putting too many stamps on your outgoing mail. Use an accurate postage scale and remember that only the first ounce requires the base rate. Additional ounces over 1 ounce go for a lower rate.

In addition to saving postage dollars, the knowledgeable medical assistant can use many special postal services. The Postal Manual, containing information on what services are available, may be purchased from the Superintendent of Documents, US Government Printing Office, Washington, DC 20402. Smaller publications that contain basic postal information are available without charge from local post offices. A summary of the most common services follows.

CLASSIFICATIONS OF MAIL

Mail is classified according to type, weight, and destination. The ounce and pound are the units of measurement. Here are the types of mail commonly handled in a medical office:

First Class Mail—sealed or unsealed handwritten or typed material, such as letters, postal cards, postcards, and business reply mail. Postage for letters weighing 12 ounces or less is based on weight, in ounce increments. First class mail weighing over 12 ounces is classified as priority mail, and the postage is calculated on the basis of weight and destination, with the maximum weight being 70 pounds. Envelopes larger than the standard #10 business envelope should have the green diamond border to expedite first class delivery.

Second Class Mail—newspaper and periodical publications. Publishers who mail in bulk lots and who have been granted second class mail privileges pay a special second class rate. Copies mailed unsealed by the public go by transient rate, or the fourth class rate, whichever is lower.

Third Class Mail—printed matter or merchandise weighing up to but not including 16 ounces, and not included in first or second class. Third class mail includes such items as catalogs, circulars, books, photographs, and other printed matter, and even seeds, bulbs, keys, and so forth. Pieces should be sealed or secured, so that they can be handled by machine, but must be clearly marked with the two words "Third Class." Mailing of sealed articles at the third class rate carries the implied consent of the mailer to postal inspection of the contents.

Fourth Class Mail (Parcel Post)—merchandise, books, printed matter, and so forth, not included in the first or second class and weighing 16 ounces or more but not exceeding 70 pounds. There are also size limitations on fourth class mail; check with your post office regarding regulations on very large parcels. Rates are determined on the basis of weight

10

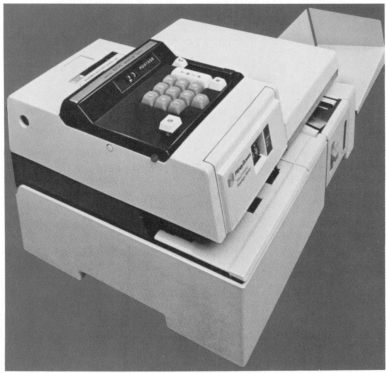

Figure 10–8
Example of one type of postage meter-mailing machine. (Courtesy of Pitney Bowes Company.)

and destination. Such mail may be sealed or unsealed.

Combination Mailing. A first class letter may be sent along with a parcel, either by placing the letter in an envelope and attaching it to the outside of the package or by enclosing it within the parcel and writing on the outside, just below the space for postage, "Letter Enclosed." In either case, separate postage is paid for the letter. This method is often used in the physician's office when mailing x-rays and an accompanying letter. This type of mailing travels with the appropriate class for the package, not with first class letters.

Educational Materials. A special rate, lower than regular fourth class, is applicable for educational materials. This includes bound books of 24 or more pages, manuscripts for books, sound recordings and films, and printed tests. The package must be marked "Educational Materials." This was formerly called the book rate.

SIZE STANDARDS FOR DOMESTIC MAIL

Nonstandard Mail. It is important to use the correct-sized envelope. The Postal Service assesses a surcharge on each piece of nonstandard mail in addition to the applicable postage and fees. Envelope sizes were standardized when the Postal Service began sorting mail by machine. The following material is considered nonstandard mail: first class mail weighing 1 ounce or less, or single-piece third class mail weighing 2 ounces or less, that:
1. Exceeds any of the following:
   Height—6⅛ inches
   Length—11½ inches
   Thickness—¼ inch
2. Has a height-to-length ratio that does not fall between 1:1.3 and 1:2.5 inclusive.

Minimum Mail Sizes. All mail must be at least 0.007 of an inch thick, and mail that is ¼ inch or less in thickness must be:
1. At least 3½ inches in height and at least 5 inches long, and
2. Rectangular in shape

PRIVATE MAIL SERVICES

Not all mail is delivered by the United States Postal Service. There are many private services that will pick up and deliver mail overnight; among these are Federal Express, Emory, and Purolator, which are highly advertised and competitive. United Parcel Service (UPS) has been available for many years and is increasing its services. All large cities and many smaller communities have centralized points where you may drop off your packages for the service of your choice. These are often more convenient than standing in line at a post office, and the services provided are more varied.

ELECTRONIC MAIL

Computer-to-computer communications systems are available for transmitting messages and documents. Some offer delivery within 2 hours. CompuServe, MCI Mail, Federal Express Corporation's ZapMail, and Western Union's EasyLine are examples of providers of these services. The transmitting and receiving computers may be located on the user's own premises or on the service provider's premises. The messages and documents may be received electronically or on paper.

E-COM (electronic computer-originated mail) service permits mailers to enter computer-generated messages into the postal service at designated serving post offices by electronic means. Messages are submitted in electronic form to one or more serving post offices, where they are transformed into printed letters, inserted into special marked envelopes, and delivered as first class mail.

Mailers may submit messages into private E-COM access service companies or directly to the USPS through dial-up access facilities. Service companies may perform a variety of data processing and transmission services in connection with E-COM service, including the collection of messages from many small mailers.

A list of companies providing E-COM access services can be obtained by writing the Director, Office of E-COM Operations, 475 L'Enfant Plaza SW, Washington, DC 20260-7140, or from your post office.

POSTAL SERVICES

Different types of mail require different handling by the post office. Make sure you classify your mail appropriately. Mail traveling long distances may be given special treatment.

Air Mail. All domestic first class mail outside the local area travels by air, and it is no longer necessary to use special air mail postage.

International Mail. Letters to distant points of the globe will in almost all cases be sent air mail and can be expected to reach their destination within a very few days. First class mail to Canada and Mexico travels at the same postal rates as within the United States. A table of other international rates can be obtained from your local post office. The rates for international mail are based on one-half ounce. Aerogrammes, thin air mail–weight sheets of paper that can be folded for mailing and do not require an envelope, can be purchased at the post office and used for sending messages anywhere in the world. In some cases this is a considerable saving. Writing can be on only one side of an aerogramme, and no enclosures are permitted. Aerogrammes are convenient as well as inexpensive. If you wish to supply a foreign correspondent with reply postage, international reply coupons may be purchased at the post office and sent to other countries.

Special Delivery. Any class mail that has been marked special delivery will be charged the special delivery rate. Such pieces may be regular first or second class mail, registered, insured, or COD (Collect on Delivery) pieces. Special delivery instruction generally does not speed up the normal travel time between two cities but does assure immediate delivery of the item when it arrives at the designated post office. Special delivery stamps may be purchased at the post office, or the equivalent value in regular stamps may be placed upon the envelope, which should always be clearly marked "Special Delivery." Use Special Delivery when you need delivery the same day the item is received at the addressee's post office, including weekend delivery not available with regular mail. Do not use for mail addressed to a Post Office Box or military installation.

Special Handling. For a small additional fee, third and fourth class mail will receive the fastest handling and ground transportation practicable, about the same as first class mail. This does not include insurance or special delivery at the destination, but special delivery, if desired, is available at an added fee. If a parcel is sent by priority mail, special handling is of no additional advantage, because it is already traveling at the greatest possible speed. Fees are determined according to weight.

Express Mail Service. This service is based on a high-speed delivery network linking all major cities in the United States as well as many smaller communities. One of its features is a Downtown-to-Downtown service, which guarantees that if you mail by 5 PM at the designated window, your urgent communication or parcel will be ready for pickup at the receiving post office at 10 AM the next business day or will be delivered by 3 PM. There are also special curbside pickup mailboxes for prepaid Express Mail in metropolitan areas. Five other service options are available on a contract basis under Express Mail:
1. Door to door
2. Your door to a destination airport
3. Originating airport to addressee
4. Airport to airport
5. United States to England

Check with your local post office for the availability of Express Mail service in your area.

Mailgram. A popular service offered jointly by the Postal Service and Western Union, the mailgram is described in Chapter 9 under Telegraph Services.

ENSURING PROPER DELIVERY

There are also ways to ensure proper delivery of valuable or important pieces of mail.

Certificate of Mailing. If a sender needs proof of mailing but is not especially concerned with proof of receipt of an item, the most economical method is to obtain a Certificate of Mailing. Fill in the required information, attach a stamp for the current fee, and hand it to the postal clerk along with the piece of mail. The clerk will postmark the receipt, initial it, and hand it back as acknowledgment of having received the piece of mail at the post office. This is sometimes used when mailing income tax reports or other items that must be posted by a certain date.

Certified Mail. Anything without intrinsic value that you wish to mail, on which postage is paid at the first class rate, will be accepted as certified mail. Such items as contracts, deeds, mortgages, bank books, checks, passports, insurance policies, money orders, and birth certificates, which are not valuable intrinsically but would be hard to duplicate if lost, should be certified. Certified mail is also often used as an aid in collections. Regular postage plus a Certified fee must be attached. For an additional fee, a receipt of delivery can be requested. Certified mail can be sent special delivery if the prescribed special delivery fees are paid. A record of delivery of certified mail is kept for 2 years at the post office of delivery. However, no record is kept at the post office of origin, and this type of mail does not provide insurance coverage. The medical assistant should keep a supply of certified mail forms and return receipts on hand (Figs. 10–9 and 10–10). These may be obtained at any post office. Full instructions are included on the forms. Fees and postage may be paid by ordinary postage stamps, meter stamps, or permit imprint. Certified mail can be mailed at any post office, station, or branch, or can be deposited in mail drops or in street letter boxes if you follow specific instructions.

Registered Mail. All classes of mail, particularly those of unusually high value, can be given additional protection, together with evidence of having been delivered, if registered. Registering mail also helps to trace delivery. When sending a registered letter it is necessary to go to the post office and fill in the required forms. All articles to be registered must be thoroughly sealed with Postal Service ap-

10

P04 9527980

RECEIPT FOR CERTIFIED MAIL

NO INSURANCE COVERAGE PROVIDED—
NOT FOR INTERNATIONAL MAIL
(See Reverse)

SENT TO

W B SAUNDERS

STREET AND NO.

W. WASHINGTON SQUARE

P.O., STATE AND ZIP CODE

PHILADELPHIA PA 19105

POSTAGE				$	
CONSULT POSTMASTER FOR FEES	CERTIFIED FEE				¢
	OPTIONAL SERVICES	SPECIAL DELIVERY			¢
		RESTRICTED DELIVERY			¢
		RETURN RECEIPT SERVICE	SHOW TO WHOM AND DATE DELIVERED X		¢
			SHOW TO WHOM, DATE, AND ADDRESS OF DELIVERY		¢
			SHOW TO WHOM AND DATE DELIVERED WITH RESTRICTED DELIVERY		¢
			SHOW TO WHOM, DATE AND ADDRESS OF DELIVERY WITH RESTRICTED DELIVERY		¢

TOTAL POSTAGE AND FEES	$
POSTMARK OR DATE	

PS Form 3800, Apr. 1976

CERTIFIED

P04 9527980

MAIL

Figure 10–9
Receipt for certified mail. Attach to front of envelope on left of address.

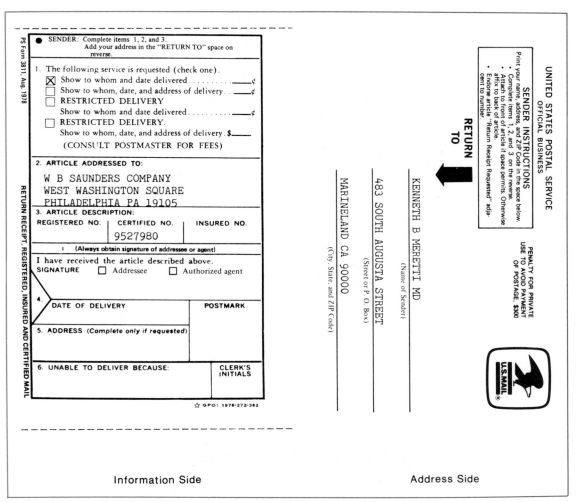

Figure 10–10

Receipt for delivery of certified, registered, or insured mail. Attach to front of article if space permits. Otherwise, attach to back of article and endorse front of article with return receipt requested *adjacent to the number.*

proved tape (do not use cellophane tape) and have postage paid at first class rates. Upon receipt of the item, the recipient is required to sign a form, acknowledging receipt of delivery. A registered letter may be released to the person to whom it is sent or to his agent. For an additional fee, a personal receipt may be requested. This assures that the letter will be released only to the individual to whom it is addressed. Such pieces bear the label "To Addressee Only." Registered mail is accounted for by number from time of mailing until delivery and is transported separately from other mail under a special lock. In case of loss or damage, the customer may be reimbursed up to $10,000, provided the value of the registered article has been declared at the time of mailing and the appropriate fee has been paid.

Insured Mail. Third or fourth class mail may be insured against loss. All packages valued at more than $25 and not registered should be insured. Parcel post packages may be registered with postage paid at the first class rate, but generally they are insured instead of registered. Indemnity on insured mail is limited.

Postal Money Orders. Postal money orders are a convenient way of mailing money, especially for the individual who does not have a personal checking account. Postal money orders may be purchased in amounts as high as $700. If a sum greater than $700 is needed, additional money orders must be purchased in increments of $700 or less. The rates are reasonable.

Money orders may also be sent via Western Union.

HANDLING SPECIAL PROBLEMS

Forwarding Mail. First class mail only may be forwarded from one address to another without payment of additional postage. Simply cross out the printed address and write in the address to which it should be delivered.

Obtaining Change of Address. If the mailer wants to know an addressee's new address, this service can be obtained from the post office by placing the words "Address Correction Requested" beneath the return address on the envelope. This can be handwritten, stamped, typewritten, or printed. The post office will charge a postage-due fee for this service. For first class mail, the post office will forward the piece of mail and return a card to the sender showing the forwarding address of the addressee. The card will have a postage due stamp on it for the amount of the required fee.

Recalling Mail. If you have dropped a letter in the mailbox and want it back, do not ask the mail collector to give it to you; he is not permitted to do this. Mail can be recalled, however, by making written application at the post office, together with an envelope addressed identically to the one being recalled. If your letter has already left the local post office, the postmaster, at the sender's expense, can telephone or telegraph the postmaster at the destination post office to return the letter.

Returned Mail. If a letter is returned to the sender after an attempt has been made to deliver it, it cannot be remailed without new postage. It is best simply to prepare a new envelope with the correct address, affix the proper postage, and remail.

Tracing Lost Mail. Receipts issued by the post office, whether for money orders, registered mail, certified mail, or insured mail, should be retained until receipt of the item has been acknowledged. If, after an adequate time elapses, no acknowledgment of receipt for such mailing arrives, notify the post office to trace the letter or package. Regular first class mail is not easily traced, but the post office will make every attempt to find it for you. In tracing a lost letter or package, the post office requires that a special form be filled out, on which data from any original receipt should be written, along with any other identifying information.

INCOMING MAIL

Each day a great variety of mail will be received at the doctor's office and must be processed. There will be:

- General correspondence
- Payments for services
- Bills for office purchases
- Laboratory reports
- Hospital reports
- Medical society mailings
- Professional journals
- Promotional pieces and samples from pharmaceutical houses
- Advertisements
- Insurance claim forms to be completed

In large clinics and centers the mail is opened by specially designated persons in some central department, to speed up this daily task. But in the average professional office, the medical assistant opens the mail, using the ordinary letter-opener method.

Procedure for Processing. Before opening any mail, the medical assistant should have an agreement with the physician as to what procedure to follow regarding incoming mail. In other words, what letters should be opened and what pieces does the doctor prefer to open personally? For instance, the physician may prefer to open any communications from an attorney or accountant, even when they are not marked Personal. If there is any doubt in your mind in regard to opening a letter, the best rule to follow is, Don't! Treat your doctor's mail with the same consideration you expect others to exercise toward your own.

Before tackling the mail, assemble the equipment and supplies you will need:

- Letter opener
- Paper clips
- Stapler
- Transparent tape
- Date stamp

Sorting. Sort the mail according to importance and urgency:

1. Mailgrams or special delivery letters
2. Checks from patients
3. Doctor's personal mail
4. Ordinary first class mail
5. Periodicals and newspapers
6. All other classes, including drug samples

Opening. Even such a simple procedure as opening the day's mail can be done with more efficiency if a good system is followed (Fig. 10–11). Have a clear working space on your desk or counter, and proceed as follows:

1. Stack the envelopes so that they are all facing in the same direction.
2. Pick up the top one and tap the envelope so that when you open it you will not cut the contents.
3. Open all envelopes along the top edge for easiest removal of contents.
4. Remove the contents of each envelope and hold the envelope to the light to see that nothing remains inside.
5. Make a note of the postmark when this is important.
6. Discard the envelope after you have checked to see that there is a return address on the message contained inside. (Some offices make it a policy to attach the envelope to each piece of correspondence until it has received attention.)
7. Date stamp the letter and attach any enclosures.
8. If there is an enclosure notation at the bottom of the letter, check to be sure the enclosure was included. Should it be missing, indicate this on the notation by writing the word "no" and circling it. It may be that this is as far as your employer will want you to proceed with handling the correspondence.

Annotating. If **annotating** the mail is within your duties, you can perform an additional service by reading each letter through, underlining the significant words and phrases, and noting in the margin any action required. This is called annotating. If it is a letter that needs no reply, you can code it for filing at this time. A non-print pencil that does not

10

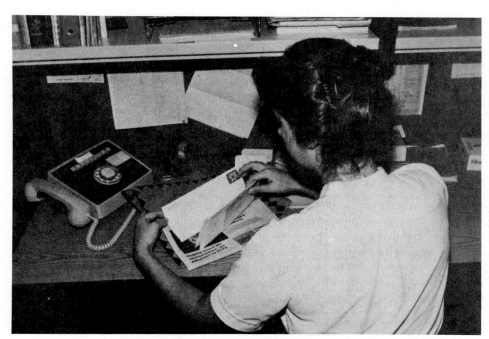

Figure 10–11
Medical assistant opening the mail. (Courtesy of Ferris State College, Big Rapids, MI.)

photocopy may be used for the annotating if desired.

When mail refers to previous correspondence, obtain this from the file and attach it. Or if a patient's chart is needed in replying to an inquiry, pull the chart and place it with the letter.

A specific place should be agreed upon for placing the opened and annotated mail. This will probably be some spot on the physician's desk. When you have completed the sorting, opening, and annotating of mail, place those items that the doctor will wish to see in the established place, with the most important mail on top. Personal mail, of course, is unopened. Should you in error open a piece of personal mail addressed to your employer, fold and replace it inside the envelope, and write across the outside "Opened in error," followed by your initials. Use the same procedure with a piece of mail addressed to another office that may have been opened in error. In that case, reseal the envelope with transparent tape, and hand it to your carrier.

Responding to the Mail. In some offices the doctor and the medical assistant go over the mail together. As you gain confidence, you will find that you can draft a reply to some inquiries. Most doctors are very pleased to delegate this responsibility, especially on matters that do not relate to patient care.

Letters of referral from other physicians should be carefully noted so that an answer may be sent after the doctor has seen the patient and can give a report. If considerable time may pass before such information can be sent, it is a courteous gesture to write a thank-you note to the referring physician advising that a detailed letter will follow. Some physicians send printed cards expressing thanks for referrals; others prefer to write thank-you letters to professional colleagues.

MAIL THE ASSISTANT CAN HANDLE

Cash Receipts and Insurance Forms. There will be some mail that the medical assistant can handle alone; for instance, payments from patients and insurance forms to be completed. All cash and checks should be separated and recorded immediately in the day's receipts. Insurance forms for completion should be put in a predetermined place for handling at the appropriate time. If there is an insurance clerk or other individual who processes the claims, they should be passed along to that person immediately.

Drug Samples. There may be sample drugs and related literature in the mail. Determine from the physician what types of literature and samples should be saved. Most physicians keep pertinent new samples in their desks, along with the accompanying literature for immediate reference. Other drug samples are categorically stored. Drugs should never be tossed into the trash. (See Chapter 18.)

VACATION MAIL

When the doctor is away from the office, it is generally the responsibility of the medical assistant to handle all mail. In this event, all pieces should be studied carefully. The medical assistant can then make a decision in regard to handling each piece on the basis of the following questions:

- Is this important enough that I should phone or telegraph the doctor?
- Shall I forward this for immediate attention?
- Shall I answer this myself or send a brief note to the correspondent explaining that there will be a slight delay because the doctor is out of the office?
- Can this wait for attention until the doctor returns without appearing negligent?

If you are unable to contact the physician or to forward important mail, always answer the sender immediately, explaining the delay and asking cooperation. Most offices have some kind of copy machine as part of the office equipment. Instead of forwarding an original piece of mail and risking possible loss, make a copy for forwarding. Then, if the physician wishes you to answer the letter, notations can be made on the copy and returned to you without defacing the original letter.

If your employer is traveling from place to place, the envelope on each communication should be numbered consecutively. Doing this enables the doctor to easily determine whether any mail has been lost or delayed. By keeping your own record of each piece of mail sent out, with its corresponding number, anything that might be lost can be identified and remailed if necessary.

Correspondence that does not require immediate action, but which the medical assistant is unable to answer until the doctor returns, should be placed in a special folder on the doctor's desk, marked "Requires Attention." Mail that the medical assistant can answer, but which requires the doctor's approval before mailing, should be put into another special folder, marked "For Approval." When the doctor returns, these letters can be rapidly checked and signed.

Any letters marked "Personal" that you hesitate to open and are unable to forward may be acknowledged to the return address on the envelope. The brief acknowledgment should state that the doctor is out of town for a certain length of time and will attend to the letter immediately upon returning. Your acknowledgment should also offer your help in any way possible in the meantime.

Discard any mail that you are sure the doctor

would not wish to see. Some promotional literature will fall into this category. (Make certain, however, that mailings from professional organizations, whether they are first, second, third, or fourth class, are saved.)

There may be rare periods when the entire office is closed. In such cases, the local post office should be notified to forward all first class mail to an address supplied by the doctor, if possible. Your postal carrier cannot accept an oral request to leave the mail with the person next door for a few days. A formal request must be made. If forwarding is out of the question, place a request with the post office to hold the mail until a specified date when someone will again be on duty. Never leave mail unattended to gather outside a mailbox or clutter up a doorway in a hall. Even mail slots may become filled or magazines may become stuck in them, causing important mail to pile up outside the slot. There is far too much money and mail of a confidential nature sent to doctors' offices to take chances on mail theft or destruction.

Systematizing your routine for processing all incoming and outgoing mail can put you in control of the paper blizzard!

REFERENCES AND READINGS

Jennings, L. M.: *Secretarial and Administrative Procedures*, 2nd ed. Englewood Cliffs, NJ, Prentice-Hall, 1983.

Kutie, R., and Rhodes, J.: *Secretarial Procedures for the Electronic Office*, 2nd ed. New York, Wiley, 1985.

Popham, D., et al.: *Secretarial Procedures and Administration*, 6th ed. Cincinnati, South-Western Publishing Co., 1983.

Sabin, W.: *The Gregg Reference Manual*, 5th ed. New York, Gregg Division/McGraw-Hill, 1984.

Strunk, W., Jr., and White, E. B.: *The Elements of Style*, 3rd ed. New York, Macmillan, 1979.

The Postal Manual. Superintendent of Documents, US Government Printing Office, Washington, DC.

10

CHAPTER OUTLINE

Reasons for Medical Records
Style and Form of Records
Contents of the Complete Case History
    Subjective Information
    Objective Information

Problem-Oriented Medical Record
Obtaining the History
Making Additions and Corrections
Keeping Records Current
Transfer of Files
Retention and Destruction of Records
    Case Histories
    Business Records

Protection of Records
Storage of Records
Filing Equipment

Supplies
    Procedure 11–1: Initiating a Medical File
    for a New Patient

Filing Procedures
Rules for Indexing
Filing Systems
    Alphabetic Filing
    Numeric Filing
    Subject Filing
    Color Coding
    Procedure 11–2: Color Coding Patient
    Charts

Organization of Files
    Procedure 11–3: Filing Supplemental
    Material in Established Patient
    Histories

VOCABULARY

See Glossary at end of book for definitions.

alphabetic filing	direct filing system	shelf filing
alpha-numeric	filing system	statute of limitations
caption	litigation	subject filing
chronologic order	microfilming	tab
continuity	numeric filing	tickler
correlation	pejorative	transfer
cross-reference	retention schedule	unit
demographic	sequential	

Medical Records Management

OBJECTIVES

Upon successful completion of this chapter you should be able to:

1. Define the terms listed in the Vocabulary of this chapter.
2. State three important reasons for keeping good medical records.
3. Illustrate the meaning of subjective and objective information in a medical history.
4. List four categories each of subjective and objective information contained in a complete case history.
5. List the 15 items of personal data needed on a patient history.
6. Explain the basic differences between the traditional and the problem-oriented medical record (POMR), and three advantages of the POMR.
7. Discuss changing an entry in the medical record and the importance of following correct procedure.
8. List and describe the three classifications of patient files.
9. List and discuss the basic equipment and supplies in a filing system.
10. Describe the seven sequential steps in filing a document.
11. List and discuss application of the four basic filing systems.
12. Explain how color-coding of files can be advantageous in a medical facility.

Upon successful completion of this chapter you should be able to perform the following activities:

1. Initiate a medical record for a new patient.
2. Add reports and correspondence into the patient's file in the correct manner and sequence.
3. Make a correction in a patient's chart in a manner affording legal protection.
4. Typewrite a list of names in indexing order and arrange them alphabetically for filing.
5. Arrange a group of patient numbers in filing sequence for a terminal digit filing system.
6. Using the color key in this chapter, state the tab color to be used for a given list of names.

Records management is not just a fancy name for storing information. Management of medical records includes not only assembling the medical record for each patient but also having an efficient system for the filing, retrieval, transferring, protection, retention, storage, and destruction of these records.

Some of the objectives of good records management are:

- Saving space
- Reducing filing equipment expenditures
- Reducing the creation of unnecessary records
- Faster retrieval of information
- Reducing misfiles
- Compliance with legal safeguards
- Protection of confidentiality
- Saving the physician's and the patients' time

Complete and accurate records are essential to a well-managed medical practice. They provide a continuous story of a patient's progress from the first visit to the last. The treatment and therapy prescribed are noted, along with regular reports on the patient's condition. When a patient is discharged, the degree of improvement is placed upon the record.

REASONS FOR MEDICAL RECORDS

There are three important reasons for carefully recording medical information:

1. To Provide the Best Medical Care. The doctor examines the patient and enters the findings on the patient's medical record. These findings are the clues to diagnosis. The doctor may order many types of tests to confirm or augment the clinical findings. As the reports of these tests come in, the findings fall into place like the pieces of a jigsaw puzzle. Now, with the confirmation data to support the diagnosis, the physician can prescribe treatment and form an opinion about the patient's chances of recovery, assured that every resource has been used to arrive at a correct judgment.

Keeping good medical records helps a physician provide **continuity** in the patients' medical care. Earlier illnesses and difficulties that appear on the patient's record may supply the key to current medical problems. For example, the information on the record that the patient was treated for rheumatic fever as a child can be extremely important in determining the course of treatment the doctor prescribes for that patient when an illness develops a number of years later.

2. To Supply Statistical Information. Medical records may be used to evaluate the effectiveness of certain kinds of treatment or to determine the incidence of a given disease. **Correlation** of such statistical information may result in a new outlook on some phases of medicine and can lead to revised

techniques and treatments. The statistical data from medical records also are valuable in the preparation of scientific papers, books, and lectures.

3. To Provide Legal Protection. Sometimes a physician must produce case histories and medical records in court. For example, a patient may wish to substantiate claims made to an insurance company for damages resulting from an accident in which the patient was injured and required medical treatment. A patient may involve a physician in **litigation.** The physician's records can be a help or a hindrance, depending on the care with which they are kept.

For adequate legal protection the patient record should include the following:

- Patient's medical history
- Results of examinations
- Records of treatment
- Copies of laboratory reports
- Notations of all instructions given
- Copies of all prescriptions, and notes on refill authorizations
- Documentation of informed consent when applicable
- Any other pertinent data

Specific quotes of comments made by the patient about symptoms or reasons for consulting the doctor are particularly helpful if there should ever be litigation. The doctor should also record what was told the patient.

When a patient fails to follow instructions or refuses recommended treatment, a letter to this effect should be sent to the patient by certified mail, and a copy retained in the medical record. A similar type of letter should be sent if the patient leaves the doctor's care or if the doctor feels it is necessary to withdraw from the case.

Some entries should not be made in the record. For instance, reports from consulting physicians should not be placed in the record until they have been carefully reviewed to ensure that the overall diagnostic and treatment plan is consistent with them, or to identify and justify any inconsistencies. If the report contains confidential data from another source, release of such data without authorization can lead to legal difficulties. Transferred records from past treating physicians should never be added to the patient's new record until the physician has reviewed them. The same advice would apply to records received from any outside source, e.g., hospital emergency departments or freestanding urgent care clinics. **Pejorative** or flippant comments should never be entered in the record. For example, one doctor sometimes entered only one note in the record after seeing a patient who tended toward hypochondria: "Same verse, same refrain" or "New verse, same refrain." This would not have looked good in court. In most states, patients or their representatives have the legal right to a copy of their medical records.

Sometimes a record introduced in court may be of more significance because of an omission than for what was included. If information that should have been included in a record is omitted, a jury may form the opinion that the omission was deliberate and intended to conceal the truth.

STYLE AND FORM OF RECORDS

A record is any form of recorded information. It may be on:

- Paper
- Film
- A magnetic medium such as computer tapes or disks

If a record is to be useful, it must be easily retrievable, orderly, complete, and understandable by anyone who needs to use it. To be helpful it must be completely accurate. To be good it must be brief.

Coding of information on records is sometimes a helpful shortcut, but any coding system used should be a standard one that can be understood by anyone who needs to consult the chart. If the coding does vary somewhat from the standard, an explanation of the code should be prepared and placed in the front of the files for immediate reference (Table 11–1).

The style and form selected by a physician for recording case histories will depend partly upon the nature of the practice. General practitioners and some specialists keep very detailed records. A spe-

```
                    REGISTRATION SLIP

PLEASE PRINT              DATE  April 20, 1988
NAME  Morris, Samuel Albert
ADDRESS  3810 Commonwealth Avenue
                                      ZIP
CITY  Los Angeles, CA                 CODE  90056
                          Birth
Telephone 213 862 9917    Date 04-05-40  Sex  M

   ☐ Single  ☒ Married  ☐ Widowed  ☐ Divorced

Occupation    Merchant        Phone 213 462 8122
Employed by  Morris Appliances (self)
Employer's address 5400 Hollywood Blvd,LA 90036
Name of Spouse
or Parent  Louise Marie
Occupation   Office Manager    Phone 213 462 8122
Employed by  Morris Appliances
Employer's address (see above)
Referred by  Frank Gentry, M.D.
                         Soc. Sec.
INSURANCE:               Number  012 34 5678
Medical Insurance Cert. No.  WD 4305
Company  Occidental
Hospital Insurance Cert. No.
Company
Other Health Insurance

FORM NO. 3320. COLWELL CO., CHAMPAIGN, ILL.
```

Figure 11–1
Patient registration slip. (Courtesy of Colwell Systems, Champaign, IL.)

11

cialist who sees patients only on a consultant basis, or a specialist who is likely to see a patient only once, such as a dermatologist, a radiologist, or an anesthesiologist, need not keep complex records.

The nature of the patient's complaint is also a factor in determining just how detailed a record should be. If a patient comes into a physician's office to have a foreign body removed from an eye or to have some minor injury such as a cut finger treated, a detailed past medical history or family history is unnecessary. In contrast, the patient who is being treated for cardiac, hypertensive, or diabetic symptoms will require a complete examination and a detailed history.

In some medical offices where detailed histories are not required, a simple patient registration slip (Fig. 11–1) can be used to record personal data and a plain sheet of paper used to record the complaint and treatment given. In the great majority of offices, however, a more complete record and an individual folder for each patient is preferable.

The physician who uses just a plain sheet of paper for the patient record generally develops an outline that serves as a guide to taking down the information required for a history. The physician

Table 11–1
Abbreviations Commonly Used in Patient History and Physical Examination

Abbreviation	Meaning
A & W	Alive and well
CC	Chief complaint
CNS	Central nervous system
CR	Cardiorespiratory
CV	Cardiovascular
Dx	Diagnosis
FH	Family history
GI	Gastrointestinal
GU	Genitourinary
GYN	Gynecology
HEENT	Head, ears, eyes, nose, throat
MM	Mucous membrane
PH	Past history
PI	Present illness
prn	As necessary (pro re nata)
ROS/SR	Review of systems/Systems review
TPR	Temperature, pulse, respirations
UCHD	Usual childhood diseases
VS	Vital signs
w/d	Well developed
w/n	Well nourished
WNL	Within normal limits

then dictates the history, and the medical assistant types it according to an established format and places it in the patient's folder, after having it read and initialed by the physician. In every medical arena you will find certain technical terms being used frequently in the doctor's reports. The medical assistant who types the reports should become familiar with the correct spelling and meaning of the medical terms. Because of the close similarity in sound and spelling of some medical terms, it is wise to also check the definition to be sure the word fits the context in which it is used.

For the physician who wishes to use a more structured format, there are many different types of forms available from professional stationers: forms for general practice, obstetrics, surgery, pediatrics, internal medicine, or any other of the established specialities. Some physicians design their own forms to suit their particular practice and have them printed to order. Companies that specialize in medical forms sometimes provide a planning kit for the physician to use. Local printers, too, often can be very helpful in form design. The record may be **sequential**, or it may be separated into "problems," as described later, in the section on the problem-oriented medical record. Regardless of the form it takes, the case history will contain certain basic information.

CONTENTS OF THE COMPLETE CASE HISTORY

Recordkeeping in the hospital medical records department is deemed important enough that it is entrusted only to specially trained individuals. The position of medical record librarian requires a master's degree; a medical record technician requires an associate degree with specialization in the specifics of cataloging and recordkeeping in the hospital medical records department. The medical assistant in a doctor's office does not need such extensive training, but must be familiar with the basic essentials of recordkeeping.

The medical case history is the most important record in a doctor's office. For completeness each patient's record should contain:
A. *Subjective Information Provided by the Patient*
   1. Routine personal data about the patient
   2. Patient's personal and medical history
   3. Patient's family history
   4. Patient's complaint (in the patient's own words) and date of onset
B. *Objective Information Provided by the Doctor*
   5. Physical examination and findings; laboratory and x-ray reports
   6. Diagnosis and prognosis
   7. Treatment prescribed and progress noted
   8. Condition at time of termination of treatment
If these entries are completed, the case history will

stand the test of time. No branch of medicine is exempt from the necessity of keeping records. Records aid the physician in the practice of medicine, as well as provide legal protection.

Subjective Information

Routine Personal Data About the Patient. The patient's case history begins with routine personal data, which the patient usually supplies on the first visit. The basic facts needed are:
   1. Patient's full name, spelled correctly
   2. If patient is a child, names of parents
   3. Patient's sex
   4. Date of birth
   5. Marital status
   6. Name of spouse, if married
   7. Number of children, if any
   8. Home address and telephone number
   9. Occupation
   10. Name of employer
   11. Business address and telephone number
   12. Employment information for spouse
   13. Health insurance information
   14. Source of referral
   15. Social Security number

Patient's Personal and Medical History. This portion of the medical record, which is often obtained by having the patient complete a questionnaire, provides information about any past illnesses or surgical operations that the patient may have had, and includes data about injuries or physical defects, congenital or acquired. It also furnishes information about the patient's daily health habits.

Patient's Family History. The family history comprises the physical condition of the various members of the patient's family, any past illnesses or diseases that individual members may have suffered, and a record of the causes of death. This information is important, since a definite hereditary pattern is often present in the case of certain diseases.

Patient's Complaint. This is a concise account of the patient's symptoms, explained in the patient's own words. It should include the nature and duration of pain, if any, the time when the patient first noticed symptoms, the patient's opinion as to the possible causes for the difficulties, any remedies that the patient may have applied prior to seeing the doctor, and any other medical treatment received for the same condition in the past.

Objective Information

All of the foregoing facts are provided by the patient. Objective findings, sometimes referred to as "signs," become evident from the physician's examination of the patient.

Physical Examination and Findings; Laboratory and X-ray Reports. This section of the case history varies greatly with the specialty of the physician and the complaint of the patient. After the physician has examined the patient, the physical findings are recorded on the history. Results of other tests or requests for these tests are then recorded or, if they appear on separate sheets, attached to the history.

Diagnosis. The physician, on the basis of all evidence provided by the patient's past history, the physician's examination, and any supplementary tests, places the diagnosis of the patient's condition upon the medical record. If there is some doubt, it may be termed "Provisional Diagnosis."

Treatment Prescribed and Progress Notes. The physician's suggested treatment is listed following the diagnosis. Generally, instructions to the patient to return for follow-up treatment in a specific period of time are noted here, too.

On each subsequent visit, the date must be entered on the chart, and information about the patient's condition and the results of treatment added to the history, on the basis of the physician's observations. Notations of all medications prescribed or instructions given, as well as the patient's own progress report, should be placed in the record. Any home visits are noted. If the patient is hospitalized, the name of the hospital, the reason for admission, and the dates of admission and discharge are recorded. Much of this information may be obtained from the hospital discharge summary.

Condition at Time of Termination of Treatment. When the treatment is terminated, the physician will record that information. For example:

August 18, 1987. Wound completely healed. Patient discharged.

PROBLEM–ORIENTED MEDICAL RECORD

The traditional patient record is "source-oriented"; that is, observations and data are catalogued according to their source—physician, laboratory, x-ray, nurse, technician—with no recording of a logical relationship between them. The problem-oriented medical record (POMR) is a radical departure from the traditional system of keeping patient records. It is sometimes referred to as the "Weed System" because it was originated by Lawrence L. Weed, MD, a professor of medicine at the University of Vermont's College of Medicine. The POMR is a record of clinical practice that divides medical action into four bases:

1. The *data base* includes chief complaint, present illness, and patient profile; and also a review of systems, physical examination, and laboratory reports.

2. The *problem list* is a numbered and titled list of every problem the patient has that requires management or workup. This may include social and **demographic** troubles as well as strictly medical or surgical ones.

3. The *treatment plan* includes management, additional workups needed, and therapy. Each plan is titled and numbered with respect to the problem.

4. The *progress notes* include structured notes that are numbered to correspond with each problem number.

One company, which designed the Andrus/Clini-Rec Charting System, has developed a file folder for its recommended organization of patient data. The folder is preprinted on the front for age dating and easy access to basic information. With the calendar years printed on the cover it is simple to keep track of when the patient was last seen. On the initial visit, the year, say 1985, is checked on the cover. If the patient appears again in 1987, and the year 1986 is not checked, you know immediately that more than a year has elapsed since the last visit (Fig. 11–2). The system has suggested dividers for lab reports, consultations, hospital reports, and x-ray and EKG reports (all scientific information) on the left side; and data base and progress notes (communication and supervision) on the right side.

The chart is begun by obtaining a patient-completed data base system record, which contains family and past medical history together with 135 carefully selected screening questions. It is so designed that the page that goes into the chart shows only the positive answers (Fig. 11–3). There are also questionnaires designed for screening problems in specialty practices.

The problem list is entered on the divider cover for lab reports. Special sections are provided for current major and chronic problems, and for inactive major or chronic problems. The divider cover for progress notes is a chart for listing medications and other therapeutic modalities. Progress notes follow the SOAPing approach (Fig. 11–4):

    S Subjective impressions
    O Objective clinical evidence
    A Assessment or diagnosis
    P Plans for further studies, treatment or management

The problem-oriented medical record has the advantage of imposing order and organization on the information added to a patient's medical record. The records are more easily reviewed, and the likelihood of overlooking a problem is greatly reduced. SOAPing essentially forces a rational approach to patient problems and assists in formulating a logical and orderly plan of patient care.

While the POMR was practically unheard of be-

____CREDIT____

Vol. No.: _VII_

Patient Name: _BROWNING, ELIZABETH B._

Patient Address: _1400 TIMOTHY LANE_

City, State: _BELLVIEW, MS_

Patient Telephone: _323-1609_

Doctor: _MEARS_

PATIENT CLASSIFICATION

IND. ACCIDENT	MEDICAID	MEDICARE
		XXX

ALLERGIC REACTIONS

DATE	SUBSTANCE	EFFECT
01/84	PENICILLIN	HIVES

Bibbero Systems, Inc.

ANDRUS/CLINI-REC® PRIMARY CARE

CHARTING SYSTEM

16-7100-00   BIBBERO SYSTEMS, INC., PETALUMA, CA.

1985	✗
1986	✗
1987	✗
1988	
1989	
1990	
1991	
1992	
1993	
1994	
1995	
1996	
1997	
1998	
1999	
2000	
2001	
2002	
2003	
2004	
2005	

Figure 11–2

Andrus/Clini-Rec File Folder, preprinted on the front for age dating and easy access to basic information. (Courtesy of Bibbero Systems, Inc., Petaluma, CA.)

QUESTIONNAIRE

CONFIDENTIAL

27. Do you wear eyeglasses? . . . . No___ Yes___
28. Do you wear contact lenses? . . . . No___ Yes___
29. Has your vision changed in the last year? . . . . No___ Yes___

VISION/HEARING
Wears eyeglasses
Wears contacts
Vision changed in last year

	Rarely/Never	Occasionally	Frequently	
30. How often do you have:				
a. Double vision?				Double vision
b. Blurry vision?				Blurred vision
c. Watery or itchy eyes?				Watery/itchy eyes
31. Do you ever see colored rings around lights?				Sees halos
32. Do others tell you you have a hearing problem?				Hearing problem
33. Do you have trouble keeping your balance?				Loses balance
34. Do you have any discharge from your ears?				Discharge from ears
35. Do you ever feel dizzy or have motion sickness?				Dizzy/motion sickness

36. Do you have any problems with your hearing? . . . . . No___ Yes___ Hearing problems
37. Do you ever have ringing in your ears? . . . . No___ Yes___ Ringing in ears

NOSE/THROAT/RESPIRATORY

	Rarely/Never	Occasionally	Frequently	
				Head colds
				Chest colds
				Runny nose
				Head congestion
				Sore/hoarse throat
				Coughing spells
				Sneezing spells
				Trouble breathing
				Nose bleeds
				Cough blood

No___ Yes___ Worked on a farm
No___ Yes___ Worked in a mine
No___ Yes___ Worked in a laundry/mill
No___ Yes___ Worked in high dust concentrations
No___ Yes___ Exposed to toxic chemicals
No___ Yes___ Exposed to radioactive materials
No___ Yes___ Exposed to asbestos

CARDIOVASCULAR

Rarely/Never	Occasionally	Frequently	
			Out of breath quickly when exercising
			Dizziness
			Fainted

PART C – BODY SYSTEMS REVIEW

I. **MEN**: Please answer . . .
skip to quest . . .
WOMEN: Please st . . .

MEN ONLY
1. Have you had o . . . prostate troubl . . .
2. Do you have . . . or with impo . . .
3. Have you e . . . lesions on . . .
4. Have you . . . from your . . .
5. Do you . . . or swelling . . .
Check here if you wish . . .

GENITAL
. . . rouble . . . . Yes___
. . . oblems or . . .
. . . on penis . . . . Yes___
. . . . Yes___
. . . . Yes___

		Occasionally	Frequently
6. Is it sometimes hard to start your . . .			
7. Is urination ever painful?			
8. Do you have to urinate more than 5 times a da . . .			
9. Do you get up at night to urinate?			
10. Has your urine ever been bloody or dark colored?			
11. Do you ever lose urine when you strain, laugh, cough or sneeze?			
12. Do you ever lose urine during sleep?			

WOMEN ONLY

Do you:	Rarely/Never	Occasionally	Frequent
13. a. Have any menstrual problems?			
b. Feel rather tense just before your period?			
c. Have heavy menstrual bleeding?			
d. Have painful menstrual periods?			
e. Have any bleeding between periods?			
f. Have any unusual vaginal discharge or itching?			
g. Ever have tender breasts?			
h. Have any discharge from your nipples?			
i. Have any hot flashes?			

14. How many times, if any, have you been pregnant? ____
15. How many children born alive? ____
16. Are you taking birth control pills? . . . . No___ Yes___
17. Do you examine your breasts for lumps every month? . . . . No___ Yes___
17a. What was the date of your last menstrual period? . . . . Date____
Check here if you wish to discuss any special problem with the doctor . . . .

MEN & WOMEN

	Rarely/Never	Occasionally	Frequent
18. In the past year have you had any:			
a. Severe shoulder pain?			
b. Severe back pain?			
c. Muscle or joint stiffness or pain due to sports, exercise or injury?			
d. Pain or swelling in any joints not due to sports, exercise or injury?			

19. Do you have dry skin or brittle fingernails? . . . . . No___ Yes___
20. Do you bruise easily? . . . . No___ Yes___
21. Do you have any moles that have changed in color or size? . . . . No___ Yes___
22. Do you have any other skin problems? . . . . No___ Yes___

23. In the last 3 months have you had:
   a. A fever that lasted more than one day? . . . . . . No___ Yes___
   b. Sores or cuts that were hard to heal? . . . . No___ Yes___
   c. Any cold sores (fever blisters)? . . . . No___ Yes___
   d. Any lumps in your neck, armpits or groin? . . . . . No___ Yes___
   e. Do you ever have chills or sweat at night? . . . . No___ Yes___

24. Have you traveled out of the country in the last 2 years? . . . . No___ Yes, Traveled in:___

25. Write in the dates for the shots you have had: . . . .
   Measles____ Smal____
   Mumps____ Teta____
   Polio____ Typh____

26. Have you had a tuberculin (TB) skin test? . . . . . . No___ Yes____ Date____
   If so, was it negative or positive? . . . . Neg____ Pos____

© 1979, 1983 Bibbero Systems International, Inc. **PLEASE TURN THIS PAGE** 19-711-4 5/83

Chart No. _____

ANDRUS/CLINI-REC® HEALTH HISTORY QUESTIONNAIRE Today's Date 05/25/85

Identification Information
Name BROWNING, ELIZABETH B. Date of Birth 10/31/86
Occupation Accountant Marital Status Married

PART A – PRESENT HEALTH HISTORY

I. CURRENT MEDICAL PROBLEMS
Please list the medical problems for which you came to see the doctor. About when did they begin?

Problems	Date Began
Cough	Jan. '85

What concerns you most about these problems?
Persistence of cough; Family History

If you are being treated for any other illnesses or medical problems by another physician, please describe the problems and write the name of the physician or medical facility treating you.

Illness or Medical Problem	Physician or Medical Facility	City

II. MEDICATIONS
Please list all medications you are now taking, including those you buy without a doctor's prescription (such as aspirin, cold tablets or vitamin supplements)
Vit B complex

III. ALLERGIES AND SENSITIVITIES
List anything that you are allergic to such as certain foods, medications, dust, chemicals, or soaps, household items, pollens, bee stings, etc., and indicate how each affects you.

Allergic To:	Effect	Allergic To:	Effect
Penicillin	Hives		

IV. GENERAL HEALTH, ATTITUDE AND HABITS

How is your overall health now? . . . . Health now: Poor___ Fair___ Good__X__ Excellent___
How has it been most of your life? . . . . Health has been: Poor___ Fair___ Good___ Excellent__X__
In the past year:
Has your appetite changed? . . . . Appetite: Decreased___ Increased___ Stayed same__X__
Has your weight changed? . . . . Weight: Lost___lbs Gained___lbs No change__X__
Are you thirsty much of the time? . . . . Thirsty: No__X__ Yes___
Has your overall 'pep' changed? . . . . Pep: Decreased___ Increased___ Stayed same__X__
Do you usually have trouble sleeping? . . . . . . Trouble sleeping: No__X__ Yes___
How much do you exercise? . . . . Exercise: Little or none___ Less than I need__X__ All I need___
Do you smoke? . . . . Smokes: No__X__Yes___If yes, how many years?___
How many each day? . . . . Cigarettes___Cigars___Pipesfull___
Have you ever smoked? . . . . Smoked No___Yes__X__If yes, how many years?_20_
How many each day? . . . . _20_Cigarettes___Cigars___Pipesfull___
Do you drink alcoholic beverages? . . . . Alcohol: No___Yes__X__I drink___Beers_2_Glasses of Wine___Drinks of hard liquor - per day

Have you ever had a problem with alcohol? . . . . Prior problem: No__X__ Yes___
How much coffee or tea do you usually drink? . . . . Coffee/Tea: _3_ cups of coffee or tea a day.
Do you regularly wear seatbelts? . . . . Seatbelts: No___ Yes__X__

DO YOU:	Rarely/Never	Occasionally	Frequently	DO YOU:	Rarely/Never	Occasionally	Frequently
Feel nervous?	X			Ever feel like committing suicide?	X		
Feel depressed?		X					
Find it hard to make decisions?	X			Feel bored with your life?	X		
Lose your temper?	X	X		Use marijuana?	X		
Worry a lot?	X			Use "hard drugs"?	X		
Tire easily?			X				
Have trouble relaxing?		X		Do you want to talk to the doctor about a personal matter? No__X__ Yes___			
Have any sexual problems?	X						

Created and Developed by "Medical Economics" Professional Systems
Copyright © 1979, 1983 Bibbero Systems International, Inc.

STOCK NO. 19-711-4 5/83

Page 1

CONFIDENTIAL

11

Figure 11–3

Data base self-administered general health history questionnaire. (Courtesy of Bibbero Systems, Inc., Petaluma, CA.)

OUTLINE FORMAT PROGRESS NOTES

Patient Name _____ Mrs. Evelyn _____

Prob. No. or Letter	DATE	**S** Subjective	**O** Objective	**A** Assess	**P** Plans

Page _____ 4 _____

| 1 | 9/6/87 | Patient complains of two days of severe high epigastric pain and burning, radiating through to the back. Pain accentuated after eating. |

On examination there is extreme guarding and tenderness, high epigastric region. No rebound. Bowel sounds normal. BP 110/70.

R/O gastric ulcer, pylorospasm.

To have upper gastrointestinal series. Start on Cimetidine 300 mg. q.i.d. Eliminate coffee, alcohol & aspirin. Return two days.

Start each Progress Note (Subjective, Objective,   Assessment and Plans) at the appropriate   shaded column to create an outline form. Write
through the intervening columns to the right   margin of the page.

ANDRUS/CLINI-REC® PRIMARY CARE CHARTING SYSTEM FORM NO. 26-7115, ©1976 BIBBERO SYSTEMS, INC., PETALUMA, CA.

Figure 11–4

The SOAP Progress Note form. The four columns on the left indicate **S**ubjective impressions, **O**bjective clinical evidence, **A**ssessment or diagnosis, and **P**lans for further studies. (Courtesy of Bibbero Systems, Inc., Petaluma, CA.)

fore 1970, it has become increasingly popular and is especially advantageous in clinics, group practices, and hospitals, where more than one person must be able to find essential information in the chart.

OBTAINING THE HISTORY

The medical assistant usually secures the routine personal data. The personal and medical history and the patient's family history may be secured by asking the patient to complete a questionnaire, with the physician augmenting this during the patient interview.

If the doctor delegates the taking of patients' histories to the medical assistant, care must be exercised to assure that the patient's answers are not heard by others in the reception room. If privacy is not possible, it is better to give the patient a form to fill out and then transfer this information to permanent records later. If convenient, it is time-saving to ask the patient questions and at the same time type the answers directly on the record. This method offers an opportunity to become better acquainted with the patient as you complete the necessary records. In some offices, where lengthy questionnaires are to be completed by the new patient, the questionnaire is mailed to the patient with a request that it be completed and returned to the doctor's office prior to the appointment.

The patient's chief complaint may have been indicated to the medical assistant, but the physician will question the patient in more detail on this. The majority of doctors write their own entries on the chart in longhand. Others may dictate the material, either directly to the medical assistant or by using a recording device. If the material is dictated and typed, the physician should check each entry and then initial the entry to verify accuracy. Although the physician may find this is a bother, it should be encouraged. For a chart to be admissible as evidence in court, the person dictating or writing the entries should be able to attest that they were true and correct at the time they were written. The best indication of that is the physician's signature or initials on the typed entry.

MAKING ADDITIONS AND CORRECTIONS

As long as the patient is under the physician's care, the medical history will be building. Each laboratory report, x-ray report, and progress note is added to the record, in **chronologic order**, with the latest information always on top. Although each item is important, the most recent is usually of greatest significance to the patient's care. Again,

the physician should read and initial each of these reports before they are placed in the record.

Laboratory Reports. Different colors of paper are often used for reporting different procedures. For example, urinalysis report forms may be yellow, blood count forms pink, and so forth. Laboratory slips are usually smaller than the history form and should be placed on a standard 8½ × 11 inch sheet of colored paper. Type the patient's name in the upper righthand corner, and then, with transparent tape, fasten the first report even with the bottom of the page. The second laboratory report will be taped or glued in place on top of and about ½ inch above the first slip, allowing the date to show on the first report. By this method, called "shingling," the latest report always appears on top. When checking previous reports, it is necessary only to run your finger down the slips until you find the desired date; then flip up the slips above. Fifteen to twenty slips may be kept on one sheet by using this method, which is illustrated in Figure 11–5. Laboratory report carrier forms with adhesive strips may be purchased (Fig. 11–6).

X-ray Reports. X-ray reports are usually typed on standard letter-size stationery. X-ray reports are placed in the patient's history folder, with the most recent report on top. All x-ray reports may be stapled together or kept behind a special divider in the chart.

Progress Notes. Reports on the patient's progress are continually being added to the case history. Each visit of the patient should be entered on the chart, with the date preceding any notations about the call. The medical assistant can type or stamp the date on the chart when readying the charts for the patients' visits. Every instruction, prescription, or telephone call for advice should be entered with the correct date. If there are several persons handling and making entries on a patient's record, it is advisable to initial each entry. This aids in tracing entries about which there may be some question.

Corrections. Sometimes it is necessary to make corrections on medical records. Erasing and obliteration must be avoided.

CORRECTING A HANDWRITTEN ENTRY

1. *Draw a line through the error.*
2. *Insert the correction above or immediately following.*
3. *In the margin, write "correction" or "Corr.," your initials, and the date.*

Errors made while typing are corrected in the usual way. An error discovered in a typed entry at a later

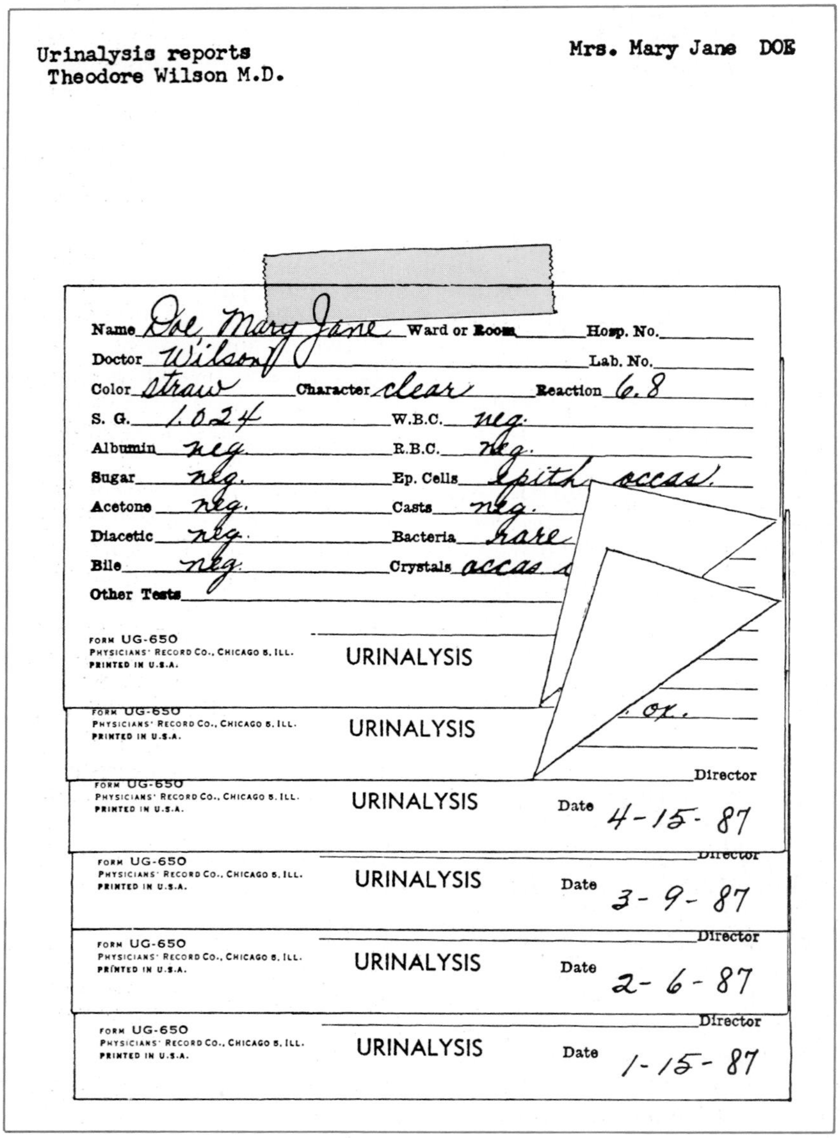

Urinalysis reports
Theodore Wilson M.D.

Mrs. Mary Jane DOE

Name *Doe, Mary Jane* Ward or Room_____ Hosp. No._____
Doctor *Wilson* Lab. No._____
Color *straw* Character *clear* Reaction *6.8*
S. G. *1.024* W.B.C. *neg.*
Albumin *neg.* R.B.C. *neg.*
Sugar *neg.* Ep. Cells *epith. occas.*
Acetone *neg.* Casts *neg.*
Diacetic *neg.* Bacteria *rare*
Bile *neg.* Crystals *occas.*
Other Tests_____

FORM UG-650
PHYSICIANS' RECORD CO., CHICAGO 6, ILL.
PRINTED IN U.S.A.
URINALYSIS

FORM UG-650
PHYSICIANS' RECORD CO., CHICAGO 6, ILL.
PRINTED IN U.S.A.
URINALYSIS

FORM UG-650
PHYSICIANS' RECORD CO., CHICAGO 6, ILL.
PRINTED IN U.S.A.
URINALYSIS
Date *4-15-87*
Director

FORM UG-650
PHYSICIANS' RECORD CO., CHICAGO 6, ILL.
PRINTED IN U.S.A.
URINALYSIS
Date *3-9-87*
Director

FORM UG-650
PHYSICIANS' RECORD CO., CHICAGO 6, ILL.
PRINTED IN U.S.A.
URINALYSIS
Date *2-6-87*
Director

FORM UG-650
PHYSICIANS' RECORD CO., CHICAGO 6, ILL.
PRINTED IN U.S.A.
URINALYSIS
Date *1-15-87*

Figure 11–5
Laboratory reports arranged chronologically on a page. (Courtesy of Physicians Record Company, Chicago, IL.)

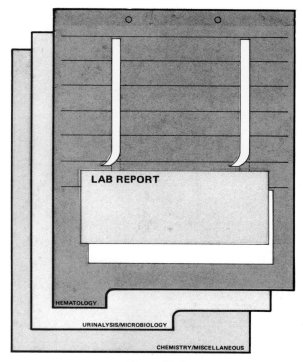

Figure 11–6
Quick-Stick color-coded lab carriers. Reports are affixed to proper carrier in chronological order by shingling from bottom of page to top. Remove zip tape from designated spot and press down on report. Be sure to indicate problem number on each report for future reference. (Courtesy of Bibbero Systems, Inc., Petaluma, CA.)

date, however, is corrected in the same manner as described above for a handwritten entry.

KEEPING RECORDS CURRENT

One of the greatest dangers to good recordkeeping is procrastination. The record must be methodically kept current. It is the medical assistant's responsibility to see that this is done.

The case histories and reports may accumulate on the doctor's or the medical assistant's desk during the day. After the last patient has gone, check each history to make certain all necessary material has been recorded and that each entry is sufficiently clear for future understanding. Give the physician all extra reports, such as laboratory and x-ray, to read and initial so that they may be filed in the patient's case history folder.

While the doctor is reviewing these reports, you can pull the histories of any patients seen outside the office that day, as well as those of patients who have been given special instructions by telephone or for whom prescriptions were ordered. These entries are made in the same manner as for an office visit, but the type of call is explained in

parentheses after the date. For example, here is what the history might include about a home visit to see a patient:

May 23, 1987 (Res.) Routine PX. Temp 98.6. Chest clear. Cont. Rx. May now eat semi-bland diet.

When a patient telephones the doctor, the entry should be made on the patient's record, for example:

June 26, 1988 (Tel.) To change Rx (Vit. B Comp) to one b.i.d. Force fluids. Feeling much better.

If tests are ordered for a patient, they should be charted in detail on the medical record:

April 10, 1987. Consultation. Scheduled with Dr. Abbot for office consultation on April 26. Bilateral mammograms scheduled at SJH on April 17.

Prescriptions should be charted:

April 25, 1987. Refill Tylenol c̄ Cod. #25.

A prescription pad, printed on no-smear, spot carbon paper, is available for a timesaving, write-it-once system. By placing the prescription blank over the patient's record, the Rx is automatically copied on the record as it is written (Fig. 11–7). Prescription carriers with adhesive strips are also available for the doctor who uses duplicate prescription blanks (Fig. 11–8).

The patient record should not leave the office. A Physician's Pocket Call Record, as shown in Figure 11–9, can be used for outside calls, and the information transferred to the chart in the office.

Also, at the end of the day, notations should be made of any unkept appointments or of refusals to cooperate with instructions.

After all records have been reviewed, they should be placed in a file tray and locked away for the night, if there is insufficient time to file them the same day. Do not leave histories out in view at night, especially if the office has a night cleaning service.

On arrival the next morning, the medical assistant can index the histories for filing. Attach extra reports and information sheets; don't just drop them into the folders. It is best to attach them to the case histories with tape or rubber cement. When this is done, the records are ready for filing.

The doctor may prefer to dictate progress notes rather than write them in longhand. At appropriate moments during the day everything is dictated: patient histories, physical examination findings, medications prescribed, follow-up findings, summaries of telephone conversations. At the end of

11

THOMAS A. SCOTT, M.D.
General Practice
135 SO. ELM STREET
SACRAMENTO, CALIFORNIA 94106
TELEPHONE: (916) 344-5550

CAL. LIC. #6099914
DEA #AK08888888   DATE___2/12/87___

PATIENT___John W. Bates_____

ADDRESS___723 North Avenue_____

___Crossville_____

	Rx Drug	Strength	Qty.	Rep.	Directions
1.	Esidrix	25 mgm	100	2x	1 tab. p.c. bid
2.					
3.					
4.					

☐ Total Drugs

☐ Please label unless checked here

Strength is Mg. Units or %; Quantity is total amount to be dispensed. Rep. is number of refills.

Authority is given for dispensing by non proprietary name (generic equivalent) unless checked here. ☐

*Thomas A Scott*_____ M.D.
Thomas A. Scott, M.D.

FORM #25-8296

Figure 11–7
Prescription pad for write-it-once system. (Courtesy of Bibbero Systems, Inc., Petaluma, CA.)

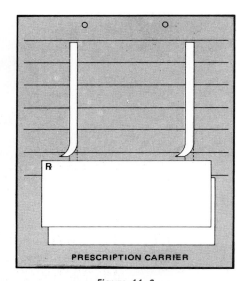

PRESCRIPTION CARRIER

Figure 11–8
Quick-Stick Prescription Carrier for shingling copies of prescriptions in patient record. (Courtesy of Bibbero Systems, Inc., Petaluma, CA.)

the day the recorded information is handed to the medical assistant for transcribing onto the records.

A great deal of time may be saved in transcribing these notes by using a continuous roll or pages of self-adhesive strips (Fig. 11–10). When the transcription is completed, the doctor may wish to check the notes, underline important points, and initial each entry before returning the notes to the medical assistant for insertion in the charts. The use of self-adhesive strips saves removing the sheet from a chart which may be bound with metal fasteners, inserting the sheet into the typewriter, and putting the sheet back into the folder. It also simplifies the doctor's part in checking and initialing the notes, because only the transcribed material is handled, not the bulky charts.

PHYSICIANS POCKET CALL RECORD		DATE				
NAME	ADDRESS OR REMARKS	SYMBOL	MONEY RECEIVED		HOME CHARGES	HOSPITAL CHARGES
Donald Jones	out time	H.				5.—
Mrs. Mary L. Lint	Chest exam inj	Res	15	00	15	
John James	Chickenpox (report to P.H.D)	"			7.—	
Mrs. Ronald White	Surgery St. Luke's Blue Cross # 512-8669	H.				350 —

After posting totals to Office Book file this card by date in BANCO PROFESSIONAL SYSTEM filing box.

Post these TOTALS to office book daily ☞

FORM 924 BANCO-PRINTERS S.F.   REG. U. S. PAT. OFF.

Figure 11–9
Physician's Pocket Call Record for patient visits outside office. (Courtesy of Banco Printers, San Francisco, CA.)

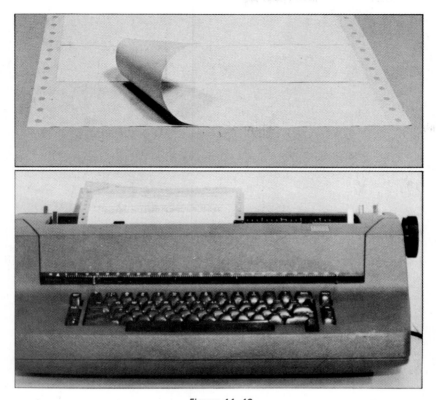

Figure 11-10
Adhesive transcription strips. Simply insert this continuous form of pressure-sensitive, adhesive-backed strips into the typewriter for easy dictation typing. Then peel off the strip and affix on Progress Notes or any other form. (Courtesy of Bibbero Systems, Inc., Petaluma, CA.)

11

TRANSFER OF FILES

Some system should be established for regular **transfer** of files. In most medical offices, records are filed according to three classifications: active, inactive, or closed:

- *Active files* are those of patients currently receiving treatment.
- *Inactive files* generally are those of patients whom the doctor has not seen for 6 months or more. When such individuals return for care, their folders are replaced in the active file.
- *Closed files* are records of patients who have died, moved away, or otherwise terminated their relationship with the physician.

Charts for patients who are currently hospitalized may be kept in a special section for quick reference, then placed in the regular active file when the patient is discharged from the hospital.

In a surgical practice, there is frequently a specific date on which the patient is discharged from the doctor's care and the notation made on the chart, "Return prn." This record may safely be placed in the inactive file.

In a general practice office, the outside of the folder may be stamped with the date of the patient's visit each time he is seen. It will then be a simple matter to determine when the chart should be transferred to the inactive status. In the parlance of filing, this is called the perpetual transfer method.

RETENTION AND DESTRUCTION OF RECORDS

There is no standard rule to follow in establishing a records **retention schedule. Statutes of limitations** regarding professional liability litigation are a consideration in the retention of medical records. Tax regulations affect the retention of business records.

Case Histories

Space permitting, these will probably be kept permanently, or at least as long as the doctor is in practice. Then, if the patient is still living, the record may be made available to another doctor of the patient's own choosing. The record would not be given to the patient, because of the possibility of misinterpretation.

Business Records

Tax Records. Income tax returns are kept indefinitely; the last three returns are retained in a fireproof filing cabinet or safe; older returns are filed in dead storage.

Insurance Policies. Keep current policies in a fireproof cabinet or safe. When superseded by a new policy, throw away the old one *unless* a claim is pending. Professional liability policies are kept permanently.

Canceled Checks. Keep in a fireproof file for 3 years, then indefinitely in dead storage.

Receipts for Business Equipment. Keep until item is fully depreciated.

General Correspondence. Copies of correspondence should be reviewed periodically, as time permits, and any papers that are no longer of value destroyed. If the slightest doubt exists as to whether a paper should be destroyed, be sure to check with the doctor or retain the paper in the file.

Miscellaneous. Many papers that are filed should instead be destroyed. Examples of these are letters of acknowledgement, announcements of meetings, duplicate copies, and letters of transmittal. Any document that is superseded by another in the file should be removed. For instance, when a new catalog is filed, destroy the old one; when a new fee schedule is received, destroy the old one. Blue Cross and Blue Shield representatives say that retaining old copies of fee schedules and claim forms causes countless problems. The Army has developed the technique of discarding papers to the highest level, and every document receives a date of destruction notation before it goes into the file.

PROTECTION OF RECORDS

Occasions may arise when records are temporarily out of the office. Some physicians release case histories to their colleagues, or an original record may be subpoenaed by the courts. In such instances an OUTfolder should be substituted in place of the regular folder, and a notation made of the name, date, and to whom the record was released. Interim papers may be placed in the OUTfolder until the original is returned.

The sending out of original case histories should be avoided if possible. Instead, prepare a summary, or photocopy the materials needed for reference, and retain the original in the physician's office. Drawers and cabinets should be kept closed at all times when the office is unattended, for further protection of the records.

STORAGE OF RECORDS

Large clinics and offices may find it advisable to **microfilm** records for storage. This permits storage of a considerable number of histories in a small space, saves time in searching, offers protection, and eliminates loss and misfiling. However, the cost is high, microfilm is hard to read for prolonged study, it is difficult to produce film in court, and if a patient returns, it is too small for refiling with the folders in the active file.

Some papers that should be kept but which need not be readily accessible may be placed in storage. Sturdy storage file boxes may be obtained from your stationery supply house. These boxes should be labeled to identify their contents in case it should be necessary to reclaim a file or refer to a record. The boxes are uniform in size and are available with a lift-off lid or in a drawer model. They can be kept in some out-of-the-way place or, if no room is available in the office, they can be placed with a storage company for a low monthly rental. If the latter is done, a record of the contents of each box should be kept in the office. When selecting a commercial records center, you should determine whether:

- They will retrieve items from a carton or only the entire carton
- The speed of retrieval is satisfactory
- They will deliver records (or must you pick them up?)
- They have an on-site work area available to their clients
- Fire protection and security is adequate
- The cost is reasonable

Thus far, the medical record itself has been emphasized. But this record must be filed so that it can be easily and quickly found when needed. This is sometimes the most neglected area of management practice. A **filing system** is only as good as the "findability" of everything in the files. A modern filing system, according to Michael Silver, Practice Management Consultant ("How to Tailor Your Filing System to Your Own Needs," *Physician's Management,* November 1979) should have three key components:

1. A way to tell if the record is active or inactive from the outside of the jacket or folder, so that updating is continuous and easy
2. Safeguards to prevent misfiling
3. A filing technique that allows quick, accurate retrieval and refiling

FILING EQUIPMENT

The vertical four-drawer steel filing cabinet, used with manila folders with the patient's name on the **tab**, was the traditional system of choice for years.

The most popular system today is color-coding on open shelves. There are also rotary, lateral, compactable, and automated files. Some records are kept in card or tray files.

Some of the considerations in selecting filing equipment are:

- Space availability
- Structural considerations
- Cost of space and equipment
- Size, type, and volume of records
- Confidentiality requirements
- Retrieval speed
- Fire protection

Regardless of the type or style of equipment, the best quality is always an economy.

Drawer files should be full-suspension; they should roll easily, close securely, and be equipped with a locking device. The best cabinets have a center trough at the bottom of each drawer with a rod for holding divider guides. Floor space of twice the depth of the drawer must be allowed so that the drawer can be pulled out to its full extent. A drawback of the vertical four-drawer file is that only one person can use a file cabinet at any given time. They are also slower because the drawer must be opened and closed each time a file is pulled or filed. They are relatively easy to move, but for safety reasons they should be bolted to the wall or to each other.

Shelf files should have doors to protect the contents. A popular type of shelf file has doors that slide back into the cabinet; the door from a lower shelf may be pulled out and used for work space. About 50% more material per square foot of floor space may be filed in shelf files as compared with the four-drawer file. Open shelf units hold files sideways and can go higher on the wall because there is no drawer to pull out. File retrieval is faster because several individuals can work simultaneously.

Open shelf units without doors are the most economical but offer little protection or confidentiality to the records. They are susceptible to water and flame damage in case of fire. Shelf files are available in many attractive colors and can add a decorative note to the business office.

Special storage or shelf space should be provided for x-rays if many films are stored.

Rotary circular files can hold a large volume of records. They save space and clerical motion. The files revolve easily; some come with push-button controls. Several persons can work at one rotary file and use records at the same time. One disadvantage is that they afford less privacy and protection than files than can be closed and locked.

Lateral files are good for personal files and are especially attractive for the physician's private office. They use more wall space than the vertical file but do not extend out into the room so far. The folders are filed sideways in the lateral file, left to right, instead of front to back as in a vertical file. Some have a pull-out drawer, as the vertical file does; others have doors that slide into the cabinet, exposing the filing space.

The office with little space and a great volume of records might use *compactable files*, which are a variation of open shelf files. The files are mounted on tracks in the floor, and the units slide along the tracks so that access is gained to the needed records. They may be either automated or manual. One drawback is that not all records are available at the same time.

Automated files are very expensive initially and require more maintenance. They will probably be found only in very large installations such as clinics or hospitals. These files bring the record to the operator instead of the operator going to the record. When the operator presses a button indicating the appropriate shelf, the shelf automatically moves into position in front of the operator for record retrieval. The automated or "power" file is fast and can store large amounts of records in a small amount of space. Only one person can use the unit at one time.

Almost every office will have some occasion to use a *card file*. This may be for patient ledgers, a patient index, library index, index of surgical tray setups, telephone numbers, or numerous other records. A good-quality steel box or tray is a sound investment.

Special Items. Metal framework is available that will convert a regular drawer file into suspension-folder equipment. The assistant with a great deal of filing may wish to purchase a portable filing shelf that fits on the side of an opened drawer and can be moved from place to place as needed. A sorting file can be a great timesaver. A portable file cart for the temporary filing of unbilled insurance claims may be quite useful. Such a file cart may also be used for the preliminary sorting of charts to be refiled. This is sometimes called a suspense file.

SUPPLIES

Filing supplies include divider guides, OUT-guides or OUTfolders, folders, vertical pockets, and labels.

Divider Guides. Each file drawer or shelf should be equipped with plenty of dividers or guides. Some authorities recommend one guide for approximately each inch and a half of material, or every 8 to 10 folders. Guides should be of good-quality pressboard. "Economy" guides will soon become bent and frayed and have to be replaced. Divider guides have a protruding tab, which may be either an integral part of the card or may be made of metal or plastic. The guides reduce the area of search and serve as supports for the folders. They are available in single, third, or fifth cut (one, three, or five different positions). The guide may have a projection at the bottom edge with a ring or hole through which a rod may go. This type of guide card is used in drawers that have a trough for the projection and a rod to hold the guides in place.

OUTguides. An OUTguide is a heavy guide that is used to replace a folder that has been temporarily removed. It should be of a distinctive color for quick detection. This makes refiling simpler and alerts the file clerk that a file is missing. Several colors may be used, each color designating the temporary location of the file. The OUTguide may have lines for recording information, or it may have a plastic pocket for inserting an information card.

Folders. Most records to be filed are placed in tabbed folders. The most commonly used is a general-purpose third-cut manila folder that may be expanded to ¾ inch. These are available with a double-thickness reinforced tab that will greatly lengthen the life of the folder. Folders kept in drawers have tabs at the top; those kept on shelves have tabs at the side.

There are many variations of folder styles obtainable for special purposes:

Classification folders separate the papers in one file into six categories yet keep them all together.

OUTfolders are used like the OUTguide and provide space for temporary filing of materials.

The *vertical pocket*, which is heavier weight than the general purpose folder, has a front that folds down for easy access to contents and is available with up to 3½ inch expansion. These are used for bulky histories or correspondence.

Hanging or suspension folders are made of heavy stock and hang on metal rods from side to side of a drawer. They can be used only with files equipped with suspension drawers.

Binder folders have fasteners with which to bind papers within them. These offer some security for the papers but are time-consuming in filing the materials.

The number of papers that will fit in one folder depends on the thickness of the papers. Near the bottom edge of most folders are one or more score marks, which should be used as the contents of the folders expand. If folders are refolded at these score marks, the danger of their bending and sliding under other folders is reduced, and a neater file results. Papers should never protrude from the folder edges, and they should always be inserted with their tops to the left. When papers start to "ride up" in any folder, the folder is overloaded.

Labels. Each shelf, drawer, divider guide, and folder must have a label. The label is a necessary

"filing and finding" device. Labels may be prepared with a mechanical tapewriter or the typewriter. Paper labels may be purchased in rolls of gummed tape, or they may have adhesive backs that are peeled from a protective sheet after typing. Labels are available in almost any size, shape, or color to meet the individual needs of any office. Visit your stationer and study the catalogs to find the best product for you.

The label on the drawer or shelf identifies the nature of its contents. It should also indicate the range (alphabetic, numeric, or chronologic) of the material filed in that space. For example:

```
┌──────────────────────────────────┐
│                                  │
│   PATIENT HISTORIES (Active)     │
│              A–F                 │
│                                  │
└──────────────────────────────────┘
```

or

```
┌──────────────────────────────────┐
│                                  │
│   GENERAL CORRESPONDENCE         │
│         1986–1988                │
│                                  │
└──────────────────────────────────┘
```

The label should be easy to read. The tapewriter is probably preferable to the typewriter for these labels.

The final step in locating a record in the file is identification of the individual folder. Every reasonable filing aid should be used to ensure reaching this as speedily as possible. The folder label must be descriptive and legible.

FILING PROCEDURES

Steps in Filing. Filing of all materials will involve several steps. In the language of filing, these steps are called (1) conditioning, (2) releasing or inspecting, (3) indexing, (4) coding, (5) **cross-referencing** (if necessary), (6) sorting, and (7) storing or filing (Table 11–2).

Conditioning of papers involves removing all pins, brads, and paper clips; stapling related papers together; attaching clippings or items smaller than page size to a regular sheet of paper with rubber cement or tape; and mending damaged records.

The term *releasing* simply means that some mark is placed on the paper indicating that it is now ready for filing. This will usually be either the medical assistant's initials or a FILE stamp placed in the upper left corner.

Indexing means deciding where to file the letter or paper, and *coding* means placing some indication of this decision on the paper. This may be done by underlining the name or subject, if it appears on the paper, or writing, in some conspicuous place, the indexing subject or name. If there is more than

Procedure 11–1

INITIATING A MEDICAL FILE FOR A NEW PATIENT

PROCEDURAL GOAL

To initiate a medical file for a new patient that will contain all the personal data necessary for a complete record and any other information required by the agency.

EQUIPMENT AND SUPPLIES

Typewriter
Clerical supplies (pen, clipboard)
Information on agency's filing system
Registration form
File folder
Label for folder
ID card if using numeric system
Cross-reference card
Financial card
Routing slip
Private conference area

PROCEDURE

1. Determine that the patient is new to the agency.
2. Obtain and record the required personal data.
   Purpose: Complete information is necessary for credit and insurance claim processing.
3. Typewrite the information onto the patient history form.
4. Review the entire form.
   Purpose: To confirm that the information is complete and correct.
5. Select a label and folder for the record.
   Explanation: If color coding is used, a decision must be made regarding the appropriate color for the patient's name (see p. 165).
6. Type caption on label and apply to folder.
   Explanation: Use patient's name for alphabetic filing or appropriate number for numeric filing.
7. For numeric filing system, prepare cross-reference card and patient ID card.
   Purpose: Numeric filing is an indirect system and requires a cross-reference to patient name for locating chart. Patient will use number of ID card when arranging appointments or making inquiries.
8. Prepare financial card, or place patient name in computerized ledger.
9. Place patient history form and all other forms required by the agency into prepared folder.
10. Clip a routing slip on the outside of patient's folder.

TERMINAL PERFORMANCE OBJECTIVE

Given the listed equipment and supplies, and another student for role-play as new patient, gather all the necessary information and prepare a medical file for a new patient to the agency's standard, within 15 minutes, to a performance level of 95%.

11

one logical place to file the paper, the original is coded for the main location and a *cross-reference* sheet prepared, indicating this location and coded for the second location. Every paper placed in a patient's chart should have the name of the patient on it, usually in the upper right corner.

Sorting is arranging the papers in filing sequence. Sort papers before going to the file cabinet or shelf. Do any necessary stapling of papers at your desk or filing table. Invest in a desk sorter with a series of dividers between which papers are placed in filing sequence. One general-purpose sorter has six

Table 11–2
Steps in Filing

1. Conditioning	Removing paper clips, mending tears, mounting slips on standard-size sheets
2. Releasing	Making a notation that a record is ready for filing
3. Indexing	Choosing the **caption** under which a record is to be filed
4. Coding	The marking of materials with captions under which they will be stored
5. Cross-referencing	Placing a notation in a file that a record is stored elsewhere and stating the location
6. Sorting	Arranging papers in order of filing
7. Storing or Filing	Placing item in appropriate location in filing system

means of classification: alphabetic sections, numbers 1 to 31, days of the week, months of the year, numbers in groups of five, and space on the tabs for special captions to be taped when desired. In the preliminary sorting you will place the papers in the appropriate division in the sorter. Then it is comparatively simple to arrange these groups into the proper sequence for filing.

In *storing or filing* papers in the folder, items should be placed face up, top edge to the left, with the most recent date to the front of the folder. Lift the folder an inch or two out of the drawer before inserting material, so that the sheets can drop down completely into the folder.

If you are refiling completed folders, arrange them in indexing order before going to the file cabinets.

Preventing Accidents. File drawers are heavy and can tip over, causing serious damage, unless reasonable care is observed. Open only one file drawer at a time and close it when the filing has been completed. A drawer left even slightly open can cause injury to a passerby.

Locating Misplaced Files. Unless files are promptly replaced after use, they may become lost. Papers may be misfiled, requiring a thorough search to find them. After you have made a methodical and complete search through the proper folder, there are several places you may look for a misplaced paper: in the folder in front of and behind the correct folder; between the folders; on the bottom of the file under all the folders; in a folder of a patient with a similar name; in the sorter.

RULES FOR INDEXING

Indexing rules are fairly well standardized, based on current business practices. The American Records Management Association takes an active part in updating the rules. For the average physician's office, the following basic rules will be all that is needed (see Table 11–3 for examples).

1. Last names of persons are considered first in filing; given name (first name), second; and middle name or initial, third. Compare the names from the first letter to the last. The first letter that is different in two names is the letter that determines the order of filing. Example:

> abE
> abI
> abX
> aCl
> acM
> aDa
> adE
> adI

and so forth.

2. Initials precede a name beginning with the same letter. Example:

> Smith, J.
> Smith, Jason

This illustrates the librarian's rule, "Nothing comes before something."

3. Hyphenated names, whether first names, middle names, surnames of people, or business names, are considered to be one **unit**.

4. The apostrophe is disregarded in filing. Anderson's Surgical Supply is filed as Andersons Surgical Supply. Before the most recent revision, anything after the apostrophe was not considered in filing.

5. Unusual names of individuals, such as Truyen Nguyen, should be filed under the last name and cross-indexed. Example:

> Nguyen, Truyen
> Truyen Nguyen (see Nguyen, Truyen)

6. Names with prefixes are filed in the usual alphabetic order. DeLong is filed as Delong; LaFrance as Lafrance; von Schmidt as Vonschmidt.

7. Abbreviated names are indexed as if spelled in full: St. John as Saintjohn; Wm. as William; Edw. as Edward; Jas. as James.

8. Mac and Mc are filed in their regular place in the alphabet:

> Maag
> Mabry

MacDonald
Machado
MacHale
Maville
McAulay
McWilliams
Meacham

If your files contain a great many names beginning with Mac or Mc you may, for convenience, wish to file them as a separate letter of the alphabet.

9. The name of a married woman is indexed by her legal name (her husband's surname, her given name, and her middle name or maiden surname). For example:

Doe, Mary Jones (Mrs. John L.)
not
Doe, Mrs. John L.

10. Titles, when followed by a complete name, are disregarded in indexing:

Breckenridge, John J. (Prof.)

Titles without complete names are considered the first indexing unit:

Madame Sylvia
Sister Mary Catherine

Degrees are disregarded in filing but placed after the name, in parentheses:

Wilson, Theodore (MD)

11. Articles such as "The" or "A" are disregarded in indexing:

Moore Clinic (The)

12. Terms of seniority, such as Junior, Senior, or Second, are not considered in indexing. If two names are otherwise identical, the address is used to make the indexing decision (State, City, Street).

FILING SYSTEMS

There are four basic systems of filing: (1) **alphabetic** by name, (2) **numeric**, (3) geographic, and (4) **subject**. A fifth system, chronologic, is sometimes used. In the management of records in the physician's office, the medical assistant will probably be concerned with only three filing systems—alphabetic, numeric, and subject. These will be described more fully. Geographic filing is a specialized variation of alphabetic filing. The file is usually subdivided into a geographic hierarchy (country, state, county, city, and street), with each level alphabetized. Geographic filing is used in businesses that

11

Table 11–3
Application of Indexing Rules

Indexing Rule	Name	Unit 1	Unit 2	Unit 3
1	Robert F. Grinch	Grinch	Robert	F.
	R. Frank Grumman	Grumman	R.	Frank
2	J. Orville Smith	Smith	J.	Orville
	Jason O. Smith	Smith	Jason	O.
3	M. L. Saint-Vickery	Saintvickery	M.	L.
	Marie-Louise Taylor	Taylor	Marielouise	
4	Charles S. Anderson	Anderson	Charles	S.
	Anderson's Surgical Supply	Andersons	Surgical	Supply
5	Ah Hop Akee	Akee	Ah	Hop
6	Alice Delaney	Delaney	Alice	
	Chester K. DeLong	Delong	Chester	K.
7	Michael St. John	Saintjohn	Michael	
8	Helen M. Maag	Maag	Helen	M.
	Frederick Mabry	Mabry	Frederick	
	James E. MacDonald	Macdonald	James	E.
9	Mrs. John L. Doe (Mary Jones)	Doe	Mary	Jones (Mrs. John L.)
10	Prof. John J. Breck	Breck	John	J. (Prof.)
	Madame Sylvia	Madame	Sylvia	
	Sister Mary Catherine	Sister	Mary	Catherine
	Theodore Wilson, M.D.	Wilson	Theodore (M.D.)	
11	The Moore Clinic	Moore	Clinic (The)	
12	Lawrence W. Sloan, Sr.	Sloan	Lawrence	W. (1100 Main Street)
	Lawrence W. Sloan, Jr.	Sloan	Lawrence	W. (384 Turner Street)

are interested in information by location rather than by name, such as sales organizations, mailing houses, or real estate firms. Chronologic filing refers to filing according to date and is used in a follow-up or tickler file, as described on page 167.

Alphabetic Filing

Alphabetic filing by name is the oldest, simplest, and most commonly used system. It is the system of choice for filing patient records in the majority of physicians' offices. If you can find a word in the dictionary or a name in the telephone directory, you already know some of the rules. Some people have difficulty all their lives with remembering the sequence of letters in the alphabet. This can play havoc with alphabetic filing!

Alphabetic filing is traditional and simple to set up, requiring only a file cabinet or shelf, folders, and some divider guides. It is a **direct system** in that one need only know the name in order to find the desired file. One of the drawbacks is confusion over a name's proper spelling. There are additional drawbacks. As the files grow in number, more space will be needed for each section of the alphabet. This will require periodic shifting of folders from drawer to drawer, or shelf to shelf, to allow for expansion. As the files expand, more time is required for filing each folder, as well as for retrieving a file, because of the additional folders involved in the search. This can be greatly alleviated by color coding, which will be discussed in detail later in the chapter.

Numeric Filing

Numeric filing is an indirect system, requiring the use of an alphabetic cross-reference in order to find a given file. Some people object to this added step and overlook the advantages. Management consultants differ in their recommendations, some recommending numeric filing only if there are more than 5,000 charts, more than 10,000 charts, or in some cases more than 15,000 charts. Others recommend nothing but numeric filing. This is an individual choice.

Some form of numeric filing combined with color and **shelf filing** is used by practically every clinic or hospital of any size. In numeric filing each new patient is assigned a number, and an alphabetic cross-index card is prepared to identify the name. In a computerized office, the cross-index will probably be in the computer. It is possible to use the patient's ledger (financial) card as a cross-index by simply writing the patient's number at the top of the card. This does have the disadvantage that ledger cards customarily are taken from the active file when the account is paid in full. The use of 3 × 5 cards attached to a Rolodex or Wheelodex

system on the medical assistant's desk is usually more convenient and more efficient. Some clinics give each new patient an identification card bearing an assigned number, with instructions to give this number to the medical assistant each time the patient telephones or comes into the office.

Numeric filing allows unlimited expansion without periodic shifting of folders, and shelves are usually filled evenly. It provides additional confidentiality to the chart. The greatest advantage is the time saved in retrieving and refiling records quickly. One knows immediately that the number 978 falls between 977 and 979. By contrast, an alphabetic system, even with color coding, requires a longer search for the exact spot.

There are several types of numeric filing systems. In the *straight* or *consecutive* numeric system, patients are given consecutive numbers as they visit the practice. This is the simplest of the numeric systems and works well for files of up to 10,000 records. It is time consuming, and there is more chance for error, in filing documents with five or more digits. Filing activity is greatest at the end of the numeric series.

In the *terminal digit system*, patients are also assigned consecutive numbers, but the digits in the number are usually separated into groups of twos or threes and are read in groups from right to left instead of from left to right. The records are filed "backward" in groups.

For example, all files ending in 00 are grouped together first, then those ending in 01, etc. Next the files are grouped by their middle digits so that the 00 22s come before the 01 22s. Finally the files are arranged by their first digits, so that 01 00 22 precedes 02 00 22. Example:

$$01\ 99\ 00$$
$$00\ 73\ 01$$
$$05\ 55\ 11$$
$$01\ 68\ 21$$
$$01\ 68\ 22$$
$$88\ 34\ 23$$
$$90\ 34\ 23$$

Middle digit filing begins with the middle digits, followed by the first digit and finally by the terminal digits.

Some practices use the last four digits of each patient's Social Security number to file patient records.

Numeric filing requires more training, but once the system is mastered, fewer errors will occur than with alphabetic filing.

Subject Filing

Subject filing can be either alphabetic or **alphanumeric** (A 1–3, B 1–1, B 1–2, etc.) and is used for general correspondence. The main difficulty with subject filing is indexing, or classification—deciding where to file a document. Many papers will require **cross-referencing**. All correspondence dealing with a particular subject is filed together. The papers within the folders are filed chronologically, the most recent on top. The subject headings are placed on the tabs of the folders and filed alphabetically.

Color Coding

When a color coding system is used, both filing and finding are easier, and misfiled folders are kept to a minimum. The use of color visually restricts the area of search for a specific record. A misfiled chart is easily spotted even from a distance of several feet. In color coding, a specific color is selected to identify each letter of the alphabet. The application of the principle may be through using colored folders, adhesive colored identification labels, or various combinations of these (Fig. 11–11). Any selection of colors may be used, and the division of the alphabet determined by one's own needs. However, studies have shown that there is wide variation in the frequency with which different letters occur. The following division is one that has been used successfully. Experience has proven that this breakdown results in almost equal representation of the five colors.

Color of Label	Letters of Alphabet
Red	A B C D
Yellow	E F G H
Green	I J K L M N
Blue	O P Q
Purple	R S T U V W X Y Z

Alphabetic Color Coding. There are several ways of color coding files. One alphabetic system utilizes five different colored folders, with each color representing a segment of the alphabet. The *second* letter of the patient's last name determines the color, as in the following system:

Red Folder (second letters a, b, c, d)	Canfield Eberhart Ackerman Adams
Yellow Folder (second letters e, f, g, h)	Venable Effron Igawa Thill
Green Folder (second letters i, j, k, l, m, n)	Histed Bjork Akron Ullman Imhoff Anderson
Blue Folder (second letters o, p, q)	Gordon Epperley Aquino

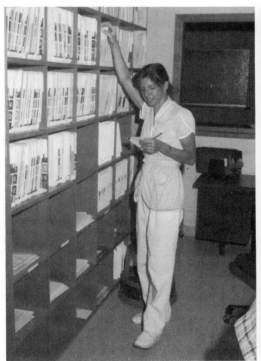
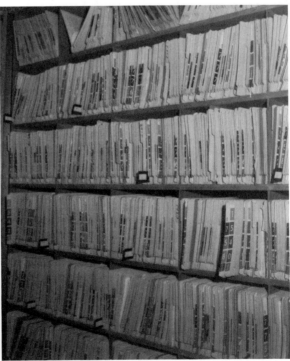

Figure 11–11
Color-coded numeric filing system. (Courtesy of Vista Medical Group, EL Toro, CA. Photos by Dan Santucci.)

Purple Folder
(second letters r, s, t, u, v, w, x, y, z)

Greiner
Osterberg
Atherton
Auer
Uvena
Owsley
Oxford
Nye
Azzaro

There are a number of ready-made systems available (e.g., Acme, Ames, Bibbero, Colwell, Remington Rand, TAB, VisiRecord). Self-adhesive colored letter blocks with either two or three letters in the specific colors are supplied in rolls. The color blocks with the appropriate letter are placed on the index tab of the folder, along with the patient's full name. The letters are in pairs so they can be seen from either side of the chart. Strong, easily differentiated colors are used, creating a band of color in the files that makes it easy to spot out-of-place folders.

Numeric Color Coding. Color coding is also used in numeric filing. Numbers 0 through 9 are each assigned a different color. In a terminal digit filing system, the colors for the last two numbers would be affixed to the tab. If the number 1 is red and 5 is yellow, all files with numbers ending in 15 will form a red and yellow band. Usually a predetermined section of the number will be color coded.

Other Color Coding Methods. There are many other ways to make color work for you. Small pressure-sensitive tabs in a variety of colors may be used to identify certain types of insured patients. For example, a patient on Medicaid may have a red tab over the edge of the folder; a Champus patient may be identified by a blue tab; a worker's compensation patient by a green tab, and so forth. Matching tabs may be attached to the ledger cards. Research cases may be identified by a special color tab. In a partnership practice, it may be desirable to use a different color folder or label for each doctor's

Procedure 11-2

COLOR CODING PATIENT CHARTS

PROCEDURAL GOAL

To color code patient charts using the agency's established coding system to effectively facilitate filing and finding.

EQUIPMENT AND SUPPLIES

20 patient charts
Information on agency's coding system
20 file folders
Full range of color labels

PROCEDURE

1. Assemble patient charts.
2. Arrange charts in indexing order.
   Purpose: When charts have been color coded they will be in filing order.
3. Pick up first chart and note second letter of patient's surname.
   Explanation: For purpose of this activity the color coding system in the text will be used.
4. Choose a folder and/or caption label of appropriate color.
5. Type patient's name on label in indexing order and apply to folder tab.
   Purpose: To identify sequence of folder in filing system.
6. Repeat steps 4 and 5 until all charts have been coded.
7. Check entire group for any isolated color.
   Purpose: If order and color of folders is correct, all charts of the same color within each letter of the alphabet will be grouped together.

TERMINAL PERFORMANCE OBJECTIVE

Given the listed equipment and supplies, color code 20 patient charts following the agency's coding system, within 20 minutes, to a performance level of 100%.

Table 11–4
Color Coding for Business Records

Main Heading:	DISBURSEMENTS	Red label
Subheading:	Equipment	Blue label
Subdivisions:	Typewriter	Yellow label
	Copier	Yellow label
	Calculator	Yellow label

patient. Self-adhesive tabs are easily removed, less bulky than metal or plastic tabs, and not so likely to be inadvertently pulled from the record.

Color can be used to differentiate dates—one color for each month or year. Brightly colored labels on the outside of a patient chart can indicate certain health conditions, such as drug allergies.

The business records may also utilize color coding. Main divider guide headings may be of one color, subheadings in a second color, and subdivisions in a third color. (See Table 11–4 for an example of this type of arrangement.) A fourth color might be used for personal items. The use of color in the files is limited only by the imagination. One word of caution, though. Every person in the office who uses the files should know the key to the coding, and the key should also be written in the agency's procedures manual.

ORGANIZATION OF FILES

Patient Records. It is very difficult for a physician to study a disorganized history. Some systematic method must be followed in placing the material in the patient folder. The content of the patient record has already been discussed. From the filing standpoint, it should be stressed that when a patient record is not in actual use, there is only one place it should be—in the filing cabinet or shelf. Many precious hours can be lost in searching for misplaced or lost records that were carelessly left unfiled. The patient's full name, in indexing order, should be typed on a label and attached to the folder tab. The patient's full name should also be typed on each sheet within the folder. A strip of transparent tape can be placed on the label to prevent smudging if this is a problem.

Medical Correspondence. Correspondence pertaining to patients' medical records should be filed with the case history. Other medical correspondence will probably be filed in a subject file.

General Correspondence. The physician's office must be operated as a business, as well as a professional service. There will be correspondence of a general nature pertaining to the operation of the office. In all likelihood a special drawer or shelf will be set aside for the general correspondence. The correspondence will be indexed according to subject matter or names of correspondents. The guides in a subject file may appear in one, two, or three positions, depending upon the number of headings, subheadings, and subdivisions. Examples are shown in Table 11–4.

Miscellaneous Folder. Papers that do not warrant an individual folder are placed in a miscellaneous folder. Within the folder, all papers relating to one subject, or with one correspondent, are kept together in **chronologic order**, the most recent on top, and then filed alphabetically with other miscellaneous material. Related materials may be stapled together. Never use paper clips for this purpose. When as many as five papers accumulate with one correspondent or subject, a separate folder should be prepared.

Business and Financial Records. The most active financial record is, of course, the ledger. In most offices this will be a card or vertical tray file, and the accounts will be arranged alphabetically by name. There will be at least two divisions: active accounts and paid accounts. Special categories may be set up, for example: (1) government-sponsored insurance; (2) worker's compensation; (3) delinquent accounts; (4) collection accounts; and so forth.

Other business files include records of income and expense, financial statements, income and payroll tax records, canceled checks, and insurance policies. These papers may be filed chronologically.

Tickler or Follow-up File. The most frequently used follow-up method is that of a **tickler** file, so called because it "tickles" the memory that something needs to be done or followed up on a particular date. The tickler file is always a chronologic arrangement. In its simplest form it consists of notations on the daily calendar. If information concerning a patient who has an appointment to come in is expected, such as an x-ray report or laboratory report, the medical assistant might make a note on the calendar or tickler file a day ahead to check on whether the report has arrived.

The tickler file is often a card file with 12 guides for the names of the months, and 31 guides printed with numbers 1 through 31 for the days of the month. The guide for the current month, followed by the 31 day guides, is placed at the front of the file. Notations of actions to be taken are placed behind the guides for specific days of the current month. Notations for future months are placed behind the guide for that month. In order to be effective, the tickler file must be checked the first thing each day. It is a useful reminder for recurring events, such as payments, meetings, and so forth.

11

Procedure 11-3

PROCEDURAL GOAL

To add supplemental documents and progress notes to patient histories, observing standard steps in filing, while creating an orderly file that will facilitate ready reference to any item of information.

EQUIPMENT AND SUPPLIES

Assorted correspondence, diagnostic reports, and progress notes
Patient histories
Typewriter
Stapler
Mending tape
FILE stamp or pen
Sorter

PROCEDURE

1. Group all papers according to patients' names.
   Purpose: Some related papers may require stapling.
2. Remove any pins or paper clips.
   Purpose: Pins in file folders are hazardous; paper clips are bulky and may become inadvertently attached to other materials.
3. Mend any damaged or torn records.
4. Attach any small items to standard-size paper.
   Purpose: Small items are easily lost or misplaced in files.
5. Staple any related papers together.
6. Place your initials or FILE stamp in upper left corner.
   Purpose: To indicate that document is released for filing.
7. Code the document by underlining or writing the patient's name in the upper right corner.
   Purpose: To indicate where the document is to be filed.
8. Continue steps 2 through 7 until all documents have been conditioned, released, indexed, and coded.
9. Place all documents in sorter in filing sequence.
   Explanation: Sorter can be taken to file cabinet or shelf for placing documents in patient folders.

TERMINAL PERFORMANCE OBJECTIVE

Given the listed equipment and supplies, prepare and add supplemental documents to patient histories according to standard filing methods and established procedures of agency, within 30 minutes, to a performance level of 90%.

On the last day in each month, all the notations from behind the next month's guide are distributed behind the daily numbered guides, and the guide for the month just completed is placed at the back of the file.

Transitory or Temporary File. Many papers are kept longer than necessary because no provision is made for segregating those that have a limited usefulness. This situation is avoided by having a transitory or temporary file. For instance, if the medical assistant writes a letter requesting a reprint, the carbon is placed in the transitory folder. When the reprint is received, the carbon of the letter is destroyed. The transitory file is used for materials having no permanent value. The paper may be marked with a "T" and destroyed when the action involved is completed.

REFERENCES AND READINGS

Battista, M. E.: "Malpractice Risks of Documentation." Physicians' Management, February 1985, pp. 232–258.

Diamond, S. Z.: *Records Management, A Practical Guide.* New York, Anacom Book Division, American Management Association, 1983.

Chabner, D. E.: *The Language of Medicine*, 3rd ed. Philadelphia, W. B. Saunders Co., 1985.

Jennings, L. M.: *Secretarial and Administrative Procedures*, 2nd ed. Englewood Cliffs, NJ, Prentice-Hall, 1983.

Johnson, M. M., and Kallaus, N. F.: *Records Management*, 3rd ed. Cincinnati, South-Western Publishing Co., 1982.

Kinn, M. E.: *Medical Terminology Review Challenge*. Albany, NY, Delmar, 1987.

Krevolin, N.: *Filing and Records Management*. Englewood Cliffs, NJ, Prentice-Hall, 1986.

Popham, E., et al.: *Secretarial Procedures and Administration*, 8th ed. Cincinnati, South-Western Publishing Co., 1983.

Stewart, J. R., and Kahn, G.: *Gregg Quick Filing Practice*. New York, Gregg Division, McGraw-Hill, 1979.

11

CHAPTER OUTLINE

Professional Fees
    How Fees are Determined
    Advance Discussion of Fees
      Procedure 12–1: Explaining Doctor's Fees
    Adjusting or Canceling Fees
    Charges to Avoid

Credit Arrangements
    Extending Credit
    Installment Buying of Medical Services
      Procedure 12–2: Making Credit
      Arrangements with a Patient
    Confidentiality

VOCABULARY

See Glossary at end of book for definitions.

assignment
fee profile
fiscal agent

medical indigent
professional courtesy
third party payer

usual, customary, and reasonable
   (UCR)

12

Professional Fees and Credit Arrangements

OBJECTIVES

Upon successful completion of this chapter you should be able to:

1. Define the terms listed in the Vocabulary of this chapter.
2. Name three values that are considered in determining professional fees.
3. Give an example of a usual and customary fee.
4. Explain how a physician's fee profile is determined.
5. List three reasons for giving patients an estimate slip.
6. Discuss the concept of professional courtesy in medical fees.
7. List four kinds of charges that should be avoided.
8. Explain what is meant by third party liability.
9. Identify the three items of information that can be released in response to a request for credit information.
10. State three items that should be excluded in replying to a request for credit information.

Upon successful completion of this chapter you should be able to perform the following activities:

1. Make financial arrangements with a patient requesting credit.
2. Prepare a Truth in Lending form.
3. Respond to a patient's request for explanation of the physician's fee.

PROFESSIONAL FEES

While service to the patient is the primary concern of the medical profession, a physician must charge and collect a fee for such services in order to continue providing medical care. The practice of medicine is a business as well as a profession, and the details of conducting the business aspects are often the responsibility of the medical assistant. The physician will determine what the fees will be. The medical assistant will usually bear the responsibility of informing the patient on financial matters, collecting the payment, and in some cases making arrangements for deferred payment.

How Fees are Determined

Setting fees is no simple matter. The physician has three commodities to sell—time, judgment, and services. Yet the value of these commodities is never exactly the same to two different individuals. Medical care has little value except to the patient, and the value to the patient may not be consistent with the ability to pay. In every case the physician must place an estimate upon the value of the services. This value may then be modified by other considerations.

Prevailing Rate in the Community. One of the bases for determining medical fees is the economic level of the community. Different communities reflect different living scales, and this situation is reflected in medical fees as well. Consequently, the prevailing rate in the community—the average composite fee—must be taken into consideration by each individual physician. Strangely enough, fees that are too low drive patients away just as quickly as do fees that are too high.

Usual and Customary Fee. Most insurance plans base their payments on what has become known as a usual and customary fee for a given procedure. Some include the word reasonable; that is, **usual, customary**, and **reasonable**.

- The physician's *usual* fee for a given service is the fee that that individual physician most frequently charges for the service.
- The *customary* fee is a range of the usual fees charged for that same service by physicians with similar training and experience practicing in the same geographic and socioeconomic area. There is now a growing tendency for fees to be determined by national trends rather than by local customs.
- The term *reasonable* usually applies to a service or procedure that is exceptionally difficult or complicated, requiring extraordinary time or effort on the part of the physician.

It should be noted that under Medicare Part B, "customary" and "prevailing" correspond to "usual" and "customary" as defined here.

To illustrate, let us suppose that Dr. Wallace usually charges private patients $60 for a first office visit. The usual fees charged for a first visit by other doctors in the same community with similar training and experience range from $35 to $75. Dr. Wallace's fee of $60 is within the customary range and would therefore be paid by an insurance plan that pays on a usual and customary basis. If, on the other hand, the range of usual fees in the community is from $35 to $55, the insurance plan would allow only the maximum within the range, or $55, to Dr. Wallace.

Doctor's Fee Profile. The **fiscal agents** for government-sponsored insurance programs as well as some private plans keep a continuous record of the usual charges submitted for specific services by each individual doctor. By compiling and averaging these fees over a given period, usually a year, the doctor's **fee profile** is established. This fee profile is then used in determining the amount of third party liability for services under the program. One of the objections voiced by doctors is the lag between the time of a private fee increase and the time it is reflected in payments by an insurance carrier. It may be as long as 2 to 3 years.

Insurance Allowance. In some individual cases, the physician may not wish to charge the patient in addition to what will be allowed by the patient's insurance. The full fee should be quoted to the patient and charged to the account, with the understanding that after the insurance allowance has been received, the balance will be discounted. If a smaller fee is quoted and charged, several problems may arise:

1. The lower fee will alter the doctor's fee profile.
2. If it should become necessary to bring suit for payment of the fee, only the reduced fee can be recovered.
3. If the insurance allowance is paid on the basis of a certain percentage of the doctor's fee and a lower fee is charged, the insurance allowance will be correspondingly lower. Also, if the physician does this with many patients, the insurance company may take the position that the reduced fee is the doctor's usual fee, and base its payments accordingly. It may even be considered fraudulent in some instances.

Advance Discussion of Fees

It is natural for the patient, particularly one new to the practice, to wonder, "How much is this going to cost?" However, some patients may be reluctant to voice this concern.

It is the responsibility of the doctor or the medical assistant to raise the discussion of fees if the patient does not do so. Clyde T. Hardy, Jr., associate dean for Private Patient Services and Director of the Department of Clinics, Bowman Gray School of Medicine, Wake Forest University, Winston-Salem, NC, writing in Medical Economics (Feb. 7, 1977), states:

> Be prepared to discuss fees with any patient who's interested, but don't assume you must do so with everyone.

Mr. Hardy suggests opening the discussion of fees with something like this: "Mr. Willardson, do you have any questions about the costs of your operation? If you do, I'll be glad to review them." On the other hand, in this preliminary discussion of fees, the doctor must not sidestep the issue by saying "Don't worry about the bill, let's just get you well first." Avoid attempting to calm a worried patient about to undergo surgery by saying, "There's really nothing to it." The patient may later complain loudly about the bill because he misunderstood the complexity of the service.

In discussing fees with the patient,
DO SAY:
  "Mrs. Patient, do you have any questions about the costs of your operation? If you do I'll be glad to review them."
DON'T SAY:
  "Don't worry about the bill, Mrs. Patient, let's just get you well first."

Even in those cases where the doctor quotes a fee, the medical assistant is often charged with the responsibility of explaining the doctor's fees to the patient. The medical assistant must know how fees are determined and why charges vary, as well as have a thorough knowledge of the physician's practice and policies in order to handle perplexing situations involving fees.

As understanding of the practice increases, the medical assistant can be something of a "salesperson" for the doctor's services by subtly convincing patients that money spent for medical care is an excellent investment in the future. It is a rare patient who understands the intricate procedures involved in diagnosis and treatment. Other points to emphasize are:

- The long years of training and study and the heavy expenses involved in securing a medical education

- That running a modern professional office is a costly process relying upon day-to-day income in return for services

Advance fee discussions help the patient to plan ahead for medical expenditures. Most patients want to pay their financial obligations but rightly insist upon an accurate estimate of those obligations before they contract for purchase of goods or services. When a doctor frankly discusses fees in advance with patients, even to the point of describing how a fee is established, misconceptions about overcharging and fee frictions are usually eliminated. One doctor wrote the American Medical Association that, with 95% of his patients, 3 minutes at the end of the visit spent in explaining the medical bill ensures financial success.

Because many physicians and patients are reluctant to broach the subject of fees, the American Medical Association sells, for a very modest price, an attractive wall plaque that encourages fee discussions, with this message:

> TO ALL MY PATIENTS—I INVITE YOU TO DISCUSS FRANKLY WITH ME ANY QUESTIONS REGARDING MY SERVICES OR MY FEES. THE BEST MEDICAL SERVICE IS BASED ON A FRIENDLY, MUTUAL UNDERSTANDING BETWEEN DOCTOR AND PATIENT.

This plaque should be placed in the physician's office, not in the reception room.

Explaining Additional Costs. Explanations of medical costs should extend beyond the doctor's own charges. For example, if a patient is to undergo surgery, the doctor should also explain the costs of the operation, the anesthetist's and radiologist's charges, the laboratory fees, and the approximate hospital bill. The importance of calling in another physician for consultation should be explained to patients when consultation becomes necessary. It should be made clear, in advance, that there will be a separate bill submitted by the consulting physician. Patients do not always understand that the consultation is for the benefit of the patient, not the physician.

Estimate Slips. Some physicians give patients an estimate of medical expenses before hospitalization (Fig. 12–1). A few medical societies cooperatively develop such estimate sheets with local hospitals. The American Medical Association includes an example of an estimate sheet in its publication, *The Business Side of Medical Practice*. Individual doctors occasionally work up their own estimate forms when a patient is embarking on long-term treatment. The doctor should, however, emphasize that it is an estimate only and that the actual cost may vary somewhat.

Estimate slips should be prepared in duplicate so that the patient may have a copy and the original can be retained in the patient file. This eliminates the possibility of misquoting the fee later or forgetting the charge originally discussed. Advance estimation and explanation of medical fees simplifies collection, since it eliminates later misunderstanding and confusion over charges.

12

Procedure 12-1

PROCEDURAL GOAL

To explain the doctor's fees so that the patient understands his or her obligations and rights for privacy.

EQUIPMENT AND SUPPLIES

Patient's statement
Copy of physician's fee schedule
Quiet private area where the patient feels free to ask questions

PROCEDURE

1. Determine that the patient has the correct bill.
   Purpose: To make certain it is this patient's bill and that the insurance numbers, the address, and the phone number are correct.
2. Examine the bill for possible errors.
   Purpose: To demonstrate that the patient's concerns are important and that you are willing to make any necessary adjustments.
3. Refer to the fee schedule for the services rendered.
   Purpose: To explain how physicians determine their fees. If an error has occurred, correct it immediately with a sincere apology.
4. Explain itemized billing:
   a. Date of each service.
   b. Type of service rendered.
   c. Fee.
   Purpose: To make certain that the patient realizes the number and extent of services rendered.
5. Display professional attitude toward the patient.
   Purpose: To reassure the patient that you have a thorough understanding of the fee schedule and show willingness to answer questions politely and completely.
6. Determine whether the patient has specific concerns that may hinder payment.
   Purpose: To provide an opportunity for making special arrangements if needed.
7. Make appropriate arrangements for a discussion between the physician and patient if further explanation is necessary for resolution of the problem.

TERMINAL PERFORMANCE OBJECTIVE

Given the listed equipment and supplies, a patient and a private area, explain your physician's charges and office policy, with professional demeanor and absolute accuracy, within 10 minutes, to a performance level of 100% (time varies with the patient and the problem).

Role-play under supervision of instructor.

Adjusting or Canceling Fees

Care for Those Who Cannot Pay. The medical profession has traditionally accepted the responsibility of providing medical care for individuals unable to pay for these services. In spite of the increased scope of government-sponsored care for the **medically indigent**, doctors still donate thousands of dollars' worth of such medical services each year.

In many instances, medical care of the indigent is available through social service agencies. The medical assistant should become acquainted with the various local organizations and agencies that can aid the patient in obtaining the necessary assistance. The doctor can provide only medical services. Other agencies must provide hospitalization, for example, or arrange for paying the costs of special therapy, rehabilitation, or medications. Unfortunately there is still a large group of working

```
                    SURGICAL COST ESTIMATE

Name of Patient_____Date_____

Procedure_____

        Your surgery has been scheduled at _____Hospital
on _____. You should report to the Admitting Office between the
hours of ____ (a.m.) (p.m.) and _____ (a.m.) (p.m.).

        Although medical and hospital expenses are seldom welcomed, knowing in
advance what expenses to expect and how to plan for them can lessen the burden.
This estimate is prepared to assist you in budgeting your surgical costs.

                        PROFESSIONAL FEES

     When you have major surgery, the surgical team includes the operating
surgeon, the assistant surgeon, and the anesthetist.  Each has an important
part in your care, and each will render a separate statement for services.
While each doctor will independently set his/her own fee, it is usually possible
to estimate in advance an approximate range of fees.  Assuming an uncomplicated
course for your surgery, the charges are estimated as follows:
             Operating surgeon           $_____ to $_____
             Assistant Surgeon            _____ to  _____
             Anesthetist                  _____ to  _____
The assistant surgeon and the anesthetist usually base their fees on the
operating time; consequently, if a surgical procedure turns out to be more
complicated than was expected, their fees may be correspondingly increased.

        The estimated duration of your hospital stay is _____ days at $_____
a day for a (semi-private) (private) room.  During your hospital stay there
will be charges for laboratory tests, medications as required, and other
services.  It is impossible to estimate in advance what these charges will
be; they will be itemized on your hospital bill.  If you have health insurance,
please take the appropriate forms and I.D. information with you on the day of
your admittance.


            PLEASE KEEP IN MIND THIS IS ONLY AN ESTIMATE
```

Figure 12–1
Form for surgical cost estimate.

poor who have no insurance but who do not qualify for any assistance programs and often go without care.

If a doctor accepts a case for which a fee will not be paid, complete records must still be kept on the patient. The only deviation in procedure is that the financial record will indicate no charge (n/c) in the debit column.

Fees in Hardship Cases. Sometimes a doctor is faced with the problem of deciding whether to reduce or cancel a fee in a hardship case. Before adjusting or canceling a fee, the doctor or the medical assistant should encourage a frank discussion of the patient's financial situation. Find out whether the patient is entitled to insurance settlement of some kind. Circumstances may qualify the patient for local or state public assistance programs. If so, the assistant may direct the patient to the appropriate agency.

If the circumstances of hardship are known before the services are rendered, thorough discussion of what the fee will be and how it will be paid should take place at that time. In most cases it is far better to adjust a fee before rather than after treatment. The doctor may suggest that a medically indigent patient seek care at a county hospital with public assistance. A doctor should be free to choose his or her form of charity and not feel obligated to substantially reduce or cancel a fee when the circumstances are known in advance.

After the doctor and patient have agreed upon a fee, special circumstances may arise that create a hardship. If the doctor then agrees to reduce the fee, the patient should be told that the reduction will be effective only after the adjusted amount is paid in full. For instance, if a fee of $300 is reduced to $200, the full amount of the $300 charge should appear on the ledger and when $200 has been received, the remainder can be written off as an adjustment.

There must be some limit put on the time, effort, and expense invested in trying to collect an uncollectible account. Under some circumstances it may be better simply to write off an unpaid account. An example of a letter that might be used to cancel the account and at the same time improve the image of the physician is shown in Figure 12–2.

Pitfalls of Fee Adjustments. Great care should be taken in reducing the fee for care of a patient who dies. The doctor's sympathy is with the family in such instances, but the doctor's generosity in reducing a fee could be misinterpreted and result in a suit for malpractice.

If the doctor agrees to settle for a reduced fee in a situation in which the patient is disputing the fee, care should be taken to make certain the negotiations are "without prejudice." By taking this precaution the doctor protects the right to collect the original sum should the patient refuse to pay the lowered fee. The offer of a discount, therefore, should be made in writing, with the insertion of the words "without prejudice," and a definite time limit for making payment stated. Make two copies of the agreement and have the signatures witnessed. Keep the original for the doctor and give a copy to the patient.

A fee should never be reduced on the basis of a poor result or as a means of obtaining payment to avoid the use of a collection agency. A reduction for these reasons degrades the doctor and the practice of medicine.

Professional Courtesy. Traditionally, doctors do not charge other doctors or their immediate dependents for medical care. Although the concept of **professional courtesy** is often attributed to Hippocrates, the foundations of professional courtesy today are actually derived from Thomas Percival's Code of 1803.

In some cases, the giving of professional courtesy represents the loss of a large amount of potential income. If there is a substantial outlay in the cost of materials, the professional colleague will probably wish to reimburse the physician for the materials used. Most doctors today subscribe to a health insurance plan. If the care they receive is covered by insurance, it is entirely ethical for the attending physician to accept the insurance benefits in payment for services.

If the services are frequent enough to involve a significant proportion of the doctor's professional time, or extend over a long period of time, the doctor may wish to charge on an adjusted basis.

If professional courtesy is offered, but the recipient insists upon paying, the physician need not hesitate on ethical grounds to accept a fee for services.

Professional courtesy is often extended beyond fellow physicians and their dependents. Most physicians treat their own medical assistants without charge, and grant discounts to nurses and medical assistants not in their direct employ. Professional courtesy is sometimes extended to others in the health care field, for instance, pharmacists and dentists. There is a growing sentiment that professional courtesy has outlived its usefulness and should be abandoned.

Charges to Avoid

Telephone Calls. It is generally considered inadvisable to charge for telephone calls. Some physicians, especially pediatricians, find they must give considerable advice over the telephone. Many of these calls, however, are fairly routine to the office (although not to the worried mother or patient), and an able medical assistant can be trained to

```
Patient Name
Street Address
City, State, ZIP

Dear Patient:

Your balance of $150 has been on our books since
March 15, 1985.

In view of the financial circumstances that make
payment on these past services difficult for you,
Dr. Johnson has instructed me to consider the debt
cancelled.  We will no longer bill you for it.

The doctor wants you to feel free, however, to call
on him for any future service you may require.

                    Sincerely yours,


                    Office Manager for
                    E. F. Johnson, M.D.
```

Figure 12–2
Example of letter canceling fee.

12

answer many of the questions, or a special time can be set aside for telephone calls.

Late Charges. Levying late charges on fees for professional services not paid within a prescribed time is usually not in the best interest of the public or the profession. However, the physician who has experienced problems with delinquent accounts may properly choose to request that payment be made at the time of treatment or add interest or other reasonable charges to delinquent accounts. The physician must comply with state and federal regulations applicable to the imposition of such charges (see Truth in Lending Act, p. 181).

Missed Appointments. Most physicians feel that charging for a missed appointment or for one not canceled 24 hours in advance, although not unethical if the patient is fully advised, is nevertheless not in the best interest of their patients or their practices.

Insurance Forms. If the patient has multiple insurance forms to be completed, the physician is justified in making a charge but should be willing to complete the first standard form without charge.

> *Avoid charging for:*
> *Telephone calls*
> *Late payments*
> *Missed appointments*
> *First insurance forms*

CREDIT ARRANGEMENTS

Extending Credit

Whenever a service is rendered before payment is received, an extension of credit has been made. If payment is collected upon completion of the service, no problem exists. But if payment is deferred, credit arrangements are best made during the patient's initial visit. Successful collection of an account may depend upon the skill and tact with which the medical assistant conducts the first interview.

Federal law (Equal Credit Opportunity Act of 1977) bars discrimination in all areas of credit, with the purpose of ensuring that credit is made available fairly and impartially, and specifies "prohibited bases" under the law.

> *The law prohibits discrimination against any applicant for credit because of race, color, religion, national origin, sex, marital status, or age; or because the applicant receives income from any public assistance program; or because he has exercised rights under consumer credit laws.*

Many medical assistants inform a patient telephoning for a first appointment that new patients are expected to pay cash for their first visit, at which time credit arrangements can be established if further care is needed. You can say, for example,

> "Mr. Barrington, your appointment is scheduled for 9:30 AM, Tuesday, September 25, with Dr. Newhouse. The usual charge for a first office visit is about XX dollars, and we ask that payment for a first visit be made at the time of service. If you wish to establish credit arrangements in case further care is needed, please plan to be here 15 minutes early so that the necessary papers can be completed."

This approach informs the patient in advance that he will be expected to complete a credit application.

Information from the Patient. Good records are essential to follow-up of collections. It is extremely important that the medical assistant get adequate information about the patient's ability to pay—on the first office visit if possible. It is neither unprofessional nor time consuming to get full credit information from patients. The public is conditioned to supplying such information, and will respect a businesslike approach if it is done tactfully and without apology. While a patient needing medical care will rarely be turned away because of a credit risk, the information provided on the initial visit may alert the medical assistant to be cautious about allowing an account to fall in arrears.

Although the registration form the patient completes in the doctor's office is usually not as detailed as an application for credit in, for example, a department store, it must establish an information base, should future collection steps become necessary. The form illustrated in Figure 12–3 is typical.

The medical assistant should check the completed form carefully, to make certain that nothing was overlooked. The new patient will view these questions as reasonable, but the established patient may resent such an inquiry. Consequently, it is important that the form be completed on the first visit.

Irrespective of the form or techniques used, the following information should be obtained:

1. *Patient's full name (first, middle, and last), correctly spelled.* J. A. Brown is not sufficient if later collection follow-up is necessary. John Allen Brown would be more helpful.

2. *Date of birth.* This will be useful as identification if there are two patients with similar names. Also, you will be able to determine the patient's exact age at any future time.

3. *Social Security number, if any.* The Social Security number is an increasingly important item of identification. In many states it is required in making collection efforts against bank accounts, wages, or any other personal property. Many insurance policies use the patient's Social Security number as the certificate number.

PATIENT INFORMATION FOR MEDICAL RECORDS (PLEASE PRINT)

□ Mr.

□ Mrs.

NAME □ Miss ___Brooks_____Marie_____Allen___
LAST   FIRST   MIDDLE INITIAL

Social Security # __000 11 2222_____

Drivers License # __315Z09A_____

HOME ADDRESS __1234 East Street_____ CITY __Cincinnati__ STATE __OH__ ZIP __45202__

HOME PHONE (513) 252-0000____ WORK PHONE (513) __212-0000___ BIRTHDATE __03 / 26 / 50__ AGE _____

MARITAL STATUS (✓): □ MARRIED □ SINGLE □ DIVORCED □ SEPARATED □ WIDOW/ER □ MINOR

EMPLOYED BY __Central Financial Management_____

WORK ADDRESS __15 Main Street, Cincinnati 45210__ OCCUPATION____CPA_____

SPOUSE/PARENT __Brooks_____Walter_____Z____ OCCUPATION___writer_____
LAST   FIRST   MIDDLE INITIAL

WORK ADDRESS __1234 East Street, Cincinnati_____ WORK PHONE (513) __252-0000_____

WHO REFERRED YOU TO THIS OFFICE? __M. A. Wilkins, M.D._____

▼ MEDICAL INSURANCE INFORMATION

HOW DO YOU INTEND TO PAY? (✓) □ Cash □ Check □ Credit Card □ Insurance □ Medicare □ Medicaid or Medi/Cal

NAME OF INSURANCE CO. __Travelers_____ ADDRESS __Columbus, Ohio_____
CITY   STATE   ZIP

POLICY NUMBER __TLC 2000_____ GROUP NAME/#_____

REASON FOR THIS VISIT: ☒ Illness □ Injury □ Job Related Injury □ Auto Accident □ Personal Injury

DATE OF INJURY OR ONSET OF PROBLEM: ___/___/___ MAJOR COMPLAINT_____

IF SOMEONE OTHER THAN PATIENT IS RESPONSIBLE FOR PAYMENT
▼ PLEASE COMPLETE THIS SECTION

NAME OF RESPONSIBLE PARTY _____
ADDRESS   CITY   STATE   ZIP

WHAT IS THEIR RELATIONSHIP TO THE PATIENT? _____ SOCIAL SECURITY NUMBER_____

EMPLOYED BY _____ WORK PHONE ( )_____ HOME PHONE ( )_____

▼ IF YOUR INJURY IS JOB RELATED

NAME OF PERSON WHO CAN AUTHORIZE TREATMENT _____

COMPANY'S INSURANCE CARRIER _____
ADDRESS

INSURANCE CARRIER PHONE NUMBER ( )_____ OK'D BY_____

▼ PLEASE SIGN AND RETURN TO RECEPTIONIST

I, the undersigned, have insurance coverage with_____ and assign directly to
Name of Insurance Carrier

_____ all surgical and/or medical benefits, if any, otherwise payable to me for
Name of Doctor

services rendered. I understand that I am financially responsible for all charges whether or not paid by insurance. I hereby authorize the doctor to release all information necessary to secure the payment of benefits.

Date_____ Signed _____

*NOTE: Please notify us if any of the above information changes during the course of your treatment.

BIBBERO SYSTEMS, INC. • PETALUMA, CA • FORM NO. #58-8408 • © 1982

12

Figure 12–3
Patient information sheet for medical records. (Courtesy of Bibbero Systems, Inc., Petaluma, CA.)

4. *Marital status and number of dependents.* This information may be useful in determining ability to pay.

5. *Current address and telephone number, and past addresses for at least two years.* Frequent changes of address sometimes indicate financial instability. If the patient has no home telephone, get the number of a telephone where he or she can be reached.

6. *Patient's occupation, employer's name, address, and telephone number.* It may be necessary to call the patient at work or contact the employer.

7. *Spouse's occupation and name and address of employer.* Employment title and name of immediate supervisor may be helpful.

8. *Name and relationship of person legally responsible for payment.* See paragraph on third party liability, below.

9. *Name, address, and telephone number of person to be notified in case of emergency.*

10. *Driver's license number,* if any.

11. *Source of referral.* If the patient was referred by another physician, you will want to send a report to that physician. If the patient was referred by another patient, the doctor may wish to thank the referring patient on his next visit to the office.

12. *Health insurance information.* See paragraph below on this page.

> *When a patient applies for credit, you may not ask the applicant's sex, race, color, religion, or national origin. You may not ask about birth control practices or plans to have children. You may collect this information when it is part of a medical history, but not when it is related to granting credit.*

Under the Equal Credit Opportunity Act, once you agree to extend credit to one patient, you must offer the same arrangement to any other patient who requests it. You can refuse to do so only on the basis of ability or inability to pay. It is interesting that one way to avoid involvement with the credit laws is to accept bank credit cards.

Third Party Liability. If financial responsibility is attributed to an individual other than the patient, spouse, or parent, be sure to obtain full name, address, employment data, and other credit information about that person. Also, contact the named individual for verification of the obligation. If a **third party payer's** agreement to pay is contingent upon the patient's failure to pay, such as agreement must be in writing to be enforceable and must be made prior to treatment. Any agreement made after completion of treatment could be considered as a moral obligation only. The guarantee of a person to pay the account of another may be very simple. It may be typewritten or handwritten, stating:

I, the undersigned, do promise to pay for the medical services rendered by Theodore Wilson,

MD, to my nephew, Robert L. Smith.
Date:
Signed:

or

I, the undersigned, promise to pay the medical bill of Robert L. Smith, if his mother, Mrs. Lydia Smith, does not pay by the 15th of July, 19xx.
Date:
Signed:

Accounts rendered to a spouse or child should always carry full data about the party responsible, which in most cases is the other spouse or the parent. Generally, a responsible spouse or parent pays the account without any follow-up collection procedures. In the case of a minor, it is generally held that the parent accompanying the child to the medical facility is responsible for paying. Any agreement between divorced or separated parents is solely between them and does not affect the obligation to the physician.

If you foresee legal difficulties in collecting an account in which divorce, legal guardianship, or the involvement of an emancipated minor complicates the matter, it is best to contact your doctor's attorney for advice. The laws governing such matters vary according to each state. One reminder, however, is that you must always have the signature of the third party responsible for the debt if he or she is not otherwise obligated by law. An oral agreement is not binding.

Health Insurance Information. The initial interview is the best time to get full information on the patient's insurance coverage. The patient registration form usually provides a place for the name of the insurance company. Ask to see the patient's identification card and make a photocopy for your records. The card usually shows the name of the subscriber and the group and member number, and often includes a service code indicating the patient's coverage. Also obtain information on any supplementary coverage—for instance, a plan in which the spouse is the subscriber and the patient is covered as a dependent. There may also be major medical or supplementary benefits to the patient's policy.

Assignment of Benefits. Many doctors ask the patient to execute an **assignment** of insurance benefits at this time. The assignment, authorizing the insurance company to pay benefits directly to the doctor, may be stamped on the insurance form or may be subsequently attached to a completed insurance form.

Consent for Release of Information. If a standard claim form is used or if the patient has brought along his own form, this is an appropriate time to have the patient sign the consent for release of the information that is necessary on most claims, so that the insurance form can be processed without delay as services are performed. Some states require a special form for release of information separate and apart from the insurance claim form itself. The medical assistant should check local regulations.

Installment Buying of Medical Services

Because installment buying is so much a part of our economic system today, the physician's office must be prepared to help patients budget for their medical care. Patients expect to use their credit resources and will appreciate businesslike assistance in establishing a payment plan. The medical profession has too long suffered a poor collection record because of its fear of appearing "too commercial." The doctor should be ready to arrange credit when medical bills will be high or when a patient for some reason is unable to pay at the time of service. In general, fees for routine office calls and small medical bills should be kept on a pay-as-you-go basis.

Credit Cards. The acceptance of credit cards, sometimes called bank cards, is becoming commonplace in medical practice. Patients appreciate the convenience, and paying by credit card may help to improve collections. The signed credit card voucher is deposited to the doctor's bank account. The card company deducts a percentage (from 1% to 5% depending upon volume) for the collection service. The patient may pay the full amount when billed by the card company or may pay a portion and be charged interest on the balance.

Special Budget Plans. If a patient appears concerned about the ability to meet his financial obligations, the doctor or the medical assistant can suggest in a tactful way:

"Mr. Elwood, if you think you will have difficulty paying for your treatments at one time, we can work out some special arrangements."

This allows the patient to ask what sort of plan you have in mind, and the discussion progresses very easily into various payment plans. Generally, it is better to let the patient decide what arrangements will be best rather than to suggest a plan. However, if the patient has no suggestion, the medical assistant can say:

"Mr. Elwood, would you be able to pay $50 each month until the account is paid in full?"

or

"Usually an account of this size can be settled in 3 to 4 months. Would you be able to pay $100 now, then $50 a month until the account is paid in full?"

When the amount of each installment has been agreed upon, it is then wise to establish definite dates on which the payments will be expected.

Truth in Lending Act. Regulation Z of the Truth in Lending Act, which is enforced by the Federal Trade Commission, requires that when there is a bilateral agreement between doctor and patient to accept payment in more than four installments, the doctor is required to provide disclosure of information regarding finance charges. Even if there are no finance charges involved, the form must be completed stating this fact. A copy of the form is retained by the doctor, and the original is given to the patient. Specific wording is required in the disclosure. The form in Figure 12–4 meets the requirements. Have the patient sign the agreement in your presence, as you must have proof of signing. The disclosure statement must be kept on file for two years. Although the disclosure statement is

LEONARD S. TAYLOR, M.D.
2100 WEST PARK AVENUE
CHAMPAIGN, ILLINOIS 61820

TELEPHONE 351-5400

FEDERAL TRUTH IN LENDING STATEMENT
For professional services rendered

Patient ___Joseph Brookhurst___

Address ___353 West Terry Lane___
___Birmingham, Alabama 35209___

Parent _____

1. Cash Price (fee for service)	$ 1200.00
2. Cash Down Payment	$ 200.00
3. Unpaid Balance of Cash Price	$ 1000.00
4. Amount Financed	$ 1000.00
5. FINANCE CHARGE	$ -0-
6. Finance Charge Expressed As Annual Percentage Rate	-0-
7. Total of Payments (4 plus 5)	$ 1000.00
8. Deferred Payment Price (1 plus 5)	$ 1200.00

"Total payment due" (7 above) is payable to ___Dr. Leonard S. Taylor___ at above office address in ___five___ monthly installments of $___200.00___ The first installment is payable on ___May 1___ 19XX, and each subsequent payment is due on the same day of each consecutive month until paid in full.

___4-15-19xx___ _____
Date ___ Signature of Patient; Parent if Patient is a Minor

FORM 9402 COLWELL SYSTEMS, INC. CHAMPAIGN, ILLINOIS

Figure 12–4
Disclosure statement. (Courtesy of Colwell Systems, Inc., Champaign, IL.)

designed as protection for the debtor, it can be a good collection tool for the creditor.

It is recognized that physicians generally permit their patients to pay in installments, and as long as there is no specific agreement on the part of the physician for payment to be made in more than four installments, and no finance charge is made, the account is not subject to the regulation. If the patient chooses to pay in installments instead of the full amount, this is considered a unilateral action

Procedure 12–2   *MAKING CREDIT ARRANGEMENTS WITH A PATIENT*

PROCEDURAL GOAL

To assist the patient in paying for services by making mutually beneficial credit arrangements according to established office policy.

EQUIPMENT AND SUPPLIES

Patient's ledger
Calendar
Truth in Lending form
Assignment of Benefits form
Patient's insurance form
Typewriter
Private area for interview

PROCEDURE

1. Answer thoroughly and kindly all questions about credit.
2. Inform the patient of office policy regarding credit:
   a. Payment at time of first visit
   b. Payment by bank card
   c. Credit application
   Purpose: To ensure complete understanding of mutual responsibilities.
3. Have the patient complete the credit application.
   Purpose: To comply with office practices on extension of credit.
4. Check the completed credit application.
   Purpose: To confirm that all necessary information is included.
5. Discuss with the patient the possible arrangements, and ask the patient to decide which of those arrangements is most suitable.
   Purpose: Better compliance can be expected when patient makes the choice.
6. Prepare the Truth in Lending form and have the patient sign it if the agreement requires more than four installments.
   Purpose: To comply with Regulation Z.
7. Have the patient execute assignment of insurance benefits.
   Purpose: To comply with credit policy.
8. Make a copy of the patient's insurance ID and have the patient sign a consent for release of information to insurance company.
   Purpose: Consent for release of information is necessary on most insurance forms before a claim can be processed.
9. Keep credit information confidential.

TERMINAL PERFORMANCE OBJECTIVE

Given the listed equipment and supplies, make credit arrangements that are agreeable to the patient and that conform to office policy, within 15 minutes, to a performance level of 100% (time will vary with patient and problem).

and the physician, in accepting such payments, probably would not be subject to the provisions of the regulation. The doctor's office, however, must be certain to bill for the full balance each time. If the statement is for only a partial payment, it then becomes a bilateral agreement and as such is subject to Regulation Z.

Helping patients budget their medical expenses is a rather new aspect of the business side of medical practice. However, it is a real service to patients and demonstrates that the doctor and the office staff are sincerely anxious to help patients pay their own way. It may also prevent many collection problems.

Confidentiality

Credit information is confidential. It should be guarded as carefully as a confidential medical history and should be disclosed to no one. When you ask for credit information from patients in the office, do so in a private area where others cannot overhear the conversation. A desk or table away from the reception area where a patient can sit in total privacy and complete a credit application is a great asset. Credit information is personal—it should be kept that way.

Credit Bureaus. Some doctors join a credit bureau, particularly in large cities where it is more difficult to gauge informally the patients' ability to pay. Credit bureaus gather credit information from many sources, pool it, and make it available to dues-paying bureau members. If you receive a request for credit information about one of your patients, it is permissible to furnish it because the debtor, by giving the doctor's name as a reference, has given implied consent; otherwise, the credit bureau would not have contacted you. According to the Fair Credit Practices Act Amendments of 1975, you can reply by giving ledger information only:

1. When the account was opened
2. How much the patient now owes
3. The highest amount of the account at any time

The doctor's office should confine information furnished to these three items and avoid any reference to character, paying habits, or credit rating.

Medical-Dental-Hospital Bureaus. The Medical-Dental-Hospital Bureaus of America (MDHBA), with headquarters in Chicago, is a national organization of agencies serving physicians, dentists, and hospitals. It seeks to maintain the highest standards among its members and is committed to following the collection methods most acceptable to physicians. Doctors who use their collection services have access to credit information on accounts assigned by other clients. Member bureaus of the MDHBA frequently assist the medical assistant by sponsoring collection seminars, as well as by providing speakers for medical assistant society meeting.

REFERENCES AND READINGS

American Medical Association: *The Business Side of Medical Practice.* Chicago, The Association, 1979.

Manning, F. F.: *Medical Group Practice Management.* Cambridge, Ballinger Publishing Co., 1977.

12

CHAPTER OUTLINE

What Is Accounting?
 Account Bases
 Financial Summaries

Cardinal Rules of Bookkeeping
Good Working Habits
Terminology of Accounts
Kinds of Accounting Records
Comparison of Common Accounting Systems
 Single Entry System
 Double Entry System
 Pegboard or Write-It-Once System

Using the Pegboard Accounting System
Special Accounting Entries
  Procedure 13–1: Posting Service Charges
   and Payments Using Pegboard System

Accounts Receivable Control
Trial Balance of Accounts Receivable
Accounts Payable Procedures
  Procedure 13–2: Accounting for Petty Cash

Periodic Summaries
Accounting with the Aid of the Computer

VOCABULARY

See Glossary at end of book for definitions.

account balance	disbursements	payables
accounting equation	general journal	posting
accounts payable	invoice	statement
accounts receivable	packing slip	

Accounting Systems

13

OBJECTIVES

Upon successful completion of this chapter you should be able to:

1. Define the terms listed in the Vocabulary of this chapter.
2. List the two bases of accounting and explain their differences.
3. State the four kinds of information that the financial records of any business should show at all times.
4. Differentiate between a debit balance and a credit balance.
5. Describe and demonstrate the entry for a credit balance.
6. List six kinds of accounting records.
7. Compare the three most common accounting systems used in the professional office.
8. State the basic accounting equation.
9. Discuss the importance of a trial balance.
10. List and state the purpose of the five common periodic accounting summaries.

Upon successful completion of this chapter you should be able to perform the following activities:

1. Prepare a ledger account for a new patient.
2. Prepare a patient charge slip.
3. Journalize service charges and payments using a single entry system.
4. Post the entries from the daily journal to patient ledger cards.
5. Prepare a daily posting proof.
6. Prepare a daily cash control proof.
7. Prepare a monthly trial balance.
8. Establish and maintain a petty cash fund.
9. Post service charges and payments using a pegboard.

A physician's business records are the key to good management practice. The medical assistant who can keep accurate financial records and who will conduct the nonmedical side of the practice in a businesslike fashion is genuinely needed and appreciated.

Financial records that are complete, correct, and current are essential for:

- Prompt billing and collection procedures
- Professional financial planning
- Accurate reporting of income to federal and state agencies

WHAT IS ACCOUNTING?

Accounting is the art or system of recording, classifying, and summarizing financial transactions.

Bookkeeping is mainly the recording part of the accounting process. The bookkeeping must be done daily and is the responsibility of the administrative medical assistant in a small practice. In a larger practice the office manager or financial manager assumes this responsibility.

Account Bases

There are two bases for accounting: the *cash basis* and the *accrual basis* (Table 13–1).

Most physicians use the cash basis of accounting. Expressed simply, this means that charges for services are entered as income when payment is received and expenses are recorded when they are paid.

Merchants, on the other hand, generally use an accrual basis of accounting. On the accrual basis, income is considered earned when services have been performed or goods have been sold, even though payment may not have been received. Expenses are recognized and recorded when incurred, even though they have not been paid.

Financial Summaries

The financial records of any business should at all times show:

- How much was earned in a given period

- How much was collected
- How much is owed
- The distribution of expenses incurred

From the daily entries, the accountant can prepare monthly and annual summaries that provide a basis for comparing any given period with another similar period.

Periodic analyses of the financial records can result in improved business practices, better management of time, curtailment or elimination of unprofitable services, and better budgeting of expenses.

CARDINAL RULES OF BOOKKEEPING

1. Enter all charges and receipts immediately in the daily record or journal.
2. Write a receipt in duplicate for any currency received. Writing receipts for checks is optional, but a consistent pattern should be followed.
3. Post all charges and receipts to the patient ledger daily.
4. Endorse checks for deposit as soon as received.
5. Deposit all receipts in the bank.
6. Verify that the total of the deposit plus the amount on hand equals the total to be accounted for in the daily journal.
7. Use a petty cash fund to pay for small unpredictable expenses. Pay all other expenses by check (a canceled check is the best proof of payment).
8. Pay all bills before their due dates, after checking them for accuracy. Place date of payment and number of check on paid bills.

GOOD WORKING HABITS

A willingness to pay attention to detail, good organizational skills, and the ability to concentrate and maintain consistency in working patterns and procedures are all necessary qualifications for the person who has the responsibility of keeping financial records. The careful bookkeeper will:

- Use good penmanship
- Use the same pen style and ink consistently
- Keep columns of figures straight
- Write well-formed figures (a careless "9" may look like a "7"; an open "0" may resemble a "6")
- Carry decimal points correctly
- Check arithmetic carefully and not put blind faith in a calculator
- Not erase, write over, or blot out figures (if an error is made, a straight line should be drawn through the incorrect figure and the correct figure written above it)

Bookkeeping procedures are not difficult or com-

Table 13–1
Accounting Bases

	Cash Basis	Accrual Basis
Income is recorded	When received	When service is performed or goods are sold
Expense is recorded	When paid	When incurred (even if not paid)

186

plicated, but they do require concentration to avoid errors. There is no such thing as *almost* correct financial records. The books either balance or they do not balance. The bookkeeping is either right or wrong. This is not the place to be creative or take shortcuts.

The medical assistant should set aside a certain time each day for bookkeeping tasks, if possible. Do not attempt to work on financial records when you are busy attending patients or when there are other distractions.

TERMINOLOGY OF ACCOUNTS

In order to understand and perform bookkeeping procedures, it is first necessary to learn some of the terminology of accounts.

A business *transaction* is the occurrence of an event or of a condition that must be recorded. For example:

- A service is performed for which a charge is made
- A patient makes a payment on account
- A piece of equipment is purchased
- The monthly rent is paid

Each is a transaction that must be recorded within the accounting system.

The *daily journal* is called the book of original entry because this is where all transactions are first recorded (Fig. 13–1).

A patient's financial record is called an *account*. All of the patients' accounts together constitute the *accounts receivable ledger*.

Account cards vary in design, but all will have at least three columns for entering figures:

- The *debit* (abbreviation: Dr) column on the left is used for entering charges and is sometimes called the charge column.
- The *credit* (abbreviation: Cr) column to the right, sometimes headed "Paid," is used for entering payments received.
- The *balance* column on the far right is used for recording the difference between the debit and credit columns.
- An *adjustment* column is available in some systems, and is used for entering professional discounts, write-offs, disallowances by insurance companies, and so forth (Fig. 13–2).

Posting means the transfer of information from one record to another. Transactions are posted from the journal to the ledger (this is accomplished in one writing in the pegboard system).

The *account balance* is normally a debit balance (charges exceed payments). A debit balance is entered by simply writing the correct figure in the balance column.

A *credit balance* will exist when payments exceed

charges; for instance, when a patient pays in advance. This is common in obstetric practices. To show a credit balance, record the figures in one of the following two ways:

1. Write the credit balance on the card in regular ink and enclose the figure in parentheses or encircle it.

2. Write the credit balance in red ink (this cannot be accomplished on the pegboard unless red carbon is inserted).

Discounts are also credit entries and are entered in the adjustment column or, if there is no adjustment column, the discount is entered in the debit column in red ink or enclosed in parentheses. By making the entry this way, it is recognized as a subtraction from the charges. In totaling columns, any figure in red or in parentheses is always subtracted.

Receipts are cash and checks taken in payment for professional services.

Receivables are charges for which payment has not been received—amounts that are owing.

Disbursements are cash amounts paid out.

Payables are amounts owed to others but not yet paid.

KINDS OF ACCOUNTING RECORDS

General Journal. The general journal (or daily journal) is the chronologic record of the practice—the financial diary. All information regarding services rendered, charges, and receipts is first recorded in the daily journal. It is important that every transaction be recorded.

In addition to professional services rendered in and out of the office, there may be income from other sources, such as rentals, royalties, interest, and so forth. Usually a special place is provided in the journal for such income. Any income that is not practice-related should be recorded separately from patient receipts.

Ledger. The accounts receivable ledger comprises all the patients' financial accounts on which there are balances. All charges and payments for professional services are posted to the ledger daily. The ledger then becomes a reliable source of information for answering all inquiries from patients about their accounts.

A separate account card or page is prepared for each patient (or each family) at the time of the first visit or service (Fig. 13–3). The heading of the account should include all information pertinent to collecting the account:

- Name and address of person responsible for payment
- Insurance identification
- Social Security number

13

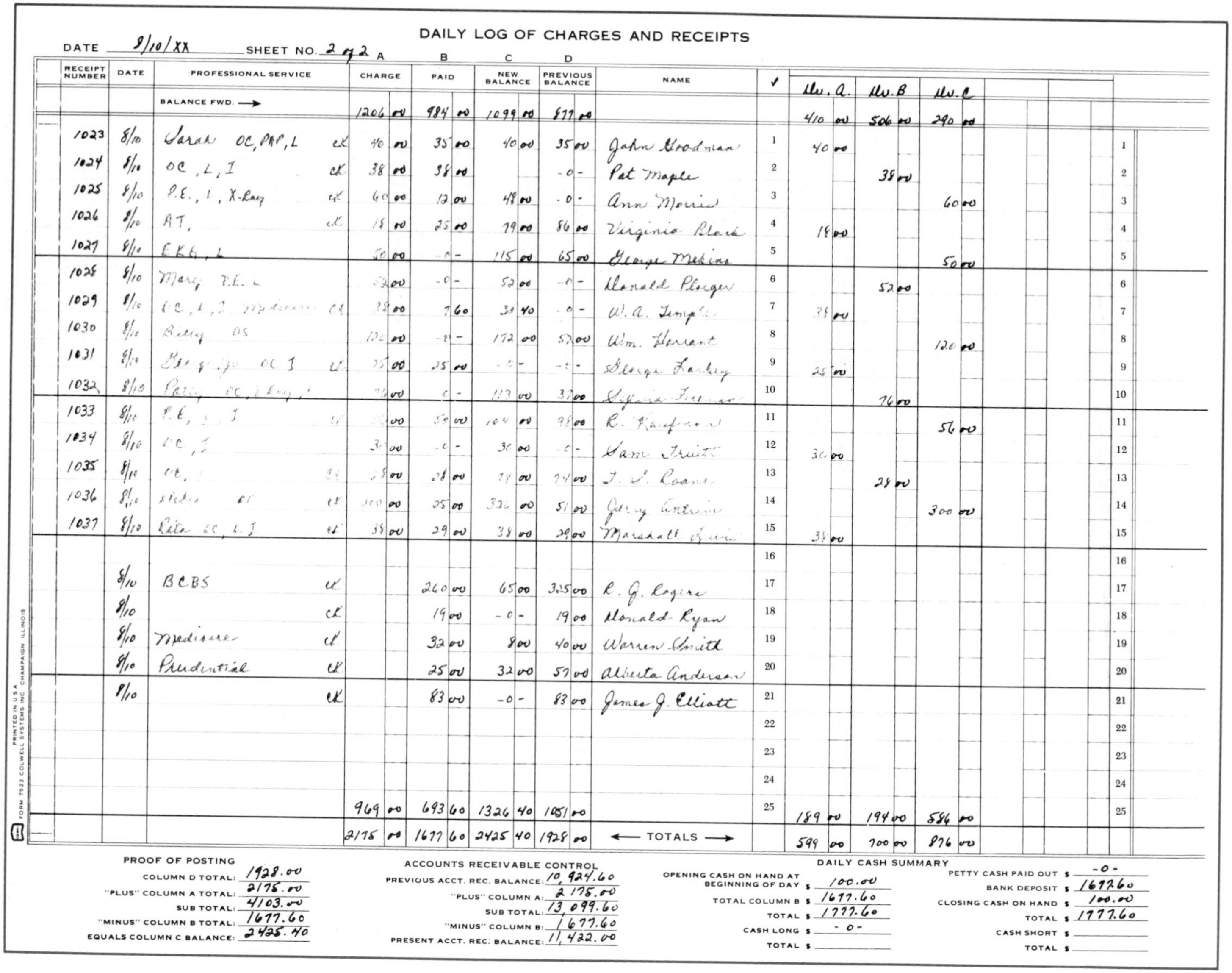

Figure 13–1

Sample day sheet for pegboard bookkeeping system, with deposit list of checks and optional business analysis summaries. (Courtesy of Colwell Systems, Inc., Champaign, IL.)

STATEMENT TO:

JANE L JONES
1211 EAST FIRST AVENUE
ANYWHERE US 10000

- -
TEAR OFF AND RETURN UPPER PORTION WITH PAYMENT

DATE	PROFESSIONAL SERVICE	FEE		PAYMENT		ADJUST-MENT		NEW BALANCE	
03/04	90060	100	00	200	00			100	00
04/20	90020	30	00	100	00			170	00
04/21						30	00	200	00
	Debit column ————————→								
	Credit column ————————→								
	Adjustment column ————————→								
	Balance column showing credit balance ————————→								

Figure 13–2
Account card/statement showing debit, credit, and credit balance. (Courtesy of Bibbero Systems, Inc., Petaluma, CA.)

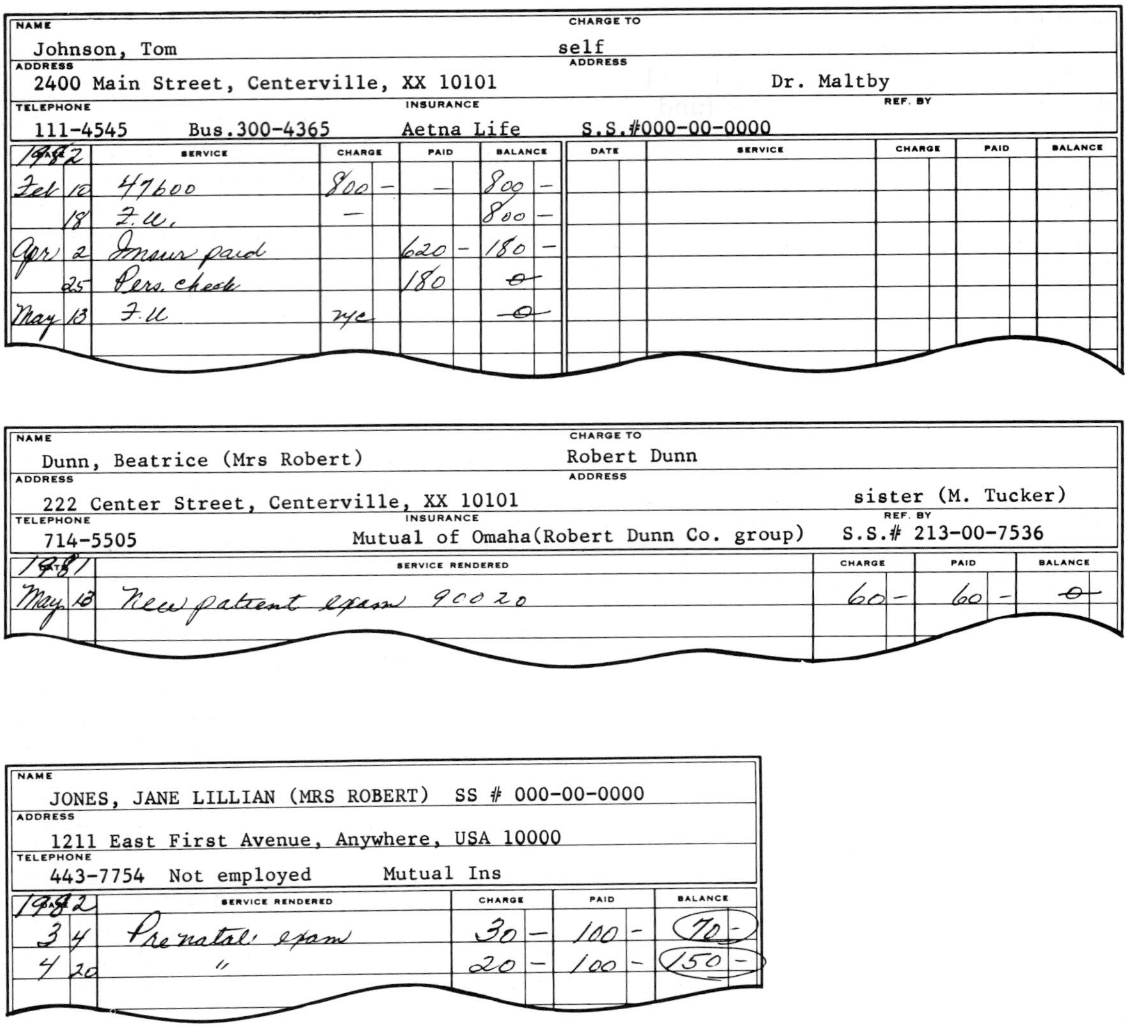

NAME: Johnson, Tom
CHARGE TO: self
ADDRESS: 2400 Main Street, Centerville, XX 10101
ADDRESS: Dr. Maltby
REF. BY
TELEPHONE: 111-4545 Bus.300-4365
INSURANCE: Aetna Life S.S.#000-00-0000

1982		SERVICE	CHARGE	PAID	BALANCE
Feb	10	47600	800 –	—	800 –
	18	F.U.	—		800 –
Apr	2	Insur paid		620 –	180 –
	25	Pers. check		180	-0-
May	13	F.U.	n/c		-0-

DATE		SERVICE	CHARGE	PAID	BALANCE

NAME: Dunn, Beatrice (Mrs Robert)
CHARGE TO: Robert Dunn
ADDRESS: 222 Center Street, Centerville, XX 10101
ADDRESS
REF. BY: sister (M. Tucker)
TELEPHONE: 714-5505
INSURANCE: Mutual of Omaha(Robert Dunn Co. group) S.S.# 213-00-7536

1981		SERVICE RENDERED	CHARGE	PAID	BALANCE
May	13	New patient exam 90020	60 –	60 –	-0-

NAME: JONES, JANE LILLIAN (MRS ROBERT) SS # 000-00-0000
ADDRESS: 1211 East First Avenue, Anywhere, USA 10000
TELEPHONE: 443-7754 Not employed Mutual Ins

1982		SERVICE RENDERED	CHARGE	PAID	BALANCE
3	4	Prenatal exam	30 –	100 –	(70 –)
4	20	"	20 –	100 –	(150 –)

Figure 13–3
Examples of patient account cards. (Courtesy of Colwell Systems, Inc., Champaign, IL.)

- Home and business telephone numbers
- Name of employer
- Any special instructions for billing

Billing statements to the patient and the patient's insurance are prepared from the ledger.

Checkbook. All receipts are deposited in the checking account, and a record of the deposit is entered on the check stub. A copy of each deposit slip should be kept with the financial records. All bills are paid by check, and a record of the payment is entered on the check stub and in the disbursements section of the general journal (Fig. 13–4).

Disbursements Journal. In simplified accounting systems, the disbursements journal usually comprises a section at the bottom of each daysheet and a check register page at the end of each month, plus monthly and annual summaries. It must show:

- Every amount paid out
- Date and check number
- Purpose of payment

Disbursements that are not practice-related should be recorded separately.

Petty Cash Record. A petty cash fund and voucher system should be established to take care of minor unpredictable expenditures such as:

- Postage due
- Parking fees
- Small contributions

In the average medical office, $25 to $50 is sufficient for the petty cash fund. If a larger sum is available there is a tendency to pay too many bills out of petty cash.

When the check for this fund is exchanged at the bank for small bills and coins, the money is placed in a cashbox or drawer that can be locked or kept in the safe at night. One person only should be in charge of the petty cash fund. This person must be able to account for the full amount of the fund at any time.

Payroll Record. The payroll record is an auxiliary disbursement record. A separate page or card for each employee, as well as a summary record, should be kept. This procedure is discussed in more detail in Chapter 19 as a management responsibility.

COMPARISON OF COMMON ACCOUNTING SYSTEMS

Success in accounting also requires a thorough understanding of the system and what it is expected to accomplish. There are many variations in accounting systems, from simple to complex, no one of which will meet the needs of every doctor. The basic principles are the same for all; only the system of recording varies.

The three most common systems found in the professional office are:

• Single entry
• Double entry
• Pegboard or write-it-once

The recording process in all of these systems can be performed by hand or by computer; the choice will probably depend on the volume.

An overview of the three systems will be presented here, followed later in the chapter by more detailed instruction for the pegboard system, which is currently the most widely used system in medical practices.

Single Entry System

Single entry accounting is inexpensive, simple to use, and requires very little training. It is the oldest and simplest of accounting systems and includes at least three basic records:

1. A general journal, which may also be called a daily log, daybook, daysheet, daily journal, or charge journal (Fig. 13–5).

2. A cash payment journal, which in its simplest form is a checkbook.

3. An accounts receivable ledger, which is a record of the amounts owed by all the doctor's patients. The accounts receivable ledger may be a

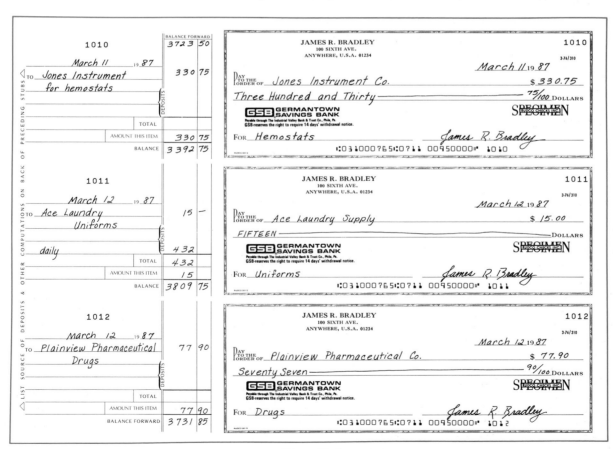

Figure 13–4

Page from a commercial checkbook with end stubs.

October 20, 19xx

HOUR	NAME	SERVICE RENDERED	√	CHARGE	PAID
9:00	Brown, John	90030		30 00	
9:20	Sullivan, Bertha	90050		40 00	
9:40	James, Ella	P.O.Dressing		n/c	
10:00	Grover, Ellen	90030		30 00	30 00
10:20	Johnson, Tom	FU		n/c	
10:40	Taylor, Theo	90050		40 00	40 00
11:00	Sorenson, Betty	90730		30 00	
11:20	Boston, Stuart	81000		20 00	20 00
11:40	Daniger, Fred	90030		30 00	
12:00					
12:20					
12:40					
1:00	Marlow, Eva	FU		n/c	
1:20	Arnold, Anne	P.O.Dressing		n/c	
1:40	Tucker, Benjamin	90015		70 00	70 00
2:00					
2:20	Thompson, Dan	90015		70 00	70 00
2:40					
3:00	Dunn, Beatrice	90020		120 00	
3:20					
3:40					
4:00	Histed, J. B.	90000		50 00	
4:20	Roberts, Victor	90020		120 00	120 00
4:40					
5:00					

Figure 13–5
Page from daily log used in single entry bookkeeping. (Courtesy of Colwell Systems, Inc., Champaign, IL.)

bound book, a loose-leaf binder, a card file, or loose pages in a ledger tray.

There may also be auxiliary records for petty cash and payroll records.

The records of charges and receipts are usually entered into a bound journal with a page for each day in the year, monthly summary pages, and an annual summary. Daily pages have columns for entering each transaction, showing the patient's name, the service performed and the charge, any payments received, and the totals for charges and receipts. The daily totals are entered on the monthly summary, and the monthly totals are carried forward to the annual summary.

The same bound book may also have space for recording cash payments, or the checkbook may be the only cash payment journal. Monthly and annual summaries would be done from the checkbook.

The accounts receivable ledger usually consists of an account card for each patient on which are entered the charges and payments from the general journal. The patients' statements are prepared from these cards (Fig. 13–6).

In a single entry system, each entry is made separately:

1. The entry is recorded on the daily journal or log.

2. A patient receipt is written if payment was made.

3. The transaction is posted to the ledger.

4. A monthly statement is generated from the ledger.

The single entry accounting system does satisfy the requirements for reporting to government agencies, but errors are not easily detected, there are no built-in controls, and periodic analyses are inadequate for financial planning. Although it was at one time widely used in physicians' offices, it is gradually being phased out for more complete accounting systems.

BILLING NAME	NAMES OF OTHER FAMILY MEMBERS

PATIENT'S NAME	
TAYLOR, THEODORE	Wife: Mary

RES PHONE 443 7840 BUS. PHONE 423 1846	
OCCUPATION Programmer	RELATIVE OR FRIEND
EMPLOYED BY IBM	REFERRED BY Dr. Coomber
INS INFORMATION Travelers	SOC. SEC. NUMBER 999 00 8888

FORM NO. MDP. 8550   1976 BIBBERO SYSTEMS, INC. · SAN FRANCISCO

GEORGE D. GREEN, M.D.
JOHN F. WHITE, M.D.
Family Practice
100 MAIN STREET, SUITE 14
ANYTOWN, CALIFORNIA 90000
TELEPHONE: (999) 399-6000

STATEMENT TO:

Theodore Taylor
6015 North Broadway
San Tomas, XX 90077

— — — TEAR OFF AND RETURN UPPER PORTION WITH PAYMENT — — —

DATE	PROFESSIONAL SERVICE	FEE	PAYMENT	ADJUST-MENT	NEW BALANCE
5/13/88	Office visit 90015	48 00			48 00

PROFESSIONAL SERVICE CODES:

1. OFFICE VISIT	9. COLLECTION OF LAB. SPEC.	17. SURGICAL
2. HOME VISIT	10. SPECIAL REPORTS	18. CASTS
3. HOSPITAL VISIT	11. OTHER SERVICES	19. LABORATORY
4. EMERGENCY ROOM	12. SPEC. DIAGNOSTIC SERVICES	20. X-RAY
5. CONSULTATION	13. SPEC. THERAPEUTIC SERV.	21. ALLERGY TEST.
6. IMMUNIZATION	14. EXTENDED CARE FACILITY	22. NO CHARGE
7. INJECTION	15. CUSTODIAL CARE	23. ADJUSTMENTS OR CORRECTIONS
8. DRUGS/SUPPLIES/MATERIALS	16. OBSTETRICAL CARE	24. TOTAL CARE

GEORGE D. GREEN, M.D.   **JOHN F. WHITE, M.D.**
CAL. LIC. # 6-2856   CAL. LIC. # G-5281

Figure 13–6
Combination account card/statement from accounts receivable ledger. (Courtesy of Bibbero Systems, Inc., Petaluma, CA.)

13

Double Entry System

Double entry accounting is also inexpensive but requires a trained and experienced bookkeeper or the regular services of an accountant. In addition to the basic journals used in a single entry system, there may be numerous subsidiary journals. The system is based on the **accounting equation**:

Assets = Liabilities + Proprietorship (Capital)

Every transaction requires an entry on each side of the accounting equation, and the two sides must always be in balance. For this reason the system is called double entry, and it is the most complete of the three systems.

Assets are the properties owned by a business, such as bank accounts, accounts receivable, buildings, equipment, and furniture. Assets are also called equities, which may be subdivided into creditors' equities and owner's equity.

Liabilities are the debts of the business, such as the mortgage on a building, installment notes on equipment purchased, any salaries payable, amounts payable to vendors, and so forth. Liabilities are also called creditors' equities. The owner's equity (*proprietorship* or *capital*) is what remains of the value of the assets after the creditors' equities (liabilities) have been subtracted.

For example, if the doctor purchased equipment for $1,000, paid $250 down, and gave a promissory note for $750, this would translate into

Assets $1,000 =	Liabilities	$ 750
	+	
	Proprietorship	250
$1,000		$1,000

The accounting terms proprietorship, capital, owner's equity, and net worth are used interchangeably.

Few medical assistants are trained in accounting. If a double entry system is used, it is usually set up by a practice management consultant or the accountant who does most of the actual bookwork and reports. The medical assistant in this instance generally maintains only the daily journal, from which the accountant takes the figures once a month.

The double entry system provides a more comprehensive picture of the practice and its effect on the doctor's net worth. Errors show up readily and there are many built in accuracy controls, but because of the time and skill required, it is not frequently used in the small practice.

Pegboard or Write-It-Once System

The initial cost of materials for the pegboard system is slightly more than for a single or double entry system but is still moderate. The system is simple to operate, and training is included in most medical assisting programs.

The system gets its name from the lightweight aluminum or masonite board with a row of pegs along the side or top that hold the forms in place. The accounting forms are perforated for alignment on the pegs. All of the forms used in any system must be compatible so that they may be aligned perfectly on the board.

The pegboard system generates all the necessary financial records for each transaction with one writing:

• Charge slip and receipt
• Ledger card
• Journal entry

It may also include a statement and a bank deposit slip.

The system provides current accounts receivable totals and a daily record of bank deposits and cash on hand, in addition to the record of income and expenses. The need for separate posting to patient accounts is eliminated, and the chance for error decreased. Pegboard accounting is the most widely used of the three systems in physicians' offices today.

USING THE PEGBOARD ACCOUNTING SYSTEM

The pegboard accounting system provides positive control over cash, collections, and receivables, and ensures that every cent is accounted for and properly entered. It provides a record of every patient, every charge, and every payment. You have a daily recap of earnings—a running record of receivables and an audited summary of cash. The

Table 13-2

Accounting Systems

	Advantages	Disadvantages
Single Entry	Inexpensive Requires little training Simple to use	Provides only simple summaries Errors difficult to locate No built-in controls
Double Entry	Provides comprehensive financial picture Built-in accuracy controls	Requires special training, more time, and greater skill
Pegboard	Generates all records with one writing Daily control on accounts receivable Daily record of bank deposits and cash on hand	Cost of supplies greater than single entry system Some training required (usually included in medical assistant programs)

system requires a minimum of time. With one writing you can:

- Enter a transaction on the daysheet
- Give the patient a receipt for payment
- Bring the patient's account up to date
- Provide a current statement of account for the patient
- Give the patient a notation of the next appointment

All of these features communicate the "money message" to patients effectively and courteously as well as generate good financial records.

Materials Required. The pegboard may be of inexpensive masonite construction with pegs down the left side, or it may be a more sophisticated aluminum sliding board that allows flexible positioning of materials. The basic forms are:

- The journal daysheet
- The patient ledger
- The patient charge slip/receipt or superbill

All of the forms must be compatible and are available from medical office supply companies. They are customized to the practice, incorporating the usual services and procedure codes of the practice.

Preparing the Board. At the beginning of each day place a new daysheet on the accounting board. Some systems have a sheet of "clean carbon" attached to the daysheet; others use special carbon with holes for the pegs; some use NCR (no carbon required) paper. The carbon goes on top of the daysheet. Over the carbon, place the charge slip/receipt or superbill. The receipt has a carbonized writing line that should align with the first open writing line on the daysheet. If the slips are shingled, lay the entire bank of receipts over the

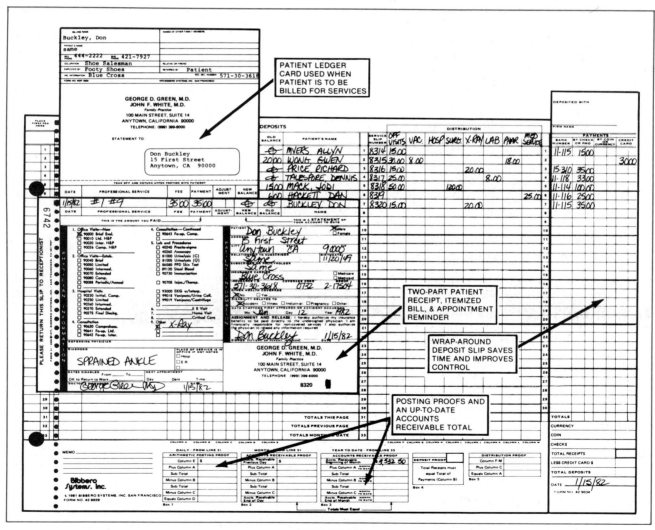

Figure 13–7
Sample daily log of charges and receipts. (Courtesy of Bibbero Systems, Inc., Petaluma, CA.)

pegs, with the top one aligned as mentioned. The remainder will be automatically in place. Receipts should be used in numeric order.

Pulling the Ledger Cards. If a great many patients are to be seen in one day, it will save time to pull the ledger cards for all the scheduled patients at the beginning of the day. Keep the cards in the order in which they are scheduled to be seen.

Entering and Posting Transactions. As each patient arrives, insert the patient's ledger card under the first receipt, aligning the first available writing line of the card with the carbonized strip on the receipt. Enter the receipt number and date, the account balance in the space labeled previous balance, and the patient's name. The information recorded on the receipt is automatically posted to the ledger and the daysheet (Fig. 13–7).

The charge slip is then detached and clipped to the patient chart to be routed to the doctor, who now has an opportunity to see how much the patient owes and can discuss the account in privacy if desired.

After the service has been performed, the doctor enters the service on the charge slip and asks the patient or the nurse to return it to the medical assistant. The assistant then has an opportunity to ask the patient whether this is to be a charge or cash transaction, before completing the posting.

Again, insert the ledger card under the proper receipt, checking the number that was previously entered to make sure you have the correct card. Record the service by procedure code, post the charge from the fee schedule, enter any payment made, and write in the current balance. If there is no balance, place a zero or straight line in the balance column. If another appointment is required, enter the date and time at the bottom of the receipt.

You have now posted the journal and the ledger and, if payment was made by the patient, automatically made a receipt. The service receipt is given to the patient; no other receipt is necessary. The ledger card is ready for refiling.

File the charge slips in numeric order for your internal audit. At the end of the month the total of the charge slips should equal the total of the charges recorded on the daysheets for the month.

Recording Other Payments and Charges. Payments will be received in the mail and may be brought in by patients some time after a service was performed. These payments are entered on the daysheet and the ledger card in the same manner as previously explained. Payments by mail do not require a receipt.

The doctor may have daily charges for visits to patients in a hospital or convalescent facility. Enter these charges on the daysheet and ledger card only.

Surgery fees are usually recorded as one entry that includes the surgery and aftercare.

End-of-Day Summarizing. At the end of the day, all columns must be totalled and proved. Although all bookkeeping is done in ink, it is a good idea to write the totals in pencil until they have been proved. If an error is discovered, you must correct the entry in which it occurred. Do not attempt to erase or write over the incorrect entry. Simply draw a line through it and make a new entry on the first open writing line. Remember that you must reinsert the ledger card for these corrections. Also, if the entry included a receipt for the patient, you must make a new receipt and notify the patient of the correction.

Pegboard accounting systems provide several ways for proving the arithmetic on the daysheet. Some examples are shown on the opposite page.

SPECIAL ACCOUNTING ENTRIES

The following special entries are necessary occasionally and may be used with pegboard or any other accounting system.

Adjustments. At times it is necessary to enter a credit adjustment. Examples are:

- Professional discounts
- Insurance disallowances
- Write-offs

If the system has an adjustment column, enter them here. Otherwise, since the adjustment is actually a subtraction from the charge, enter it in the charge column with the figure enclosed in parentheses or circled, and an explanation of the entry in the description column. When the column of figures is totaled, this figure will be *subtracted* rather than added. The learner has a tendency to ignore the circled figures. This is incorrect—they must be subtracted.

Credit Balances. A credit balance occurs when:

- A patient has paid in advance
- There has been an overpayment

For example, an overpayment will occur if the patient made a partial payment and later the insurance allowance was more than the remaining balance. The difference between the total amount of money received and the amount owed must be entered in the balance column and enclosed with parentheses or circled. This indicates a credit balance.

In actuality, the credit balance is money owed to the patient. If the patient has paid in advance or wishes to leave the overpayment in the account in

```
┌─────────────────────────────────────────────────────────────┐
│                     Posting Proof for Day                    │
│   Old balance                               $_____         │
│      Plus total charges                       _____        │
│                                    Subtotal  $_____         │
│      Less payments received                   _____        │
│                                    Subtotal  $_____         │
│      Less adjustments                         _____        │
│   New balance                               *$_____         │
└─────────────────────────────────────────────────────────────┘
```

*This figure is carried forward to next page for "old balance."

```
┌─────────────────────────────────────────────────────────────┐
│                      Cash Control Proof                      │
│   Cash on hand at beginning of day          $_____         │
│      Cash received                            _____        │
│                                    Subtotal  $_____         │
│      Less cash paid out                       _____        │
│      Less bank deposit                        _____        │
│   Cash on hand at end of day                *$_____         │
└─────────────────────────────────────────────────────────────┘
```

*This figure is carried forward to next page for "cash on hand at beginning of day."

anticipation of future charges, care must be taken in figuring the balance on future transactions. Whereas normally a charge increases the balance, it will decrease a credit balance.

Refunds. If a patient wishes to have an overpayment refunded, write a check for the amount due and enter the transaction on the daysheet as follows:

1. Place the ledger card on the daysheet.
2. Enter an explanation in the description column.
3. Show the existing credit balance within parentheses or encircled.
4. Write the amount of the refund in the payment column in parentheses or encircled to show that it is a subtraction.
5. Show a zero balance.

NSF (Nonsufficient Funds) Checks. Sometimes a patient will send in a check without having sufficient funds to cover it, which you will later deposit to the physician's account. The bank will return the check to you marked NSF. You must now perform two accounting functions:

1. Deduct the amount from your checking account balance.

2. Add the amount back into the patient's account balance by:
   a. Entering the amount in the paid column in parentheses
   b. Increasing the balance by the same amount
A brief explanation of the transaction goes into the description column (Fig. 13–8).

One-Entry Cash Transactions. For the transient patient who has no ledger card and pays at the time of service, use a receipt as previously described. Enter the amount of the fee in the charge column and in the paid column, and a zero balance. This records the transaction on the journal page and provides a receipt for the patient. There is no need for a ledger card.

Collection Agency Payments. When a collection agency recovers an account for the physician, the agency deducts a commission, usually 40% to 50% of the amount recovered. For example, if the patient has a balance of $100 and pays it in full, the agency will send you $50. The patient now has a zero balance and you have only $50. To record this transaction on the ledger card and the daysheet you will enter:

1. $100 in the previous balance

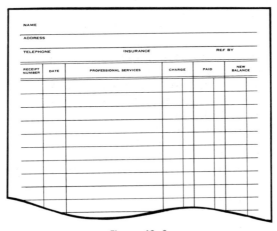

NAME					
BROWN, JOHN		S.S.# 000 00 0000			
ADDRESS					
429 West Market, Long Desert, XX 80056					
TELEPHONE					
345-6789					

1980		SERVICE RENDERED	CHARGE	PAID	BALANCE
10	20	90020	60 —	30 —	30 —
11-	15	90050	20 —	—	50 —
11-	20	Pers. check		30 —	20 —
11-	28	Check returned NSF		(30)	50 —

Figure 13–8
Entry for returned NSF check.

Procedure 13–1

POSTING SERVICE CHARGES AND PAYMENTS USING PEGBOARD SYSTEM

PROCEDURAL GOAL

To post one day's charges and payments, and complete daily accounting cycle using a pegboard.

EQUIPMENT AND SUPPLIES

Pegboard
Calculator
Pen
Daysheet
Carbon
Receipts
Ledger cards
Balances from previous day

PROCEDURE

1. Prepare the board:
   a. Place a new daysheet on the board.
   b. Cover daysheet with carbon.

Procedure continued on opposite page

c. Place bank of receipts over the pegs aligning the top receipt with the first open writing line on the daysheet.

2. Carry forward balances from previous day.
   Purpose: To keep all totals current.
3. Pull ledger cards for patients to be seen today.
4. Insert the ledger card under the first receipt, aligning the first available writing line of the card with the carbonized strip on the receipt.
   Purpose: To ensure that one writing will correctly post entry to receipt, ledger, and daysheet.
5. Enter the patient's name, the date, receipt number, and any existing balance from the ledger card.
6. Detach the charge slip from the receipt and clip it to the patient's chart.
   Purpose: The doctor will indicate the service performed on the charge slip and return it to you.
7. Accept the returned charge slip at the end of the visit.
8. Enter the appropriate fee from the fee schedule.
9. Locate the receipt on the board with a number matching the charge slip.
   Purpose: To make certain it is the correct receipt.
10. Reinsert the patient's ledger card under the receipt.
11. Write the service code number and fee on the receipt.
12. Accept the patient's payment and record the amount of payment and new balance.
    Purpose: Brings patient's account up to date and provides current statement for patient.
13. Give the completed receipt to the patient.
14. Follow your agency's procedure for refiling the ledger card.
15. Repeat steps 4 to 14 for each service for the day.
16. Total all columns of the daysheet at the end of the day.
    Purpose: To determine total amount of charges, receipts and resulting balances for the day.
17. Write temporary totals in pencil.
    Purpose: To facilitate any necessary changes.
18. Complete proof of totals and enter totals in ink.
19. Enter figures for accounts receivable control.
    Purpose: To complete daily accounting cycle.

TERMINAL PERFORMANCE OBJECTIVE

Given the listed equipment and supplies, make necessary entries to record all charges and payments for one day, account balances, daily totals, and accounts receivable control for month to date, within 30 minutes, to a performance level of 100%. (Time will vary according to number of transactions.)

13

2. $50 in the cash received or paid column
3. $50 in the adjustment column
4. Zero in the new balance column

If there is no adjustment column, the $50 commission is entered in the charge column in parentheses ($50), so that the total charge business is reduced by this amount and the transaction is reflected correctly in the accounts receivable control.

ACCOUNTS RECEIVABLE CONTROL

The accounts receivable control is a daily summary of what remains unpaid on the accounts.

This is an integral part of the pegboard and double entry systems, but is a separate operation in single entry accounting. A simple form such as the one illustrated in Figure 13–9 will be useful. Using a separate page or card for each month, proceed as follows:

1. Total the unpaid balances from your entire ledger on the last day of the preceding month and enter this figure at the top of the card or page.
2. Total the charges and receipts at the end of each day and enter these figures in columns 1 and 2.
3. Determine the accounts receivable figure as follows:

   a. If charges for the day exceed the receipts, there is an increase in the accounts receivable. Enter this figure in column 4 and add it to the balance in column 6.

   b. If receipts for the day exceed the charges, there is a decrease in the accounts receivable. Enter this figure in column 5 and subtract it from the balance in column 6.

Note that the accounts receivable figure changes at the end of any day on which there is financial activity. The balance consists of the accounts receivable figure from the previous day, plus the charges

```
Accounts Receivable Control

Total outstanding A/R balance
   (from previous day)                                        $_____

   Plus today's charges                                         _____

                                            Subtotal  $_____

   Less today's payments                                        _____

                                            Subtotal  $_____

   Less today's adjustments                                     _____

Balance outstanding                                          *$_____
```

*This figure is carried forward to the next page for "total outstanding A/R balance."

for the day, minus the day's receipts and adjustments.

The total of the entire file of ledger card balances at the end of any given day should equal the accounts receivable balance shown for that day on the control form.

TRIAL BALANCE OF ACCOUNTS RECEIVABLE

A trial balance should be done at least once a month, preferably before preparing the monthly statements. The trial balance will disclose any discrepancies between the journal and the ledger. It does not, however, prove the accuracy of the accounts. For example, if a charge or payment were posted to the wrong account, or if the wrong amount were entered in the journal and then posted to the ledger, the totals would still "balance," but the accounts would not be accurate.

It is best to use an adding machine or calculator with a tape for this process. All posting must have been completed before taking a trial balance. To begin, pull all the account cards that have a balance, enter each balance on the adding machine, and total the figures. This should equal the accounts receivable balance figure on your control. If you have not kept a daily control, you must total all the charges, payments, and adjustments for the month, and then do the computation on the opposite page.

The accounts receivable at end of month figure must agree with the figure arrived at by adding all the account card balances. The accounts are said to be in balance. If the two totals do not agree, you must locate the error.

Locating and Preventing Errors. After you have checked your tape and verified that you have not made an error in calculation, the first step in locating an error in your trial balance is to find the difference between the two totals. Then search the daily journal pages and the account cards for an entry of the identical amount. Check each one you find, to verify that it was posted correctly. Of course, there may be more than one error.

If there is only one error, and the amount of the error is divisible by 9, you may have transposed a

```
                    ACCOUNTS RECEIVABLE CONTROL
Month of  December    , 19 XX     Accounts Receivable at end
                                   of last day of preceding
                                   month: $37506
```

Day	1 Value of Services Rendered	2 Received from Patients	3 Adjust-ments	4 Increase	5 Decrease	6 Accounts Receivable Balance
1	785	1098			313	37193
2	210	630			420	36773
3	950	510	33	407		37180
4						

Figure 13–9
Accounts receivable control for single entry bookkeeping system.

Accounts receivable at first of month	$_____
Plus total charges for month	_____
Subtotal	$_____
Less total payments for month	_____
Subtotal	$_____
Less total adjustments for month	_____
Accounts receivable at end of month	$_____

figure. For example, if the difference is $81 (a number divisible by 9), you may find that you wrote $209 instead of $290. If the amount of the error is divisible by 2, you may have posted to the wrong column, reversing a debit and a credit.

A common error is made by entering the wrong amount in the "previous balance" column or in figuring the new balance. This kind of error will show up on the pegboard daily proof, but could easily go undetected in the single entry system.

Another common error is made by carrying forward a wrong total from one day to the next; for instance, carrying the beginning accounts receivable total rather than the ending accounts receivable total.

There is always a chance of sliding a number, that is, writing the first digit in the wrong column, such as writing 400 for 40, or 60 instead of 600.

Many bookkeepers avoid errors in the cents column by using a line (—) instead of writing two zeros when only even dollars are involved. For example, instead of writing $12.00, the bookkeeper will write $12.—. This eliminates the possibility of misreading zeros as other numbers. It also speeds the adding process when columns must be totaled.

If you are unable to locate any numeric error, there is the possibility that an account card was lost or overlooked, or was transferred as paid in full.

ACCOUNTS PAYABLE PROCEDURES

Invoices and Statements. When time purchases are made, that is, the item is not paid for at the time of purchase, the vendor will usually include a packing slip with delivery of the merchandise. A packing slip describes the items enclosed. The vendor may also enclose an invoice. An invoice describes the items and shows the amount due. Always check to verify that the items listed on the packing slip and invoice are included in the delivery.

Invoices should be placed in a special folder until paid. You may be making more than one purchase from the same vendor during the month. Some vendors request that payment be made from the

invoice; others expect to send a statement later. A statement is a request for payment.

Paying for Purchases. At the time of payment, compare the statement with the invoice(s) to verify accuracy, fasten the statement and invoices together, write the date and check number on the statement, and place in the "paid" file.

Recording Disbursements. Both the pegboard and the single entry accounting systems provide pages for recording disbursements. This is sometimes called a check register (Fig. 13–10). On these pages, disbursements are distributed to specific expense accounts such as:

auto expense
dues and meetings
equipment
insurance
medical supplies
office expenses
printing, postage, stationery
rent and maintenance
salaries
taxes and licenses
travel and entertainment
utilities
miscellaneous
personal withdrawals

Each check should be entered on the disbursement page, showing the date, to whom the check was written, the number and amount of the check, and the payment allocated to one or more of the expense accounts. It is important to separate personal expenditures from business expenses. Business expenses are tax deductible and are considered in determining net income from the practice, but personal expenditures are not.

Recording Personal Expenditures. Some system must be established for transferring funds from the practice account to the physician's personal account. If the practice is incorporated, the physician will be paid a salary. In the unincorporated practice,

13

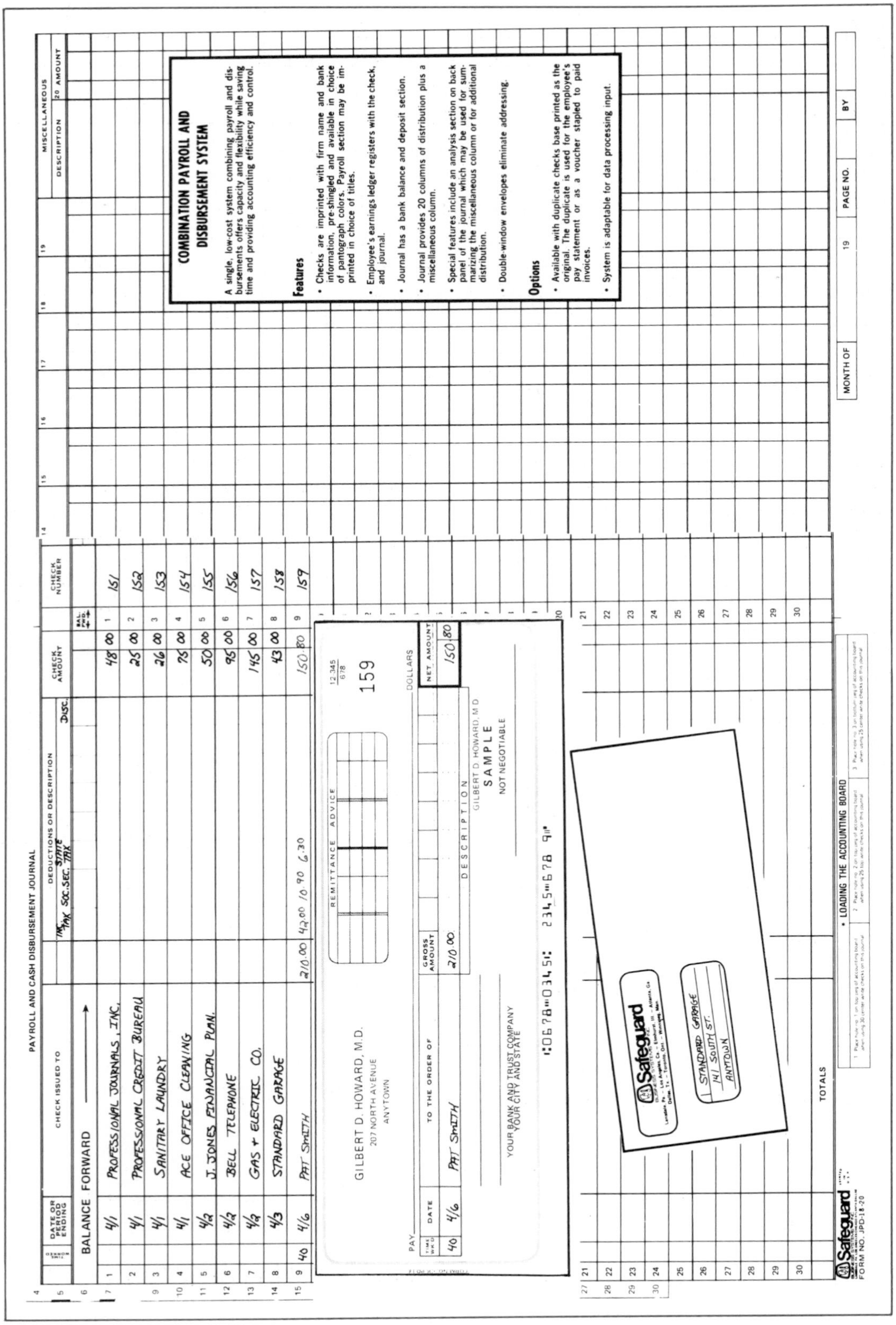

PAYROLL AND CASH DISBURSEMENT JOURNAL

DATE OR PERIOD ENDING	CHECK ISSUED TO	DEDUCTIONS OR DESCRIPTION			CHECK AMOUNT	MO. FED.	CHECK NUMBER
		TAX SOC. SEC. TAX	STATE TAX	DISC.			
	BALANCE FORWARD						
4/1	PROFESSIONAL JOURNALS, INC.				48 00	1	151
4/1	PROFESSIONAL CREDIT BUREAU				25 00	2	152
4/1	SANITARY LAUNDRY				26 00	3	153
4/1	ACE OFFICE CLEANING				75 00	4	154
4/2	J. JONES FINANCIAL PLAN.				50 00	5	155
4/2	BELL TELEPHONE				95 00	6	156
4/2	GAS + ELECTRIC CO.				145 00	7	157
4/3	STANDARD GARAGE				43 00	8	158
4/6	PAT SMITH	210.00 42.00 10.90 6.30			150 80	9	159

Combination Payroll and Disbursement System

A single, low-cost system combining payroll and disbursements offers capacity and flexibility while saving time and providing accounting efficiency and control.

Features

- Checks are imprinted with firm name and bank information, pre-shingled and available in choice of paragraph colors. Payroll section may be imprinted in choice of titles.
- Employee's earnings ledger registers with the check, and journal.
- Journal has a bank balance and deposit section.
- Journal provides 20 columns of distribution plus a miscellaneous column.
- Special features include an analysis section on back panel of the journal which may be used for summarizing the miscellaneous column or for additional distribution.
- Double-window envelopes eliminate addressing.

Options

- Available with duplicate checks base printed as the original. The duplicate is used for the employee's pay statement or as a voucher stapled to paid invoices.
- System is adaptable for data processing input.

GILBERT D. HOWARD, M.D.
207 NORTH AVENUE
ANYTOWN

12 345
6/8
159

REMITTANCE ADVICE

PAY

DATE	TO THE ORDER OF	GROSS AMOUNT		DESCRIPTION	NET AMOUNT
4/6	PAT SMITH	210 00			150 80

GILBERT D. HOWARD, M.D.
SAMPLE
NOT NEGOTIABLE

YOUR BANK AND TRUST COMPANY
YOUR CITY AND STATE

⑈06 78⑈⑈034 5⑈: 234 5⑈⑈ 678 9⑈⑈

Safeguard

STANDARD GARAGE
141 SOUTH ST.
ANYTOWN

LOADING THE ACCOUNTING BOARD

TOTALS

MISCELLANEOUS

| | 19 | 18 | 17 | 16 | 15 | 14 | DESCRIPTION | 20 AMOUNT |

MONTH OF _____ 19___   PAGE NO. ___   BY ___

FORM NO. JPD-18-20

Figure 13–10

Payroll and cash disbursement journal showing payroll check being prepared for employee, and window envelope for mailing checks. (Courtesy of Safeguard Business Systems.)

DATE	DESCRIPTION	VOUCHER NUMBER	TOTAL AMOUNT	Office Exp.	Donations	Auto				Misc.	BALANCE
4-01	Fund established										25.00
4-02	Postage due	1	.26	.26							24.74
4-05	Nurse's Benefit ticket	2	5.00		5.00						19.74
4-08	Parking fee	3	2.00			2.00					17.74
4-17	Stationery items	4	1.68	1.68							16.06
4-25	Delivery charges	5	3.12	3.12							12.94
4-29	Coffee	6	2.88							2.88	10.06
			14.94	5.06	5.00	2.00				2.88	
5-01	Bal. $10.06										
	Check #376 14.94										
	Total 25.00										

Figure 13–11
Petty cash record.

the transfer is usually accomplished through what is known in accounting terms as a drawing account.

The physician establishes a personal checking account and perhaps one or more savings accounts. Each month, or at any specified time, the medical assistant writes a check payable to the physician, which is then endorsed and deposited to the physician's personal account. In the disbursements journal, the amount of the check is posted in a special column headed "Personal" or "Drawing."

Although personal expenses are not deductible in determining net income from the practice, some will qualify as personal deductions in computing personal income tax, so a careful accounting should be kept. Deductible expenses would include property taxes, interest paid out, contributions, and so forth.

Accounting for Petty Cash. The petty cash fund is a revolving fund. It does not change in amount except to increase or decrease the established fund. To establish the petty cash fund, a check is written payable to "Cash" or "Petty Cash" and entered in the disbursements journal under Miscellaneous. This is the only time the petty cash check will be charged to Miscellaneous.

Each time the fund is replenished, the amount of the check is spread among the various accounts for which the money was used. This is determined from a record of expenditures such as that shown in Figure 13–11. The headings of the columns should correspond to headings in the disbursements journal to which they will be posted.

A pad of petty cash vouchers is kept in or near the box. For every disbursement from the fund, the

13

AMOUNT $ 5 00   NO. 2

RECEIVED OF PETTY CASH

April 5   19—

FOR Nurse's Benefit, Mercy Hospital

CHARGE TO Donations

APPROVED BY   RECEIVED BY

MK   F. Dunn, R.N.

AICO-UTILITY Line Form No. 55-061

Figure 13–12
Petty cash voucher.

petty cashier should either have a receipt or prepare a voucher similar to the one in Figure 13–12. The total of the petty cash vouchers and receipts plus the amount of cash in the box must always equal the original amount of the fund.

Receipt and voucher total	$14.94
Cash on hand	10.06
Amount of fund	$25.00

Figure 13–11 shows that $25 was received into the fund on April 1. This is entered in the Description column and in the Balance column. On April 2, postage due was paid out, a voucher prepared, the number of the voucher and the amount of 26

cents entered, and a new balance brought down. On April 5, the doctor made a cash donation to the O.R. nurse benefit at the hospital. The amount of $5 was entered in the record, $5 taken from petty cash to reimburse the doctor, and the new balance of $19.74 brought down.

At the end of the month, or sooner if the fund is depleted, a check is written to "Cash" for replenishing the fund, but instead of being charged to Miscellaneous as previously, the amount of the check is divided among the various accounts affected. Our record shows that at the end of April we have $10.06 remaining in the fund and need $14.94 to bring it back to $25.

When the check is written for $14.94, it is ac-

Procedure 13–2

ACCOUNTING FOR PETTY CASH

PROCEDURAL GOAL

To establish a petty cash fund, maintain an accurate record of expenditures for one month, and replenish the fund as necessary.

EQUIPMENT AND SUPPLIES

Form for petty cash fund
Pad of vouchers
Disbursement journal
Two checks
List of petty cash expenditures

PROCEDURE

1. Determine the amount needed in the petty cash fund.
2. Write a check in the determined amount.
   Purpose: To establish the fund.
3. Record the beginning balance in the petty cash record.
4. Post the amount to miscellaneous on the disbursement record.
   Purpose: To account for original amount of fund.
5. Prepare a petty cash voucher for each amount withdrawn from the fund.
   Purpose: Voucher will be used for internal audit.
6. Record each voucher in the petty cash record and enter the new balance.
   Purpose: To record current balance and determine need for replenishing fund.
7. Write a check to replenish the fund as necessary.
   Note: The total of the vouchers plus the fund balance must equal the beginning amount.
8. Total the expense columns and post to appropriate accounts in the disbursement record.
   Purpose: To record expenditures in correct expense category.
9. Record the amount added to the fund.
10. Record the new balance in the petty cash fund.

TERMINAL PERFORMANCE OBJECTIVE

Given the listed equipment and supplies, establish and maintain the petty cash fund for one month, with all transactions entered and fund balanced, within 20 minutes, to a performance level of 100%. (Time will vary according to number of transactions.)

counted for in the monthly distribution of expenditures by posting $5.06 as office expense, $5 as donations, $2 as auto expense, and $2.88 as a miscellaneous expense. In this way the expenditures from petty cash are charged to the actual accounts affected.

The accounted-for vouchers are clipped together and placed with paid invoices, the check for $14.94 is cashed, and the money is placed in the petty cash fund. The amount of the check is entered as being received into the fund, and the new balance of $25 is brought down.

Avoid the habit of borrowing from the petty cash fund. This admonition applies to the doctor as well as to the medical assistant. If the doctor requests cash from the fund, request a personal check or an office check in exchange for cash from the fund.

It is also poor policy to use the petty cash fund for making change. In facilities where patients frequently pay with currency, a separate change fund should be kept.

PERIODIC SUMMARIES

Financial summaries are compiled on monthly and annual bases. They may be prepared either by the medical assistant or by the accountant (or by computer). The common summary reports are:

- Statement of income and expense
- Cash flow statement
- Trial balance
- Accounts receivable trial balance and aging analysis
- Balance sheet

The *statement of income and expense* is also known as the profit and loss statement and covers a specific period. It lists all the income received and all expenses paid during the period. The total income is called gross income or earnings. The income after deduction of all expenses is the net income.

A *cash flow statement* starts with the amount of cash on hand at the beginning of the month (or for any specified period). It then lists the cash income and the cash disbursements made throughout the period, and concludes with a statement of the amount of cash remaining on hand at the end of the period.

A *trial balance* is necessary in order to determine that the books are in balance. All of the columns on the disbursements journal must be totaled at the end of the month. The combined totals of all the expense columns must be equal to the total of the checks written. If the figures do not balance, it is necessary to recheck every entry until an error is found.

The *accounts receivable trial balance* is done prior to sending out the monthly statements. First, record the total of the accounts receivable ledger at the end of the previous month; then add the charges for the current month, and subtract the adjustments and the payments received. The remainder should equal the total of the accounts receivable ledger at the end of the current month.

The *balance sheet*, also known as a statement of financial condition, shows the financial picture of the practice on a specific date. Often it is done only on an annual basis. The balance sheet is set up using the accounting equation explained on page 194. The title of the statement had its origin in the equality of the elements—the balance between the sum of the assets and the sum of the liabilities and capital.

At the end of the accounting year it is very simple to combine the monthly reports to compile the annual summaries. The annual summaries simplify the reporting of income for tax returns.

ACCOUNTING WITH THE AID OF THE COMPUTER

The office with an in-house computer and the appropriate software can accomplish all the described accounting operations and more in a fraction of the time required to do them manually. The role of the computer in the medical practice was discussed in Chapter 6. The office without a computer can still reap some of the benefits by using an outside computer service.

A computer service can relieve the office staff of the repetitive clerical procedures necessary in the recording of charges, and in the preparation and mailing of statements and insurance forms. It can produce weekly and monthly financial reports that would be too time-consuming and perhaps beyond the capabilities of the staff to do manually.

One type of computer service is based on a telephone-linked terminal on a time-share basis with other users. Another is the batch type, in which the information is picked up at the office and taken to a computer center for processing. Whether to use computer services and the selection of what service to use are highly individualized decisions that require study and analysis of the practice. It is important to choose a service that will explain what can be expected from the computer and that will provide all the instruction and supervision necessary to ensure success in using it.

13

REFERENCES AND READINGS

Anthony, R. N., and Graham-Walker, R.: *Essentials of Accounting: A Reference Guide.* Menlo Park, CA, Addison-Wesley, 1985.

Colwell Systems: *One-Write Pegboard Bookkeeping System.* Champaign, IL, 1986.

Fess, P. E., and Warren, C. S.: *Financial Accounting,* 2nd ed. Cincinnati, South-Western Publishing Co., 1985.

Moscove, S. A., *Accounting Fundamentals for Non-Accountants.* Reston, VA, Reston Publishing, 1984.

CHAPTER OUTLINE

Checks
    Types of Checks
    Advantages of Using Checks
    ABA Number
    Magnetic Ink Character Recognition (MICR)

Bank Accounts
    Common Types of Accounts
    Service Charges

Systematizing Bill Paying
    The Business Checkbook
    Checkbook Stubs
    Lost and Stolen Checks
    Writing Checks
    One-Write Check Writing
    Signing Checks
    Mailing Checks
Special Problems with Checks

Payment from Patients
Endorsement of Checks
    Necessity for Endorsement
    Kinds of Endorsement
    Endorsement Procedures

Making Deposits
    Preparing the Deposit
    Depositing by Mail
      Procedure 14–1: Preparing a Bank Deposit
    "HOLD" on Account
    Returned Checks

Bank Statement
    Reconciling the Bank Statement
      Procedure 14–2: Reconciling a Bank
        Statement
Safe Deposit Box
Medical Assistant's Position of Trust

VOCABULARY

See Glossary at end of book for definitions.

disbursements	negotiable	power of attorney
endorser	payee	teller
maker	payer	third-party check

14

Banking Services and Procedures

OBJECTIVES

Upon successful completion of this chapter you should be able to:

1. *Define the terms listed in the Vocabulary of this chapter.*
2. *State the four requirements of a negotiable instrument.*
3. *Discuss six advantages of using checks for the transfer of funds.*
4. *Explain why it is important to complete the check stub before writing a check.*
5. *State how you would handle mistakes made in preparing a check.*
6. *List and discuss eight precautions to observe in accepting checks.*
7. *State the purpose of a check endorsement.*
8. *Name and compare four kinds of endorsements.*
9. *Cite five reasons for depositing checks promptly.*
10. *Discuss the action necessary when a deposited check is returned.*

Upon successful completion of this chapter you should be able to perform the following activities:

1. *Prepare a bank deposit.*
2. *Correctly write a check.*
3. *Pay office bills by check.*
4. *Reconcile a bank statement with the checkbook balance.*

Financial transactions in the professional office nearly always involve banking services and the use of checks. Therefore, the medical assistant must understand the responsibilities involved in accepting payments, in endorsing and depositing checks, in writing checks, and in regularly reconciling bank statements.

CHECKS

A check is a draft or an order upon a bank for the payment of a certain sum of money to a certain person therein named, or to the bearer, and is payable on demand. It is considered to be a negotiable instrument.

A Negotiable Instrument Must:
- *Be written and signed by a maker*
- *Contain a promise or order to pay a sum of money*
- *Be payable on demand or at a fixed future date*
- *Be payable to order or bearer*

Types of Checks

You are probably already familiar with the standard personal check, but there are many additional types of checks in use in business transactions. You should be familiar with the following:

Bank Draft. A check drawn by a bank against funds deposited to its account in another bank.

Cashier's Check. A bank's own check drawn upon itself and signed by the bank cashier or other authorized official. It is also known as an officer's or treasurer's check. A cashier's check is obtained by paying the bank cashier the amount of the check, in cash or by personal check. Some banks charge a fee for this service. Cashier's checks are often issued to accommodate the savings account customer who does not maintain a checking account.

Certified Check. This is the depositor's own check, upon the face of which the bank has placed the word "CERTIFIED" or "ACCEPTED" with the date and a bank official's signature. Because the bank deducts the amount of the check from the depositor's account at the time it certifies the check, the bank can guarantee that the amount is available. A certified check, like a cashier's check, can be used when an ordinary personal check would not be acceptable. If not used, a certified check should be redeposited promptly, so that the funds previously set aside will be credited back to the depositor's account.

Limited Check. A check may be limited as to the amount written on it and as to the time during which it may be presented for payment. The limited check is often used for payroll or insurance checks.

Money Orders. Domestic money orders are sold by banks, some stores, and the United States Postal Service. The maximum face value varies according to the source. International money orders may be purchased for limited amounts, indicated in US dollars, for use in sending money abroad.

Traveler's Check. Traveler's checks are designed for persons traveling where personal checks may not be accepted or for use in situations in which it is inadvisable to carry large amounts of cash. Traveler's checks are usually printed in denominations of $10, $20, $50, and $100, and sometimes $500 and $1,000. They require two signatures of the purchaser, one at the time of purchase and the other at the time of use. They are available at banks and some travel agencies.

Voucher Check. A voucher check is one with a detachable voucher form. The voucher portion is used to itemize or specify the purpose for which the check is drawn. It is used for the convenience of the **payer,** showing discounts and various other itemizations. This portion of the check is removed before presenting the check for payment and provides a record for the **payee** (Fig. 14–1).

Warrant. A warrant is a check that is not considered to be negotiable but which can be evidence of a debt due because of certain services rendered, and the bearer is entitled to certain payment for this service. Government and civic agencies often issue such warrants. A claim draft on an insurance claim is a warrant issued by the insurance adjuster as evidence that the claim is valid. It authorizes the insurance company to pay the claim.

Advantages of Using Checks

Using checks for the transfer of funds has many advantages:

- Checks are both safe and convenient, particularly for making payments by mail.
- Expenditures are quickly calculated.
- Specific payments can be easily located from the check record.
- A stop-payment order can protect the payer from loss due to lost, stolen, or incorrectly drawn checks.
- Checks provide a permanent reliable record of disbursements for tax purposes.
- The deposit record provides a summary of receipts.
- Checking accounts protect the money while on deposit.

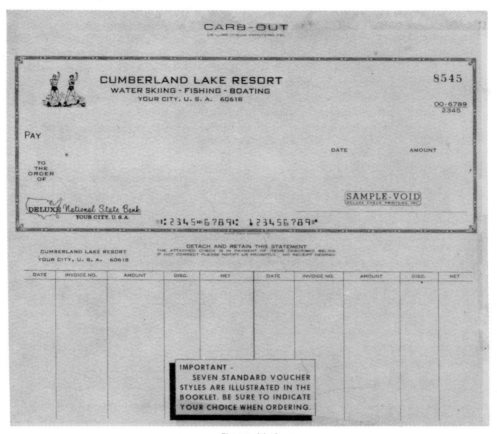

Figure 14–1
Page from bank order book showing sample voucher check.

ABA Number

The ABA number is part of a coding system originated by the American Bankers Association. You will see it in the upper right area of a printed check. It is used as a simple way to identify the area where the bank upon which the check is written is located and the particular bank within the area. The code number is expressed as a fraction: $\frac{90\text{-}1822}{1222}$ (Fig. 14–2). In the top part of the fraction, before the hyphen, the numbers 1 to 49

14

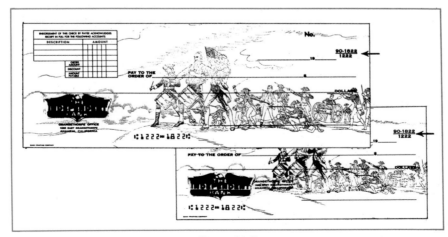

Figure 14–2
Sample checks. Arrow indicates ABA number.

designate cities in which Federal Reserve banks are located or other key cities; the numbers from 50 to 99 refer to states or territories. The part of the number after the hyphen is a number issued to each bank for its own identification purposes. This whole ABA number is used in preparing deposit slips, to identify each check. The bottom part of the fraction includes the number of the Federal Reserve District in which the bank is located and other identifying information.

Magnetic Ink Character Recognition (MICR)

Characters and numbers printed in magnetic ink are found at the bottom of checks. They represent a common machine language, readable by machines as well as by humans. When a check is deposited, the amount of the check can also be printed in magnetic ink below the signature. MICR identification facilitates processing through a high-speed machine that reads the characters, sorts the checks, and does the bookkeeping.

BANK ACCOUNTS

Common Types of Accounts

Checking Account. By placing an amount of money on deposit in a bank, a depositor can set up a checking account. Simply stated, a checking account is a bank account against which checks can be written. Many variations in checking accounts have been developed in recent years. Instead of a straight non–interest bearing account, one might have an insured money market checking account, which bears interest at the daily money market rate if a certain minimum balance is retained (Fig. 14–3).

Savings Accounts. Money that is not needed for current expenses can be deposited in a savings account (Fig. 14–4). In most cases, savings accounts earn interest upon the amounts deposited; that is, the bank pays the depositor a certain percentage monthly or quarterly for the use of the money in the savings account.

The ordinary savings account, called a passbook account, draws interest at the lowest prevailing rate, has no minimum balance requirement, and no check-writing privileges.

An insured money market account requires a minimum balance, frequently $2500, draws interest at money market rates, and allows the writing of a specified number of checks (frequently three) per month. There may be a minimum amount for each transaction. Such checks are usually written for transfer of funds to a checking account.

Service Charges

In all types of accounts, the bank may charge a fee for services rendered in bookkeeping. Usually in the case of an individual account, it is a flat fee; in a business account the fee is based on services rendered. If the average or minimum balance is maintained at an established level, the bank may forego a service charge.

SYSTEMATIZING BILL PAYING

A systematic plan should be established for the writing of checks and the paying of bills. Check writing usually is done on the 10th or 15th of each month. An exception sometimes arises when it is possible to realize a good discount if payment of a bill is made within a specified time, for instance 10 days. Such discounts usually are indicated at the bottom of invoices or billing statements.

When a check is written in payment of a statement or invoice, it is good practice to write on the invoice the number of the check and the date it was paid. Then if any question arises about whether or when the bill was paid, you can readily locate the check stub.

The Business Checkbook

The checkbook most generally used in the professional office has three checks per page with a perforated stub at the left end of the check (Fig. 14–5). The checks may be in a bound soft cover or punched for a ring binder. The check and matching stubs will be numbered in sequence, preprinted with the depositor's name and account number and any additional optional information such as address and telephone number. From 100 to 300 checks are usually ordered at one time and the cost charged against the account.

Numbered deposit slips are also supplied to the depositor.

Checkbook Stubs

The checkbook stub, the part that remains in the book after the check has been written and removed, is your own record of the checks written, date, amount, payee, and purpose. It is important that the stub be completed before the check. This prevents the possibility of writing a check and neglecting to complete the stub. If the stub is not completed and the check is sent out, you will have no record of the payee and the amount taken from the account until the canceled check is returned at a later date. Consequently, you will be unable to balance your account or determine the amount on hand until you receive those canceled checks.

STATEMENT OF ACCOUNT

FOR CHECKING ACCOUNT INQUIRIES
CALL: 1-800-482-8800

Great American
First Savings Bank

SAN CLEMENTE
601 N. EL CAMINO REAL
SAN CLEMENTE, CA 92672

Divisions
San Diego Savings • Laguna Savings • San Joaquin First Savings
Peoples Savings • First Savings Bank of South Pasadena • Riverside Savings
Kaweah Savings • Sonoma County Savings
105-000-3803

PAYMENT ENCLOSED
$

TO MAKE A PAYMENT, DETACH ABOVE PORTION AND MAIL WITH CHECK TO ADDRESS ON REVERSE

STATEMENT OF ACCOUNT

INSURED MONEY-
MARKET CHECKING

LAST STATEMENT
01/28/85

THIS STATEMENT
02/25/85

PAGE 001
ENCLOSURES 9

CURRENT YEAR
INTEREST EARNED
55.13

ACCOUNT 105-000-3803 SUMMARY

BEGINNING BALANCE AS OF......01/28/85...........5,139.40
TOTAL ADDITIONS(001)..........................600.00
TOTAL INTEREST EARNED..........................30.48
TOTAL DEDUCTIONS(009).........................363.56
ENDING BALANCE AS OF........02/25/85...........5,406.32

ACCOUNT ACTIVITY

NUMBER	DATE	AMOUNT	NUMBER	DATE	AMOUNT	NUMBER	DATE	AMOUNT
516	01-29	13.95	521	01-31	115.00	524	02-11	41.89
519*	02-08	12.35	522	02-04	60.30	525	02-22	7.95
520	02-04	14.12	523	02-07	78.00	526	02-20	20.00

DATE	DEDUCTIONS	ADDITIONS	
01-31		600.00	ACCOUNT CREDIT-DIRECT DEPOSIT
02-25		30.48	ACCT CREDIT - CURRENT PERIOD INTEREST

DAILY BALANCE AND INTEREST RATE INFORMATION

START DATE	ENDING DATE	BALANCE	INTEREST RATE	START DATE	ENDING DATE	BALANCE	INTEREST RATE
01-29	01-30	5,125.45	7.30	02-11	02-19	5,403.79	7.30
01-31	02-03	5,610.45	7.30	02-20	02-21	5,383.79	7.30
02-04	02-06	5,536.03	7.30	02-22	02-24	5,375.84	7.30
02-07	02-07	5,458.03	7.30	02-25	02-25	5,406.32	7.30
02-08	02-10	5,445.68	7.30				

AVERAGE BALANCE FOR THE PERIOD   5,429.00

INTEREST EARNED LAST YEAR: 507.69

BASED ON THE ABOVE DAILY RATES, THE AVERAGE ANNUAL RATE FOR
INSURED MONEY-MARKET CHECKING FROM 01-29 THROUGH 02-25 WAS 7.30

MONEY LINE PERMITS YOU TO TRANSFER FUNDS BETWEEN ACCOUNTS
AND TO PRE-AUTHORIZE PAYMENTS TO YOUR LOAN AND CREDIT CARD
ACCOUNTS. APPLY TODAY. CALL 1-800-423-8ANK, EXTENSION 1500.

NOTICE: See reverse side for important information.   *Indicates a break in check number series.

14

Figure 14-3
Example of Insured Money Market Checking Account Statement.

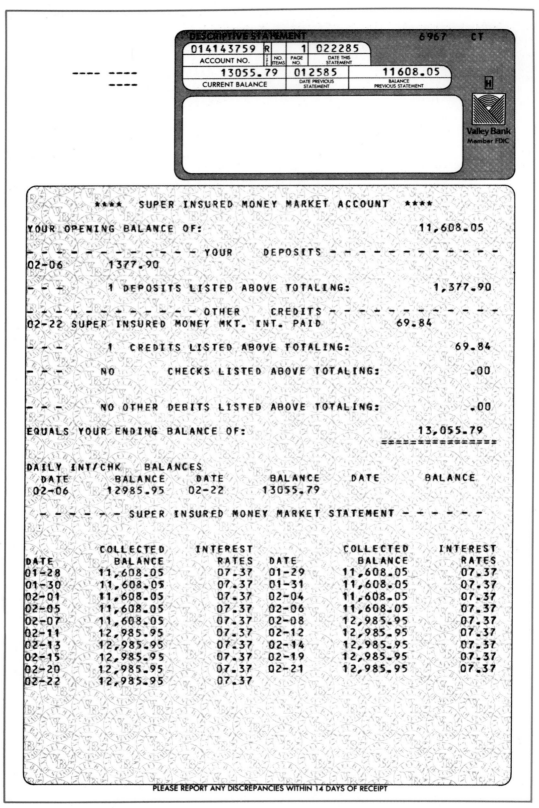

Figure 14–4
Example of Super Insured Money Market Savings Account Statement. Limited Check Writing Privilege.

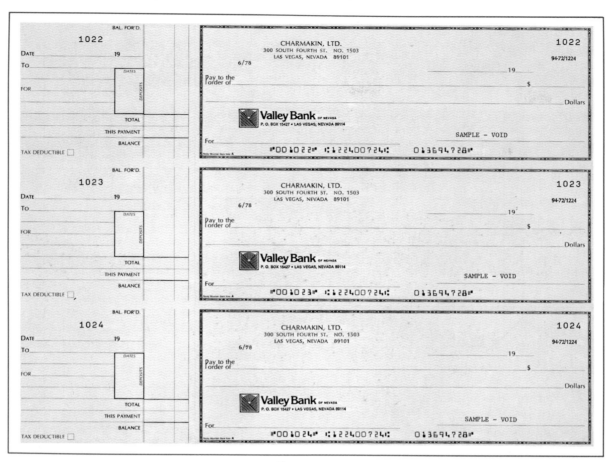

Figure 14-5
Example of business check with stub.

Lost and Stolen Checks

If you lose any of your checks, report this to your bank promptly. The bank will place a warning on your account, and signatures on incoming checks will be carefully inspected to detect possible forgeries.

If you suspect that your checks have been stolen, first make a report to the police in the city or town where the theft took place. Then notify your bank and tell them the time, date, and place the police report was made. A warning will be placed on your account. In some cases, you may be asked to close your account and open a new one under a different number.

As long as you have reported your checks missing or stolen to the proper authorities, you usually will not be held responsible for losses due to forgery. The bank or merchant who accepts the forged checks will be charged for the loss. For this reason, anyone accepting a check from a person who is not known personally must be very careful about establishing the person's identity.

Writing Checks

The handling and writing of checks must be done with extreme care.

1. Before you write the check, fill out the stub or the place designated for recording your expenditures (Fig. 14–6). This will include the date, name of payee, amount of check, the new balance to be carried forward, and usually the purpose of the check.

2. Both the check and the stub should be written in ink or typewritten. The typewritten check has a more professional look.

3. Date the check the day it is written (do not postdate).

4. Write the name of the payee after the printed words, ''pay to the order of.'' Always try to write the name of the payee correctly. When paying bills, you will usually find a notation on the invoice stating ''Make check payable to _____'' with the necessary information following. Do not use abbreviations unless so instructed.

14

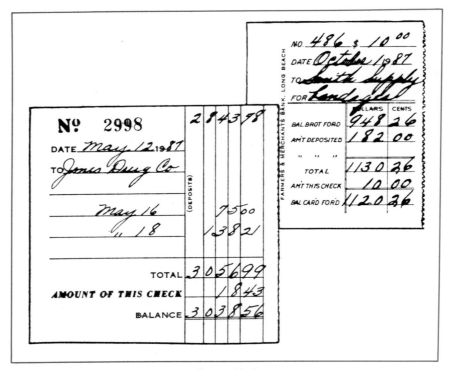

Figure 14–6
Methods of filling out check stubs.

5. Leave no space before the name, and follow it with three dashes if there is space remaining.

6. Omit personal titles from the names of payees.

7. If a payee is receiving a check as an officer of an organization, the name of the office should follow the name. For example, John F. Jones, Treasurer, or Margaret F. Brown, President.

8. Double-check your figures to verify that the amount of the check is recorded correctly on the stub, in the box for the dollar ($) amount, and on the line where the amount is written in words.

9. Start writing at the extreme left of each space. Leave no blank spaces. Keep the cents notation close to the dollars figure, to prevent alteration.

10. If necessary, a check can be written for less than one dollar, but be very careful to emphasize the amount. The figures by the $ sign may be circled to assure proper attention, as ($.65) or enclosed in parentheses, as $-(65¢). When writing out the amount of money, write "only sixty-five cents–". The word dollars should not be crossed out. Figures 14–7 and 14–8 show examples of correct and incorrect check writing.

Handling Corrections and Mistakes. Do not cross out, erase, or change any part of a check. Checks are printed on sensitized paper so that erasures are easily noticeable, and the bank has the right to refuse to pay on any check that has been altered.

If a mistake is made, write the word "VOID" on the stub and the check, but do not throw out or destroy the check. It should be filed with the canceled checks so that it is available for auditing purposes.

Writing "Cash" Checks. A cash check is a check made payable to cash or bearer. Such checks are completely negotiable. Since these checks are easily cashed without positive identification, it is poor policy to write cash checks unless they are to be cashed at the time they are written. Banks may require that the person receiving the cash endorse the check.

One-Write Check Writing

A one-write system of writing checks can save time and minimize errors in medical office **disbursements**. The office with a pegboard bookkeeping system (see Chapter 13) may wish to include one-write check writing. By using a combination check writing system such as the one illustrated in Fig. 14–9, one check and one record of checks drawn handle both bill paying and payroll check writing.

When the check is written, a permanent record is created through the carbonized line of the check onto the record of checks drawn and the employee's payroll record, including a record of all deductions.

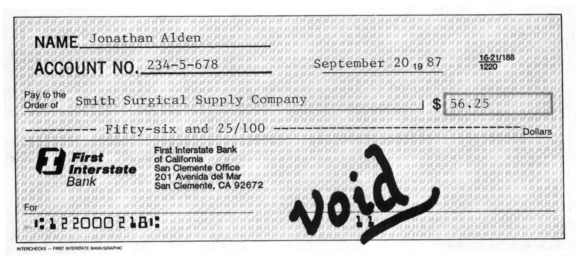

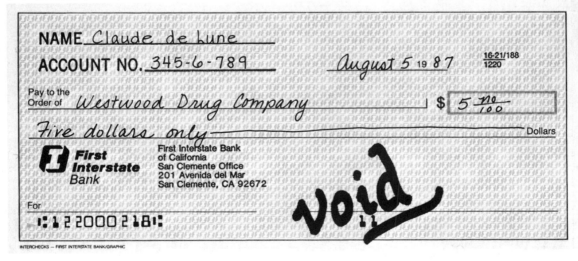

Figure 14–7
Correct methods of writing checks.

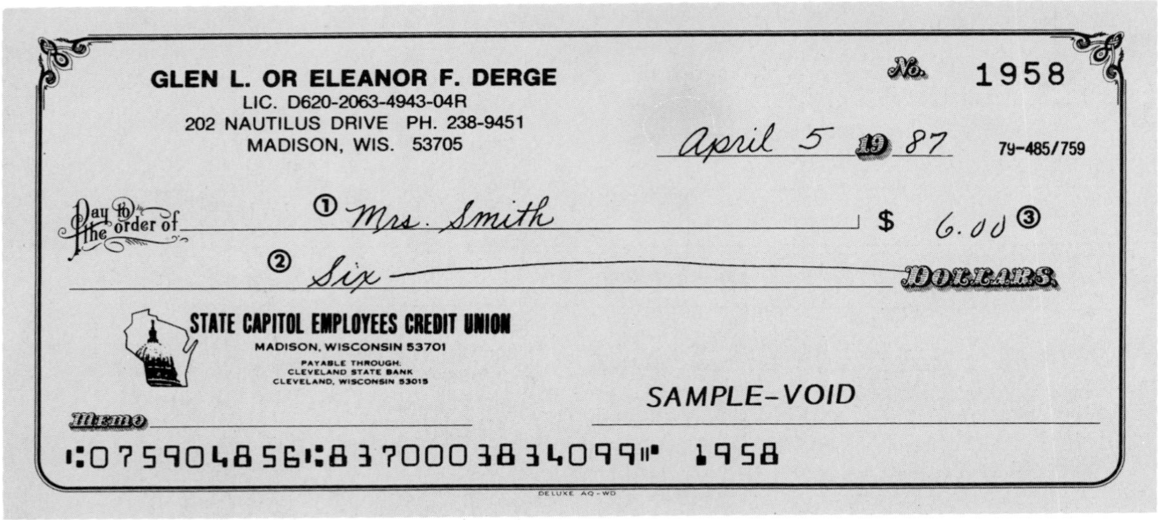
GLEN L. OR ELEANOR F. DERGE
LIC. D620-2063-4943-04R
202 NAUTILUS DRIVE PH. 238-9451
MADISON, WIS. 53705

No. 1958

April 5 19 87 79-485/759

Pay to the order of ① Mrs. Smith $ 6.00 ③

② Six ———— DOLLARS

STATE CAPITOL EMPLOYEES CREDIT UNION
MADISON, WISCONSIN 53701
PAYABLE THROUGH CLEVELAND STATE BANK CLEVELAND, WISCONSIN 53015

SAMPLE-VOID

MEMO

⑆075904856⑆837000383409⑈ 1958

DELUXE AQ-WD

701

MARY E. KINN
MARY L. HISTED
259 WEST MARQUITA
SAN CLEMENTE, CA 92672

June 28 19 87 90-7101/3222

PAY TO THE ORDER OF Mary Louise Jones $ 75/100

Seventy five cents only DOLLARS

Great American
First Savings Bank
601 North El Camino Real
San Clemente, California 92672

SAMPLE-VOID

MEMO

⑆322271012⑆0701⑈105000380 3⑈

BALBOA ISLAND

Figure 14–8

Top, *Incorrect method of writing a check:* 1, *incomplete name;* 2, *check could be made into $26 very easily;* 3, *the "00" could be made into 88.* Bottom, *Correct method of writing a check.*

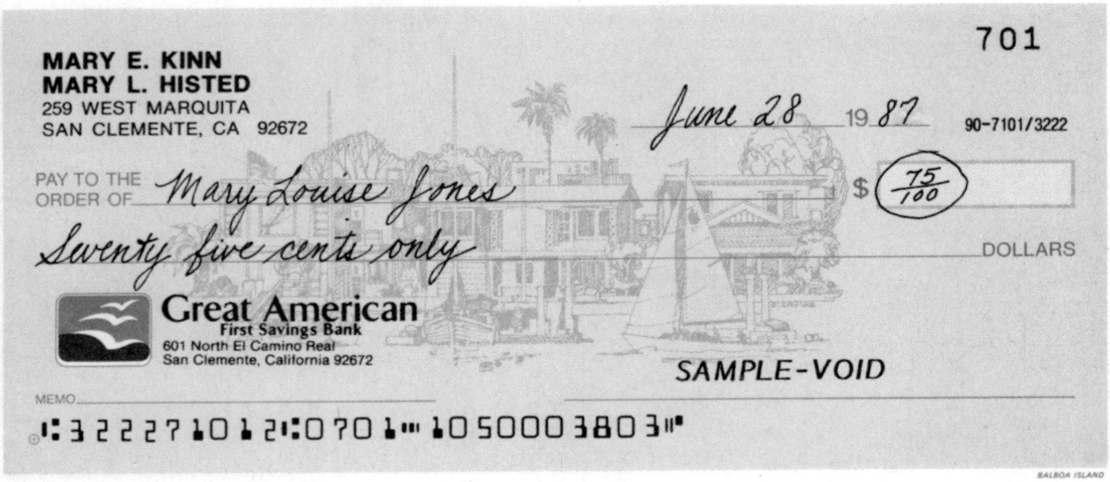

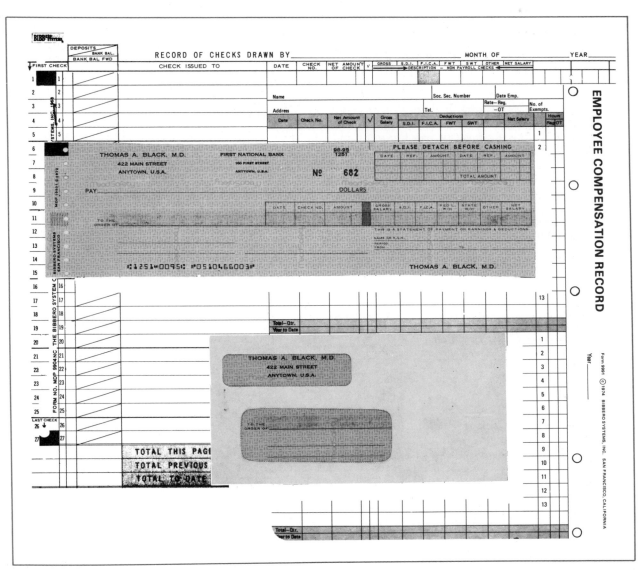

Figure 14–9
Pegboard system for check writing. (Courtesy of Bibbero Systems, Inc., Petaluma, CA.)

14

Space is provided for the payee's address so that the check can be mailed in a window envelope. This not only saves time but ensures that the check goes to the right address. Suppliers of basic pegboard systems can also provide a check-writing system such as the one described.

Signing Checks

After all checks have been written, place them, along with the invoices or other verifying information, on the physician's desk for signature. In some facilities, the medical assistant who has charge of the financial matters is also allowed to sign the checks. This is accomplished by filing a **power of attorney** at the depositor's bank (Fig. 14–10). The power of attorney may limit the check-signing authorization to a certain amount, or to a limited time period.

Mailing Checks

When checks are sent through the mail, the check should not be visible through the envelope. Either place the check within a letter or fold it into a plain sheet of paper. Checks may be folded at the right end to conceal the amount of money written.

Make certain the envelopes are sealed before mailing, and mail all checks yourself as soon as possible after writing.

SPECIAL PROBLEMS WITH CHECKS

Special problems may arise when a check is written on nonexistent funds or when a payer wishes, for a legitimate reason, to prevent the payee from cashing a check.

Account Overdrawn or Overdraft. When a depositor draws a check for more than the amount on deposit in the account, the account becomes overdrawn. In most states it is illegal to issue a check for more than the amount on deposit in the bank. Should this happen through error or oversight, the bank may refuse to honor the check and will return it to the bank that presented it for payment. Such a check is said to "bounce."

If the check is written by an established depositor, the bank may honor the check and notify the depositor that the account is overdrawn. If the bank thus pays or "covers" the check, it issues an overdraft on the depositor's account.

Stop-Payment Order. A depositor or maker of a check who wishes to rescind or stop payment of that check has the right to request the bank to stop payment on it. Stop-payment orders should be used only in emergencies. Reasons for stop-payment requests are:

- Loss of a check
- Disagreement about a purchase
- Disagreement about a payment

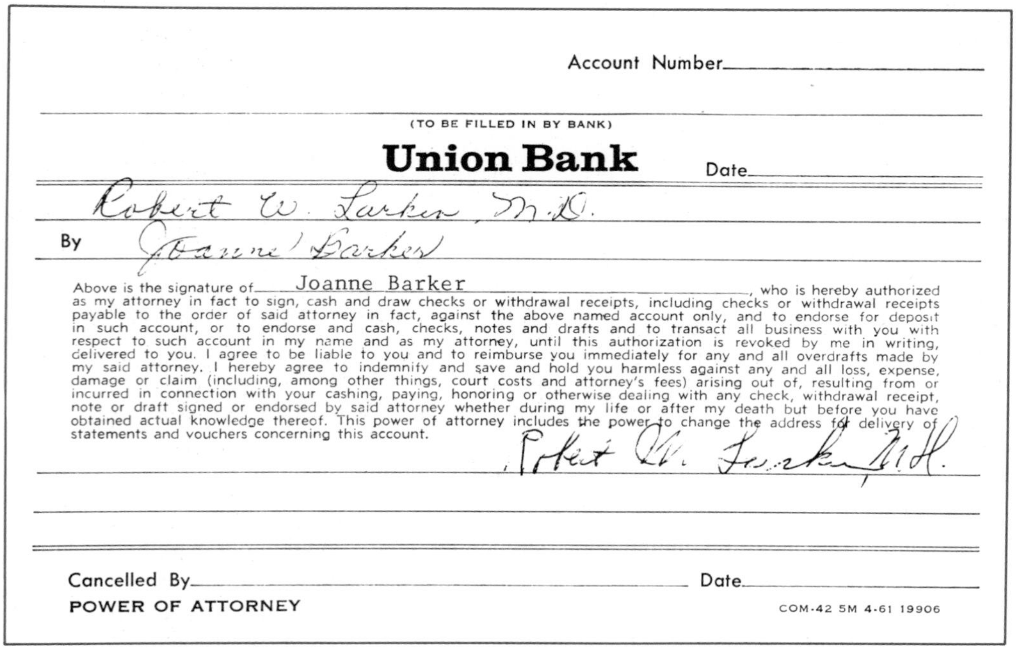

Account Number________

(TO BE FILLED IN BY BANK)

Union Bank Date________

Robert W. Larker, M.D.

By Joanne Barker

Above is the signature of Joanne Barker, who is hereby authorized as my attorney in fact to sign, cash and draw checks or withdrawal receipts, including checks or withdrawal receipts payable to the order of said attorney in fact, against the above named account only, and to endorse for deposit in such account, or to endorse and cash, checks, notes and drafts and to transact all business with you with respect to such account in my name and as my attorney, until this authorization is revoked by me in writing, delivered to you. I agree to be liable to you and to reimburse you immediately for any and all overdrafts made by my said attorney. I hereby agree to indemnify and save and hold you harmless against any and all loss, expense, damage or claim (including, among other things, court costs and attorney's fees) arising out of, resulting from or incurred in connection with your cashing, paying, honoring or otherwise dealing with any check, withdrawal receipt, note or draft signed or endorsed by said attorney whether during my life or after my death but before you have obtained actual knowledge thereof. This power of attorney includes the power to change the address for delivery of statements and vouchers concerning this account.

Robert W. Larker, M.D.

Cancelled By________ Date________

POWER OF ATTORNEY

COM-42 5M 4-61 19906

Figure 14–10
Application for power of attorney.

PAYMENT FROM PATIENTS

Acknowledging Payment in Full. If payment in full is to be recognized in regard to a given check, the statement "Payment in Full to Date" must appear on the back of the check, above the endorsement, not on the face of the check. Canceled checks are a receipt for the **maker** of the check, not for the payee.

Precautions in Accepting Checks. The medical assistant is frequently presented with checks in payment for the physician's services. In most cases these will be personal checks. The following guidelines should be observed:

- Scan the check carefully for the correct date, amount, and signature.
- Do not accept a check with corrections on it.
- If you do not know the person presenting a personal check, ask for identification and compare signatures.
- Accept an out-of-town check, government check, or payroll check only if you are well acquainted with the person presenting it, and it does not exceed the amount of the payment.
- Acceptance of "third-party" checks is generally unwise. A **third-party check** is one made out to your patient by a party unknown to you. A check from the patient's health insurance carrier is an exception.
- When accepting a postal money order for payment, make certain it has only one endorsement. Postal money orders with more than two endorsements will not be honored.
- Do not accept a check marked "Payment in Full" unless it does pay the account in full up to and including the date on which it is received. If a check so marked is less than the amount due, you will be unable to collect the balance on the account once you have accepted and deposited such a check. It is illegal for you to scratch out the words "Payment in Full."
- Accepting checks written for more than the amount due is poor policy because, first, you will have to return cash for the difference between the amount of the check and the amount owed. If the check is not honored by the bank, your office will suffer the loss not only of the amount of the check but also of the amount returned in cash. Second, the canceled check could be used by the patient to indicate the amount paid on account.

ENDORSEMENT OF CHECKS

An endorsement is a signature plus any other writing on the back of a check by which the **endorser** transfers all rights in the check to another party. Endorsements are made in ink, with either pen or rubber stamp, on the back of the check across the left, or perforated, end.

Necessity for Endorsement

The Uniform Negotiable Instrument Act, applicable in all states, explains the need of an endorsement as follows:

> An instrument is negotiated when it is transferred from one person to another in such a manner as to pass title to another party. If payable to bearer, it is negotiated by delivery. If payable to order, it is negotiated by the endorsement of the holder completed by delivery.

The name of the last endorser of the check shows who last received the money. If a check is cashed for someone who did not endorse it and is returned for some reason, the bank will charge the check to the last endorser, not to the last person receiving the money. For this reason, it is not wise to cash a check made payable to another party without having the endorsement of the person who delivered the check to you for cashing.

Kinds of Endorsements

The four principal kinds of endorsements are:

- Blank
- Restrictive
- Special
- Qualified

Blank and restrictive endorsements are the ones most commonly used.

Blank Endorsement. The payee signs only his or her name. This makes the check payable to the bearer. It is the simplest and most common type of endorsement on personal checks, but should be used only when the check is to be cashed or deposited immediately.

Restrictive Endorsement. This specifies the purpose of the endorsement. You will use a restrictive endorsement in preparing checks for deposit to the physician's checking account. An example is shown in Figure 14–11.

Special Endorsement. This endorsement includes words specifying the person to whom the endorser makes the check payable. For instance, a check naming Helen Barker as payee may be endorsed to the physician by writing on the back of the check

Pay to the order of
Theodore F. Wilson, M.D.
Helen Barker

14

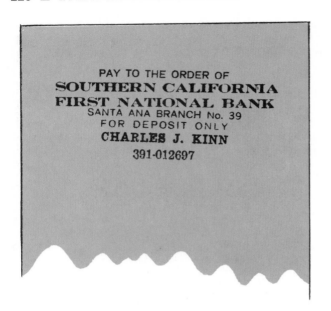

PAY TO THE ORDER OF
**SOUTHERN CALIFORNIA
FIRST NATIONAL BANK**
SANTA ANA BRANCH No. 39
FOR DEPOSIT ONLY
CHARLES J. KINN
391-012697

*Figure 14–11
Example of restrictive endorsement.*

The check is still negotiable but requires Dr. Wilson's signature or endorsement.

Qualified Endorsement. The effect of the endorsement is qualified by disclaiming or destroying any future liability of the endorser. Usually the words "Without Recourse" are written above by an attorney who accepts a check on behalf of a client but who has no personal claim in the transaction.

Endorsement Procedures

The medical assistant may use a blank endorsement when cashing a check to replenish the petty cash fund. This endorsement should be made only at the time of exchanging the check for cash.

As checks from patients and other sources arrive, they should be recorded on the ledger and immediately stamped with the restrictive endorsement "For Deposit Only." This is a safeguard against lost or stolen checks.

Any endorsement should agree exactly with the name on the face of the check. If the name of the payee is misspelled, it is usually necessary for the payee to endorse the check the way the name is spelled on the face, followed by the correctly spelled signature. The Uniform Commercial Code, Section 3-203, states:

> Where an instrument is made payable to a person under a misspelled name or one other than his own, he may endorse in that name or his own or both; but signature in both names may be required by a person paying or giving value for the instrument.

Most banks will accept routine stamp endorsement that is restricted to "Deposit Only," if the customer is well known and maintains an established account.

Some insurance checks or drafts require a personal signature endorsement; a stamped endorsement is not acceptable. This will be stated on the back of the check. In such cases, ask the payee to endorse the check, then stamp immediately below the signature the restrictive endorsement "For Deposit Only."

MAKING DEPOSITS

Financial duties of the medical assistant include depositing checks and reconciling the bank statements with the checkbook.

Checks should be deposited promptly because:

- There is the possibility of a stop-payment order.
- The check may be lost, misplaced, or stolen.
- Delay may cause the check to be returned because of insufficient funds.
- The check may have a restricted time for cashing.
- It is a courtesy to the payer.

Preparing the Deposit

Deposit slips are itemized memoranda of cash or other funds that a depositor presents to the bank with the money to be credited to the account. All deposits must be accompanied by a deposit slip. A carbon or photocopy of the deposit slip should be kept on file.

There are several types of deposit slips, sometimes called deposit tickets. The commercial slip (Fig. 14–12) is used for the office checking account. The deposit slips are printed with the number of the account in magnetic ink characters to correspond with the checks. Preprinted deposit slips are ordered along with the checks.

Some write-it-once accounting systems include a deposit slip that the bank will accept as the itemization if it is attached to the customer's numbered deposit slip. The deposit slip should be prepared before you go to the bank, with the money organized and ready to present to the bank teller.

Payment on patient accounts is generally made by check, but some payments will be in currency (paper money). Each type of funds is recorded separately on the deposit slip. The currency is usually listed first. Organize the currency so that all of the bills are facing in the same direction—that is, the black side up and the portrait right side up. Place the larger bills on top, graduating down to the smallest ones.

The coin amount is listed next. Count the coins

1427

DEPOSIT STUB

DATE OF DEPOSIT ____________

ADDED IN AND NEW BALANCE
BROUGHT FORWARD ON STUB NO. ____________

TOTAL AMOUNT OF DEPOSIT ____________

ITEM(S) DEPOSITED ____________

LC 128 (REV 5-84)

DEPOSIT SLIP

CHARMAKIN, LTD. 6/78
300 SOUTH FOURTH ST. NO. 1503
LAS VEGAS, NEVADA 89101

Date ____________ 19____

A HOLD FOR UNCOLLECTED FUNDS MAY BE PLACED ON CHECKS OR SIMILAR INSTRUMENTS YOU DEPOSIT. ANY DELAY WILL NOT EXCEED THE PERIOD OF TIME PERMITTED BY LAW.

Valley Bank OF NEVADA
P. O. BOX 15427 • LAS VEGAS, NEVADA 89114

RM 565 (05 84)

CURRENCY	
COIN	
CHECKS	
TOTAL FROM OTHER SIDE	
TOTAL	

94-72/1224

PLEASE IDENTIFY ATTACHED TAPES WITH YOUR ACCOUNT NUMBER

⑈001427⑈ ⑆122400724⑆ 013694728⑈ 20

Figure 14–12
Business deposit slip.

and place them in an envelope. If there is a large quantity of a certain coin, place it in rolls provided by the bank. The depositor should sign these rolls, since the rolled coins are usually not counted by the **teller**.

Checks are recorded individually by the ABA number. If the checks are arranged alphabetically by the names of the patient accounts, with these names included on your office copy of the deposit slip, you will have a ready reference of checks deposited should a question arise regarding a patient's payment.

Money orders, either postal, express, or others, are identified by "PO Money Order," or "Exp. MO." Remember that money orders cannot have more than two endorsements.

The deposit slip should be carefully totaled and the total entered in the checkbook. Any torn bills should be mended with transparent tape. Clip the currency together, and clip the checks in a separate packet. Then place the entire amount in a heavy envelope for taking to the bank. Deposit daily if possible.

Depositing by Mail

Depositing by mail will save time and is easily accomplished if the deposit consists of checks only. Banks usually supply their customers with special mailing deposit slips and envelopes upon request (Fig. 14–13). Some mailing deposit slips have an attached portion that the bank will stamp and return as your receipt. Others may provide the customer with a receipt card that is sent along with the deposit each time for the bank's notation. These deposits are prepared in the same manner as the regular deposits, but certain precautions should be observed:

- Do not send cash or currency by mail. If this is absolutely necessary, then send it by registered mail.

VALLEY BANK OF NEVADA

1. Checking Accounts — Please use only YOUR personalized deposit ticket to insure proper credit.
2. Savings Accounts — Please use only a savings deposit ticket.
3. Endorse check in this way:
   Pay to the order of
   VALLEY BANK OF NEVADA
   Signature, as check is drawn
   Your correct signature (if necessary)
   Your Account Number
4. This card, validated mailing receipt, and new mailing envelope will be returned to you ready for your next deposit.
5. Registered mail should be used if currency is included.

Please Indicate Any Change of Address

STREET

CITY STATE ZIP

Checking Account No.	Savings Account No.

EN-21

USE THIS HANDY TWO-WAY CARD FOR SPEEDY SERVICE

Figure 14–13
Example of bank-by-mail deposit ticket.

14

- Use only a restrictive endorsement; use a deposit stamp or write the notation "For deposit only to the account of xxxx ."
- If you have not obtained mailing deposit slips or your bank does not provide them, make duplicate slips and mail them with your deposit. Ask the bank to stamp one copy and return it to you as a receipt.

"Hold" on Account

Under certain circumstances, money that is deposited may not be immediately available for use. A "Hold for Uncollected Funds (UCF)" may be placed for the full amount of a check you deposit if it is:

- For a sizable amount

- Drawn on another bank or another branch of your bank
- Issued by a person or organization not known to the bank

The hold means that you cannot use the funds until the check has cleared (been processed and paid to your account).

You will be told if a hold has been placed on your account. The teller will note the hold in your deposit record by writing "UCF" and the number of days the hold will be in effect; this will appear next to the date of deposit. If the deposit was made by mail, you will be either telephoned or notified of the hold by return mail.

The hold will be for a specified number of business days and for the full amount of the check. After that time, you can begin to draw against the funds. If for some reason the check does not clear, you will be notified.

Procedure 14-1

PREPARING A BANK DEPOSIT

PROCEDURAL GOAL

To prepare a bank deposit for the day's receipts and complete appropriate office records related to the deposit.

EQUIPMENT AND SUPPLIES

Currency
Six checks for deposit
Deposit slip
Endorsement stamp (optional)
Typewriter
Envelope

PROCEDURE

1. Organize currency.
   Purpose: To arrange currency in best order for speedy and accurate presentation to teller.
2. Total the currency and record the amount on the deposit slip.
3. Place restrictive endorsement on checks, using an endorsement stamp or the typewriter.
   Purpose: To transfer title and protect checks from loss or theft.
4. List each check separately on deposit slip by ABA number and amount of check.
5. Total the amount of currency and checks and enter on deposit slip.
6. Enter amount of deposit in checkbook.
   Purpose: To record current balance in account.
7. Prepare copy of deposit slip for office record, including names of payers.
   Purpose: For verification of checks deposited, if necessary.
8. Place currency, checks, and deposit slip in envelope for transporting to bank.

TERMINAL PERFORMANCE OBJECTIVE

Given the listed equipment and supplies, prepare a deposit of the day's receipts according to the agency's standard procedures, within 10 minutes, to a performance level of 100%.

The Complete Statement®

DIRECT INQUIRIES TO

(397) ACCT NO.
(PER)   ITM023199

5
X

F1 First Interstate Bank

CG
09
1 B
PAGE   1
THIS STATEMENT DATE   AUGUST 13, 1986
NEXT STATEMENT DATE SEPTEMBER 12, 1986

USE YOUR RED OR GOLD FIRST INTERSTATE BANCARD AT HUNDREDS OF RETAIL STORES
DISPLAYING THE INTERLINK SYMBOL AND GET THE CONVENIENCE OF PAYING FOR YOUR
PURCHASE WITH NO CHECKS TO WRITE!

CHECKING ACCOUNT 188-3-18049   SUMMARY

BALANCE FORWARD AS OF 07-14-86	3,110.80
TOTAL DEPOSITS/CREDITS.	.00
TOTAL CHECKS/DEBITS	363.58
SERVICE CHARGES	.00
ENDING BALANCE	2,747.22
MINIMUM BALANCE ON 08-13	2,747.22
AVERAGE BALANCE.	3,000.00

CHECKING ACCOUNT TRANSACTIONS

CHECKS

CHECK NO	DATE	AMOUNT	CHECK NO	DATE	AMOUNT	CHECK NO	DATE	AMOUNT
933	07-15	55.73	935	07-28	60.10	941*	08-13	200.00
934	07-17	11.00	936	08-11	36.75			

A FIRST INTERSTATE MASTERCARD OR VISA CARD MEANS MORE CASH FOR YOUR VACATION.

PLANNING NEXT YEAR'S VACATION? START WITH A FIRST INTERSTATE SAVINGS ACCOUNT.

BALANCE PLUS LINE OF CREDIT   ACCOUNT 188-3-18049
                      SUMMARY

PREVIOUS BALANCE	.00
AMOUNT BORROWED THIS PERIOD	.00
** FINANCE CHARGE ** THIS PERIOD THRU 08-13-86	.00
TOTAL PAYMENTS AND CREDITS.	.00
NEW BALANCE.	.00
** FINANCE CHARGE ** PAID YEAR-TO-DATE THRU 08-13-86. . . .	.00
CREDIT LINE	500.00
CREDIT AVAILABLE	500.00
MINIMUM PAYMENT NOW DUE.	.00
NEXT STATEMENT DATE. . . . . SEPTEMBER 12, 1986	
DAILY PERIODIC RATE % .05479 X 365 = ** ANNUAL PERCENTAGE RATE ** OF	20.00%

BALANCE PLUS GIVES YOU FINANCIAL SECURITY WHILE YOU'RE ON VACATION.

14

Note: An asterisk (*) next to any check listed above means there has been a break in the
numerical sequence of your checks.

Notice: Please see reverse side and any accompanying statement(s) for important information.
Examine this statement carefully and report any irregularities promptly.

Figure 14–14
Example of regular checking account statement.

Returned Checks

Occasionally the bank may return a deposited check because of some irregularity such as a missing signature or missing endorsement. More often it will be because the payer has insufficient funds on deposit to cover the check.

If the check is stamped "NSF," indicating non-sufficient funds, do not delay in contacting the person who gave you the check. If you are unable to contact the maker of a bad check, waste no time in tracking down all leads, such as referrals, numbers you obtained from credit cards, driver's license, and so forth. There are several places to which bad checks may be reported. Credit associations are often a great help when such a problem arises. Turn the account over to a qualified collection agency if you do not succeed in collecting on the account yourself within a short time.

If a check is returned to your office marked "No Account," and it is a check that you had deposited promptly, you have obviously been swindled. This check should be given to the police, the local Better Business Bureau, or your collection agency.

BANK STATEMENT

A statement is periodically sent by the bank to the customer, showing the status of the customer's account on a given date. This statement indicates the beginning balance, deposits received, checks paid, bank charges, and ending balance at the time the statement is prepared (Fig. 14–14). The bank statement is usually accompanied by the customer's canceled checks.

Some banks are now microfilming canceled checks and storing the information in the bank's computer. The customer is asked for permission to use this procedure, and has the privilege of requesting a copy of any check when needed. Bank statements are prepared at regular intervals, usually once a month. The bank statement is also known as a bank reconciliation.

Reconciling the Bank Statement

The bank statement balance and the customer's checkbook balance will usually be different, except in a relatively inactive account. The two balances must be reconciled. The reconciliation will disclose any errors that may exist in the checkbook or, on rare occasions, in the bank statement (Fig. 14–15). Most banks ask to be notified within 10 days of any error found in the statement. The bank statement should be reconciled as soon as it is received. You will usually find a form to follow in carrying out this procedure on the back of the bank statement.

The reconciliation procedure may be put in a formula, as shown below:

Bank statement balance	$_____
Less outstanding checks	$_____
Plus deposits not shown	$_____
CORRECTED BANK STATEMENT BALANCE	$_____
Checkbook balance	$_____
Less any bank charges	$_____
CORRECTED CHECKBOOK BALANCE	$_____

If these balances agree, you may stop here. If they do not agree, *subtract* the lesser from the greater; the difference will usually give you a clue to locating the error.

In searching for a possible error, ask yourself these questions:

- Did you forget to include one of the outstanding checks?
- Is your arithmetic correct?
- Did you fail to record a deposit or did you record it twice?
- Do all stubs and checks agree?
- Have you carried your figures forward correctly?
- Have you transposed a figure? (If the amount of your error is divisible by nine, you probably did.)
- Did your employer write a check without your knowledge?
- Did you fail to correct your checkbook balance at the time of the previous statement?

Many people find the reconciliation process confusing at first, but after a few times it will become easier and fairly routine.

SAFE DEPOSIT BOX

Most commercial banks and many savings institutions have safe deposit boxes that may be rented by their customers. Safe deposit boxes provide protection for valuable papers and personal property for a moderate fee. They are obtainable in various sizes to suit the need of the customer. Chapter 11 (Medical Records Management) lists certain items that might be placed in a safe deposit box. The medical assistant may be asked to keep a perpetual inventory of the contents of the safe deposit box.

The box provides protection in several ways. The box itself is a metal container that is locked with

BALANCING YOUR ACCOUNT

1. First, review this statement and mark off (✓) the corresponding entries in your account register.

2. **Add** to your register balance the amount of any deposits, interest credited, or other credits on this statement which you have not previously added.

3. **Subtract** from your register balance the amount of any checks or other charges recorded on this statement which you have not already subtracted. (For example, service charges, automated teller machine withdrawals, automatic loan or bill payments, transfers to other accounts, check printing charges, etc.)

4. List below all **outstanding** items (checks, automated teller machine withdrawals, automatic deductions, etc.) from your register that are not reflected on this statement and total them.

5. Using the Account Summary below, enter the ending balance as shown on the front of this statement.

6. Enter any deposits to your account after the statement date and add them to your ending balance.

7. Subtract the total amount of the outstanding items. The remaining balance should agree with your register balance. If it does not, use the check list at the bottom of this page to find the error.

Outstanding Items Not Charged On This Statement

NO.	AMOUNT	NO.	AMOUNT
	$		$
	TOTAL $		

Account Summary

Ending Balance Shown
On This Statement $_____

ADD: Deposits Not
      Credited On
      This Statement
      (if any) $_____

      _____

      _____

                        TOTAL $_____

SUBTRACT: Total
           Outstanding Items $_____

                        BALANCE $_____

14

IF YOUR ACCOUNT DOES NOT BALANCE, PLEASE CHECK THE FOLLOWING:

_____ Have you checked all addition and subtraction in your register?

_____ Have you correctly entered all items in your register?

_____ Have you carried the correct balance forward from one register page to the other?

_____ Have you deducted all fees and charges?

_____ Have you added any interest credited to your register?

Figure 14–15
Reverse side of bank statement. Use for reconciling your checking account.

Procedure 14-2

PROCEDURAL GOAL

To reconcile a bank statement with the checking account.

EQUIPMENT AND SUPPLIES

Ending balance of previous statement
Current bank statement
Canceled checks for current month
Checkbook stubs
Calculator
Pen

PROCEDURE

1. Compare the opening balance of the new statement with the closing balance of the previous statement.
   Purpose: To determine that balances are in agreement.
2. Compare the canceled checks with the items on the statement.
   Purpose: To verify that they are your checks and that they are listed in the right amount.
3. Arrange the canceled checks in numeric order and compare with the checkbook stubs.
4. Place a checkmark (√) on each stub for which a canceled check has been returned.
   Purpose: To locate any outstanding checks.
5. List and total the outstanding checks.
6. Subtract the total of outstanding checks from the bank statement balance.
   Note: Do not include any certified checks as outstanding, because the amount has already been deducted from the account.
7. Add to the total in Step 6 any deposits made but not included in the bank statement.
   Purpose: To correct the credits in the bank statement balance.
8. Total any bank charges that appear on the bank statement and subtract them from the checkbook balance. Such charges may include service charges, automatic withdrawals or payments, and NSF checks.
   Purpose: To correct the checkbook balance.
9. If the checkbook balance and the statement balance do not agree, repeat the process.

TERMINAL PERFORMANCE OBJECTIVE

Given the listed information, equipment and supplies, determine that the bank statement and the checkbook are in balance, within 15 minutes, to a performance level of 100%.

two keys into a compartment in the bank's vault. One key is in the possession of the customer; the second key is held by the bank. The bank is very strict about giving access to the safe deposit boxes. The customer must register on a special form when requesting access to the box. After signatures have been compared, the customer is admitted to the vault, accompanied by a bank attendant. The attendant opens one lock with the bank key and opens the other lock with the customer's key. The box may then be removed and taken to a private room, or, if the customer merely wishes to place something in the box, this can be done and the box can be immediately replaced and locked.

The customer is given two identical keys upon renting the box. These must be guarded carefully because they cannot be duplicated, and the customer must return both keys to the bank when the box is relinquished. If a key is lost, the bank will charge a fee; if both keys are lost, the fee is considerably higher because the lock must be changed.

MEDICAL ASSISTANT'S POSITION OF TRUST

The medical assistant who manages the financial responsibilities of a medical practice is in a position of great trust. Conscientious and reliable attention to detail in this position can be a great source of job satisfaction and an attribute toward job security.

14

CHAPTER OUTLINE

VOCABULARY

See Glossary at end of book for definitions.

accounts receivable ratio
age analysis
collection ratio

invasion of privacy
statute of limitations

subsidize
superbill

Billing and Collecting Procedures

15

OBJECTIVES

Upon successful completion of this chapter you should be able to:

1. Define the terms listed in the Vocabulary of this chapter.
2. Name the three ways by which payment for medical services is accomplished.
3. List nine items that should be addressed in developing a credit policy.
4. State three reasons for itemizing billing statements.
5. Describe cycle billing and its advantages.
6. Discuss the significance of determining the collection ratio and the accounts receivable ratio.
7. List the three most common reasons for patients' failure to pay accounts.
8. Discuss the do's and don'ts of telephone collection procedures.
9. Name five sources of information in tracing skips.
10. State the procedure to follow upon receiving notice of a debtor's bankruptcy.
11. List three advantages of using a small claims court for collecting delinquent accounts.
12. Discuss five appropriate follow-up actions after assigning accounts to a collection agency.

Upon successful completion of this chapter you should be able to perform the following activities:

1. Prepare patients' monthly statements.
2. Calculate a collection ratio and an accounts receivable ratio.
3. Prepare an age analysis of accounts receivable.
4. Initiate proceedings to collect delinquent accounts.
5. Demonstrate telephone collection techniques.

In Chapter 12 we discussed how fees are determined, the importance of advance discussion of fees, the adjusting or canceling of fees in hardship cases, and the legal aspects of credit arrangements. We also addressed the importance of getting adequate information on the first visit when it appears that an extension of credit will be necessary.

The collection of fees and financial management of the medical practice is often entrusted to the medical assistant. To be an effective financial manager, the medical assistant must:

- Believe that the doctor and the office have a right to charge for the services provided
- Not be embarrassed to ask for payment for the value of the service
- Possess tact and good judgment
- Give individual attention and personal consideration to each situation
- Be courteous and show a sincere desire to help the patient who has financial problems
- Try to find out the patient's reason for nonpayment when this occurs

The payment for medical services is accomplished in three ways:
1. Payment at time of services
2. Billing when extension of credit is necessary
3. Using outside collection assistance

PAYMENT AT TIME OF SERVICE

Every practice in which there are patient visits should stress time-of-service collection. This is especially important in an office-based primary care practice because many of these office visits are uninsured and may be difficult to collect later. If patients get into the habit of paying their current charges before they leave the office, there are no further billing and bookkeeping expenses, and there is not time for inflation to decrease the value of the account.

If patients are informed when making an appointment that payment will be expected at the time of service, they are not surprised when you say at the end of the visit, "Your charge for today, Mrs. Casey, is $xx. Will that be cash or check?" Many patients are hesitant to ask about charges and are unsure whether to offer to pay or to wait until asked. You will make it easier for the patients by offering to accept their payments, since most people are prepared to meet small bills on a cash basis.

Even if a patient requests to be billed, you can say that an exception is being made at this time, but the normal procedure is to pay at the time of service. For patients who may have forgotten their checkbook, you may hand them a self-addressed envelope with the charge slip, and ask them to send the payment in the next mail.

BILLING AFTER EXTENSION OF CREDIT

In some types of medical practice, particularly those involving large fees for surgery or long-term care, it becomes necessary to extend credit and establish a regular system of billing. This requires informing the patient of:

- What the charges will be
- What professional services these charges cover
- The credit policy of the office

Credit Policy

Many offices do not have a true credit policy; thus, each account continues to be evaluated individually. It is almost impossible to judge accounts objectively and equitably under such circumstances.

The doctor and the staff should think through their situation, decide what they expect of patients with respect to payments, and how they will inform the patient. Although there will always be exceptions to any rule, there must *be* a rule, which should be in writing and conveyed to the patient at the outset of the relationship.

In many medical practices, an information booklet is prepared that includes the payment policy. New patients are given a copy of the booklet. Any patient who needs special consideration can be counseled by the medical assistant.

Some of the issues to be addressed in the credit policy are:

- When payment is due from patients
- When the practice requires payment at time of service
- When or if assignment of insurance benefits is accepted
- Whether insurance forms will be completed by the office staff
- Billing procedures
- Collection protocol
- How long an account will be carried without payment
- Telephone collection protocol
- Sending accounts to a collection agency

The medical assistant who has the guidance of an established credit policy can perform with confidence in handling patient accounts.

Billing Methods

Computerized Billing. The medical office that "has gone on computer" for accounts receivable management will be completing statements and insurance forms by computer. These procedures were discussed in Chapter 6.

Microfilm Billing. Recommended by many management consultants, microfilm billing is particularly useful to offices with large volume billings. On a specified day of the month, a representative of the billing service brings portable camera equipment to the office and microfilms each ledger that has a balance due. This requires very little time, and the ledgers remain under the control of the office. The film is processed by the billing service, and a copy of the ledger is mailed to the patient. The mailing can include a self-addressed envelope for direct payment to the physician. An extra benefit of microfilming is that a duplicate set of ledger cards is generated, which would be useful in case of loss of the office records by fire or other causes.

Copy Van or Centralized Photocopying. In some areas you may find a billing service with a copier mounted in a van that will call at the doctor's office once a month. The representative takes the ledger tray from the office to the van, runs the ledgers through a high-speed copier, and returns the ledgers to the doctor's office in a matter of minutes. The service can include inserting the copy in an envelope, stamping, and mailing. For the office without a photocopy machine, this may be the most inexpensive method of outside billing.

BILLING NAME: Paul Allan
PATIENT'S NAME: same
RES PHONE 492 3737 BUS PHONE 551 1797
OCCUPATION: teacher
EMPLOYED BY: Anytown Unified School District
INS. INFORMATION: California General
FORM NO. MDP 8510

NAMES OF OTHER FAMILY MEMBERS: Wife: Thelma A.; Daughter: April
RELATIVE OR FRIEND
REFERRED BY: David Bucher, M.D.
SOC. SEC. NUMBER: 111 00 2222
© 1965 BIBBERO SYSTEMS, INC. - SAN FRANCISCO

ADAM J. BROWN, D.C.
ROBERT F. BLACK, D.C.
PALMER CHIROPRACTORS
100 MAIN STREET, SUITE 10
ANYTOWN, CALIFORNIA 90000
TELEPHONE: 399-4000

STATEMENT TO:

Mr. Paul Allan
123 Main Street
Anytown, XX 00000

TEAR OFF AND RETURN UPPER PORTION WITH PAYMENT

DATE 1987	PAYMENTS: BANK NUMBER	PAYMENTS: BY CHECK OR P.M.O.	PAYMENTS: BY COIN OR CURRENCY	PROFESSIONAL SERVICE		FEE	LAST AMOUNT IN THIS COLUMN IS BALANCE DUE
05 29				90050	Office call	25 00	25 00
				85010	CBC	10 00	35 00
06 05				90040	Office call	20 00	55 00

PROFESSIONAL SERVICE CODES:
1. CONSULTATION
2. EXAMINATION
3. DIAG. EXAM., MAJOR
4. CHIROPRACTIC ADJUSTMENT
5. ADJUSTMENT, PROLONGED
6. COMPLETE FULL SPINE X-RAYS
7. SPINE CERVICAL A-P AND LAT.
8. SPINE, CERVICAL COMP. (DAVIS)
9. SPINE, THORACIC, TWO VIEWS
10. SPINE, THORACO — LUMBAR, A-P AND LAT.
11. SPINE, LUMBOSACRAL COMPLETE
12. PELVIS, COMPLETE
13. PELVIS, SACRUM AND COCCYX, A-P AND LAT.
14. KNEE SERIES
15. SHOULDER SERIES
16. URINALYSIS
17. CERVICAL PILLOW AND CASE
18. CERVICAL COLLAR AND CASE
19. LUMBOSACRAL SUPPORT
20. NARRATIVE REPORT
21. OTHER
22. NO CHARGE
23. ADJUSTMENTS OR CORRECTIONS

ADAM J. BROWN, D.C. - LIC. #56372 ROBERT F. BLACK, D.C. - LIC. #32780

Figure 15–1
Example of itemized statement.

Internal Billing by the Medical Assistant

In a practice in which the number of accounts is not too great, the medical assistant will handle the preparation and mailing of statements. This may be accomplished by:

- Superbill
- Typewritten statement
- Photocopied statement

The appearance of the statement carries a visual impact just as a letter does, so the statement heads should be carefully chosen and the typing clean and accurate. Statement heads usually are imprinted with the same information as the doctor's letterhead. They should be of good quality and large enough to allow itemization of charges. Envelopes should be imprinted with "Address Correction Requested" under the return address, to maintain up-to-date mailing lists. A self-addressed return envelope included with the bill will encourage prompt payment. This is mainly for the convenience of patients who do not always have stationery available for sending a return payment or who are less likely to return a payment immediately if they must address an envelope.

The Superbill. The **superbill** is a combination charge slip, statement, and insurance reporting form. There are variations in styles, and they are usually personalized for the practice. Figure 15–2 on page 233 is an example of a form used in an Ob-Gyn office. It has space for all the elements required in submitting medical insurance claims:

1. Name and address of patient
2. Name of insurance carrier
3. Insurance identification number
4. Brief description of each service by code number
5. Fee for each service
6. Place and date of service
7. Diagnosis
8. Doctor's name and address
9. Doctor's signature

The superbill can be used as a charge slip for office treatments if the doctor checks the services performed at the completion of the visit and asks the patient to hand it to the medical assistant upon leaving. Either the doctor or the medical assistant may write in the amount of the fee. The doctor indicates at the bottom of the sheet when the patient should return, and the assistant can fill in the date and time. If a payment is made, it can be so indicated. Instructions to the patient for filing insurance claims are on the bottom left. The doctor's office keeps one copy; the patient is given the original and one copy for filing with the insurance company.

Statements must be correct and must include the patient's name and address as well as the balance owed. If statements are photocopied or microfilmed, special care must be taken with the ledger card because it will be duplicated in the billing process.

Typewritten Statements. The use of continuous form billing statements is a timesaver. The statements are printed in a roll with perforated edges for separation. The roll is fed into the typewriter for the first statement and remains until the last statement is typed, eliminating the time and energy necessary for inserting and removing each statement form from the typewriter.

Another timesaver is the multiple copy statement. The Colwell Company calls its version "E-Z Statements." The E-Z Statement features three monthly statements plus one patient's ledger card in each set, all in NCR (no carbon required) paper.

Services and payments are posted during the month, and at billing time the top sheet is removed, folded, and mailed in a window envelope. If more than three mailings are required, a new set must be headed and the balance forwarded.

Photocopied Statements. Photocopy equipment is almost as standard as the typewriter in today's offices. The production of photocopied statements is a natural consequence. Coordinated ledger cards and copy paper are used, and a perfect statement is ready for mailing in minimum time. Extra care must be used in posting the ledgers, however. A black pen should be used in making entries on the ledger card. Other ink colors do not reproduce well. Writing must be clear and legible. There should be no personal notes made on the ledger cards unless it is something you wish conveyed to the patient. (It is possible to get pencils with nonreproducible lead if you feel this is necessary for making collection entries.) Usually a window envelope is used for mailing, which means that the name and address on the ledger must be neat, correct, and in the right position for the window.

Billing System

Itemizing the First Statement. If the medical fee has been explained in advance, as discussed in Chapter 12, the monthly statement is merely a confirmation of what is owed, and there should be no misunderstanding. However, it is good business practice—and a courtesy to the patient—to itemize the charges. This is absolutely essential if the statement is to be used for billing the patient's insurance. Patients are entitled to an understanding of the doctor's statement for services (Fig. 15–1).

Itemizing statements is not difficult. The simplest method is merely to allow space on the original statement, below the "For Professional Services" line, on which to list the separate charges for office, house, or hospital calls, or for treatments or tests done in the doctor's office.

Many doctors have devised their own itemized charge slips, which are given to the patient when payment is made at the time of service, or later mailed in a combination statement-reply envelope. Use of such charge slips simplifies the itemization procedure, since filling out the slips is usually just a matter of checking the procedures listed. An itemized charge slip is shown in Figure 15–3.

Although the itemization of bills may seem an unnecessary waste of time, in the long run you will spend less time explaining services provided, clearing up misunderstanding with patients, and following up on delinquent accounts if you routinely itemize all bills.

Time and Frequency of Billing. A regular system of rendering statements should be put into operation. Most people expect to receive statements from their creditors, and they plan their budgets around first-of-the-month bills received. Punctuality in billing encourages prompt payment.

Statements should be sent at least once each month. Some offices send bills immediately after treatment; others bill all patients on the same day each month. Mailing statements twice a month— for example, half of the accounts on the 10th and the remaining half on the 25th—is also common practice.

When a billing date for an account has been established, the date of mailing the statement must not, according to the Fair Credit Practices Act Amendments of October 1975, vary more than five days without notification to the debtor. If the balance due is over one dollar, the account must be billed every 30 days.

Once-a-Month Billing. If a monthly pattern is followed, bills should leave your office in time to reach the patient no later than the last day of each month and preferably by the 25th of the month. Planning ahead for the preparation of statements can lighten the burden of once-a-month billing. The statement can be prepared at the time of service (or during slack periods), postdated, and mailed at the end of the month.

Cycle Billing. Many physicians prefer to use the cycle billing system, which calls for the billing of certain portions of the accounts receivable at given times during the month instead of preparing all statements at the end of each month. Cycle billing has been used for some time in large businesses

RICHARD W. LANGERT, M.D.
Obstetrics, Gynecology, Infertility
647 CAMINO DE LOS MARES, SUITE 221
SAN CLEMENTE, CALIFORNIA 92672
TELEPHONE: (714) 661-0543

CAL. LIC. # G-41043
TAX ID # 95-3419518
PROVIDER # OOG-410430

N⁰ 33

☒ PRIVATE	☐ BLUE CROSS	☐ BLUE SHIELD	☐ IND.	☐ MEDI-CAL	☐ MEDICARE	☐ GOV'T.

PATIENT INFORMATION

PATIENT'S LAST NAME	FIRST	INITIAL	BIRTHDATE	SEX	TODAY'S DATE
Albertson	Margaret	O	05 04 60	☐ MALE ☒ FEMALE	10 11 81

ADDRESS	CITY	STATE	ZIP	RELATIONSHIP TO SUBSCRIBER
143 W. Osborn	Anytown	XX	00000	spouse

SUBSCRIBER OR POLICYHOLDER	INSURANCE CARRIER
Donald W. Albertson	Travelers Insurance Company

ADDRESS	CITY	STATE	ZIP	INS. I.D.	COVERAGE CODE	GROUP
same				975 00 333		049

OTHER HEALTH COVERAGE	IDENTIFY	DISABILITY RELATED TO:	DATE SYMPTOMS APPEARED, INCEPTION OF PREGNANCY,
☐ NO ☐ YES		☐ ACCIDENT ☐ INDUSTRIAL ☒ PREGNANCY ☐ OTHER	OR ACCIDENT OCCURRED: LMP 08 07 81

ASSIGNMENT: I HEREBY AUTHORIZE MY INSURANCE BENEFITS TO BE PAID DIRECTLY TO THE UNDERSIGNED PHYSICIAN. I AM FINANCIALLY RESPONSIBLE FOR NON-COVERED SERVICES.

SIGNED (Patient or Parent, if Minor) *Margaret Albertson* Date 10/11/81

RELEASE: I HEREBY AUTHORIZE THE UNDERSIGNED PHYSICIAN TO RELEASE ANY INFORMATION ACQUIRED IN THE COURSE OF MY EXAMINATION OR TREATMENT.

SIGNED (Patient or Parent, if Minor) *Margaret Albertson* Date 10/11/81

PHYSICIAN INFORMATION

A. PROFESSIONAL SERVICE CODES

	1 OFFICE VISIT		2 HOSPITAL VISIT		3 EMERGENCY ROOM		4 CONSULTATION	FEE
TYPE OF PATIENT ▶	NEW	ESTAB.	INITIAL	REPEAT	NEW	ESTAB.	ALL	
Minimal Service		90030				90530		
Brief Service	90000	90040	90200	90240	90500	90540		
Limited Service	90010	90050	90250	90250	90510	90550	90600	
Intermediate Service	(90015)	90060	90215	90260	90515	90560	90605	35.00
Extended Service		90070		90270		90570	90610	
Comprehensive	90020	90080	90220				90620	
Other		90088		90275		90589	90630	

✓	DESCRIPTION	CODE	FEE	✓	DESCRIPTION	CODE	FEE	✓	DESCRIPTION	CODE/MD	FEE
	B. OFFICE PROCEDURES				**C. LABORATORY (CONT.)**				**D. HOSPITAL PROCEDURES (CONT.)**		
	Total OB Care & Delivery	59400			Serology	86592			Abdominal Hysterectomy	58150	
	Total OB Care & repeat C/S	59501			Pregnancy Test - Urine	82996			Vaginal Hysterectomy	58260	
	IUD Insertion	58300			Pregnancy Test - Serum	82998			Anterior-Posterior Repair	57260	
	IUD Removal	58301			Wet Mount	87210			Vaginal Hyst. w/Repair	58265	
	Diaphragm	57170			Pap Smear	88150			Marshall - Marchetti	51840	
	Culdocentesis	57020			SMA—12	80112			Cold Cone, D & C	57521	
	Treatment, Condylomata	56500			Thyroid Panel	84251			Salpingo - Oophorectomy	58720	
	I & D, Bartholin's Abscess	56420			Rubella Titer	86171			Oophorectomy	58940	
	Biopsy, Vulva	56600			C/S - Cervix, Vagina	87070			Partial Ovarian Resection	58900	
	Biopsy, Cervix	57500			C/S - Urine	87088			Diagnostic Laparoscopy	58980	
	Biopsy, Endometrium	58100			C/S - Throat	87060			Lararoscopic Tubal Ligat.	58982	
	Cryotherapy, Cervix	57511			F.B.S.	82947			Exploratory Laparotomy	49000	
	Colposcopy	57452			Biopsy Tissue Evaluation	88304			SAb D & C	59804	
	Post-Coital Test	89300							Circumcision	54150	
	Hydrotubation	58350							Assist Surgeon	-80	
	H.A.I.	58999			**D. HOSPITAL PROCEDURES**						
	Pessary Insertion	57160			Amniocentesis	59000			**E. MISCELLANEOUS**		
					Non-Stress Test	58999			Special Supplies, Mat'ls	99070	
					Contraction Stress Test	58999			Injection, Therapeutic	90730	
	C. LABORATORY				Post-Partum Tubal Ligation	58605			Immunization	90721	
	Urinalysis	81000	7.00		Primary C/S	59500			Collection-Lab, Spec.	99007	
	CBC	85022			Tubal Ligation @ C/S	59550			Special Reports	99080	
	Sed. Rate	85651			Marsupialization,	56440					
	Hematocrit	85014			Bartholin's Abscess						
	Rh & Type	86082									
	Prenatal Ab Screen	86016	15.00		Diagnostic D & C	58120					

DIAGNOSIS:
1. *Pregnancy*
2.
3.

SERVICES PERFORMED AT:		ADMIT	
☐ MISSION COMMUNITY HOSP. ☒ OFFICE	☐ SAN CLEMENTE GEN. HOSP. ☐		
27802 PUERTA REAL	654 CAMINO DE LOS MARES	DISCHARGE	
MISSION VIEJO, CA 92691	SAN CLEMENTE, CA 92672		

REMARKS:

DOCTOR'S SIGNATURE/DATE
Richard W. Langert MD

RETURN APPOINTMENT INFO.:
DAYS ____ WKS. ____ MONS. 1 MINS. ____

NEXT APPOINTMENT
DAY *Thursday* DATE 11-12 TIME 10

INSTRUCTIONS TO PATIENT FOR FILING INSURANCE CLAIMS:

1. Complete upper portion of this form; sign and date.
2. Mail this form directly to your insurance company. You may attach your own insurance company's form if you wish, although it is not necessary.

PLEASE REMEMBER that our charges are due at the time the service is performed and payment is your obligation regardless of insurance or other third party involvement.

RECEIVED BY: *MK*		
☐ CASH	TODAY'S FEE	57.00
☒ CHECK	Amount Received Today	57.00
☐ CREDIT CARD	BALANCE THIS VISIT	-0-
	OLD BALANCE	
	NEW BALANCE	-0-

15

Figure 15-2
Example of a superbill. (Courtesy of Bibbero Systems, Inc., Petaluma, CA.)

Figure 15–3
An itemized charge slip. (Courtesy of Bibbero Systems, Inc., Petaluma, CA.)

such as department stores, banks, and oil companies. The system of cycle billing has become increasingly popular in the physician's office. Its many advantages include avoiding once-a-month peak workloads and stabilizing the cash flow. In a small office in which billing is done only once a month, the unexpected illness or absence of the medical assistant for any emergency can leave the doctor in a financial bind if the statements do not go out.

This is how the cycle billing system works: The accounts are separated into fairly equal divisions, the number of divisions depending upon how many times you wish to do billing during a month. For example, if you expect to bill twice a month, divide the accounts into two equal sections; for weekly billing, divide into four groups; for daily billing, divide into 20 groups.

Small alphabetic groups can be combined to keep your divisions nearly equal in the number of statements to prepare on each billing day. If your files are color-coded, you may wish to use the same alphabetic breakdown in billing. Regardless of constant changes in the accounts themselves, the mailing dates for accounts in each section remain the same. A schedule for processing and mailing of accounts is thus established, apportioning the load of work throughout the entire month.

Cycle billing allows the medical assistant to continue all routine duties each day, handling the statements on a day-to-day or weekly schedule rather than in one intensive period at the end of the month. This means that whole days need not be sacrificed from other duties in order to get statements into the mail. By spacing the billing throughout the month, more time and consideration can be given to each statement, the itemization of bills will be less burdensome, and the likelihood of error will be decreased.

Patients generally accept the cycle billing system quickly, often with enthusiasm. However, if your office decides to change from a once-a-month billing to a cycle billing system, patients should be notified in advance and the new plan explained to them. To explain the new system to established patients, enclose a notice in each statement 2 months prior

to the transfer, describing the plan and indicating the future dates on which each patient will receive the bill.

Before a doctor, particularly one in a small community, adopts the cycle billing system, several factors should be taken into consideration:

• What is the general income level of the community, and how and when does the average patient receive his pay?
• Do local companies pay employees at various times during the month, or are most paychecks handed out at the beginning of the month?
• Would cycle billing benefit patients as well as the overall operation of the office?

Procedure 15-1

PREPARING MONTHLY BILLING STATEMENTS

PROCEDURAL GOAL

To process monthly statements and evaluate accounts for collection procedures in accordance with the agency's credit policy.

EQUIPMENT AND SUPPLIES

Typewriter
Patient Accounts*
Agency's Credit Policy*
Statement Forms

PROCEDURE

1. Assemble all accounts with outstanding balances.
2. Separate accounts that need special attention in accordance with the agency's credit policy.
   Explanation: Routine statements should be prepared first, after which special attention can be given to delinquent accounts.
3. Prepare routine statements, including:
   a. Date statement is prepared
   b. Name and address of person responsible for payment
   c. Name of patient if different from "b"
   d. Itemization of dates, services, and charges for month
   e. Any unpaid balance carried forward (may or may not be itemized, depending on office policy)
4. Determine action to be taken on acounts separated in Step 2.
5. Make note of necessary action on ledger card (telephone call, collection letter series, small claims court, or assignment to collection agency).
   Purpose: For guidance in executing action and for later follow-up when necessary.

TERMINAL PERFORMANCE OBJECTIVE

Given the listed equipment and supplies, process the monthly statements and evaluate accounts for collection procedures in accordance with agency's credit policy, within 30 minutes, to a performance level of 100%. (Time will vary with number of accounts and difficulty of analysis.)

---

*From student workbook or instructor.

15

Billing Third Party Payers and Minors. Collection problems may arise if the medical assistant fails to get the necessary insurance information, particularly Medicare and Medicaid information (see Chapter 12, section on Credit Arrangements).

In some instances the insurance forms are not completed correctly, and the claim is denied because of minor infractions such as failing to name the responsible party or omitting Social Security information, the policy number, or the group number.

Time limits must also be observed in billing third party payers. In cases of Medicare patients with a terminal illness, it may be best to accept assignment of benefits. If the doctor does not take assignment, sometimes the doctor will receive nothing, because the family is not obligated to pay and Medicare will not pay after a certain time or if the claim has not been correctly filed.

Bills for minors must be addressed to a parent or legal guardian. If a bill is addressed to a minor, the parent or parents could take the attitude that they are not responsible because a bill was never received. If the parents are separated or divorced, the parent who brings the child in for treatment is responsible for payment. Whatever financial agreement exists between the parents is strictly their personal business and should not concern the medical office. The responsible parent should be so informed from the beginning. Minors cannot be held responsible for payment of a bill unless they are emancipated (see Chapter 5).

If an emancipated minor appears in the office and requests treatment and you can ascertain that the person is not living at home, the minor is responsible for the bill. It may be wise to make a determination either with the business manager or with the physician as to whether your office wishes to treat this emancipated minor.

Collection Goals

Management consultants for the medical profession say that if good financial practices are followed, the accounts receivable on a doctor's books should equal no more than 2 to 3 months' gross charges, but if the receivables start falling below the average of 1 month's total charges, perhaps the collection procedures are too stringent.

Evaluation of collections is based on the collection ratio and the accounts receivable ratio.

Collection Ratio. The **collection ratio** (Table 15–1) measures the effectiveness of the billing system. The basic formula for figuring the collection ratio is:

$$\text{Collection Ratio} = \frac{\text{Total Collections}}{\text{Net Charges}}$$

Table 15–1
Figuring the Collection Ratio

Gross Charges		$125,000
Less:		
Courtesy discounts	$5,000	
Third party insurance allowance	6,000	
Other adjustments	1,000	
Total Adjustments		12,000
Net Charges		$113,000
Total Collections		110,000
Collection Ratio $\left(\dfrac{110,000}{113,000}\right)$		97%

A minimum of 6 to 12 months' data should be used in computing the collection ratio.

Accounts Receivable Ratio. The **accounts receivable ratio** (Table 15–2) measures how fast outstanding accounts are being paid. The formula is:

Accounts Receivable Ratio =

$$\frac{\text{Current Accounts Receivable Balance}}{\text{Average Gross Monthly Charges}}$$

A desirable accounts receivable ratio is less than 2 months. It is the medical assistant's responsibility to keep both the accounts receivable and collections within normal limits.

Importance of Collecting Delinquent Accounts

The reasons for pursuing collections go beyond the obvious one that a physician must be paid for services in order to pay expenses and continue to treat patients.

Failure to collect can result in the loss of a patient. A person who owes the doctor money and is not prodded gently into payment may stay away in embarrassment or may even change doctors.

Noncollection of medical bills may also imply guilt. A patient may infer that the doctor felt that the patient received inadequate or improper care, and a malpractice suit may result.

Table 15–2
Figuring the Accounts Receivable Ratio

Annual Gross Charges	$125,000
Average Monthly Gross Charges $\left(\dfrac{125,000}{12}\right)$	10,417
Current Acc/Rec Balance	16,000
Acc/Rec Ratio $\left(\dfrac{16,000}{10,417}\right)$	1.54 months

Nor is it fair to the paying patients to make no attempt to collect from nonpaying patients. Abandoning accounts without collection follow-up encourages nonpayers and, as a result, the paying patients indirectly **subsidize** the cost of medical care for those who can pay but do not.

Most patients are honest; it is estimated that probably fewer than 4% never intend to pay. There may be a larger percentage who are financially "shipwrecked" and temporarily unable to pay. Also, a certain percentage of patients irresponsibly live beyond their incomes.

According to the American Medical Association, the three most common reasons for patients' failure to pay are:
1. Negligence
2. Inability to pay
3. Unwillingness to pay

Aging Accounts Receivable

Aging is a term used for the procedure of classifying accounts receivable by age from the first date of billing, and should be done on a regular basis. Aging of accounts helps collection follow-up, since it enables the medical assistant to tell at a glance which accounts need attention in addition to a regular statement. Computer billing programs usually include this feature. With sufficient time, an age analysis may be accomplished manually (Fig. 15–4).

If the patient is billed on the day of service, the aging begins on that day; if the first billing is 30 days after service, the aging begins at 30 days. Some systems use a breakdown of Current, 30 days, 60 days, 90 days, and 90-plus days.

Looking at Figure 15–4 you see that:
- Patient A has a balance of $450. Unless regular payments are being made, this account may be heading toward a collection problem because $350 of the balance is over 3 months old.
- Patient B presents no problem because the entire balance is current.
- Patient C definitely is a potential problem even though the account is small. The entire balance is over 3 months old, and one-fourth of it is over 6 months old.
- Patient D's account should never have been allowed to reach this stage of delinquency. If there had been a good collection policy established, it would not have.

The **age analysis** is simply a tool to show at a glance the status of each account. There is no need to do this every month if time is at a premium. If you age the accounts quarterly you will stay on top of the problem. Usually a coding system with metal clip-on tabs or adhesive peel-off labels on the ledger cards is used in conjunction with the age analysis system.

For example, after two statements have been sent, a green tab is placed on the record, indicating that a courteous reminder was sent with the last statement.

The following month the green tab is replaced with a yellow tab, showing that a second payment request was sent in the form of a polite letter or printed request.

An orange tab is substituted the next month, indicating that the patient received a letter requesting prompt attention to the account.

Red tabs may be reserved for the accounts of patients who, as a last resort, have been notified of a specific time limit in which payment must be

ACCOUNTS RECEIVABLE AGE ANALYSIS

Dr. _____

Address _____   Date _____

PATIENT'S NAME	TOTAL ACCOUNT RECEIVABLE	DISTRIBUTION OF ACCOUNTS RECEIVABLE BY AGE				REMARKS
		1-2-3 MONTHS	4-5-6 MONTHS	7-8-9-10-11-12 MONTHS	OVER 1 YEAR	
A	450.00	100.00	350.00			
B	50.00	50.00				
C	100.00		75.00	25.00		
D	200.00		10.00	150.00	40.00	
E	550.00		550.00			
F	42.50	42.50				
G	65.00	20.00	45.00			
H	325.00	325.00				

Figure 15–4
Form for accounts receivable age analysis.

15

made, after which sterner measures will be taken. If you reach this stage in pursuing a particular account, make certain you record the date of the time limit on the patient's ledger.

The law requires that once you have made a statement in regard to a particular collection procedure, you must follow through or be liable for the consequences under the law. If you say, for example, "I am going to turn your·account over for collection unless it is paid within 10 days," then you must do so. If you state in a collection letter that you are going to take the debtor to small claims court if the account is not paid by a certain date, then you must do as you say. The intent of the law is to prevent the collector from making idle threats or harassing a debtor. A patient may sue for harassment if such idle threats are made.

> *Fair Debt Collection Practices Act 1977 (Federal) states that the following conduct is a violation:*
>
> *Section 807 (5) The threat to take any action that cannot legally be taken or that is not intended to be taken.*

Collection Program

Persuasive collection procedures include:

- Telephone calls
- Collection reminders and letters
- Personal interviews

Telephone Collection Techniques. A telephone call at the right time, in the right manner, is more effective than a collection letter. The personal contact of a telephone call will bring in more money. In the absence of time to make calls, the collection letter is the next best avenue. If collections are a serious problem, it may pay to hire an extra person to do the telephoning. Written notification is a must, however, if it is a final demand for payment before collection or legal proceedings are started.

GENERAL RULES TO FOLLOW IN TELEPHONE COLLECTIONS

1. *Call the patient when you can do so in privacy.*
2. *Call between 8 AM and 9 PM*
3. *Determine the identity of the person with whom you are speaking. If you ask, "Is this Mrs. Noble?" and she answers "Yes," it could be the patient's mother-in-law or daughter-in-law, who is also "Mrs. Noble." Use the person's full name.*
4. *Be dignified and respectful in·your attitude. You can be friendly and formal at the same time.*
5. *Ask the patient if it is a convenient time to talk with you. Unless you have the attention of the called party, there is little to be gained by continuing. If you are told that you have called at an inopportune time, ask for a specific time when you may call back, or get a promise for the patient to call you at a specified time.*
6. *After a brief greeting, state the purpose of your call. Make no apology for calling but state your reason in a friendly, businesslike way. You expect payment and are interested in helping the patient meet the financial obligation. "This is Alice, Dr. Brown's financial secretary. I'm calling about your account." A well-placed pause at this point in the call sometimes gets an immediate response from the debtor in regard to the nonpayment.*
7. *Assume a positive attitude. For example, convey the impression that you know the patient intends to pay, and it is only a matter of working out some suitable arrangements.*
8. *Keep the conversation brief and to the point, and avoid threats of any kind.*
9. *Try to get a definite commitment—payment of a certain amount by a certain date.*
10. *Follow up on promises. This is best accomplished by a tickler file or a note on your calendar. If the payment does not arrive by the promised date, remind the patient with another call. If you fail to do this, your whole effort has been wasted.*

There are no hard and fast rules for pursuing collections by telephone. You must handle each case individually on the basis of your own acquaintance or experience with the person concerned.

ACTIONS TO AVOID

1. *Calling between 9 PM and 8 AM. To do so may be considered harassment.*
2. *Making repeated phone calls.*
3. *Calling at the debtor's place of work if you know that the employer prohibits personal calls.*
4. *If you do call the debtor at work and the person cannot take the call, you can leave a message asking to "call Mrs. Black at 727-9238" without revealing the nature of the call—that is, do not state that the call is from "Dr. Jones's office" or "Dr. Jones's medical assistant."*
5. *Losing your temper or showing hostility. An angry patient is a poor-paying patient. Insulted patients often do not pay at all.*

Collection Letters. Some consultants believe that a printed collection letter or reminder enclosed with a statement is more effective than a personal letter, the theory being that a patient may be embarrassed by a personal letter and feel that he has been singled out, whereas he may be nudged into sending a payment in response to a printed message without the personal connotation. The printed form is a timesaver and is sometimes recommended if lack of time is contributing to poor collection follow-up. Commercially printed forms can be obtained, or you can compose your own and have them printed locally.

Letters that are friendly requests for an explanation of why payment has not been made are still effective in many cases. These letters should indicate that the doctor is sincerely interested in the patient's story and wants to help straighten out the financial obligations. The patient should be invited to visit the doctor's office to explain the reasons for nonpayment so that, if possible, special arrangements can be worked out. To give the patient an opportunity to save face, these letters can suggest that the patient may have overlooked previous statements.

Upon receipt of such a letter, most patients will make some effort to explain their failure to make payment. If a patient really is in dire financial straits, the doctor may be able to get public assistance for him or her. Or, if it is a temporary financial difficulty, the doctor and the patient may together be able to work out a satisfactory installment plan type of payment program.

The medical assistant often is given a free hand in designing collection patterns and composing collection letters. Many medical assistants compose a series of collection letters, using letters that they have found to be effective as models. Such a series usually includes at least five letters, ranging through varying degrees of forcefulness. One would never use the same type of collection letter for a patient with good paying habits as for one who is known to neglect financial obligations. Never use a postcard or put an overdue notice of any kind on the outside of an envelope. This is an **invasion of privacy**.

Who Signs Collection Letters? The question sometimes arises as to who should sign collection letters. In most medical offices the medical assistant signs them with the identification "Assistant to Dr. Brown" or "Financial Secretary" below the typewritten signature. Some physicians may wish to personally sign these communications, but generally the medical assistant who handles the accounts also signs the collection letters.

Sample Letters. Following are some ideas for reminders and collection letters. These can serve as a guide for composing your own letters to suit the circumstances involved.

A gentle reminder often brings results:

> Your account has always been paid promptly in the past, so this must be an oversight. Please accept this note as a friendly reminder of your account due for $_____ .

> Since your care in this office in March we have had no word from you in regard to how you are feeling or your account due.
> If it is impossible for you to pay the full amount of $_____ at this time, please call this office before June 15 so that satisfactory arrangements can be worked out.

> Medical bills are payable at the time of service unless special credit arrangements are made.
> Please send your check in full or call this office before June 30.

> If you have some question about your statement we will be happy to answer it for you. If not, may we have a payment before the end of this month?

> Unless some definite arrangement is made to reduce your balance of $_____ we can no longer carry your account on our books.
> Delinquent accounts are turned over to our collection agency on the 25th of the month.

15

When a payment plan has been established, it can be reinforced by recognizing the first remittance with a letter of acknowledgement:

> Thank you for the recent payment of $_____ on your account. We are glad to cooperate with you in this arrangement for clearing your account.
> We will look for your next check at about the same time next month, and your final payment the following month.

When a payment schedule has been arranged by a telephone call, it can be confirmed by letter:

> As agreed upon in our telephone conversation today, we will expect you to mail a payment of $50 on February 10; $50 on March 10; and the balance on April 10.
>
> If some emergency should prevent your making one of these payments on time, please notify us immediately by telephone.

It is important to remember that you should:

- Individualize letters to suit the situation
- Design your early letters as merely reminders of debt
- Always imply that the patient has good intentions to pay, until lack of response over a period of time proves otherwise
- Send letters with a firmer tone only after you have sent one or two friendly reminders

Sometimes even the person with poor paying habits will pay the bill if treated with respect and consideration. See Figure 15–5 for a suggested collection program.

The medical assistant should never go beyond the authority granted by the physician in pursuing collections. If you have questions about special collection problems, always check with the doctor before proceeding. This is particularly important with patients whom you do not know personally—for example, patients the doctor has seen in the hospital or at home, and others for whom you have no credit history. It is difficult to say whether pressing collections too hard loses more good will of patients than not pursuing collections diligently enough. The doctor and the medical assistant together should agree upon general collection policies as outlined earlier in this chapter, and then the policies should be followed. In all cases in which an account is assigned for collection, be sure that the doctor is aware of it.

Personal Interviews. Personal interviews with patients can sometimes be more effective than a whole series of collection letters. By talking to a patient face to face, you can come to an understanding of the problem more quickly and reach an agreement about future payment plans.

Occasionally, a patient may undergo a long course of treatment and yet make no attempt to pay anything on account. Perhaps such a patient is only waiting for the doctor or the medical assistant to suggest that a payment be made. When there is advance knowledge that the patient will require extensive treatment, the matter of payment should be discussed early in the course of treatment, the credit policy explained, and some agreement reached as to a payment plan.

Since the fee for medical services is far more intangible than any commercial account, collection efforts must not be delayed too long. Any responsible, sincere patient will call or write the doctor's office after receiving a second statement and explain why payment has not been made, or ask for a payment plan.

If it becomes necessary to refer the account to a collector, a good agency should have a 50% to 60% recovery rate with an account that is assigned within 4 or 5 months. This may drop to 25% if the account is held only a few more months.

The value of medical accounts diminishes in direct proportion to the length of time that has elapsed since service was rendered. Do not fight the law of diminishing returns. All collection activity is costly. Know when to stop and call on the services of a professional agency.

Special Collection Problems

Tracing "Skips." When a statement is returned marked "Moved—no forwarding address," you may consider this account as a "skip." This generally is accepted as an indication that the patient is attempting to avoid liability for debts. Some so-called skips are innocent errors. The person may have been careless in not leaving a forwarding address. Or the mistake may have occurred in the doctor's office; the wrong name or address may have been placed on the statement. However, immediate action should be taken in regard to returned statements. Do not wait until the next billing time to attempt to trace the debtor.

SOME SUGGESTIONS FOR TRACING SKIPS

1. *Examine the patient's original office registration card.*
2. *Call the telephone number listed on the card. Occasionally a patient may move without leaving a forwarding address but will transfer the old telephone number. Or the new telephone number will be given when you call the old number.*
3. *If you are unable to contact the individual by telephone, make a few discreet calls to the references listed on the registration card to get leads.*
4. *Check the city directory to secure the name and telephone number of neighbors or the landlord, and contact these persons to secure information about the debtor's whereabouts.*

1. Inform the patient, before or at the time of service, what charges he may expect.

2. For smaller fees, give him an opportunity to pay at the time of service.

3. 30 days: Send itemized statement

4. 60 days: Send statement:

   For Professional Services

   March services $ _____

5. 75 days: If there has been no response, telephone patient or send brief note.

   (Suggested wording)

   If you are unable to pay your account this month, please telephone this office (776-4900) before June 15 and let us know how you plan to take care of it.

   Balance due $100

6. 90 days: Send reminder letter requesting prompt attention

7. 120 days: Send final letter, certified mail, return receipt.

   (Suggested wording)

   Every courtesy has been extended to you in arranging for payment of your long over-due account. Our auditor suggests that it no longer be carried on our books.

   Unless we hear from you by August 15 the account will be turned over to _____ for collection.

8. 15th of next month
   or date mentioned
   in final letter: Account to collector

Figure 15–5
A suggested collection program.

Procedure 15-2

PROCEDURAL GOAL

To initiate proceedings to collect delinquent accounts.

EQUIPMENT AND SUPPLIES

Typewriter
Telephone
Delinquent accounts*
Stationery
Collection letter series
Agency's credit policy*

PROCEDURE

1. Assemble delinquent accounts.
2. Separate accounts according to action required.
   Purpose: It is more efficient to process as a group all accounts requiring the same activity.
3. Make telephone calls to those so designated.
4. Record responses on ledger card.
   Purpose: For further action as necessary.
5. Review accounts requiring collection letters.
6. Choose appropriate letter from collection series and individualize for account in question.
   Purpose: Form letters may be used as a guide, but should be individualized to suit the situation.
7. Typewrite collection letter(s).
8. Make notation of action taken on ledger card.
   Purpose: To avoid repetition of same letter if further action is necessary.

TERMINAL PERFORMANCE OBJECTIVE

Given the listed equipment and supplies, initiate proceedings to collect delinquent accounts using telephone and collection letter techniques in accordance with the agency's credit policy, within 30 minutes, to a performance level of 90%. (Time will vary with number and difficulty of accounts.)

---

*From student workbook or instructor.

---

5. *Do not inform a third party that the person owes you money. Simply state that you are trying to locate or verify the location of the individual.*
6. *Check the debtor's place of employment for information. If the person is a specialist in his or her field of work, the local union or similar organizations may be contacted. Although they may not give you the person's current address, they will relay the message that you are seeking to contact him or her. Often people will be stirred into paying a bill if they think that their employer may learn of their payment failure.*

7. *Do not communicate with a third party more than once. This is specifically forbidden by law (Public Law 95-109, Sec. 804) unless the third party requests the collector to do so.*

The tracing of skips is a challenge to any medical assistant. A certified letter can be sent; by paying additional fees, you can request the postal service to obtain a receipt including the address where the letter was delivered. The certified letter may be sent in a plain envelope so that the patient will not refuse to accept the letter because of the letterhead.

If all your attempts fail, turn the account over to

your collection agency without delay. Do not keep a skip account too long, since the trail may become so cold as time elapses that even collection experts will be unable to follow it.

Claims Against Estates. A bill owed by a deceased patient may be handled a little differently from regular bills. Courtesy dictates that a bill not be sent during the initial period of bereavement, but do not delay more than 30 days. The person responsible for settling the affairs of the estate will be assembling outstanding accounts and will expect to receive the medical bills along with all others. Address the statement to:

> Estate of (name of patient)
> c/o (spouse or next of kin, if known)
> Patient's last known address

Do not address the statement to a relative unless you have a signed agreement that that person will be responsible. If for some reason the statement cannot be addressed as suggested above—for instance, if the patient was in a convalescent home and you do not know the name of a relative—you may seek information from the county seat in the county in which the estate is being settled. A will is usually filed within 30 days of a death. A request to the Probate Department of the Superior Court, County Recorder's Office, will usually provide you with the name of the executor or administrator. The time limits for filing an estate claim are determined by the state in which the decedent resided.

After the name of the administrator or executor of the estate has been obtained, a duplicate itemized statement of the account should be sent to that person by certified mail, return receipt requested, so that you will know who received it. If no response is received in 10 days, you should contact the executor or the county clerk where the estate is being settled and obtain forms for filing claim against the estate. (Some states do not have special claim forms but will accept simple itemized statements.) This claim against the estate must be made within a certain length of time, varying from 2 to 36 months depending upon the state in which it is filed.

The executor of the estate will either accept or reject the claim and, if it is accepted, will send an acknowledgment of the debt. Payment is often delayed, owing to the legal complications in settling an estate, but if the claim has been accepted you will receive your money in due time. If the claim is rejected and you have full justification for claiming the bill, you must file claim against the executor within a limited time, according to state laws. The time limit in such cases starts with the date on the letter of rejection that was sent you in response to your original claim.

Because of the various state time limits and statutes in regard to such matters, it is advisable for the medical assistant to contact the doctor's attorney or the local court for the exact procedure to follow.

Bankruptcy. Bankruptcy laws are federal and are applicable in all states. When you are notified that a patient has declared bankruptcy, you should no longer send statements or make any attempt to collect the account.

Bankruptcy laws were passed to secure equal distribution of the assets of an individual among the individual's creditors. There are two types of bankruptcy: a straight petition in bankruptcy and a wage earner's bankruptcy. In both cases, the debtor becomes a ward of the court and has its protection. A creditor who continues collection proceedings against a bankrupt debtor can be fined for contempt of court.

In a *straight petition in bankruptcy* you should file a claim on the appropriate form, which can be obtained from a stationery store or by writing the referee in bankruptcy. Although you may be notified of a creditors' meeting, it is usually a waste of time to attend. A doctor's fee is an unsecured debt and, therefore, one of the last to be paid.

In a *wage earner's bankruptcy*, the debtor pays a fixed amount, agreed on by the court, to the trustee in bankruptcy. This is then passed on to the creditors. During this period, none of the creditors can attach the debtor's wages or otherwise attempt to collect the debt.

Statutes of Limitations

A **statute of limitations** assigns a certain time after which rights cannot be enforced by action.

Malpractice Statutes. In many states there are statutes of limitations in regard to malpractice lawsuits, which set a limit to the time during which malpractice actions can be filed. It is usually best to wait until this time has passed before pressing the account of a patient who may feel he is entitled to sue the doctor. However, this should not be made a blanket policy; each case should be judged on its own merit.

Collection Statutes. Statutes of limitations in regard to collections prescribe the time within which a legal collection suit may be rendered against a debtor; the term "outlaw" is sometimes used to refer to debts on which the time limit has passed. This legal time limit varies according to the state in which a doctor practices. Table 15–3 lists the time limits for collections in the various states. It should be noted that if the debtor moves out of state, either temporarily or permanently, the time spent out of state is not included in the time limit. Only the

Table 15–3
*Statute of Limitations**

Location	Open Accounts (Years)	Contracts in Writing (Years)
Alabama	3	6
Alaska	6	6
Arizona	3	6
Arkansas	3	5
California	4	4
Colorado	6	6
Connecticut	6	6
Delaware	3	6
District of Columbia	3	3
Florida	4	5
Georgia	4	6
Hawaii	6	6
Idaho	4	5
Illinois	5	10
Indiana	6	10
Iowa	5	10
Kansas	3	5
Kentucky	5	15
Louisiana	3	10
Maine	6	6
Maryland	3	3
Massachusetts	6	6
Michigan	6	6
Minnesota	6	6
Mississippi	3	6
Missouri	5	10
Montana	5	8
Nebraska	4	5
Nevada	4	6
New Hampshire	6	6
New Jersey	6	6
New Mexico	4	6
New York	6	6
North Carolina	3	3
North Dakota	6	6
Ohio	6	15
Oklahoma	3	5
Oregon	6	6
Pennsylvania	6	6
Rhode Island	6	6
South Carolina	6	6
South Dakota	6	6
Tennessee	6	6
Texas	4	4
Utah	4	6
Vermont	6	6
Virginia	3	5
Washington	3	6
West Virginia	5	10
Wisconsin	6	6
Wyoming	8	10
Puerto Rico	15	—

*From Summary of Collection Laws published in the American Collectors Association, Inc., 1986 Membership Roster. (Reprinted with permission of American Collectors Association, Inc., Minneapolis, MN.)

time during which the debtor resides within the state is included in the statute.

The time limit may vary according to the class of account. Generally, accounts may be placed in one of three classes: open book accounts, written contracts, or single entry accounts.

Open Book Accounts. Open book accounts are accounts on the books that are open to charges made from time to time. The bill for each illness or treatment is computed separately, and the last date of entry—debit or credit—for that particular illness is the time designated by the statute of limitations for starting that specific debt. As you can see, it is almost impossible to have a time limit on an account of a patient with a chronic condition, since there is no actual termination of the illness or treatment unless the patient changes physicians or dies. When legal time limits are set, they usually refer to these "open book accounts."

Written Contracts. Written contracts often have the same time limit as open book accounts, but in some states have a longer time limit. The time limit on written contracts starts from the date due.

Single Entry Accounts. Single entry accounts are accounts that have only one entry or charge. These accounts are usually short-lived and are for small amounts. Some states, such as California, place a shorter statute of limitations span on such accounts.

In many states, even though the legal time limit set by the statutes has passed, the account may be reopened and the date extended if you are able to obtain a written acknowledgment of the debt due. For instance, a letter from the patient stating "Yes, I know I owe you $150, but I do not intend paying Dr. Brown" is an acknowledgment of the debt. If this letter is signed and dated, keep it and contact your collector; on the basis of this letter, the collector can then proceed with collection. Also, a small payment on account will extend the date. Photocopy these small checks for proof of payment, should proof become necessary.

USING OUTSIDE COLLECTION ASSISTANCE

When you have done everything possible in your office to follow up on an outstanding account and have not received payment, the question arises as to what step to take next.

- Should the doctor sue for the amount?
- Should the account be turned over to a collection agency?
- Should the account be written off as a bad debt?

Before forcing an account, you must first consider the time element. Has the patient been given a fair chance to pay this bill? Have you sent statements regularly and used a systematic method of following the account? Ask yourself if there might be a misunderstanding in regard to the fee charged. Did you fully itemize the first statement? A large unexplained bill may frighten a patient into making no payments at all because the whole thing looks too big.

If you have used correct registration forms to secure advance credit information, you should know the financial abilities of the patient in regard to payment. However, illness may have caused a loss of salary and resulted in temporary inability to pay. A little investigation will reveal any such troubles.

Could the patient have been dissatisfied with the care received? For some unknown reason a patient may feel that he or she was not treated correctly. Perhaps the patient expected a complete cure too soon. Only an explanation of the condition, prognosis, and care can enlighten such patients, and this is best handled by the doctor. If a bill is pressed too hard and the patient is dissatisfied for some reason, a malpractice suit may be filed by the patient to "get even."

Collecting Through the Court System

Should We Sue? Will a doctor lose more good will by suing for a bill than by writing it off as a loss? One management official has related that, strangely enough, when a doctor-client sued two patients for large sums, the patients lost the cases, paid up, and were back in the office for treatment very shortly! However, most physicians feel it is unwise to resort to the court to collect medical bills unless there are extraordinary circumstances.

An account must be considered a 100% loss to you before legal proceedings are started. Remember that you should never threaten to instigate legal proceedings unless you are prepared to carry out the threat and have the doctor's consent to issue such a warning.

If your employer decides in favor of a lawsuit, investigate thoroughly before taking action. Litigation to collect a bill is generally in order in the following instances:

1. When a patient can afford to pay without hardship.
2. When the physician can produce office records that support the bill.
3. When the physician can justify the size of the bill by comparison with fee practices in the community.
4. When the patient's general condition after treatment is satisfactory.
5. When the persuasive powers of an ethical collection agency have been exhausted, and the agency advises suing.
6. When the patient can be given ample warning of the physician's intention to sue.
7. When the defendant (whether a patient or a parent or legal guardian) is legally liable for the services rendered to the patient.

8. When the defendant is not judgment-proof.
9. When the statute of limitations has ruled out any possible malpractice action.
10. When the physician is not bubbling over with indignation and is not in a "he-can't-do-this-to-me" frame of mind.

The experienced practitioner ticks off these ten "whens" before plunging into costly litigation.

Small Claims Court. Many doctors' offices find the small claims court a satisfactory and inexpensive way to collect delinquent accounts. The law places a limit on the amount of the debt for which relief may be sought in the small claims court. Since this varies from state to state, and in some instances even within a state, this limit should be checked locally before seeking recovery in this manner.

Parties to small claims actions may not be represented by an attorney at the trial, but may send another person to court in their behalf to produce records supporting the claim. Doctors often send their bookkeeper or medical assistant with records of unpaid accounts to show the judge.

In addition to the judgment for the amount owed, the plaintiff in small claims court may also recover the costs of the suit. This rarely exceeds $20. For a very small investment in time and money, the doctor who uses this method:

- Has saved the time of a regular court action
- Has had no attorney's fee to pay
- Has not sacrificed the commission charged by a collection agency

Remember, though, that the court has awarded only a judgment. You still must collect the money. Also, the only person in a small claims action who has the right of appeal is the defendant. An appeal by the defendant may have the judgment set aside. The plaintiff (doctor) cannot file an appeal in a small claims action; the decision of the court is final.

The forms for filing action and full instructions on the course to follow may be obtained from the clerk of the small claims court. The medical assistant who has never appeared in the court would probably be wise to attend once as a spectator only, in order to preview the procedure and feel more at ease when appearing for the doctor.

A collection agency, to whom an account may have been assigned, may not file or handle a small claims action. It must either sue in the regular municipal or justice court or attempt to collect the debt in some other way.

Using a Collection Agency

The medical assistant should try every means possible to collect accounts before they become delinquent. But as soon as the account is deter-

15

mined uncollectible through your office—that is, the patient has failed to respond to your final letter or has failed to fulfill a second promise on payment—send the account to the collector without delay. Skips should be assigned immediately.

Even though collection by an agency will mean sacrificing from 40% to 60% of the amount owed, further delay will only reduce the chances of recovery by the professional collector. If the agency finds that the case deserves special consideration, it will seek the physician's advice before proceeding further.

Selecting a Collection Agency. There are a number of agencies either owned and operated as an integral part of the county medical society or operated separately from the medical society but supervised by the medical profession. These bureaus provide specialized medical collection services.

Another type of collection agency is a division of the local credit association, recognized by the National Retail Credit Association. If the local credit association does not maintain a collection department, it will be able to recommend a reputable one. A nationally recognized credit association has considerable responsibility and a high standard to maintain. These factors act as monitors to its reliability.

The most common type of collection agency throughout the United States is the privately owned and operated agency. Many of these work with the local professional societies and strive to keep their work on a high ethical standard. Because a few bureaus are unethical and unscrupulous in their tactics, care should be taken to be sure that the one you choose is reliable and ethical. For the sake of comparison, many health care facilities use two or three agencies.

The following guidelines should assist you in choosing a collection agency:

1. The best sources of referral for a collection agency are the doctor's colleagues, other doctors in the same specialty, and associates in the hospitals.

2. For references of local agencies, you may check with the Medical-Dental-Hospital Bureaus of America, 111 East Wacker Drive, Chicago, IL 60601; the American Collectors Association, 4040 West 70th Street, Minneapolis, MN 55434; or the Associated Credit Bureaus of America, Collection Division, 6767 Southwest Freeway, Houston, TX 77074.

3. Investigate the methods of collection used. Ask to see any letters, reminder notices, or follow-up literature used.

4. Investigate to determine if the agency has contacts with other services to aid in the collection of out-of-town accounts.

5. Find out the agency's collection ratio and the fees for various kinds of accounts assigned to them (large or small accounts, out-of-town accounts, skips). Its fees should be in line with the amount of effort expended to collect your accounts.

6. The agency should rely heavily on a persuasive approach rather than being "suit-happy."

7. Find out whether the agency will report cases deserving special consideration back to the physician's office.

8. Generally speaking, one should not sign a contract.

Responsibilities to the Collection Agency. When the physician selects a reputable agency and decides to make use of its services, you must be prepared to provide the agency with all the necessary data to enable it to begin prompt collection procedures on overdue accounts. The agency should receive:

- Full name of the debtor
- Name of the spouse
- Last known address
- Full amount of the debt
- Date of the last entry on account (debit or credit)
- Occupation of the debtor
- Business address
- Any other pertinent data

After an account has been turned over to a collection agency, your office makes no further collection attempts. Once the agency has begun its work, follow these guidelines and procedures:

1. Send no more statements.

2. Mark the patient's ledger or stamp it so that you know it is now in the hands of the collector.

3. Refer the patient to the agency if he or she contacts you in regard to the account.

4. Promptly report any payments made directly to your office (a percentage of this payment is due the agency).

5. Call the agency if you obtain any information that will be of value in tracing or collecting the account.

6. Do not push the agency with frequent calls. The representatives of the agency will report to you regularly and keep you posted on collection progress.

ACCOUNTS RECEIVABLE INSURANCE PROTECTION

The potential income represented by the doctor's accounts receivable ledger is probably considerable, and the patient ledgers may be the only record the doctor has of what is owed. This potential income deserves insurance protection. The doctor's general insurance representative can obtain insurance protection for these records. Most insurance companies require that the ledgers be kept in a safe place, such as an insulated file cabinet. This is a good practice to follow in any case. They will also require that the accounts receivable balance be reported monthly, for the cost of the insurance is usually based on the average balance during the year. The premium for this type of insurance is nominal. Anyone who has ever lost important records through fire or flood would say it is priceless.

In conclusion, we point out that to the best of our ability we have checked and verified all statements made in this chapter about collection law and legal procedures. However, laws do change, and it is recommended that you check with your local state regulations and laws to verify points pertinent to your special area. State law will take precedence over federal law if the state law is stronger. For a general instruction manual of this nature, it is impossible to check each of these state requirements to determine which are stronger and which would prevail over Federal Public Law 95-109.

15

CHAPTER OUTLINE

Brief History of Health Insurance
Purpose of Health Insurance
Availability of Health Insurance
Types of Insurance Coverage
Payment of Benefits
Kinds of Plans
    Blue Cross and Blue Shield
    Foundations for Medical Care
    Independent Insurers
    Government Plans
    Life Insurance

Coding
    Coding Systems

Guidelines for Claims Processing
    Gathering the Information and Materials
    Claim Forms

Superbill
Assignments
Establishing a System
Completing the Form
Claim Rejection

Billing Requirements
    Blue Plans
    Medicare
      Procedure 16–1: Completing Insurance Forms
    Medicaid
    Medi/Medi
    CHAMPUS and CHAMPVA
    Worker's Compensation

Health Care and Cost Containment

VOCABULARY

See Glossary at end of book for definitions.

assignment of insurance benefits
beneficiary
claim
coinsurance/copayment
deductible
disability

fee schedule
indemnity
medical indigent
member physician
pre-existing condition

premium
professional standards review
   organization
rider
subscriber

16

Health and Accident Insurance

OBJECTIVES

Upon successful completion of this chapter you should be able to:
1. Define the terms listed in the Vocabulary of this chapter.
2. Review the history of health insurance in the United States, including the origin of the Blue Plans, CHAMPUS, Medicare, and prepaid plans.
3. Cite three advantages of group insurance over individual policies.
4. Name seven major types of health insurance coverage.
5. State the basic differences between indemnity and service benefit plans.
6. Identify four purposes for numeric diagnostic and procedural coding.
7. Name the principal coding systems that link the medical profession and the insurance system.
8. List 10 reasons for possible rejection of insurance claims.
9. State the maximum billing period for Medicare claims.
10. Explain why a patient's care under worker's compensation should be recorded separately from care as a private patient.
11. Compare closed-panel and open-panel prepaid care.
12. Discuss the provisions of the Prospective Payment System and the reasons for its development.

Upon successful completion of this chapter you should be able to perform the following activities:
1. Identify and complete the appropriate insurance forms for patients covered by:
   a. Medicare
   b. CHAMPUS
   c. Worker's compensation
   d. Blue Cross and Blue Shield
2. Calculate the billing for patients whose insurance includes deductibles and coinsurance.

Health insurance is an important factor in the practice of medicine. As a medical assistant you will need to understand insurance terminology, types of insurance coverage, the importance of obtaining consent for release of information, the effect of **assignment of insurance benefits**, and how to handle **claims.** You must also be able to communicate with patients about processing their insurance.

You may be expected to:

- Prepare insurance claim forms
- Maintain an insurance claims register
- Trace unpaid claims
- Evaluate claims rejection
- Report procedures to prepaid care plans
- Translate medical terminology into procedural and diagnostic codes

Fifty years ago health insurance as we know it now was very uncommon, but today most patients who come into a health care facility will have some kind of health insurance coverage, either privately or through government-sponsored programs. Although the rapid growth of health insurance coverage is a recent phenomenon brought about by economic necessity, the concept of health insurance is not new.

BRIEF HISTORY OF HEALTH INSURANCE

The first company organized specifically to write health insurance was founded in 1847. The nation's earliest accident insurance company came into being in 1850 in response to public demand for coverage against frequent rail and steamboat accidents of the mid-nineteenth century. By the turn of the twentieth century, 47 American companies were issuing accident insurance.

In its early stages, the emphasis of health insurance was directed toward replacement of income rather than toward hospital or surgical benefits. The early insurance company policy protected the policyholder against loss of earned income due to a limited number of diseases, including typhus, typhoid, scarlet fever, smallpox, diphtheria, diabetes, and a few others. Emphasis on the income aspects of the insurance continued until 1929, the start of the Great Depression.

At this time a group of school teachers banded together to form an arrangement with Baylor Hospital in Dallas, Texas, to provide themselves with hospital care on a prepayment basis. This was the origin of the Blue Cross service concept for provision of hospital care.

A further major change occurred during World War II. The freezing of industrial wages made the fringe benefit a significant element of collective bargaining. Group health insurance became a large part of the fringe benefit package.

In 1956 government became a major insurer with passage of Law 569, which authorized dependents of military personnel to receive treatment by civilian physicians at the expense of the government. We know this today as CHAMPUS (Civilian Health and Medical Program of the Uniformed Services).

Title XIX of Public Law 89-97, under the Social Security Amendments of 1965, provided for agreements with states for assistance from the federal government in providing health care for the **medically indigent**, and is known as Medicaid.

Medicare under Social Security for the patient over 65 went into effect on July 1, 1966. The law was expanded in 1973 to cover disabled persons under 65 who had been receiving Social Security or railroad retirement checks for two or more years. This included disabled workers, persons who became incapacitated before age 22, disabled widows, and disabled dependent widowers.

The passage of the Health Maintenance Organization (HMO) Act in 1973 provided for federal aid to health insurance prepayment plans that met certain criteria. This brought about an accelerated growth of HMOs, organizations that provide for comprehensive health care to an enrolled group for a fixed periodic payment.

Title VI of the Social Security Amendments Act of 1983 contained the prospective payment system (PPS) for hospitals, which would begin the radical restructuring of the payment system to hospitals for Medicare inpatient services.

PURPOSE OF HEALTH INSURANCE

Voluntary health insurance is designed primarily for those who can take care of the costs of routine illnesses but to whom a major illness may prove a real financial burden. Minor bills for preventive injections, routine office calls, and treatment of ailments of short duration such as colds should be considered a predictable expense in a family budget. Covering such items in an insurance program boosts administrative costs of the insurance plan out of proportion to the small benefits received.

Cost of Coverage. Few insurance policies pay all expenses resulting from accident or illness. The basic cost of health care coverage is an annual **premium** for which the insurer agrees to provide certain benefits. The real cost to the individual includes additional costs that occur at the time of treatment:

- Deductibles
- Copayment
- Services not covered

The **deductible** is that portion of the bill that a **subscriber** must pay before insurance coverage is effective. The amount of the deductible is stated in the contract.

A **copayment** is a contribution the subscriber must make to cover some portion of each bill. This could be as low as $2 to $3 for each office visit or, more commonly, 20% of the total cost. Services not covered, such as eye examinations or dental care, are also a part of the total cost.

A coordination of benefits or nonduplication of benefits provision is included in many group contracts. In many families both husband and wife are wage earners, and frequently both are eligible for health insurance benefits through their own employment and that of their spouse. With a coordination of benefits provision, the patient's plan is the primary carrier and will pay the full benefits of its policy. Any remaining covered expenses will be paid by the spouse's plan.

In the case of a child with two parents enrolled in such plans, the father's insurance is usually considered the primary carrier. In the case of an employed person who is eligible for Medicare benefits, the employer's plan is the primary carrier and Medicare is the supplemental carrier.

AVAILABILITY OF HEALTH INSURANCE

Health insurance may be purchased under a group policy or an individual policy. Many people are covered by government plans.

Group Policies. Insurance written under a group policy covers a group of people under a master contract, which is generally issued to an employer for the benefit of the employees. The individual employee may be given a certificate of insurance containing information regarding the master policy and indicating that the individual is covered under the policy. Professional associations also frequently offer group insurance as a benefit of membership.

Group coverage usually provides greater benefits at lower premiums, and a physical examination is seldom required for the enrollees. Every person in a group contract has identical coverage.

Individual Policies. Some individuals do not qualify for inclusion in a group policy, but most companies that write group insurance also offer individual policies. The applicant may be required to have a physical examination before acceptance and, if there is an unusual risk, may be denied insurance or may have to accept a **rider** or limitation on the policy. In any event, the individual premium will probably be greater and the benefits less than in a group policy.

Government Plans. The over-65 patient will probably be covered by Part B of Medicare under Social Security. The medically indigent patient may be eligible for Medicaid with or without Medicare. Dependents of military personnel are covered by CHAMPUS (Civilian Health and Medical Program of the Uniformed Services); surviving spouses and dependent children of veterans who died as a result of service-connected disabilities are covered by CHAMPVA (Civilian Health and Medical Program of the Veterans Administration). Many wage earners are protected against the loss of wages and the cost of medical care resulting from occupational accident or disease through worker's compensation insurance.

All of these plans are dealt with in further detail later in this chapter.

TYPES OF INSURANCE COVERAGE

An insurance package is tailored to the needs of each individual or group policy, and the combinations of benefits are limitless. A policy may contain any one or any combination of the following kinds of coverage.

Hospitalization. Hospital coverage pays the cost of all or part of the insured person's hospital room and board and special hospital services. Hospital insurance policies frequently set a maximum amount payable per day and a maximum number of days of hospital care. Some insurance companies require that the hospital be an accredited or a licensed hospital. Most hospital plans exclude admission for diagnostic studies.

Surgical. Surgical coverage pays all or part of the surgeon's fee; some plans also pay for an assistant surgeon. Surgery includes any incision or excision, removal of foreign bodies, aspiration, suturing, and reduction of fractures. The surgery may be accomplished in the hospital, in a doctor's office, or elsewhere. The insurer frequently provides the subscriber with a surgical fee schedule that sets forth the amount payable for commonly performed procedures.

Basic Medical. Medical coverage pays all or part of the physician's fee for nonsurgical services, including hospital, home, and office visits, depending upon coverage. It may include provision for diagnostic laboratory, x-ray, and pathology fees. Many medical plans do not cover a routine physical examination when the patient does not have a specific complaint or illness.

Major Medical (formerly called Catastrophic Coverage). Major medical insurance provides protection against especially heavy medical bills resulting from catastrophic or prolonged illnesses. It may be a supplement to basic medical coverage or a comprehensive integrated program providing both basic and major medical protection.

16

Disability (Loss of Income) Protection. Weekly or monthly cash benefits are provided to employed policyholders who become unable to work owing to an accident or illness. Many policies do not start payment until after a specified number of days or until a certain number of sick leave days have been used. Payment is made directly to the patient and is intended to replace loss of income resulting from illness. It is not intended for payment of specific medical bills.

Dental Care. Dental coverage is included in many fringe benefit packages. Some policies are based on a copayment and incentive program, with the company's copayment increasing each year until 100% coverage is reached.

Vision Care. Vision care insurance is the latest development in the total health package. It may include reimbursement for all or for a percentage of the cost for refraction, lenses, and frames.

Senior Citizen Policies. These are contracts insuring persons 65 years of age or over, in most cases supplementing the coverage by Medicare.

Special Class Insurance. Applicants for health insurance who cannot qualify for a standard policy by reason of health may be issued special class insurance with limited coverage.

Special Risk Insurance. This insurance protects a person in the event of a certain type of accident, such as automobile or airplane crashes, or for certain diseases, such as tuberculosis or cancer. There is usually a maximum benefit.

Liability Insurance. There are many types of liability insurance, including automobile, business, and homeowners' policies. Liability policies often include benefits for medical expenses payable to individuals who are injured in the insured person's home or car, without regard to the insured person's actual legal liability for the accident.

Life Insurance. Life insurance policies sometimes provide monthly cash benefits if the policyholder becomes permanently and totally disabled. Sometimes the proceeds from life insurance are used to meet the expenses of the insured person's last illness.

Overhead Insurance. A self-employed individual may carry overhead insurance that becomes effective during a period of illness or disability. Overhead insurance reimburses the insured person for specific fixed monthly expenses that are normal and customary in the operation and conduct of the person's business or office.

PAYMENT OF BENEFITS

Insurance benefits may be determined and paid in one of several ways:

- By indemnity schedules
- By service benefit plans
- By determination of the usual, customary, and reasonable fee

Indemnity Schedules. In **indemnity** plans, the insurer agrees to pay the subscriber a set amount of money for a given procedure or service. The insured person is given a schedule of indemnities (**fee schedule**) when the policy is purchased.

Indemnity plans do not agree to pay for the complete services rendered. Many times there is a difference in the amount paid by the insurance company and the amount of the physician's fee. For example, the insurer may agree to pay up to $1000 for an appendectomy, with no consideration for the time or complications of the surgery. If the physician charges $1200, the difference of $200 is the responsibility of the patient.

This type of plan takes the major expense out of medical bills and helps to keep the premiums down. The amount of the premium often determines the schedule of benefits. Indemnity benefits are usually paid to the person insured unless that person has authorized payment direct to the provider.

Service Benefit Plans. In service benefit plans, the insuring company agrees to pay for certain surgical or medical services without additional cost to the person insured. There is no set fee schedule. Service benefit plans are usually sponsored by medical societies or groups.

In a service benefit plan, a surgery with complications would warrant a higher fee than an uncomplicated procedure. Premiums are sometimes higher for this type of coverage, but often payments are larger. Frequently the payment for benefits is sent directly to the physician and is considered full payment for the services rendered.

Usual, Customary, and Reasonable Fee. Some insurance companies agree to pay on the basis of all or a percentage of the physician's usual, customary, and reasonable fee. (See Chapter 12.)

KINDS OF PLANS

Blue Cross and Blue Shield

In the early 1930s, hospitals introduced Blue Cross plans to provide protection against hospital costs. Today there are local Blue Cross plans operating in all states of the union, the District of Columbia, Canada, Puerto Rico, and Jamaica.

In 1939, state medical societies in California and Michigan began sponsoring health plans to provide medical and surgical services; these became known as Blue Shield plans. Other states soon followed, and today Blue Shield is the largest medical prepayment system in the country.

Early in its development, Blue Shield was often known as "the doctor's plan." **Member physicians** agreed to bill Blue Shield for services to subscribers and abide by other prearranged procedures. Under many Blue Shield contracts, physicians will accept Blue Shield's payment as payment in full for covered services. Blue Shield and its member physicians agree on methods of reimbursement in advance of the service performed.

In many plans Blue Shield provides the medical and surgical coverage and Blue Cross provides hospital coverage. However, in some areas Blue Cross plans write medical and surgical insurance in addition to providing hospital coverage. Conversely, some Blue Shield plans offer hospital insurance as well as medical and surgical coverage.

Blue Cross benefits are normally paid to the provider of service. In some cases a check issued jointly to the provider and the person insured is sent to the latter, who must then endorse and forward it to the provider.

Blue Shield makes direct payment to member physicians. For services of a nonmember physician, the payment is sent to the subscriber.

Blue Shield Reciprocity. Blue Shield reciprocity is an agreement among Blue Shield plans to provide benefits to subscribers who are away from home. It means the subscriber can receive benefits almost anywhere in the country. The identification card of subscribers having reciprocity has a double-end red arrow symbol with an "N" followed by three digits (Fig. 16–1). When the reciprocity **beneficiary** receives covered care outside his or her own district, the physician bills the local Blue Shield plan using the local Blue Shield form. For those who do not have the double-end red arrow, the subscriber's home plan must be billed.

Foundations for Medical Care

A foundation for medical care is a management system for community health services. It takes the form of an organization created by local physicians through their medical society, and it concerns itself with the quality and cost of medical care. Under the foundation concept the following procedure occurs:

- An insurance company sells and negotiates the policy. It collects the premiums, assumes all the risks, and reimburses the foundation for the cost of the claims office.

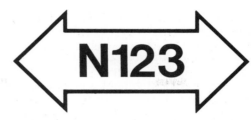

Figure 16–1
Blue Shield reciprocity symbol. (From Fordney, M.: Insurance Handbook for the Medical Office, 2nd ed. Philadelphia, W. B. Saunders Co., 1981.)

- The foundation sets policy standards; receives, processes, reviews, and pays claims to doctors; sets maximum fees based on current fees in the area; elects doctor-members yearly; and continually studies local medical-economic problems.
- Member doctors agree to accept foundation fees as full payment under foundation-approved policies.
- The local medical society legally controls the foundation and selects foundation trustees.
- The patient selects the doctor of his or her own choice; the patient or the patient's union or employer pays the premium directly to the insurance company.

Independent Insurers

More than half of those covered by some form of health insurance are covered by private (commercial) insurance companies. Physicians and medical societies control neither the premiums paid nor the benefits received from such policies. Payment is normally made to the subscriber unless the subscriber has authorized that payment be made directly to the physician.

Government Plans

MEDICARE UNDER SOCIAL SECURITY

There are two distinct parts (A and B) to the Medicare program.

Part A: Hospital Insurance. Any person who is receiving monthly Social Security or railroad retirement checks is automatically enrolled for hospital insurance benefits, and pays no premiums for this insurance. Part A is financed by special contributions paid by employed individuals as deductions from their salary, with matching contributions from their employers. These sums are collected along with regular Social Security contributions from wages and self-employment income earned during a person's working years.

16

There is a sizable deductible that the hospitalized patient must pay toward the hospital expenses.

Part B: Medical Insurance. Those persons who are eligible for Part A are eligible for Part B, but must apply for this coverage and pay a monthly premium. Some federal employees and former federal employees who are not eligible for Social Security benefits and Part A may still enroll in Part B. Certain disabled persons under the age of 65 are also eligible for Medicare (Fig. 16–2).

The patient with Medicare Part B will have to meet an annual deductible before benefits become available, after which Medicare will pay 80% of the covered benefits. The patient must pay the remaining 20% plus any amount not allowed by Medicare.

Many Medicare enrollees also carry private supplemental insurance that pays the deductible and the 20% copayment.

MEDICAID

Title XIX of Public Law 89–97, under the Social Security Amendments of 1965, provides for agreements with states for assistance from the federal government in providing health care for the medically indigent. All states and the District of Columbia have Medicaid programs, but there may be wide variations among them.

Eligibility for benefits is determined by the respective states. The state also determines the type and extent of medical care that will be covered. A card showing proof of eligibility is usually issued to the beneficiary on a monthly basis. The dates of issuance will vary, but the medical assistant should always check the patient's card or coupon to establish the fact of current coverage.

At the federal level the administration of the Medicaid program is handled by the Social and Rehabilitation Service of the Department of Health and Human Services. Direction at the state level is usually in the Department of Social Welfare.

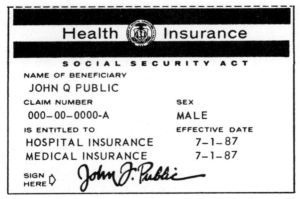

Figure 16–2
Identification card for a Medicare patient.

MEDI/MEDI

Some patients who qualify for Medicare will still be unable to pay the portion for which they are responsible and may qualify for both Medicare and Medicaid. Medicare will be the primary coverage and any residual will be paid by the Medicaid assistance program.

MILITARY MEDICAL BENEFITS

CHAMPUS. In 1956 the passage of Law 569 authorized dependents of military personnel to receive in-hospital treatment by civilian physicians at the expense of the government. This program was first called Medicare, but was later changed to CHAMPUS (Civilian Health and Medical Program of the Uniformed Services).

On September 30, 1966, the Military Medical Benefits Amendment Act of 1966 became law. This act added outpatient care benefits, including prescription drugs, to the in-hospital benefits previously allowed. The patient pays an out-of-pocket deductible (now $50, not to exceed $100 per family) each fiscal year (October 1 to September 30), plus 20% of the balance for outpatient care. Families of active duty members pay at least $25 or a small fee for each day in a civilian hospital—whichever is greater.

Military retirees and their dependents and dependents of deceased members became eligible for outpatient benefits in January 1967, except that their copayment amount is 25% after the deductible.

CHAMPVA. In 1973 a program similar to CHAMPUS was established for the spouses and dependent children of veterans suffering total, permanent, service-connected disabilities and for the surviving spouses and dependent children of veterans who have died as a result of service-connected disabilities. This is called CHAMPVA (Civilian Health and Medical Program of the Veterans Administration).

Eligibility is determined, and identification cards are issued, by the nearest VA Hospital. The insured persons then are free to choose their own private physicians. Benefits and cost-sharing features are the same as those for CHAMPUS beneficiaries who are military retirees or their dependents, and dependents of deceased members of the military. Retirees, their families, and the families of service members who have died pay 25% of the cost of care in a civilian hospital.

Further information regarding these military medical benefit programs may be obtained by writing to CHAMPUS, Aurora, CO 80045.

WORKER'S COMPENSATION

All state legislatures have passed worker's compensation laws to protect wage earners against the loss of wages and the cost of medical care resulting from occupational accident or disease. State laws differ as to the classes of employees included and the benefits provided.

None of the states' worker's compensation laws cover all employees. However, if a patient says that he or she was injured in the workplace or is suffering from a work-associated illness, the medical assistant should check with the patient's employer to verify the insurance coverage.

Compensation benefits include medical care benefits, weekly income replacement benefits for temporary disability, permanent disability settlements, and survivor benefits where applicable. The provider of service (doctor, hospital, therapist, and so forth) accepts the worker's compensation payment as payment in full and does not bill the patient.

Time limitations are set forth for the prompt reporting of worker's compensation cases. The employee is obligated to promptly notify the employer; the employer in turn must notify the insurance company and must refer the employee to a source of medical care. In some states the employer and the insurance company have the right to select the physician who will treat the patient. In essence, the purpose of worker's compensation laws is to provide prompt medical care to the injured or ill worker so that the person may be restored to health and return to full earning capacity in as short a time as possible.

Life Insurance

When an individual whom the physician is treating or has treated in the past makes application for life insurance, the insuring company naturally wants to know the current state of the applicant's health and any significant past medical history.

In order to get an account of the applicant's current state of health, the insurance company authorizes one or more physicians in each community to perform physical examinations of prospective clients.

The insurance company's agent arranges the applicant's appointment for the physical examination and supplies the necessary forms for completion. The examining physician makes a report to the insurance company following the examination. The company may require that the forms be completed in the doctor's own handwriting. The physician is paid a stipulated fee by the insurance company upon receipt of the report.

For a summary of the applicant's past medical history, the agent asks the applicant to supply the names and addresses of any physicians consulted in the past. The company, in turn, will request reports from these physicians. Your physician may receive a request for such information concerning a current or previous patient. Before completing the form, make certain the applicant has signed an authorization for release of information.

The request form usually has a voucher check for a minimal fee attached. The physician may accept the proffered fee or, if it is inadequate, may bill the insurance company for "balance of fee." If the bill is reasonable it will be paid without question.

CODING

In recent years it has become necessary to identify diagnoses and services by code. Transforming verbal descriptions of diseases, injuries, and procedures into numeric designations is the essence of coding. Numeric diagnostic and procedural coding was developed for a number of reasons:

- Tracking disease processes
- Classification of medical procedures
- Medical research
- Evaluation of hospital utilization

However, this transference of words to numbers also facilitated the use of computers in claims processing. Without the use of computers it would be impossible to take care of the 60 to 65 thousand claims processed each day in an average mid-sized claims processing center.

Coding Systems

Relative Value Scales (RVS). The RVS was pioneered by the California Medical Association in 1956 to help physicians establish rational, relative fees, and other states soon followed suit. Hundreds of the most commonly performed procedures were compiled, assigned procedure numbers similar to those in the AMA's *Current Procedural Terminology*, and assigned a unit value. The assigned unit value represented the value of that procedure in relation to other procedures commonly performed. Although no monetary value was placed on the units, many insurance companies used the RVS to determine benefits by applying a conversion factor to the unit values. In 1978 the Federal Trade Commission interpreted the California RVS as a fee-setting instrument and prohibited its publication and distribution. The FTC was attempting to make medical practice more competitive by ruling against the setting of fees and by encouraging physicians to advertise. Interest in relative value schedules has been renewed, and attempts are being made by several professional groups to reestablish and na-

16

tionalize a relative value schedule. Code books no longer include unit values.

Two coding systems, one for classifying diagnoses and one for naming medical procedures, have emerged as the standard communications link between the medical profession and the insurance system. These are:

1. *Physicians' Current Procedural Terminology,* Fourth Edition *(CPT-4).* American Medical Association, 1985.

2. *International Classification of Diseases, Ninth Revision, Clinical Modification (ICD-9-CM).*

CPT-4 Coding. *Physicians' Current Procedural Terminology (CPT-4)* is a listing of descriptive terms and identifying codes for reporting medical services and procedures performed by physicians. The purpose of the terminology is to provide a uniform language that will accurately designate medical, surgical and diagnostic services, and will thereby provide an effective means for reliable, nationwide communication among physicians, patients, and third parties. *CPT* was developed initially in 1966 by the American Medical Association; it has undergone several revisions and is updated yearly.

CPT-4 is organized in five sections: Medicine, Anesthesiology, Surgery, Radiology, and Pathology and Laboratory. An alphabetic index of procedures is located at the back. Guidelines are found at the beginning of each section, explaining items unique to that section that should be reviewed by the coder. Explanations as to the content of subsections, headings, and individual codes are found in the form of "notes." A number of specific code numbers have been designated for reporting unlisted procedures. Use of an unlisted code requires a special report. Two-digit modifiers may be attached to the five-digit code to indicate that the service or procedure has been altered. For instance, − 50 indicates multiple or bilateral procedures; − 80 indicates surgical assistant services; − 62 indicates two surgeons.

CPT-4 is available from

> Order Department
> American Medical Association
> PO Box 10946
> Chicago, Illinois 60610

Medicare's HCPCS Coding System. Most Medicare carriers have converted or will be converting to the *Health Care Financing Administration Common Procedure Coding System (HCPCS). HCPCS,* which is based on the current edition of *CPT,* is a five-digit alpha-numeric coding system with the possibility of addition of modifiers. There are three levels of codes assigned and maintained by the Medicare carriers:

• Level 1, which comprises approximately 95–98% of all Medicare Part B procedural coding, contains only *CPT* codes, excluding anesthesiology, which is currently designated by surgery codes.

• Level 2 codes are assigned by the Health Care Financing Administration (HCFA) and are consistent nationwide. These codes are for physician and nonphysician services not contained in the *CPT* system, and are alpha-numeric, ranging from A0000 to V9999.

• Level 3 codes are assigned and maintained by each local fiscal intermediary. These codes represent services that are not included in the *CPT* system and are *not* common to all carriers. These codes range from W0000 to Z9999.

ICD-9-CM. *International Classification of Diseases, Ninth Revision, Clinical Modification (ICD-9-CM)* is published in three volumes:

• Volume 1—*Diseases*: *Tabular List*
• Volume 2—*Diseases*: *Alphabetic Index*
• Volume 3—*Procedures*: *Tabular List and Alphabetic Index*

It is used by hospitals and other health care providers in coding and reporting clinical information required for participation in Medicare and Medicaid programs, and for statistical tabulation.

Each single disease entity has been assigned a three-digit category. A fourth-digit has been added to provide specificity to the diagnosis regarding etiology, site, or manifestations. In certain cases a fifth-digit level has been added which, when provided, is not optional.

Volumes 1 and 2 are used in physicians' offices to complete insurance claims. Volume 3 is used primarily in hospitals.

ICD-9-CM may be ordered from:

> Superintendent of Documents
> US Government Printing Office
> Washington, DC 20402

> or

> Edwards Brothers Printers
> PO Box 991
> Ann Arbor, Michigan 48106

GUIDELINES FOR CLAIMS PROCESSING

Gathering the Information and Materials

Anyone in the medical facility who makes appointments, does the bookkeeping, treats the patient, or keeps records plays a role in insurance claims.

When the first appointment is made, the medical assistant should ask the patient for all insurance information. If the patient has an identification card, it should be checked to determine that the coverage is current and then photocopied for the office record. If more than one insurance policy is involved get the information for each of the companies. The initial information necessary for the patient record (see Chapter 11) will be required for processing the insurance claim. Additionally, you will need the name of the subscriber if it is someone other than the patient.

Make sure that the physician enters a diagnosis on the patient's chart along with the service performed. It may be the medical assistant's responsibility to properly code the diagnosis and procedure for insurance reporting.

The medical assistant who does the bookkeeping must post the charges promptly and accurately.

Claim Forms

Universal Health Insurance Claim Form. The Health Care Financing Administration Health Insurance Claim Form (HCFA-1500) has been designed to answer the needs of many health insurers (Fig. 16–3). It is the basic form designed by HCFA for the Medicare and Medicaid programs for claims from physicians and suppliers, except for ambulance companies, who will continue to use the HCFA-1491. The HCFA-1500 has also been adopted by CHAMPUS and has received the approval of the AMA Council on Medical Services. The HCFA-1500 claim form is available in a single sheet, two-part snap-out and in two-part computer pin-feed continuous forms. Only the two-part snap-out forms are available with the preprinted provider name and address format.

Superbill

Private insurance companies often send their own form to the patient. One method of supplying insurance information to the patient is by the superbill, discussed in Chapter 15. If billing is done by the physician's office, a copy of the superbill can simply be attached to the insurance form. Many providers totally eliminate insurance billing by preparing the superbill in multiple copies that are either handed to the patient upon completion of service or mailed with instructions for the patient to use this form in billing for his insurance.

Assignments

Some insurance companies honor requests for assignment of benefits to the physician. The medical assistant should request that the patient complete an Assignment of Benefits form (Fig. 16–4). This is an authorization to the insurance company to make payment of any benefits directly to the physician.

It is the patient's responsibility to pay any balance that is not covered by the insurance.

All claims for government-sponsored insurance ask whether the physician will accept assignment. The physician must check either Yes or No in an appropriate box. Checking the Yes box means that the physician will accept the fee determination of the plan and the insurance carrier will pay 80% of the fee directly to the physician. The patient is responsible for the remaining 20%.

Establishing a System

Keeping current with insurance information and changes is no small part of the medical assistant's responsibility. The procedure manual should be updated as changes occur (Fig. 16–5). Government programs are frequently modified, and these changes are reported in bulletins sent to all physicians. Read these bulletins carefully and save those that contain pertinent information.

Watch for workshops offered to medical assistants and physicians in your area and keep the information in a notebook or folder.

Keep a log of insurance claims as they are received and processed (Fig. 16–6). Date-stamp the forms as they are received and enter the information on the log. This log will enable you to determine immediately whether or not a claim form has been completed and mailed.

- If possible, set aside a definite time for completing insurance claims.
- Have a central location for all insurance forms.
- Have readily available the necessary manuals, code books, and other references needed.
- Make it a practice to complete the forms as soon as possible after service is rendered.
- Use the superbill or Universal Claim Form as often as possible.
- Complete the forms by category (all Blue Cross, all Medicare, and so forth).
- Set the tabulator stops on the typewriter for the form being completed. Make a note of these stops so they can be easily set up when doing the same kind of form again.

Completing the Form

1. If you plan to mail the form directly to the insurance company, be sure that the patient has signed the Authorization to Release Information (Fig. 16–7).
2. Have Medicare patients sign an Extended Signature Authorization Form (Fig. 16–8).
3. Typewrite all claim forms and keep a carbon or photocopy of each.
4. Use accepted diagnostic and procedure codes,

Text continued on page 262

16

PLEASE DO NOT STAPLE IN THIS AREA →

FORM APPROVED
OMB NO. 0938-0008

HEALTH INSURANCE CLAIM FORM

(CHECK APPLICABLE PROGRAM BLOCK BELOW)

| [X] MEDICARE (MEDICARE NO.) | [ ] MEDICAID (MEDICAID NO.) | [ ] CHAMPUS (SPONSOR'S SSN) | [ ] CHAMPVA (VA FILE NO.) | [ ] FECA BLACK LUNG (SSN) | [ ] OTHER (CERTIFICATE SSN) |

PATIENT AND INSURED (SUBSCRIBER) INFORMATION

1. PATIENT'S NAME (LAST NAME, FIRST NAME, MIDDLE INITIAL)	2. PATIENT'S DATE OF BIRTH	3. INSURED'S NAME (LAST NAME, FIRST NAME, MIDDLE INITIAL)
Switzer, Arthur O.	06 06 14	Switzer, Arthur O.

4. PATIENT'S ADDRESS (STREET, CITY, STATE, ZIP CODE)	5. PATIENT'S SEX	6. INSURED'S I.D. NO. (FOR PROGRAM CHECKED ABOVE, INCLUDE ALL LETTERS)
4705 Waring Place Los Angeles, CA 90033	MALE [X] FEMALE [ ]	066 11 7865 A

7. PATIENT'S RELATIONSHIP TO INSURED
SELF [X] SPOUSE [ ] CHILD [ ] OTHER [ ]

8. INSURED'S GROUP NO. (OR GROUP NAME OR FECA CLAIM NO.)

[ ] INSURED IS EMPLOYED AND COVERED BY EMPLOYER HEALTH PLAN

TELEPHONE NO.

9. OTHER HEALTH INSURANCE COVERAGE (ENTER NAME OF POLICYHOLDER AND PLAN NAME AND ADDRESS AND POLICY OR MEDICAL ASSISTANCE NUMBER)
------

10. WAS CONDITION RELATED TO:
A. PATIENT'S EMPLOYMENT YES [ ] [X] NO
B. ACCIDENT AUTO [ ] [X] OTHER

11. INSURED'S ADDRESS (STREET, CITY, STATE, ZIP CODE)
4705 Waring Place
Los Angeles, CA 90033
TELEPHONE NO.

11.a. CHAMPUS SPONSOR'S:
STATUS [ ] ACTIVE DUTY [ ] RETIRED [ ] DECEASED BRANCH OF SERVICE

12. PATIENT'S OR AUTHORIZED PERSON'S SIGNATURE (READ BACK BEFORE SIGNING) I AUTHORIZE THE RELEASE OF ANY MEDICAL INFORMATION NECESSARY TO PROCESS THIS CLAIM. I ALSO REQUEST PAYMENT OF GOVERNMENT BENEFITS EITHER TO MYSELF OR TO THE PARTY WHO ACCEPTS ASSIGNMENT BELOW.
SIGNED *Arthur O. Switzer* DATE 9/11/86

13. I AUTHORIZE PAYMENT OF MEDICAL BENEFITS TO UNDERSIGNED PHYSICIAN OR SUPPLIER FOR SERVICE DESCRIBED BELOW.
SIGNED (INSURED OR AUTHORIZED PERSON) *Arthur O. Switzer*

PHYSICIAN OR SUPPLIER INFORMATION

14. DATE OF: ILLNESS (FIRST SYMPTON) OR INJURY (ACCIDENT) OR PREGNANCY (LMP)	15. DATE FIRST CONSULTED YOU FOR THIS CONDITION	16. IF PATIENT HAS HAD SAME OR SIMILAR ILLNESS OR INJURY, GIVE DATES	16.a. IF EMERGENCY CHECK HERE
07 21 86 ◄	07 21 86	----	[ ]

17. DATE PATIENT ABLE TO RETURN TO WORK: NA

18. DATES OF TOTAL DISABILITY FROM NA THROUGH NA

DATES OF PARTIAL DISABILITY FROM NA THROUGH NA

19. NAME OF REFERRING PHYSICIAN OR OTHER SOURCE (e.g. PUBLIC HEALTH AGENCY)
------

20. FOR SERVICES RELATED TO HOSPITALIZATION GIVE HOSPITALIZATION DATES
ADMITTED 07/21/86 DISCHARGED 09/11/86

21. NAME AND ADDRESS OF FACILITY WHERE SERVICES RENDERED (IF OTHER THAN HOME OR OFFICE)
St. Vincent's Hospital, Los Angeles

22. WAS LABORATORY WORK PERFORMED OUTSIDE YOUR OFFICE?
YES [X] NO CHARGES:

23. A. DIAGNOSIS OR NATURE OF ILLNESS OR INJURY. RELATE DIAGNOSIS TO PROCEDURE IN COLUMN D BY REFERENCE NUMBERS 1, 2, 3, ETC. OR DX CODE
1. Subacute bacterial endocarditis
2.
3.
4.

B.
EPSDT YES [ ] [ ] NO
FAMILY PLANNING YES [ ] [ ] NO
PRIOR AUTHORIZATION NO.

24. DATE OF SERVICE FROM — TO	B. PLACE OF SERVICE	C. PROCEDURE CODE (IDENTIFY)	FULLY DESCRIBE PROCEDURES, MEDICAL SERVICES OR SUPPLIES FURNISHED FOR EACH DATE GIVEN (EXPLAIN UNUSUAL SERVICES OR CIRCUMSTANCES)	D. DIAGNOSIS CODE	E. CHARGES	F. DAYS OR UNITS	G. T.O.S.	H. LEAVE BLANK
07/21/86	1	90220		1	200 00	1		
07/22–08/13/86	1	90250		1	805 00	23	1	
08/14/86	1	90270	Complete cardiac re-evaluation	1	100 00	1		
08/15–09/11/86	1	90250		1	945 00	27	1	

25. SIGNATURE OF PHYSICIAN OR SUPPLIER (INCLUDING DEGREE(S) OR CREDENTIALS) (I CERTIFY THAT THE STATEMENTS ON THE REVERSE APPLY TO THIS BILL AND ARE MADE A PART THEREOF)
9-11-86
DATE *Robert O. Elam. MD*

26. ACCEPT ASSIGNMENT (GOVERNMENT CLAIMS ONLY) (SEE BACK)
YES [X] NO [ ]

30. YOUR SOCIAL SECURITY NO.
222 33 4444

27. TOTAL CHARGE	28. AMOUNT PAID	29. BALANCE DUE
$2050.00	-0-	$2050.00

31. PHYSICIAN'S, SUPPLIER'S, AND/OR GROUP NAME, ADDRESS, ZIP CODE AND TELEPHONE NO.
ROBERT O ELAM MD 213-111-2222
300 NO BROADWAY
LOS ANGELES CA 90005
I.D. NO.

32. YOUR PATIENT'S ACCOUNT NO.

33. YOUR EMPLOYER I.D. NO.
00 0000000

*PLACE OF SERVICE AND TYPE OF SERVICE (T.O.S.) CODES ON THE BACK
REMARKS:

APPROVED BY AMA COUNCIL ON MEDICAL SERVICE 6/83

Form HCFA-1500-C2-SC(1-84) Form OWCP-1500
Form CHAMPUS-501 Form RRB-1500

Figure 16–3
Medicare billing form.

ASSIGNMENT OF INSURANCE BENEFITS

I, the undersigned represent that I have insurance coverage with and do hereby

authorize_____to pay and assign directly
(NAME OF COMPANY)

to_____all surgical and/or medical benefits, if any, other-
(NAME OF DOCTOR)

wise payable to me for services as described on the attached forms hereof, but not to exceed the charges for those services. I understand that I am financially responsible for all charges whether or not paid by said insurance. I hereby authorize said assignee to release all information necessary to secure the payment of said benefits.

Date_____Signed_____

Figure 16–4
Assignment of Benefits form.

INSURANCE CARRIER Name & Address	Department and Individual to Contact	POLICYHOLDER Indiv to Contact	Group or Policy Number	SPECIAL NOTES
BLUE SHIELD P O BOX 12345 Anytown, USA	Tom Jones Professional Relations 123–456–7890	Aerospace Industries Joan Crawford 123–888–3030	AI–89037	Tom Jones will speak to groups or give personal assistance in office
		Bell Burgers Nancy Donovan 123–465–2210	BB–3415Z	Scheduled Benefits
OCCIDENTAL P O BOX 42873 Anytown, USA	Cathy Redding Claims Dept. 213–440–3131	Town School Dist. Mary Embers 312–055–3210	Group No. 4414	Does not pay for assistant surgeon

16

Figure 16–5
A page from the procedure manual. Insurance problems can be diminished by knowing who to contact at the insurance carrier and the policyholder.

INSURANCE CLAIM FORMS			
PATIENT	INSURANCE CO.	DATE IN	DATE OUT
James Bush	Continental Casualty	3-14	3-15
Virginia Ellis	Aetna Life	3-14	3-15
Robert Haskell	Occidental	3-15	3-15
Mary Blodgett	Travelers	"	3-15
Stan Wilson	Prudential	"	3-15
" "	State Disability	"	3-15
Wm. Price	County Employees Group	3-16	3-18 returned to pt.
Earl Jacoby	Fireman's Fund	"	3-17
Mary Frederick	Aetna Casualty	"	3-17

Figure 16–6
Insurance log.

RECORDS RELEASE DATE_____

TO_____
DOCTOR

_____
ADDRESS

I HEREBY AUTHORIZE AND REQUEST YOU TO RELEASE

TO_____
DOCTOR

_____
ADDRESS

THE COMPLETE MEDICAL RECORDS IN YOUR POSSESSION, CONCERNING MY ILLNESS

AND/OR TREATMENT DURING THE PERIOD FROM_____TO_____

SIGNED_____
(PATIENT OR NEAREST RELATIVE)

RELATIONSHIP_____

_____
WITNESS

FORM 122 - EASTMAN, INC.

Figure 16–7
Authorization to release medical information form.

NAME OF BENEFICIARY _____

HEALTH INSURANCE CLAIM NUMBER _____

I request that payment of authorized Medicare
benefits be made either to me or on my behalf
to (name of physician or supplier) for any
services furnished me by that
physician/supplier. I authorize any holder
of medical information about me to release to
the Health Care Financing Administration and
its agents any information needed to
determine these benefits or the benefits
payable for related services.

Signature of Patient _____

Date _____

Figure 16–8
Patient's Extended Signature Authorization.

16

and be certain that the procedures are consistent with the diagnoses.

5. List all procedures performed, one procedure per line. Be specific. If a laceration is treated, give location, length and depth, number of sutures required, and time of treatment involved. If a sterile surgical tray was used for office surgery, itemize and bill as a separate fee. If a treatment injection was given, state injected material and amount given.

6. Attach a copy of the x-ray report, hospital report, and/or consultant's report in complicated cases.

7. State the usual and customary fee on all claim forms, regardless of what payment is expected.

8. Never alter a claim as to services performed, date of service, or fees established.

9. If more than one visit per day was required, state the times of day so that the claims processor will know they were separate procedures.

10. Fill in all blanks. Type DNA (does not apply) or NA (not applicable) or simple dash lines (---) rather than leave an item blank. This is confirmation that the item was not overlooked.

Claim Rejection

The claim form must be sufficiently detailed, complete, and accurate. Some of the reasons for claim rejection are:

1. Diagnosis is missing or incomplete.
2. Diagnosis is not coded accurately.
3. Diagnosis does not correspond with treatment.
4. Charges are not itemized.
5. Patient's group, member, or policy number is missing or incorrect.
6. Patient's portion of form is incomplete or signature is missing.
7. Patient's birth date is missing.
8. Fee is not listed.
9. Dates are incorrect or missing.
10. Doctor's signature or address is missing.

BILLING REQUIREMENTS

Blue Plans

Claims should be submitted as soon after service as possible. Many of the Blue Plans have adopted use of the Universal Health Insurance Claim Form. Check with the local office or representative for your area. Blue Shield representatives frequently call at physicians' offices to answer any questions. They also conduct workshops and speak at medical assistants' meetings in order to keep billing and reporting procedures current.

Medicare

Form HCFA-1500 is used for Medicare. Billing for services may be accomplished in any one of three ways:

1. If the doctor accepts assignment, ask the patient to sign the Patient and Insured Information part of the billing form on the first visit (Fig. 16–9). Itemize the services on the claim form, have the physician sign it, check Item 26 indicating that the physician accepts assignment, and submit the claim to the Medicare carrier. When the charge determination has been made, you then will bill the patient for the remaining 20% plus the deductible if this has not already been met for the current year.

2. If the doctor does not accept assignment, you may bill the patient directly. The patient then must submit the billing form to the Medicare carrier. In order to do this, the patient will need from the doctor either an itemized bill that can be attached to the claim form, or an itemization of services on the form.

3. If the doctor does not accept assignment, you can still submit the claim for Medicare for the patient, and check "No" under Item 26. Medicare determines the allowed amount, the carrier sends an Explanation of Benefits (EOB) to the patient. The patient who carries a supplemental policy that pays the deductible and the copayment can then send the EOB to that insurance carrier for processing.

Claims for Medicare must be filed by December 31 of the year following that in which services were rendered. Care rendered in 1987 must be billed no later than December 31, 1988. If the patient had the first covered services during the last 3 months of any year, the cost of these services may be applied to the deductible for the following year.

Medicare patients are particularly appreciative of your assistance in preparing claim forms. In addition to the public relations value, an advantage of submitting claims directly is that supportive documents, such as operation reports, x-ray reports, and so forth, may be attached.

Medicaid

A physician is free to accept or to refuse to treat a patient under Medicaid. However, if the patient is accepted, requirements for rendering service and billing for services are strict and must be closely followed:

- The patient's identification card must be current. Some include labels that must be attached to the billing form.
- Proper authorization may be required for the service for which a form is completed. For an emergency situation, authorization may be secured by telephone but must be followed up with the appropriate form.

50529

☆ U.S. GOVERNMENT PRINTING OFFICE: 1983-685-252

PLEASE DO NOT
STAPLE IN
THIS AREA

FORM APPROVED
OMB NO. 0938-0008

HEALTH INSURANCE CLAIM FORM

(CHECK APPLICABLE PROGRAM BLOCK BELOW)

| □ MEDICARE (MEDICARE NO) | □ MEDICAID (MEDICAID NO.) | □ CHAMPUS (SPONSOR'S SSN) | □ CHAMPVA (VA FILE NO.) | □ FECA BLACK LUNG (SSN) | □ OTHER (CERTIFICATE SSN) |

PATIENT AND INSURED (SUBSCRIBER) INFORMATION

1 PATIENT'S NAME (LAST NAME, FIRST NAME, MIDDLE INITIAL)

2 PATIENT'S DATE OF BIRTH

3 INSURED'S NAME (LAST NAME, FIRST NAME, MIDDLE INITIAL)

4. PATIENT'S ADDRESS (STREET, CITY, STATE, ZIP CODE)

5 PATIENT'S SEX

MALE □ FEMALE □

6. INSURED'S I.D. NO. (FOR PROGRAM CHECKED ABOVE, INCLUDE ALL LETTERS)

7 PATIENT'S RELATIONSHIP TO INSURED

SELF □ SPOUSE □ CHILD □ OTHER □

8. INSURED'S GROUP NO. (OR GROUP NAME OR FECA CLAIM NO)

TELEPHONE NO.

□ INSURED IS EMPLOYED AND COVERED BY EMPLOYER HEALTH PLAN

9. OTHER HEALTH INSURANCE COVERAGE (ENTER NAME OF POLICYHOLDER AND PLAN NAME AND ADDRESS AND POLICY OR MEDICAL ASSISTANCE NUMBER)

10. WAS CONDITION RELATED TO:

A. PATIENT'S EMPLOYMENT

YES □ NO □

B. ACCIDENT

AUTO □ OTHER □

11. INSURED'S ADDRESS (STREET, CITY, STATE, ZIP CODE)

TELEPHONE NO.

11.a. CHAMPUS SPONSOR'S:

STATUS: □ ACTIVE DUTY □ DECEASED □ RETIRED

BRANCH OF SERVICE

12. PATIENT'S OR AUTHORIZED PERSON'S SIGNATURE (READ BACK BEFORE SIGNING) I AUTHORIZE THE RELEASE OF ANY MEDICAL INFORMATION NECESSARY TO PROCESS THIS CLAIM. I ALSO REQUEST PAYMENT OF GOVERNMENT BENEFITS EITHER TO MYSELF OR TO THE PARTY WHO ACCEPTS ASSIGNMENT BELOW.

SIGNED X _____ DATE _____

13. I AUTHORIZE PAYMENT OF MEDICAL BENEFITS TO UNDERSIGNED PHYSICIAN OR SUPPLIER FOR SERVICE DESCRIBED BELOW

SIGNED (INSURED OR AUTHORIZED PERSON)

PHYSICIAN OR SUPPLIER INFORMATION

14. DATE OF ◄ ILLNESS (FIRST SYMPTOM) OR INJURY (ACCIDENT) OR PREGNANCY (LMP)

15. DATE FIRST CONSULTED YOU FOR THIS CONDITION

16. IF PATIENT HAS HAD SAME OR SIMILAR ILLNESS OR INJURY, GIVE DATES

16.a. IF EMERGENCY CHECK HERE □

17. DATE PATIENT ABLE TO RETURN TO WORK

18. DATES OF TOTAL DISABILITY

FROM _____ THROUGH _____

DATES OF PARTIAL DISABILITY

FROM _____ THROUGH _____

19. NAME OF REFERRING PHYSICIAN OR OTHER SOURCE (e g PUBLIC HEALTH AGENCY)

20 FOR SERVICES RELATED TO HOSPITALIZATION GIVE HOSPITALIZATION DATES

ADMITTED _____ DISCHARGED _____

21. NAME AND ADDRESS OF FACILITY WHERE SERVICES RENDERED (IF OTHER THAN HOME OR OFFICE)

22. WAS LABORATORY WORK PERFORMED OUTSIDE YOUR OFFICE?

YES □ NO □ CHARGES

23. A. DIAGNOSIS OR NATURE OF ILLNESS OR INJURY RELATE DIAGNOSIS TO PROCEDURE IN COLUMN D BY REFERENCE NUMBERS 1, 2, 3 ETC. OR DX CODE _____

1.
2.
3.
4.

B.

EPSDT YES □ NO □

FAMILY PLANNING YES □ NO □

PRIOR AUTHORIZATION NO.

24. A. DATE OF SERVICE FROM TO	B.* PLACE OF SERVICE	C. FULLY DESCRIBE PROCEDURES, MEDICAL SERVICES OR SUPPLIES FURNISHED FOR EACH DATE GIVEN PROCEDURE CODE (IDENTIFY) (EXPLAIN UNUSUAL SERVICES OR CIRCUMSTANCES)	D. DIAGNOSIS CODE	E. CHARGES	F. DAYS OR UNITS	G.* T.O.S.	H. LEAVE BLANK

25. SIGNATURE OF PHYSICIAN OR SUPPLIER (INCLUDING DEGREE(S) OR CREDENTIALS) (I CERTIFY THAT THE STATEMENTS ON THE REVERSE APPLY TO THIS BILL AND ARE MADE A PART THEREOF)

DATE

26. ACCEPT ASSIGNMENT (GOVERNMENT CLAIMS ONLY) (SEE BACK)

YES □ NO □

30. YOUR SOCIAL SECURITY NO

27. TOTAL CHARGE

28. AMOUNT PAID

29. BALANCE DUE

31. PHYSICIAN'S SUPPLIER'S AND OR GROUP NAME, ADDRESS, ZIP CODE AND TELEPHONE NO.

BOUCH MCL   G4955
DR MC L BOUCHELLE
1781 W ROMNEYA #D
ANAHEIM CA 92801-1861

32. YOUR PATIENT'S ACCOUNT NO

33. YOUR EMPLOYER I D NO

I.D. NO

* PLACE OF SERVICE AND TYPE OF SERVICE (T.O.S.) CODES ON THE BACK

REMARKS

APPROVED BY AMA COUNCIL ON MEDICAL SERVICE 6/83

Form HCFA-1500 (9) (SC) (1 84)
Form CHAMPUS-501 RRB-1500
Form OWCP-1500

Figure 16–9
Health insurance claim form for patient's signature.

16

Procedure 16–1

PROCEDURAL GOAL

To complete insurance claim form for services to Medicare patient with physician accepting assignment.

EQUIPMENT AND SUPPLIES

Patient chart
Patient ledger
HCFA-1500 claim form
Typewriter

PROCEDURE

1. Ask for patient's identification card.
   Purpose: To determine whether the patient is insured under Medicare Part B.
2. Photocopy card and place in patient's file.
3. Have patient sign an Extended Signature Authorization Form.
   Purpose: Grants lifetime signature authorization for the physician to submit assigned or unassigned claims in the beneficiary's behalf (must be canceled upon patient's request).
4. Complete the following entries on the HCFA-1500 form:
   1. Name of patient
   2. Six-digit birth date
   3. Patient's full name
   4. Patient's full address
   5. Check box for male or female
   6. Number from ID card, including letter
   9. Insured person's address and telephone number
   12. Type "Patient's request for payment on file"
   14. Date illness began
   15. Date patient first consulted physician for this condition
   20 & 21. Name of hospital and dates, if applicable
   23. Each diagnosis on separate line
   24. Columns A–G using appropriate codes and listing each service separately
   25. Physician's personal or stamped signature
       Explanation: Stamped signature is acceptable on Medicare claims.
   26. Checkmark in Yes box.
       Explanation: Must be marked for assignment.
   27–29. Total charge, amount paid, and balance due
       Purpose: No payment will be made unless charge is entered on form.
   30. Physician's Social Security number
   31. Physician's name, address, and telephone number
   33. Employer's ID number

TERMINAL PERFORMANCE OBJECTIVE

Given the listed equipment and supplies, complete a Medicare form, within 10 minutes, to a performance level of 100%.

- There will be a time limit for billing, after which the claim may be rejected.

It is important that the medical assistant check the local regulations and keep current on requirements.

Medi/Medi

The HCFA-1500 form is used, and the physician must always accept assignment. Failure to indicate acceptance of assignment will result in Medicare payment going to the patient, and rejection of the claim by Medicaid. A label from the patient's ID card or a photocopy of the current card may be required.

The claim form is first processed through Medicare and then automatically forwarded to Medicaid. It is not necessary to prepare two claim forms.

CHAMPUS and CHAMPVA

Use Form HCFA-1500 for the covered portion of the fee. Bill the patient directly for the deductible and coinsurance portion. The claim must be filed no later than December 31 of the year following that in which services were provided (Fig. 16–10).

Worker's Compensation

Records for the worker's compensation case (sometimes referred to as an industrial case) should be kept separate from the physician's regular patient histories. If the patient who is seen for an industrial injury has previously been treated as a private patient, a new chart and ledger should be started that will be used only for the treatment rendered under conditions of the Worker's Compensation law.

The insurance carrier may request and is entitled to receive copies of all records pertaining to the industrial injury but not the records of a private patient. Information in the records of a private patient is privileged information and may be released only with the patient's consent. There could be a lawsuit or a hearing before a referee or Appeals Board for which records are subpoenaed. If separate records are kept, there is no question of privilege involved.

The physician who sees the injured or ill worker first will complete what may be called the Doctor's First Report of Work Injury within the time limit imposed by state regulations (Fig. 16–11). The medical assistant should make a minimum of five copies of this report. The insurance company will usually require at least two copies, one copy will go to the state regulatory body, the employer may get a copy, and one file copy should remain with the physi-

cian's record. This report must be personally signed by the physician and should contain the following information:

1. The history of the case as obtained from the patient, noting any **pre-existing condition** (injuries or diseases).
2. The patient's symptoms and physical complaints.
3. The complete physical findings, including laboratory and x-ray results.
4. A tentative diagnosis.
5. An estimate of the type and extent of the disability. In cases in which permanent disability has resulted, there should be a careful survey, and the extent of disability given in detail.
6. Treatment indicated, including type, frequency, and duration. It may be necessary to attach a letter giving more detailed information to assist in making an evaluation of the case.
7. Whenever possible, the date the patient may be able to return to work, if he or she has been totally disabled.

The insurance company may supply its own billing forms. Payment is usually made on the basis of a fee schedule. Any charges in excess of the fee schedule must be fully explained and documented.

In billing for the service, use the coding system specified in your state. Itemize the statement, including any drugs and dressings used.

In severe or prolonged cases, supplemental reports and billing should be sent to the insurance carrier at least once a month (Fig. 16–12).

At the termination of treatment, a final report and bill are sent to the insurance carrier. Do not bill the patient.

HEALTH CARE AND COST CONTAINMENT

As mentioned earlier, since World War II, group insurance has become a significant fringe benefit in collective bargaining. It is believed by some that this has been a factor in increasing cost and overuse of medical care, because when the cost of care is borne by insurance, the patient loses awareness of the financial aspect. Attempts to meet the need for cost containment are being made by the medical profession, health insurance providers, and the federal government by modifying the delivery of medical care.

Fee-for-Service Payment. In the fee-for-service concept the patient sees the doctor, receives care, and then gets a bill for the service. Insurance programs were first designed simply to pay those bills. The patient who had insurance paid an annual premium and in return the insurance company paid at least a portion of the bills. This is still the most common system. Much of the fee-for-service care has been provided by Medicare, Medicaid, and the

16

PLEASE DO NOT
STAPLE IN
THIS AREA

→

HEALTH INSURANCE CLAIM FORM

FORM APPROVED
OMB NO. 0938-0008

(CHECK APPLICABLE PROGRAM BLOCK BELOW)

| ☐ MEDICARE (MEDICARE NO.) | ☐ MEDICAID (MEDICAID NO.) | X CHAMPUS (SPONSOR'S SSN) | ☐ CHAMPVA (VA FILE NO.) | ☐ FECA BLACK LUNG (SSN) | ☐ OTHER (CERTIFICATE SSN) |

PATIENT AND INSURED (SUBSCRIBER) INFORMATION

1. PATIENT'S NAME (LAST NAME, FIRST NAME, MIDDLE INITIAL)

Carter, Elaine

2. PATIENT'S DATE OF BIRTH

07 | 16 | 53

3. INSURED'S NAME (LAST NAME, FIRST NAME, MIDDLE INITIAL)

Carter, Scott W.

4. PATIENT'S ADDRESS (STREET, CITY, STATE, ZIP CODE)

337 Peppertree Drive
Baldwin, NY 11510

TELEPHONE NO. 516 323 0897

5. PATIENT'S SEX

MALE ☐   X FEMALE

7. PATIENT'S RELATIONSHIP TO INSURED

SELF ☐   SPOUSE X   CHILD ☐   OTHER ☐

6. INSURED'S I.D. NO. (FOR PROGRAM CHECKED ABOVE, INCLUDE ALL LETTERS)

S12345

8. INSURED'S GROUP NO. (OR GROUP NAME OR FECA CLAIM NO.)

☐ INSURED IS EMPLOYED AND COVERED BY EMPLOYER HEALTH PLAN

9. OTHER HEALTH INSURANCE COVERAGE (ENTER NAME OF POLICYHOLDER AND PLAN NAME AND ADDRESS AND POLICY OR MEDICAL ASSISTANCE NUMBER)

10. WAS CONDITION RELATED TO:

A. PATIENT'S EMPLOYMENT

YES ☐   X NO

B. ACCIDENT

AUTO ☐   OTHER ☐

11. INSURED'S ADDRESS (STREET, CITY, STATE, ZIP CODE)

HHC 2nd Batt., 24th Infantry
APO New York NY 10026

TELEPHONE NO.

11.a. CHAMPUS SPONSOR'S

STATUS   X ACTIVE DUTY   ☐ DECEASED   ☐ RETIRED

BRANCH OF SERVICE

USA

12. PATIENT'S OR AUTHORIZED PERSON'S SIGNATURE (READ BACK BEFORE SIGNING) I AUTHORIZE THE RELEASE OF ANY MEDICAL INFORMATION NECESSARY TO PROCESS THIS CLAIM I ALSO REQUEST PAYMENT OF GOVERNMENT BENEFITS EITHER TO MYSELF OR TO THE PARTY WHO ACCEPTS ASSIGNMENT BELOW.

SIGNED   DATE

13. I AUTHORIZE PAYMENT OF MEDICAL BENEFITS TO UNDERSIGNED PHYSICIAN OR SUPPLIER FOR SERVICE DESCRIBED BELOW.

SIGNED (INSURED OR AUTHORIZED PERSON)

PHYSICIAN OR SUPPLIER INFORMATION

14. DATE OF: ILLNESS (FIRST SYMPTOM) OR INJURY (ACCIDENT) OR PREGNANCY (LMP)

05 27 87

15. DATE FIRST CONSULTED YOU FOR THIS CONDITION

05 28 87

16. IF PATIENT HAS HAD SAME OR SIMILAR ILLNESS OR INJURY, GIVE DATES

16.a. IF EMERGENCY CHECK HERE

X

17. DATE PATIENT ABLE TO RETURN TO WORK

07 07 87

18. DATES OF TOTAL DISABILITY

FROM 05 27 87   THROUGH 06 12 87

DATES OF PARTIAL DISABILITY

FROM 06 13 87   THROUGH 07 06 87

19. NAME OF REFERRING PHYSICIAN OR OTHER SOURCE (e.g. PUBLIC HEALTH AGENCY)

----

20. FOR SERVICES RELATED TO HOSPITALIZATION GIVE HOSPITALIZATION DATES

ADMITTED 05 28 87   DISCHARGED 06 03 87

21. NAME AND ADDRESS OF FACILITY WHERE SERVICES RENDERED (IF OTHER THAN HOME OR OFFICE)

Island Hospital, 50 Kenmore Parkway, Garden City, NY 11530

22. WAS LABORATORY WORK PERFORMED OUTSIDE YOUR OFFICE?

YES   X NO   CHARGES

23. A. DIAGNOSIS OR NATURE OF ILLNESS OR INJURY. RELATE DIAGNOSIS TO PROCEDURE IN COLUMN D BY REFERENCE NUMBERS 1, 2, 3, ETC. OR DX CODE

1. Acute cholecystitis with cholelithiasis
2.
3.
4.

B.

EPSDT   YES ☐   NO ☐

FAMILY PLANNING   YES ☐   NO ☐

PRIOR AUTHORIZATION NO.

24. A. DATE OF SERVICE FROM — TO	B. PLACE OF SERVICE	C. FULLY DESCRIBE PROCEDURES, MEDICAL SERVICES OR SUPPLIES FURNISHED FOR EACH DATE GIVEN — PROCEDURE CODE (IDENTIFY)	(EXPLAIN UNUSUAL SERVICES OR CIRCUMSTANCES)	D. DIAGNOSIS CODE	E. CHARGES	F. DAYS OR UNITS	G. T.O.S.	H. LEAVE BLANK
05 28 87	1	47610		1	1200 00	2		

25. SIGNATURE OF PHYSICIAN OR SUPPLIER (INCLUDING DEGREE(S) OR CREDENTIALS) (I CERTIFY THAT THE STATEMENTS ON THE REVERSE APPLY TO THIS BILL AND ARE MADE A PART THEREOF)

Clifford Z. Turner, MD

DATE 6-3-87

32. YOUR PATIENT'S ACCOUNT NO.

26. ACCEPT ASSIGNMENT (GOVERNMENT CLAIMS ONLY) (SEE BACK)

YES X   NO ☐

30. YOUR SOCIAL SECURITY NO.

000 00 0000

33. YOUR EMPLOYER I.D. NO.

00 0000000

27. TOTAL CHARGE

$1200.00

28. AMOUNT PAID

–

29. BALANCE DUE

$1200.00

31. PHYSICIAN'S, SUPPLIER'S, AND/OR GROUP NAME, ADDRESS, ZIP CODE AND TELEPHONE NO.

Clifford Z. Turner, MD
94 Kenmore Parkway
I.D. NO. Garden City, NY 11530   516 445 8394

*PLACE OF SERVICE AND TYPE OF SERVICE (T.O.S.) CODES ON THE BACK
REMARKS:

APPROVED BY AMA COUNCIL ON MEDICAL SERVICE 6/83

Form HCFA-1500-C2-SC(1-84)   Form OWCP-1500
Form CHAMPUS-501   Form RRB-1500

Figure 16–10
CHAMPUS claim form.

DOCTOR'S FIRST REPORT OF WORK INJURY

STATE OF CALIFORNIA
DEPARTMENT OF INDUSTRIAL RELATIONS
DIVISION OF LABOR STATISTICS AND RESEARCH
P. O. Box 965, San Francisco, Calif. 94101

Immediately after first examination mail one copy **directly** to the Division of Labor Statistics and Research. Failure to file a report with the Division is a misdemeanor. (Labor Code, Sections 6407-6413.) Answer all questions fully.

A. INSURANCE CARRIER State Compensation Insurance Fund

	Do not write in this space
1. **EMPLOYER** Jones Hardware	
2. Address (No., St. & City) 750 Tenth Street, San Francisco, CA 94100	
3. Business (Manufacturing shoes, building construction, retailing men's clothes, etc.) retail store	

4. **EMPLOYEE** (First name, middle initial, last name) John J. Doe   Soc. Sec. No. 000-00-0000
5. Address (No., St. & City) 234 -11th Street, San Francisco, CA 94100
6. Occupation   clerk   Age 40   Sex M
7. Date injured 10/13/82   Hour 3 P.M. Date last worked same
8. Injured at (No., St. & City) 750 Tenth Street, San Francisco   County San Francisco
9. Date of your first examination 10/13/82   Hour 5 P.M. Who engaged your services? employer
10. Name other doctors who treated employee for this injury none

11. **ACCIDENT OR EXPOSURE:** Did employee notify employer of this injury? yes   Employee's statement of cause of injury or illness:

Fell from ladder a distance of four feet to the floor. Twisted right ankle.

12. **NATURE AND EXTENT OF INJURY OR DISEASE** (Include all objective findings, subjective complaints, and diagnoses. If occupational disease state date of onset, occupational history, and exposures.)

Simple fracture lateral malleolus rt. ankle - undisplaced.

13. **X-rays:** By whom taken? (State if none) St. Martha's Hospital
Findings: as above

14. **Treatment:** Short leg cast applied - no anesthesia

15. Kind of case (Office, home or hospital) office   If hospitalized, date   Estimated stay
Name and address of hospital
16. Further treatment (Estimated frequency and duration) weekly
17. Estimated period of disability for: Regular work 3 months   Modified work 6 weeks
18. Describe any permanent disability or disfigurement expected (State if none) none

19. If death ensued, give date
20. **REMARKS** (Note any pre-existing injuries or diseases, need for special examination or laboratory tests, other pertinent information.)

Name Friend Hunton   Degree M.D. [PERSONAL SIGNATURE OF DOCTOR] *Friend Hunton, M.D.*
(Type or print)
Date of report 10/14/82   Address (No., St. & City) 450 Sutter Street, San Francisco, CA 94100

FORM 5021   *Use reverse side if more space required*   87939-607 10-85 600M ① Ⓑ OSP

16

Figure 16-11
First report of work injury.

DOCTOR'S FINAL (OR MONTHLY) REPORT AND BILL

Itemized bills, IN DUPLICATE, are to be submitted at the termination of the case.
Monthly statements are POSITIVELY required on cases under treatment.
Mail to....State Compensation Insurance Fund....Address..525 Golden Gate Avenue, San Francisco
Services beginning late in month and extending into succeeding month may be itemized on one statement.

EMPLOYER....Jones Hardware, 750 Tenth Street, San Francisco, CA 94100
EMPLOYEE....John J. Doe..Social Security #...000-00-0000
DATE OF INJURY...10/13/82..............SERVICES FOR MONTH OF....October...................., 19..82.

Patient refused treatment....................--, 19......   Patient able to return to work.........--...., 19......
Patient stopped treatment   Patient discharged as cured.............--...., 19......
    without orders..................--...., 19......   Condition at time of last visit...convalescent
Patient entered hospital...............--...., 19......

Any other charges authorized such as Drugs?....--....Hospital?....--..
                                          (Check)   (Check)

Code: O—Office; V—Home Visit; H—Hospital Visit; N—Night Visit; S—Operation; X—X-Ray.

Month	1	2	3	4	5	6	7	8	9	10	11	12	13	14	15	16	17	18	19	20	21	22	23	24	25	26	27	28	29	30	31
Oct													S														O				

                                                                  Totals

First aid treatment (describe)..$.........

Office Visits....10/27/82..............CRVS #90060.........................$...12.00
Home Visits...$.........
Hospital Visits..$.........
Operations ......10/13/82 Short leg walking cast CRVS #29425 $...40.00
MATERIAL (Itemized at cost)...$.........

                                                TOTAL $...52.00

Any charges shown above which are in excess of the minimum fee must be explained below regarding nature
of such services, indicating the date rendered.

Make check payable to:

Doctor..Friend Hunton..........................   Signature *Friend Hunton M.D.*

Address..450 Sutter Street, San Francisco   Date..October 31, 1982

*Figure 16–12
Monthly statement for Worker's Compensation.*

Blue Plans, but all of these are beginning to take steps toward cost containment and alternatives to fee-for-service insurance.

Preferred-Provider Organizations (PPOs). One strategy that preserves the fee-for-service concept, desirable in the eyes of many physicians, is the PPO. The insurer, representing its clients, contracts with a group of providers who agree on a predetermined list of charges for all services, including complex and unusual procedures. Then the insurer pays that rate.

A doctor who joins a PPO does not need to alter the manner of providing care. The doctor continues practicing on a fee-for-service basis, treating and billing the regular patients. When a patient comes from the PPO group, the physician treats the patient and then bills the PPO. The care is not prepaid.

Prepaid Plans. Prepaid plans are usually called health maintenance organizations (HMOs). The HMO may be closed-panel or open-panel.

A *closed-panel HMO* employs a staff of physicians and pays each one a salary. The HMO charges each patient a predetermined amount, which is usually negotiated through a group contract, and in addition may charge a small copayment for each visit.

An *open-panel HMO* is known as an independent practice association (IPA). Instead of maintaining its own staff and clinic buildings, the IPA contracts with independently practicing physicians who continue to practice in their own offices. The IPA may pay each doctor a set amount per patient in advance, or the fees for members may be billed directly to the IPA rather than to the patient. Fees for nonmember patients are handled the same as any fee-for-service.

Peer Review Organizations (PROs). Peer review organizations are an outgrowth of a 1972 amendment to the Social Security Act that brought about the formation of federal **professional standards review organizations** (PSROs), whose purposes were to monitor the validity of diagnoses and quality of care and to evaluate the appropriateness of hospital admissions and discharges of patients covered by government-sponsored health insurance. The effectiveness of PSROs was continually debated, and the PSROs were gradually phased out.

In 1982, PROs were legislated in as part of the Tax Equity and Fiscal Responsibility Act (TEFRA). The purpose of a PRO is identical to that of the PSROs. The primary difference is that the PROs are mostly limited to a single group within a state. PRO contracts are awarded by the Health Care Financing Administration to physician-based organizations within each state, and the mechanics of PROs vary slightly from state to state. In an attempt to control costs, an insurance carrier may require prior authorization from the PRO before a patient is hospitalized for elective medical or surgical care. If the patient's condition can be adequately and safely treated on an outpatient basis, payment for hospitalization will not be approved. It is important that the medical assistant be aware of the types of admission cases that require previous authorization and that the authorization be obtained prior to the admission date.

Prospective Payment System (PPS). In April 1983 the Social Security Amendments Act of 1983 (P.L. 98-21) was signed into law. Title VI of this law contained the prospective payment system (PPS) for hospitals, which would begin the radical restructuring of the payment system to hospitals for Medicare inpatient services.

> As identified by the Health Care Financing Administration (HCFA), a major objective of the prospective payment system (PPS) is to establish the government as a "prudent buyer" of health care while maintaining beneficiaries' access to quality care. The "prudent buyer" objective is to be accomplished by paying Medicare providers a predetermined specific rate per discharge rather than on the basis of reasonable costs. Access to quality care is to be ensured through reviews by Peer Review Organizations of the validity of diagnoses, quality of care and appropriateness of admissions and discharges.*

If a hospital does not contract with a PRO it will be ineligible for payment from the Medicare program. The law provides authority to grant waivers from the PPS if a state has an approved hospital

---

*American Medical Association: *DRGs and the Prospective Payment System: A Guide for Physicians*. Chicago, The Association, 1984.

reimbursement control system. Four states (Maryland, Massachusetts, New Jersey, and New York) currently have such a waiver.

Physician Prospective Payment System. Probability is high that HCFA will set up a PPS for physicians. Every claim form you file with Medicare or any other third party payer becomes part of a permanent computerized record that may be used in the future as the basis of your physician's fee profile if the PPS is expanded to include reimbursement of physician charges. Your coding must be performed accurately and precisely if meaningful profiles are to be established. The two more likely approaches to a PPS for physicians are diagnosis related groups (DRGs) (see below) and relative value scales (RVSs), discussed earlier in this chapter.

Diagnosis Related Groups (DRGs). The DRG classification forms the basis for payment under the prospective payment system, as opposed to the traditional method of payment based on actual costs incurred in the provision of care. Payment to the hospital of a DRG amount will, generally, constitute payment in full for services rendered to Medicare patients.

The DRG system classifies patients on the basis of diagnosis, and was developed by Yale researchers in the 1970s as a mechanism for utilization review. DRGs are derived from taking all possible diagnoses identified in the ICD-9-CM system, classifying them into 23 major diagnostic categories (MDCs) based on organ system, and further breaking them into 467 distinct groupings, each of which is said to be "medically meaningful."

In all, there are actually 470 DRGs. The first 467 are based on the principal diagnosis or procedure performed. Number 468 is assigned when the principal procedure performed does not conform with the principal diagnosis. Numbers 469 and 470 are codes that reflect coding errors and are automatically returned to the hospital for correction or verification. The principal diagnosis is the most critical factor in the assignment of DRGs. All diagnoses must reflect information contained in the patient's medical record.

In order to assign a case to a DRG, five pieces of information are necessary:

- The patient's principal diagnosis and up to four complications or comorbidities
- The treatment procedures performed
- The patient's age
- The patient's sex
- The patient's discharge status

PHYSICIAN'S RESPONSIBILITY. The major factor determining the assignment of a DRG is the physician's assessment of the principal diagnosis. It is the physician's responsibility to record the principal

16

diagnosis, as well as the other determining factors, on a discharge face sheet. It is extremely important that the principal diagnosis, as stated by the physician, correspond to the various tests, procedures, and notes contained within the complete medical record.

Once the discharge face sheet has been completed by the physician, the chart is forwarded to the hospital's medical records department for review and coding. The codes contained in the ICD-9-CM are used for determining the DRG and therefore must be entered in the appropriate section of the discharge face sheet.

From the medical records department the information is forwarded to the financial office for completion of the bill to be submitted to the fiscal intermediary. The fiscal intermediary, through use of a grouper computer program, will determine the appropriate DRG and then calculate the payment to the hospital.

GLOSSARY OF PROSPECTIVE PAYMENT TERMS

Any discussion of the prospective payment system requires an acquaintance with the terminology involved.

capitation A method of payment for health services in which an individual or institutional provider is paid a fixed, per capita amount for each person served without regard to the actual number or nature of services provided to each person.

comorbidity A pre-existing condition that will, because of its presence with a specific principal diagnosis, cause an increase in length of stay by at least 1 day in approximately 75% of the cases.

complication A condition that arises during the hospital stay that prolongs the length of stay by at least 1 day in approximately 75% of the cases.

diagnosis related groups (DRGs) A system developed by Yale University for classifying patients into groups that are clinically coherent and homogeneous with respect to resources used. There are 467 DRGs.

DRG creep Inflating diagnoses to obtain a higher payment rate.

DRG weight An index number that reflects the relative resource consumption associated with each DRG.

discharge face sheet (may also be called **discharge summary** or **discharge abstract**) A summary of the admission, prepared at the time of the patient's discharge from the hospital. Information contained on the discharge face sheet includes demographic information, source of payment, length of stay, principal diagnosis, secondary diagnoses or complications, procedures per-

formed, services provided, and other information that may be relevant to a particular hospital.

grouper Computer software program that is used by the fiscal intermediary in all cases to assign discharges to the appropriate DRGs using the following information abstracted from the inpatient bill: patient's age, sex, principal diagnosis, principal procedures performed, and discharge status.

ICD-9-CM (International Classification of Diseases, Ninth Revision, Clinical Modification) A system for classifying diseases and operations to facilitate collection of uniform and comparable health information.

major diagnostic category (MDC) An MDC is a broad clinical category that is differentiated from all others based on body system involvement and disease etiology. The 23 MDCs cover the complete range of diagnoses contained in the ICD-9-CM.

outliers (atypical cases) Cases involving an extremely long length of stay (day outlier) or extraordinarily high costs (cost outlier) when compared with most discharges classified in the same DRG.

peer review organization (PRO) An entity that is composed of a substantial number of licensed doctors of medicine and osteopathy engaged in the practice of medicine or surgery in the area, or an entity that has available to it the services of a sufficient number of physicians engaged in the practice of medicine or surgery, to assure the adequate peer review of the services provided by the various medical specialties and subspecialties.

principal diagnosis That condition which after study is determined to be chiefly responsible for occasioning the admission of the patient to the hospital.

principal procedure One that was performed for definitive treatment rather than for diagnostic or exploratory purposes, or one necessary to take care of a complication. It is that procedure most related to the principal diagnosis.

Prospective Payment Assessment Commission (ProPAC): A 15-member commission of independent experts with experience and expertise in the provision and financing of health care who are appointed to review and provide recommendations on: the annual inflation factor; DRG recalibration; new and existing medical and surgical procedures and services.

sole community hospital (SCH) Those hospitals that, by reason of factors such as isolated location, weather conditions, travel conditions, or absence of other hospitals (as determined by the Secretary), are the sole source of inpatient hospital services reasonably available to individuals in a geographic area.

Tax Equity and Fiscal Responsibility Act (TEFRA) Signed into Federal law in 1982. Contains provisions for major changes in Medicare reimbursement.

uniform hospital discharge data set (UHDDS) A minimum data set required to be collected for each Medicare patient on discharge.

weight (DRG) An HCFA-derived figure intended to reflect the relative resource consumption of each DRG. The payment rate is multiplied by the appropriate DRG weight to determine the reimbursement amount for each patient.

REFERENCES AND READING

American Medical Association: *DRGs and the Prospective Payment System: A Guide for Physicians.* Chicago, The Association, 1984.

American Medical Association: *Physician's Current Procedural Terminology,* 4th ed. Chicago, The Association, 1984.

Blue Shield of California: *Medicare Bulletin,* August 1984.

CHAMPUS Handbook 6010-46-H, January 1983.

Fordney, M.: *Insurance Handbook for the Medical Office,* 2nd ed. Philadelphia, W. B. Saunders Co., 1981.

16

CHAPTER OUTLINE

VOCABULARY

See Glossary at end of book for definitions.

agenda	lexicographic	periodical
colloquialism	monograph	prognosis
galley proofs	order of business	treatise

Editorial Duties and Meeting and Travel Arrangements

17

OBJECTIVES

After successful completion of this chapter you should be able to:

1. Define the terms listed in the Vocabulary of this chapter.
2. Originate and maintain a card catalog for a personal library.
3. Discuss the nature and importance of an abstract.
4. List the four items to include on a cross reference card for a general reference file.
5. Name five items of information to include on a diagnostic file card.
6. Name the library classification system that uses decimal numbers.
7. Identify the classification system that uses a combination of letters of the alphabet and numerals.
8. Cite three indexes available in medical libraries for use in locating various periodical references.
9. Name two of the largest medical data bases for electronic retrieval of information.
10. List the seven items of information needed for each reference in a bibliography.
11. Briefly outline the general procedure for preparing a manuscript for publication in a periodical.
12. List the five items that should be included in the first paragraph of the minutes of a meeting.

After successful completion of this chapter you should be able to perform the following activities:

1. Typewrite a speech in correct format and estimate the time necessary for delivery.
2. Prepare cards for an abstract file.
3. Set up a diagnostic file, including subject cards and the necessary subheadings to accommodate the patient charts.
4. Retype a manuscript that has been edited using proofreader's marks.
5. Make travel arrangements for a proposed trip.
6. Prepare a typewritten itinerary.
7. Make arrangements for a group meeting.
8. From a rough draft, typewrite the minutes of a meeting in correct form, including the secretary's signature.

EDITORIAL DUTIES

The medical profession is unique in that the physician traditionally shares with others, through writing and speaking, the discoveries, information, and observations gained in practice, research, and private study. The medical assistant who becomes proficient in maintaining the physician's personal library and in assisting with the preparation of articles and speeches can be of immeasurable help in these endeavors.

The Physician's Library

The books that a physician acquires while in medical school will become the nucleus of a personal library that will grow over the years. New books reflecting the changes in medicine and the physician's special interests will be added (Fig. 17–1). The physician may accumulate a file of professional journals such as the *Journal of the American Medical Association* (JAMA), the journal of the state medical society, specialty journals, trade journals, and even informative material provided by pharmaceutical companies.

Journals should be bound at regular intervals,

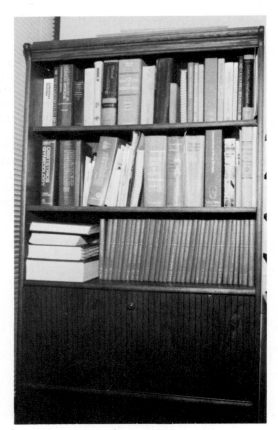

Figure 17–1
Typical basic library in physician's office. (Courtesy of Vista Medical Group, El Toro, CA. Photo by Dan Santucci.)

generally by volume, in order to preserve the individual copies. The medical assistant may be responsible for having the journals bound regularly and consistently. Most journals in the medical field publish indexes, annually, semiannually, or quarterly. The index should be bound with the journal pages. In most cities the binding of **periodicals** can be done locally. The hospital librarian is a good source of information for locating a bookbinder.

Organizing the Library. While the physician's library may not be large, it must be systematically organized so that information is readily accessible.

In setting up or rearranging a small library, books should be classified by subject groupings that reflect medical specialties. Those dealing with related topics should be placed together. Journals and periodicals are usually arranged alphabetically.

Card Catalog of Books. The books should be indexed in a card catalog or looseleaf binder. A 3 × 5 inch card file is practical. Generally, three or more cards should be prepared for each book:

- Title card
- Subject card
- Author card(s)

Here's how to index a book in this manner, using the book you are reading as an example:

1. Prepare a title card with the heading *The Medical Assistant: Administrative and Clinical*.
2. Prepare a subject card with the heading "Medical Assisting."
3. Prepare the author cards (Fig. 17–2).
4. The four cards should then be filed either in a **lexicographic** file (all entries alphabetized together) or in a file divided into sections for title, subject, and author. With such a file and cross-reference system, any book can be located very quickly.

The computerized office will undoubtedly store this information on disk for ready retrieval.

Periodical File. One of the physician's greatest difficulties is in keeping up with medical literature, particularly the articles appearing regularly in the periodicals. It is unlikely that the physician will want to maintain a complete index of all articles in these periodicals, but most doctors want to keep track of articles that are of particular interest. Abstracts are of great value in the continuing task of keeping abreast of scientific developments.

Preparation of an Abstract. An abstract is a kind of summary or epitome of a book, paper, or case history. It is brief, indicating the nature of the article and summarizing the most important points and conclusions. Abstracts prepared by professionals are found in many medical journals as a service to the individual physician.

Many physicians prepare abstracts of the articles that they find of particular value, and in some offices the medical assistant is trained to do abstracting for the doctor. A medical assistant who

---

Medical Assistant: Administrative and Clinical, The

6th edition
Mary E. Kinn and Eleanor F. Derge
Philadelphia, W. B. Saunders Company, 1988

Textbook and reference covering all phases of medical assisting in the physician's office

---

TITLE CARD

Medical Assisting

The Medical Assistant: Administrative and Clinical
6th edition
Philadelphia, W. B. Saunders Company, 1988

Mary E. Kinn and Eleanor F. Derge

SUBJECT CARD

Kinn, Mary E.

The Medical Assistant: Administrative and Clinical
6th edition
Philadelphia, W. B. Saunders Company, 1988

1. Medical Assisting   2. Derge, Eleanor F., joint author

Derge, Eleanor F.

The Medical Assistant: Administrative and Clinical
6th edition
Philadelphia, W. B. Saunders Company, 1988

1. Medical Assisting   2. Kinn, Mary E., joint author

AUTHOR CARDS

Figure 17–2
Title, subject, and author cards for referencing a book in the personal library.

can prepare a good abstract of an article can save the doctor from reading 10 to 20 pages of the original article and can help focus attention upon information of particular interest in the article.

Abstracts must clearly indicate the nature of the information contained in the article. Each should note:

- Any new procedures
- Results of studies and experiments
- Conclusions noted

The length and character of the article will determine the type and length of the abstract. In most scientific articles, the conclusions of the writer will be summarized at the end of the piece. This summary is of great help in preparing an abstract.

These abstracts are typed on cards, with the text of the abstract preceded by the following information:

- Title of article
- Surname and initials of the author
- Name of publication
- Volume
- Inclusive page numbers
- Month and year

The cards are then filed. If abstract cards are kept, it is not necessary to clip and file the actual articles separately. The journals in which they appear can be kept in the usual alphabetic order.

Reprints. When physicians write articles or present papers before scientific meetings, their work is often published in a periodical and reprints of it made available to their colleagues. A portion of each doctor's library is usually composed of a collection of such reprints. The doctor may ask the medical assistant to write for a particular reprint. Sometimes the doctor may have a special postcard made up for ordering reprints (Fig. 17–3).

Other physicians prefer to write personal letters in which they compliment the author upon the excellence of the article and request copies of it for their files. Reprints often present a filing problem in the office because they are not of uniform size. This problem can be solved by placing references to these reprints in the library card file, and placing the reprints in a separate drawer.

Other Reference Files. Physicians frequently need a variety of miscellaneous medical information in addition to book collections, periodicals, and their indexes. For this reason they may accumulate a separate reference file. Often this consists of pages photocopied from journals or reference books.

Organization of Reference Files. The physician and the medical assistant together may set up (1) a subject index for filing the material, and (2) a cross reference card file for locating the material easily. Begin by tabbing file dividers with the main topics and folders with subheadings. When an article or item is photocopied, a card is made up with:

- The title of the article or chapter
- Its author
- The periodical or book in which it appeared
- The date of publication

The copy of the reference material is filed in the appropriate folder and the card filed by subject for easy reference. As new developments occur, later articles may be filed and outdated material discarded.

Diagnostic Files. Physicians often draw material for their writing and speaking from the case histories of their own patients. For this reason, many doctors like to set up diagnostic files so that they

17

Please send me _____ copies of your article,
_____ ,
(title)
which appeared in _____ (publication) _____
_____ , 19 _____ .

_____
(Doctor's signature)

Figure 17-3
Typical card for ordering reprints.

can quickly pull out information on, for example, the incidence of certain side effects among patients treated with a particular medication. The medical assistant will have to be familiar with medical terminology to maintain such a file.

Organization of the Diagnostic File. The system used will vary from office to office, but subject cards generally will have:

- A main heading with the name of the disease or surgical procedure
- Subheadings for various aspects of the disease or procedure
- The patient's name, diagnosis, and type of treatment listed below

For example, one subject entry with subheadings might be:

BLOOD DISEASES
    Anemia
    Granulocytosis
    Hemophilia
    Leukemia
    Polycythemia
    Thalassemia
    Toxemia

Patient cards will be headed with the patient's name and diagnosis, treatment, **prognosis**, and miscellaneous information below.

By keeping such a file a physician can readily obtain the charts of all patients with a particular condition from the history files. This is particularly valuable to physicians who do a great deal of teaching, writing, or research. The physician's office equipped with a computer will find it very easy to keep a detailed diagnostic file using these same principles.

Library for Patients

Many doctors keep a small library of educational information for patients. This library generally contains some books written in language that the average patient can understand, and a number of pamphlets and reprints that the patient can take home. This might include information on such subjects as diabetes, heart disease, skin conditions, danger signals of cancer, lung disease, first aid, and other subjects of interest to many patients. The specialist may have information dealing specifically with the doctor's specialty. A library service such as this saves the physician considerable time in repeating simple educational information and is generally welcomed by the patients.

Helping To Gather Information

The medical assistant who is employed by a doctor who teaches, writes, or speaks frequently may be called upon to assist with the preparation of papers. The duties might include:

- Making up a list of references for a talk or paper for publication
- Doing actual research
- Preparing abstracts

Any medical assistant who is called upon to assume such responsibilities must know how to make the best use of the available library and reference facilities.

USING LIBRARY FACILITIES

Almost all doctors, even those practicing in rural areas, have access to medical libraries. The doctor who practices in a metropolitan area or near a medical center such as a university is particularly fortunate, since these offer outstanding library facilities.

All general hospitals maintain medical libraries comprising a basic collection of carefully selected, authoritative medical textbooks and reference works of the latest edition and files of current journals. The Medical Library Association sets standards for member libraries.

A physician usually has access to a county society library or can use the package library services of the state society. In addition, extension library facilities can be used to obtain information from special supplemental collections. The American

Medical Association, for example, and some specialty societies, offer periodical lending services and package library services to their members.

The National Library of Medicine has established a system whereby doctors may get materials from a Regional Medical Library Program when information is not available locally. In those instances when the Regional Program cannot satisfy the need, the request is channeled to the National Library of Medicine.

All libraries systematically organize the books, periodicals, and other materials in a fairly uniform manner in order that the information can be easily located and accessible. The medical assistant who finds it necessary to go to a library to do special work should seek out the librarian or an assistant and get an idea of what the library has to offer in the way of materials, the arrangement of materials, privileges, rules, and regulations for use of the library. After a brief discussion, the trained medical librarian usually can suggest shortcuts that are of great help in locating references or doing research.

Card Catalog of Books. All books, **monographs, treatises,** handbooks, dictionaries, and encyclopedias contained in a library are indexed by author and subject and sometimes by title in the card catalog. This catalog is really an index of the book contents of the library. Cards are arranged alphabetically, with subject, author, and title cards alphabetized in one series, or are alphabetized within separate sections for subject, author, or title.

Classification Systems. There are a number of systems for classifying library books. In library procedure, classification means putting together materials on a given subject with related materials placed nearby. Medical libraries use various classification systems.

The Dewey decimal system, used not only in medical but in all types of libraries, is sometimes used for arranging medical library collections. This system uses decimal numbers to indicate particular subjects and arranges the book collection in numeric sequence for easy location. For example, 616 indicates Pathology, Diseases, Treatment. Here's an example of how the Dewey decimal system works:

616.1   Diseases of the cardiovascular system
616.9   Communicable and other diseases
616.96   Parasitic diseases
616.99   Other general diseases
616.992   Neoplasms and neoplastic diseases

The Library of Congress classification system is also used. This consists of a number of separate, mutually exclusive classifications based upon combination of letters of the alphabet and numerals:

QR: Bacteriology
RD: Surgery
RC 321-431:   Diseases of the nervous system

The National Library of Medicine classification system is replacing the Library of Congress system in many medical libraries.

There are other systems, such as the Boston Medical Library Classification, the Cunningham Classification, and the Barnard Classification, that are used by some medical libraries. A brief discussion with the librarian and a quick look at the card catalog will generally help acquaint you with the system used.

How the Card Catalog Can Help You Locate Books. No matter what system of classification is used, the main purpose is to help those who use the library to locate volumes quickly. The symbol for the particular book, whether it be a numeral, a letter, or a combination of numerals and letters, appears on the card for the book in the card file. This symbol is called a classification mark. It also appears on the spine of the volume.

To locate a volume, check the classification mark on the card and if an open shelf system is used, find that shelf in the library where corresponding symbols appear. If a closed shelf system is used in the library, give the number of the book and its title to a librarian who will locate it for you.

Periodical Indexes. The bulk of current medical literature appears in medical journals, and some reference system for these thousands of articles is necessary. The majority of journals publish their own indexes, one for each volume, with sometimes an annual index. If you know the name of the journal that published the article you are looking for, this is the fastest way to locate it. Otherwise, composite indexes may be consulted.

Clinical Medicine. The monthly *Index Medicus* and the annual *Cumulated Index Medicus,* published by the National Library of Medicine, include author and subject indexes for over 3000 periodicals. They are international in scope, with foreign publications and languages being represented as well as publications in English.

The monthly *Abridged Index Medicus* and the annual *Cumulated Abridged Index Medicus* are smaller versions of *Index Medicus* and *Cumulated Index Medicus,* and are limited to indexing 100 major periodicals in the medical field. These periodicals are readily available in the majority of medical libraries. The computer equivalent of both the *Index Medicus* and the *Abridged Index Medicus* is MEDLINE.

Nursing and Allied Health. The *Cumulative Index to Nursing & Allied Health Literature* is published by Glendale Adventist Medical Center. This index is very comprehensive and is the only thorough source for coverage of allied health. It is published bimonthly with an annual cumulation. The computer equivalent is Nursing & Allied Health Index on Bibliographic Retrieval System (BRS) and Dialog.

The *International Nursing Index* is published quarterly, with an annual cumulation, by the *American*

17

Journal of Nursing. The computer equivalent is MED-LINE.

Hospital and Healthcare. *Hospital Literature Index* is published quarterly, with annual cumulations, by the American Hospital Association (AHA). Before 1978 the AHA produced a biannual index entitled "Cumulative Index to Hospital Literature," but this is no longer in print. The computer equivalent to *Hospital Index* is MEDLINE/Health file.

Bibliography Search. Information for bibliographies may be produced by either a manual search through indexes, or a computer search.

For a manual search you must look under the subject closest to the one on which you need information, then copy down all the information (author, title of journal, and complete bibliographic information, including volume number, pages, and date).

Most of the world's literature is now accessible through various vendors who provide computer access to specialized files. There are thousands of these databases. The major vendors in healthcare facilities are:

- National Library of Medicine
- Dialog Information Services, Inc.
- Bibliographic Retrieval System (BRS)
- Systems Development Corporation (SDC)

The National Library of Medicine is the least expensive of these four vendors.

Electronic Retrieval of Information. Two of the largest medical databases are MEDLINE and EMBASE, each of which includes citations and abstracts from thousands of publications.

MEDLINE is produced by the National Library of Medicine and covers materials from 1966 and later. *Index Medicus* is produced from this computer file.

EMBASE is produced by Excerpta Medica, and the *Excerpta Medica Index* is produced from this database. There is a great deal of overlap between the two databases, but EMBASE does include some literature not indexed in *Index Medicus*.

Computer access to MEDLINE is available in the majority of hospital libraries and is often provided as a free service to affiliates of the hospital. Many hospitals subscribe to at least one additional vendor from either Dialog, BRS, or SDC's Orbit. With the aid of a computer, a researcher in a library may rapidly locate wanted information by using search terms such as topic, author, and publication. The computer search will generate a bibliography of literature. The searcher must then locate a copy of the article. Some files provide abstracts available on-line. Articles not available from a local health care library can usually be requested through that library as an interlibrary loan.

The individual physician or health care facility with a computer, a modem, telecommunications software, and a telephone line may subscribe to one or more information utilities. Some of the medically oriented utilities are:

- GTE Medical Information Network (MINET)
- BRS Colleague Medical
- DIALOG

Through GTE, access may be made to EMPIRES (Excerpta Medica Physician Information Retrieval and Education Service), the American Medical Association's clinical literature database containing current and historic citations and abstracts from over 300 key medical journals.

The development of databases and electronic retrieval systems has provided an invaluable service to the medical profession by making possible easy access to references on an unlimited number of medical subjects. It is also possible for subscribers to read the complete text of books, journals, and other publications.

Other Reference Sources. There are a number of other specialized reference volumes that a medical librarian may use to locate literature. The Monthly Catalog of U.S. Government Publications, for example, contains certain medical listings and is sometimes valuable in research work. Or, in securing biographic information about physicians or other professionals, it is often necessary to turn to such books as the *Directory of Medical Specialists, American Men of Science,* the *American Medical Directory,* or *Who's Who Among Physicians and Surgeons.* Encyclopedias such as *Encyclopedia Britannica* and the *Practical Medicine* series also are sometimes helpful in obtaining basic information.

PREPARING A BIBLIOGRAPHY

Utilizing the various reference sources of the medical library, you can make up a bibliography or list of references on a specific topic with comparatively little difficulty. It does take time, since the list of references must be accurate. Many researchers recommend listing each reference separately on a card or in a small looseleaf notebook (Fig. 17–4). This simplifies the actual preparation of the formal bibliography that always accompanies any published medical paper. Take down the following information for each reference:

- Subject
- Author
- Title of book or article
- Publisher or periodical
- Volume
- Date of publication
- Page numbers

Sometimes card catalogs and other periodical references will list brief summaries of the specific reference cited; this information is also helpful in research and should be noted.

Author.. Subject..

Title... Available at:......................................

.... Call No...

Publisher/Journal... Reference: Excellent, Good, Fair

Copyright Date.................. Volume:.............. Pages:.............. Illustrated:.............................

Student's Name:..

(Summary, including problem, source of data, method, results, quotations, references.)

Summary:...

....

....

....

....

....

Figure 17–4
Card for reporting bibliographic data.

Some libraries prepare medical bibliographies free of charge or for a small fee. Some also abstract or review literature, translate articles, and collect case reports. The library of the American College of Surgeons, for example, offers this service at a modest fee to its members. The American Medical Association also offers this service to its members.

Manuscript Preparation

In most cases the medical assistant's tasks in connection with the preparation of a talk or a manuscript for publication are mainly mechanical; the doctor is responsible for the actual writing. However, since many physicians ask their medical assistants to serve in the capacity of editorial assistants, smoothing out and actually editing their copy before submitting it for publication, a basic understanding of the style, format, and characteristics of medical papers is helpful.

Writing Style. Each medical journal has its own style for publishing papers. The individual hoping to publish in a specific journal should request a copy of the journal's guidelines for manuscripts in advance and then prepare the manuscript accordingly in order to minimize editorial changes. There are certain fairly uniform procedures, however, in the preparation of a manuscript to be submitted for publication.

A good medical paper must present established new facts, modes, or practices; principles of value; results of suitable original research; or a review of facts on a subject from which the reader can draw a legitimate conclusion. The subject should be limited to a definite area or problem before writing is begun, and the purpose should be determined in advance.

The typical medical article begins with an introductory section outlining the nature of the material or problem to be covered, follows with actual discussion of the subject, and concludes with a summary in which conclusions are usually noted in numeric form. The format for case reports is somewhat similar. Case reports based on clinical information should be written clearly in smooth narrative style and should not read like a collection of telegraphic notes. There should be a clear presentation of sequence of events. A brief abstract may appear at the beginning or end of any article. This summary should be rigidly condensed and should contain the deductions as well as clearly reflect the author's viewpoint. Only the actual conclusions reached should be numbered.

The writing in a scientific paper should be simple and straightforward. Excess words should be ruthlessly pared from the article. Grammatic construction must facilitate direct, clear expression. The paper should be well organized and proceed smoothly from beginning to end in a direct fashion. Slang, **colloquialisms,** personal allusions, and reminiscences should generally be avoided in papers for publication, although they are often acceptable and add a friendly tone to a paper to be delivered in person before a medical meeting.

Typing the Manuscript. Many drafts of a paper may be made before the final copy. Using an electronic word processor or computer can greatly reduce the laborious retyping of manuscripts, but the author may still want a printout of each revision. Sometimes different colors of paper are used to distinguish between each draft. Double- or triple-space drafts to allow plenty of room for revisions by the author.

Revising the Manuscript. An important step in the preparation of any manuscript is a careful revision of copy. This is a duty sometimes delegated to the secretary or medical assistant. Revisions should be made with these specific objectives in mind.

- Organization
- Accuracy
- Content
- Conciseness
- Correct sentence and grammatic construction
- Clarity and smoothness

Check for correct spelling, using a medical dictionary as well as a standard dictionary.

Preparing Final Copy. Use good quality white paper. Type on one side of the paper only. Double-space the copy, allowing a margin of at least one inch at each side and at the bottom. Double-spacing provides space for the editor who receives the manuscript to make corrections or insert instructions for the printer. Number each page, either in the center of the top or bottom margin or in the upper right- or left-hand corner.

The original manuscript is submitted to the publisher, and the author should retain one or more copies. If the manuscript is on disk or tape, one printout is sufficient to retain in the file.

Footnotes. When a paper is based upon a study of the writing of others, it is necessary to acknowledge the sources used. In medical and scientific papers, footnotes usually provide exact references to sources of material. Forms of footnotes differ slightly, depending upon the style of the particular periodical, but in general a footnote contains the following:

- Author's name
- Title of the work cited
- Facts of publication
- Exact page from which the citation was taken

The first time a book or article is mentioned in a footnote, all the information about publication should appear in the footnote; after that, references to the same source can be shortened to the author's last name and the page number cited. When a periodical is concerned, a later reference need contain only the author's name, the journal name, and the page number.

Detailed information about footnote preparation can be obtained from *The Chicago Manual of Style* or one of several published reference manuals for office workers.

Final Bibliography. All scientific papers should carry a complete bibliography of source materials. List only those sources that directly pertain to the paper and were used in its preparation. The form of bibliographies is fairly uniform.

A periodical listing includes:

- Author's name and initials
- Title of article
- Name of periodical
- Volume number
- Pages cited
- Date of publication

A book reference includes:

- Author's name and initials
- Title of book
- Edition (only after first edition)
- Place of publication
- Name of publisher
- Year of publication

Bibliographies may be arranged alphabetically according to authors' names or numerically as the references appear in the text. Whatever form and punctuation are used should be consistent throughout the entire listing.

Illustrations. All drawings, photographs, and other illustrative material submitted with a manuscript should be placed on separate sheets and keyed to the manuscript. In other words, illustrations should be numbered and indications noted in the manuscript as to where each illustration should be placed. Do not include such materials in the body of the manuscript. The explanation of the drawing or illustration should appear in a caption or legend.

Glossy black and white photographs reproduce best. Captions for photos should be typed on separate sheets or may be attached with rubber cement below the photo. On the back of the photograph the author's name and the number of the illustration should be penciled lightly. Do not use paper clips on photos. Credit lines should be given for copyrighted or commercial photos or illustrations. If x-ray films are submitted, make sure the prints are shiny; indicate on the back where they may be cropped, but leave localizing landmarks.

Charts and line drawings must be carefully prepared in order to get good reproduction. Such drawings preferably should be done with India or black ink on heavy white bond paper. Charts should be condensed and simplified as much as possible. Letters and identifying numerals can be placed on the face of the chart with the explanation in the legend below.

Tables should be typewritten on separate sheets in a uniform style; each table should be numbered consecutively and have a descriptive heading.

Mailing the Manuscript. Generally, manuscripts should not be folded but should be mailed flat in a large envelope. Sometimes a paper of fewer than four pages can be folded twice and mailed in a regular business envelope, or a manuscript of four to eight pages can be folded once and mailed in a 6 by 9 envelope. A letter stating that the manuscript is being submitted for publication should be enclosed. Photos and illustrations should be mailed flat, between protective cardboards.

Proofreading. A paper accepted for publication will be set in type, and proofs of the article will usually be returned by the editor to the author for checking. Since changes in a manuscript once it is set in type are costly, revisions should be limited to correction of errors and minor changes.

If possible, work as a team when checking **galley proofs**, with one person holding the proofs and the other person reading from the original copy. Check for typographic errors, omitted lines and words, and so forth. When correcting proofs, use a different-colored pencil from the one used by the proofreader on the publication. Corrections should be entered in the margins of the proof, next to the line with the error to be corrected. A knowledge of proofreader's marks is helpful (Fig. 17–5).

One corrected set of galley proofs should be returned to the editor and one set of proofs should be retained by the author. If a second set of proofs is sent later, check the first corrected set against the second set to make sure all corrections have been made.

Indexing. Often it is necessary to provide an index for a long paper or a book. An author and subject index can be made from page proofs. One system for indexing is to use slips of paper or 3×5 cards. Each index entry is listed on a separate card or slip; this simplifies alphabetizing under major headings later. The whole index can then be typed from the alphabetized cards. Manuscripts prepared by computer can be indexed quickly and accurately with the necessary software.

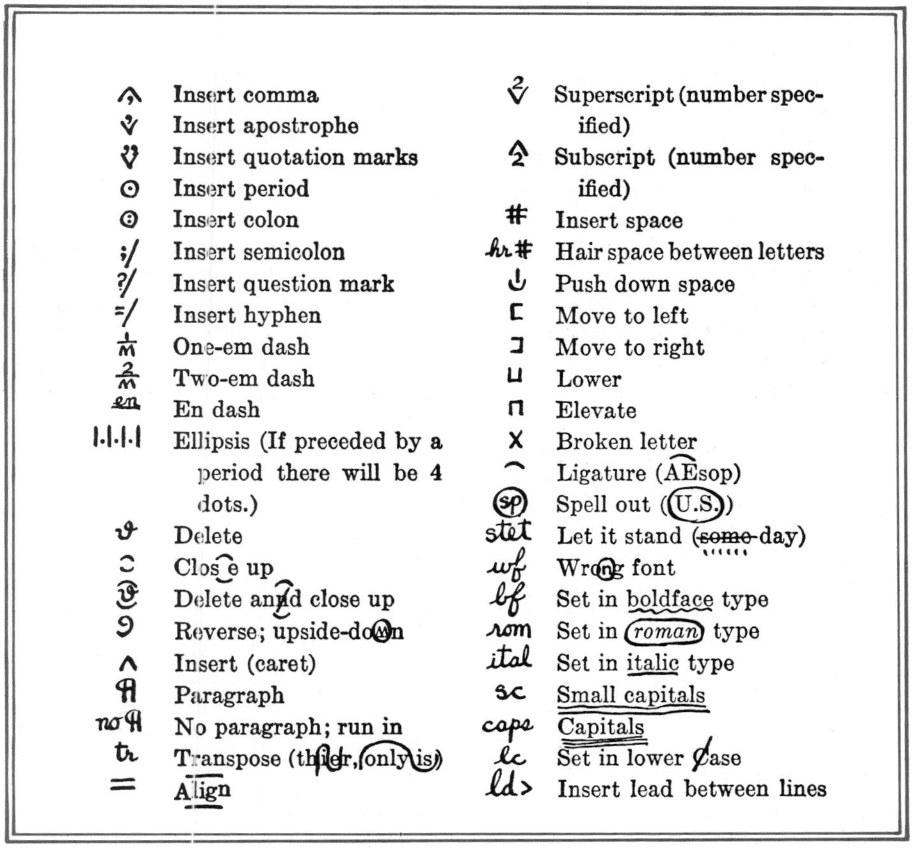

Figure 17–5
Proofreader's marks.

Reprints. At the time an article is set in type the physician should order all reprints needed, since type is often destroyed after the original press run. Most doctors send copies of their articles to colleagues, to physicians who have evidenced an interest in their work, and to hospitals and teaching institutions with which they have had contact. They will probably maintain a card file of names and addresses of those to whom they want to send reprints.

The medical assistant will generally handle the ordering of the reprints, which may be as many as 500 copies or more. The order should be adequate to cover any future needs. Addresses in the card file should be checked from time to time in the *American Medical Directory* or by scanning membership and request lists. Some record of reprint mailing should be kept and acknowledgments checked. A person who does not acknowledge two or three reprints should be taken from the mailing list.

An enclosure card, printed in advance, is sent by some authors with a copy of the reprint. Others prefer to enclose a short letter stating that the reprint is a complimentary copy.

Speeches. Not all papers are intended for publication. Some are prepared for presentation before medical and scientific meetings. Speeches should be typed double-space; in some offices a jumbo or magnatype machine is used so that the speech is easy to read. Special large-type elements, such as the IBM Orator, are available for single element typewriters.

At the bottom of each page, in the lower right-hand corner, type the first two or three words that appear at the beginning of the next page. The final draft of the paper should be carefully checked for typographic errors.

At large meetings a speaker is usually allotted from 10 to 20 minutes to present a paper; at county society and small meetings the speaker may have from 30 minutes to an hour for the presentation. Check in advance to find out exactly how much time will be allowed. The doctor or the medical assistant should time the speech. On the average it takes about 2 minutes to read a page of copy on which there are about 200 to 250 words. If slides or other illustrations are planned, arrangements for showing this material must be made in advance and the necessary time allowed.

MEETING AND TRAVEL ARRANGEMENTS

Meeting Calendar

A calendar of all meetings that the physician plans to attend should be kept by the medical assistant, with both the physician and the medical assistant retaining a copy. The calendar can be merely a sheet of paper but should include the following for each event:

- Name of meeting
- Date
- Place
- Time

Any changes or additions to the calendar should be made on both copies as notices are received. A reminder to the physician a few days in advance of each meeting is usually appreciated.

Transportation and Hotel Arrangements

The medical assistant may also have the responsibility of making transportation and hotel arrangements for the doctor for out-of-town meetings. Although the doctor who is located in a metropolitan area will probably use a travel agent for most travel arrangements, the medical assistant may be responsible for working with the travel agent and preparing the detailed itinerary.

The medical assistant who does not deal with a travel agent may be expected to personally make the hotel and transportation arrangements. Keep a file of the telephone numbers of railroads, airlines, and buses, and descriptions and telephone numbers of hotels. Ask for confirmation of all hotel arrangements. The doctor who is a member of an auto club can use membership privileges to obtain names of good hotels and motels, road maps, and other vital travel information.

Itinerary

When all arrangements are final, typewrite the itinerary. Keep one copy in the office file. Give the doctor the original and several copies for distribution to family members or other individuals. Since it is sometimes necessary to reach the doctor while traveling, it is important that the itinerary be carefully prepared, including locations and telephone numbers.

Meeting Responsibilities

The physician often accepts official responsibilities in his or her professional society or on the hospital board. The administrative medical assistant for this physician may be expected to assist in arranging meetings, preparing an agenda, and typing minutes of the meeting dictated by the physician.

The medical assistant who takes an active part in a professional society for medical assistants will have personal use for these skills as well.

Procedure 17–1

MAKING TRAVEL ARRANGEMENTS

PROCEDURAL GOAL

To make travel arrangements for physician from city of residence to Toronto, Canada.

EQUIPMENT AND SUPPLIES

Travel plan
Telephone
Telephone directory
Typewriter
Typing paper

PROCEDURE

1. Verify details of planned trip:
   a. Desired date and time of departure
   b. Desired date and time of return
   c. Preferred mode of transportation
   d. Number in party
   e. Preferred lodging and price range
2. Telephone travel agency to arrange for transportation and lodging reservations.
3. Arrange for travelers cheques if desired.
4. Pick up tickets or arrange for their delivery.
5. Check tickets to confirm conformance with travel plan.
   Purpose: To avoid any error due to misunderstanding and to check on compliance with requests.
6. Check to see if hotel reservations are confirmed.
7. Prepare itinerary, including all the necessary information:
   a. Date and time of departure
   b. Flight numbers or identifying information of other modes of travel
   c. Mode of transportation to hotel(s)
   d. Name, address, and telephone number of hotel(s), with confirmation numbers if available
   e. Date and time of return
8. Place one copy of itinerary in office file.
   Purpose: It may be necessary to contact the doctor or to forward mail.
9. Give several copies of itinerary to physician.
   Purpose: Physician may wish to have extra copies for family or friends.

TERMINAL PERFORMANCE OBJECTIVE

Given the listed equipment and supplies, make arrangements for physician's trip from city of residence to Toronto, Canada, and prepare detailed itinerary, within 1 hour, to a performance level of 95%. (Time will vary.)

17

Arranging a Meeting. You will need to have advance information of:

- The purpose of the meeting
- How many will be expected to attend
- Whether a meal is to be included
- The expected duration of the meeting
- The date, time, and place
- To whom notices are to be sent

Choosing the Location. Some groups meet regularly, using the same facility each time. In this case it is necessary merely to confirm the date and time with the facility. If a meal will be served, the menu, price, and approximate number expected to attend will need to be determined. If a new location is being used, you will need to determine that:

- The space is adequate

- Parking facilities are available if needed
- Lighting and ventilation are adequate
- Menus are available if a meal is to be included

Notice of Meeting. Meeting notices are usually mailed to all members of the group. For a small committee meeting, the notice may be made by telephone. If there is to be a speaker, the name of the speaker and the topic will be included in the meeting notice. The notice must include the date, time, and place.

Preparing the Agenda. Organizations whose by-laws specify *Robert's Rules of Order, Newly Revised,* as the parliamentary authority, and which have not adopted a special order of business, use the following prescribed **order of business:**

1. Reading and approval of minutes
2. Reports of officers, boards, and standing committees
3. Reports of special (select or ad hoc) committees
4. Special orders
5. Unfinished business and general orders
6. New business

Procedure 17–2

ARRANGING GROUP MEETINGS

PROCEDURAL GOAL

To arrange a breakfast meeting for the physician's hospital committee.

EQUIPMENT AND SUPPLIES

Directory of committee members
Meeting plan
Telephone
Typewriter
Post cards

PROCEDURE

1. Verify the proposed date and time for the meeting.
2. Gather details for meeting arrangements:
   a. Purpose of meeting
   b. Expected attendance
   c. Name of speaker, if any, and program topic
   d. Expected duration of meeting
3. Arrange meeting room based on requirements.
4. Mail notice of meeting to members and invited guests. Include:
   a. Date
   b. Time
   c. Place
   d. Name of speaker and topic
   e. Cost, if any
   f. Registration information
5. Arrange for any necessary equipment (microphone, projector, screen, etc.).
6. Notify meeting place of number of reservations, if required.
7. Arrange for registration check-in.
8. Prepare agenda.
9. Give required number of copies of agenda to physician.

TERMINAL PERFORMANCE OBJECTIVE

Given the listed equipment and supplies, arrange all details of a breakfast meeting for the physician's hospital committee according to the agency's standards, within 1 hour, to a performance level of 95%. (Time will vary according to number of details and notices to prepare.)

The order of business lists the different divisions of business in the order in which each will be called for at business meetings.

An **agenda** is a list of the specific items under each division of the order of business that the officers or board plan to present to a meeting. The medical assistant who is expected to prepare the agenda should determine what topics are to be discussed, type them in the prescribed order, and duplicate enough copies for the meeting. For a large group the program is usually printed. For the smaller group, photocopies are satisfactory.

Preparing Minutes. The record of the proceedings of a meeting is called the minutes. The minutes contain mainly a record of what was done at the meeting, not what was said by the members.

The first paragraph of the minutes should contain the following information:

- The kind of meeting (regular, special, and so forth)
- The name of the association
- The date, time, and place of the meeting
- The fact that the regular chairman and secretary were present or, in their absence, the names of the persons who substituted for them
- Whether the minutes of the previous meeting were read and approved

The body of the minutes should contain a separate paragraph for each subject matter. It should include all main motions including:

- The wording in which each motion was adopted or otherwise disposed of
- The disposition of the motion
- The name of the mover

The name of the seconder of the motion should not be entered in the minutes unless ordered by the assembly. The body of the minutes should also include any points of order and appeals, whether they were sustained or lost, and the reasons given by the chair for the ruling. The minutes may include the name and subject of a guest speaker, but no attempt should be made to summarize the speech.

The last paragraph should state the hour of adjournment.

The minutes should be signed by the secretary. In some organizations the president also signs the minutes. The practice of including the words "Respectfully submitted" is obsolete and should not be used.

The medical assistant who might be expected to type the minutes of meetings should consult an authoritative book on the subject and prepare a model to follow in typing the minutes of each meeting so that every set of minutes will be in the same style.

REFERENCES AND READINGS

Robert's Rules of Order, Newly Revised. Glenview, IL, Scott, Foresman and Co., 1981.

Strunk, W., Jr., and White, E.B.: *The Elements of Style,* 3rd ed. New York, Macmillan, 1979.

University of Chicago Press: *The Chicago Manual of Style,* 12th ed. Chicago, The Press, 1982.

Valancy, J.: Information at your fingertips: Tapping the resources. Physician's Management, April 1984, pp. 29–32.

17

CHAPTER OUTLINE

Planning and Organizing Facilities
    General Environment
    Area Utilization and Care

Maintenance
Furniture and Equipment

Supplies
    Procedure 18–1: Establishing and
        Maintaining a Supply Inventory
        and Ordering System

Doctor's Bag
Safety and Security Considerations

VOCABULARY

See Glossary at end of book for definitions.

Capital purchase	Caustics	Inventory
Categorically	Expendable	Reputable

18

Facilities and Supplies: Organization and Care

OBJECTIVES

Upon successful completion of this chapter you should be able to:

1. Define the terms listed in the Vocabulary of this chapter.
2. List seven areas of concern in the general environment of the medical facility.
3. Discuss the utilization of various areas of the medical facility.
4. Describe how the medical assistant would arrange for and supervise a maintenance service.
5. Explain the inventory process.
6. Explain the importance of the instructions and warranties accompanying new equipment purchases.
7. Cite precautions to be observed in storing poisons, narcotics, acids and caustics, and flammable items.
8. Discuss the procedure for storing supplies and drug samples.
9. List six possible safety hazards in a medical facility.
10. Discuss the importance of and procedures in routine office security.

Upon successful completion of this chapter you should be able to perform the following activities:

1. Write instructions for a maintenance service.
2. Set up an equipment inventory.
3. Organize and dispose of drug samples.
4. Establish and maintain a supply inventory and ordering system.

PLANNING AND ORGANIZING FACILITIES

The same principles of organization and planning that guide the business management of a medical office are essential in the organization and care of the facilities and supplies. A comfortable, attractive, clean environment lifts the spirits of patients and contributes to the efficiency and enthusiasm of the staff.

General Environment

Temperature. The ideal temperature for a reception room is about 74°F. Working areas can be somewhat cooler. There should be a constant change of air by means of open windows or air conditioning. However, you should guard against drafts, as people who are ill are very susceptible to chills.

Lighting. Working areas need to be well-lighted. Fluorescent lights are usually preferred because the lighting is uniform and does not give off heat. Lamps in the reception area can be decorative, but they are useful only if carefully chosen and properly placed. They should be at reading height; if they are too high they will shine into the eyes of others in the waiting room. Lighting, furnishings, and comfort of the reception room are fully discussed in Chapter 7.

Walls and Floor Coverings. Carpeting is usually the choice for floor covering in the reception area and often in the physician's consultation room. Unsecured rugs should never be used in a medical facility. In the clinical areas, a smooth washable floor covering such as vinyl or tile is generally more satisfactory. If wax is used on the floor covering, specify that it be the nonskid variety.

Wallpaper can add a pleasant atmosphere in the reception area. In the administrative and clinical areas a good quality wall paint in soft colors is attractive, easily cleaned, and long-lasting.

Traffic Control. The furnishings in the entrance and reception areas should be arranged to allow easy traffic without crowding in any one area. The reception desk must be placed so that anyone coming into the office can easily spot the desk, and so that the medical assistant at the desk can view the entire reception area (see Chapter 7). In the inner office the doctor and the other members of the staff should be able to pass from one station to another without creating a roadblock.

Sound Control. Walls should be soundproof if possible, to prevent voices and conversation from being heard from one room to another.

Privacy. Treatment rooms should be arranged so that the patient is out of view if it should be necessary to open the door to a hallway.

Efficiency. The physician and medical assistant must be able to move easily within each room and have access to equipment and supplies as needed.

Area Utilization and Care

The medical facility, whether large or small, is separated by utilization into these areas:

- Reception
- Administration
- Clinical activities
- Lavatories
- Storage and utility

The overall cleaning and maintenance of these areas will probably be done by an outside service under the direction of the medical assistant or office manager. However, additional individual attention will be required by the staff. In some instances, particularly in rural areas, it may be the sole responsibility of the medical assistant.

Good housekeeping begins with having a place for everything, and keeping everything clean and ready for use. Good housekeeping saves time and energy, conserves property, and eliminates incorrect use of materials. Poor housekeeping holds potential dangers for patients, physicians, and assistants alike.

RECEPTION AREA

The importance of a neat, attractive reception room was discussed in Chapter 7, Patient Reception. Draperies, carpet, and upholstery should be cleaned at regular intervals in addition to the daily maintenance.

ADMINISTRATION AREA

The administration area includes the reception desk, the records storage, telephone equipment, business machines such as typewriters, computer, calculators, photocopier, and so forth. This area should be separated from the reception room by a locked door. Records and business papers on the reception desk should be placed in desk trays where they will be safe and out of sight of visitors during the day, and in locked files at night. Personal items should be put away in a drawer or locker.

CLINICAL AREA

The clinical area includes the physician's consultation room, which is used for patient interviews and for the physician's private study; patient examination and treatment rooms; the laboratory; and a recovery room where patients may rest after therapy or minor surgery.

Consultation Room. The physician's consultation room should always be kept neat and clean. Give this room a quick once-over after each patient visit and remove any evidence of the departing patient. Follow the preferences of the physician with respect to straightening the desk or other furnishings.

Examination and Treatment Rooms. Examination/treatment rooms are designed for utility; only necessary equipment and supplies should be found here. Instruments, medications, and other supplies are in cabinets or drawers (Fig. 18–1). Supply cabinets should be checked daily before the first patient arrives (Fig. 18–2). The room must be straightened and all counter tops and the sink wiped clean after each patient; disposable gowns, towels, and tissues disposed of and fresh linens provided; and the room left spotless. The temperature in these rooms is crucial to the comfort of the patients, who are often asked to disrobe and put on a gown.

Laboratory. The laboratory may be anything from a small closet to a large room. It must be kept clean, with everything in its place, in order for accurate work to be accomplished. Sterility must be maintained in the laboratory just as in the examination/treatment rooms. Laboratory table tops should be scrubbed after contact with any contaminated material, and the contaminated material properly disposed of by wrapping it in paper or plastic bags and placing it in a plastic-lined waste container. Autoclave any contaminated articles that are not disposable. Adequate ventilation in the laboratory is especially important. There are many odors from the laboratory that the office staff becomes accustomed to but which may be disagreeable to patients.

Recovery Room. The recovery room should be comfortable, clean, and quiet. Provide facilities so that patients can relax and keep warm. Interesting reading material will help the time pass more pleasantly. If the patient wishes to sleep, see that no one enters the room.

LAVATORIES

In the small solo practice office, the lavatory may be shared by staff and patients. In this situation every member of the staff should be instructed to leave the room meticulously clean. Most medical facilities provide a separate lavatory for patients. This room must be checked by the medial assistant after each use to be certain it is left clean and that all supplies are replenished as needed.

STORAGE AND UTILITY ROOMS

There must be storage space for office and medical supplies, cleaning equipment and supplies, staff lockers or coat hooks, and so forth. The size of these spaces will vary, but whatever area is available must be kept organized and supplies and other items kept in order. Storage and utility rooms are generally closed to all except the staff.

MAINTENANCE

Responsibilities of Staff. One member of the staff, often the administrative medical assistant, is delegated the responsibility of overseeing the maintenance of the premises. The details should be

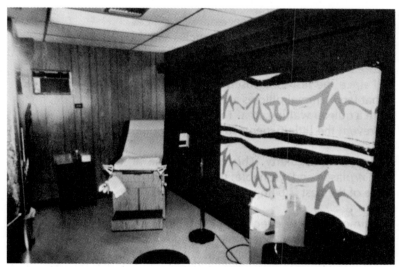

Figure 18–1
A clean, neat, and orderly patient examination room.

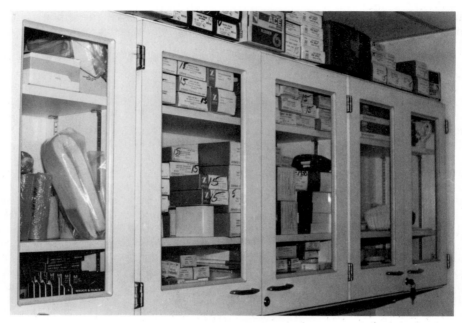

Figure 18–2
An example of a neat cabinet for orthopedic supplies.

outlined in the office policy and procedure manual (see Chapter 19).

Each member of the staff will probably wish to tidy and dust his or her own desk or work station, with the administrative medical assistant taking care of the physician's desk.

The clinical medical assistant will usually be the one who periodically cleans the interior of cabinets and drawers in the examination/treatment rooms. This should be done only when there is time to complete the job. Do one shelf at a time, starting at the top.

1. *Remove all items from the shelf and place on a table in the same order as on the shelf.*
2. *Wash the shelf and rinse well. Dry.*
3. *Clean and polish the instruments and check for faults. Examine hinges and blades.*
4. *Check all labels on containers for clarity. Reglue labels, if necessary. Examine supplies for expiration dates, quantity, and deterioration. Make a list of those items that should be reordered.*
5. *Replace the supplies in their original places on the shelf.*

Clean the tops of cabinets and the undersides of towel and tape dispensers as necessary. These areas are frequently overlooked in the daily cleaning.

Maintenance services do not usually include as part of their service such tasks as cleaning mirrors, replacing light bulbs, cleaning the refrigerator, daily cleaning of sinks, straightening magazines, and watering plants. These and numerous other occa-sional as well as daily jobs are performed by the office staff.

Instructions to Maintenance Service. Every member of the staff must be alert to any problem of cleanliness or safety that might be overlooked by the maintenance service, and report the condition to the medical assistant in charge. The staff member who has the responsibility for instructing the maintenance service must be able to plan and be explicit in giving instructions:

- Prepare a written list of the services that you expect.
- Go over it with the service people.
- Be specific about any areas that are not to be entered or disturbed.
- Set up a regular schedule.
- Evaluate the service regularly.
- Communicate your pleasure or displeasure promptly to the person in charge of performing the service.

FURNITURE AND EQUIPMENT

The physician, individually or as a member of a group practice, has a large investment in the furnishings and equipment necessary to carry on a medical practice. The medical assistant has a responsibility to properly use and care for any piece of equipment in order to preserve its useful life.

Acquisition. When a new piece of equipment is acquired, read the instructions thoroughly and carefully. Do not attempt to assemble or use items that you have not first studied. Keep the purchase invoice on file. The date of purchase and the cost are required for insurance and for depreciation credit on income tax.

Warranty Requirements. If there is a warranty card with the item, copy the code number, fill in the blanks, and mail as instructed.

Service. Keep a service file for equipment that needs regular servicing. This file should contain:

- Warranty dates
- Frequency of service
- When and by whom the item was last serviced
- Cost of service

File all instructions in a special folder and save them for future reference or for your successors.

Inventory. It is good business to **inventory** all equipment and supplies once a year. If you have an office computer, keep the inventory on disk for easy access and updating.

First, list all **capital purchases**, such as furniture, medical and surgical instruments, sterilizers and autoclaves, laboratory equipment, business machines, and any major pieces of artwork or artifacts. These items are permanent and usually expensive. List the date of purchase for each item, along with the original price.

Next, list the smaller, less costly items that are considered **expendable**, such as small instruments, syringes, and thermometers.

Last, estimate the usable supplies and drugs on hand. Keep this inventory to check against the inventory for the coming year. An inventory is valuable in preparing income tax, and especially in case of office burglary or loss from other causes.

SUPPLIES

Selection of Supplies and Suppliers. Supplies are those items that are expendable and must be ordered more or less frequently. In the administrative functions of the practice, these will include:

- Stationery and filing supplies
- Appointment books and cards
- Accounting supplies
- Small desk items such as paper clips, staples, typewriter ribbons, pens and pencils

In the clinical area, expendable supplies will include:

- Examination/treatment items such as disposable scopes, specula, lubricants, tongue blades, applicators, syringes and needles, dressings, and bandages
- Paper gowns, drapes, towels
- Autoclaving and sterilizing supplies

For general usage, you will need to order:

- Soap and towels for lavatories
- Cleaning supplies
- Tissues
- Items for staff lounge

In general, the person who will use the item is the best person to select what is to be ordered, but it is probably best for one person only to be in charge of ordering all supplies. The purchasing agent in the local hospital is a good soure of information on supplies and their sources.

Since there is such a variety of supplies needed, you will have to use more than one supplier. Study the market and find the items that are best suited to the practice with respect to quality and packaging, and order from the suppliers who offer the best service and prices. You should make periodic price checks, but do not sacrifice convenience and service for the sake of saving a few pennies.

Ordering Supplies. There should be an established method for ordering supplies. Keep a list or running inventory from which you can note diminishing supplies and determine when to re-order. Representatives of supply houses regularly call at physicians' offices and are often very helpful in suggesting new items and answering questions about what is available to meet your needs. Mail-order houses also send catalogs describing a great variety of equipment and supplies that can be ordered by mail.

It is advisable to establish good credit with several **reputable** supply companies, both local and mail-order, to provide a choice of vendors. However, do not shift your purchases from company to company without good reason. The loyal customer usually receives better service and may enjoy special privileges, such as being given the option of trying out a piece of equipment before actually agreeing to purchase it.

Attention to detail in ordering will speed delivery and assure greater accuracy. Use the actual title of the supply being ordered, including any special name, size, color, and so forth. The order should state whether payment is enclosed or whether the purchase is to be charged to the physician's account.

Prevention of Waste. In some cases the unit cost of an item may be reduced by purchasing in larger quantities, but this is not always a saving. Make this decision only after considering the following questions:

1. Will the supply be used in a reasonable length of time?
2. Will it spoil or deteriorate?
3. Is there sufficient space for storage?
4. Will the practice continue to use the product?

Receiving and Storing. All orders should be placed in the storage area and opened only when

18

Procedure 18-1

ESTABLISHING AND MAINTAINING A SUPPLY INVENTORY AND ORDERING SYSTEM

PROCEDURAL GOAL

To establish an inventory of all expendable supplies in the physician's office and follow an efficient system of order control using a card system.

EQUIPMENT AND SUPPLIES

File box
Inventory and order control cards
List of supplies on hand
Metal tabs
Re-order tags
Pen or pencil

PROCEDURE

1. Write the name of each item on a separate card.
   Purpose: To establish a record of all items in inventory.
2. Write the amount on hand of each item in the space provided.
   Purpose: To establish beginning inventory.
3. Place a re-order tag at the point where the supply should be replenished.
   Purpose: Tag will serve as an alert that supply is low.
4. Place a metal tab over the *order* section of the card.
   Purpose: Metal tab will be reminder to include this item in next order.
5. When the order has been placed, note the date and quantity ordered and move the tab to *on order* section of the card.
6. When the order is received, note the date and quantity in the appropriate column, remove the tab, and refile the card.
   Note: If the order is only partially filled, let the tab remain until order is complete.

TERMINAL PERFORMANCE OBJECTIVE

Given the listed equipment and supplies, establish and maintain a supply inventory and ordering system according to agency's needs, to a performance level of 100%. (Time will vary according to number of items.)

you have time to check the contents. Compare the items in the package with your original purchase order and the invoice included with the shipment. Check for correct items, sizes, and styles as well as the number or amount received. Note any back orders and discrepancies. When you are satisfied that the order is correct and complete, make the necessary notations on the inventory and order cards and place the items in their designated storage areas.

If you have any questions regarding the order or if you have a complaint to make, gather the following information before contacting the supplier:
• Invoice number
• Date ordered
• Name of person who placed order

List on paper your questions and the information you desire. If a catalog was used in placing the order, open your copy to the correct page and secure any additional pertinent information. With all this information at hand you can make a professional inquiry by letter or telephone.

Follow good housekeeping standards in storing supplies. Place supplies where they are most accessible yet protected from damage and exposure to moisture, heat, light, and air.

Most drugs and solutions should be stored in a cool, dark cupboard, because direct light and sunlight cause drug deterioration.

Poisons should be stored in a locked compartment and kept separate from products used routinely. Have a distinct label or cap for poisons. A

ORDER | (ITEM NAME) 3-ply Disposable Drape Sheets (white) 7459 | **ON ORDER**

ORDER QUANTITY __300__   REORDER POINT __100__

ORDER	QTY	REC'D	COST	PREPAID	ON ACCT	ORDER	QTY	REC'D	COST	PREPAID	ON ACCT
1/25	300	2/10	64.95	X							

INVENTORY COUNT

	JAN	FEB	MAR	APR	MAY	JUNE	JULY	AUG	SEPT	OCT	NOV	DEC
19 _87_	200											
19 ____												

ORDER SOURCE   UNIT PRICE

The Colwell Company   100 – $23.95

201 Kenyon Road   300 – $64.95

Champaign, IL 61820

FORM 2450 COLWELL CO., CHAMPAIGN, ILLINOIS

**RED FLAG
RE-ORDER TAG**

when this inventory
point is reached,
its time to reorder

Product
Identification

The Colwell Company
Champaign, Illinois

18

bright red color for their labels or caps may be useful.

Narcotics must be stored in a secure place out of sight.

Acids and **caustics** should have special resistant lids; never use metal lids for these substances. Do not store strong acids next to alkalis.

Inflammable items must be stored away from heat.

If drugs and solutions are to be stored for some time, the stoppers should be dipped in paraffin to seal them from the air. Do not fill these bottles to the very top; leave a little room for expansion.

Labels. If a bottle is to be used for a long time, the label should be indestructible. The original label should be treated for preservation when it is first received. When using the contents of the bottle, pour away from the label side to prevent any dripping on the label. Plastic screw caps protect the lip of the bottle and keep it clean.

When a label shows signs of wear or mutilation, or is difficult to read, replace the entire bottle and solution for safety purposes.

Drug Samples. Samples of drugs and medications that are suitable to the physician's practice should be organized **categorically** in a sample cupboard or drawer.

Place all similar drugs together, preferably in boxes of similar size and shape, with the tops open and plainly labeled on the outside. Clear plastic boxes are excellent for this type of storage. Color-coded labels are an additional help in identification.

Keep all the sedative samples in one box, all stimulant samples in another, and so forth. It is good practice to band together drug samples that have the same code number or expiration date. Rotate the drugs by placing the most recently received items in back of those that were previously on hand. At regular intervals check all samples for expiration dates, and properly dispose of those that have expired.

THE DOCTOR'S BAG

Minutes may mean the difference between life or death in a medical emergency. The doctor's bag must be completely fitted and ready for use at any hour of the day or night. Any medical assistant who is given this responsibility must regard it seriously and give it close and continual attention.

The items that are included in the bag will depend upon professional requirements, the kinds of emergencies that are responded to, and the personal preferences of the person using it. That person could be the physician, a physician's assistant, a nurse practitioner, or an emergency medical technician.

Following is a basic inventory of items commonly found in a physician's bag:

Blood pressure set	Sterile hemostatic forceps
Stethoscope	Sterile syringes and
Thermometers (oral and rectal)	needles (preferably disposable)
Flashlight or penlight	Sterile swabs
Sterile gloves and lubricant	Sterile dressings
Wooden applicators	Tongue depressors
Assorted bandages	Scissors
Adhesive tape (assorted widths)	Sterile dressing forceps
Safety pins	Aspiration equipment
Towel	Microscopic slides and fixative
Ballpoint pens	Containers for specimens
Prescription pads	Culture tubes for throat cultures
Sterile suture set	Medications:
Sterile scalpel	Adrenalin
Probe	Digitalis
Tourniquet	Antibiotics
Percussion hammer	Antihistamines
Illuminated diagnostic set (otoscope and ophthalmoscope)	Alcohol and/or skin disinfectant
Sterile tissue forceps	Sterilizing solution
	Spirits of ammonia

As a guide, keep an inventory of the bag's contents posted inside a cupboard above the place where you check and clean the bag. When checking the bag after a patient has been tended to, remove any specimens and see that they are properly labeled with the patient's full name, the date, and the type of test if the specimen is to be sent out for examination.

If any instruments or gloves have been used, remove them and replace with sterile ones. Even if this equipment has not been used, it should be sterilized weekly. Keep the containers of alcohol, germicides, and other substances filled, and check containers often for any leakage. Allow a small space for heat expansion in containers of fluid.

SAFETY AND SECURITY CONSIDERATIONS

Detection of Hazards. The physician and every member of the staff should continually monitor possible hazards to themselves and the patients.

The reception room and public areas of the facility are particularly vulnerable. Are the chairs in the reception room safe for children? . . . for an exceptionally heavy patient? . . . for a physically disadvantaged patient? Are there any exposed telephone or light cords that someone could trip on? . . . lamps that could tip?

In the examining rooms, be especially careful to put away any sharp instruments, hazardous liquids, or medications. Any spills on the floor should be wiped immediately to prevent a fall or slipping. Keep prescription pads out of sight.

Are the stairways and entrances to the facility well lighted and safe? Are there any known hazards in the parking area?

Drug Enforcement Administration (DEA) Regulations. A physician who has controlled substances (narcotics) stored on the premises must keep these drugs in a locked cabinet or safe. Any loss of controlled drugs by theft must be reported to the regional office of the DEA at the time the theft is discovered. The local police department and the State Bureau of Narcotic Enforcement should also be notified.

Smoke Alarms and Fire Extinguishers. Smoke alarms are required in all new buildings and should be installed in every existing medical facility. Their functioning must be checked regularly to ensure effectiveness if they should be needed. There should be a fire extinguisher readily accessible to any part of the facility.

Fire Exits. Fire exits should be clearly marked and the staff instructed on evacuation proceedings in case of fire.

Contact with Security Systems. If the doctor's office is located in a multiple unit building or medical complex, know whom to contact if a security emergency should occur. Have the telephone number handy for local fire and police departments (911 in many areas).

Routine Office Security. Within the office all valuables should be kept out of sight. A frequent target of thieves is the medical assistant's handbag, which is often left under a desk or table, where it can be easily spotted by an intruder.

It is most important to secure all entrances—windows as well as doors. Have good double locks put on by a reliable locksmith. It may be well worth the cost to consult a professional security service and follow their advice. Making an office burglar-proof is impossible, but entry can be made difficult, and this in itself will usually discourage the amateur.

---

warning

WE HAVE JOINED
OPERATION IDENTIFICATION
ALL ITEMS OF VALUE
ON THESE PREMISES
HAVE BEEN INDELIBLY MARKED
FOR READY IDENTIFICATION
BY LAW ENFORCEMENT AGENCIES

Figure 18–3
Sign for office window indicating that valuables have been marked for purposes of identification.

Outside sensor lights with unbreakable shields are extremely helpful. Leaving a light burning and a radio playing inside the office are additional deterrents. Tell the local police or the building security force which lights will always be left on.

Alarms can be helpful if they are reliable and are not easily disconnected by an expert. Loud local alarms are usually sufficient to frighten off a prowler. It is possible, if greater security is needed, to install an alarm system that will ring in the local police station or at a special security office.

Police departments urge that all valuables be protected by etching them with personal identification, such as the owner's name or social security number. This is easily done with an electric engraving tool that cuts into the equipment, and the marking is practically impossible to eradicate. Even if an attempt is made to scratch it off, a sufficient impression will be left so that police, with the aid of a special chemical, can bring the engraved characters up again (Fig. 18–3).

The most effective step in protecting your premises against break-ins is to remember to check carefully at the end of every day to make certain that all doors and windows are doubly locked.

18

CHAPTER OUTLINE

Purpose of Management
Qualities of a Supervisor
Management Duties
Personnel Management
    Office Policy Manual
    Recruiting
    Orientation and Training
    Performance and Salary Review
    Dismissal

Office Management
    Staff Meetings
    Office Procedure Manual

Practice Development
    Patient Education

Financial Management
    Payroll Records
    Income Tax Withholding
    Federal Unemployment Tax (FUTA)
    State Unemployment Taxes
    State Disability Insurance

Special Duties
    Moving a Practice
    Closing a Practice

VOCABULARY

See Glossary at end of book for definitions.

ancillary
appraisal
candid
circumvention
discrimination

disseminate
insubordination
meticulous
motivation

orientation
philosophy
probationary
recruit

Management Responsibilities

19

OBJECTIVES

Upon successful completion of this chapter you should be able to:

1. Define the terms listed in the Vocabulary of this chapter.
2. State the purpose and goals of medical office management.
3. Discuss the desirable qualities of an office manager and their importance in the selection of a supervisor.
4. Identify the goals of an office policy manual and how they may be achieved.
5. Discuss the steps in the hiring and dismissal of employees.
6. List five kinds of staff meetings.
7. Explain how a procedure manual differs from a policy manual.
8. Discuss the concept of practice development and its importance.
9. List at least 10 features of a patient information folder.
10. State two advantages of patient instruction sheets.
11. Discuss the supervisor's role in financial management.
12. Identify the source of reference for information on employer taxes and deposit requirements.

Upon successful completion of this chapter you should be able to perform the following activities:

1. Interview an applicant for a position, utilizing the guidelines in this chapter.
2. Prepare an outline of contents for a basic office policy manual.
3. Write a procedure sheet for a specific task.
4. Outline a patient information folder.
5. Outline a financial policies folder.
6. Write a patient instruction sheet.
7. Complete an Employer's Quarterly Federal Tax Return.

PURPOSE OF MANAGEMENT

The purpose of management in a medical practice is to provide a quiet, functional environment in which the physician(s) can see and treat patients, provide competent medical care, safely store medical records, and bill and collect for services in order to continue practicing medicine. We have learned that the daily functioning of a medical office involves a multitude of details and that good management does not just happen.

The lone medical assistant in a solo practice must be able to assume many of the management responsibilities with cooperation from the doctor. An office with three or more employees should have one person designated as supervisor or office manager. Other employees will answer to the supervisor; the supervisor will answer to the physician(s). This sets up an orderly way for:

- The office staff to consult with the doctor regarding administrative or technical problems, complaints, or grievances
- The doctor to check on the operation of the office, **disseminate** information on policy changes, and correct errors or grievances

Management problems can often be avoided by carefully defining the areas of authority and responsibility of each employee. Many physicians say that friction between workers is their most common personnel problem. A definite chain of command must be established, and the physician must not undermine the supervisor's authority by **circumvention**. When employees know what is expected of them, they can plan both their daily and long-term work more effectively.

QUALITIES OF A SUPERVISOR

What qualities should a supervisor have? Job experience may be important, but the supervisor should also possess:

- Leadership ability
- Good judgment
- Good health
- Ability to organize
- Ability to learn and improve
- Original ideas
- A sense of fairness
- Strength to stand firm on policy, but enough flexibility to recognize when an exception should be made

The selection of the right person to supervise the employees is critical. The supervisor may come from within the ranks or may be selected as a new member of the staff. Some employees do not wish to assume management responsibilities; others may not have the necessary qualifications.

Running the administrative side of a medical

practice is a complex job that is getting more complex every day. The American Medical Association's Department of Practice Management offers workshops designed to help medical assistants hone their office skills. One workshop called "Team Building—A Better Way to Supervise" is especially designed to sharpen the supervisory skills needed by the medical office manager. Some practice management consultants conduct seminars for medical office personnel. These are often arranged through a chapter of the American Association of Medical Assistants or the local medical society.

MANAGEMENT DUTIES

Medical office routines fall into three broad categories: patient scheduling, medical recordkeeping, and business management. We have dealt in detail with the first two categories in previous chapters. It is the third category, management processes, that concerns us here. The duties of an office manager or supervisor will of necessity vary with the practice, but may involve:

1. Personnel management
   a. Preparing and updating the office policy manual
   b. Recruiting
   c. Hiring
   d. Orientation and training
   e. Performance and salary review
   f. Dismissal
2. Office management
   a. Planning staff meetings
   b. Maintaining staff harmony
   c. Preparing procedure manual
   d. Establishing work flow guidelines
   e. Improving office efficiency
   f. Supervising purchase and care of equipment
   g. Patient education
   h. Eliminating time wasters for physician
   i. Practice marketing
3. Financial management
   a. Supervising cash transactions
   b. Maintaining payroll records
   c. Taking care of employee benefits

PERSONNEL MANAGEMENT

Office Policy Manual

An office policy manual serves as a training guide for the new employee, a ready reference for the temporary employee, and a reminder of policies for the regular employee. A policy manual accomplishes several goals:

- It solidifies what may have been vague thoughts into definite statements of policy.

- It communicates these statements in exactly the same way to every employee.
- It provides a permanent record of these policies.

This does not mean that the policies can never be changed, but a well-formulated policy may be the difference between order and chaos. The manual must be:

- Designed for a specific office
- Comprehensive but flexible
- Easy to read
- In conformance with professional ethics

The manual must be reviewed frequently and kept up-to-date as changes in policy occur.

Content of Policy Manual. What should be included in the policy manual? It should probably start with a statement of the **philosophy** of the practice and any general office policies, followed by a personnel chart showing the line of authority and stating who has authority to enforce the policies. The manual should also include professional information regarding the physician's education and specialty boards, hospital staff memberships, memberships in professional societies, state license number, and narcotic registry number.

Expectations regarding the personal appearance of employees should be set forth so that there is no misunderstanding. Guidelines regarding proper dress, use of make-up, nail polish, and perfume, cleanliness, grooming, and hygiene are difficult to discuss on a personal basis but can be matter-of-fact in an office manual.

Describe the work week, listing the daily office hours and any days off, the daily appointment schedule, and where the doctor can be reached with messages or emergencies. Specify the time allowed each day for lunch and breaks, and whether they must be taken at a specific time. Discuss the vacation policy, including how much vacation time the employee is allowed in terms of number of working days, who authorizes it, and whether there are any restrictions as to when vacation time may be taken.

What provision is there for sick leave, emergency leave, and any other absences? When is the employee eligible for benefits? Are medical services provided by the staff? What holidays does the office observe? What are the overtime policies?

Is there a policy for performance reviews, salary reviews, and merit increases? (See Fig. 19–1.) When is payday? Are there annual bonuses? If so, on what are they based? Are there other benefits for employees, such as payment of professional dues, health insurance, uniform allowances, pension plan, profit sharing, free parking? How much notice is expected if an employee wants to quit? What are grounds for immediate dismissal?

To whom should employees go with problems or suggestions? Is time off given for education courses or for attending professional organization conventions or seminars? If so, is this time counted as paid time or as vacation time? Does the office pay for courses, professional memberships, and expenses for professional conventions?

Recruiting

The office manager can be expected to initiate the **recruiting** and screening of prospective employees.

Name _____ Soc. Sec. No._____
Job Classification_____
Employment Date _____ Starting Salary_____

    Salary checks are issued every (week) (two weeks) (semi-monthly) (month) on_____(day or date).
    Increase-in-pay review will be conducted six months after the completion of three-month probationary period and each six months thereafter.
    Date of first pay review _____
    Current maximum salary for this job classification $_____
        Revised_____ $_____
        Revised_____ $_____

SALARY SCHEDULE

Date	Amount of Increase	Total Salary
_____	_____	_____
_____	_____	_____
_____	_____	_____
_____	_____	_____

Figure 19–1
Example of a page from an office policy manual.

19

Careful judgment and objectivity must be used in the search for an employee who will be suitable for the practice.

Preliminary Steps. Before interviewing any applicant, one should determine the following:

- What personal qualifications the applicant should have
- What the duties of the position are
- Salary range
- How soon the position will be open

Add any other specifications for the position. Then, after reviewing the policy manual, prepare an outline to guide you in selecting prospective applicants. Here are a few suggested guidelines:

- Do the applicant's appearance and personal grooming meet the standards set forth in the policy manual?
- Has the applicant been previously employed? What duties were performed?
- If previously employed, how long was the applicant in the last position? Why did the applicant leave?
- In what skills is the applicant proficient? Do these meet the requirements for the position as set forth in the office procedure manual? Does the applicant seem to accept and enjoy responsibility?
- What is the applicant's formal education? Certified Medical Assistant? If not certified, is the applicant interested in taking the certifying examination? Is the applicant a member of a professional organization? Does he or she attend meetings?

Arranging the Personal Interview. If the applicant sent a letter asking for an interview, note whether the letter was correctly typed, included the essential information, and provided a personal data sheet (see Chapter 20). Forget the applicant who sends a letter handwritten in pencil. By telephoning the applicant you will have an opportunity to judge the telephone voice. If it is poor, you may not wish to consider the applicant further.

Set a time for the personal interview when you most likely will be able to give the applicant your undivided attention. However, an applicant who is being considered for employment should have an opportunity to see your office when there is a fairly normal amount of activity. The prospective employee who is interviewed in a peaceful, quiet office on the doctor's day out may not be prepared for the activity on a normal working day.

The Interview. Before interviewing any applicant, make certain you are thoroughly familiar with the federal, state, and local fair-employment practice (FEP) laws affecting hiring practice. The pur-

pose of such laws is to prevent **discrimination** in the hiring of minority-group members, women, older people, the handicapped, and others. Unless you are up-to-date on these regulations, you could find yourself involved in an expensive lawsuit or settlement with a disappointed applicant claiming discrimination. These laws also determine what information you may request on an employment application. Check with the Department of Labor for current regulations.

Either send the applicant an application form to be completed and brought in at the time of the interview, or allow ample time for its completion on the day of the interview. The application form can serve as a check of the applicant's penmanship and thoroughness as well as a permanent record for your files. If you wish it completed in the applicant's own handwriting, be sure to state this on the instructions. The applicant should be **meticulous** about following instructions and filling in all the blanks (Fig. 19–2).

As you speak with the applicant, make a mental note of whether the applicant:

- Converses easily
- Is a good listener
- Is free of annoying mannerisms
- Has a ready smile
- Is interested enough to ask as well as to answer questions
- Appears interested in the office and the doctor's specialty

An interview should be a two-way exchange of information between applicant and interviewer. If the applicant appears to be one who will receive serious consideration, you have the responsibility of explaining what will be expected in the way of duties; office policies regarding appearance, working hours, overtime, time off, and vacations; what initial salary is offered, any fringe benefits, and the office policy on increases. Often the interviewer fails to mention these items, and the applicant may be hesitant to inquire.

Discuss the job description for the position being filled. This is essential if you are to be certain that the person being interviewed understands the required duties and responsibilities.

During the hiring proceedings, the interviewer may wish to invite the prospective employee to lunch with the staff, or for coffee in the more relaxed atmosphere of the employee lounge. This permits an opportunity to discover whether the applicant's personality will mesh with the atmosphere of the office.

Follow-up Activities. When the interview is over, take a few moments to immediately rate the applicant on your checklist. Jot down some notes to refresh your memory when you refer this applicant to the doctor for the final interview. Do not trust to memory, especially if several applicants will be interviewed. The following is a suggested checklist that may be modified to suit your own circumstances:

```
Name _____ Date _____ Time _____
                        Above
            Superior Average Average Poor Remarks
Appearance
   and groom-
   ing
General health
Voice and dic-
   tion
Mannerisms
Poise
Friendliness
Interest in
   work
Did applicant
   ask ques-
   tions?
Overall
   impression
```

If your employer is a member of a credit bureau, it may be advisable to request the applicant's permission to check his or her credit rating, especially if handling office finances will be one of the responsibilities. It can be safely assumed that one who is unable to handle personal financial affairs will be a poor risk in handling office finances.

Checking References. It is always advisable to carefully check all references, and follow through on any leads for information. It is best to use the telephone in checking references because people are sometimes less than **candid** in a letter; furthermore, letter writing is time-consuming and you may not get a reply.

Prepare a checklist before you place the call, and then when you talk with the person called be sure to "listen between the lines." Note the tone of the replies to your questions. Here are some questions you might ask in your inquiry:

```
Applicant's name _____
Name of reference called _____
Telephone No. _____
1. When did _____ work for you?
   How long? _____
2. What were the duties?
3. Why did the employee leave?
4. Would you rehire this person under the right
   circumstances?
5. Was there frequent absenteeism or tardiness?
6. Did the employee assume responsibility well?
7. Was there good rapport with other staff mem-
   bers?
8. Do you have any suggestions or advice about
   hiring this person?
```

Hiring. When a decision has been reached to hire someone, notify the applicant of your decision and state when the applicant will be expected to report for work.

Remember to notify all others who have applied. They may have hesitated to accept other interviews in the hope of hearing from you. It is unfair to keep individuals who are seeking employment "on the string." Good etiquette requires that you drop them a note or call by telephone, and say the position is filled. Thank the individual for applying, and say that you will keep the application on file.

Orientation and Training

Recruitment does not end with the hiring. Some preliminary **orientation** and training will help new employees to understand what is expected and to develop their full potential. Introduce the new employee to:

- The rest of the staff
- The physical environment by a tour of the entire facility
- The nature of the practice and specialty by explaining what type of patients will be dealt with and how the staff is expected to interact with them
- The office policies by having the employee read the policy manual and then discussing it
- Your long-range expectations, but not expecting that they will all be handled efficiently on the first day

Performance and Salary Review

A new employee should be granted a **probationary** period. Sixty to 90 days has been traditional, but many employers feel that 2 weeks is sufficient to determine whether the employee will be able to learn and adapt to the position.

A definite date for a performance review at the end of the probationary period should be set at the time of employment. This review should not be squeezed in between patient visits, or be given a token few minutes at the end of a day. There should be ample time to relax and talk. At this time the new employee is told how well expectations have been met and whether there are any deficiencies. Then give the employee an opportunity to ask questions. Sometimes an employee fails to perform because of never having been told what was expected.

The performance **appraisal** will include a judgment of both the quality and quantity of work, personal appearance, attitudes and team spirit, dependability, self-discipline, **motivation**, attendance, and any other qualities essential to satisfactory performance of the job in question.

Although the probationary period does not always allow time to fully train an individual for a

19

EMPLOYMENT APPLICATION

Prospective employees will receive consideration without discrimination because of race, creed, color, sex, age, national origin or handicap.

PERSONAL INFORMATION

Last Name	First	Middle	Date

Street Address	Home Phone ( ) —

City, State, Zip	Business Phone ( ) —

Have you ever applied for employment with us? ☐ Yes ☐ No If Yes: Month and Year _____ Location _____	Social Security No.

Position Desired	At what salary do you expect to start?

Apart from absence for religious observance, are you available for full-time work? ☐ Yes ☐ No If not, what hours can you work? _____	

Are you legally eligible for employment in the United States?	When will you be available to begin work? _____

Other special training or skills (languages, machine operation, etc.)	Whom to notify in emergency:

How did you learn of our organization?	

EDUCATIONAL BACKGROUND

SCHOOL	NAME AND LOCATION OF SCHOOL		NO. OF YEARS COM-PLETED	DID YOU GRADUATE?	DEGREE
College				☐ Yes ☐ No	
High				☐ Yes ☐ No	
Elementary				☐ Yes ☐ No	
Other				☐ Yes ☐ No	

MEMBERSHIP IN PROFESSIONAL OR CIVIC ORGANIZATIONS

Figure 19–2
Example of application used in a medical facility. (Courtesy of Medical Consultants, Anaheim, CA.)

PREVIOUS EMPLOYMENT

1

Company Name	Telephone ( ) –
Address	Employed (State Month and Year) From To
Name of Supervisor	Weekly Pay Start Last
State Job Title and Describe Your Work	Reason for Leaving

2

Company Name	Telephone ( ) –
Address	Employed (State Month and Year) From To
Name of Supervisor	Weekly Pay Start Last
State Job Title and Describe Your Work	Reason for Leaving

3

Company Name	Telephone ( ) –
Address	Employed (State Month and Year) From To
Name of Supervisor	Weekly Pay Start Last
State Job Title and Describe Your Work	Reason for Leaving

HOBBIES & OUTSIDE INTERESTS

_____

_____

Can you handle?

1. Medicare and Medi-Cal billing forms?_____

2. Compensation first reports and final billings?_____

3. All other insurance billings?_____

4. Disability Reports?_____

Typing speed:_____Bookkeeping abilities:_____

Computer experience_____Dictating equipment_____Transcription_____

Medical terminology_____Ability to complete neat, properly spaced,

and properly spelled letters_____

How long do you plan to work full time?_____

Date:_____   Signature_____

Figure 19–2 Continued

19

specific position, it is fair to assume that the potential for being a satisfactory employee can be judged at this time. Now is the time to talk out any problems and make suggestions for improvement.

The supervisor is responsible for an ongoing performance appraisal of all employees, complimenting whenever possible and appropriate, and offering helpful criticism when necessary. A formal performance appraisal at the end of the probationary period and at regular 6-month intervals thereafter, with a report to the physician employer, is helpful in the employee's salary review.

Dismissal

The necessity of having to dismiss an employee is unpleasant at best, but if the ground rules are decided upon in advance, written into the policy manual, and explained to all employees, the problem is partially solved. The policies must be applied equally and impartially to all. The final decision for dismissal will probably be made by the physician but may be based on the recommendation of the office manager/supervisor. The person who does the hiring should do the firing.

Probationary Employee. The probationary employee who does not prove satisfactory should be dismissed at the end of the probationary period with tact and a full explanation of the reasons for dismissal. In all fairness, an individual should be told why the employment is ended, and not be given weak excuses or untruths that do not help to correct deficiencies. If you are not straightforward in telling an employee the reason for dismissal, you are not helping that person to grow.

Long-term Employee. An employee who has been in service for some time and is giving unsatisfactory performance should be warned and given an explanation of the specific improvements expected. If a second chance does not produce improvement in performance or attitude, then dismissal must follow. It should be done privately, with tact and consideration.

Most practice consultants believe that firing should come close to the end of the day, after all other employees have left, and that the break should be clean and immediate. If the office policy provides for 2 weeks' notice, give 2 weeks' pay. A fired employee should not be allowed to train or influence a replacement.

The exit meeting should be planned just as carefully as the employment interview. Be honest with the employee. Discuss the employee's assets as well as liabilities, and give the reasons for the termination before you announce the dismissal. There is no need to dwell upon the employee's deficiencies. These should have been thoroughly discussed at the warning interview, and the employee need only be told that the necessary improvements have not been made. Do listen to the employee's feedback, however. This may reveal some important administrative problems that need correction.

After you dismiss an employee, do not leave that person in the office unattended. Request and get the office keys before giving a dismissed employee the final paycheck. And don't offer to give the employee a good reference unless you can do it sincerely.

Certain breaches of conduct, such as embezzlement, blatant **insubordination** or violation of patient confidentiality, are grounds for immediate dismissal without warning.

Occasionally an employee will voluntarily terminate a job without giving a valid reason. The physician or office manager may wish to follow up with a letter to the former employee to seek out any problem that may have prompted the resignation (Fig. 19–3).

OFFICE MANAGEMENT

Staff Meetings

There must be some formal mechanism for keeping the office manager and other key employees current on the daily business affairs of the practice. One of the most common complaints from office personnel is that of being unable to discuss problems with the doctor. The solution to this problem may be to hold regular staff meetings, which may be scheduled as frequently as weekly but should be no less often than quarterly. Some of the best ideas for improvement come from the office staff, and this should be encouraged.

The simplest technique is to set aside a specific time for regular meetings at an hour when the most people can attend with the least disruption. The meetings need not be long or overly formal, but in order to be effective they must be planned and organized. There must be a leader, and a secretary should be appointed to take notes. The effectiveness of the leader, a person who can balance firmness with fairness, is an important aspect of the meeting. This is usually either the physician or the office manager/supervisor. All members of the staff should be encouraged to submit ideas for discussion.

Draw up a simple outline of the issues you want to discuss and prepare any supporting data needed for the meeting. There are many kinds of staff meetings. They may be purely informational, or problem solving, or brainstorming; they may be work sessions for updating manuals; training seminars, or whatever is necessary to that practice. The staff should meet to discuss new ideas and any changes in office procedures, and to resolve any

Dear_____:

　　Since your decision to leave our employ a few weeks ago, I have been concerned about your reasons for doing so. There may have been more than one reason—and one of them may have been dissatisfaction with the working conditions.

　　If there was in fact some reason for dissatisfaction that influenced your decision to leave our employ, I would appreciate your passing it along to me, so that I may avoid losing other valuable employees in the future.

　　Please drop me a note, telephone, or come in if you wish. I assure you that any comments you care to make will be treated with respect and appreciation.

Cordially yours,

Figure 19–3
Example of a letter from physician to an employee who resigns suddenly.

problems. The staff meeting must not be allowed to deteriorate into a gripe session. Individual complaints should be handled privately.

The meeting must have a set agenda, with time for topics that need discussion on a regular basis, as well as time to handle any current problems. The agenda might be similar to that of any business meeting:

1. Reading of the last meeting's minutes
2. Discussion of any unfinished business
3. Discussion of any problems in the clinical area
4. Discussion of any problems in the administrative area
5. Discussion of any problems in common areas
6. Adjournment

Some physicians like to combine the staff meeting with a breakfast or lunch. The time or place is not important as long as it is "neutral," suits the practice, and the meetings are conducted regularly, democratically, and without interruption (Fig. 19–4).

There must be follow-up to the items discussed; otherwise, the only result will be frustration and a reluctance to discuss problems at future meetings.

Office Procedure Manual

The office procedure manual supplements the office policy manual. Sometimes the two are com-

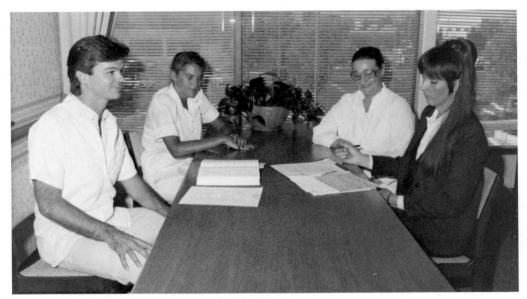

Figure 19–4
Setting for staff meeting. (Courtesy of Vista Medical Group, El Toro, CA. Photo by Dan Santucci.)

19

bined. The policy manual is informational; the procedure manual is a "how to" manual, containing a job description for each position in the practice and detailed steps for carrying out each task. Unfortunately, too few practices take the time to develop such a manual, and even those that do will often neglect to use it and keep it up to date.

Job Descriptions. A job description is a detailed account of the duties and the qualifications for a specific position (Fig. 19–5). In some cases it should state both primary and secondary duties, emphasizing that the employee must be flexible. Job descriptions may change with personnel changes. No two people have the same capabilities and interests; and there's no need to try to mold a person to a job description when a simple shift in duties may accomplish a happier result. For instance, an administrative assistant might normally be expected to complete the computer sheets at the end of the day, but if a clinical assistant has a special aptitude for this and really enjoys the task, there is no reason this change in responsibility should not be made. Note it on the job description so that there is no confusion about who is responsible. Following the list of duties there should be a procedure sheet for each task.

Procedure Sheets. A procedure sheet is a verbal flow chart that lists step-by-step the logical sequence of activities involved in a given task. An employee should be able to perform the task by following the written instructions (Fig. 19–6). Procedure writing is sometimes difficult because we tend to take for granted many of the simpler steps involved in performing a task once we become proficient. After a task has been learned it is unnecessary to refer to the procedure sheet for instructions, but it is invaluable in training the new recruit and in assisting the temporary employee.

Benefits and Contents of the Procedure Manual. Job descriptions and procedure sheets help the employee achieve expectations. Practice management specialists say that the most common remark from a discharged employee is "I didn't know I was supposed to . . ." A written job description may also help avoid legal problems with an employee who is dismissed for not meeting performance standards.

A great deal of instruction can be incorporated into a procedure manual. Preferred performance procedures, both administrative and clinical, should be spelled out in detail, including the following information:

POSITION: Office Manager
RESPONSIBLE TO: Physician

The office manager is responsible for the coordination of all office activities, including recruitment and training of personnel, accounting and financial procedures.

SPECIFIC TASKS:

1. Preparation of annual budget
2. Preparation of monthly profit and loss statement
3. Approval of all expenditures
4. Review and disposition of delinquent accounts
5. Approval of all write-offs
6. Liaison with accountant
7. Recruiting, hiring, and firing
8. Conducting performance appraisals and reporting to physician
9. Arrange personnel vacations and keep records of leave days
10. Assist in improving work flow and office efficiencies
11. Supervise purchase and repair of equipment
12. Purchase and storage of supplies
13. Arrange for practice insurance
14. Supervise regular staff meetings
15. Keep office policy manual current
16. Prepare patient education materials as needed

JOB QUALIFICATIONS: CMA-A or degree in business administration
Previous medical office experience
Supervisory experience helpful

Figure 19–5
Example of a job description.

PROCEDURE SHEET   PROCESS INCOMING MAIL

1. Assemble all necessary tools and supplies: letter opener, paper clips, stapler, mending tape, date stamp.

2. Open all mail except letters marked *personal*.

3. Check to be sure writer's address is on letter before destroying envelope. Staple envelope to letter if address is missing.

4. Paper clip enclosures to letter (or note their absence if they are not enclosed).

5. Date stamp the letter or piece of mail.

6. Set aside cash receipts for processing.

7. Route insurance claim forms and inquiries to insurance clerk.

8. Arrange mail with second and third class on bottom, then first class, with any personal mail on top.

9. Place entire stack in mail tray on right side of doctor's desk.

Figure 19–6
Example of a procedure sheet.

- A checklist of daily, weekly, monthly, quarterly, and yearly duties.
- How much time is allotted for new patients? Established patients? Postoperative patients?
- How are records prepared and filed? A description of the filing system may save the day if a temporary employee needs to find something in the file during the regular medical assistant's absence.
- How is the telephone to be answered? Which calls are put through to the doctor immediately, and which may the medical assistant handle? Include a list of the names and telephone numbers of persons you call often—for example, consulting physicians, hospitals, laboratories, and the physician's spouse.
- Billing and collection procedures. Is billing done weekly, twice monthly, monthly? Are the statements prepared in the office? By what method? Is a collection agency used? Which one?
- Completed samples of forms that need to be filled out and samples of correspondence (these provide excellent visual instruction).
- What kind of setup does the doctor prefer for office surgeries or treatments? Is there a card index showing these setups? If so, where is it kept?
- Where and how are supplies ordered and stored? Include the name, address, and telephone number of each supplier. Also include an inventory of major equipment with serial numbers, where and when purchased, and a telephone number for servicing.
- Any special duties the doctor expects of the medical assistant, such as organizational activities or making travel arrangements.

Management studies indicate that, in the multiple-employee office, it is good practice to have an understudy for each position who can substitute in an emergency. A well-documented procedure manual that is kept current ensures continuity when one employee must on occasion fill in for or assist another.

Development of a procedure manual is a good discussion item for staff meetings; the cooperation of the staff is essential if the project is to be successful. Keep it simple to update by using a three-ring binder. Include date of revision. Be sure to destroy old pages when revisions are made. One complete master copy should remain in the custody of the office manager and one with the physician. Each employee should have a copy of the portion that pertains to his or her particular job.

Practice Development

The office manager may play a large role in practice development, or practice marketing as it is often referred to. Practice development techniques are the outcome of a conscious need to improve the professional image, to increase exposure to the public, and to attract and keep patients.

As health costs continue to rise, and patients become more demanding and selective in choosing their health care providers, practice survival may depend on good marketing techniques.

It may become necessary to make slight changes in office hours to accommodate the patient population, including, in some cases, providing for evening and weekend hours or even house calls.

The medical assistant with management respon-

19

sibilities can encourage the physician to participate in community affairs, such as by offering to give mass inoculations when needed, serving as a consultant in area health fairs, or speaking on health topics to civic and professional groups. Some physicians gain public exposure by writing articles or a question-and-answer column for an area newspaper. Local events may suggest other ways of promoting the practice.

Communication with the patient is essential. The practice with a computer or word processor can easily generate a newsletter several times a year containing information pertaining to the practice specialty or advances in health care in general. Letters to the patient and the patient's referring physician after a consultation are greatly appreciated by both and are easily and quickly accomplished with electronic equipment. Holiday and birthday remembrances are another easy way of keeping the patient aware of the practice and conveying your concern.

The first, last, and most important rule of marketing a medical practice, of course, is to treat the patients well, because the best source of patients consists of referrals from existing satisfied patients.

Patient Education

Patients have many common concerns about the doctor's policies, such as office hours, what is included in the doctor's specialty, directions for reaching the office, parking facilities, emergency services, answering service, cancelations, house calls, prescription renewals, payment of fees, and so forth. You can satisfy the patients' concerns and save your own time by putting these policies in writing and giving a copy to every new patient.

Many management experts recommend that two separate folders or pamphlets be prepared—one devoted to general office information and another to financial policies.

Patient Information Folder. Only an estimated 10% of practices have a booklet that explains the information basic to the operational and service aspects of the practice. Yet a patient information folder can easily be compiled by the physician and staff cooperatively in a staff meeting. Experience has shown that if such a folder is given to every new patient, the number of incoming phone calls can be reduced by an average of 20 to 30%. It can also reduce misunderstanding and forgotten instructions. The folder must of necessity be tailored to the specific practice, but guidelines may be obtained free of charge from the American Medical Association's Department of Practice Management.

The patient information folder should be an introduction to the practice and, if possible, mailed to a new patient prior to the first visit. A supply may also be left with referring physicians' offices to be given to patients coming to your office. It should be designed to easily fit into a #10 business envelope. Consider using a photo of the medical building for easy identification by the new patient.

What should be included in the folder? The practice name, of course, and the practice logo if there is one. A statement of philosophy is frequently included in the introduction (see Office Policy Manual, p. 298). List all physicians in the practice, their education, training, and board certifications, and define their specialties. List the key clinical and administrative staff members, such as RNs and nurse practitioners, medical assistants, office managers, business manager, and so forth.

Show the practice address, a map of how to get there, and the parking facilities. List the telephone number(s) and explain the function of the answering service. If a separate "business only" telephone line is available, be sure to include this.

List what days and hours of the week the practice is open and the days it is closed. State if you close for lunch. Outline the appointment and cancellation policies, and your policy on house calls. Describe any **ancillary** or laboratory services provided, how test results are reported, and your policy on prescription renewals. Patients need to know the provisions for emergency procedures: What hospitals does the practice use regularly? What is the night and weekend coverage? Hospitalization procedures and postoperative care and follow-up may be included.

Financial Policies Folder. A small folder covering the financial policies of the office can eliminate many questions and possible misunderstanding. Keep it small enough to fit into the billing envelope and send it out with the first monthly statement. The folder should include answers to the following questions:

- Are office visits payable at the time of service?
- How can payment be made?—for instance, are VISA and MasterCard acceptable? Can time payments be arranged?
- Is there a charge for missed appointments?
- Is there a charge for completing insurance and disability forms? How much? Are there any exceptions?
- Are there charges for other services such as telephone prescriptions, year-end statements, returned checks?

The financial policies folder should also clearly state that the ultimate responsibility for payment lies with the patient.

Patient Instruction Sheets. In most medical offices there are patient procedures that occur over and over again. Instead of attempting to orally instruct a patient each time, why not develop clearly stated instruction sheets that you can review with the patient and then give the patient the written instructions to take home. The instruction sheets can include such procedures as:

- Preparation for x-ray or laboratory tests
- Preoperative and postoperative instructions
- Diet sheets
- Taking an enema
- Dressing a wound
- Taking medications
- Using a cane, crutches, walker, or wheelchair
- Care of casts
- Exercise therapy

In fact, anything for which patients are repeatedly given instructions can be written on these sheets.

FINANCIAL MANAGEMENT

The physician in a solo practice or small partnership may prefer to handle most financial aspects of the practice personally or may place that responsibility in the hands of a certified public accountant (CPA) or management consultant. In this situation the medical assistant's involvement may be limited to the billing and bookkeeping activities discussed in previous chapters.

The medical assistant who is able to handle more responsibility will probably have the opportunity to do so. This could be the most challenging part of the position and may include any or all of the following activities:

- Supervising cash receipts:
    Banking
    Billing
    Collection
- Preparing periodic profit and loss statements
- Computing collection ratios
- Making provision for:
    Practice insurance
    Professional liability
    Worker's compensation
    Employee's health benefits
    Disability insurance
    Unemployment insurance
- Writing payroll checks
- Paying bills
- Preparing reports for governmental agencies
- Acting as a liaison with the accountant

Payroll Records

Handling payroll records, whether for one employee or dozens of employees, involves frequent reporting activities. If it were necessary only to write a check to each employee for the agreed upon salary for a given pay period, no discussion of payroll records would be necessary. But government regulations require the withholding of income taxes and payment of certain other taxes by both employee and employer.

In order to comply with government regulations, complete records must be kept for every employee. Such records will include the following:

- Social Security number of employee
- Number of exemptions claimed
- Amount of gross salary
- All deductions for Social Security taxes, federal, state, and city or other subdivision withholding taxes, state disability insurance, and state unemployment tax, where applicable

Preliminary Activities. Each employee and each employer must have a tax identification number. The Social Security number (000-00-0000) is the employee's tax identification number. Any person who does not have a Social Security number should apply for one using Form SS-5 available from any Internal Revenue Service or Social Security office and from most post offices.

The employer applies for a number for federal tax accounting purposes (00-0000000) from the Internal Revenue Service, using Form SS-4. In states that require employer reports, a state employer number must also be obtained.

Before the end of the first pay period, the employee should complete an Employee's Withholding Exemption Certificate (Form W-4) showing the number of exemptions claimed (Fig. 19–7). Otherwise the employer must withhold on the basis of a single person with no exemptions.

The employee should complete a new form whenever changes occur in marital status or in the number of exemptions claimed. Each employee is entitled to one personal exemption and one for each qualified dependent. The employee may elect to take no exemptions, in which case the tax withheld will be greater and a refund may be due when the employee's annual tax report is filed.

A supply of all the necessary forms for filing federal returns, preinscribed with the employer's name, will be furnished to an employer who has applied for an employer identification number. Extra forms may be obtained from the Internal Revenue office.

Accounting for Payroll. The simplest way to prepare the payroll checks and generate the necessary accounting records is by using a write-it-once combination check-writing system such as the one illustrated in Figure 19–8. This includes an employee compensation record (Fig. 19–9). The employee's compensation record is aligned with the first open line on the record of checks drawn, and

19

Form **W-4** (Rev. January 1986)	Department of the Treasury—Internal Revenue Service **Employee's Withholding Allowance Certificate**	OMB No. 1545-0010 Expires: 11-30-87

1 Type or print your full name	2 Your social security number

Home address (number and street or rural route)

City or town, state, and ZIP code

3 Marital Status
☐ Single ☐ Married
☐ Married, but withhold at higher Single rate
Note: If married, but legally separated, or spouse is a nonresident alien, check the Single box.

4 Total number of allowances you are claiming (from line F of the worksheet on page 2) . . . .

5 Additional amount, if any, you want deducted from each pay . . . . $

6 I claim exemption from withholding because (see instructions and check boxes below that apply):
  a ☐ Last year I did not owe any Federal income tax and had a right to a full refund of **ALL** income tax withheld, **AND**
  b ☐ This year I do not expect to owe any Federal income tax and expect to have a right to a full refund of **ALL** income tax withheld. If both a and b apply, enter the year effective and "EXEMPT" here ▶ | Year 19
  c If you entered "EXEMPT" on line 6b, are you a full-time student? . . . . ☐ Yes ☐ No

Under penalties of perjury, I certify that I am entitled to the number of withholding allowances claimed on this certificate, or if claiming exemption from withholding, that I am entitled to claim the exempt status.

Employee's signature ▶   Date ▶   , 19

7 Employer's name and address (Employer: Complete 7, 8, and 9 only if sending to IRS)	8 Office code	9 Employer identification number

- Detach along this line. Give the top part of this form to employer; keep the lower part for your records. - - - - - - - - - - - - - - - - - -

Figure 19–7
Employee's Withholding Allowance Certificate.

a check with a carbonized strip is placed upon it. All information written on the check is automatically transferred to the compensation record, and the record of checks is drawn in one writing. The checks have a place for the address of the payee and can be mailed in a window envelope.

In practices with a number of employees, the summarization of the different categories for tax and reporting purposes is simplified, as the separate columns for different kinds of taxes on the record of checks drawn can simply be totaled at the end of the month (Fig. 19–10). If regular bank printed checks are used, the information for each employee must be posted to a separate record each time a payroll check is issued.

Income Tax Withholding

Employers are required by law to withhold certain amounts from employees' earnings and to report and forward these amounts to be applied toward payment of income tax. The amount to be withheld is based on the following:

- Total earnings of the employee
- Number of exemptions claimed
- Marital status of the employee
- Length of the pay period involved

The Federal Employer's Tax Guide includes tables to be used in determining the amount to be withheld. Sample pages are shown in Figure 19–11. There is one table for single persons and unmarried heads of households, and one for married persons.

The tables cover monthly, semimonthly, biweekly, weekly, and daily or miscellaneous periods.

Employer's Income Taxes. The physician who is practicing as an individual is not subject to withholding tax but will be expected to make an estimated tax payment four times a year. The accountant will prepare four copies of Form 1040-ES, Declaration of Estimated Tax for Individuals, for the ensuing year when the annual income tax return is prepared. The first form and one-quarter of the estimated tax for the next year will be filed at the same time as the tax return. The remaining three forms, with the estimated tax due, must be filed on June 15, September 15, and January 15. It may be the office manager's duty to see that these returns are filed when due.

The employer will also contribute to Social Security in the form of a self-employment tax. The rate is slightly higher than that of an employee but less than the combined employee-employer contribution. This is computed and paid as a part of the income tax return.

Social Security Taxes. Social Security taxes are imposed on both employers and employees under the Federal Insurance Contributions Act (FICA). The tax rate is reviewed frequently and is subject to change by Congress.

Three programs are included under the FICA umbrella:

- The retirement benefits program called old-age survivors' insurance (OASI)

Text continued on page 316

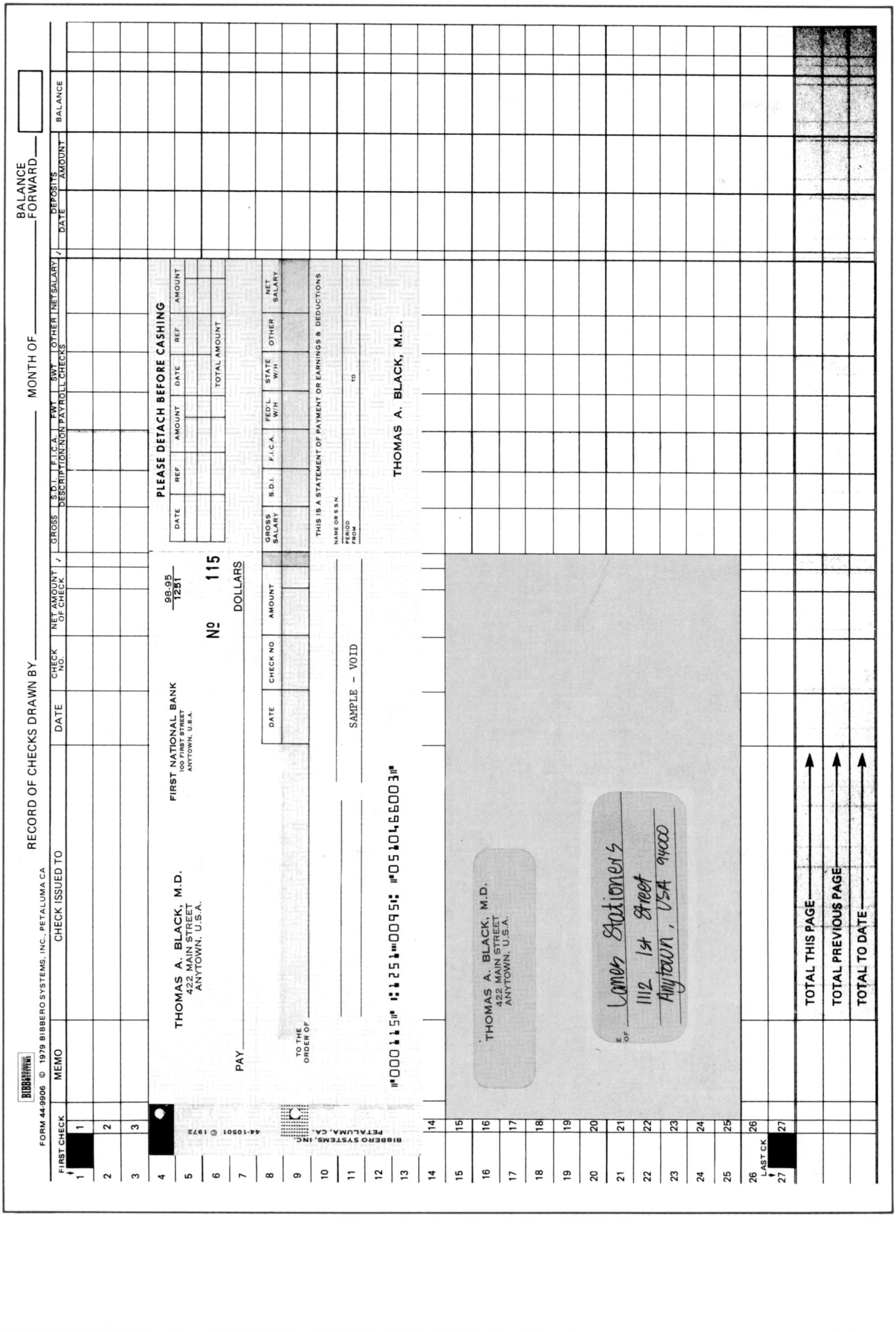

Figure 19–8

Write-it-once checkwriting system. (Courtesy of Bibbero Systems, Inc., Petaluma, CA.)

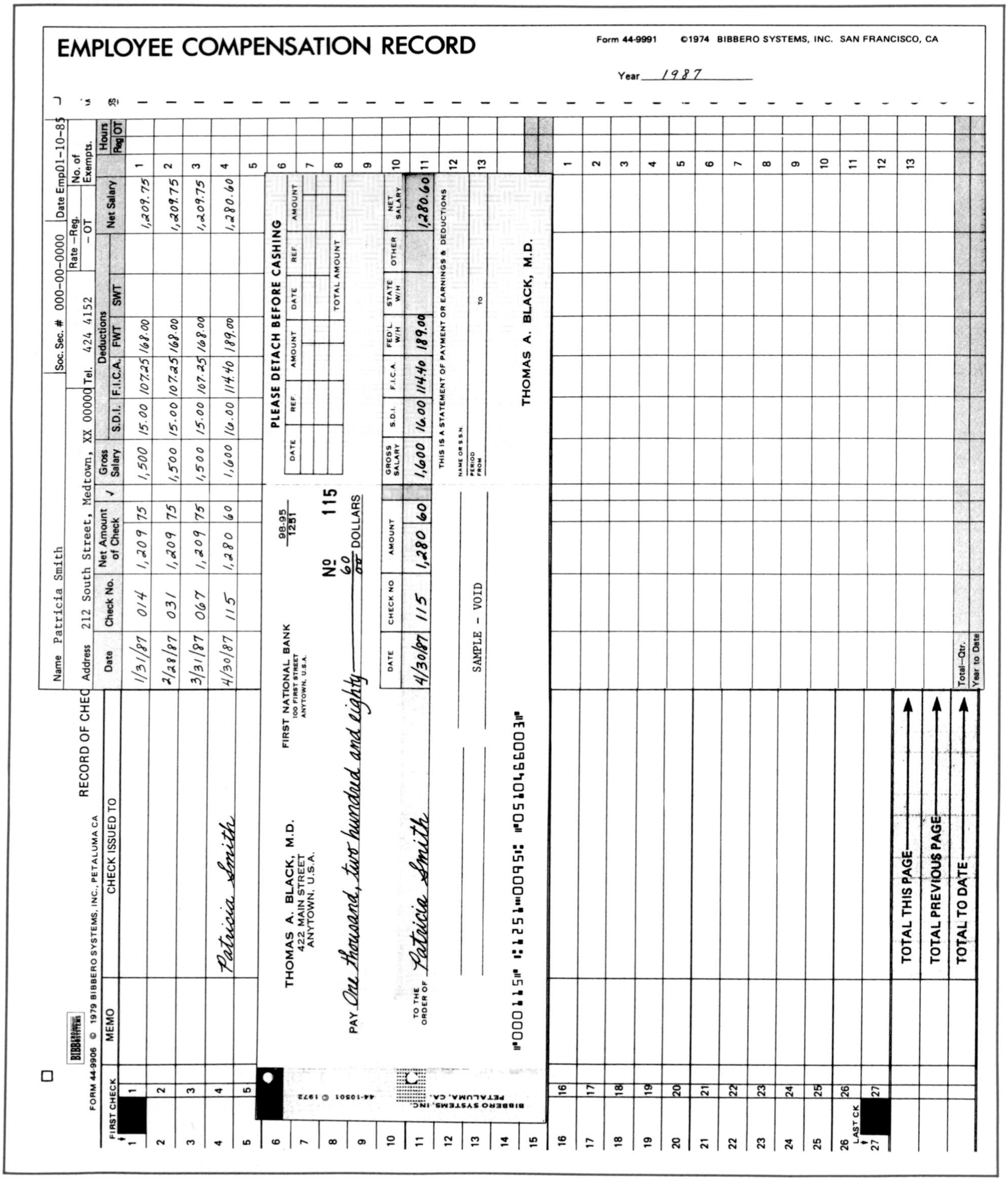

EMPLOYEE COMPENSATION RECORD

Form 44-9991   ©1974 BIBBERO SYSTEMS, INC. SAN FRANCISCO, CA

Year 1987

Name Patricia Smith   Soc. Sec. # 000-00-0000   Date Emp 01-10-85

Address 212 South Street, Medtown, XX 00000   Tel. 424 4152

RECORD OF CHECKS

Date	Check No.	✓	Net Amount of Check	Gross Salary	S.D.I.	F.I.C.A.	FWT	SWT	Net Salary	Reg/OT Hours
1/31/87	014		1,209.75	1,500	15.00	107.25	168.00		1,209.75	1
2/28/87	031		1,209.75	1,500	15.00	107.25	168.00		1,209.75	2
3/31/87	067		1,209.75	1,500	15.00	107.25	168.00		1,209.75	3
4/30/87	115		1,280.60	1,600	16.00	114.40	199.00		1,280.60	4

PLEASE DETACH BEFORE CASHING

DATE	REF	AMOUNT	REF	DATE	AMOUNT

TOTAL AMOUNT

GROSS SALARY	S.D.I.	F.I.C.A.	FED'L. W/H	STATE W/H	OTHER	NET SALARY
1,600	16.00	114.40	189.00			1,280.60

THIS IS A STATEMENT OF PAYMENT OR EARNINGS & DEDUCTIONS

NAME OR S.S.N.
PERIOD
FROM   TO

THOMAS A. BLACK, M.D.

CHECK ISSUED TO   MEMO

Patricia Smith

FIRST NATIONAL BANK
100 FIRST STREET
ANYTOWN, U.S.A.

98-95
1251

No. 115

No. 60
DOLLARS

DATE	CHECK NO	AMOUNT
4/30/87	115	1,280.60

SAMPLE – VOID

THOMAS A. BLACK, M.D.
422 MAIN STREET
ANYTOWN, U.S.A.

PAY One thousand, two hundred and eighty

TO THE ORDER OF Patricia Smith

⑈000 115⑈ ⑆1251⑆0095⑆ ⑈05 1046600 3⑈

44-10501 © 1972
BIBBERO SYSTEMS, INC.
PETALUMA, CA.

FORM 44-9906 © 1979 BIBBERO SYSTEMS, INC., PETALUMA CA

FIRST CHECK

LAST CK

TOTAL THIS PAGE
TOTAL PREVIOUS PAGE
TOTAL TO DATE

Total-Qtr.
Year to Date

Figure 19-9

Employee compensation record for write-it-once checkwriting system. (Courtesy of Bibbero Systems, Inc., Petaluma, CA.)

EMPLOYEE COMPENSATION RECORD

Name Patricia Smith   Soc. Sec. # 000-00-0000   Date Emp 01-10-85

Address 212 South Street, Medtown, XX 00000 Tel. 424 4152

Rate —Reg. / — OT

No. of Exempts.

Date	Check No.	Net Amount of Check	✓	Gross Salary	S.D.I.	F.I.C.A.	FWT	SWT	Net Salary		Hours Reg	OT
1/31/87	014	1,209 75		1,500	15.00	107.25	168.00		1,209.75	1		
2/28/87	031	1,209 75		1,500	15.00	107.25	168.00		1,209.75	2		
3/31/87	067	1,209 75		1,500	15.00	107.25	168.00		1,209.75	3		
4/30/87	115	1,280 60		1,600	16.00	114.40	189.00		1,280.60	4		
										5		
										6		
										7		
										8		
										9		
										10		
										11		
										12		
										13		
Total—Qtr.												
Year to Date												
										1		
										2		
										3		
										4		
										5		
										6		
										7		
										8		
										9		
										10		
										11		
										12		
										13		
Total—Qtr.												
Year to Date												

Year 1987

Form 44-9991   ©1974 BIBBERO SYSTEMS, INC. SAN FRANCISCO, CA

19

Figure 19–10
Payroll record for first quarter of year, one employee. (Courtesy of Bibbero Systems, Inc., Petaluma, CA.)

MARRIED Persons–MONTHLY Payroll Period
(For Wages Paid After December 1985)

And the wages are–		And the number of withholding allowances claimed is–										
At least	But less than	0	1	2	3	4	5	6	7	8	9	10
		The amount of income tax to be withheld shall be–										
$0	$220	$0	$0	$0	$0	$0	$0	$0	$0	$0	$0	$0
220	224	1	0	0	0	0	0	0	0	0	0	0
224	228	1	0	0	0	0	0	0	0	0	0	0
228	232	2	0	0	0	0	0	0	0	0	0	0
232	236	2	0	0	0	0	0	0	0	0	0	0
236	240	2	0	0	0	0	0	0	0	0	0	0
240	248	3	0	0	0	0	0	0	0	0	0	0
248	256	4	0	0	0	0	0	0	0	0	0	0
256	264	5	0	0	0	0	0	0	0	0	0	0
264	272	6	0	0	0	0	0	0	0	0	0	0
272	280	7	0	0	0	0	0	0	0	0	0	0
280	288	7	0	0	0	0	0	0	0	0	0	0
288	296	8	0	0	0	0	0	0	0	0	0	0
296	304	9	0	0	0	0	0	0	0	0	0	0
304	312	10	0	0	0	0	0	0	0	0	0	0
312	320	11	1	0	0	0	0	0	0	0	0	0
320	328	12	2	0	0	0	0	0	0	0	0	0
328	336	13	3	0	0	0	0	0	0	0	0	0
336	344	14	4	0	0	0	0	0	0	0	0	0
344	352	15	5	0	0	0	0	0	0	0	0	0
352	360	15	6	0	0	0	0	0	0	0	0	0
360	368	16	6	0	0	0	0	0	0	0	0	0
368	376	17	7	0	0	0	0	0	0	0	0	0
376	384	18	8	0	0	0	0	0	0	0	0	0
384	392	19	9	0	0	0	0	0	0	0	0	0
392	400	20	10	0	0	0	0	0	0	0	0	0
400	420	21	11	2	0	0	0	0	0	0	0	0
420	440	24	14	4	0	0	0	0	0	0	0	0
440	460	26	16	6	0	0	0	0	0	0	0	0
460	480	29	18	8	0	0	0	0	0	0	0	0
480	500	31	20	10	0	0	0	0	0	0	0	0
500	520	33	23	13	3	0	0	0	0	0	0	0
520	540	36	25	15	5	0	0	0	0	0	0	0
540	560	38	27	17	7	0	0	0	0	0	0	0
560	580	41	30	19	9	0	0	0	0	0	0	0
580	600	43	32	21	11	2	0	0	0	0	0	0
600	640	47	36	25	15	5	0	0	0	0	0	0
640	680	53	41	30	19	9	0	0	0	0	0	0
680	720	58	46	35	24	14	4	0	0	0	0	0
720	760	64	51	39	29	18	8	0	0	0	0	0
760	800	70	57	44	33	23	13	3	0	0	0	0
800	840	75	63	50	38	27	17	7	0	0	0	0
840	880	81	68	56	43	32	21	11	2	0	0	0
880	920	86	74	61	49	37	26	16	6	0	0	0
920	960	92	79	67	54	42	31	20	10	0	0	0
960	1,000	98	85	72	60	47	36	25	15	5	0	0
1,000	1,040	104	91	78	65	53	41	30	19	9	0	0
1,040	1,080	110	96	84	71	58	46	35	24	14	4	0
1,080	1,120	117	102	89	77	64	51	39	29	18	8	0
1,120	1,160	123	109	95	82	70	57	44	33	23	13	3
1,160	1,200	130	115	101	88	75	63	50	38	27	17	7
1,200	1,240	136	122	107	93	81	68	56	43	32	21	11
1,240	1,280	142	128	114	99	86	74	61	49	37	26	16
1,280	1,320	149	134	120	106	92	79	67	54	42	31	20
1,320	1,360	155	141	126	112	98	85	72	60	47	36	25
1,360	1,400	162	147	133	118	104	91	78	65	53	41	30
1,400	1,440	169	154	139	125	110	96	84	71	58	46	35
1,440	1,480	177	160	146	131	117	102	89	77	64	51	39
1,480	1,520	184	168	152	138	123	109	95	82	70	57	44
1,520	1,560	191	175	159	144	130	115	101	88	75	63	50
1,560	1,600	198	182	166	150	136	122	107	93	81	68	56
1,600	1,640	205	189	173	157	142	128	114	99	86	74	61
1,640	1,680	213	196	180	164	149	134	120	106	92	79	67
1,680	1,720	220	204	187	171	155	141	126	112	98	85	72
1,720	1,760	227	211	195	178	162	147	133	118	104	91	78
1,760	1,800	236	218	202	186	169	154	139	125	110	96	84
1,800	1,840	245	225	209	193	177	160	146	131	117	102	89
1,840	1,880	254	234	216	200	184	168	152	138	123	109	95
1,880	1,920	263	243	223	207	191	175	159	144	130	115	101
1,920	1,960	271	252	232	214	198	182	166	150	136	122	107
1,960	2,000	280	260	241	222	205	189	173	157	142	128	114
2,000	2,040	289	269	249	230	213	196	180	164	149	134	120
2,040	2,080	298	278	258	238	220	204	187	171	155	141	126
2,080	2,120	307	287	267	247	227	211	195	178	162	147	133
2,120	2,160	316	296	276	256	236	218	202	186	169	154	139

Figure 19–11
Pages from 1986 withholding tax table.

SINGLE Persons–MONTHLY Payroll Period
(For Wages Paid After December 1985)

And the wages are–		And the number of withholding allowances claimed is–										
At least	But less than	0	1	2	3	4	5	6	7	8	9	10
		The amount of income tax to be withheld shall be–										
$0	$120	$0	$0	$0	$0	$0	$0	$0	$0	$0	$0	$0
120	124	1	0	0	0	0	0	0	0	0	0	0
124	128	1	0	0	0	0	0	0	0	0	0	0
128	132	1	0	0	0	0	0	0	0	0	0	0
132	136	2	0	0	0	0	0	0	0	0	0	0
136	140	2	0	0	0	0	0	0	0	0	0	0
140	144	3	0	0	0	0	0	0	0	0	0	0
144	148	3	0	0	0	0	0	0	0	0	0	0
148	152	4	0	0	0	0	0	0	0	0	0	0
152	156	4	0	0	0	0	0	0	0	0	0	0
156	160	5	0	0	0	0	0	0	0	0	0	0
160	164	5	0	0	0	0	0	0	0	0	0	0
164	168	5	0	0	0	0	0	0	0	0	0	0
168	172	6	0	0	0	0	0	0	0	0	0	0
172	176	6	0	0	0	0	0	0	0	0	0	0
176	180	7	0	0	0	0	0	0	0	0	0	0
180	184	7	0	0	0	0	0	0	0	0	0	0
184	188	8	0	0	0	0	0	0	0	0	0	0
188	192	8	0	0	0	0	0	0	0	0	0	0
192	196	9	0	0	0	0	0	0	0	0	0	0
196	200	9	0	0	0	0	0	0	0	0	0	0
200	204	9	0	0	0	0	0	0	0	0	0	0
204	208	10	0	0	0	0	0	0	0	0	0	0
208	212	10	0	0	0	0	0	0	0	0	0	0
212	216	11	1	0	0	0	0	0	0	0	0	0
216	220	11	1	0	0	0	0	0	0	0	0	0
220	224	12	2	0	0	0	0	0	0	0	0	0
224	228	12	2	0	0	0	0	0	0	0	0	0
228	232	13	3	0	0	0	0	0	0	0	0	0
232	236	13	3	0	0	0	0	0	0	0	0	0
236	240	14	3	0	0	0	0	0	0	0	0	0
240	248	14	4	0	0	0	0	0	0	0	0	0
248	256	15	5	0	0	0	0	0	0	0	0	0
256	264	16	6	0	0	0	0	0	0	0	0	0
264	272	17	7	0	0	0	0	0	0	0	0	0
272	280	18	8	0	0	0	0	0	0	0	0	0
280	288	19	9	0	0	0	0	0	0	0	0	0
288	296	20	9	0	0	0	0	0	0	0	0	0
296	304	21	10	0	0	0	0	0	0	0	0	0
304	312	22	11	1	0	0	0	0	0	0	0	0
312	320	23	12	2	0	0	0	0	0	0	0	0
320	328	24	13	3	0	0	0	0	0	0	0	0
328	336	25	14	4	0	0	0	0	0	0	0	0
336	344	26	15	5	0	0	0	0	0	0	0	0
344	352	28	16	6	0	0	0	0	0	0	0	0
352	360	29	17	7	0	0	0	0	0	0	0	0
360	368	30	18	7	0	0	0	0	0	0	0	0
368	376	31	19	8	0	0	0	0	0	0	0	0
376	384	32	20	9	0	0	0	0	0	0	0	0
384	392	33	21	10	0	0	0	0	0	0	0	0
392	400	34	22	11	1	0	0	0	0	0	0	0
400	420	36	24	13	3	0	0	0	0	0	0	0
420	440	39	26	15	5	0	0	0	0	0	0	0
440	460	42	29	17	7	0	0	0	0	0	0	0
460	480	45	32	20	9	0	0	0	0	0	0	0
480	500	47	35	22	11	1	0	0	0	0	0	0
500	520	50	38	25	14	4	0	0	0	0	0	0
520	540	53	40	28	16	6	0	0	0	0	0	0
540	560	56	43	31	19	8	0	0	0	0	0	0
560	580	59	46	33	21	10	0	0	0	0	0	0
580	600	62	49	36	24	13	3	0	0	0	0	0
600	640	67	53	40	28	16	6	0	0	0	0	0
640	680	73	59	46	33	21	10	0	0	0	0	0
680	720	79	65	52	39	26	15	5	0	0	0	0
720	760	86	71	58	45	32	20	9	0	0	0	0
760	800	92	78	64	50	38	25	14	4	0	0	0
800	840	98	84	70	56	43	31	19	8	0	0	0
840	880	105	90	76	62	49	36	24	13	3	0	0
880	920	112	97	82	68	55	42	29	17	7	0	0
920	960	119	103	89	74	61	47	35	22	11	1	0
960	1,000	126	110	95	81	67	53	40	28	16	6	0
1,000	1,040	133	117	102	87	73	59	46	33	21	10	0
1,040	1,080	140	124	108	94	79	65	52	39	26	15	5
1,080	1,120	148	131	115	100	86	71	58	45	32	20	9

Figure 19–11 Continued

- The hospital insurance program (HI) that provides hospitalization under Medicare
- The public disability insurance program (DI) that provides benefits to disabled workers

Deposit Requirements. Generally, the employer must deposit withholding and Social Security taxes in an authorized financial institution or a Federal Reserve Bank. The amount of taxes owed determines the frequency of the deposits. The rules are subject to change and are set forth in the Employer's Tax Guide previously referred to (Table 19–1).

Quarterly Reports. The Employer's Quarterly Federal Tax Return (Form 941) must be filed on or before the last day of the first month after the end of the quarter (Fig. 19–12). Due dates for this return and full payment of tax are April 30, July 31, October 31, and January 31. If deposits in full payment of taxes due have been made, the due date for the return is extended 10 days. The return must show the following:

- Number of employees
- Names of all employees with their Social Security numbers
- Total wages paid
- Amount of withholding tax
- Amount of wages subject to FICA

Table 19–1
Summary of Deposit Rules for Social Security Taxes and Withheld Income Tax

Deposit Rule	Deposit Due
(1) If at the end of the quarter your total undeposited taxes for the quarter are less than $500:	(1) No deposit is required. You may pay the taxes to IRS with Form 941 (or 941E), or you may deposit them by the due date of the return.
(2) If at the end of any month your total undeposited taxes are less than $500:	(2) No deposit is required. You may carry the taxes over to the following month.
(3) If at the end of any month your total undeposited taxes are $500 or more but less than $3,000:	(3) Within 15 days after the end of the month. (No deposit is required if you made a deposit for an eighth-monthly period during the month under rule 4. However, if this occurs in the last month of the quarter, deposit any balance due by the due date of the return).
(4) If at the end of any eighth-monthly period (the 3rd, 7th, 11th, 15th, 19th, 22nd, 25th, and last day of each month) your total undeposited taxes are $3,000 or more:	(4) Within 3 banking days after the end of the eighth-monthly period.

- FICA taxes paid
- Total deposits for the quarter
- Any undeposited taxes due

Annual Reports. Form W-2, Wage and Tax Statement, should be given to employees by January 31. Form W-2 must show the following:

- Employer's identification number
- Employee's Social Security number
- Total wages and other compensation paid (whether or not they are subject to withholding)
- Amounts deducted for income tax and Social Security tax, including hospital insurance
- Total amount of advance earned income credit payment, if any

The employer is required to furnish two copies of Form W-2 to each employee from whom income tax or Social Security tax has been withheld, or from whom income tax would have been withheld if the employee had claimed no more than one withholding exemption.

If employment ends before December 31, the employer may give the W-2 to the terminated employee any time after employment ends. If the employee asks for Form W-2, the employer should give the employee the completed copies within 30 days of the request or the final wage payment, whichever is later (Fig. 19–13).

Employers must file Form W-3, Transmittal of Income and Tax Statement, annually, to transmit wage and income tax withheld statements (Forms W-2) to the Social Security Administration. These forms are processed by the Social Security Administration, which then furnishes the Internal Revenue Service with the income tax data that it needs from those forms. Form W-3 and its attachments must be filed separately from Form 941 on or before the last day of February following the calendar year for which the W-2 Forms are prepared (Fig. 19–14).

Federal Unemployment Tax

Employers also contribute under the Federal Unemployment Tax Act (FUTA). Generally, credit can be taken against the FUTA tax for amounts paid into a State unemployment fund up to a certain percentage.

Employers are responsible for paying the FUTA tax; it must not be deducted from employees' wages.

FUTA Deposits. For deposit purposes, the FUTA tax is figured quarterly, and any amount due must be paid by the last day of the first month after the quarter ends. The formula for determining the amount due is set forth in the Federal Employer's Tax Guide.

FUTA Annual Return. An annual FUTA return

Form **941**
(Rev. April 1986)
Department of the Treasury
Internal Revenue Service 4141

Employer's Quarterly Federal Tax Return
▶ **For Paperwork Reduction Act Notice, see page 2.**
Please type or print

Your name, address, employer identification number, and calendar quarter of return. (If not correct, please change.)

		OMB No. 1545-0029 Expires: 8-31-88
Name (as distinguished from trade name)	Date quarter ended	T
Trade name, if any	Employer identification number	FF
		FD
Address and ZIP code		FP
		I
		T

If address is different from prior return, check here ▶ ☐

IRS Use

1 1 1 1 1 1 1 1 1 1 1 1   2 2 2 2 2 2 2 2 2 2   3 3 3 3 3 3
4 5 5 5 6 6 6 7 8   9 9 9 9 9 9 10 10   11 11 11 11 11 11 11 11 11 11 11 11

If you are not liable for returns in the future, check here . . . ▶ ☐   Date final wages paid . . . . ▶

Complete for First Quarter Only

1a Number of employees (except household) employed in the pay period that includes March 12th . . ▶	1a	
b If you are a subsidiary corporation AND your parent corporation files a consolidated Form 1120, enter parent corporation employer identification number (EIN) . . ▶	1b	–
2 Total wages and tips subject to withholding, plus other compensation . . . . ▶	2	
3 Total income tax withheld from wages, tips, pensions, annuities, sick pay, gambling, etc. . . . ▶	3	
4 Adjustment of withheld income tax for preceding quarters of calendar year (see instructions) . . ▶	4	
5 Adjusted total of income tax withheld	5	
6 Taxable social security wages paid . . . . . $ _____ X 14.3% (.143) . .	6	
7a Taxable tips reported . . . . $ _____ X 7.15% (.0715) . .	7a	
b Tips deemed to be wages (see instructions) . . $ _____ X 7.15% (.0715) . .	7b	
c Taxable hospital insurance wages paid . . . . $ _____ X 2.9% (.029) . .	7c	
8 Total social security taxes (add lines 6, 7a, 7b, and 7c)	8	
9 Adjustment of social security taxes (see instructions for required explanation) . . . . . ▶	9	
10 Adjusted total of social security taxes (see instructions)	10	
11 Backup withholding . . . . ▶	11	
12 Adjustment of backup withholding tax for preceding quarters of calendar year	12	
13 Adjusted total of backup withholding	13	
14 Total taxes (add lines 5, 10, and 13) . . . . ▶	14	
15 Advance earned income credit (EIC) payments, if any (see instructions)	15	
16 Net taxes (subtract line 15 from line 14). **This must equal line IV below** (plus line IV of Schedule A (Form 941) if you have treated backup withholding as a separate liability.)	16	
17 Total deposits for quarter, including overpayment applied from a prior quarter, from your records . ▶	17	
18 Balance due (subtract line 17 from line 16). This should be less than $500. Pay to IRS	18	

19 If line 17 is more than line 16, enter overpayment here ▶ $ _____ and check if to be:
☐ Applied to next return or   ☐ Refunded.

Record of Federal Tax Liability (Complete if line 16 is $500 or more) See the instructions under rule 4 for details before checking these boxes.
Check only if you made eighth-monthly deposits using the 95% rule ▶ ☐   Check only if you are a first time 3-banking-day depositor ▶ ☐

Date wages paid	Tax liability (**Do not show Federal tax deposits here.**)					
	First month of quarter		Second month of quarter		Third month of quarter	
1st through 3rd	A		I		Q	
4th through 7th	B		J		R	
8th through 11th	C		K		S	
12th through 15th	D		L		T	
16th through 19th	E		M		U	
20th through 22nd	F		N		V	
23rd through 25th	G		O		W	
26th through the last	H		P		X	
Total liability for month	I		II		III	

IV Total for quarter (add lines *I*, *II*, and *III*) . . . . ▶

Under penalties of perjury, I declare that I have examined this return, including accompanying schedules and statements, and to the best of my knowledge and belief it is true, correct, and complete.

Signature ▶   Title ▶   Date ▶

Figure 19–12
Employer's Quarterly Federal Tax Return.

19

must be filed on Form 940 on or before January 31 following the close of the calendar year for which the tax is due. Any tax still due is payable with the return. Form 940 may be filed on or before February 10 following the close of the year, if all required deposits were made on time and if full payment of the tax due is deposited on or before January 31 (Fig. 19–15).

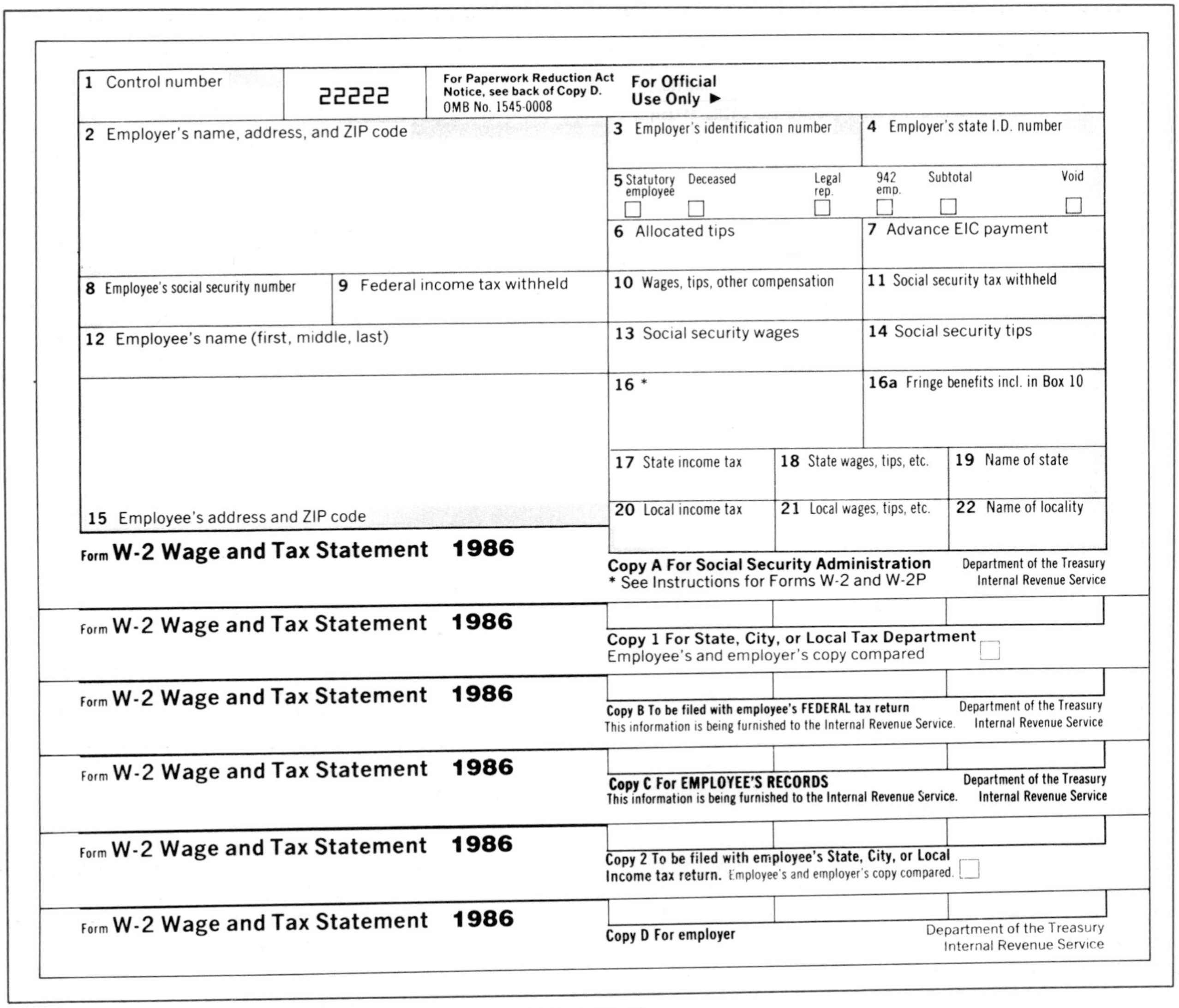

1 Control number		22222	For Paperwork Reduction Act Notice, see back of Copy D. OMB No. 1545-0008	For Official Use Only ▶		
2 Employer's name, address, and ZIP code				3 Employer's identification number	4 Employer's state I.D. number	
				5 Statutory employee ☐ Deceased ☐	Legal rep. ☐	942 emp. ☐ Subtotal ☐ Void ☐
				6 Allocated tips	7 Advance EIC payment	
8 Employee's social security number		9 Federal income tax withheld		10 Wages, tips, other compensation	11 Social security tax withheld	
12 Employee's name (first, middle, last)				13 Social security wages	14 Social security tips	
				16 *	16a Fringe benefits incl. in Box 10	
				17 State income tax	18 State wages, tips, etc.	19 Name of state
15 Employee's address and ZIP code				20 Local income tax	21 Local wages, tips, etc.	22 Name of locality

Form **W-2 Wage and Tax Statement** **1986**
Copy A For Social Security Administration
* See Instructions for Forms W-2 and W-2P
Department of the Treasury Internal Revenue Service

Form **W-2 Wage and Tax Statement** **1986**
Copy 1 For State, City, or Local Tax Department
Employee's and employer's copy compared

Form **W-2 Wage and Tax Statement** **1986**
Copy B To be filed with employee's FEDERAL tax return
This information is being furnished to the Internal Revenue Service.
Department of the Treasury Internal Revenue Service

Form **W-2 Wage and Tax Statement** **1986**
Copy C For EMPLOYEE'S RECORDS
This information is being furnished to the Internal Revenue Service.
Department of the Treasury Internal Revenue Service

Form **W-2 Wage and Tax Statement** **1986**
Copy 2 To be filed with employee's State, City, or Local Income tax return. Employee's and employer's copy compared.

Form **W-2 Wage and Tax Statement** **1986**
Copy D For employer
Department of the Treasury Internal Revenue Service

Figure 19–13
Form W-2 Wage and Tax Statement.

State Unemployment Taxes

All of the states and the District of Columbia have unemployment compensation laws. In most states the tax is imposed only on the employer, but a few states require employers to withhold a percentage of wages for unemployment compensation benefits.

An employer may be subject to federal unemployment tax and not subject to state unemployment tax. In some states, for instance, the employer with fewer than four employees is not subject to the state unemployment tax. The regulations for the individual state should be checked.

State Disability Insurance

Some states require that employees be covered by disability or sick-pay insurance. The employer may be required to withhold a certain amount from the employee's salary to pay for this insurance.

SPECIAL DUTIES

Before closing the chapter, we should mention certain events that do not occur with regularity but which may confront the office manager at some time.

Moving a Practice

The thought of moving into a shiny new spacious office can be exciting. Unless the move is planned in advance, however, moving day—and the weeks that follow—can be a nightmare.

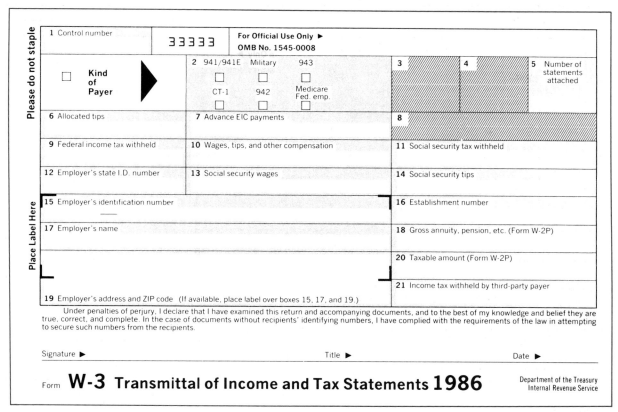

Figure 19–14
Form W-3 Transmittal of Income and Tax Statements.

Planning the New Quarters. Do some careful measuring to see how the furniture and equipment you plan to move will fit into the new quarters. If possible, draw the rooms to scale and show where each item is to be placed by the mover. Include the location of available electrical outlets in your floor plan. If new furniture, carpets, or equipment will be needed, try to have them in place before moving day. Don't expect to have the new carpet installed the day of your move.

Establishing a Moving Date. Decide what day you will move and whether you will close the office for one day or several. Select a mover and confirm the date. Patients must be notified of the move. As soon as the moving date is established, post a notice in the office and draw the patients' attention to it. You may want to send announcement cards to the active patients. Many doctors place a notice in the local newspapers.

Notifying Utilities and Mailers. At least 60 days in advance of the move, start a change-of-address notification campaign. Notify publishers of journals and suppliers of catalogs. (Cards for changes of address are available from the post office.) Six weeks' notice is generally required on all subscriptions, and postage due on forwarded journals can be very expensive. Notify the telephone company

and utility companies well in advance so that there will be no break in service. File a change of address card with the local post office. Order stationery and business cards with the new address.

Packing. The moving company will supply packing cartons for you to use. Have each employee be responsible for packing and labeling the items from his or her own work area. Tag each carton with a number and keep a master list of what is in each numbered carton. This will help you find items that you need. Also, if a carton should be lost or mislaid, you will have a record of what was in it. If time allows, just before moving is a good time to cull material from the files and discard old journals, supply catalogs, and any obsolete supplies or equipment.

Moving Day Strategy. Prepare a written outline of the moving day strategy, indicating each person's responsibility, and give each member of the office staff a copy. It may be wise to work in shifts to avoid confusion, but have one person stationed at the new address to direct the movers when they arrive.

Follow-up. After the move, be sure to mention the new address when patients call for appoint-

19

Form **940**		**Employer's Annual Federal Unemployment (FUTA) Tax Return**			OMB No. 1545-0028	
Department of the Treasury Internal Revenue Service		► **For Paperwork Reduction Act Notice, see page 2.**			19**85**	

		T	
		FF	
If incorrect, make any necessary change. ►	Name (as distinguished from trade name) Calendar Year **1985**	FD	
	Trade name, if any Employer identification number	FP	
	Address and ZIP code	I	
		T	

A Did you pay all required contributions to your state unemployment fund by the due date of Form 940? (If none required, check "No.") . . . ☒ **Yes** ☐ **No**

If you checked the "Yes" box, enter amount of contributions paid to your state unemployment fund . . . . . . ► $ ___3453.24___

B Are you required to pay contributions to only one state? . . . . . . ☒ **Yes** ☐ **No**

If you checked the "Yes" box, (1) Enter the name of the state where you are required to pay contributions . . . . . . ► ___Calif.___
(2) Enter your state reporting number(s) as shown on state unemployment tax return . . . . . . ► ___154 2192 8___

Part I Computation of Taxable Wages and Credit Reduction (To Be Completed by All Taxpayers)

1	Total payments (including exempt payments) during the calendar year for services of employees	1	176,793 87
2	Exempt payments. (Explain each exemption shown, attaching additional sheets if necessary) ► *Amount paid*	2	
3	Payments for services of more than $7,000. Enter only the excess over the first $7,000 paid to individual employees not including exempt amounts shown on line 2. Do not use the state wage limitation	3 94,573 67	
4	Total exempt payments (add lines 2 and 3)	4	94,573 67
5	**Total taxable wages** (subtract line 4 from line 1). (If any part is exempt from state contributions, see instructions) ►	5	82,220 20
6	Credit reduction for unpaid advances to the states listed (by 2-letter Postal Service abbreviations). Enter the wages included on line 5 above for each state and multiply by the rate shown. (See the instructions.)		

(a) CT ____ x .007 ____	(e) OH ____ x .008 ____	**Outside the United States**
(b) IL ____ x .009 ____	(f) PA ____ x .009 ____	(i) PR ____ x .006 ____
(c) LA ____ x .006 ____	(g) VT ____ x .006 ____	(j) VI ____ x .012 ____
(d) MN ____ x .011 ____	(h) WV ____ x .008 ____	

7	Total credit reduction (add lines 6(a) through 6(j) and enter in Part II, line 2 or Part III, line 4). . . . ►	7	

Part II Tax Due or Refund (Complete if You Checked the "Yes" Boxes in Both Questions A and B Above)

1	FUTA tax. Multiply the wages in Part I, line 5, by .008 and enter here	1	657 76
2	Enter amount from Part I, line 7	2	
3	**Total FUTA tax** (add lines 1 and 2)	3	
4	Less: Total FUTA tax deposited for the year, including any overpayment applied from a prior year (from your records). .	4	
5	**Balance due** (subtract line 4 from line 3—if over $100, see Part IV instructions). Pay to IRS	5	657 76
6	**Overpayment** (subtract line 3 from line 4). Check if it is to be: ☐ Applied to next return, or ☐ Refunded . . . ►	6	

Part III Tax Due or Refund (Complete if You Checked the "No" Box in Either Question A or B Above. Also complete Part V)

1	Gross FUTA tax. Multiply the wages in Part I, line 5, by .062	1	
2	Maximum credit. Multiply the wages in Part I, line 5, by .054	2	
3	Enter the smaller of the amount in Part V, line 11, or Part III, line 2	3	
4	Enter amount from Part I, line 7	4	
5	**Credit allowable** (subtract line 4 from line 3) (If zero or less, enter 0.)	5	
6	**Total FUTA tax** (subtract line 5 from line 1).	6	
7	Less: Total FUTA tax deposited for the year, including any overpayment applied from a prior year (from your records). .	7	
8	**Balance due** (subtract line 7 from line 6—if over $100, see Part IV instructions). Pay to IRS . . . . . . ►	8	
9	**Overpayment** (subtract line 6 from line 7). Check if it is to be: ☐ Applied to next return, or ☐ Refunded. . . . ►	9	

Part IV Record of Quarterly Federal Tax Liability for Unemployment Tax (Do not include state liability)

Quarter	First	Second	Third	Fourth	Total for Year
Liability for quarter	295.60	232.52	82.90	46.74	657.76

If you will not have to file returns in the future, write "Final" here (see general instruction "Who Must File") and sign the return ► _____

Under penalties of perjury, I declare that I have examined this return, including accompanying schedules and statements, and to the best of my knowledge and belief, it is true, correct, and complete, and that no part of any payment made to a state unemployment fund claimed as a credit was or is to be deducted from the payments to employees.

Signature ► *Robert Lander*   Title (Owner, etc.) ► Pres.   Date ► 1/28/86

Form **940** (1985)

Figure 19–15
Form 940 Employer's Annual Federal Unemployment Tax Return.

ments. This is often neglected, especially after a few months have passed, and is very upsetting to the patient who tries to check in at the former address.

Closing a Practice

A medical practice may be closed because of retirement, death, a change in geographic location, or a change in profession. If the closing is unexpected, as in the case of sudden death of the physician, much of the burden falls on the staff. If the closing is voluntary and planned for, the physician may wish to consult an attorney or the local medical society for guidelines. The following information will be useful in either event.

Advance Notice to Patients. The physician who anticipates retirement can begin cutting back the practice months in advance. Patients can be notified as they come in that the practice will be closing on a specified date and asked to begin arrangements for care from another physician. The physician can also ask that patients pay at the time of service, to minimize accounts receivable at the time of retirement.

Avoiding Abandonment Charge. To avoid a charge of abandonment, the physician should notify active patients by letter that the practice is being discontinued. The letter should be sent out at least 3 months in advance, if possible. If a patient has been discharged or has not been in to see the doctor for at least 6 years, there is no obligation to send the notice.

Public Announcement. About 1 month after the physician begins telling patients of the closing, an announcement should be placed in a local newspaper, giving the closing date of the office, explaining any arrangements made for continuing care, and thanking patients for their support in prior years.

Other Notices. Hospital affiliations should be informed early, particularly if the doctor will be leaving the community. If the office space is being rented, be sure to notify the landlord in observance of the rental contract if there is one. Insurance carriers must be advised of the change. The state medical licensure board should be contacted. If the practice is incorporated, an attorney should be consulted about disincorporation.

Patient Transfer and Patient Records. If another doctor is taking over the practice, tell the patient about the new doctor. However, be sure to explain that the patient's records will be transferred to any doctor the patient chooses and that the request for transfer of records must be in writing. For convenience, the doctor can have a form available that needs only the patient's signature.

Although the records belong to the physician, they can legally be transferred to another physician only with the consent of the patient. Any records not transferred should be stored, either in bulk or on microfilm, until the statutes of limitations for malpractice and abandonment have run out.

Financial Concerns. Income tax returns and supporting documents should be kept for at least 3 years after the tax return was filed. Appoint someone to take care of any remaining outstanding accounts receivable.

Disposition of Controlled Substances. Check with the Drug Enforcement Administration for current regulations on disposal of controlled substances and the physician's certificate of registration. Do not simply toss them out. The certificate will have to be sent to the DEA for cancellation and then it will be returned. It may be necessary to produce an inventory of all controlled substances on hand when the practice is terminated, along with duplicate copies of the official order forms that were used to obtain them. Return any unused forms to the DEA. Don't use leftover prescription blanks for note pads. Burn them to avoid misuse.

Professional Liability Insurance. The physician who is discontinuing active medical practice altogether can safely drop the professional liability insurance. However, do not destroy any of the previous policies. Most professional liability claims are covered by the policy that was in effect at the time the alleged act of negligence took place. The suit may be filed many years later and it is important that the old policy be available.

Furnishings and Equipment. Unfortunately, used office furniture and equipment do not bring much in the marketplace. If another physician is taking over the practice, the value of the furnishings and equipment can be negotiated. Many doctors donate their libraries to the local hospital and declare the gift as a deduction on their income tax. This is something to check with the accountant.

Some physicians reward loyal employees with severance pay. On the average this equals at least 1 month's salary plus prorated compensation for any unused vacation time. A letter of reference is usually offered.

There are many details to take care of in closing a practice. Contact the local medical society for further guidance.

REFERENCES AND READINGS

American Medical Association: The Business Side of Medical Practice, Chicago, The Association, 1979.
Cotton, H.: Medical Practice Management. 2nd ed. Oradell, NJ, Medical Economics Books, 1977.
Department of the Treasury, Internal Revenue Service: Circular E, current edition.

For general information and Equal Employment Opportunity Commission publications, contact:

Office of Public Affairs
Equal Employment Opportunity Commission
2041 E Street N.W., Room 412
Washington, D.C. 20507

19

CHAPTER OUTLINE

Externship
  What is Externship?
  Duration and Time of Externship
  Student Responsibilities
  Externship Sites
  Benefits from Externship

Finding the Right Position
  Preparation for the Interview
    Procedure 20–1: Preparing a Resumé
  Locating Prospective Employers
  The Interview
    Procedure 20–2: Answering a Help-Wanted
      Advertisement

VOCABULARY

See Glossary at end of book for definitions.

avocational	extracurricular	personal inventory
chronologic	format	resumé
externship	objective	seminar

20

Externship and Finding the Right Position

OBJECTIVES

Upon successful completion of this chapter you should be able to:

1. Define the terms listed in the Vocabulary of this chapter.
2. Explain the essentials of an externship.
3. Briefly explain four responsibilities of the student during externship.
4. Describe the responsibilities of an externship office or agency.
5. Explain how a student will benefit from the externship experience.
6. List the three steps in applying for a position.
7. Identify the five essential parts of a personal inventory.
8. List seven basic items that should be included in every resumé.
9. Specify five items that must not be inserted in a resumé.
10. Cite five sources of leads for employment as a medical assistant.
11. List three avenues of evaluation that an interviewer may use in selecting an employee.

Upon successful completion of this chapter you should be able to perform the following activities:

1. Prepare a personal inventory.
2. Prepare two examples of a resumé.
3. Demonstrate a telephone request for an interview.
4. Write a letter in response to a newspaper help-wanted ad.
5. Compose a follow-up letter of thanks following an interview for a position.

EXTERNSHIP

As you progress in your training you will be giving thought as to just how and where you will fit into the health care arena, and you will undoubtedly have acquired certain preferences.

One aid in defining and focusing your interests is an **externship** program that provides practical experience in a variety of qualified physicians' offices, accredited hospitals, or other health care facilities. Externship experience is included by most schools and colleges that have a complete curriculum for medical assistants. In those programs accredited by the Committee on Allied Health Education and Accreditation (CAHEA) in collaboration with AMA and AAMA, an externship is mandatory. A minimum of 160 hours is recommended.

What is Externship?

The externship phase of your training may also be known as work experience or on-the-job training (Fig. 20–1). During these very important weeks you will have an opportunity to apply your administrative and clinical skills under the supervision of a practicing medical assistant. The medical assistant and the physician who supervise your practical experience will be responsible for an ongoing evaluation of your performance, which will be given to your instructor and become a part of your student records.

Duration and Time of Externship

The duration of the externship and the time at which it is introduced into the program will vary, depending upon the school or college. Some schools have the student spend a day or two in a health facility near the beginning of the training, to provide a frame of reference for later instruction. Some programs combine work experience with classroom instruction throughout the training period. The majority of schools prefer a concentrated period of externship near the conclusion of the education process.

Student Responsibilities

During your externship, both your looks and actions must be professional. You will report to

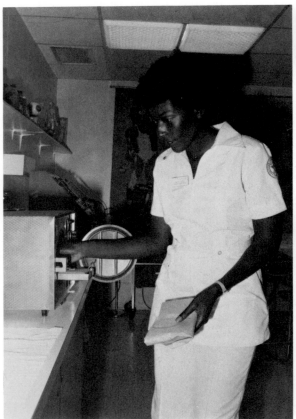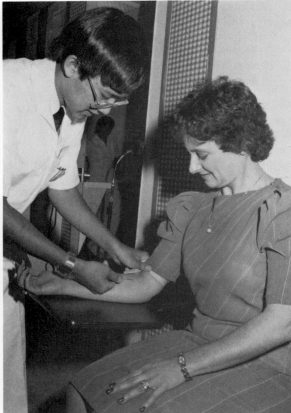

Figure 20–1

Students in externship. (Courtesy of Southern California College of Medical and Dental Careers, Anaheim, CA. Photo by Dan Santucci.)

324

work at a specified time on specified days, just as if you were a regular employee, but you will not be paid by the training facility. You may spend all your externship in one facility, but it is usually preferable to rotate among several types of practice for a well-rounded experience. Do not be surprised if you are expected to apply and be interviewed for the position just as you will later on when you are seeking employment. This is valuable experience and should be welcomed.

You, as a student, should recognize that a health care agency that cooperates with your education is accepting a great responsibility. You will require continual supervision and your questions must be answered. You must be aware of ethical and legal concerns and the potential for a claim of medical malpractice. One large concern is that of patient privacy. You must reveal no information concerning a patient or the practice to persons outside the facility. Some agencies may ask you to sign an oath of privacy while in that facility.

Externship Sites

The school or college will designate a specific individual to be your externship coordinator, who will carefully choose and screen suitable training facilities. The supervising staff at the health care facility must agree to provide ample opportunity for you to practice your skills, and to complete an evaluation of your performance. Quite often the coordinator will seek out offices where former graduates of the program are employed. This ensures greater understanding and cooperation as well as the assurance that work habits and procedures meet the standards promoted in the classroom. In rare instances a student may feel that the training facility is taking advantage of a situation and simply using the student to perform menial tasks. If you do have such an experience, it should be reported to your instructor.

The value of the externship is enhanced when the training program includes a weekly **seminar** where all the students serving externship and their instructor may share experiences, problems, and solutions.

Benefits from Externship

All three parties to the agreement—the school, the externship office or facility and the trainee—benefit from the experience.

The school has a line of communication to the community, and is better able to assess the needs and requirements of the public for which it is training prospective employees.

The externship agency benefits from the new ideas and methods that the trainee may introduce.

If the facility is looking for additional help, this is an ideal way to evaluate the performance of a trainee without involvement in the hiring process.

You, the trainee, benefit most of all by exposure to practical experience in a variety of settings. This practical experience in the "real world" will remove a great deal of the anxiety that you might otherwise have in a first employment situation. If you perform well during the externship you may be offered a permanent job with the facility where you trained, but you should not depend upon this happening. The externship facility may also be used as a reference when you are seeking a permanent position. When you know that you have performed well and have a comfortable relationship with the supervisory staff in the training facility, you may ask for a reference to be used later on when interviewing for employment.

FINDING THE RIGHT POSITION

After you have completed your classroom training and externship, the next step will be that of finding the right position. Your aptitudes and skills must be matched with the requirements of a physician or facility in need of an employee. Whether you are seeking your first position or are returning to the field after an absence of several years, or even if you are an experienced medical assistant preparing to change employers, the steps in applying for a position are essentially the same:

Step 1—Preparation for the interview
Step 2—Locating prospective employers
Step 3—The interview

Looking for work is a job in itself. Establish a schedule and stick to it.

PRELIMINARY STEPS

Before seeking an interview, ask yourself some pertinent questions:

- What type of work do I really want?
- Where can I function best?
- Do I prefer clinical or administrative duty?
- What are my skills?
- Do I prefer to work in a solo practice or in a large medical group?
- Would I enjoy the variety of a general practice or the concentration of a specialty practice?
- How important to me are salary, hours, and location?

In your externship experience you may have formed some rather definite preferences, or you may feel absolutely certain of some things that would cause you to be dissatisfied.

20

Preparation for the Interview

PERSONAL INVENTORY

It sometimes happens that your first position is so ideally suitable that you will accept and stay in it for the remainder of your working years. More likely, though, you will have to make several changes of employment during your lifetime.

A **personal inventory**, to which you will add as you gain additional experience and education, will prove invaluable to you later as well as now. The personal inventory is for your own information and reference. It will be a ready source of information in preparing and updating your **resumé**. The *personal inventory* is complete information about yourself; a *resumé* is selected information tailored to the position you are seeking.

1. Start with a page for biographic data: your name, birth date, Social Security number, address, and telephone number.

BIOGRAPHIC DATA

Name _____ Birth Date _____
_____ Soc. Sec. No. _____
Address _____
_____ Tel. No. _____

---

2. Prepare a separate page for your employment history. If you have never been employed but have done volunteer work requiring personal responsibility, list that here. The employment history should include dates of employment, name of employer, type of business, your position title, and major duties. Because this will be a continuing record that you will add to as you gain experience, it is prepared in **chronologic** order, starting with the first major job you held. When you use this information in a resumé, however, it will be listed in reverse chronologic order, beginning with the latest position.

EMPLOYMENT HISTORY

June 1978 to June 1980 Employer Looking Good
Month Year Month Year

Type of Business _____ Women's clothing _____
Position Held _____ Part-time sales clerk _____

Major Duties: Assisting customers in their selections, registering sales, closing out register at end of day

Satisfactions: Enjoyed personal contacts
Learned to accept responsibility

Dissatisfactions: Not related to my goals

---

3. Next, record your educational data, beginning with high school. List the dates, the institution attended, and the year of graduation, plus the diploma or degree earned. Make note of the areas of study you enjoyed most and list special competencies, awards, or honors. As time goes by it may be difficult to recall these details, and you never know what will be important to an employer in the future. Remember, you are starting a permanent record for your own information and as a handy reference tool when needed. As with the employment history, the educational data is listed here in chronologic order but will appear in reverse chronologic order in a resumé, starting with the highest degree or certificate.

EDUCATIONAL DATA

Dates	Institution Attended	Yr Graduated/Degree
1982–1985	Valley High School Ola Vista	1985 Diploma
1985–1987	Ola Vista Community College	1987 Associate in Science, Medical Assisting

Special Competencies:
Typing Certificate (70 WPM)
Limited X-ray permit, 1987
CPR Certificate, 1987, renewed annually
Fluency in Spanish

Awards:
Dean's List, all four semesters in college

---

4. You may wish to include a page for your extracurricular interests and activities. List organization memberships and activities and any positions of leadership you held. Your volunteer activities might be included here if they are not in your employment record. Also include any significant hobbies.

EXTRACURRICULAR INTERESTS AND ACTIVITIES

Organization Memberships	Year	Personal Participation
Associated Women Students	1985–1986	Secretary
American Association of Medical Assistants	1985–	Student member Page, 1985 convention
Girl Scouts of the U.S.A.	1978–	Brownie group leader, 1984

Hobbies

Oil painting, backpacking

---

5. Finally, have a page for your personal goals. What are your immediate goals? your long-term goals? What concessions are you willing to make in order to reach your goals?

```
                    PERSONAL GOALS

  Date    Immediate Goals          Long-Term Goals
  1987    Medical assistant position,   Bachelor of Science
          preferably in pediatric        in Business
          practice                       Administration

                                   Administrative position
                                     in large group practice
                                     or HMO
```

RESUME

The final and most important step in preparing for an interview is producing a resumé that will arouse the interest of a prospective employer.

If you do not feel confident in doing this yourself, get help. If you are a student in a two-year college there is probably a career center on campus where you can ask for assistance. There are also many guidebooks in the public library and in bookstores where you can find ideas galore. See the references at the end of this chapter.

Purpose of the Resumé. The purpose of the resumé is to get an interview, not to get a job. Keep this in mind as you decide what to include. Using your personal inventory, select the information that applies to the position you have in mind. Choose an attractive format, and type the information on one sheet of paper with absolutely no errors or misspelled words (Figs. 20–2 and 20–3). Tinted

```
THERESA O'SULLIVAN, CMA-AC          Certified Medical Assistant
233 West Wentworth Street            Administrative and Clinical
San Diego, CA  92184

Telephone: 619-239-2345

EDUCATION:          Associate in Science and
                    Certificate in Medical Assisting
                    Ola Vista Community College        June 1986

                        Dean's List, 4 semesters

                    Diploma, Valley High School        June 1984


SPECIAL             Speak Spanish fluently
COMPETENCIES:       Hold Limited X-ray Permit
                    CPR Certificate (renewed
                       annually since 1983)


EMPLOYMENT:         William O. Madden, M.D.            June 1985
                       Part-time Medical Assistant        to
                    Duties included: preparing         June 1986
                    patients for examination in
                    general practice office; taking
                    height, weight, and vital signs;
                    telephone, reception, and
                    appointment scheduling, four
                    afternoons a week


                    Baxters Department Store           June 1983
                       Part-time Salesperson              to
                    Duties included: assisting         June 1985
                    customers in their selections;
                    registering sales; closing out
                    register at end of day.


AVOCATIONAL         Student member, American
INTERESTS:             Association of Medical Assistants
                    Secretary, Associated Women
                       Students OVCC


REFERENCES          Furnished upon request
```

Figure 20–2
Sample chronologic resumé.

20

```
                    THERESA O'SULLIVAN, CMA-AC
                  STATEMENT OF EMPLOYMENT ASSETS
                         FOR A CAREER IN
                         MEDICAL  ASSISTING

     233 West Wentworth Street, San Diego CA 92184          619-239-2345

     SKILLS

     Administrative      Appointment scheduling, filing, pegboard and electronic
                         billing systems, account collections, insurance billing,
                         coding, recordkeeping, bank deposits and statement
                         reconciliation, patient histories, medical terminology,
                         machine transcription, word processing.


     Clinical            Specialized knowledge of medical ethics, symptoms and
                         diseases, collecting and handling laboratory specimens,
                         procedures for assisting with physical examination,
                         emergency first aid and CPR, injections, sterile
                         techniques, EKG, inventory and supplies.


     References          Furnished upon request
```

Figure 20–3
Sample skills resumé.

paper will make the resumé more distinctive, but avoid using bright colors or arty headings. The resumé gives you an opportunity to display the qualifications that enhance your appeal to prospective employers. Omit anything that cannot help you or anything that would detract from your image. Once you are in the interview, you can clarify any item not entirely explained on the resumé.

Writing the Resumé. There is no standard format for a resumé, but it should be typewritten on 8½ × 11 good quality paper. It should be concise, honest, and have a professional look.

Heading. At the top of your paper, so that it stands apart (may be centered), place the necessary personal information: name, address, and telephone number. Display this prominently for easy identification.

Objective. The modern trend is to omit reference to an objective, particularly if your qualifications are vocationally specific. If you do include an objective, avoid such words as "challenge" or "opportunity," as this focuses on what the applicant wants instead of showing understanding of what the employer wants and needs.

Education and Experience. If you are a recent graduate with little or no experience, list your education first and then your employment, if any. College graduates need not include high school backgrounds. If you have a good history of recent employment, make this the first item, followed by

education. In both cases, start with your most recent position and list the rest in reverse time order.

Professional Licenses. Include any professional licenses or certificates, and memberships in professional organizations.

Extracurricular Activities. List any **extracurricular** or **avocational** interests that would be applicable to the position sought.

References. State on your resumé that references will be furnished upon request. (Do not list names and addresses of references on the resumé.) Be prepared to furnish the names of at least three references at the time of your interview. These should have been typewritten on a separate page in the same style as your resumé. Don't forget to obtain permission from the persons you are listing.

Do not include: your photograph, names of spouse and/or children, reasons for terminating previous position, past salaries or present salary requirements, or the names and addresses of references.

Locating Prospective Employers

If you are a student in an accredited school, your instructor or the school may be able to give you names of prospective employers. Other good sources for leads are the local medical society, other medical assistants, branches of the United States Employment Service, and state-operated employment offices. You may also wish to check the classified advertisements in your local newspaper, or place your name with an employment agency. Private employment agencies generally charge a fee equivalent to 2 to 4 weeks' salary to successful applicants. This fee is sometimes paid by the employer.

The Interview

REQUESTING AN INTERVIEW

If you are responding to an advertisement that lists a telephone number, *telephoning to request an interview* is preferable to writing a letter, but an unsolicited telephone call may be disruptive and destroy the opportunity for an interview. If no telephone number is included in the advertisement, there will be an address listed (usually a box number) to which you may direct a letter requesting an interview.

Letter in Response to Advertisement. A *cover letter responding to an advertisement* should include:

1. A reference to the advertisement, including name of newspaper, date of publication, and position title. The employer may be running more than one recruitment ad.

Procedure 20–1

Preparing a Resumé

PROCEDURAL GOAL

To prepare a resumé of education and experience that will be informative to a prospective employer and create interest in arranging an interview for employment.

EQUIPMENT AND SUPPLIES

Summary of personal data
Quality stationery
Typewriter

PROCEDURE

1. Assemble all personal data necessary for resumé.
2. Arrange in reverse chronologic order.
   Purpose: To enable you to proceed in orderly fashion in preparing the resumé and to check accuracy of dates.
3. Typewrite heading that includes your name, address, and telephone number.
   Purpose: For easy identification by reader.
4. List highest education degree or diploma, including name of institution and year. Include high school if you are not a college graduate.
   Purpose: Training may be important to your employability.
5. List all work experience in reverse chronologic order.
   Purpose: To demonstrate transferable experiences toward future employment.
6. Include any professional licenses, certificates, and memberships in professional organizations.
   Purpose: Indicates employability and personal interest in profession.
7. List any extracurricular or avocational interests applicable to the position sought.
8. State that references will be furnished upon request.
   Purpose: Prospective employers may wish to verify your experience and character.
   Note: Obtain permission prior to listing anyone as a reference.
9. Review resumé for accuracy, completeness, and attractive format.

TERMINAL PERFORMANCE OBJECTIVE

To prepare a resumé that will project a positive image of employability and provide necessary introductory information in seeking an interview for employment, within 30 minutes, to a performance level of 100%. (Time may vary.)

20

2. An enthusiastic expression of interest in the position.

3. A comparison of your own qualifications with those of the position to be filled.

4. Information about where you can be contacted.

5. A request for a response or interview.

6. Thanks for considering your request.

Unsolicited Interview Request. You may decide to canvas a number of medical facilities to determine whether there are openings for a medical assistant. Write a letter such as the one shown in Figure 20–4

and enclose your resumé. Then follow up with a telephone call in about a week.

DAY OF THE INTERVIEW

Your appearance is extremely important. Clothing should be conservative, neat, and well-pressed. Women should wear a dress or suit with a skirt. Slacks or pantsuits and open sandals are considered inappropriate for job interviews. Men should wear a suit and tie, and appropriate dress shoes. The man or woman who is still actively in a student

```
                233 West Wentworth Street
                San Diego, CA 92184
                June 1, 19xx


                Arthur M. Blackburn, M.D.
                2200 Broadway
                Anytown, US 98765

                Dear Doctor Blackburn:

                In a few weeks I will complete my formal training in medical
                assisting, with an Associate in Science Degree from Ola Vista
                Community College.

                The medical assisting program at Ola Vista has included theory
                and practical application in both administrative and clinical
                skills.  My six weeks supervised externship gave me additional
                practical experience in two specialty practices.

                While studying at Ola Vista I have also worked part-time for a
                busy physician in family practice, while maintaining a 3.5 grade
                point average.  My experience as Dr. Madden's employee is
                outlined on the enclosed resume.  I have enjoyed my work in
                Dr. Madden's office but am now seeking full-time employment.

                If you will require a replacement or addition to your staff in
                the near future, may I be considered as an applicant?  My
                telephone number is 619-239-2345.  I will follow up with a
                telephone call within a week.

                Sincerely yours,



                Theresa O'Sullivan

                Enc. Resume
```

Figure 20–4
Sample cover letter.

Procedure 20-2

ANSWERING A HELP-WANTED ADVERTISEMENT

PROCEDURAL GOAL:

To write a letter in response to a newspaper advertisement that will relay your qualifications and generate interest in arranging an interview.

EQUIPMENT AND SUPPLIES

Recent newspaper with classified employment ads.
Stationery
Typewriter
Pen

PROCEDURE

1. Review letter writing information in Chapter 10, Written Communications.
2. Draft a letter to include:
   a. Name of newspaper, date of publication and title of position for which you are applying.
      Purpose: Employer may be running more than one advertisement.
   b. Information about where you can be contacted.
      Purpose: To enable interested employer to reach you.
3. Express enthusiastic interest in the position offered, and state your qualifications.
4. Request a response to your letter by telephone or letter.
   Purpose: So that an interview can be arranged if position is still open and employer is interested in your qualifications.
5. End the letter with an expression of thanks for considering your request.
   Purpose: To demonstrate your knowledge of courtesy.
6. Review the letter for content and accuracy.
   Purpose: To make certain that you have included all essential information and that the letter is free of errors.

TERMINAL PERFORMANCE OBJECTIVE

To produce a persuasive letter in response to a newspaper advertisement that will result in an interview for employment, within 15 minutes to a performance level of 95%.

---

program may wish to go to the interview in a fresh, clean uniform bearing the school insignia (Fig. 20–5).

Hair should be well-groomed and worn in a professional looking style. Keep jewelry to a minimum and avoid heavy scents of perfume or antiperspirants. Women should be careful and conservative in applying makeup and should carry a modest purse that is not bulging with unnecessary items.

Take a critical look at yourself in the mirror before leaving home and again just before entering the prospective employer's office.

Arrive promptly for the interview. Under no circumstances should you be even so much as a minute late and then have to make a weak excuse.

Go alone. You may want moral support, but you will be more relaxed if there is no one waiting for you.

Enter the office confidently, without appearing rushed.

Introduce yourself to the receptionist, then express appreciation when you are asked to be seated.

If you must wait, try to relax, but avoid slouching in your chair.

Do not smoke or chew gum!

When you prepared your resumé you listed your job skills and/or education. The interviewer already knows how well you ought to be able to do the job. However, you will be judged in at least two other areas of evaluation:

1. *What kind of co-worker you will be.* Work in a

20

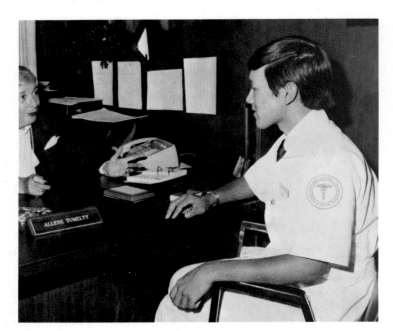

Figure 20–5
Student being interviewed for a job. (Courtesy of Southern California College of Medical and Dental Careers, Anaheim, CA. Photo by Dan Santucci.)

health care facility is a team effort, and your ability to work in cooperation and coordination with others will bear heavily on how well you will do your job, apart from how good your specific job skills may be.

2. *What kind of employee you will be.* Dependability, trustworthiness, dedication, loyalty, and other personal characteristics are always important to an employer.

EMPLOYMENT APPLICATION

Completing an employment application is not standard procedure in smaller medical practices, but you should be prepared for this if asked. Larger health agencies such as hospitals and HMOs will definitely ask you to fill out their application form.

Make notes in advance of your Social Security number, driver's license, and telephone numbers where you can be reached. Your resumé should have the information you will need regarding education and employment. Be prepared to furnish telephone numbers for previous employers if asked, and have available the names, addresses, and telephone numbers of three references who have given you their permission to list them.

The appearance and completeness of your filled-in application will be considered in your overall evaluation. By law, employers cannot require you to answer questions regarding your place of birth, ethnic origin or religious preference, or about your age, marital status, or number of children. If these questions are on the application you may choose to leave them blank, but all allowable questions should be answered honestly and completely. Print your answers or write as plainly as possible. Having your own favorite pen with you may help.

DURING THE INTERVIEW

When you are ushered into the interviewer's room, wait to be seated until you are invited to do so. Let the interviewer lead the conversation. Be prepared to answer such questions as "Tell me about yourself," and "Why do you want to work here?" One reason for an opening such as this is to provide a little time to relax and get acquainted. You might start out by reviewing your professional background and training, and then progress to personal interests, hobbies, and so forth.

Remember that the interviewer will be observing your manners, poise, speech, alertness, and ability to give direct answers. A relaxed, friendly manner with good eye contact is important. You must look directly at the person to whom you are speaking. Your sense of humor may be tested as well, and questions may be directed to you that will test your common sense and frankness. You can promote yourself honestly and graciously by showing that you enjoy others, are willing to work and accept responsibility, and that you have an open mind about the position and are willing to learn.

Recent legislation in fair employment practices has influenced hiring practices nationwide. Employers are restricted in the information that can be required on an application or asked in an interview.

But while you may not be required to answer questions regarding your age, birthplace, marital status, and so forth, a prospective employer might appreciate your mentioning any such pertinent information in conversation. Remember your objective—a position.

At the end of the interview, if the interviewer has not mentioned hours and salary, you may properly inquire at this time. If you are not really interested in the position, do not bother to ask, but if the position sounds satisfactory and is one that you would like to accept, you may then ask if the interviewer wishes to discuss the salary. This should be enough of a lead, since it was probably an oversight on the interviewer's part. If the interviewer seems reluctant to discuss it, though, do not press the issue, as this may be an indication that your qualifications do not fit the position and there is no reason to pursue the interview further.

If you have been given a tour of the office (Fig. 20–6), you may make some pleasant observations and comments, but do not be falsely overenthusiastic. When you are introduced to the staff be gracious and friendly. Try to remember their names so that you can thank them later. Show enthusiasm, but do not overdo it, because it may appear to others that you are "putting on an act."

CLOSING THE INTERVIEW

The interviewer will usually take the initiative in closing the interview, perhaps by sliding back the chair and asking whether you have further questions. Do not show disappointment if the position is not offered to you at the time of the interview.

There may be other applicants to see, or the interviewer may wish to check your references before making a commitment. Express your thanks for the interview as you leave, and remember, too, to thank the receptionist and say a friendly goodbye.

FOLLOW-UP ACTIVITIES

A brief, well-worded letter of thanks sent to the interviewer immediately after the interview could be crucial in deciding whether you will be hired. This is one of the most essential steps in the whole job-seeking process—and the one most overlooked by job-seekers. Simply write a brief note expressing appreciation for the interview and interest in the position (Fig. 20–7).

After a few days you may call the office and ask if the position has been filled, and tell them you are interested because you enjoyed your interview and the office. If the position is still open, ask whether you may inquire again in a few days. Be brief and thank the person with whom you are speaking.

If you don't get the job, ask yourself some pertinent questions:

- Did I look my best?
- Did I show enthusiasm for the job?
- Did I listen carefully during the interview?
- Did I say or do something I shouldn't have?

Even if you are not hired, you should never feel that an interview is a waste of time. You learn from each experience, and with experience you are better able to promote your qualifications in future interviews.

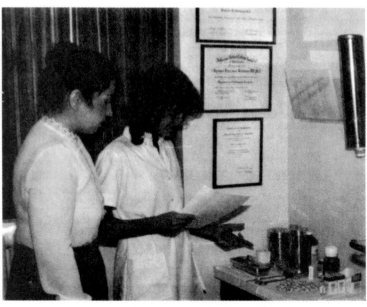

Figure 20–6
The medical assistant is often required to give a prospective employee a tour of the facilities.

20

```
233 Wentworth Street
San Diego, CA 92184
June 15, 19xx


Arthur M. Blackburn, M.D.
2200 Broadway
Anytown, US 98765

Dear Doctor Blackburn:

Thank you for taking the time to talk with me today
about the medical assistant position in your office,
and for considering my qualifications for filling that
position.

I would be pleased to accept your offer if you should
decide that I meet your requirements.

Sincerely yours,


Theresa O'Sullivan
```

Figure 20–7
Thank-you letter following an interview.

REFERENCES AND READINGS

Beatty, R. H.: *The Resume Kit.* New York, John Wiley & Sons, 1984.

Bolles, R. N. : *The Three Boxes of Life, and How to Get Out of Them.* Berkeley, CA, Ten Speed Press, 1983.

Bolles, R. N.: *What Color Is Your Parachute?* Berkeley, CA, Ten Speed Press, 1987.

Bostwick, B.: *Resume Writing.* New York, John Wiley & Sons, 1980.

Camden, T. M., and Green, F.: *How to Get a Job in Los Angeles—The Insider's Guide.* Chicago, IL, Surrey Books, 1985. (This is one of a series available for large cities in the U.S. and contains excellent information.)

Claypool, J.: *How to Get a Good Job.* New York, Franklin Watts, 1982.

Elsman, M.: *How to Get Your First Job.* New York, Crown Publishers, 1985.

Gootnick, D.: *Getting a Better Job.* New York, McGraw-Hill Paperbacks, 1978.

Holtz, H.: *Beyond the Resume: How to Land the Job You Want.* New York, McGraw-Hill, 1984.

Jackson, T.: *The Perfect Resume.* Garden City, NY, Anchor Press Doubleday, 1981.

Lewis, A.: *How to Write a Better Resume.* Woodbury, NY, Barron's Educational Series, 1983.

Reed, J. (Editor, Resume Service): *Resumes That Get Jobs.* New York, Arco Publishing, 1981.

20

SECTION III THE CLINICAL ASSISTANT

CHAPTER OUTLINE

Normal Nutrition
  Nutrition and Dietetics
  Food
  Energy
  Dietary Evaluation
  Nutrients
    Carbohydrates
    Fats
    Proteins

Vitamins
Minerals
Water
Fiber

Clinical Nutrition
  Modifying a Diet
  Prescribing a Diet
  Seven Dietary Guidelines for Americans

VOCABULARY

See Glossary at end of book for definitions.

anorexia nervosa
atherosclerosis
bulimia
diabetes

endogenous
exogenous
glycogen

obesity
phenylketonuria
scurvy

21

Assisting With Nutrition and Diet Modification

OBJECTIVES

Upon successful completion of this chapter you should be able to
1. Define and spell the words listed in the Vocabulary for this chapter.
2. Describe normal nutrition.
3. List the four basic food groups.
4. Discuss what is meant by Recommended Dietary Allowance.
5. Calculate the caloric value of carbohydrates, fats, and proteins.
6. Describe the appearance of saturated fats and unsaturated fats.
7. Differentiate between fat-soluble and water-soluble vitamins.
8. Describe the role of carbohydrates in the diet.
9. State the causes of the following deficiency diseases: beriberi, pellagra, scurvy, anemia, pernicious anemia, rickets, and diabetes.
10. Explain the need for calcium, sodium, potassium, and iodine in the daily diet.
11. List the 7 dietary guidelines for Americans.

Upon successful completion of this chapter you should be able to perform the following activities:
1. Write a personal diet history for two weeks.
2. Calculate the total daily calories in your personal diet.
3. Determine whether your daily food intake includes the four basic food groups, in the recommended servings.
4. Adjust your daily diet to meet the recommended daily allowances for nutrients.

NORMAL NUTRITION

Good health is the state of emotional and physical well-being that is determined to a large extent by a person's diet. We are, quite literally, what we eat, since the food we consume is used to build and repair every part of our bodies. Consequently, it is important that the food choices made are based on sound information and knowledge. A person who is well nourished will probably be more alert in every way and emotionally better balanced. The well-nourished person is also better able than the poorly nourished individual to ward off infections.

The physician, the medical assistant, and the dietitian all are closely involved in the nutritive care of the patient. The physician prescribes the diet, and, ideally, the dietitian instructs the patient in how to follow it. Frequently, however, such professional aid is not available. In this case, it is often necessary for the assistant to discuss the diet with the patient, answer questions, and explain certain aspects of the modifications involved. Many patients may hesitate to ask the physician details about the diet, or questions may arise after the patients leave the office. Such concerns typically include methods of preparation, sources of information, and interpretation of labels, and the medical assistant is the one the patient turns to for answers. Consequently, the assistant should be able to answer basic questions on normal nutrition and should have a fundamental knowledge of the diets that physicians prescribe most often.

Nutrition and Dietetics

Nutrition refers to all the processes involved in the intake and utilization of nutrients. *Nutrients* are the organic and inorganic chemicals in food that supply the energy and raw materials for cellular activities. *Metabolism* refers to the cellular activities that occur inside and outside the cells. *Digestion* is a series of reactions occurring in the mouth, stomach, and small intestine that results in reducing large food molecules into simple absorbable forms. These absorbed nutrients are then carried by the bloodstream to all parts of the body, where they are metabolized.

The word nutrition is also used to indicate nutritional status, or the condition of the body resulting from the utilization of the essential nutrients available to the body. Public interest in nutrition has increased in recent years owing to the growing concern about physical fitness.

We gratefully acknowledge the contributions of Lee Weller Callaway, R.D., M.P.H., Ph.D., to previous editions of this chapter.

Dietetics is the practical application of nutritional science to individuals. It is "the combined science and art of feeding individuals or groups under different economic or health conditions according to the principles of nutrition and management." The dietitian is the individual who is concerned with this promotion of good health through proper diet and with the therapeutic use of diet in the treatment of disease.

Food

Food is defined as any material that meets the nutritive requirements of an organism for the maintenance of growth and physical well-being. To be classified as a food, a substance must perform one or more of three basic functions in the body: provide a source of fuel, or energy; supply nutrients to build and repair tissues; and supply nutrients to regulate body processes (Fig. 21–1). Most foods supply both fuel and nutrients; however, no one food supplies all the nutrients required for proper metabolism. Consequently, a combination of different foods is necessary. With a little planning, a well-balanced diet supplying all the body's needs can be obtained. A deficient or inadequate diet results in malnutrition and may lead to a variety of diseases. Good nutrition is particularly critical for pregnant women and young children, since malnutrition during development and growth may result in physical and mental retardation.

Energy

Every bodily action, whether voluntary or involuntary, requires energy. Even when asleep, the body still needs a source of energy to keep the heart beating, the lungs breathing, and other vital organs functioning. The involuntary activities of digestion and respiration also require energy even though they are not consciously controlled. *Basal metabolism* is the term used for this energy expenditure when the body is at rest.

There are basically two energy sources available to the body: **exogenous** and **endogenous**. When the quantities of food (exogenous) consumed are insufficient to furnish the required fuel, the body begins to break down its fat reserves (endogenous) in an attempt to supply the necessary energy. Generally, it is desirable for the daily food intake to equal the total energy needs of the body (number of calories needed for both voluntary and involuntary activities).

Quantities of energy are expressed in units of heat energy called calories. A *calorie (cal)* is the amount of heat needed to raise the temperature of

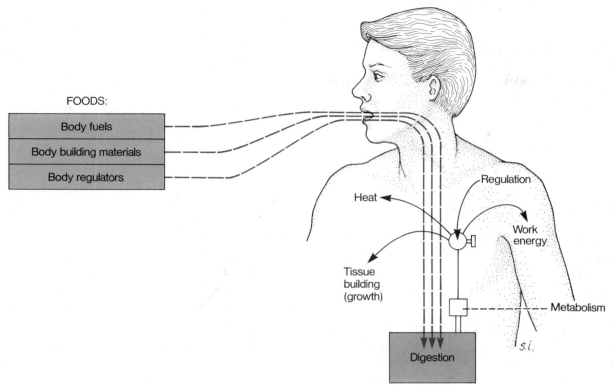

FOODS:

| Body fuels |
| Body building materials |
| Body regulators |

Regulation

Heat

Work energy

Tissue building (growth)

Metabolism

s.i.

Digestion

Figure 21–1

Diagram summarizing the functions of food. To qualify as a food, an item must offer substances that act as body fuel to provide energy, serve to build or maintain body tissues, or act as regulators of body processes. Many foods contain substances that serve all three purposes.

1 gm of water one degree centigrade. Since this unit represents a relatively small amount of energy and metabolism involves much larger quantities of energy, the *large calorie (Cal)*, or *kilocalorie (kcal)*, is commonly used. A kilocalorie is defined as the amount of heat required to raise the temperature of 1 kg of water one degree centigrade. Of the seven food constituents (carbohydrates, proteins, fats, water, minerals, vitamins, and fiber), only carbohydrates, proteins, and fats are capable of furnishing the body with energy. Carbohydrates and proteins yield 4 kcal/gm, whereas 1 gm of fat provides 9 kcal. The amount of energy needed by a given individual varies considerably according to activity level and basal requirements; however, most adults require 1800 to 3300 kcal a day (Table 21–1).

Dietary Evaluation

Nutritional requirements based on average daily amounts of the nutrients considered necessary have been established by international and national committees. *The Food and Nutrition Board* has established the *recommended dietary allowances (RDA)* (Table 21–2) for maintenance of good nutrition of healthy persons. Even though a diet may be adequate in calories, it may not be adequate in nutrients. A *balanced diet* includes adequate amounts of the essential food constituents. To meet the body's nutritional requirements, the daily diet should include food from the four main groups: milk and dairy products; meats, eggs, nuts, peas, or beans; fruits and vegetables; and breads and cereals (Table 21–3).

Foods within a group supply similar nutrients, although the foods differ in caloric level. If the Four Basic Food Groups plan is followed and no other foods are included, the average diet will supply 1200 kcal. If the foods from each group are chosen wisely, a person can meet all of the nutrient requirements (with the possible exception of iron for women). Additional calories are easily obtained by either increasing the total quantity of food eaten from the Basic Four or adding sugars and fats to these foods (Table 21–2).

In planning daily menus, a person should try to schedule regularly spaced meals. It is not an absolute necessity that three meals be consumed; however, it is extremely difficult to meet all of the nutrient and caloric requirements with fewer meals. Each meal should supply about one third of the total daily requirements. This means that something from each group should be included at every meal.

Table 21-1
Mean Heights and Weights and Recommended Energy Intake*

Category	Age (years)	Weight (kg)	Weight (lb)	Height (cm)	Height (in)	Energy Needs (with range) (kcal)	(MJ)
Infants	0.0–0.5	6	13	60	24	kg × 115 (95–145)	kg × .48
	0.5–1.0	9	20	71	28	kg × 105 (80–135)	kg × .44
Children	1–3	13	29	90	35	1300 (900–1800)	5.5
	4–6	20	44	112	44	1700 (1300–2300)	7.1
	7–10	28	62	132	52	2400 (1650–3300)	10.1
Males	11–14	45	99	157	62	2700 (2000–3700)	11.3
	15–18	66	145	176	69	2800 (2100–3900)	11.8
	19–22	70	154	177	70	2900 (2500–3300)	12.2
	23–50	70	154	178	70	2700 (2300–3100)	11.3
	51–75	70	154	178	70	2400 (2000–2800)	10.1
	76+	70	154	178	70	2050 (1650–2450)	8.6
Females	11–14	46	101	157	62	2200 (1500–3000)	9.2
	15–18	55	120	163	64	2100 (1200–3000)	8.8
	19–22	55	120	163	64	2100 (1700–2500)	8.8
	23–50	55	120	163	64	2000 (1600–2400)	8.4
	51–75	55	120	163	64	1800 (1400–2200)	7.6
	76+	55	120	163	64	1600 (1200–2000)	6.7
Pregnant						+300	
Lactating						+500	

Slightly adapted from Recommended Dietary Allowances, revised 1980, Food and Nutrition Board, National Academy of Sciences–National Research Council, Washington, D.C.

*The data in this table have been assembled from observed median heights and weights of children, together with desirable weights for adults for the mean heights of men (70 inches) and women (64 inches) between the ages of 18 and 34 years as surveyed in the U.S. population (HEW/NCHS data).

The energy allowances for the young adults are for men and women doing light work. The allowances for the two older groups represent mean energy needs over these age spans, allowing for a 2% decrease in basal (resting) metabolic rate per decade and reduction in activity of 200 kcal/day for men and women between 51 and 75 years, 500 kcal for men over 75 years, and 400 kcal for women over 75. The customary range of daily energy output is shown in parentheses for adults, and is based on a variation in energy needs of ±400 kcal at any one age, emphasizing the wide range of energy intakes appropriate for any group of people.

Energy allowances for children through age 18 are based on median energy intakes of children of these ages followed in longitudinal growth studies. The values in parentheses are 10th and 90th percentiles of energy intake, to indicate the range of energy consumption among children of these ages.

Table 21-2
Recommended Daily Dietary Allowances, Revised 1980*

	Age (years)	Weight (kg)	Weight (lb)	Height (cm)	Height (in)	Protein (g)	Fat-Soluble Vitamins — VITAMIN A (μg RE)†	VITAMIN D (μg)‡	VITAMIN E (mg α TE)§	Water-Soluble Vitamins — VITAMIN C (mg)	THIAMINE (mg)
Infants	0.0–0.5	6	13	60	24	kg × 2.2	420	10	3	35	0.3
	0.5–1.0	9	20	71	28	kg × 2.0	400	10	4	35	0.5
Children	1–3	13	29	90	35	23	400	10	5	45	0.7
	4–6	20	44	112	44	30	500	10	6	45	0.9
	7–10	28	62	132	52	34	700	10	7	45	1.2
Males	11–14	45	99	157	62	45	1000	10	8	50	1.4
	15–18	66	145	176	69	56	1000	10	10	60	1.4
	19–22	70	154	177	70	56	1000	7.5	10	60	1.5
	23–50	70	154	178	70	56	1000	5	10	60	1.4
	51+	70	154	178	70	56	1000	5	10	60	1.2
Females	11–14	46	101	157	62	46	800	10	8	50	1.1
	15–18	55	120	163	64	46	800	10	8	60	1.1
	19–22	55	120	163	64	44	800	7.5	8	60	1.1
	23–50	55	120	163	64	44	800	5	8	60	1.0
	51+	55	120	163	64	44	800	5	8	60	1.0
Pregnant						+30	+200	+5	+2	+20	+0.4
Lactating						+20	+400	+5	+3	+40	+0.5

Slightly adapted from the Food and Nutrition Board, National Academy of Sciences–National Research Council, Washington, D.C.

*The allowances are intended to provide for individual variations among most normal persons as they live in the United States under usual environmental stresses. Diets should be based on a variety of common foods in order to provide other nutrients for which human requirements have been less well defined.

†Retinol equivalents. 1 Retinol equivalent = 1 μg retinol or 6 μg β-carotene.

‡As cholecalciferol. 10 μg cholecalciferol = 400 IU vitamin D.

§α-tocopherol equivalents, 1 mg d-α-tocopherol = 1 α-TE.

Table continued on opposite page

Nutrients

CARBOHYDRATES

Carbohydrates are chemical organic compounds composed of carbon, hydrogen, and oxygen. They are divided into three groups based on the complexity of the molecule: monosaccharides, disaccharides, and polysaccharides.

Monosaccharides and disaccharides are also called simple sugars; that is, they are made of one (mono) or two (di) units (saccharides). They are water-soluble and sweet to the taste. The three most important monosaccharides in our diet are glucose, fructose, and galactose. Sucrose, lactose, and maltose are examples of disaccharides. Glucose (also called dextrose) and fructose (fruit sugar) are widely distributed in fruits and vegetables. During the process of digestion, disaccharides and the polysaccharide, starch, are broken down into monosaccharides and absorbed into the bloodstream. Once absorbed, they are transported to the liver, where fructose and galactose are converted to glucose. Glucose, then, is an especially important sugar, since it is the form of carbohydrate used by the body for energy and the only form of carbohydrate used in the brain and nervous system for fuel. Galactose is not found free in foods but is one of the two monosaccharides found in the disaccharide lactose.

Lactose is the major carbohydrate in milk and is the only common sugar not found in plant sources. It is not as sweet as many sugars and, therefore, is frequently used to sweeten formulas for tube feedings or to increase the caloric value of juices without appreciably changing the sweetness. Sucrose is granulated, or table, sugar obtained from either sugar cane or sugar beets. Maltose is produced mainly as an intermediate product of starch breakdown during the process of digestion. Some maltose is also found in cereal grains, malted drinks, and sprouting grains.

Polysaccharides are complex sugars, composed of many units of simple sugars. They are neither water-soluble nor sweet to the taste. Sources of polysaccharides are starches, **glycogen,** and cellulose. Starches are found in grain products such as rice and wheat, in vegetables, and in smaller amounts in fruits. Glycogen is not found in the food supply to any appreciable degree. Its importance is that it is formed during the metabolism of glucose and is the storage form of carbohydrate in the body. As such, it is stored in liver and muscle tissue. To use glycogen for energy, the body breaks it down to glucose in the liver. Cellulose is the structural component of plants. In humans, diges-

Table 21–2
Recommended Daily Dietary Allowances, Revised 1980 Continued

| | *Water-Soluble Vitamins* Continued | | | | *Minerals* | | | | | |
RIBO-FLAVIN (mg)	NIACIN (mg NE)‖	VITAMIN B₆ (mg)	FOLACIN¶ (μg)	VITAMIN B₁₂ (μg)	CALCIUM (mg)	PHOSPHORUS (mg)	MAGNESIUM (mg)	IRON (mg)	ZINC (mg)	IODINE (μg)
0.4	6	0.3	30	0.5**	360	240	50	10	3	40
0.6	8	0.6	45	1.5	540	360	70	15	5	50
0.8	9	0.9	100	2.0	800	800	150	15	10	70
1.0	11	1.3	200	2.5	800	800	200	10	10	90
1.4	16	1.6	300	3.0	800	800	250	10	10	120
1.6	18	1.8	400	3.0	1200	1200	350	18	15	150
1.7	18	2.0	400	3.0	1200	1200	400	18	15	150
1.7	19	2.2	400	3.0	800	800	350	10	15	150
1.6	18	2.2	400	3.0	800	800	350	10	15	150
1.4	16	2.2	400	3.0	800	800	350	10	15	150
1.3	15	1.8	400	3.0	1200	1200	300	18	15	150
1.3	14	2.0	400	3.0	1200	1200	300	18	15	150
1.3	14	2.0	400	3.0	800	800	300	18	15	150
1.2	13	2.0	400	3.0	800	800	300	18	15	150
1.2	13	2.0	400	3.0	800	800	300	10	15	150
+0.3	+2	+0.6	+400	+1.0	+400	+400	+150	††	+5	+25
+0.5	+5	+0.5	+100	+1.0	+400	+400	+150	††	+10	+50

¶The folacin allowances refer to dietary sources as determined by *Lactobacillus casei* assay after treatment with enzymes ("conjugases") to make polyglutamyl forms of the vitamin available to the test organism.

**The RDA for vitamin B₁₂ in infants is based on average concentration of the vitamin in human milk. The allowances after weaning are based on energy intake (as recommended by the American Academy of Pediatrics) and consideration of other factors such as intestinal absorption.

††The increased requirement during pregnancy cannot be met by the iron content of habitual American diets nor by the existing iron stores of many women; therefore the use of 30–60 mg of supplemental iron is recommended. Iron needs during lactation are not substantially different from those of nonpregnant women, but continued supplementation of the mother for 2–3 months after parturition is advisable in order to replenish stores depleted by pregnancy.

‖1 NE (niacin equivalent) is equal to 1 mg of niacin or 60 mg of dietary tryptophan.

Table 21–3
The Four Basic Food Groups

Food Group	Average Amount/Serving	Average Servings/Day	Major Nutrients
Milk and dairy products	8 oz fluid milk ⅔ cup ice cream 1 oz cheddar cheese	Children, 4 Adults, 2	Calcium, phosphorus, protein, riboflavin
Meats (beef, lamb, poultry, fish, veal); eggs; and meat alternatives (dry beans, peas, lentils, nuts, or peanut butter)	3 oz meat (cooked weight) 1 cup dry beans or nuts 5 tsp peanut butter	2	Protein, iron, thiamine, niacin
Fruits and vegetables	½ cup	4 (1 citrus daily, 1 dark-green leafy or deep-yellow vegetable every other day)	Vitamin A, vitamin C
Breads and cereals	1 slice bread ½ cup cooked cereal ¾ cup dry cereal	4 (whole grain or enriched)	Thiamine, iron, protein, niacin, riboflavin

tion of cellulose is limited, so cellulose has little nutritive value. It is, however, important as a source of bulk, or roughage, which aids in proper elimination. Cellulose and other indigestible carbohydrates will be discussed later in this chapter.

In the body, the main functions of carbohydrates are to

• Provide a source of energy, supplying between 45 and 50 percent of the calories in the American diet.
• Aid in metabolism of fat (without a source of carbohydrate, the metabolism of fat cannot go to completion).
• Spare protein from being used as a source of energy (protein is needed for specific functions in the body and cannot be replaced by any other nutrient.

FATS

Also composed of carbon, hydrogen, and oxygen, fats differ from carbohydrates in the proportions of each of these elements. Fats can be classified in several different ways: by their source, by their physical appearance, or by their chemical structure.

Source: Animal or Vegetable. Animal fats are found in dairy products, meat, fish, and eggs. They are usually solid at room temperature. Vegetable fats are found in plants. Sources include corn, olives, cottonseed, nuts, and beans. They are generally liquid at room temperature and are called oils.

Physical Appearance: Visible or Invisible. Visible fats are those having a fatty appearance, such as butter or the fat around meat. Fats such as those in avocados or eggs are labeled invisible, since they are not discernible.

Chemical Structure: Saturated or Unsaturated. Saturated fats are those fatty acids that contain all the hydrogen possible. They are usually from animal sources and are solid at room temperature. Examples of saturated fats are lard, butter, meat fat, and **hydrogenated** fats. Unsaturated fatty acids can take on more hydrogen under the proper conditions. They are found in plants and are usually liquid at room temperature. Examples are the oils from corn and safflower. Some fats, such as those of the soft-type margarines, are partially hydrogenated. That is, an unsaturated fat is treated so that it takes up a predetermined quantity of hydrogen, resulting in a product that exhibits properties of both a saturated and an unsaturated fat. These fats are usually soft at room temperature.

Cholesterol is a lipid commonly found with saturated fats. It is also made by the body. If the levels of cholesterol in the blood are abnormally high (above 250 mg/100 ml), the risk of deposition of this compound on the walls of blood vessels becomes greater. Such a condition may increase the individual's chances of having a fatal heart attack. For such individuals, a low-cholesterol diet is usually prescribed. Foods such as egg yolk, organ meats, shellfish, whole dairy products, and meat fat are restricted, since they are high in cholesterol and saturated fats.

Fats make up about 35 to 40 percent of the total calories in the American diet. Since fats supply 9 kcal/gm, they are the most concentrated source of energy in our diet.

The major functions of fat in the body are to

• Provide a source of energy.
• Carry fat-soluble vitamins A and D.

21

- Supply those fatty acids essential for growth and life.
- Slow down emptying time of the stomach, thus increasing the satiety value of the diet.

When fat is stored in the body as adipose tissue, it acts as a reserve energy supply and as insulation and padding for the body and its vital organs.

Provide padding for vital organs

PROTEINS

The word protein comes from a Greek word meaning "to take first place," and rightly so, for protein is necessary to all living cells. Chemically, proteins are made of carbon, hydrogen, and oxygen, similar to the composition of carbohydrates and fats. However, they also contain nitrogen and several other elements, such as sulfur, phosphorus, and iron. It is the nitrogen that distinguishes proteins from other molecules.

Proteins are very large, complex molecules. They are composed of units known as amino acids, which are the materials that our bodies use to build and repair tissues. It is in the form of amino acids that proteins are absorbed into the system and metabolized. There are 23 amino acids, of which ten are essential in the adult for normal growth and maintenance of tissues. These ten essential amino acids must come from food.

Proteins are classified according to whether or not they contain all essential amino acids in good proportions to one another. A *complete protein* is one that contains a well-balanced mixture of all ten essential amino acids. If it is the only source of protein in the diet, it will support life and normal growth. A *partially complete protein* is one that supplies an imbalanced mixture of essential amino acids. If it is the sole protein source, it will maintain life but will not support normal growth. An *incomplete protein* will support neither life nor normal growth. It must not be the sole protein source, for it is missing, or extremely low in, one or more of the essential amino acids. Food sources of these proteins are as follows:

Complete Proteins: meat, fish, poultry, eggs, and dairy products.
Partially Complete Proteins: grains and vegetables.
Incomplete Proteins: corn and gelatin.

Fortunately, most foods have a mixture of proteins that supplement each other. Since there is little, if any, storage of amino acids in the body, it is important that a source of protein be included at each meal. If incomplete or partially complete proteins are used, attempts should be made to balance them. That is, a protein deficient in one amino acid should be eaten with one that is high in the same amino acid.

Vegetarianism has become increasingly popular, and many different forms exist. Some vegetarians consume no red meats but will eat fish and poultry.

Some include eggs and/or dairy products in their diets. Others (classified as vegans) consume no animal proteins at all, relying solely on vegetable foods for protein. Those who eat some animal protein in the form of fish, eggs, and milk are generally not at risk nutritionally. Vegetarians must include a variety of foods to ensure the nutritional adequacy of their diets. To supply sufficient protein, vegetables that complement each other must be eaten together. Vegetarians must compensate for the deficiencies in their diets by properly combining foods to get the correct proportion of amino acids. This is customarily done in the diets of different cultures. For example, in Mexico, beans are combined with rice, and in Middle Eastern countries, wheat bread is combined with cheese.

The recommended intake of proteins is 0.8 gm per kilogram of weight (Table 21–2). Of this, at least one third should be obtained from complete proteins. However, if the individual is a strict vegetarian, as already mentioned, care must be taken to balance the proteins consumed.

The average American diet is about 12 to 15 percent protein. Protein deficiency is the most common form of malnutrition and exists throughout the world. Almost one half of preschool-age children in developing countries are malnourished. A condition called *kwashiorkor* afflicts young children whose protein intake is deficient despite adequate caloric intake. Their diets are very poor in protein and consist mainly of carbohydrates and polished rice. The syndrome is characterized by edema, hypopigmentation, sparse and silky reddish hair, and a pathetic, fretful look. Another deficiency syndrome, called *marasmus*, results from a total decrease in both proteins and calories. It occurs in infants and young children and is characterized by emaciation, loose skin in folds, large sunken eyes, loss of flesh, and the general appearance of old age.

Of the numerous functions of protein in the body, the major ones are to

- Build and repair body tissue (this cannot be accomplished with any other nutrient). *The only Nutrient*
- Aid in the body's defense mechanisms against disease.
- Regulate body secretions and fluids.
- Provide energy.

VITAMINS

Vitamins are defined in the *Handbook of Diet Therapy* as organic substances "occurring in minute quantities in plant and animal tissues; essential for specific metabolic functions or reactions to proceed normally." They do not supply calories in our diets. Rather, they function as catalysts and help or allow metabolic reactions to proceed. Originally, they were lettered or numbered as they were discovered.

However, as they have been identified chemically, they have been given more specific names. In many cases, their chemical names are as well known as their letter designations.

Vitamins are divided into two groups: fat-soluble (A, D, E, and K) and water-soluble (C and the B complex). Deficiencies of a vitamin cause illness. However, there is no good evidence that large intakes of vitamins are useful in the healthy individual. Vitamins will not cure a disease or illness other than one caused by the lack of that nutrient. For example, vitamin C will not cure bleeding gums unless the condition is specifically caused by a lack of ascorbic acid, the chemical name for vitamin C. It should also be noted that toxic symptoms from excessive ingestion of vitamins A and D are proven clinical entities, and large intakes of some water-soluble vitamins may cause adverse effects.

Functions of Vitamin A	Deficiency Symptoms
Required for healthy skin and mucous membranes in the nose, throat, eyes, gastrointestinal (GI) tract, and genitourinary (GU) tract	Tissues become dry, cracked, and unable to resist infection
Necessary for proper vision	Night blindness—ability to adapt to darkness is impaired
Required for normal growth functions	Skeletal retardation

Fat-Soluble Vitamins (Fig. 21–2)

Vitamin A, or Retinol. We can obtain vitamin A by two methods: (1) as a vitamin or (2) from a compound called carotene, which the body converts to vitamin A. Carotene is known as a precursor of vitamin A. It is probably a more important source of the vitamin than the preformed compound, since vitamin A, as such, is present in very few foods.

HUMAN REQUIREMENTS. The recommended daily dietary allowance for the adult is 800 to 1000 RE* (see Table 21–2). This can be supplied by many different foods; for example, half an ounce of beef liver, half a large potato, a third of a cup of cooked spinach, or three medium tomatoes.

SOURCES. The sources of vitamin A are limited to animal products. The best sources are liver, fish liver oils, egg yolk, butter, and cream. Carotene is much more widely distributed in nature and is found in foods that have a deep yellow or dark green color. Food such as carrots, yellow squash, pumpkin, dark green leafy vegetables, sweet potatoes, apricots, peaches, and cantaloupes are excellent sources.

---

*RE = retinol equivalents. This term was introduced in 1967 so that utilization of the different forms of vitamin A could be taken into account when suggesting individual vitamin A allowances. By definition, 1 RE = 1 gm retinol or an equivalent amount of other compounds, corrected for efficiency of utilization. Since most food composition tables do not distinguish sources of vitamin A, the International Unit requirement may be more useful until transition to use of this new unit is complete.

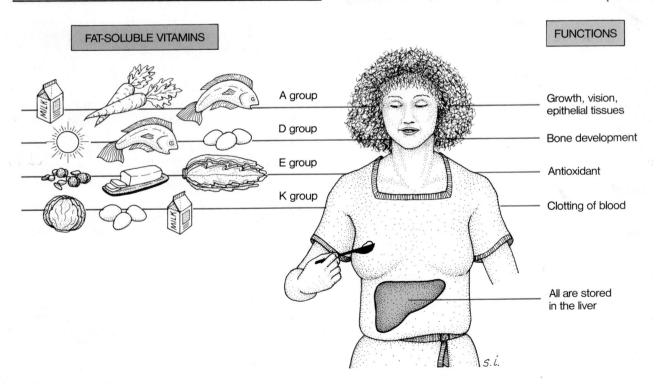

| FAT-SOLUBLE VITAMINS | | FUNCTIONS |

A group — Growth, vision, epithelial tissues

D group — Bone development

E group — Antioxidant

K group — Clotting of blood

All are stored in the liver

Fat-soluble vitamins (A, D, E, and K) and some foods high in each one. Functions of these vitamins are also shown. These vitamins are stored in our bodies.

STABILITY. Vitamin A and carotene are not water-soluble and are resistant to heat if not in prolonged contact with it. Consequently, they are not lost through most cooking methods. However, fats will become rancid when in contact with warm air, and once this occurs, the major portion of vitamin A and carotene present is destroyed.

TOXICITY. It is possible to get too much vitamin A. Toxic reactions are characterized by joint and bone pain, loss of appetite, loss of hair, and jaundice. The Council on Foods and Nutrition of the American Medical Association warns that 50,000 IU of this vitamin taken for a prolonged period of time can be dangerous.

Vitamin D, or Cholecalciferol. Vitamin D may be obtained from a few foods, but the most significant source is produced in the body upon exposure to sunlight. The preformed vitamin is not widely distributed. However, through enrichment processes, it is added to a number of foods, mainly dairy products.

Functions of Vitamin D	Deficiency Symptoms
Required for absorption of calcium and facilitates absorption of phosphorus. Necessary for metabolism of calcium and phosphorus in normal nourishment and formation of bones and teeth	Rickets—bones bend easily and do not form correctly, since calcium is not absorbed adequately. Teeth are also malformed

HUMAN REQUIREMENTS. The recommended daily dietary allowance for the adult is 5 μg, which should be readily supplied by exposure to sunlight (Table 21–2). The level for children and pregnant or lactating women is 10 μg per day. This latter could be supplied by half a teaspoon of cod-liver oil, three and a half ounces of tuna, or two cups of fortified milk.

SOURCES. Fortified milk and milk products, egg yolk, liver, butter, cream, and fish-liver oils. For most adults, the best source is probably sunlight.

STABILITY. Vitamin D is stable to heat and is not affected by most cooking methods.

TOXICITY. Excesses of this vitamin can cause toxicity symptomized by nausea, diarrhea, loss of appetite, and calcium deposits in tissues and joints. No exact figure can be given for an overdose, since exposure to sunlight varies greatly among individuals.

Vitamin E, or Tocopherol. Vitamin E is the vitamin that is still looking for a disease. Over the years, there have been numerous attempts to link this vitamin with many illnesses in humans, but efforts largely have failed. However, it does have several very important functions that are linked with its ability to combine with oxygen and thus protect various substances that would otherwise be subject to oxidation.

Functions of Vitamin E	Deficiency Symptoms
Protects red blood cells from breakdown by such substances as hydrogen peroxide	Anemia in infants
Protects structure and function of muscle tissue	Some forms of muscle degeneration have been seen in patients with low levels of vitamin E in the blood

HUMAN REQUIREMENTS. The recommended daily dietary allowance for the adult is 8 to 10 mg TE* (Table 21–2). This adult allowance could be met by one tablespoon of safflower, corn, or soybean oil, or three ounces of wheat germ.

SOURCES. The best sources of this vitamin are vegetable oils and wheat germ. Other sources include milk, eggs, grains, and leafy vegetables.

TOXICITY. None identified. This vitamin, unlike other fat-soluble vitamins, is stored in adipose tissue.

Vitamin K. The major function of this vitamin in the body has to do with the formation of *prothrombin*, which is a clotting agent in the blood. Consequently, the vitamin is often used to treat certain types of hemorrhages. Deficiency is rare and is usually due to absorption problems rather than inadequate supply of the vitamin.

Function of Vitamin K	Deficiency Symptoms
Required for formation of the protein prothrombin by the liver	Blood does not clot; hemorrhages occur

HUMAN REQUIREMENTS. There is no RDA for this vitamin. However, estimated safe and adequate daily intakes have been established (Table 21–2) for adults at 70 to 140 μg day. Probably one half to two thirds of this is supplied by bacterial synthesis in the intestines. The remainder can be supplied by half a cup of broccoli, three ounces of beef liver, or one eighth of a head of lettuce.

SOURCES. Good food sources include green leafy vegetables, egg yolk, cauliflower, and organ meats. A form of vitamin K is produced by intestinal bacteria.

TOXICITY. In large doses, vitamin K can produce a hemolytic anemia and jaundice in infants.

Water-Soluble Vitamins

Vitamin C, or Ascorbic Acid. Vitamin C was first used to treat **scurvy** in British sailors during the

*TE = alpha tocopherol equivalent. Alpha tocopherol is the chemical form of vitamin E that is the most common and the most biologically active. One mg of d-α-tocopherol has been designated as 1 α-tocopherol equivalent.

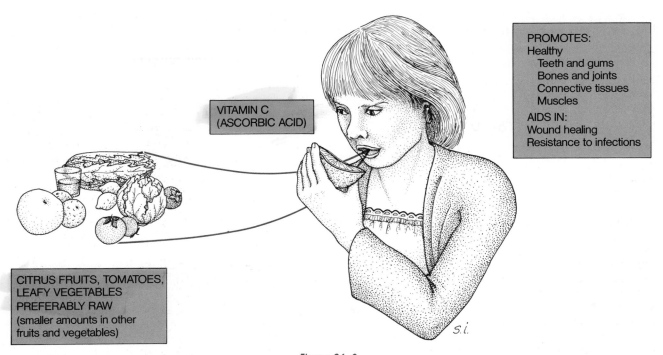

VITAMIN C
(ASCORBIC ACID)

PROMOTES:
Healthy
  Teeth and gums
  Bones and joints
  Connective tissues
  Muscles
AIDS IN:
Wound healing
Resistance to infections

CITRUS FRUITS, TOMATOES,
LEAFY VEGETABLES
PREFERABLY RAW
(smaller amounts in other
fruits and vegetables)

s.i.

Figure 21–3
Water-soluble vitamin C, its functions, and food sources. Water-soluble vitamins cannot be stored by the body, so they must be included in our diets each day.

eighteenth century (Fig. 21–3). Of course, at the time, the curative factor in the limes each sailor was required to consume daily while at sea was unknown. However, they did know that a lime daily seemed to prevent the dread disease. As a result, the British sailors were nicknamed "limeys," a term that is still used today.

Functions of Vitamin C	Deficiency Symptoms
Required for proper wound healing and promotes resistance to bacterial infection	Minor illnesses, general listlessness
Necessary for the structure and maintenance of capillary walls	Gums bleed, small pinpoint hemorrhages appear under the skin. If deficiency continues, the disease scurvy develops. Patients with this disease have skeletal malformations that are irreversible

HUMAN REQUIREMENTS. The recommended daily dietary allowance for adults is 60 mg. This amount of ascorbic acid would be supplied by six ounces of orange or grapefruit juice, one cup of strawberries, or three spears of fresh or frozen broccoli, cooked.

SOURCES. The best sources of this nutrient are citrus fruits, cabbage, dark-green leafy vegetables, and strawberries. Some sources, such as potatoes, are relatively low in vitamin C but are consumed in quantities sufficient to make them an important source.

STABILITY. Vitamin C is very easily destroyed by both heat and exposure to air. Since it is water-soluble, care must be used in cooking fruits and vegetables that contain vitamin C. Small amounts of water should be used and cooking times should be short. An alkaline medium will speed up the loss of vitamin C.

TOXICITY. Because ascorbic acid is water-soluble and is easily excreted from the body, toxic effects of this vitamin were previously believed to be unlikely. Symptoms typical of gastrointestinal tract irritation (such as nausea and diarrhea) were observed at doses of several hundred milligrams of vitamin C daily, but it has only been in recent years that larger doses (1 to 10 gm per day) have been shown to have potentially serious side effects in some individuals. For example, evidence shows that high intakes may cause kidney stones and gout in susceptible individuals. In addition, there are some studies that indicate that prolonged intake of high doses of vitamin C may lead to nutritional dependency.

Vitamin B₁, or Thiamine

HUMAN REQUIREMENTS. Need for the vitamin depends on caloric intake; generally, 0.5 mg per 1000 calories is adequate (Fig. 21–4). The level set by the National Research Council (NRC) is 1.0 to 1.4 mg per day, depending on sex (Table 21–2). To obtain this amount of thiamine, an individual must eat one tablespoon of brewers' yeast, four ounces of lean pork, or two cups of 40 percent bran flakes.

Functions of Vitamin B_1	Deficiency Symptoms
Necesssary for healthy appetite and proper functioning of the digestive tract	Loss of appetite, diminished gastric secretions, fatigue, irritability
Required for the metabolism of carbohydrates in the body and for normal functioning of the nervous system	Edema, footdrop, **beriberi**

SOURCES. Meats are not as good a source of thiamine as they are of most of the other B vitamins. However, pork and organ meats, such as liver, can contribute good amounts if consumed in large enough quantities. Although not concentrated sources of thiamine, whole-grain or enriched breads and cereals and potatoes are the most practical sources of vitamin B_1 because of the quantity of these products consumed. Legumes, wheat germ, and brewers' yeast are excellent sources, but the latter two are not included in the usual American diet.

STABILITY. Thiamine is destroyed by heat and alkaline mediums. Since it is water-soluble, small amounts of water should be used in cooking in order to preserve this nutrient.

TOXICITY. None.

Vitamin B_2, or Riboflavin

HUMAN REQUIREMENTS. The National Research Council established 1.2 to 1.6 mg per day (Table 21–2). Foods supplying this would be one and a half ounces of calf liver, cooked; three cups of yogurt or milk; or three cups of 40 percent bran flakes.

Functions of Vitamin B_2	Deficiency Symptoms
Necessary for all tissues, particularly for healthy skin and lips	Cheilosis, cracking of the mouth
Required for maintaining healthy eyes	Itching and burning of eyes, sensitivity to light, headaches
Essential for proper growth Vital as a coenzyme in energy metabolism	

SOURCES. The major source of this vitamin is milk, since one quart supplies 2 mg. Other sources include meats and enriched grains.

FOOD SOURCES AND USES IN THE BODY

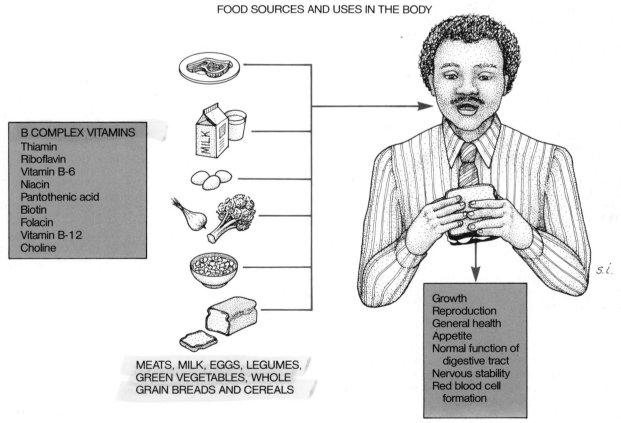

B COMPLEX VITAMINS
Thiamin
Riboflavin
Vitamin B-6
Niacin
Pantothenic acid
Biotin
Folacin
Vitamin B-12
Choline

MEATS, MILK, EGGS, LEGUMES, GREEN VEGETABLES, WHOLE GRAIN BREADS AND CEREALS

Growth
Reproduction
General health
Appetite
Normal function of digestive tract
Nervous stability
Red blood cell formation

Figure 21–4
Sources of B-complex vitamins and their uses in our bodies. B vitamins are important for a normally functioning nervous system. They, too, are water soluble and must be contained in our daily diets.

STABILITY. Riboflavin is very unstable in light. Consequently, milk should be stored in either dark glass or plasticized paper containers. Riboflavin from foods other than milk can also be lost in cooking water or drippings since it is water-soluble.

TOXICITY. None.

Niacin. Niacin is obtained either from preformed niacin or from conversion of its precursor, *tryptophan*, in the body. Tryptophan is an essential amino acid, and the body converts it to niacin. About 1 mg of niacin is produced from approximately 60 mg of tryptophan.

Functions of Niacin	Deficiency Symptoms
Composes part of some enzymes and is required for proper growth and metabolism of carbohydrates	**Pellagra**: characterized by the three D's (dermatitis, dementia, diarrhea)
Necessary for proper functioning of the GI tract and the nervous system	

HUMAN REQUIREMENTS. The recommended dietary allowance is 13 to 18 mg per day (Table 21–2). This amount of niacin would be found in six ounces of round steak or one and a half cups of pinto beans.

SOURCES. Probably one third to one half of our niacin comes from tryptophan, which is obtained from meat and other complete sources of protein. Flour and cereal products are also good sources.

STABILITY. Niacin is fairly stable to heat and air, but it can be lost in the cooking water.

TOXICITY. In large amounts, niacin causes vasodilation, which is evidenced by facial flushing and tingling sensations in the extremities. Massive doses (3 gm or more daily) cause liver damage.

Vitamin B_6, or Pyridoxine

HUMAN REQUIREMENTS. The National Research Council recommends 2 to 2.2 mg per day for adults (Table 21–2). No single food is an outstanding source of vitamin B_6. However, it is widely distributed in foods, and eating a variety of foods easily supplies adequate amounts. The NRC allowance

Functions of Vitamin B_6	Deficiency Symptoms
Many generalized functions in relation to muscle and nervous system function	Microcytic anemia, muscle weakness, difficulty in walking. Generally produced experimentally by using an antagonist. Induced symptoms include nausea, skin rash, oral lesions. Convulsions have been reported in cases of extreme deficiency in infants
Functions as a coenzyme in protein metabolism	

could be supplied by four bananas, two avocados, or twelve ounces of beef liver, fried.

SOURCES. Vitamin B_6 occurs in many foods, mainly meats and vegetables.

TOXICITY. At doses up to 150 mg, mild side effects and sleepiness have been reported. Over 200 mg, nutritional dependency has been shown, and deficiency symptoms are seen when large intakes are discontinued. Toxic effects are seen at doses over 300 mg per day.

Folic Acid, or Folacin

HUMAN REQUIREMENTS. The established allowance is 400 μg per day for adults (Table 21–2).

SOURCES. Best sources are green leafy vegetables, liver, and whole grains.

STABILITY. Folacin is destroyed by heat and is frequently lost in cooking water. Storage and cooking losses are usually high irrespective of methods.

TOXICITY. No toxic effects are known, but excessive folacin may interfere with the effectiveness of anticonvulsant drugs. Because folacin may mask early B_{12} deficiency symptoms, supplementation of folacin over the NRC allowance should not be taken unless the possibility of a B_{12} deficiency has been ruled out.

Vitamin B_{12}, or Cobalamin. Deficiency of this vitamin produces an anemia identical to that produced by a folic acid deficiency. However, if a deficiency of vitamin B_{12} is allowed to continue untreated, serious neurologic symptoms will result. (For this reason, folic acid cannot legally be added to multi-vitamin capsules except at very low levels. This is to prevent the folic acid from inadvertently masking the early symptoms of a vitamin B_{12} deficiency.

HUMAN REQUIREMENTS. For adults, 3 μg per day is recommended (Table 21–2). This is easily supplied by a quarter of an ounce of beef liver, fried; a quarter of a cup of frozen peas, cooked; or a quarter of a cup of canned pineapple.

SOURCES. Liver and muscle meats are the best sources.

Functions of Folic Acid	Deficiency Symptoms
Essential for all cells, particularly important in the formation of red blood cells	Smooth, red tongue; diarrhea; megaloblastic anemia; retarded growth

STABILITY. Vitamin B_{12} is stable under most conditions, since it is attached to a protein in foods.

TOXICITY. None.

Other B Vitamins. Other vitamins that belong to the B complex, but for which no requirements have been established, are biotin, pantothenic acid, and choline. *Biotin* is synthesized by bacteria in the gastrointestinal tract and is important in several enzyme systems. Raw egg white contains a protein, avidin, which is capable of binding biotin, thus

21

making it unavailable to the body. Avidin is changed by heating, so it will not function in this manner in cooked egg whites. The estimated safe and adequate intake of biotin is 100 to 200 μg, which could be supplied by four ounces of beef liver or two cups of cooked oatmeal. *Pantothenic acid* is involved in carbohydrate and fatty acid metabolism. It is present in almost all foods, and deficiency should not be seen if a mixed diet is consumed. The Food and Nutrition Board suggests an intake of 4 to 7 mg per day. An equivalent of this amount would be found in three ounces of beef liver, four to six eggs, or one quart of milk. *Choline* is important in the body mainly as a constituent of compounds known as phospholipids (primarily lecithin). Besides performing other functions, choline is involved in the transport and metabolism of fats. Choline is found in whole grains, meats, egg yolks, and legumes. No deficiency has been demonstrated in humans.

MINERALS

Minerals are inorganic chemical elements that make up about 4 percent of body weight. Of the many that are used by the body, only 14 are felt to be essential. Of those, allowances have been established for only six. Most minerals are required in relatively small amounts, but even so, they are absolutely essential for life.

Minerals contribute to the body's water-electrolyte balance and acid-base balance, and some are cofactors for enzymes. The largest proportion of inorganic elements is found in the skeleton. Minerals present in the largest amount include sodium, potassium, chlorine, calcium, phosphorus, magnesium, and sulfur. Those present in very small amounts, the *trace elements*, include iron, zinc, copper, cobalt, manganese, iodine, and fluorine.

The minerals that are needed only in trace amounts seem either to behave as part of hormone or enzyme systems or to work with vitamins in various metabolic reactions throughout the body. For example, iodine is part of the thyroid hormone *thyroxine*, and another hormone, *insulin*, has zinc as part of its structure. Cobalt, on the other hand, is an essential part of the B$_{12}$ molecule.

Like vitamins, these minerals can be obtained from common foods in a well-balanced diet. With the exception of iodine and iron, mineral deficiencies are rare in the average American diet.

Major Minerals

Calcium. In the American diet, calcium is the mineral that is the most likely to be deficient. The body requires calcium at all ages, but the highest requirements are during pregnancy, lactation, and childhood.

Osteoporosis is a condition in which the bones become increasingly porous and brittle because of a loss of calcium. This common condition of aging causes bones to fracture more easily. When the spine is involved, the vertebrae collapse, causing curvature and backache as well as a decrease in stature. In women, osteoporosis is associated with the postmenopausal decrease in estrogen. Many physicians are recommending additional dietary supplements of calcium to forestall this condition.

Functions of Calcium	Deficiency Symptoms
Forms the body's skeleton and teeth	Rickets: characterized by retarded growth and malformations of the bones
Aids in the formation of blood clots	Delayed blood clotting, hemorrhages
Required for normal muscle activity, especially the heart muscle	Tetany, abnormal twitching of the muscles

HUMAN REQUIREMENTS. The calcium requirements are 800 mg per day (Table 21–2) and can be supplied by two to three cups of milk or yogurt, or four ounces of cheese.

SOURCES. The major source of calcium is milk of any kind (skim, whole, low-fat, buttermilk, and chocolate milk) or milk products, such as ice cream or cheese. Other sources include dark-green leafy vegetables and shellfish (for example, clams and oysters).

Phosphorus. Phosphorus is a constituent of every living cell and, as such, has numerous functions in the body. In many cases, it works in very much the same manner as calcium. However, in addition, it is required for protein, fat, and carbohydrate metabolism, in energy metabolism, and in various buffering systems in the body. It is also involved in a number of vitamin and enzyme reactions. No specific disease is associated with a deficiency of this nutrient, but excessive and prolonged use of antacids containing aluminum hydroxide can produce symptoms of phosphorus deficiency (weakness, anorexia, and bone demineralization).

HUMAN REQUIREMENTS. The requirement is 800 mg per day (Table 21–2) and can be supplied by two to three cups of milk or yogurt, or four ounces of cheese or tuna fish.

SOURCES. Phosphorus is present in most foods, particularly in milk and meat products. Other good sources are cereals and legumes.

Magnesium. Most magnesium is found in combination with calcium and phosphorus in bone tissue. In addition to its role in bone metabolism, magnesium functions mainly in carbohydrate and amino acid reactions in the body. With other minerals, it is also important in nervous activity and muscle contractions. A deficiency of this element results in nervous irritability and, eventually, in convulsions similar to those seen in cases of *tetany (hypocalcemia).*

HUMAN REQUIREMENTS. The magnesium requirements are 300 to 350 mg per day for adults, depending on sex (Table 21–2). No single food, eaten in normal amounts, is an outstanding source of magnesium, but a combination of a half a cup of peanuts and three bananas would supply the NRC allowance.

SOURCES. Magnesium occurs in many foods, particularly dairy products, cereal grains, legumes, and dark-green vegetables.

Sodium. This mineral is required mainly for control of fluid volume in the body; an increase in the level of sodium in the serum leads to water retention. One compartment expanded as a result of fluid retention is the vascular system. Sodium, then, is directly related to blood pressure. It functions in acid-base balance and is involved in both carbohydrate and protein metabolism. Deficiencies of sodium can result from inadequate production of adrenocortical hormone or from excessive perspiration. Symptoms of deficiency include nausea, vomiting, and muscle cramps. Extreme cases may lead to heart failure.

Excessive sodium may cause an effective increase in blood volume and hence an increase in blood pressure. Although many other factors besides sodium and water retention are involved in causing high blood pressure (hypertension), it appears reasonable to suggest that sodium intake be closely monitored. Estimates place sodium consumption at roughly ten times the level actually required. Therefore, at least those persons who are predisposed to hypertension should probably try to use the salt shaker less frequently and should avoid obviously salty foods such as potato chips and broth. Salt substitutes, however, should not be used without medical supervision.

HUMAN REQUIREMENTS. The Food and Nutrition Board set the safe and adequate intake for this mineral at 1100 to 3300 mg daily. One teaspoon of table salt supplies 2000 mg of sodium, but 12 green olives or four ounces of ham could also supply over 1000 mg of sodium.

SOURCES. Sodium is found naturally in a wide variety of foods and is also added extensively to many foods during commercial production. Meats and dairy products are naturally high sources, but salt is added to foods such as soups, butter, and potato chips for flavor.

Potassium. This mineral functions in much the same way as sodium except that potassium is concentrated within the body cells. In addition to its involvement in fluid volume, potassium plays a multitude of roles in carbohydrate and protein metabolism. Deficiencies of potassium are rare and are usually related to either severe vomiting or diarrhea or to the use of diuretics (drugs that cause excretion of sodium and potassium, frequently used in treating hypertension). Symptoms of a potassium deficiency include nausea, vomiting, and muscle weak-

ness. Severe losses of potassium result in rapid contractions of the heart and, eventually, death due to heart failure.

Too much potassium can also be dangerous. Usually, *hyperkalemia* (high potassium blood level) is due to kidney failure or to the combination of a reduced ability to excrete potassium along with overingestion of potassium, either from supplements or salt substitutes.

HUMAN REQUIREMENTS. The safe and adequate intake is set at 1875 to 5625 mg per day. No single food source can supply this amount. However, many fruits and vegetables supply 300 to 400 mg per serving, so a variety of foods from these groups should adequately supply potassium in the American diet.

SOURCES. Bananas, oranges, and raisins are good sources of potassium, as are most other fruits. Potatoes in the skin and avocados are excellent sources; milk and meat contain smaller amounts.

Chlorine. As the ion chloride, this mineral acts as a companion to sodium. It is primarily involved in acid-base and fluid balance and is a component of hydrochloric acid in the stomach. Deficiencies are unusual and are generally related to sodium losses or to excessive vomiting and diarrhea. Toxicities of dietary chlorine are unknown, since it is readily excreted by the kidney. Chlorine in its gaseous form, however, is lethal.

HUMAN REQUIREMENTS. Safe and adequate intake of chlorine has been established to be 1700 to 5100 mg per day for adults. The amount of salt in the diet supplies more than enough of this nutrient.

SOURCE. Table salt.

Sulfur. Sulfur is utilized by the body in protein synthesis and in reactions in the liver. The amount of sulfur is normally adequate in diets in which the complete protein content is adequate. Deficiency of this mineral can result in dermatitis and imperfect development of hair and nails.

Trace Minerals

Iron. Although required in small amounts in comparison with such nutrients as phosphorus and calcium, iron is a vitally important element. It is an essential part of *hemoglobin* (the protein that is the oxygen-carrying substance in the blood) and is responsible for the color of red blood cells. The body is very conservative with iron, and it reuses it again and again. However, deficiencies do occur, particularly in premenopausal women or during pregnancy or hemorrhagic conditions. A deficiency of iron results in a microcytic anemia.

HUMAN REQUIREMENTS. The RDA allowance is 18 mg per day for adult women. Unless a woman eats liver and other rich sources of iron frequently, the ordinary diet may not supply a sufficient quantity of iron. In this case, an iron supplement may be desirable. For men, 10 mg per day is recommended (Table 21–2). This lower amount for men can be supplied by one cup of 40 percent bran flakes or four ounces of beef liver.

SOURCES. The best sources are liver and other organ meats, egg yolks, whole-grain products, and green leafy vegetables. Some other products, such as raisins, dried fruits, and molasses, are good sources of iron if eaten in sufficient quantities. Eating foods containing ascorbic acid along with iron-containing foods will increase the availability of iron to the body.

TOXICITY. In some cases, overdoses of iron may be a problem. Although unusual in the United States except in instances of excessive use of supplements, iron accumulation can occur because the body has no mechanism for excreting excess iron. Consequently, iron is deposited in soft tissues (liver, pancreas, and lungs) causing cell death, and may lead to complications such as **diabetes** and liver damage.

Iodine. Iodine's only function in the body is as a part of the thyroid gland hormone *thyroxine.* Although the requirement for iodine is small, the thyroid gland fails to function properly without it, and the condition known as *goiter* occurs. Iodine deficiency in a pregnant woman can result in *cretinism* in the infant. This disease is characterized by dwarfing and retarded physical and mental growth.

HUMAN REQUIREMENTS. The requirement is 150 μg per day for adults (Table 21–2). One teaspoon of iodized salt supplies 420 μg of iodine, much more than the RDA. Three glasses of milk will supply 150 μg of iodine.

SOURCES. The iodine content of plants is determined by the amount of iodine in the soil in which they are grown. Generally, vegetables grown in the Atlantic coastal area or regions around the Gulf of Mexico have the highest iodine content. Fish, seafood, and seaweed are excellent sources of iodine but are usually not eaten frequently enough to be considered dependable sources. The most reliable source of iodine is iodized table salt.

Zinc. Zinc is necessary for growth and *gonadal* development in humans. Zinc is part of the hormone insulin, which regulates carbohydrate metabolism. It is also a component of several enzyme systems in the body. A deficiency of this nutrient retards skeletal growth and sexual maturation. Additional symptoms include decreased ability to taste and delayed wound healing.

HUMAN REQUIREMENTS. Requirements are 15 mg per day for adults (Table 21–2). This could be supplied by one oyster. One milligram of zinc is found in one ounce of most meats.

SOURCES. The best sources of zinc are oysters, herring, whole grains, meats, milk, and egg yolk.

Fluoride. The major function of fluoride is in hardening bones and teeth. As a result, it is beneficial in reducing the amount of dental decay in infancy and childhood. Some evidence indicates that fluoride may also benefit adults who take it throughout life in protecting them against osteoporosis. In areas of the country where water is naturally fluoridated in excess of 6 to 8 ppm, *mottling* (brown staining) of the tooth enamel is observed. However, at levels used in artificial fluoridation programs, no health hazard has been documented.

HUMAN REQUIREMENTS. The safe and adequate intake is set at 1.5 to 4 mg per day for adults. This would be supplied by 1.5 liters (L) of fluoridated water.

SOURCES. Food sources of fluoride are unreliable. Soil content varies, so vegetables and grains are sometimes good sources. Seafood and seaweed are excellent sources. Water, when fluoridated, contains 1 ppm (1 mg per L).

Copper. Copper contributes to iron absorption and metabolism and is involved in the formation of hemoglobin. Copper deficiencies are unusual and are generally linked to genetic defects. The safe and adequate intake is established at 2 to 3 mg per day for adults. The richest sources of this mineral are shellfish, liver, legumes, and raisins.

WATER *H20*

Water is the most important nutrient, yet it is all too often overlooked when the average person considers nutritional status. It has a wide variety of functions in the body: (1) plays a key role in the maintenance of body temperature, (2) acts as a solvent and a medium for most biochemical reactions, (3) acts as a vehicle for transport of substances such as nutrients, hormones, antibodies, and metabolic wastes, and (4) acts as a lubricant for joints and mucous membranes. Approximately two thirds of the total body weight is water. It is lost daily from the body in urine, feces, and sweat and is expired in the air. Extensive water losses due to diarrhea, vomiting, burns, or perspiration can lead to electrolyte losses and resultant life-threatening imbalances. Drinking too much water (water intoxication) can also be dangerous.

Most of the daily requirements for water are satisfied by ingested fluids and foods and by water released by the metabolism of carbohydrates, fats, and proteins. All food contains some water. Most vegetables and fruits are more than 80 percent water, and meats are 40 to 60 percent water.

HUMAN REQUIREMENTS. None is set, but an adequate daily allowance for adults is 2 L (about eight glasses). *2qt*

FIBER

Fiber, or "roughage," is composed of many different substances. Three polysaccharides (cellulose, pectin, and hemicellulose) as well as the noncarbohydrate *lignin* contribute roughage to the diet. Fiber is not found in animal foods but comes only from plants. Dietary tables generally show "crude fiber" or dietary fiber, which is estimated to be 20 to 50 percent lower than the actual fiber content of the diet. Much work is needed to clarify this area of nutrition.

Fiber absorbs water easily and, consequently, functions to carry waste products from the gastrointestinal tract. Lack of sufficient fiber in the diet has been linked to many problems, including hiatus hernia, diverticulosis, and cancer of the colon.

HUMAN REQUIREMENTS. No requirement has been established, but the average fiber content of the American diet (4 to 5 gm per day) is believed to be low. This may result in reduced movement of waste material through the colon, leading to increased irritation and eventual damage to the tissues. It is generally suggested that society increase the fiber content of the diet to 12 to 20 gm per day.

SOURCES. Whole grains, fruits, and vegetables are excellent sources. Bran is a concentrated source of fiber and, if added to the diet, should be added in small amounts. It can absorb up to 200 times its dry weight in water and so may cause blockage of the intestinal tract. Increased fiber content of the diet should always be accompanied by increased water consumption.

CLINICAL NUTRITION

Although the majority of patients a physician sees will be treated medically without using a therapeutic diet, there are some illnesses and diseases that can be cured and patients whose recovery can be facilitated by the use of a special diet. In such cases, the normal (sometimes referred to as house or regular) diet is used as a basis of planning. The two major reasons for this are

1. The closer the special diet is to a normal one, the fewer changes the assistant will be asking the person to accept, and the easier it will be for the patient to adhere to the diet.

2. It is easier to be certain that the patient's diet supplies adequate amounts of the essential nutrients if a regular diet pattern is used as a baseline.

Modifying a Diet

The normal diet can be modified with regard to the following features (or combination thereof) to create a therapeutic diet:

- Consistency.
- Caloric level.
- Levels of one or more nutrients.
- Bulk.
- Spiciness.
- Levels of specific foods.
- Feeding intervals.

Consistency. Changes in consistency are sometimes ordered for individuals who have problems with their mouth, teeth, or esophagus. A texture restriction is also frequently called for in cases of illnesses of the gastrointestinal tract.

Soft or Light Diet. Foods with roughage are eliminated (no raw fruits or vegetables). No strongly flavored or gas-forming vegetables are allowed (onions, beans, broccoli, and cauliflower). In many cases, spices are limited.

Table 21–4
1983 Metropolitan Height and Weight Tables*

Men				Women			
HEIGHT FEET INCHES	SMALL FRAME	MEDIUM FRAME	LARGE FRAME	HEIGHT FEET INCHES	SMALL FRAME	MEDIUM FRAME	LARGE FRAME
5 2	128–134	131–141	138–150	4 10	102–111	109–121	118–131
5 3	130–136	133–143	140–153	4 11	103–113	111–123	120–134
5 4	132–138	135–145	142–156	5 0	104–115	113–126	122–137
5 5	134–140	137–148	144–160	5 1	106–118	115–129	125–140
5 6	136–142	139–151	146–164	5 2	108–121	118–132	128–143
5 7	138–145	142–154	149–168	5 3	111–124	121–135	131–147
5 8	140–148	145–157	152–172	5 4	114–127	124–138	134–151
5 9	142–151	148–160	155–176	5 5	117–130	127–141	137–155
5 10	144–154	151–163	158–180	5 6	120–133	130–144	140–159
5 11	146–157	154–166	161–184	5 7	123–136	133–147	143–163
6 0	149–160	157–170	164–188	5 8	126–139	136–150	146–167
6 1	152–164	160–174	168–192	5 9	129–142	139–153	149–170
6 2	155–168	164–178	172–197	5 10	132–145	142–156	152–173
6 3	158–172	167–182	176–202	5 11	135–148	145–159	155–176
6 4	162–176	171–187	181–207	6 0	138–151	148–162	158–179

Source of basic data 1979 Build Study, Society of Actuaries and Association of Life Insurance Medical Directors of America, 1980.
*Weights at ages 25–59 based on lowest mortality. Weight in pounds according to frame (in indoor clothing weighing 5 lbs. for men and 3 lbs. for women; shoes with 1" heels).
Courtesy of Metropolitan Life Insurance Company.

Mechanical Soft Diet. A regular diet in which the food is either chopped, ground, or pureed, depending upon the degree of texture change required. No foods or spices are restricted.

Liquid Diet. There are two types of liquid diets. The clear liquid diet includes only broth soups, tea, coffee, and gelatin. In some cases, apple juice and cranberry juice may be allowed. The full liquid diet includes all foods allowed on a clear liquid diet plus milk, custards, strained cream soups, refined cereals, eggnogs, milkshakes, and all juices.

The soft and mechanical diets should supply all the nutrients required by an individual. The clear liquid diet is not adequate and should be used for very brief periods of time. Full liquid diets can be made adequate, but they are usually not–and so should also be used only for short periods.

Calorie Level. Calories may be either increased or decreased. Increased calories are ordered in cases of chronic underweight, as in the eating disorders **anorexia nervosa** and **bulimia;** following an illness; for malnutrition and hyperthyroidism; during times of growth, such as infancy and childhood; and during pregnancy and lactation. Under such circumstances, the total amounts of foods on the regular diet are increased, and the diet is usually higher in fats (since fat supplies more calories per gram than either carbohydrates or proteins). The number of meals eaten may also be increased from three to six or more.

Calories are restricted in cases of **obesity** and **diabetes**. The quantities of food consumed should be decreased, but no one food group should be eliminated. For diabetes, food containing carbohydrates, particularly the simple sugars, are controlled. Lists of foods that enable diabetics to plan their diets more easily have been prepared by the American Diabetic Association. (The lists are known as Exchange Lists, and various modifications of them are frequently used for calorie-restricted diets in general.)

High-calorie diets should be adequate in all nutrients. Low-calorie diets can usually be made adequate. However, diets supplying less than 1800 kcal will probably be inadequate.

Levels of One or More Nutrients. A large number of therapeutic diets modify the levels of one or more nutrients. This type of diet is used to treat specific deficiency diseases (for example, high-iron diet) or when a patient has had a toxic reaction to a specific vitamin or mineral (for example, low–vitamin A diet). Many inborn errors of metabolism are treated by eliminating or limiting the ingestion of a nutrient (for example, **phenylketonuria** is treated by limiting the quantities of the essential amino acid phenylalanine). In cases of hypertensive heart disease, sodium is restricted. For patients with **atherosclerosis,** a low-fat or low-cholesterol diet

may be prescribed. Protein levels are changed for kidney and liver disease therapy. Fat is also restricted for gallbladder or liver disease.

In general, the normal diet is modified by restricting foods that are sources of the nutrient involved. Except for the nutrient in question, the RDA allowances can usually be met. However, if several restrictions are ordered for the same patient, a nutrient supplement may be necessary.

Bulk. Bulk or residue is changed when treating problems of the colon or large bowel. In some cases, high-residue diets are ordered; in others, low-residue diets. In either case, foods high in cellulose are considered to be high in residue, because the body does not digest this carbohydrate well, and a residue is left in the colon. In some instances, a low-residue diet is distinguished from a low-fiber diet. In this case, a low-fiber diet eliminates those foods with a high cellulose content, and a low-residue diet restricts milk, in addition to fiber content. Either diet should supply all the nutrients needed; however, if milk is restricted drastically, the calcium level must be watched carefully.

Spiciness. A bland diet restricts those dietary components that are classified as gastrointestinal irritants. Such a diet limits any foods that are chemically (for example, caffeine, pepper, chili, nutmeg, and alcohol) or mechanically (high-fiber) irritating. No fried foods or highly concentrated sweets are included. Gas-forming vegetables belonging to the onion and cabbage family are also eliminated. The diet is commonly used for problems occurring in the gastrointestinal tract (such as ulcers). The bland diet should supply sufficient nutrients for the individual to meet the RDA allowances, unless fruits and vegetables are eliminated (in which case, a supplement may be necessary).

Levels of Specific Foods. Diets that modify the levels of specific foods are most frequently used to treat allergies of various kinds. There are two basic elimination-type regimens. A simple elimination diet removes only one or two foods that are suspected of causing the allergy. The *Rowe* elimination diet involves a more extensive program. Using this method, the basic diet consists of a few hypoallergenic foods such as rice cereal, apples, pears, carrots, sweet potatoes, lamb, and milk substitutes. If no allergic reaction is observed, single food-family groups are added slowly in periods of about ten days. In children, the most common allergies are to chocolate, wheat, eggs, and milk. *Celiac disease* (an intestinal malabsorption syndrome characterized by diarrhea, hypocalcemia, bleeding, and malnutrition) is treated by eliminating foods that contain a protein called *gliadin* (found in wheat). In some cases, it may be difficult to meet the RDA allowances for all nutrients. When this situation occurs, supplements should be ordered.

Feeding Intervals. Feeding intervals can be changed. Usually, more meals are ordered rather than fewer. Generally, the increase is from three meals to six or eight meals. Feeding intervals are shortened for treating problems dealing with the gastrointestinal tract, malnutrition, or underweight. An individual who has had part or all of the stomach removed surgically (*surgical bypass of the intestine* or *gastric partitioning*) requires more meals. In some cases, the total food consumed per day is the same, but it is fed in smaller quantities at any given time. In other cases, more food is added at the extra meals. Unless the number of meals is reduced severely, the RDA allowances should be met.

Prescribing a Diet

Since there are so many different types of therapeutic diets, it is frequently impossible for the physician to stay abreast of all the restrictions and other considerations involved. For this reason, the physician will often rely on either a local dietitian or a nutritional consultant to plan the therapeutic diet and instruct patients on the modifications they should follow.

Basically, diet therapy involves a problem-solving process. First, data concerning the nutritional status of the patient must be collected. This information is generally accumulated by a variety of health professionals (headed by the physician), including in some cases medical assistants, and is expanded and coordinated by the registered dietitian. The second step is the planning phase, during which the collected data are analyzed, the nutrition-related problems are delineated, and the possible solutions are outlined. The proposed dietary measures are then implemented as a planned dietary program. (Some of the most common nutrition-related problems and the dietary modifications used to treat them are shown in Table 21–5.) Last, the program, or diet, being used is evaluated in terms of the medical problem to see if the nutrition-related disorder is being or has been corrected. If necessary, the entire process is repeated. At all times, it is preferable to involve the patient as much as possible in order to maximize results and maintain long-term dietary modifications.

If it is not feasible to use professional dietetic assistance, the physician may wish to use a service offered by some firms that develop diets, printed with the physician's name on them, that can be given to the patient. Numerous pharmaceutical or medical suppliers also supply diet lists, which usually are used as additional advertising for the products of the manufacturer. If such diets are employed, remember that one list is frequently used for more than one type of diet (for example, several different calorie levels may be listed in chart form), and it is left to the patient to decipher the information. Diets of this nature must be as clear and concise as possible so that the patient is not unduly confused or frightened.

It is important that the patient return home with written instructions after leaving the office. Many questions will arise after the diet has first been introduced in the office. A written list is the easiest method of answering these questions.

The medical assistant may be called upon to discuss the diet with the patient. It is extremely important that the assistant have a thorough knowledge of diet therapy in order to talk with the patient in a convincing manner. It is important that the patient understand the diet and the rationale behind its use. If patients feel uneasy or have many unan-

Table 21–5
Common Diet-Related Disorders

Disorder	Major Dietary Components	Corrective Dietary Measures
Allergies	Wide variety of foods as possible allergens: wheat, milk, eggs, chocolate most common	Eliminate or restrict food sources of allergen
Anemia	Deficiency of iron, B_{12}, or folacin	Increase amount of deficient nutrient
Anorexia nervosa	Starvation; fear of becoming fat; altered body image	High-calorie diet, psychotherapy, behavior modification
Atherosclerosis	High cholesterol, high saturated fat, excessive calories	Control calories, decrease total fat in diet to 30 to 35 percent of calories, change to more unsaturated fats, lower cholesterol content of diet, stress complex carbohydrates rather than simple sugars
Bulimia	Binge eating, self-induced vomiting	Regular diet; behavior modification, psychotherapy
Cancer of the colon	Low fiber	Increase dietary fiber, increase fluids
Cirrhosis of the liver	Excessive ingestion of alcohol or nutrients such as iron, lead, vitamin A or D	Reduce dietary level of excessive nutrient or substance
Constipation/ diverticulosis	Poor fiber intake, poor fluid intake	Increase dietary fiber and fluids
Diabetes mellitus	Obesity, excessive sugar consumption	Control calories and carbohydrates
Hypertension	Obesity, high salt intake	Control calories, decrease sodium intake
Obesity	Excessive calorie intake, inadequate physical activity	Decrease calories, increase activity; behavior modification, group therapy

swered questions, they will be far less motivated to follow the diet. The medical assistant can be a very valuable asset to the physician, the dietitian, and particularly, the patient. A sound understanding of nutrition and, especially, of diet therapy enables the assistant to function most effectively.

Seven Dietary Guidelines For Americans*

As previously stated, the American diet is too high in proteins. Fatty foods, sugary foods, and salty foods are consumed in volume by young and old. The American Heart Association and the U.S. Department of Agriculture advise the population to cut fats, salt, and sugar from their diets in order to reduce the risks of heart disease. At the same time, physicians are advising that people increase the quantities of starch and fiber in their daily diets.

The seven dietary guidelines for Americans are good general rules to follow whether one is on a prescribed modified diet or is just maintaining a normal weight level.

1. *Eat a Variety of Foods.* The daily diet should include all the foods listed in the basic four food groups, and in the recommended amounts.

2. *Maintain Desirable Weight.* Obesity is associated with hypertension, heart disease, and diabetes. To avoid ill health, maintain a desirable weight based on height.

3. *Avoid Excessive Fat, Saturated Fat, and Cholesterol.* The American diet is dangerously high in saturated fat. Americans have far greater risks of heart attacks than people from countries where diets contain less fats. Foods to avoid are animal fats, coconuts, and palm oils.

4. *Eat Foods with Adequate Starch and Fiber.* Complex carbohydrates (starches) contain less than half

---

*For more information, write to Human Nutrition Information Service, U.S. Department of Agriculture, Room 325A, Federal Building, Hyattsville, Maryland 20782.

the calories of fats. Furthermore, starches such as breads, cereals, fruits, and vegetables contain fiber.

5. *Avoid Excessive Sugar.* Simple sugars contain empty calories, that is, calories without essential nutrients. Most foods contain some sugar, so avoid white, brown, and raw sugar, honey, soft drinks, candies, and cakes. These sugars contain no nutrients or vitamins and encourage tooth decay.

6. *Avoid Excessive Sodium.* Sodium is an essential nutrient. However, in populations such as that of the United States, in which large amounts of sodium are consumed, there are more reported cases of hypertension. Use a variety of spices other than salt. Limit salty foods such as snack foods, canned soups, cured meats, and certain cheeses. Read labels of foods for the sodium content.

7. *If Alcoholic Beverages Are Consumed, Do So in Moderation.* Alcohol is the oldest and most widely consumed addicting psychotropic (affecting mind and behavior) drug. It is used by nearly half of all Americans and is abused by 1 in 20. Complications of alcoholism can affect many body organs. Many of these complications are due to the toxic effects of alcohol, but the majority are caused by nutritional deprivation. Alcoholic beverages are high in calories but low in nutrients. In addition, the National Institute of Alcohol Abuse and Alcoholism advises pregnant women to refrain from using alcohol because of possible birth defects.

REFERENCES AND READINGS

Guthrie, H. A.: *Introductory Nutrition.* St. Louis, C. V. Mosby, 1983.

Long, J., and Shannon, B.: *Nutrition, an Inquiry Into the Issues.* Englewood Cliffs, N.J., Prentice-Hall, 1983.

Suitor, C. W., and Hunter, M. F.: *Nutrition: Principles and Application in Health Promotion.* Philadelphia, J. B. Lippincott, 1980.

Whitney, E. N., and Cataldo, C. B.: *Understanding Normal and Clinical Nutrition.* St. Louis, West Publishing Co., 1983.

Williams, S. R.: *Nutrition and Diet Therapy,* 5th ed. St. Louis, C. V. Mosby Co., 1985.

CHAPTER OUTLINE

VOCABULARY

See Glossary at end of book for definitions.

    agar
    serum
    spore
    toxin

Basic Concepts of Asepsis

without contamination

22

OBJECTIVES

Upon successful completion of this chapter you should be able to

1. Define and spell the words listed in the Vocabulary for this chapter.
2. List six conditions that favor the growth of microorganisms and state one preventive measure for each condition.
3. Define each of the five links in the "chain of infection."
4. Differentiate between direct and indirect transmission of disease and provide examples of each.
5. List the eight steps in the inflammatory process.
6. Distinguish between the nonspecific and specific defense mechanisms of the body.
7. Compare active and passive immunity, providing examples of each.
8. List six classifications of microorganisms.
9. Name one disease example for each subclassification of bacteria.
10. Explain what special precautions are required when treating patients with hepatitis B or acquired immune deficiency syndrome (AIDS).
11. Differentiate between medical asepsis and surgical asepsis.

Upon successful completion of this chapter you should be able to perform the following activities:

1. Demonstrate the proper hand wash for assisting with medical aseptic procedures.
2. Demonstrate the proper hand wash (scrub) for assisting with surgical aseptic procedures.

Medical microbiology and the principles of asepsis focus on the study of microorganisms that are disease-producing (pathogenic) and the aseptic practices used for their control. This chapter includes concepts of disease transmission, the body's response to infection, the natural defense mechanisms of the body, the immune system, and an introduction to some of the more common pathogenic microorganisms that may invade the body. These concepts form the basis for understanding the importance of the first line of defense in preventing disease—the medical hand wash and the surgical hand scrub.

First, let's review a little background material. *Biology* is the science of living things; therefore *micro-* (small, or minute) *biology* is the science of small living things. *Microorganisms* (*microbes*) were first seen by Antonj van Leeuwenhoek, a Dutch scientist who, in about 1664, perfected a magnifying glass strong enough to see bacteria, which he called "animalcules" (little animals) (Figs. 22–1 and 22–2). He carefully described and drew what he saw but did not disclose how he made his lens. Therefore, it was not until 1820 that a truly useful microscope was perfected.

Microbiology became a science in its own right with the work of such men as Louis Pasteur, Robert Koch, Joseph Lister, and many others. Pasteur was a French chemist. In about 1837, he was asked by the wine makers to try to find out what was turning their wine sour. He discovered that it was a microorganism. This led him to work in other microbiologic areas. He perfected a treatment that prevented rabies in persons bitten by rabid animals. Later, he discovered the means for controlling anthrax, a disease of sheep.

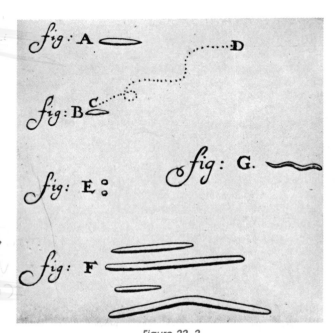

Figure 22–2

Leeuwenhoek's drawings of bacteria. Here may be seen cocci, bacilli, and (probably) a spirochete. (From Fuerst, R.: Frobisher and Fuerst's Microbiology in Health and Disease, 15th ed. Philadelphia, W. B. Saunders Co., 1983.)

Koch was a German physician who studied the causes and transmission of disease. He discovered the organism responsible for tuberculosis and developed techniques still used today for culturing (growing) and staining microorganisms for identification.

Lister, a Scottish surgeon, experimented with disinfection and sterilization techniques, especially for surgeons and operating room personnel. He proved that simple procedures, such as careful hand washing and the use of disinfectants, control the spread of disease-producing microorganisms. His principles for surgical asepsis have helped reduce surgical mortalities (deaths) from 50 percent to less than 3 percent and are still practiced.

After many years of research, medical microbiology now includes many classifications of disease-producing organisms. The last, viruses, are the smallest known microorganisms. They were not discovered until the powerful electron microscope, which uses a stream of electrons rather than light rays, was developed a few decades ago.

INFECTIOUS DISEASES

Disease may be defined as any sustained, harmful alteration of the normal structure, function, or metabolism (biochemistry) of an organism or cell. We recognize and categorize many different types of diseases: hereditary (genetic), drug-induced, structural, degenerative, and infectious, to name a few.

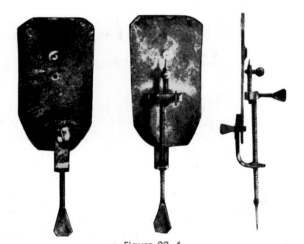

Figure 22–1

One of Antonj van Leeuwenhoek's microscopes: front, back, and side views. (From Fuerst, R.: Frobisher and Fuerst's Microbiology in Health and Disease, 15th ed. Philadelphia, W. B. Saunders Co., 1983.)

Table 22–1

Simplified Explanation of Selected Diseases, with the Abnormality and Consequences

Category and Disease	Abnormality	Consequences
HEREDITARY		
Hemophilia	Defective blood-clotting mechanism; one or more chemical factors missing or defective	Prolonged bleeding without coagulation factor; bleeding to death, if not corrected
Baldness	Loss of hair	Increased heat loss via scalp and changed appearance of head
Down syndrome	Affected individuals have one extra chromosome (47 instead of 46)	Changes in metabolism and function lead to distorted physical features (mongolism) and lowered mental processes (IQ)
METABOLIC		
Diabetes	Inability to use glucose effectively inside the body	High levels of sugar in blood and urine. If uncorrected, formation of ketone bodies, acidosis, followed by coma and death
Hyperthyroidism	Excessive secretion of thyroxine and thyronine, two hormones of the thyroid	Nervousness, irritability, muscle weakness, weight loss despite good appetite
Addison's disease	Adrenocortical hormone insufficiency	Fatigue, weakness, pigmentation of skin in pressure areas and sometimes face; postural hypotension. Delayed excretion of water, loss of sodium via urine
INFECTIOUS		
Trichomoniasis	Growth and multiplication of the flagellate, *Trichomonas vaginalis*, in urinary tract of females or males	Itching, burning of urethra
Gonorrhea	Growth and multiplication of the bacterium *Neisseria gonorrhoeae* in the genitourinary tract of males and females	Inflammation, pus; in males, burning on urination with release of pus; females may be asymptomatic
Infective osteomyelitis	Growth and multiplication usually of the bacterium *Staphylococcus aureus* in bone marrow	Bone pain and ache; bone destruction; fever

22

Sometimes, a specific disease may fit two or more categories. Table 22–1 lists some diseases that fit into these sample categories.

Infectious diseases are caused by infection; that is, the entrance of a living microbe into a cell or organism. *Infection* itself is not disease, for until the infected cell or organism shows a harmful alteration of its structure, physiology, or biochemistry, disease is either not detected or not considered present. In fact, a living microbe may be ingested, injected, or inhaled and never cause an infectious disease in that person. An unaffected person, however, could still transmit the infection to another person. In this case, we call the unaffected person a *carrier*.

Microbes that cause disease are called **pathogens**. The study of pathogens and their effects on the defense systems of the body is complex. Many factors determine the role of microbes in disease, the identification of microbes in the laboratory, and the ability of the body to maintain or recover health.

Microorganisms are almost everywhere. We carry them on our skin, in our bodies, and on our clothing. They are in ice, boiling water, the soil, and the air. The only places that are free of microorganisms are the insides of sterilized containers; inside fresh, unbruised fruits; and in certain internal body organs and tissues. Organs and tissues that do not connect with the outside by means of mucous-lined membranes are, in the normal state, free from all living microorganisms.

Conditions That Favor Growth of Pathogenic Microorganisms

Most pathogens prefer a fluid nutrient environment and an atmosphere full of oxygen. Pathogens that thrive in oxygen are called *aerobes*. Aerobes grow best when the following six conditions are present:

1. Oxygen.
2. Moisture (water).
3. Nutrients from a living source, called a host (sometimes at the expense of the host), or from dead or decaying material.
4. Temperature of 98.6° Fahrenheit (F), or 37° centigrade (C).
5. Darkness.
6. Neutral to slightly alkaline pH environment.

Other pathogens prefer an environment without oxygen. These organisms are referred to as *anaerobes*. Anaerobes thrive in the dark, damp, warm, airless places inside the body. For example, the anaerobic bacterial pathogen *Clostridium tetani* causes tetanus (lockjaw). Found in the soil or street dust, it is dormant and protected by a hard coating in what is called the **spore** stage. However, once inside human tissue, the protective spore becomes a living bacterium releasing **toxins**. The puncture wound that closes over and blocks out air (oxygen) is the perfect medium for growth. The bacterium rapidly multiplies and spreads through the bloodstream, causing the disease. In the same family of spore-forming bacteria is the *Clostridium perfringens* bacterium, which causes *gas gangrene*. The cycle is the same as for tetanus, except the infection is localized, often necessitating the amputation of a limb. Gas gangrene can result from contaminated surgical wounds. The third in this group of rod-shaped, spore-forming bacilli (bacteria) is the *Clostridium botulinum*. This organism grows in the oxygenless atmosphere of canned goods; when the can is opened, released toxins cause the disease known as *botulism*. Organisms that produce spores and release toxins are extremely dangerous, and these three diseases can be deadly.

The Chain of Infection

The life and growth of pathogens is a cycle, or chain. Break the chain, and you break the infectious process.

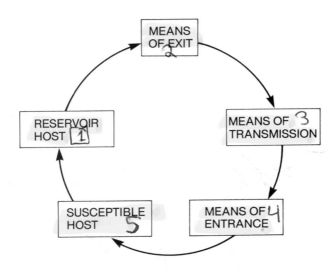

The chain of infection starts at the *RESERVOIR HOST*. A reservoir host may be an insect, animal, or human. Most pathogens must gain entrance into a host or die. The reservoir host supplies nutrition to the organism, allowing it to multiply. The pathogen either causes infection in the host or exits from the host in great enough numbers to allow its transfer to another host.

The chain of infection continues with the *MEANS OF EXIT*. This is how the organism escapes. Exits include the mouth, nose, eyes, ears, intestines, urinary tract, and reproductive tract and open wounds.

After exiting the reservoir host, organisms spread by *MEANS OF TRANSMISSION*. Transmission is either direct or indirect. *Direct transmission* is by contact with an infected person or the discharges

of an infected person, such as the feces or urine. *Indirect transmission* occurs from *droplets* in the air expelled from coughing, speaking, or sneezing; insects (called *vectors*) that harbor pathogens; contaminated food or drink; and contaminated objects (called *fomites*). The following are examples of direct and indirect means of transmission:

Direct Transmission	Indirect Transmission
Contact with infected person	Contact with droplets (cough or sneeze) of infected person
Contact with infected person's discharges or excretions	Fomites (inanimate objects such as infected instruments, paper tissue, pens, forks, equipment, or clothes)
Sexual transmission	
Contact with infected blood through a break in the skin or with blood products	Vectors (e.g., bites from ticks, lice, and mosquitos)
	Contaminated food or drink

The next step is the *MEANS OF ENTRY*. Now the transmitted organism will gain entry into a new host. The means of entry, like the means of exit, may be the mouth, nose, eyes, intestines, urinary tract, or reproductive tract or an open wound.

If the host is a *SUSCEPTIBLE HOST*, that is, one that is capable of supporting the growth of the infecting organism, the organism will multiply. Factors affecting susceptibility include the location of entry, the dose of organisms, and the condition of the individual. If the conditions are right, the organisms reach infectious levels, the susceptible host becomes a *RESERVOIR HOST*, and the cycle begins again.

PREVENTION OF DISEASE TRANSMISSION

The best way to stop the growth and transmission of pathogens is to break the chain of infection. For example, with aerobes, remove the oxygen; or if pathogens thrive at 98.6°F, raise the temperature and most of them will die. If pathogens thrive in the dark, expose them to light. Many chemicals kill pathogens, provided the pathogens are exposed to the chemicals for a sufficient period of time. Spores are very resistant to chemicals, but some chemicals can even kill spores after ten hours or more of exposure. Temperatures of 250°F (121°C) maintained for 20 minutes with at least 15 pounds of pressurized steam will kill all life forms, including spores. This is the basis of the autoclave method of sterilization, which is discussed in Chapter 23. Good sanitization and housekeeping, sunshine and ventilation, universal blood and body-fluid precautions (see Appendix C, Recommendations for Prevention of AIDS Transmission) and isolation techniques, and disinfection and sterilization are necessary to control and break the chain of infection in the medical office.

The Inflammatory Response

When pathogenic organisms invade through our protective mechanisms, our bodies respond in a predictable manner, called *inflammation* (Fig. 22–3). To defend itself, the body initiates the following eight specific reactions that destroy and remove pathogenic organisms and their by-products or, if this is not possible, limit the extent of damage caused by pathogenic organisms and their by-products: *inflammation occurs*

1. The blood vessels at the site of injury or invasion dilate, and the number of white blood cells in the area increases, causing redness.

2. The white blood cells overpower and consume *eat*

the pathogenic microorganisms in a process called *phagocytosis*.

3. Fluids in the tissues increase, creating *edema*, *swelling* which puts pressure on the nerves and causes pain.

4. An increased blood supply to the area produces heat.

So far, this process characterizes the four classic symptoms of inflammation: redness (rubor), swelling (tumor), pain (dolor), and heat (calor). If the process is not reversed, it will continue through its course as follows:

5. Destroyed pathogens, cells, and white blood cells collect in the area and form a thick, white substance called *suppuration* (pus).

6. If the pathogenic invasion is too great for the

22

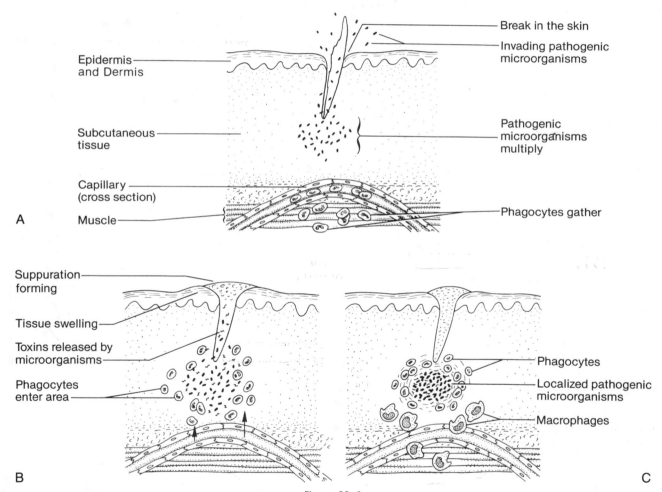

Epidermis and Dermis

Subcutaneous tissue

Capillary (cross section)

Muscle

Break in the skin

Invading pathogenic microorganisms

Pathogenic microorganisms multiply

Phagocytes gather

A

Suppuration forming

Tissue swelling

Toxins released by microorganisms

Phagocytes enter area

Phagocytes

Localized pathogenic microorganisms

Macrophages

B

C

Figure 22–3

*How the body defends itself against infection. **A**, Infection Stage. A break in the skin allows pathogenic microorganisms to enter and multiply within the tissues. As a defense, the body prepares to send phagocytes (white blood cells) to fight the invading pathogenic microorganisms. **B**, Inflammation Stage. As the pathogenic microorganisms multiply and die, toxins are released that destroy human tissue. Phagocytes have entered the infected area. Suppuration (liquified dead tissue, pathogenic microorganisms, and phagocytes, called pus) causes swelling and pain. **C**, Phagocytosis. Phagocytes engulf and ingest the invading microorganisms, localizing the infection. Macrophages (specialized phagocytes) now enter the area to ingest and clean up all the dead tissue debris. When all the debris has been enveloped and digested, swelling and pain will subside, and the wound will close and heal.*

white blood cells to control, the infection may collect in the body's lymph nodes, where more white blood cells are present to help fight the battle. This creates swollen glands.

7. If the body is too weak, or the dose of pathogens is too great in number, the infection may spread to the bloodstream. This causes a systemic condition that could ultimately affect the entire body, called *septicemia* or blood poisoning.

8. When the entire body is invaded, the condition is called general septicemia, or *pyemia*. Without appropriate medical intervention, death can occur. Antibiotics must be used to help the white blood cells bring the pathogenic invasion under control.

Nonspecific Defense Mechanisms

If microorganisms are everywhere, how do we avoid being ill most of the time? Fortunately, most microorganisms are not pathogenic. Most coexist with us, causing no harm. Some microorganisms are beneficial: microorganisms are responsible for fermenting wine and beer, the rising of bread, the manufacture of antibiotics, and the processing of waste in sewage treatment plants. Through the process of genetic engineering, bacteria are used to manufacture human insulin, human growth hormone, and other drugs in short supply, much less expensively than the older, traditional processes.

While some pathogenic microorganisms dwell on people and the human organism provides the perfect conditions for the growth and multiplication of pathogenic organisms, the human body has protective mechanisms to prevent the entry of microorganisms and disease.

The protection of the skin, mucous membranes, hair, and saliva; the washing effect of tears and stomach acid; and the lymphatic system all are parts of the *nonspecific defense system*. Transmission of disease depends on microorganisms finding entry through one of these barriers, and some pathogens cannot cause disease unless they gain entry by a specific route. As examples, the polio virus must enter through the gastrointestinal tract, and the gonococcus must enter through one of the mucous membranes to cause gonorrhea. The nonspecific defense system is our best defense against disease transmission; as long as it is working, pathogens are usually unable to make us ill.

Specific Defense Mechanisms

Immunity is the means of *specific defense*. It is called specific because a separate immune process takes place for each disease-producing organism that enters the body. However, the body is not able to build an immunity to every disease-producing organism, which is why it may be infected with some diseases again and again. The common cold is an example.

Immunity comes from antibody formation and can be *active* (the body produces the antibodies itself) or *passive* (the body borrows antibodies from others), and acquired either naturally or artificially.

Antibody Formation. Immunity means protection from disease and exists after the body forms substances called *antibodies*. Antibodies are formed in reaction to the presence of foreign substances, such as pathogens, in the blood. A foreign substance that stimulates the formation of an antibody is called an *antigen*. When an antigen is introduced into the body, special white blood cells called *B lymphocytes* are programmed to produce antibodies. The antibodies then combine with the antigens and neutralize them, so that disease is arrested or, if early enough, prevented. In this process, a specific antibody always fights a specific antigen—they are paired.

Antigens can be living bacteria, viruses, or other microorganisms that gain entrance through a break in one of the body's protective barriers or mechanisms. Toxins, pollens, and drugs can also be considered antigens if the body reacts to them by forming antibodies. In addition, antigens include killed or *attenuated* (diluted) bacteria or viruses and attenuated toxins or pollens purposely introduced into the body through inoculations, commonly called immunizations.

Active Immunity. If long-term or permanent immunity is needed, the body must be stimulated to produce its own antibodies. This is called active immunity because the body is actively producing its own antibodies. The stimulus must come from the presence in the body of a disease-producing microorganism acting as a foreign substance. The stimulus can naturally occur from transmitted microorganisms gaining entrance into the body or from inoculation, which is the artificial means. Inoculations contain microorganisms that have been killed or attenuated in a laboratory process. Their potency has been lessened so that they stimulate antibody formation but do not overpower the body and cause disease. Following immunization, a person frequently experiences inflammation at the site of the injection and generalized fever. This is because a less *virulent* disease process is going on in the body. Although the person may feel some of the effects of the disease, they are minimal. Some immunizations do not last a lifetime; in these cases, "boosters" are needed to restimulate ("boost") the B lymphocytes to produce antibodies again. Immunizations made from organisms are called *vaccines*. Immunizations made from the toxins of microorganisms are called *toxoids*.

Routinely given immunizations are listed in Table

Table 22–2
Schedule for Active Immunization of Normal Infants and Children in the United States

2 mo.	DTP[1]; TOPV[2]
4 mo.	DTP; TOPV
6 mo.	DTP; TOPV
1 yr.	Tuberculin test[3]
15 mo.	MMR[4]
18 mo.	DTP; TOPV
5–6 yr.	DTP; TOPV
14–16 yr.	Td[5]; TOPV, and given every 10 years thereafter

Adapted from The Report of the Committee on Infectious Diseases, ed. 19, Evanston, IL, American Academy of Pediatrics 1982.

[1]DTP—diphtheria and tetanus toxoids combined with pertussis vaccine

[2]TOPV—trivalent oral polio virus vaccine

[3]Frequency of repeated tuberculin tests depends on risk of exposure of the child and on the prevalence of TB in the population group.

[4]MMR—measles, mumps, rubella vaccines

[5]Td—combined tetanus and diphtheria toxoids (adult type) for those over six years of age, in contrast with diphtheria and tetanus toxoids (DT) containing a larger amount of diphtheria antigen. Tetanus toxoid at time of injury: For clean, minor wounds, no booster is needed unless ten years have elapsed since the last dose. For contaminated wounds, a booster dose should be given if more than five years have elapsed since the last dose. Routine smallpox vaccination is no longer recommended.

22–2. Others are given when exposure to a particular disease is suspected or possible. For example, typhoid-paratyphoid vaccine is suggested for persons traveling to certain foreign countries. The vaccine should be given so that there is enough time for the protection to develop. Veterinarians and others who handle animals may decide to receive rabies immunizations.

Passive Immunity. Passive immunity results when antibodies that have been produced externally are introduced into the body, either across the placenta from mother to child (natural) or through inoculation (artificial). Passive immunity lasts only a short time: what we borrow, we cannot keep. Babies are born with immunity to many of the same diseases to which their mothers are immune. However, if these infants do not receive immunizations and actively produce their own antibodies, their passive immunity will gradually fade, and they will become susceptible to these diseases.

When people have been exposed to serious diseases and there is not enough time to wait for them to produce their own antibodies, preparations made from human or animal **serum** containing known antibodies can be administered for temporary protection. These products are called *antisera* or *immune serum globulins*. If the disease is caused by bacterial toxins rather than the bacteria itself, the products administered are called *antitoxins*.

One product, *immune human serum gamma globulin*, is most often administered to persons exposed to hepatitis. *Tetanus immune globulin (TIG)*, or *tetanus antitoxin*, is administered to persons exposed to tetanus (lockjaw) organisms. TIG is made from human serum; tetanus antitoxin is manufactured from horse serum, which may cause serious reactions in people allergic to horses or horse hair. Antisera and antitoxins must be used with caution and are usually reserved for infectious diseases that could threaten life. Patients can be allergic to the derivatives in animal antisera and antitoxins, which is why human sera is preferred. *Antivenins* are also available for treating snake bites; the principle is the same.

CLASSIFICATIONS OF MICROORGANISMS

Microbes range in size from being visible to the naked eye, such as the tapeworm, to being visible only with the use of a microscope (e.g., bacteria and yeasts), to being so small that they are visible only with the use of the electron microscope (viruses). All microorganisms belong to one of the following six classifications. Some, such as bacteria, have subclassifications.

Helminths

Helminths are animal *parasites* called worms. A parasite is a plant or animal that lives upon or within another living organism and nourishes itself at the expense of the host organism. Helminths may live in animals or humans. They are usually transmitted through the soil or by infected clothing or fingernails, contact with infected persons, or contaminated food or water. Helminths go through the same life cycle as other worms. The adult worm lays eggs (ova). The ova develop into larvae. Larvae grow into adult worms, which lay eggs, and the cycle begins again. Examples of helminthic diseases are *tapeworm* (Fig. 22–4), *pinworm* (Fig. 22–5), and *Trichinella* (*pork worm*). Diagnosis is usually based on microscopic examination of feces for ova and parasites and on patient signs and symptoms.

Prevention of Disease. Break the infection cycle through cleanliness, proper preparation of foods, and isolating infected persons or animals.

Protozoa

Protozoa (s. protozoon) are single-celled animals ranging in size from microscopic to *macroscopic* (vis-

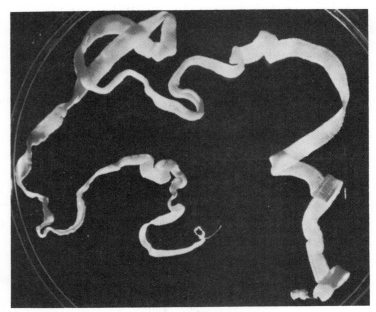

Figure 22–4
An entire tapeworm—Hymenolepis diminuta. (Photograph by Zane Price.)

They are found

ible to the naked eye). Protozoa are present in moist environments and in bodies of water such as lakes and ponds. Most are free-living (not parasitic); only a few cause disease in humans. Protozoa are transmitted through contaminated feces, food, or drink. The protozoon causing malaria, however, is transmitted to the human bloodstream by infected mosquitos (Fig. 22–6). Some pathogenic protozoa inhabit the bloodstream, others inhabit the intestines and genital tract. Pathogenic protozoa include the *Plasmodium* species, the cause of human *malaria;*

Toxoplasma gondii, a disease transmitted to a fetus or an infant from a mother infected by house cats; and *Entamoeba histolytica*, the cause of *amebic dysentery* (severe diarrhea) often seen in travelers returning home from one of the less developed countries (Table 22–3). Diagnosis is usually based on patient signs and symptoms and microscopic examination of stool and blood.

Prevention of Disease. Break the infection cycle by hand washing and precautions handling feces.

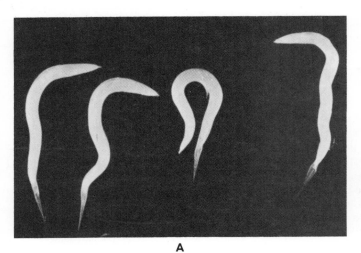

A

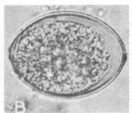

Figure 22–5
*Pinworm and ova. **A**, Adult pinworm—Enterobius vermicularis. Note the shapes and the clear, attenuated, and pointed posterior ends. (Courtesy of Louisiana State University School of Medicine. From Markell, E. K., Voge, M., and John, D. T.: Medical Parasitology, 6th ed. Philadelphia, W. B. Saunders Co., 1986.) **B**, Pinworm ova. (From Markell, E. K., Voge, M., and John, D. T.: Medical Parasitology, 6th ed. Philadelphia, W. B. Saunders Co., 1986.)*

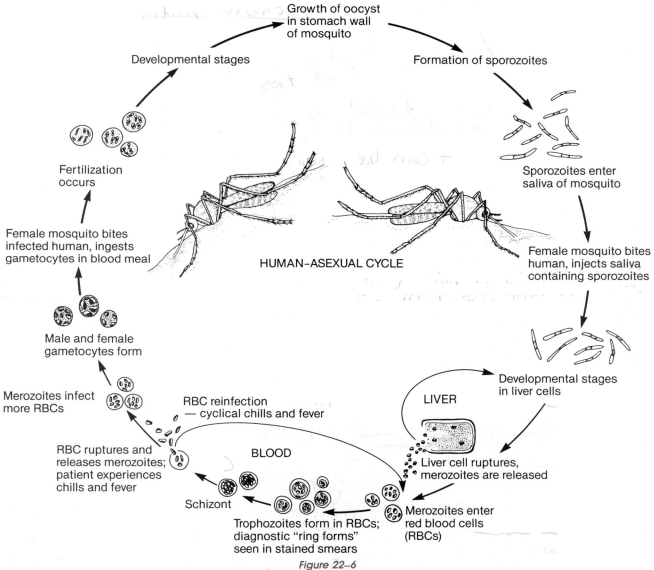

Figure 22–6

Cycle of malaria. Cycle of the parasite from human to vector (Anopheles mosquito) and back to human.

Table 22–3

Diseases Caused by Protozoa and Other Parasites

Disease	Organism	Transmission	Symptoms	Tests/Specimens
Malaria	*Plasmodium* sp. (protozoa)	Bite of the *Anopheles* mosquito	Chills, fever (cyclic)	Blood: examination of stained film for parasites
Toxoplasmosis	*Toxoplasma gondii* (protozoa)	Fecal contamination (cat litter); congenitally	Febrile illness, rash; congenital: jaundice, enlarged liver and spleen, brain abnormalities	Skin test
Amebic dysentery	*Entamoeba histolytica* (protozoa)	Fecal contamination of food and water	Bloody diarrhea, cramping, fever	Stool for ova and parasites (O & P)
Giardiasis	*Giardia lamblia* (protozoa)	Common in intestinal tract opportunist. Contaminated surface water	Asymptomatic to severe diarrhea and abdominal discomfort	Stool for O & P; intestinal biopsy; string test
Interstitial plasma cell pneumonia	*Pneumocystis carinii*	Widely prevalent in animals. Occurs in debilitated persons, immunosuppressed; common in AIDS	Pneumonia-like	Biopsy
Trichinosis	*Trichinella spiralis* (roundworm)	Ingestion of undercooked pork, bear meat	Nausea, fever, diarrhea, muscle pain and swelling, edema of face	Biopsy; blood tests
Tapeworm	*Taenia* sp.	Undercooked meats (beef and pork)	Abdominal discomfort, diarrhea, weight loss	Stool for O & P
	Diphyllobothrium latum	Undercooked fish; common in Norwegians, Japanese	As above; may become anemic	Stool for O & P
Pinworm	*Enterobius vermicularis* (roundworm)	Fecal-oral	Severe rectal itching, restlessness, insomnia	Scotch tape applied to perianal region for ova
Scabies	Itch mite: *Sarcoptes scabiei*	Direct contact; clothing, bedding	Nocturnal itching; skin burrows	Skin scrapings for parasites
Lice	*Pediculus humanus; Pthirus pubis* (crab)	Direct contact; clothing, bedding, furniture (can transmit other diseases via bite)	Intense itching; skin lesions	Finding adult lice or eggs (nits) on body or hair

Table courtesy of Kathleen Moody
Abbreviations: sp: species; O & P: ova and parasites

Fungi

Fungi (s. fungus) are vegetable organisms and include *yeasts* and *molds* (Fig. 22–7). Fungi are present in the soil, air, and water, but only a few species cause disease. Fungi thrive in warm, moist, dark places. They are transmitted by direct contact with infected persons, by prolonged exposure to a moist environment, or by inhalation of contaminated dust or soil. Fungal diseases (*mycoses*) usually are not serious, but they can be a nuisance and very difficult to cure. The *Candida* species causes *thrush* in the mouth and "yeast infection" in the vagina. The skin conditions called *tinea pedis* (*athlete's foot*) (Fig. 22–8), *tinea cruris* (*jock itch*), and *tinea capitis* (*ringworm*; although it is not a worm) are also fungal diseases. *Histoplasma capsulatum* causes a systemic fungal disease associated with bird or bat droppings (Table 22–4). Diagnosis is usually based on the culturing or testing of skin scrapings, hair samples, or samples of sputum or mucous membranes.

Prevention of Disease. Break the infection cycle by isolating contaminated persons or animals and avoiding places with contaminated dust and feces.

Bacteria

Bacteria (s. bacterium), like plants, have cell walls, but unlike plants, they lack chlorophyll. Usually, pathogenic bacteria grow best at 98.6°F (37°C), in a moist, dark environment. Bacterial infections can be spread by any means of transmission. Bacteria live and reproduce in nutrients supplied by the body or in a laboratory culture medium, which is an **agar** preparation that simulates the body's condition. Since bacteria are the most commonly encountered pathogens, most of the laboratory procedures performed in the medical office deal with the isolation and identification of these microbes (see Chapter 34).

Humans host a variety of bacteria, both harmful

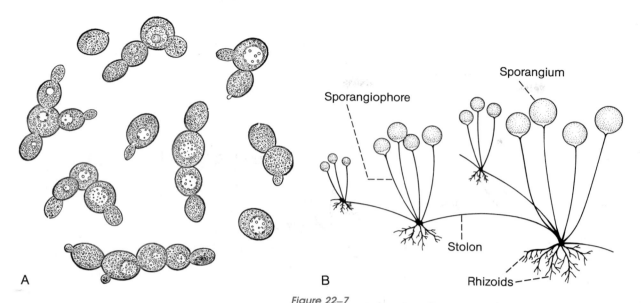

Figure 22–7

Yeast and mold. **A,** *Yeast cells. Brewers' yeast actively multiplying by budding. This species is called* Saccharomyces cerevisiae. *(Highly magnified. Sedgwick and Wilson. From Fuerst, R.: Frobisher and Fuerst's Microbiology in Health and Disease, 15th ed. Philadelphia, W. B. Saunders Co., 1983.* **B,** *A species of* Rhizopus, *a coenocytic mold.*

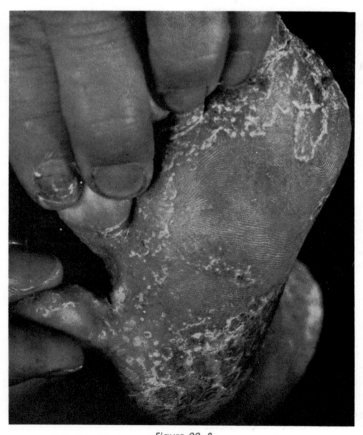

Figure 22–8

Chronic intertriginous type of tinea pedis, showing maceration and fissure between fourth and fifth toes. (From Conant, N. F., Smith, D. T., Baker R. D., et al.: Manual of Clinical Mycology, 3rd ed. Philadelphia, W. B. Saunders Co., 1971.)

Table 22–4
Selected Fungal Diseases

Disease	Organism	Predisposing Conditions and Transmission	Symptoms	Tests/Specimens
Thrush (oral yeast) Candida (vaginal yeast)	Candida species (yeast)	Oral: during birth; other: following antibiotic therapy, oral birth control, severe diabetes	White, cheesy growth	Swab for KOH prep, culture
Athlete's foot, jock itch, ringworm (tinea)	Several species of dermatophytes (skin fungi)	Opportunist; direct contact; clothing; prolonged exposure to moist environment	Hair loss, thickening of skin, nails; itching; red, scaly patches	Skin scraping for KOH prep; skin, hair for culture
Histoplasmosis	Histoplasma capsulatum	Inhalation of dust contaminated with bird or bat droppings	Mild, flu-like to systemic	Serologic
Cryptococcosis	Cryptococcus neoformans	Contact with poultry droppings	Cough, fever, malaise; can become systemic	Sputum culture
Sporotrichosis	Sporothrix schenckii	Farmers, florists, people exposed to soil	Skin lesions that spread along lymphatics; can become systemic	CSF culture, India ink direct examination, scrapings; serologic

Table courtesy of Kathleen Moody

and harmless, at all times. The skin, respiratory tract, and gastrointestinal tract are inhabited by a great variety of harmless bacteria, called *normal flora*. They are beneficial and protect the human host by aiding in metabolism and interfering with the harmful bacteria that may gain entrance. Occasionally, normal flora may become *opportunistic*, that is, cause infection. This occurs when one type of normal flora overgrows, usually as the result of an imbalance between it and the other normal flora, or when flora that is normal to one area invades another area, where it becomes pathogenic. One common example is *cystitis*, a urinary tract infection caused by contamination with *Escherichia coli*, a bacterium that is normal flora in the intestine.

 One way of classifying bacteria is by *morphology* (size and shape). Spherical bacteria are called *cocci*, rod-shaped bacteria are called *bacilli*, and those shaped like threads are called *spirilla* or *spirochetes*. If any of these groups grow in pairs, the prefix *diplo* is used, as in *diplococci*; if in chains, the prefix *strepto* is used, as in *streptococci*. If they grow in clusters, like grapes, the prefix *staphylo* is used, as in *staphylococci* (Fig. 22–9).

Different kinds of bacteria tend to affect the various organs of the body in different ways, producing diseases, each with its own symptoms and effects (Tables 22–5 and 22–6).

Staphylococcus. The staphylococcus (pl. staphylococci) organism is a normal flora of the skin. *Staphylococcus albus* is a resident bacterium found on the hands, and *Staphylococcus aureus* is frequently found in the nasopharynx. However, when these organisms invade the body, through a break in the skin for instance, they produce local infection with inflammation and pus, called an abscess or boil. Staphylococci affecting more than a local area are rare.

Streptococcus. The streptococcus (pl. streptococci) bacterium is found in the mouth, but if it gains entrance into the bloodstream, it can cause diseases such as *streptococcal sore throat*; *tonsillitis*, leading to *otitis media*; *impetigo*; *rheumatic fever* (subacute bacterial endocarditis, abbreviated *SBE*); *scarlet fever*; and severe postoperative wound infection. Streptococci usually cause the more serious systemic infections and commonly gain entrance through air droplets, direct contact with a contaminated source, or breaks in the skin.

Diplococcus. The diplococcus (pl. diplococci) bacterium causes *pneumonia*, *meningitis*, and *gonorrhea*. The *pneumococcus* and the *meningococcus* may reside in the nasopharynx and throat, but if they gain entrance to the bloodstream through the respiratory tract, they can cause pneumonia or meningitis. The gonococcus is not a resident bacterium and gains entrance through sexual contact. Diplococci are transmitted by droplet or direct contact with the contaminated source.

Spirillum. Spirillum (pl. spirilla) infections include *necrotizing ulcerative gingivitis* (*trench mouth*), *cholera*, and *syphilis*.

Bacillus. Bacillus (pl. bacilli) infections include *plague, diphtheria, tuberculosis,* and *typhoid fever*.

Chlamydia and Mycoplasma. These are separately classified bacteria. Chlamydia are *obligate* parasites (unable to survive without a host) and the smallest of all bacteria. They are important because of their role in *sexually transmitted disease* (*STD*). *Chlamydia trachomatis* is the most frequent cause of *pelvic inflammatory disease* (*PID*) and is considered the most prevalent STD today. Flies can also carry Chlamydia trachomatis and cause *trachoma*, the

Cocci

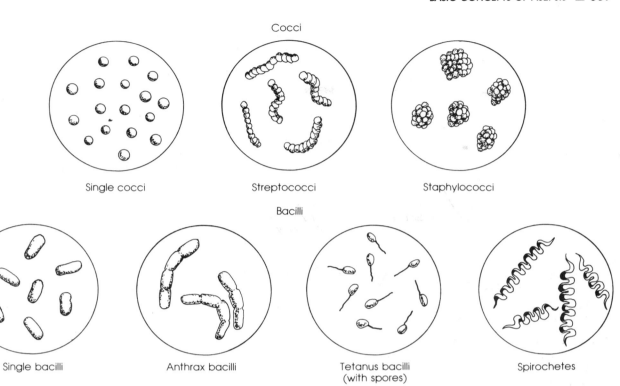

Figure 22–9
Drawings of various pathogenic microorganisms as they appear under the microscope.

Table 22–5
Common Diseases Caused by Cocci

Disease	Organism	Description	Transmission	Symptoms	Specimen	Tests
Pneumonia	*Streptococcus pneumoniae*	Gram-positive cocci in pairs	Direct contact, droplets	Productive cough, fever, chest pain	Sputum; bronchoscopy secretions	Culture, Gram stain
Strep throat	*Streptococcus pyogenes* (group A strep)	Gram-positive cocci in chains	Direct contact, droplets, fomites	Severe sore throat, fever, malaise	Direct swab	Direct agglutination; culture; WBC and differential
Wound infection, abscesses, boils	*Staphylococcus aureus*	Gram-positive cocci in clusters	Direct contact, fomites, carriers; poor hand washing	Area red, warm, swollen; pus; pain; ulceration or sinus formation	Deep swab; aspirate of drainage	Culture and sensitivity (aerobic and anaerobic)
Staphylococcal food poisoning	*Staphylococcus aureus*	Gram-positive cocci in clusters	Poor hygiene + improper refrigeration of foods	Vomiting, abdominal cramps, diarrhea	Suspected food, stool	Culture
Toxic shock	*Staphylococcus aureus*	Gram-positive cocci in clusters	Use of absorbent packing materials (e.g., tampons, nasal packs)	Fever, headache, nausea, vomiting, delirium, low blood pressure (BP)	Swab, blood	Culture and serology
Gonorrhea	*Neisseria gonorrhoeae*	Gram-negative cocci in pairs; intracellular in WBC	Sexually transmitted	*Females*: pelvic pain, discharge. May be asymptomatic *Males*: urethral drip, pain on urination	Swab of cervix, urethra; rectal and pharyngeal swabs in homosexuals	Gram stain; culture
Meningococcal meningitis	*Neisseria meningitidis*	Gram-negative diplococci	Respiratory tract secretions	High fever, headache, projectile vomiting, delirium, neck and back rigidity, convulsions, petechial skin rash	Nasopharyngeal swabs, cerebrospinal fluid, blood	Gram stain; culture; cell counts and chemistries

Table courtesy of Kathleen Moody

Table 22–6
Selected Diseases Caused by Bacilli and Spirilla

Disease	Organism	Description	Transmission	Symptoms	Tests/Specimens	Prevention and Immunization
Tuberculosis	Mycobacterium tuberculosis	Acid-fast beaded bacilli	Inhalation	Pulmonary: cough, hemoptysis, sweats, weight loss. May affect other systems	Sputum for culture; X ray; skin tests	BCG vaccine
Urinary tract infections	Escherichia coli, Proteus sp., Klebsiella sp., Pseudomonas aeruginosa	Gram-negative bacilli	Ascends urethra; catheterization	Cystitis: frequency, burning, bloody urine. Pyelonephritis: flank pain, fever	Clean-catch urine for culture and analysis	Good personal hygiene; always wipe from front to back
Syphilis	Treponema pallidum	Spirochete	Sexually; congenitally	Primary: painless sore. Secondary: generalized rash involving palms and soles of feet. Congenital: birth defects	Blood for serologic tests: VDRL, RPR, FTA	Avoidance of infected persons; use of condoms
Lyme disease	Borrelia	Spirochete	Tick bite	Fever, joint pain, red annular rash	Swab for culture	Eliminating animal vectors
Cholera	Vibrio cholerae	Gram-negative spirillum	Fecal contamination of food and water (warm climates)	Severe vomiting and diarrhea; dehydration	Stool for culture	Cholera vaccine; boiling water; cooking foods
Legionnaires' disease	Legionella pneumophila	Gram-negative bacillus (stains poorly with usual methods)	Grows freely in water (air conditioning systems)	Pneumonia-like symptoms	Sputum; blood	Isolation
Tetanus (lockjaw)	Clostridium tetani	Gram-positive spore-forming bacilli, anaerobic	Open wounds, fractures, punctures	Toxin affects motor nerves; muscle spasms, convulsions, rigidity	Blood	DPT in childhood; T or Td every ten years
Gas gangrene	Clostridium perfringens	Gram-positive spore-forming bacilli, anaerobic	Wounds	Gas and watery exudate in infected wound	Swab, aspirate of wound for culture	Proper wound care
Botulism	Clostridium botulinum	Gram-positive spore-forming bacilli, anaerobic	Improperly cooked canned foods	Neurotoxin affects speech, swallowing, vision; paralysis of respiratory muscles, death	Contaminated food; blood	Botulinus antitoxin; boil canned goods 20 minutes before tasting or eating
Diphtheria	Corynebacterium diphtheriae	Gram-positive bacilli, club-shaped	Respiratory secretions	Sore throat, fever, headache, gray membrane in throat	Swabs; Gram stain, culture; Schick test for immunity	DPT in childhood
Whooping cough	Bordetella pertussis	Gram-negative bacilli	Respiratory secretions	Upper respiratory tract symptoms; high-pitched, crowing whoop	Swabs for culture	DPT in childhood
Typhoid and paratyphoid fevers	Salmonella sp.	Gram-negative bacilli	Contaminated food, water, poor hygiene; carriers	Fever, headache, diarrhea, toxemia, rose spots on skin	Stool for culture	Typhoid/paratyphoid A and B vaccine (TAB)
Plague	Yersinia pestis	Gram-negative bacilli	Via flea bite from infected rodents	Fever and chills, delirium, enlarged, painful lymph nodes	Sputum for culture; blood	Vaccine available; rodent control
Nonspecific vaginitis	Gardnerella vaginalis, with anaerobes	Gram-variable bacillus	Sexual	Vaginal irritation, itching, fishy-smelling malodorous discharge	Swab; wet prep for "clue cells"	Avoidance of infected persons; good personal hygiene

Table courtesy of Kathleen Moody

leading cause of infectious blindness. *Mycoplasma* is another obligate parasite belonging to the bacterium family. *Mycoplasma pneumoniae* causes a type of pneumonia called *atypical pneumonia*.

Prevention for All Types of Bacterial Infections. Break the infection cycle through immunizations, proper sanitary conditions, isolation, and aseptic procedures.

Table 22–7

Diseases Caused by Rickettsia, Chlamydia, *and* Mycoplasma

Disease	Organism	Transmission	Symptoms	Tests/Specimens
Rocky Mountain spotted fever	*Rickettsia rickettsii*	Tick bite	Headache, chills, fever, characteristic rash on extremities and trunk	Blood for serologic tests; skin biopsy for direct fluorescent microscopy
Typhus	*Rickettsia prowazekii*	Tick bite	Fever, rash, confusion	Blood for serology
Atypical pneumonia	*Mycoplasma pneumoniae*	Respiratory secretions	Fever, cough, chest pain	Blood, sputum
Nongonococcal urethritis and vaginitis	*Chlamydia trachomatis*	Sexual	May be asymptomatic	Swabs for culture and serologic testing
Inclusion conjunctivitis, pneumonia		Congenital	Severe conjunctivitis in newborns Afebrile pneumonia in newborns	

Table courtesy of Kathleen Moody

Rickettsiae

Rickettsiae (s. rickettsia) are microscopic parasites that are insect-borne and fever-producing. Rickettsiae are transmitted from rodents or other animals to humans by the bites of lice, fleas, ticks, and mites. These parasites attack the linings of small blood vessels. The diseases they cause are classified in groups, the two most common being the *spotted fever group* and the *typhus group* (Table 22–7). Usually, diagnosis is based on patient signs and symptoms and blood testing.

Prevention of Disease. Break the infection cycle with control of rodent and insect populations and high sanitation standards.

Viruses Colds flus

Medical science has not yet conquered the control of viruses. Very few antiviral drugs have been introduced, and those that are used have limited effectiveness on specific viruses only. Invading viruses are difficult to treat chemically because the chemicals that effectively attack viruses also seriously damage human tissues.

Viruses can be treated easily in the external environment. Widely used chemicals such as chlorine (bleach), iodine, phenol, and formaldehyde (see Chapter 23) easily and effectively destroy viruses on surfaces and objects coming into contact with the infected patient. These agents, however, are too toxic to be used internally.

Viruses can be seen only with the electron microscope. Each virus is an organism made up of a nucleic acid core covered with a coating of protein; but the nucleic acid core of the virus is unique in nature because it has either RNA (ribonucleic acid) or DNA (deoxyribonucleic acid), but never both.

All other organisms have both RNA and DNA, which together form pairs of chromosomes that contain all the genetic codes necessary for protein synthesis and reproduction. Viruses, on the other hand, have a complete set of hereditary factors in half the number of chromosomes and, therefore, can reproduce only within living cells and only after a living host cell's enzymes dissolve the outer protein coating. A virus enters a host cell, and the host's enzymes wash away the virus's outer coating. Then the virus's nucleic acid is released into the cell's cytoplasm, where it mixes, and the virus is able to replicate itself. Once infected, the parasitized host cells die, while the multiplying viruses continue to "swarm" from the dying cells to invade and attack new cells and tissues.

Because these obligate parasites are deficient in enzymes that would enable them to grow alone, clinical and research laboratories must grow them in tissue cultures or cell systems. Most facilities do not have the resources for the isolation and identification of viruses, and specimens are usually processed at state or federal laboratories. However, there are a few rapid screening tests available for the medical office (see Chapter 35).

Viruses cause many clinically significant diseases in humans. Unfortunately, most viral diseases can be treated only *symptomatically*, that is, for the symptom and not the infective cause. General antibiotics are ineffective in preventing or curtailing viral infections, and even the few drugs that are effective against some specific viruses have limitations because viruses often produce different types of infections in host cells.

Prevention of Disease. Avoidance of the infection is the best approach. This includes staying away from public areas during the flu season and isolating patients known to be infected with a virus. Patients must be vaccinated against polio (Sabin vaccine),

Table 22–8
Viral Diseases

Disease	Transmission	Symptoms	Tests	Prevention
Smallpox	Direct contact; fomites	Vesicles on entire body, including soles and palms		Eradicated (vaccine is still available)
Herpes I (cold sores, fever blisters)	Direct contact; fomites	Recurrent painful blisters on lips, mouth	Serologic	Avoid contact with active lesions
Herpes II (genital)	Sexual contact	Recurrent painful blisters on labia, penis, rectum	Serologic	Avoid sexual contact with persons having active lesions
Infectious mononucleosis	Direct and airborne	Sore throat, fever, malaise, lymph gland involvement; hepatitis, enlarged spleen	Blood for Monospot	Avoid direct contact with known cases
Influenza	Droplet and fomites	Fever, body aches, cough		Immunization for old, young, debilitated
Warts	Direct and indirect contact	Circumscribed outgrowths on skin; most common on hands and feet		
Rabies	Contact with saliva of infected animal (dog, cat, skunk, fox, bat are usual)	Fever, uncontrollable excitement, spasms of throat, profuse salivation	Animal's brain tissue examined for Negri bodies	Vaccine available. Vaccinate pets
Mumps	Direct contact	Pain, swelling of salivary glands, fever	Acute and convalescent titers	MMR* vaccine
Measles	Direct contact; droplets	Fever, nasal discharge, red eyes; Koplik spots, rash	Serologic	MMR vaccine
Rubella	Direct contact; droplets. Congenital	Rash, swollen lymph glands; causes severe birth defects	Serologic	MMR vaccine
Common cold	Direct; droplets; fomites	Headache, fever, runny nose, congestion		Good hygiene (hand washing)
Hepatitis A (infectious hepatitis)	Fecal-oral; contaminated food and water	Nausea, fever, weakness, loss of appetite, jaundice	Serologic	Good hygiene (hand washing)
Hepatitis B (serum hepatitis)	Blood and blood products; accidental needle sticks	Similar to hepatitis A, but more severe	Serologic	Vaccine is available. Avoid contact with blood from infected persons
AIDS	Sexual; drug abuse (needles); blood and body fluids	Poor immunity, resulting in disseminated viral, fungal, and protozoan infections; Kaposi sarcoma	Serologic	Avoid casual sexual contact. Use extra caution when drawing and/or handling specimens
Polio	Direct contact; carriers. Enters via mouth	Fever, headache, stiff neck and back, paralysis of muscles		Trivalent oral polio vaccine (TOPV)

Table courtesy of Kathleen Moody
*MMR, measles, mumps, rubella

German measles (rubella vaccine), measles (rubeola vaccine), and mumps (epidemic parotitis vaccine). High-risk patients can be vaccinated against some other viruses, such as smallpox, flu, and hepatitis. This is especially important for the elderly and the chronically ill (Table 22–8).

Acute Infection. In the acute viral infection, the host cell typically dies within a period of hours or days. Symptoms appear after the tissue damage begins to occur. Usually, the virus can be isolated only shortly before or after the first symptom appears. In most acute infections, such as the common cold, the body's defense mechanisms eliminate the virus within two to three weeks.

Chronic Infection. Persistent viral infections are those in which the virus is present for a long period of time; some may persist for life. The person may be asymptomatic and the virus undetectable; or, as in chronic viral *hepatitis B*, the patient is asymptomatic, but the virus may be detected and transmissible. Hepatitis B, or *serum hepatitis*, may be transmitted by blood or blood products and is a hazard to health care personnel. Once unpreventable, blood tests now can determine the presence of certain antigens that identify a person as a carrier of hepatitis B, and a vaccine is available for protection against the disease.

Latent Infection. A latent infection is a persistent infection in which the symptoms and the virus come and go. Cold sores (oral herpes simplex) and *genital herpes* are latent viral infections. The virus first enters the body and causes the original lesion. It then lies dormant, away from the surface, in a nerve cell, until certain provocation (illness with fever, sunburn, or stress) causes the virus to leave the nerve cell and seek the surface again. Once the virus reaches the superficial tissues, it becomes detectable for a short time and causes another outbreak at that site. Another herpesvirus, *herpes zoster*, causes *chickenpox*. This virus then may lie dormant and later erupt as the painful disease *shingles.*

Slow Infection. Slow infections progress over very long periods of time. These conditions include the degenerative neurologic diseases, some with fatal outcomes. Generally, cures are not available; however these diseases may enter remission for extended periods.

Viruses and Cancer. More and more, viruses are being implicated in cancer and other tumors. A virus enters a normal cell and incorporates itself into the cell's DNA, causing the uncontrolled growth that is characteristic of tumors. *Oncogenes* (*onco,* tumor), either inherited by the person or carried in the virus's genetic coding, may be responsible for the transformation of a normal cell into a tumor cell. Host cells infected with viruses may produce a substance called *interferon,* which protects nearby cells from invasion. The use of interferon in viral disease and cancer therapy has gained much attention lately as a possible treatment or prevention for viral diseases. Research continues to identify new cancer-related viruses and to work toward cures and vaccines.

MALFUNCTIONS OF THE IMMUNE SYSTEM

Allergy

Diseases of the immune system include allergy, autoimmune phenomena, and immune deficiencies. Allergy is the most common malfunction. In allergies, the usual antigen-antibody reaction is accompanied by harmful effects on the body, ranging from sneezing, coughing, and itching to anaphylactic shock and can occur for the first time at any age. The allergen can be inhaled, ingested, injected, or applied to the skin.

Anaphylactic Shock. *Anaphylaxis* is a life-threatening allergic reaction that can occur within minutes following the introduction of an allergen. Bee stings and medications are the usual causes. In the medical office, care must be taken to ascertain each patient's allergies and to keep the patient in the office 10 to 30 minutes after certain injections and inoculations.

Anaphylactic reactions are possible in any patient following the administration of animal-derivative inoculations, certain injectable drugs such as penicillin, or allergy desensitization serum.

Symptoms include swelling, itching or burning of the throat and skin, choking, difficulty in breathing, hives, and a drop in blood pressure. If a reaction occurs, get the physician immediately and be prepared to administer basic life support (cardiopulmonary resuscitation). Anaphylactic shock is treated with intravenous epinephrine. Antihistamines or intramuscular corticosteroids may be administered in minor reactions (see Chapter 39).

Autoimmune Diseases

Autoimmune diseases occur when the body fails to recognize its own constituents (*autoantigens*) and produces antibodies to fight them. *Rheumatoid arthritis* (*RA*) and *systemic lupus erythematosus* (*SLE*) are two examples. In rheumatoid arthritis, the antibodies cause joint inflammation and bone and muscle deformity and may cause dysfunction of many organs, including the joints, heart, and kidneys. Systemic lupus erythematosus is an autoimmune disease of connective tissue. A defect in the body's regulatory mechanisms is suspected. The body is not able to control a high level of autoantibodies, which attack the body's own cells. SLE is characterized by fever and injuries to the skin, mucous membranes, joints, kidneys, and the nervous system. It is found most often in women between 30 and 40 years of age.

Diagnosis of lupus and rheumatoid arthritis is based on laboratory identification of the antibody. The tests are performed on blood serum in a special laboratory. Some rheumatoid arthritis tests are simple and are performed in the medical office by the medical assistant.

Immune Deficiency Syndromes

Immune deficiency syndromes may be either inherited or acquired. The inherited deficiencies range from the inability to fight certain types of infections to the total inability to produce antibodies of any kind. Bone marrow transplants are helpful for some patients.

Acquired Immune Deficiency Syndrome (AIDS). Acquired immune deficiency syndrome is a major health threat. AIDS is caused by HIV (human immunodeficiency virus; formerly HTLV III), which is transmitted through blood and semen and may be present in other body fluids and tissues. AIDS was first recognized in 1979 among sexually active homosexual men living in the cities of New York, Los

Angeles, and San Francisco. AIDS was originally confined to certain "H" groups: homosexuals, Haitians, hemophiliacs, and hypo abusers (drug addicts). However, it has now spread to the heterosexual population, throughout the United States and the world. Diagnosed cases have doubled every year since 1980, and health experts predict that, by 1991, the number of victims will be more than double the 1986 count. Certain groups remain at high risk, including homosexual and bisexual males who have multiple sex partners, native Haitians who have recently emigrated from their country, individuals sharing drug injection needles, persons with hemophilia or others who are receiving large quantities of blood transfusions, and patients with renal disease being treated by machine dialysis.

The virus affects a key white cell in the immune system. The body becomes deficient in fighting infections caused by certain other viruses, bacteria, fungi, and protozoa that live harmlessly on or around healthy persons. *Pneumocystis carinii* infections are common. Usually tolerable infections ravage the body. In addition, AIDS victims often develop *Kaposi sarcoma*, a rare skin cancer. AIDS kills all who acquire it, making it the most deadly illness of modern times.

Researchers have developed a test to detect the antibodies to HIV virus in blood. All blood collected for the purpose of transfusion is now routinely tested. Intensive research is concentrating on a treatment and the development of a vaccine.

Characteristics of the disease include profound fatigue, weight loss, swollen glands, loss of appetite, a dry cough, persistent fever and diarrhea, and a white coating on the tongue or throat. Diagnosis is made by the presence of symptoms and by the existence of other diseases or infections.

As in hepatitis B, all medical personnel must use extreme caution to avoid accidental needle sticks or contamination of open cuts with the patient's blood or body fluids. Medical assistants must use extreme caution when assisting the physician with patients: Use strict aseptic procedures when coming into direct contact with all body secretions (see Appendix C).

ASEPSIS

Medical Asepsis

Asepsis means freedom from infection or infectious material. Medical asepsis is defined as the destruction of organisms *after they leave the body*. When we practice the principles of medical asepsis, we are directing our efforts at preventing reinfection of the patient or cross-infection of other patients or ourselves. The goal is to isolate microorganisms by following universal blood and body-fluid precautions (see Appendix C), and disinfecting or steriliz-

ing objects as soon as possible after they have been contaminated. This creates a nonsterile but clean environment.

As previously stated, the most effective barrier against infection is the unbroken skin. If the skin and mucous membranes are intact, medical asepsis can be practiced for most noninvasive (not penetrating through human tissues) procedures such as pelvic and proctologic examinations. Instruments and objects not breaking the skin must be sterilized before being used on another patient but then they may be stored and used under clean, nonsterile conditions. Clean hands and objects may touch the patient (although the routine use of nonsterile examination gloves is gaining in popularity). Gowns and masks may be used, but they are not presterilized; they are worn to protect the operator more than the patient. Hands are washed according to the principles of the medical aseptic hand wash.

Washing the hands is the first line of defense in the practice of medical asepsis.

Hands must be washed, using the correct technique, before and after each patient. It is not necessary to do an extended scrub each time, but the first scrub in the morning should be extensive. Subsequent hand washings may be brief unless your hands become excessively contaminated. A good surgical soap with chlorhexidine, such as Hibiclens, which has antiseptic residual action that will last several hours, should be used. Buy a good quality surgical soap that is gentle to the hands; purchasing inexpensive soap may be false economy. Each office sink should be equipped with two dispensers; one with surgical soap and the other with a good grade of hospital hand lotion. Dry, cracked skin can be a source of contamination.

Proper hand washing depends on two factors: running water and friction. Water should be tepid; water that is too hot or too cold will chap the skin. Friction means the firm rubbing of all surfaces of the hands and forearms. Remember that your fingers have four sides and fingernails. For the medical hand wash, all jewelry except a plain wedding band is removed. Your hands are washed under running water, with the fingertips pointing downward. Soap and friction are applied only to the hands and wrists. Allow the water to wash away debris from your hands.

This procedure is used when you are performing medical procedures with patients. Your goal is to prevent cross-contamination of microorganisms from one patient to another. Use this procedure after you finish with one patient and before you go to attend another patient; after you finish handling one specimen and before you handle another specimen; before and after you use toilet facilities; whenever you touch something that causes your hands to become contaminated; and before you leave the office at the end of the day.

Procedure 22-1

HAND WASHING FOR ASSISTING WITH MEDICAL ASEPTIC PROCEDURES

22

PROCEDURAL GOAL

To wash your hands with soap, using friction and running water to sanitize your skin before and after assisting with nonsurgical procedures and whenever you have contaminated your hands.

EQUIPMENT AND SUPPLIES

A sink with running water
Soap in a dispenser (bar soap is not acceptable)
Hand lotion dispenser
Paper towels in a dispenser

PROCEDURE

1. Remove all jewelry except your wrist watch and a plain gold ring.
2. Turn on the faucet and regulate the water temperature.
3. Allow your hands to become wet, apply soap, and lather with friction while holding your fingertips downward. Rub well between your fingers for 30 seconds (below left).
   Purpose: Friction removes soil and contaminants from your hands and wrists.
4. Rinse well, holding your hands so that the water flows from your wrists downward to your fingertips (below right).
   Purpose: Soil and contaminants will wash off you and down the drain.

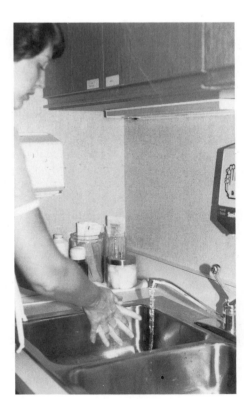 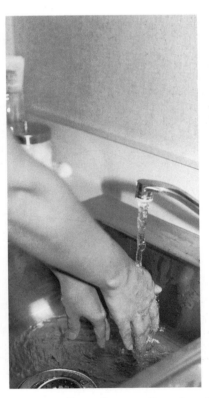

Procedure continued on following page

11000 — 21000

5. Wet your hands again and repeat the scrubbing with soap for 15 seconds (below left).
6. Rinse your hands a second time and take time to inspect them (below right).
   Purpose: To ensure that the hands are really clean.

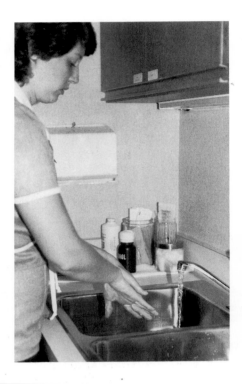 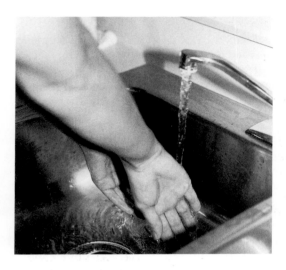

7. Dry your hands with a paper towel.
8. Turn off the water faucet with the paper towel.
   Purpose: The faucet is dirty and will contaminate your clean hands.
9. Apply hand lotion (below).

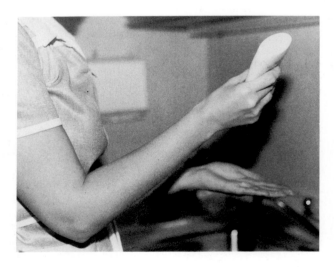

Procedure continued on opposite page

10. Cover any hangnails or open wounds with Band-Aids. *put on Gloves*
You should not perform any procedures coming in contact with a patient's blood or body fluids when you have open cuts on your hands.

TERMINAL PERFORMANCE OBJECTIVE

Given the appropriate equipment and supplies, perform a medical hand wash according to medical aseptic principles, within two minutes, without missing a step or incorrectly performing a step, as determined by your evaluator.

22

Surgical Asepsis

Surgical asepsis is defined as the destruction of organisms *before they enter the body*. This technique is used for any procedure that invades the body's skin or tissues, such as surgery or injections. Any time the skin or mucous membrane is punctured, pierced, or incised (or will be during a procedure), surgical aseptic techniques are practiced. The surgical hand wash (scrub) must be used. Everything that comes into contact with the patient should be sterile, such as gowns, drapes, instruments, and the gloved hands of the surgical team. Minor surgery, urinary catheterizations, injections, and some specimen collections, such as blood and biopsies, are performed using surgical aseptic technique.

Because it is not possible to sterilize your hands, the goal of the hand scrub is to reduce skin bacteria by the use of mechanical friction, special surgical soaps, and running water. Normally, there are two types of bacteria on your skin:

1. *Transient bacteria*. These are surface bacteria that are introduced by fomites and remain with you a short time. *on the skin for a short period.*

2. *Resident bacteria*. These are found under fingernails, in hair follicles, in the openings of the sebaceous glands, and in the deeper layers of the skin.

Resident bacteria in the deeper skin layers come to the surface with perspiration, which is why sterile gloves are used in addition to the surgical hand scrub. Some agencies recommend that you scrub for a specific number of minutes; others count the number of scrub strokes. Follow the guidelines of your employer and take periodic cultures from your scrubbed hands to determine whether or not your technique is effective (Table 22–9).

Table 22–9
How to Distinguish Between Medical and Surgical Asepsis

	Medical Asepsis	Surgical Asepsis
Definition	Destruction of organisms *after* they leave the body	Destruction of organisms *before* they enter the body
Purpose	Prevent reinfection of the patient. Avoid cross-infection from one person to another	Care for open wounds. Use in surgery
Technique	Universal blood and body-fluid precautions (Appendix C) Isolation techniques	Sterile technique
Procedure	Clean objects are kept from contamination Clean gloves and clean barriers used Objects disinfected as soon as possible after contact with the patient	Objects must be sterile Sterile gloves and articles used Objects must be sterilized before contact with the patient
When used	For examinations that do not involve open wounds or breaks in the skin or mucous membranes but do involve patient blood or body fluids. Isolating infected persons from others	Surgery, biopsy, wound treatment, insertion of instruments into sterile body cavities
Hand wash technique	Hands and wrists washed for 1–2 minutes; soap, water, and plenty of friction used to remove oil and microorganisms from fingers Hands held downward, running water allowed to drain off fingertips, hands dried with paper towels	Hands and forearms scrubbed for 3–10 minutes; surgical soap, running water, friction, and sterile brush used; fingernails must be cleaned Hands held up, under running water, to drain off elbows. Hands dried with sterile towels

Procedure 22–2

HAND WASHING FOR ASSISTING WITH SURGICAL ASEPTIC PROCEDURES

PROCEDURAL GOAL

To wash your hands with surgical soap, using friction, running water, and a sterile (optional) brush to sanitize your skin before assisting with any procedure that requires surgical asepsis.

EQUIPMENT AND SUPPLIES

A sink with a foot or arm control for running water
A nail file
Surgical soap in a dispenser
A sterile or nonsterile brush
Towels

PROCEDURE

1. Remove all jewelry.
   Purpose: Jewelry harbors bacteria and is not permitted in surgical asepsis.
2. Inspect your fingernails for length and your hands for skin breaks.
3. Turn on the faucet and regulate the water to a comfortable temperature.
4. Keep your hands upright and held at or above waist level (below left).
   Purpose: Water running from the nonscrubbed area above the elbow down to the hands will drag bacteria back onto the hands. All areas below the waist are considered contaminated during all surgical procedures.
5. Allow water to run over your hands, apply acceptable solution, lather while holding your fingertips upward, and remember to rub between the fingers (below right).   *30 seconds*
   Purpose: The surfaces of the fingers have four sides.

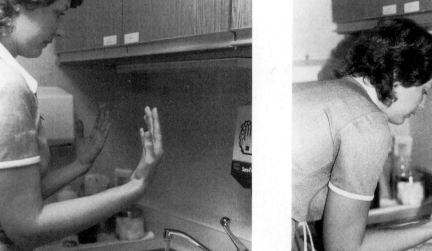
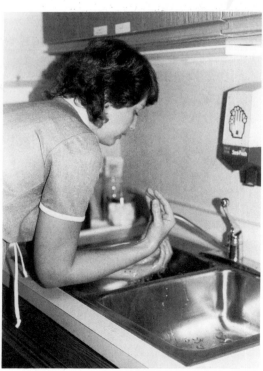

Procedure continued on opposite page

6. Clean your fingernails with a file, discard it, and rinse your hands under the faucet without touching the faucet or the insides of the sink basin (below left).
   Purpose: The sink basin and fixtures are always considered contaminated.
7. Apply more solution and repeat the scrub, remembering to wash and use friction between each finger with a firm, circular motion.
8. Wash forearms and wrists while holding your hands above waist level (below right).

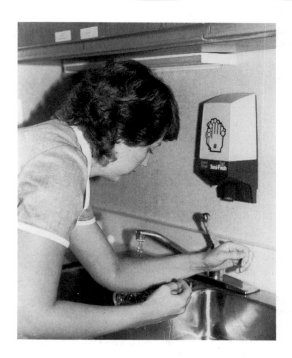 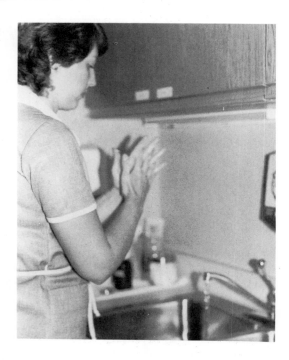

9. Scrub all surfaces with a brush, being careful not to abrade your skin. The second washing process should take at least three minutes.
10. Rinse thoroughly, keeping your hands up and above waist level (below).

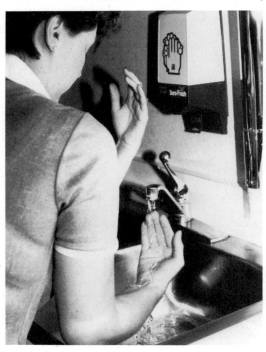

Procedure continued on following page

11. Dry your hands with a sterile towel or paper towel (below).
    Purpose: To keep your clean hands from touching the part of the towel that comes into contact with your forearms, which are not as clean as your hands. If you are to gown and glove for a procedure, you will be required to use a sterile rather than a paper towel.

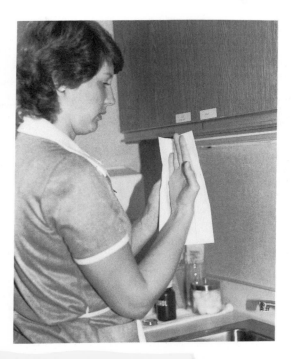

12. Using a patting motion, continue to dry the forearms (below left).
13. Turn off the faucet with the foot or forearm lever, if available, or with the towel if it is a hand faucet (below right).
    Purpose: To separate the clean hand(s) from the contaminated faucet handle(s).

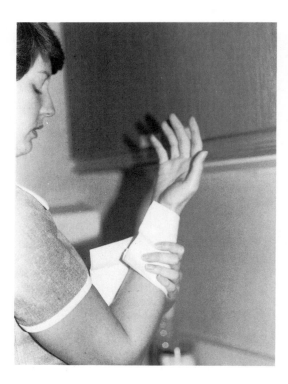
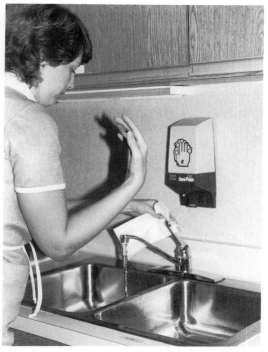

Procedure continued on opposite page

TERMINAL PERFORMANCE OBJECTIVE

Given the necessary equipment and supplies, perform a three-minute hand scrub without missing a step or incorrectly performing a step, as determined by your evaluator.

22

REFERENCES AND READINGS

Auerbach, P., and Geehr, E.: *Management of Wilderness and Environmental Emergencies.* New York, Macmillan Publishing Co., 1983.

Bonewit, K.: *Clinical Procedures for Medical Assistants,* 2nd ed. Philadelphia, W. B. Saunders Co., 1984.

Feingold, S., and Baron, E.: *Bailey and Scott's Diagnostic Microbiology.* St. Louis, C. V. Mosby Co., 1986.

Fuller, J. R.: *Surgical Technology Principles and Practice,* 2nd ed. Philadelphia, W. B. Saunders Co., 1986.

Koneman, E. W., et al.: *Clinical Microbiology Educational Series.* Bethesda, MD, Health and Education Resources, 1977.

Koneman, E. W., and Allen, S. D.: *Color Atlas and Textbook of Diagnostic Microbiology,* 2nd ed. Philadelphia, J. B. Lippincott Co., 1983.

Nester, E., and Roberts, C. E.: *Microbiology,* 3rd ed. Philadelphia, Saunders College Publishing, 1983.

Perkins, J. J.: *Principles and Methods of Sterilization in Health Sciences,* 2nd ed. Springfield, IL, Charles C Thomas Publisher, 1983.

Peter, J., and Wolde-Miriam, W.: *AIDS: Putting the Puzzle Together.* Diagnostic Medicine, vol. 7, no. 2, Feb. 1984.

Pittiglio, D. H.: *Modern Blood Banking and Transfusion Practices.* Philadelphia, F. A. Davis Co., 1983.

CHAPTER OUTLINE

VOCABULARY

See Glossary at end of book for definitions.

anhydrous	desiccation
causative	permeable
coagulable	pyogenic
corporeal	viable

Sanitization, Disinfection, and Sterilization

OBJECTIVES

Upon successful completion of this chapter you should be able to

1. Define and spell the words listed in the Vocabulary for this chapter.
2. List the criteria for choosing when each of the following procedures is required: sanitization, disinfection, and sterilization.
3. List the special precautions during sanitization that protect the medical assistant from cross-infection.
4. Recall four physical methods for achieving sterilization.
5. Name five types of disinfectant agents.
6. Recall the one chemical agent that is capable of achieving sterilization.
7. Compare the advantages and disadvantages of moist heat sterilization to those of dry heat sterilization.
8. State the minimum time, temperature, and pressure for autoclaving instruments, surgical gloves, and items in an emergency.
9. Describe the acceptable types of wrapping materials for steam sterilization.
10. List 11 causes of incomplete steam sterilization.
11. List some special problems associated with sterilizing selected items in the specialty offices.

Upon successful completion of this chapter you should be able to perform the following activities:

1. Wash and scrub contaminated articles in preparation for disinfection or sterilization.
2. Disinfect or sterilize instruments, using a chemical disinfectant or sterilant.
3. Wrap instruments and supplies for steam sterilization with the autoclave.
4. Sterilize instruments and supplies, using the autoclave.
5. Sanitize and sterilize rubber gloves.

Sterilization and the attempts to reach and understand sterility are as old as recorded history. Many practices and theories have been tried and then discarded, but with each, something has been added to the total knowledge.

Cremation was known centuries ago. It has also been known that **desiccation** sometimes preserves body tissue, and prevents the spread of sepsis. Moses, in about 1250 BC, gave the ancient Hebrews the first recorded sanitation laws. In a sense, Moses was our first "public health officer." The ancient Greeks used forms of fumigation to combat epidemics. Hippocrates (460–370 BC), who separated philosophy and medicine, realized the value of boiling water, washing hands, and using certain medications while dressing an infected wound. The next contribution of significance was the discovery of bacteria in 1683, chiefly by Anton van Leeuwenhoek. Then Joseph Lister (1827–1912), Louis Pasteur (1822–1895), and others started the world on the miraculous path of sterilization. Pasteur said on April 30, 1878, in a lecture to the Académie de Médecin:

If I had the honor of being a surgeon, convinced as I am of the dangers caused by germs of microbes scattered on the surface of every object, particularly in hospitals, not only would I absolutely clean instruments, but, after cleansing my hands with great care and putting them quickly through a flame (an easy thing to do with a little practice), I would only make use of charpie, bandages, and sponges which had previously been raised to a heat of 130°C to 150°C; I would only employ water which had been heated to a temperature of 110°C to 120°C. All that is easy in practice, and, in that way, I would still have to fear the germ suspended in the atmosphere surrounding the bed of the patient; but observation shows us every day that the number of those germs is almost insignificant compared to that of those which lie scattered on the surface of objects, or in the clearest ordinary water.

Joseph Lister was the first surgeon to use chemicals. One of his principles, which was the basis for antisepsis, was that "all instruments, dressings and everything else in contact with operations, including the hands of the surgeon and the assistant, should be rendered antiseptic." Lord Lister has been given full honor for introducing the sterile instruments, dressing, and glassware used in the operating room. He gave this advice to his fellow surgeons:

In order, gentlemen, that you may get satisfactory results from this sort of treatment, you must be able to see with your mental eye the septic ferments as distinctly as we see flies or other insects with the **corporeal** eye. If you can really see them in this distinct way with your intellectual eye, you can be properly on your guard against them; if you do not see them you will be constantly liable to relax your precautions.

BASIC CONCEPTS

Antisepsis. The process of applying substances that render microorganisms harmless either by killing them or preventing their growth, according to the agent or method of application. Antiseptics are agents made to prevent sepsis by inhibition or destruction of the **causative** organism, especially for application to living tissue. If the substance only prevents the growth of bacteria, it may be referred to as a *bacteriostatic agent*. The term *antiseptic* is sometimes used to include disinfectants, although disinfectants are usually too strong to be applied to living tissue. Antiseptics are used in the treatment of wounds and infections and are applied to the skin before surgery. Antibiotics are not classified as antiseptics because they are taken internally. by mouth

Concurrent Disinfection. Immediate disinfection and disposal of body discharges and infective matter by which a disease may be passed during the course of its progression. This process is being carried on constantly in medical offices and hospitals.

Contamination. The state of an article or surface that may have become soiled through contact with nonsterile material, especially with the introduction of disease-producing or infectious organisms. If an object is not sterile, it is considered to be contaminated.

Disinfection. The destruction of pathogenic organisms by chemical or physical means, but commonly reserved for use only with chemical agents. A disinfectant is an agent that destroys infectious organisms. As ordinarily employed, the disinfection process may or may not be adequate for the destruction of all pathogens, such as the tubercle bacilli, spores, or certain viruses. Disinfectants should be used only on inanimate objects and should not be confused with antiseptics that are applied to living tissue.

Fumigation. The process by which the microorganisms of insects and vectors are destroyed, usually by the use of gaseous agents. It is also defined as exposure to disinfecting fumes.

Fungicidal. An action that destroys fungi.

Germicidal. An action that destroys pathogenic organisms. Common usage involves the application of chemical agents to kill disease-producing organisms but not necessarily bacterial spores. Germicides are applied to living tissues as well as to inanimate objects. Another commonly used term, with a similar definition, is *bactericidal*.

Sanitization. Reducing the number of microorganisms to a level that is relatively safe by washing and scrubbing with detergents and water.

Sterilization. The complete destruction of all forms of microbial life. Objects that are free of all living organisms may be called *sterile*. Technically, there is no such thing as partially or nearly sterile; an object is either sterile or it is contaminated.

Vermicidal. An action that destroys parasitic worms or intestinal animal parasites.

SANITIZATION

Detergents and Water

Instruments and other items used in office surgery, examination, or treatment must be carefully cleaned *before* proceeding with the steps of disinfection or sterilization. Sanitization is the careful scrubbing of materials, using brushes and specially formulated, blood-dissolving laboratory detergents that have a neutral pH and are low-etching and low-sudsing. Detergents that are very alkaline are corrosive to aluminum and will also erode ground-glass surfaces. Strong alkaline detergents are also harmful to rubber. Most detergents are slightly alkaline and may be used for general purposes, but it is best to use the specially formulated laboratory detergents for cleaning glassware and rubber goods.

Detergents are mainly wetting agents that increase penetration and wetting power; they are sometimes called "soapless" soaps. Because of their ability to emulsify fats and oils, they aid in the mechanical removal of bacteria and tissue debris. Blood and debris must be removed so that later disinfection with chemicals or sterilization with steam, heat, or gases can penetrate to all the instrument's surfaces.

After washing, all items must be thoroughly rinsed in hot, running water, then in distilled water. Hot water is better for rinsing away detergent film; distilled water helps prevent mineral deposits from accumulating on instruments. Next, the items are placed on toweling or racks to dry, or they are hand-dried with a towel. Sanitization is a very important step, and it cannot be overlooked or done carelessly.

During a surgical procedure, a special receptacle is used to receive contaminated instruments. This is usually a basin of disinfectant solution placed within your reach. If a metal basin is used, you may want to line the bottom with gauze squares to prevent damage as you drop the instruments into the solution. After each procedure, immediately remove the basin to the cleaning and sterilization room.

Never allow blood or other **coagulable** substances to dry on an instrument. If immediate sanitization is not possible, leave the instruments soaking in the disinfecting solution, or rinse them with cold tap water and place them to soak in a solution of detergent and cold water. You must know the manufacturers' recommendations for sanitizing the various types of instruments. For instance, stainless steel instruments should be sanitized immediately after use, or they may acquire a tarnish that is difficult to remove. Also, chrome-plated instruments may rust where there are minute breaks in the plating, if left to soak too long. If rust and stains develop, they may become a source of bacterial deposits and contamination, and the instruments must be discarded.

When you are ready to sanitize instruments, drain off the solution and rinse each instrument in cold, running water. Separate the sharp instruments from the others; other metal instruments may damage the cutting edges, or the sharp instruments may injure the other instruments or you. Clean all the sharp instruments at one time, when you can concentrate on avoiding the dangers of injury to yourself. Open all hinges, and scrub serrations and ratchets with a small scrub brush or toothbrush. Rinse the items, then check the instruments carefully for proper working order.

Rubber and plastic items may discolor some metals, so sanitize these items last. Some rubber and plastic items should not be soaked because they may discolor, become porous, or lose their glossy surfaces. These items must be sanitized immediately without soaking or cleaned by wiping dry with alcohol.

Because it is not possible to know whether or not every patient is free of hepatitis B or HIV (AIDS virus), extreme care must be taken when handling any item that has penetrated a patient's tissues. Whenever possible, you should minimize the need for sanitization and sterilization by using *disposable* instruments, needles, and syringes when working with human blood or giving injections. A few instruments are now available in the disposable form, but most are too expensive to throw away and must be sterilized for reuse. Reusable syringes and needles have become obsolete, and medical practice is discouraged from using them unless there is no other alternative. However, some medications still must be given with glass syringes. Therefore, the procedure for sanitizing instruments includes caring for glass syringes.

Procedure 23–1 SANITIZING INSTRUMENTS AND REUSABLE SYRINGES

PROCEDURAL GOAL

To wash, scrub, and rinse contaminated articles in preparation for disinfection or sterilization.

Procedure continued on following page

EQUIPMENT AND SUPPLIES

Blood and body-fluid protection barriers (goggles, masks, and aprons or gowns), as necessary (see Appendix C, Recommendations for Prevention of AIDS Transmission)
A large basin for soaking
A laboratory detergent (low-sudsing and blood-solvent type)
Cleaning brushes
Small laboratory bottle brush or toothbrush
Nonsterile gloves
Running water and distilled water
Towel for drying
Drying rack (optional)

PROCEDURE

1. Immediately following a procedure and while still gloved, disassemble any multiunit items, rinse all items in cold water, then place them in a cool solution using a low-sudsing laboratory detergent (below and above right).
Purpose: Rinsing in cold water immediately removes some surface contaminants and prevents blood from coagulating. Soaking in a cool detergent solution further prevents the blood and other materials from coagulating.

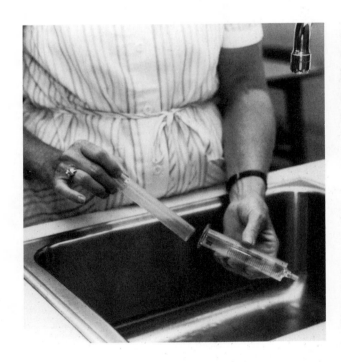

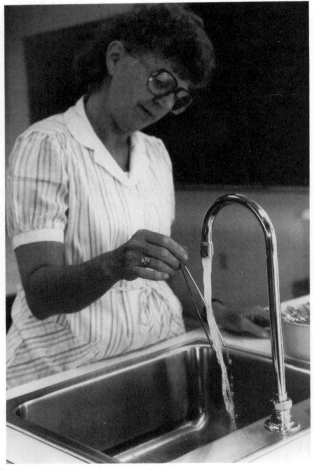

Procedure continued on opposite page

23

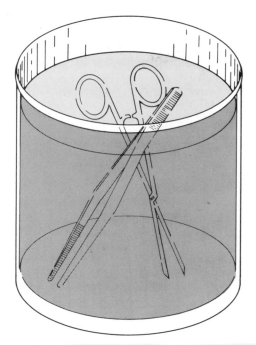

2. As soon as possible, you should return to the soaking items to sanitize them.
3. Put on gloves to further protect yourself from cross-infection.
   Purpose: Gloves provide a surgical aseptic barrier against contaminated materials.
4. Drain off the solution and rinse the items under cold, running water.
   Purpose: To wash away as much of the contaminated material and disinfectant as possible before you touch any items.
5. Work carefully to avoid cutting yourself on any sharp edges or points.
   Purpose: Hepatitis B and AIDS viruses are present in human blood and are transmitted through breaks in the skin.
6. Separate sharp-edged materials from the rest of the items.
   Purpose: To protect one instrument from the other. It also is safer for you to concentrate on all sharp instruments at the same time.
7. In an instrument basin, make a new solution with the detergent.
   Purpose: Instruments should not be cleaned in the general sink area.
8. Open hinged instruments, and with a brush, scrub all surfaces, one instrument at a time. Scrub both the inside and the outside of syringes. Use the small brush to reach all inside surfaces of syringes.
   Purpose: To remove coagulated substances and blood, which may harbor pathogens and block the sterilization process.
9. Aspirate (draw up) and flush solution through each syringe with a plunger (below).

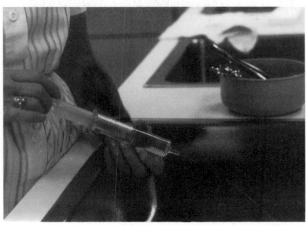

Procedure continued on following page

10. Inspect all surfaces of each item for damage, working order, or any evidence of residual contaminants.
11. Rinse or flush all items with hot water, then in distilled water.
    Purpose: Detergent film will block the sterilization process.
12. Towel or rack-dry all items (below).
    Purpose: Items must be free of water before they are wrapped or immersed in chemical solutions. Water may tear paper wrappers or soak cloth wrappers. Water on immersible items will dilute the chemicals.

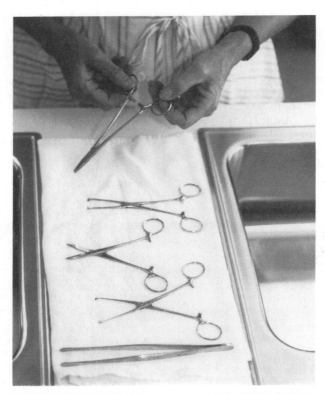

13. If any instrument needs lubricant, spray it with a silicone-based product following the manufacturer's directions. Never use an oil-based or petroleum product (below).
    Purpose: Oil-based products block disinfectants or the sterilization process from reaching the surfaces of instruments.

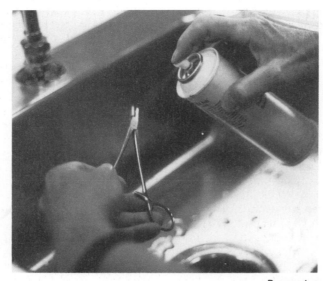

Procedure continued on opposite page

14. When the items are dry, they are ready for wrapping for steam sterilization or submersion in chemicals.

TERMINAL PERFORMANCE OBJECTIVE

Given an assortment of instruments and syringes, sanitize them within five minutes, or to other specific instruction, by correctly completing every step of the procedure in the correct order and adhering to the principles of medical asepsis, as determined by your evaluator.

23

Ultrasonics

Sound waves can be used for sanitization of instruments by placing the instruments in a bath of ultrasonic cleaner and water, then passing ultrasonic waves through it. The sound vibrates and causes bubbling, which loosens the materials attached to the instruments. Ultrasonic cleaners will not damage even the most delicate instruments.

Refrigeration

A few species of bacteria are killed by freezing temperatures. This method is not used for sterilization but rather for the preservation and sanitation of foods. It prevents the growth of bacteria. Upon thawing, however, growth and multiplication can resume, and foods may spoil more quickly.

Filtration

When fluid substances cannot be subjected to heat without causing injury to them, they may be filtered through unglazed porcelain with pores so minute that most of the bacteria are held back while the fluid passes through. This method is used for the sterilization of some drugs, bacterial toxins, antitoxins, and certain culture media. Viruses and rickettsiae that pass through these filters are known as *filterable organisms*. The water supply of some cities is purified by the filtration method.

DISINFECTION

Disinfection is the freeing of an item from infectious materials. Disinfection is not always effective against spores, the tubercle bacilli, and certain viruses. In the medical office, the term usually refers to disinfecting instruments with chemicals or boiling water. Boiling water or very strong chemicals may kill microbes within a short time but are usually very hard on the instruments. When disinfecting with chemicals, time and strength cannot be separated. Temperature is somewhat a factor, but most chemicals are used at room temperature. Some chemicals are effective enough to kill all organisms, but the usual immersion time for these sterilants is ten or more hours. When disinfecting with boiling water, time and temperature cannot be separated; strength is only a factor if chemicals are added to the boiling water. There are various methods of disinfection with varying degrees of effectiveness. It is important to know how to properly use each method, as well as its advantages, disadvantages, and the possible sources of error.

Chemical Disinfection

Chemical disinfectants and sterilants are convenient and often the agent of choice for materials that are damaged by heat. A good chemical disinfectant should be effective in a moderately low concentration and within a reasonable length of time. It should retain its potency in the presence of some dead organic matter, and it should not be too volatile (that is, rapidly evaporate).

Disinfectants are applied to inanimate objects, since they are too strong to be used on human tissues. Items that will *not* enter human tissue, the circulatory system, or a sterile body cavity may be disinfected. Items that will come into contact with the skin or mucous membrane are immersed for longer periods of time in chemicals that are considered *sterilants*.

Chemicals used for disinfecting have limitations (Table 23–1). Disinfection is very difficult to verify, since there are no convenient indicators to ensure destruction of the organisms. Most commercial disinfectants kill staphylococci. Some claim to kill the tubercle bacilli, fungi, and even spores and viruses. Because you and the physician are not experts on chemical disinfectants, you should rely upon established manufacturers, who have rigid tests and standardization for their products and do not make false advertising claims. Reliable manufacturers state on the label the organisms that can be expected to be killed by the solution at a specified concentration and time. They should also state which organisms will not be killed by the use of the solution. Each chemical must be used according to its manufacturer's directions.

Even when the manufacturer's directions for chemical strength and immersion times are followed, the following four common errors can cause chemicals to lose their effectiveness:

1. Instruments are not thoroughly sanitized, and attached organic matter changes the action of the

Table 23–1
Comparison of Chemicals for Disinfection and Sterilization

Chemical	Representative Effective Concentrations	EPA Registered		Microbiocidal Activity					Virucidal		Properties					Material Compatibility			
		Disinfectant	Sterilant	Bactericidal	Pseudomonacidal	Tuberculocidal	Sporicidal	Fungicidal	Lipophilic	Hydrophilic	Approximate pH	Requires Activation	Shelf Life After Activation	Wetting and Penetration Properties	Active in Presence of Organic Matter	Carbon Steel	Plated Metals	Rubber and Plastic	Rigid and Flexible Endoscopes
Neutral glutaraldehyde (glutarex)	2%	Yes 10 Min.	Yes 10 Hrs.	Yes	Yes	Yes	Yes	Yes	Yes	Yes	7.0	Yes	28 Days	Yes	Yes	Yes	Yes	Yes	Yes
Alkaline glutaraldehyde	2%	Yes 10 Min.	Yes 10 Hrs.	Yes	Yes	Yes	Yes	Yes	Yes	Yes	8.5	Yes	14 Days	No	Yes	Yes	Yes	Yes	Yes
Acid glutaraldehyde	2%	Yes 10 Min.	Yes 1 Hr. (60°C)	Yes	Yes	Yes	Yes	Yes	Yes	Yes	3.5	No	N/A	Yes	Yes	No	No	Yes	No
Quaternary ammonium compounds	.04–.15%	Yes	No	Yes	Yes	No	No	Yes	Yes	No	7.0	No	N/A	Yes	No	Yes	Yes	Yes	Yes
Iodophors	.045%	Yes	No	Yes	Yes	Yes	No	Yes	Yes	Yes	3.0–5.0	No	N/A	Yes	No	No	No	No	No
Chlorines	N/A	Yes	No	Yes	Yes	Yes	No	Yes	Yes	Yes	11.0	No	N/A	No	No	No	No	Yes	No
Alcohols	70–90%	No	No	Yes	Yes	Yes	No	Yes	Yes	No	7.0	No	N/A	No	Yes	Yes	Yes	No	No
Aqueous formaldehyde	10%	Yes	No	Yes	Yes	Yes	No	Yes	Yes	Yes	3.5	No	N/A	No	Yes	No	Yes	Yes	No
Phenolics	.01–.03%	Yes	No	Yes	Yes	Yes	No	Yes	Yes	No	5.5	No	N/A	Yes	No	No	Yes	No	No

Courtesy of Medical Products Division 3M, St. Paul, MN

disinfectant. No chemical can kill unless it reaches the instrument's surfaces; therefore, complete sanitization is absolutely necessary.

2. Sanitized instruments are not dried, and the wet instruments placed in the solution dilute it beyond the effective concentration.

3. A solution is left in an open container, and evaporation changes its concentration.

4. Solutions are not changed after the recommended period for use has expired.

Some of the more commonly used chemicals follow.

Soap. For many years, soap was considered the "all-purpose" disinfectant, but studies have shown that soap has very limited killing power. It is the scrubbing action and the running water that have real value, as in hand washing and sanitizing. The average household soap has limited effect, but since soap is not a single chemical, there are additives that do have lethal power. Although considerable controversy surround "germicidal" or "surgical" soaps, there are some germicidal soaps that do kill organisms, mainly staphylococci, which are the greatest offenders on our skin. These germicidal soaps leave a film of disinfectant on the skin that will last for several hours. Hexachlorophene is virtually insoluble in water but soluble in alcohol. Thus, it will remain on the skin and will not be removed by a routine hand wash, but it is removed if the hands are rinsed in alcohol. Chlorohexophene is the preferred soap currently; it is more effective than the hexachlorophenes.

Alcohol. Alcohol is the most widely used disinfectant. Ethyl alcohol had been widely used in the past, but isopropyl alcohol has become more frequently used. It exhibits slightly greater germicidal action than does ethyl alcohol. It is an excellent fat solvent and, therefore, good for cleansing the skin, but continued use is hard on the hands. Iodine and other chemicals are sometimes added to alcohol to increase its lethal powers. Alcohol may be used to disinfect delicate instruments, but it tends to rust them. Care should be used in cleansing lensed instruments with alcohol because it may dissolve the cement around the lenses. It is a good cleanser, but any excess should be wiped off or allowed to evaporate before using the instruments.

Acids. Acids in concentrated form are excellent germicides but are corrosive. The more they are diluted to decrease these hazards, the less valuable they are as disinfectants. Boric acid is a very weak antiseptic, even in saturated solutions. On the other hand, nitric acid is extremely caustic.

Phenol (carbolic acid) was first used as an antiseptic in 1865 by Joseph Lister. It is toxic to tissues in strong dilutions but is often added to other agents. Phenol is used as a standard for testing disinfectants. This standardization is the lethal quality of an agent as compared with that of phenol acting for the same length of time, on the same organisms, and at the same dilutions. This procedure is useful but has limitations, because of the various requirements an antiseptic should meet. These comparisons are carefully set according to the specifications of the United States Food and Drug Administration. Hexachlorophene is a phenolic derivative. *a tissue preservative*

Formaldehyde. Formaldehyde (formalin) has strong disinfectant properties and is used as a preservative of tissue (10 percent solution). A 5 percent solution is actively germicidal and sporicidal in the presence of organic matter. It is irritating to tissue, and any instrument disinfected with it must be thoroughly rinsed with sterile or distilled water before use. It should be used at room temperature, because cooling reduces its effectiveness.

Alkalies. A popular product that is used frequently today is plain household bleach. When mixed with water to form a 10 percent solution, it is an effective and noncaustic disinfectant. *No caustic* It is used to wipe laboratory table tops where human blood and other body fluid samples are handled. It can be used for soaking reusable rubber goods before sanitizing. Bleach is used to disinfect dialysis equipment and is an effective disinfectant for surfaces that have come into contact with viruses, including the HIV (AIDS virus). *against Aids*

Ultraviolet Disinfection

Ultraviolet rays, found in sunlight and ultraviolet lamps, are used to prevent airborne bacteria from spreading in operating rooms, classrooms, bacteriologic laboratories, beauty salons, and barber shops. The destructiveness of the ray varies greatly with the distance from the source, the air it passes through, and the surface of the article it hits. This form of radiation is not considered a method of sterilization because of its limitations and lack of penetrating power.

Desiccation

Desiccation, or drying, is used to inhibit or preserve, especially bacterial cultures and foods, respectively. Often, freeze-drying is performed rapidly for preservation. Spores are highly resistant to this method. Therefore, it is extremely limited for sterilization and should be thought of as a disinfectant.

Disinfection by Boiling (Moist Heat)

Boiling (212°F, or 100°C) kills most vegetative forms of pathogenic bacteria, but bacterial spores and some viruses associated with infectious hepa-

titis are resistant to temperatures of 212°F and below. No matter how much heat is applied or how vigorous the boil, water will reach only 212°F at sea level. The higher the elevation, the lower the temperature required to obtain a boil (for example, in Denver, Colorado, water boils at 202°F). Because of these limitations, boiling does not sterilize and is used for disinfection only. Boiling may be used for nonsterile objects that do not come in contact with patients (Fig. 23–1). *it will not get hotter than 212°F*

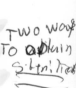

23

STERILIZATION

In the medical office, cleanliness takes the extreme form of sterilization. Sterilization reduces the perpetual threat of contamination to patients, to the physician, and to the medical assistant. To ensure proper sterilization as the end product of aseptic procedures, an area should be set aside in each office for just this purpose. The area should be divided into two sections. One section is used for receiving contaminated materials. This area should have a sink, as well as receiving basins, proper cleaning agents, brushes, sterilizer wrapping paper, envelopes and tape, sterilizer indicators, and disposable gloves. The other section should be reserved for receiving the sterile items after they are removed from the sterilizer. Clear, clean plastic bags in which to store sterile packs may be kept in the sterile area. Both areas should be spotlessly clean and well organized. Wear disposable gloves when handling contaminated items. If you have an open cut or wound on your hands, you should not clean or prepare instruments for sterilization. *purpose of holding the sterile item*

As previously mentioned, sterilization is the complete destruction of all living organisms. Sterilization can be achieved by physical methods, such as radiation, dry heat, and steam heat, or by chemical methods, such as the gas sterilizer or the chemical glutaraldehyde. *two ways to obtain sterilization*

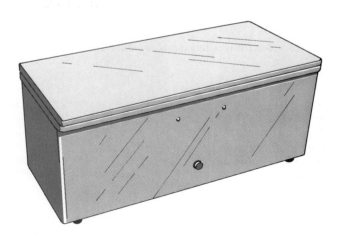

Figure 23–1
A medical office boiler. This is currently employed in some offices for articles that do not come in contact with patients. Boiler water disinfects; it does not sterilize.

Cobalt Radiation

A few medical-surgical manufacturers use cobalt radiation to achieve sterilization. Many commercially packaged sterile items are *irradiated* with cobalt. If the presterilized package states "radiation sterilized," this was the method used. Hospitals do not have their own cobalt sterilization facilities.

X-Radiation

The x-ray, or *roentgen* ray, has lethal powers. These rays penetrate deeply and rapidly. Many authorities predict that x-rays will be used for sterilization in the near future, but techniques must still be perfected.

Chemical Sterilization

True chemical sterilization is recommended for instruments that are not thermally stable at high heats or may be dulled by heat sterilization. Many chemicals are believed to be sterilants, but in reality very few are. The glutaraldehydes, such as Cidex (The 3 M Company) or Glutarex (Surgikos), will sterilize non–heat-resistant equipment, provided the items are submerged for at least ten hours. Instruments sterilized by this method must be rinsed with sterile water or sterile, distilled water before use on human tissues. For sterile use, instruments sterilized in this manner must be used immediately. Instruments that need not be sterile should be rinsed under hot running water and dried, then stored in a clean, dry area.

Procedure 23–2

STERILIZING OR DISINFECTING INSTRUMENTS WITH CHEMICALS

PROCEDURAL GOAL

To clean or sterilize instruments by placing them in the appropriate chemical disinfectant or sterilant (sterilizing agent) in a covered tray for an appropriate length of time.

EQUIPMENT AND SUPPLIES

Blood and body-fluid precaution barriers (goggles, masks, and aprons or gowns), as necessary (see Appendix C, Recommendations for Prevention of AIDS Transmission)

Assorted instruments
A chemical disinfectant or sterilant
Sterile water or sterile distilled water

A closed container (chemical sterilizer)
Nonsterile gloves

PROCEDURE

1. Put on gloves, and assemble the instruments and make sure they are clean and dry.
   Purpose: Water will dilute the chemical. Coagulants and oils will inhibit the chemical action on the microorganisms.
2. Open hinged instruments and disassemble multiunit instruments (below).
   Purpose: All surfaces must receive maximum exposure to the chemical.

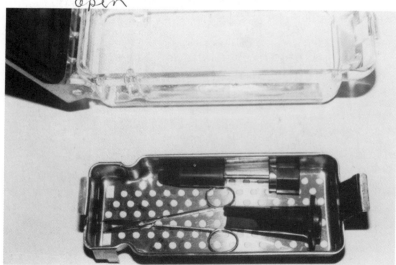

Procedure continued on opposite page

3. Read the manufacturer's directions and prepare the chemical as directed.
   Purpose: Each product varies in preparation.
4. Place the instruments in the tray and cover them completely with the chemical (below left).
   Purpose: All surfaces must receive maximum exposure to the chemical.
5. Close the lid (below right).
   Purpose: Chemicals may have harmful or annoying fumes. These chemicals are harmful to the tissues of the body, and the lid helps to isolate the chemical by preventing spills and splashes.

23

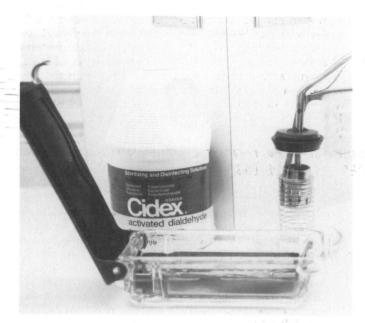

6. Label the container with the name of the chemical.
   Purpose: To notify others of its contents.
7. Identify the instruments and the time of immersion on a clipboard.
   Purpose: Some disinfectants complete their action in 20 minutes; others, such as glutaraldehydes, require 10 hours to sterilize.
8. At the end of the immersion period, transfer the items with transfer forceps to a sterile tray. Rinse the items thoroughly in sterile water or sterile distilled water, and use immediately (below).
   Purpose: The chemicals are harmful to the skin and mucous membranes of both the medical assistant and the patient.

Types of water

faucet tap water

Distilled water
when Minerals is taken out

Sterile water distilled
To Free from all
Living Microbes

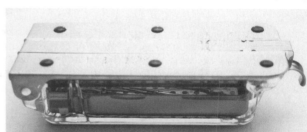

function of tape
when things has been sterilized
Seals it
can be written on.

Procedure continued on following page

9. Or rinse the items under hot running water, then dry with a towel or on a rack and store in a clean, covered area. *used for anything that doesn't go into the skin*

TERMINAL PERFORMANCE OBJECTIVE

Given appropriate supplies and equipment, disinfect or sterilize instruments using safety precautions and correct immersion times, within 30 minutes to 10 hours (as determined by the manufacturer's directions), by correctly completing every step of the procedure in the correct order, as determined by your evaluator.

Heat Sterilization

When you hang the clothes out in summer that drys

Heat is a widely used method for both disinfection and sterilization. The temperature at which an organism is killed is known as the *thermal death point*. The average organism is killed by heat of 145°F (65°C). But thermal death does not occur by temperature alone; the point of death is determined by a temperature and time formula. A certain temperature must be reached within a set period of time, and then the materials must be exposed to the heat for a particular amount of time. In some cases the formula ratios may vary: If the temperature is increased, the time may be decreased, or the reverse.

Dry Heat. *Incineration*, or burning by direct flame, destroys an organism immediately. Bacteriologic loops are flamed until the wire glows; and for years, mothers have flamed needles for the removal of splinters. Incineration is used to destroy disposable items as well as contaminated dressings, swabs, sputum cups, and other hospital supplies.

The use of *dry heat ovens* is an alternative method when direct contact with saturated steam is impractical or harmful to sharp instruments. Dry heat penetrates slowly and unevenly, so a long exposure time is required. Dry heat ovens should not be overloaded, and items should be kept away from the sides of the oven so air can freely circulate. Glassware should not touch other objects, or they may break. Wrapping items in fabric is not satisfactory, since the wrap may turn brittle. Aluminum foil is an excellent wrap for dry heat and has a long shelf life.

Most dry heat sterilizers are insulated and electrically heated with blowers to circulate air for even distribution of heat. A thermometer, located on the top of the sterilizer, is used to determine that the proper temperature is reached and sustained. Indicators should be used on every item, since there can be a variation of 40° to 60° in any oven (Fig. 23–2). It is advisable to heat the oven slowly and cool it slowly. Overheating can cause damage to sharp instruments. There are many variations of temperature and time, depending on the load, but the following are suggested:

- 340°F (170°C) for one (1) hour
- 320°F (160°C) for two (2) hours
- 250°F (121°C) for six (6) hours

The great variance found in temperature and time may also be influenced by the condition in which an item is being sterilized. For example, the destruction of some spores in **anhydrous** oil requires a temperature of 320°F for 160 minutes (2 hours 40 minutes); but with a small amount of water added (less than 0.5 percent), the same degree of sterilization can be achieved in 20 minutes at the same temperature.

Remember that organisms, both **viable** and spore forms, are more resistant to dry heat. This is the major reason that dry sterilization is not as efficient as moist heat (steam) under pressure. However,

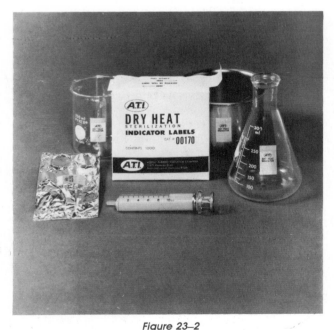

Figure 23–2
A dry heat indicator. (Courtesy of Aseptic-Thermo Indicator Co.)

Table 23–2
Sterilization Chart

Article	Method	Temperature	Time
Gauze, small, loosely packed	Autoclave	250°F	30 min
Gauze, large, loosely packed	Autoclave	270°F	30 min
Gauze, small, tightly packed	Autoclave	250°F	40 min
Gauze, large, tightly packed	Autoclave	270°F	40 min
Gauze, tightly packed	Dry heat	320°F	3 hr
Gauze, loosely packed	Dry heat	320°F	2 hr
Glass syringes in tubes	Autoclave	250°F	30 min
Glass syringe in muslin	Dry heat	320°F	1 hr
Instruments on tray, muslin under and over	Dry heat	320°F	1 hr
Instruments on tray, muslin under and over	Autoclave	250°F	15 min
Solutions in flasks with gauze plug	Autoclave	250°F	30 min
Glassware unwrapped	Dry heat	320°F	1 hr
Glassware wrapped	Autoclave	250°F	30 min
Petroleum jelly, 1-oz jar	Dry heat	340°F	1 hr
Petroleum jelly, 1-oz jar	Dry heat	320°F	2 hr
Petroleum gauze in instrument tray	Dry heat	320°F	150 min
Powder, 1-oz jar	Dry heat	320°F	2 hr
Powder, small glove packs	Autoclave	250°F	15 min

Remember to always place an indicator in areas where there is doubt that the steam will penetrate.
Do not measure by chamber pounds. A thermometer and indicator are the reliable methods of judging a killing temperature.

dry sterilization is the preferred method for sterilizing petroleum oil (for petroleum jelly and mineral oil), certain powders, and glassware (Table 23–2).

Moist Heat. Steam under pressure is the best and most accepted method of sterilization. It is the principal operation of the *autoclave* (Fig. 23–3). Steam under pressure is fast, convenient, and dependable. The pressure allows a higher heat, and when combined with moisture, these two factors create a very effective mechanism for killing all microorganisms. When steam is admitted into the autoclave chamber, it simultaneously heats and wets the object, coagulating the proteins present in all living organisms. When the cycle is complete and the chamber cooled, the steam condenses and "explodes" the cells of microorganisms, thus destroying them. To be effective, all surfaces must be contacted by the moisture. Steam under pressure is capable of much faster penetration of fabrics and textiles than is dry heat, but it has definite limitation if the proper techniques are not followed.

Incorrect operation of an autoclave may result in *superheated* steam. If steam is brought to too high a temperature, it is literally dried out, and the advantage of a higher heat is diminished. *Wet* steam is another cause of incomplete sterilization. Wet steam results from failing to preheat the chamber, which results in excessive condensation in the interior of the chamber. Condensation is necessary, but too much will prevent the sterilization process from coming to a proper completion. It can be compared to taking a hot shower in a cold bathroom, which results in heavily steamed mirrors, tile walls, and towels. If fabric packs become too saturated to dry during the drying cycle, the packs will pick up and absorb bacteria from the air or any surface they are placed on. Cold instruments placed in a hot chamber will also increase condensation. Other causes of wet steam include opening the door too wide during the drying cycle or allowing a rush of cold air into the chamber. Also, overfilling the water reservoir may produce this same effect.

The main cause of incomplete sterilization in the autoclave is the presence of residual air. Without the complete elimination of air, an adequately high temperature cannot be reached. Air and steam do not mix. Since air is heavier than steam, it will pool wherever possible. One tenth of 1 percent residual

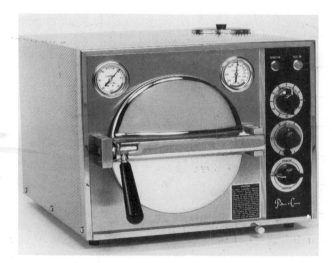

Figure 23–3
The office autoclave. A dual-purpose office sterilizer, which may be used as a steam-producing autoclave or a dry-heat sterilizer. It is a manual model and thus must be carefully monitored to ensure that minimum temperature and pressure are maintained during the timing period. (Courtesy of Pelton and Crane, Charlotte, NC.)

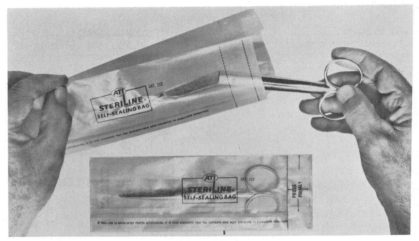

Figure 23–4
Instrument indicator bags have strips that change color when a minimum temperature is reached for a certain period of time. The translucency allows easy identification. (Courtesy of Aseptic-Thermo Indicator Co.)

air trapped around an instrument will prevent complete sterilization. This is especially dangerous in older autoclaves that do not have a chamber thermometer separate from the pressure gauge. A certain chamber pressure does not guarantee a proper chamber temperature. All release valves and discharge lines must be kept clean and free from dirt and lint.

Wrapping Materials. The maintenance of sterility is completely dependent upon the wrapper and its porosity as well as on the method of wrapping. The wrapping material must be **permeable** to steam but impervious to contaminants such as dust and insects. Muslin should be of 140-thread count, and a double thickness should be used. Canvas or duck fabric is not advisable because steam cannot penetrate it properly.

ACCEPTABLE WRAPPING MATERIALS FOR AUTOCLAVING

- *Muslin fabric that has been laundered and is double-faced*
- *A nonwoven disposable material such as Kim wrap*

- *Clear plastic with permeable paper facing envelope*
- *Permeable paper envelopes*
- *Rigid containers manufactured for autoclaving*

The nonwoven disposable material is currently the best choice for the medical office. It is permeable to steam, resists contamination, and does not become brittle during storage. It can be used one time only. Transparent envelopes or clear plastic wrappers may be used, provided one side is made of a permeable paper that allows steam penetration. They are convenient because they allow for the visibility of their contents (Fig. 23–4). Regardless of which wrapping material is used, it should be folded in such a way that it may be opened easily without contaminating the contents. Chapter 30 contains instructions on how to open sterile packages.

Rigid containers, which were originally designed for hospital instrument sets, are becoming popular. They are expensive initially, but they pay for themselves by eliminating the need for costly wrapping materials.

Procedure 23–3

WRAPPING INSTRUMENTS AND SUPPLIES FOR STEAM STERILIZATION WITH THE AUTOCLAVE

PROCEDURAL GOAL

To place dry, sanitized supplies and instruments inside appropriate wrapping materials for sterilization and storage without contamination.

Procedure continued on opposite page

EQUIPMENT AND SUPPLIES

Blood and body-fluid protection barriers (goggles, masks, and aprons or gowns), as necessary (see Appendix C, Recommendations for Prevention of AIDS Transmission)

Dry, sanitized items
Nonsterile gloves
Assorted wrapping materials
Autoclave tape
A waterproof pen

[handwritten note: Put a cotton ball between sharp hinges To keep it in place. Lay diagnally]

23

PROCEDURE

1. Put on gloves, and place the item(s) diagonally at the approximate center of the wrapping material. Make sure the size of the square is large enough for the items.
Purpose: Each of the four corners must fold over and completely cover the item(s), with a few extra inches overlap for folding back a flap (below).

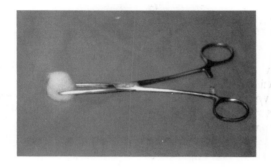

2. With the squares that are cloth fabric, use two pieces if the cloth is single-layered, or one piece if the cloth is sewn together as a double layer.
3. If the square is paper or a synthetic product, follow the manufacturer's recommendation.
4. Open slightly any hinged instruments. If the instrument is sharp, its teeth or tip should be shielded with cotton or gauze.
Purpose: To prevent puncture of the package or the operator.
5. Place a commercial sterilization indicator inside the package at the approximate center.
Purpose: To ensure that the autoclave is reaching effective levels of heat and pressure.
6. Bring up the bottom corner of the wrap, and fold back a portion of it (below).
Purpose: You will use this flap as the "handle" to open the pack. This folded-back flap is the only part of each wrapper corner that can be touched when opening a sterile package.

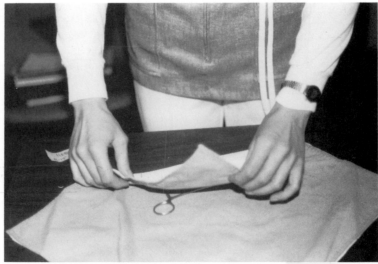

Procedure continued on following page

7. Fold over the right corner, and turn back a portion of it (below, top left).
8. Fold over the left corner, and turn back a portion of it (below, top right).
9. Fold the covered area in half (below, bottom left).
10. Bring down the top corner, and continue folding it around the pack as far as it will go.
11. Secure with autoclave tape (below, bottom right).
12. Label the package with the date, contents, and your initials, or as instructed.

    Purpose: To know what is in the pack at a later date, whether or not the shelf life has expired (expiration date), and who performed the task. As a general rule, most office autoclaved packs are considered sterile (usable) for 30 days.

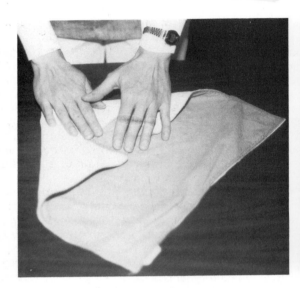
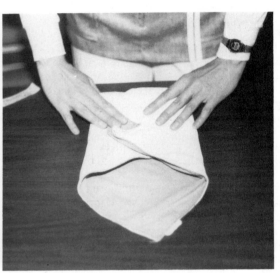
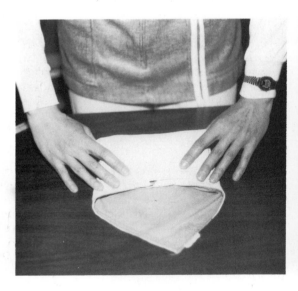
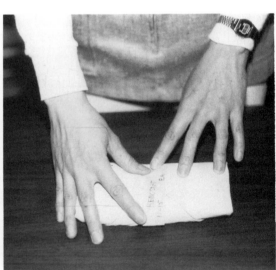

TERMINAL PERFORMANCE OBJECTIVE

Given the appropriate items and supplies, wrap and label the items for steam sterilization within three minutes, completing each step of the procedure correctly and in the correct order, as determined by your evaluator.

Gives you the indicating when things are sterilizeds

Indicators. In 1881, Robert Koch tried using anthrax spores to see if the items had been sterilized, but this method was difficult to use and gave unreliable results. Also in the 19th century, a British physician used raw eggs in a load. If the eggs were hard at the end of exposure, he considered the load to be sterile. Even with these extremely poor and unreliable methods, it was realized that there was a need to determine sterility. To eliminate the constant doubt of complete sterilization, *indicators* should be used. These indicators show, by melting or by changing color, that a certain temperature for a given period of time has been reached, irrespective of pressure. An indicator should be placed with each load, buried deep in packs, placed in constriction tubes, put in the bottoms of containers that cannot be turned on their sides, or located in any other places that might be inaccessible to the flow of steam. Many feel that an indicator is not necessary if the chamber has a thermometer, but this tells you the temperature only where the tip of the thermometer is located and not in the aforementioned places. An indicator should also be placed in the lower front near the air exhaust valve.

Read the accompanying instructions for the indicator you use. The dangers of incomplete sterilization are too great for you to be lax in your technique or in the care of the equipment.

A popular indicator that is easy to use is the OK Strip (Fig. 23–5). When the OK Strip has been exposed to 250°F for at least 15 minutes, the "OK"

will change from tan to deep black. You must remember that this test is not a true indication of sterility. It merely means that the minimum temperature has been maintained. There is no assurance of sterility of the load.

An example of an excellent system for testing the effectiveness of your office autoclave is the Attest system, manufactured by the 3M Company (Fig. 23–6A). It is a bioindicator that consists of a double-walled tube, which when broken, releases a microorganism into a culture medium. If the sterilization cycle is defective and the microorganism still lives, growth should occur within 24 hours. It can be cultured in an office water bath or a dry block incubator. Another method for determining the efficiency of sterilization processes is the indicator that contains dried bacterial spores of established, heat-resistant organisms (Fig. 23–6B). These bacterial spore strips are available commercially from reliable suppliers, but the indicators are not always practical for a physician's office because the strip, after autoclaving, must be sent to a bacteriology laboratory for sterility testing.

Autoclave or sterilizer tapes frequently have some form of indicator on them that changes after exposure to sterilization procedures. These tapes are excellent for securing packages and bags, but they are not to be used as sterilizer indicators. They never were intended for this purpose; they only indicate that the package has been processed, not that sterility has been reached.

Sterilization indicator bags are also very convenient. They are made of disposable paper or thermostable plastic, in which syringes, tubing, and many other items can be sterilized and stored. The paper or transparent material is permeable to steam and provides a barrier against airborne bacteria during storage. Each bag has an indicator printed on it, similar to the sterilizer tape, which shows that the bag has been autoclaved but does not prove that it is sterile.

The Autoclave. The office autoclave is similar to the home pressure cooker. It operates on the principle of steam under pressure. Water in an outer chamber, or jacket, is heated to produce steam. The pressure in this outer jacket builds and forces steam into the inner chamber. As steam is forced in, air is forced out (Fig. 23–7). Visualize the air flowing out of the chamber as water flowing down a sink drain. Read the manufacturer's instructions carefully. An autoclave usually has three gauges: (1) the jacket pressure gauge, which indicates the steam pressure in the outer chamber; (2) the chamber pressure gauge, which indicates the steam pressure in the inner chamber; and (3) the temperature gauge, which indicates the temperature in the inner chamber, where the items are sterilized. When the temperature gauge reaches 250°F (121°C) and the

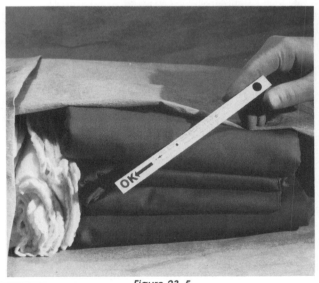

Figure 23–5
The "OK strip" is often used to indicate whether minimum temperatures have been maintained in the autoclave. It should be placed in the center of a pack. If minimum temperature has been maintained for a minimum time, the "OK" will turn from light tan to dark black. (Courtesy of Propper, Inc.)

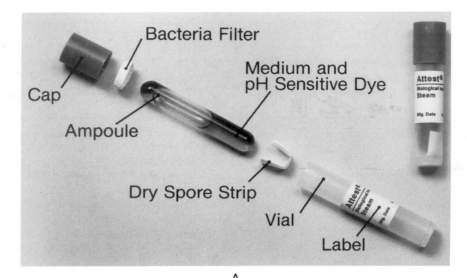

A

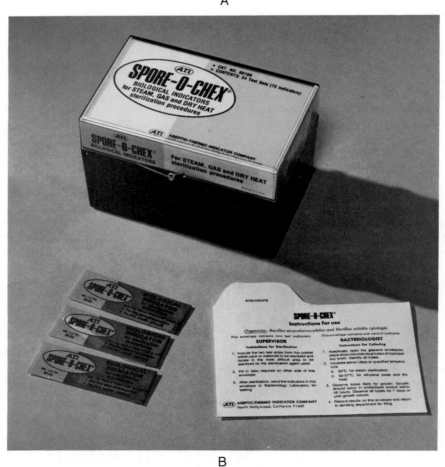

B

Figure 23–6

*Biologic indicators that confirm sterility. **A,** The Attest system assures sterilization. The tube is cultured after the autoclaving cycle; if no organisms grow, sterility is assumed. (Courtesy of Medical Products Division: 3M, St. Paul, MN.) **B,** Spore-O-Chex, which contains bacilli spores. (Courtesy of Aseptic-Thermo Indicator Co.)*

23

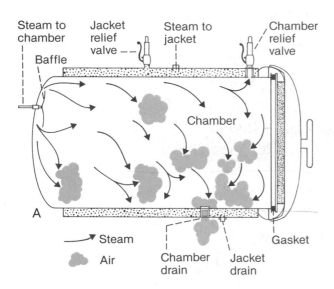

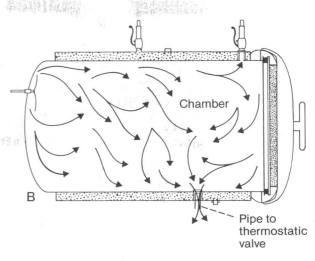

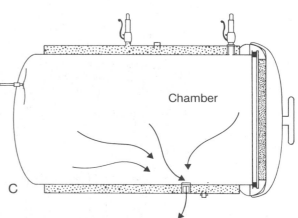

Figure 23–7
*How the sterilizer displaces air with steam. **A,** As the cycle begins, heated water turns into steam, which is forced into the chamber, pushing air out. **B,** The chamber fills with pure steam. **C,** When the cycle is completed, the steam is exhausted from the chamber, is condensed back to water, and is returned to the jacket. (Concept courtesy of Jean Hodge, RN, Supervisor, Central Supply, Methodist Hospital, Madison, WI.)*

pressure gauge indicates 15 pounds of steam pressure, the load of articles to be sterilized can be timed for 20 to 30 minutes.

The autoclave chamber must be cleaned before each loading. If there has been boiling over of solutions, the water reservoir must be drained and thoroughly cleaned and rinsed. On many models, there is no access to the reservoir, and it must be cleaned by a local manufacturer representative. Check the manufacturer's instructions carefully and do not use a commercial cleaner unless advised by the manufacturer. A mild detergent may be used in the chamber, but make certain it is very thoroughly rinsed after any type of cleaner has been used. Many manufacturers will not honor a guarantee if anything other than distilled water is used or if any type of cleaner has been put through the reservoir tank.

The trays must also be kept clean and free of lint. Be sure to re-place the bottom (chamber) tray after cleaning; it must be in place for proper steam circulation. The air exhaust valve is one of the most important parts of the autoclave and must be clean and free of lint, otherwise the air will not exhaust from the chamber. Unless proper care is taken of the autoclave, the dressings and instruments will have been *well heated but not sterilized.*

Loading the Autoclave. When loading the autoclave, prepare all packs and arrange the load in such a manner to allow maximum circulation of steam and heat. Articles should be placed so that they rest on their edges, to permit proper permeation of the materials with moisture and heat (Fig. 23–8*A*). Tiers should be alternately placed. Under no conditions, permit crowding of packs into tight masses. Jars and containers should be placed on their sides. When a container is upright, even without a lid, the air is trapped within the container and there is no circulation of steam (Fig. 23–8*B*). Instruments may be autoclaved unwrapped if they are to be used immediately or do not need to be sterile when used later. Perforated trays are used for sterilizing unwrapped instruments. Place a layer of muslin under and over the instruments to facili-

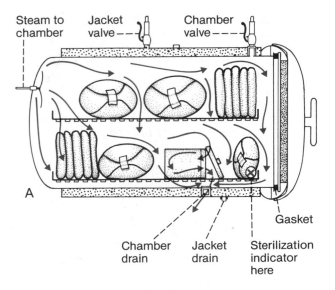

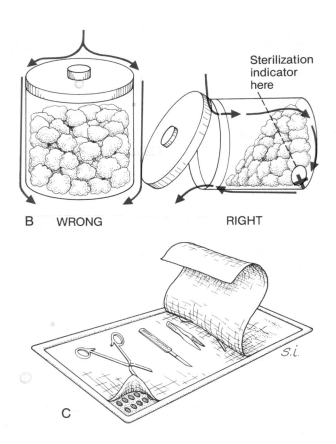

Figure 23–8
*Loading the autoclave. **A,** Place the indicator near the exhaust valve (X). Load without crowding the packs, with space between the top and bottom shelves. Note that the container is placed on its side. **B,** The correct way to load a container: Steam will flow through the correctly positioned container but cannot even enter the "incorrect" one. Place the indicator as shown with the "X." **C,** An example of how to sterilize instruments on an open tray in the autoclave.*

tate drying and to prevent contamination when removing them from the autoclave (Fig. 23–8C).

Unloading the Autoclave. When the sterilization cycle is complete, release the pressure with the control setting. Standing away from the door and with oven mits, slightly open the door about a quarter of an inch. Allow the load to dry for at least five minutes (this will vary according to the type of autoclave and the size of the load). *Capillary attraction* is the term describing the force that draws moisture through surfaces of materials. Materials act like a sponge. Any moisture outside the pack contains microorganisms, which, in turn, are drawn into the pack with the moisture. Touching a wet load will allow the microorganisms on your hands to penetrate the wrappings and to render the contents nonsterile. Dry, wrapped packs may be removed with clean, dry hands, but it is safer to wear oven mits to reduce the possibility of burns from the hot instruments inside the packs. Place the packs on a dry, dust-free surface for storage. Avoid cold surfaces, because the hot packs may cause condensation, and moisture will contaminate the contents.

Storage of Wrapped Supplies. Although experts do not agree upon the length of time that wrapped

supplies remain sterile, the following shelf-life rules are fairly standard.

- Double-wrapped muslin and double-wrapped paper packs are considered sterile up to 28 days from the date of sterilization.
- Nonpermeable plastic-wrapped packs are considered sterile up to six months from the date of sterilization. (Most medical offices do not have the equipment to sterilize supplies in nonpermeable packages. Purchased nonpermeable packs will have expiration dates printed on the outside.)

All supplies should be stored on dry, dust-free, covered shelves or in drawers. Fabric wrappers must be relaundered. A damaged pack or a broken seal renders the package nonsterile. Spills of any fluid onto a package render the pack nonsterile. When a pack is no longer sterile because of a broken seal or an expiration date that has passed, the contents must be reprocessed starting with the sanitization process.

Sterilization in an Emergency. The only method available for sterilizing instruments quickly is to autoclave them at 270°F with a minimum of 27 pounds of pressure for six minutes. Chemical methods do not sterilize. They disinfect and should be used only in a life-threatening, emergency situation when nothing else is available. Prevent such situations by having your instruments sterile and ready for use.

MECHANICAL AND PHYSICAL CAUSES OF INCOMPLETE STERILIZATION

1. Inadequate sanitization. Steam cannot penetrate to the instrument surfaces in the presence of foreign substances such as soap film, blood, feces, or tissue debris.
2. Improper wrapping.
3. Using nonpermeable wrapping materials.
4. Failure to preheat the chamber if the autoclave is cold.
5. Incorrectly loading the autoclave chamber by
   a. Overloading the chamber.
   b. Not placing jars on their edges.
   c. Blocking steam with small trays that do not have holes for circulation.
   d. Not placing thick packs vertically.
   e. Not using the autoclave bottom shelf.
6. Starting the timer before correct temperature is reached.
7. Too short an exposure time.
8. Reading the gauges incorrectly or confusing one gauge for another.
9. Too low a chamber pressure.
10. Temperature too high (superheated steam) or not high enough (wet steam).
11. Excessive condensation.
12. Not allowing items to dry completely before removal from the chamber.
13. Placing hot sterilized packages on a cold surface, causing condensation after sterilization and contamination of the packages.
14. An unreliable autoclave.
15. A dirty autoclave chamber or clogged exhaust lines.
16. Resterilizing items in used wrappers.

Table 23–3
Tips for Improving Your Autoclaving Techniques

LINENS	
Too Damp	
Clogged chamber drain	Remove strainer; free openings of lint.
Goods removed from chamber too soon following cycle	Allow goods to remain in sterilizer an additional 15 minutes with door slightly open.
Improper loading	Place packs on edge; arrange for least possible resistance to flow of steam and air.
Stained	
Dirty chamber	Clean chamber with Calgonite solution. Never use strong abrasives, steel wool, and so forth.
	Rinse thoroughly after cleaning.
INSTRUMENTS	
Corroded	
Poor cleaning; residual soil	Improve cleaning. Do not allow soil to dry on instruments. Sanitize first.
Exposure to hard chemicals (e.g., iodine, salt, and acids)	Do not expose instruments to these chemicals. If exposure occurs, rinse immediately.
Inferior instruments	Use only top-quality instruments.
Spotted or Stained	
Mineral deposits on instruments	Wash with soft soap and detergent with good wetting properties.
Residual detergents from cleaning	Rinse instruments thoroughly.
Mineral deposits from tap water	Rinse with distilled water.
Stiff Hinges or Joints	
Corrosion or soil in joint	Clean with warm, weak acid solution (10% nitric acid solution). Rinse thoroughly after.
Jaws and shanks out of alignment	Realignment by qualified instrument repairman
SOLUTIONS	
Ebullition, or Caps Blow Off	
Exhausting chamber too rapidly	Use slow exhaust, cool liquids, or turn autoclave off and let cool at its own speed. That is, let the pressure decrease at its own rate.
MECHANICAL	
Steam Leakage	
Worn gasket	Replace
Door closes improperly	Reopen door and shut carefully. Have serviced if unable to close door properly.
Chamber Door Will Not Open	
Vacuum in chamber (check chamber pressure gauge)	Turn on controls to starting steam pressure, and wait until equalized, then vent and open door.

Procedure 23–4

STERILIZING WITH THE STEAM AUTOCLAVE

PROCEDURAL GOAL

To sterilize supplies and instruments, using the autoclave.

EQUIPMENT AND SUPPLIES

An autoclave
Wrapped items, such as:
  a hemostat
  a thumb dressing forceps
  a glass syringe
  cotton balls
  applicators
  gauze sponges
A jar containing gauze
A basin that can be autoclaved

PROCEDURE

1. Check the water level in the reservoir and add distilled water as necessary.
   Purpose: Too much or too little water may alter the effectiveness of the equipment. Tap water will leave lime deposits in the chamber.
2. Adjust the control to "fill" to allow water to flow into the chamber. The water will flow until you turn the control to its next position. Do not let the water overflow.
3. Load the chamber with wrapped items, then space them for maximum circulation and penetration.
4. Close and seal the door. The door must be closed or the heated water in the chamber will evaporate.
5. Turn the control setting to "on" or "autoclave" to start the cycle.
6. Watch the gauges until the temperature gauge reaches at least 250°F (121°C) and the pressure gauge reaches 15 pounds of pressure.
7. Set the timer for the desired time, usually between 20 and 30 minutes.
8. At the end of the timed cycle, turn the control setting to "vent."
   Purpose: This releases the steam and pressure. The water at the bottom of the chamber will drain back into the reservoir.
9. Wait for the pressure gauge to reach zero.
10. Open the chamber door a quarter of an inch.
    Purpose: To allow steam to escape faster.
11. Leave the autoclave control at "vent" to continue producing heat.
    Purpose: To dry the items faster.
12. Allow complete drying of all articles.
13. Using heat-resistant gloves or pads, remove the items from the chamber.
14. Place the sterilized packages on dry, covered shelves.
15. Turn the control knob to "off," and keep the door slightly ajar.

TERMINAL PERFORMANCE OBJECTIVE

Given appropriate supplies and equipment, load, operate, and unload the autoclave, within 60 minutes, completing each step of the procedure correctly and in the correct order, as determined by your evaluator.

Gas Sterilization

Gas as a sterilizing agent has been used since ancient times. Gases were used for killing insects by the ancient Greeks and Romans: Homer referred to the use of sulfur for fumigation in about 850 BC. In 473 BC, the Athenians attempted to use this method to stop a plague. In 1384, Chaucer used the term "fumigacioun" in English. This early use of fumigation was adequate only on exposed areas and required considerable airing before a site was tolerable again for human use.

Even some of the more modern methods required airing and presented problems of safety. Formaldehyde came into use over 70 years ago to fumigate the sickroom, but it too is a very potent and dangerous chemical. After World War II, the Army Chemical Corps started a search for a new sterilizing agent that would be bactericidal and sporicidal at moderately low temperatures, would penetrate porous substances, and would not damage metals, plastics, rubber, leather, wood, or wool. Additional goals included developing an agent that would be easily removed by aeration and that would be low in toxicity, nonflammable, and easy to store and use. *Ethylene oxide gas* fit all these qualifications, except that it was explosively flammable. Then, in 1949, it was discovered that carbon dioxide or Freon could be mixed with ethylene oxide to lessen the problem of flammability.

Many researchers now report that gas sterilization could be the exclusive method of sterilization in the future, thereby eliminating the need for other methods. There is no doubt that gas sterilization has many advantages over all other methods in use today.

There are considerable differences between the various gas sterilizers on the market, and each manufacturer has its own set of conditions necessary to achieve sterilization. The major disadvantages with the use of gas sterilization are time and the general hazards connected with using gas. The length of exposure time is usually one and a half to two hours, although exposure times sometimes can be lessened by slightly increasing the temperature. Another disadvantage is the time required for aeration after sterilization. Sterilizers must be properly vented to reduce human exposure to the gas. In August 1984, standards were issued by the United States Occupational Safety and Health Administration (OSHA). If you work with ethylene oxide gas, you should have a copy of these standards on the premises. The human hazards of gas sterilization include the possibility of damage to the reproductive organs of the operator as well as the development of cancer from prolonged exposure to high concentrations of ethylene oxide.

Preparation and Wrapping of Items for Gas Sterilization. As for any type of sterilization, items are sanitized with care, and moisture is removed from all surfaces. Be sure that all surfaces of the items are exposed in the sterilizer; do not pack them too tightly. Almost all forms of wrapping materials are acceptable for gas sterilization, but the combination paper-plastic wrapper is preferred because the contents are visible and the package is easy to open under aseptic conditions (Fig. 23–9). Wrapping materials that have a low ethylene oxide gas permeability also have a low air permeability and, therefore, may tend to burst when used in a sterilizer that has a vacuum cycle. To reduce this possibility, it is essential that as much air as possible be removed from the bag before sealing. A wrapping material that is suitable for one type of gas sterilizer may not be suitable for another. Again, check the manufacturer's instructions.

Indicators for Gas Sterilization. Gas indicators also include materials that change color or small test tubes of bacteria that are placed through the sterilization cycle with the materials to be sterilized. The color indicators provide a visual confirmation that a package has been through the process of sterilization, and the bacterial cultures show whether or not the process was able to kill the bacteria in the small tube. There are several excellent indicators on the market for gas sterilization, but the bacterial cultures are the superior method of checking that sterilization has, in fact, taken place. Ethylene oxide indicator labels and strips are reliable if they are buried deep within the pack (Fig. 23–10A). Indicator bags and tape are useful only in indicating that the outside of the package has been exposed to the gas; they are not indicators of com-

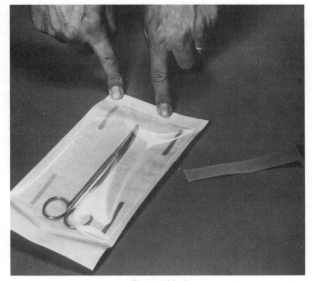

Figure 23–9

A clear transparent bag that has a paper side for steam penetration. (Courtesy of Propper, Inc., New York, NY.)

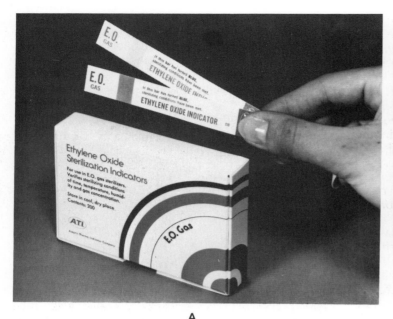

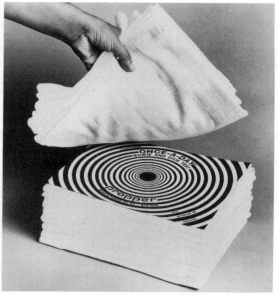

A   B

Figure 23–10

Indicators for gas sterilizers. **A,** Ethylene oxide indicators. (Courtesy of Aseptic-Thermo Indicator Co.) **B,** The Bowie and Dick Test. (Courtesy of Propper, Inc., New York, NY.)

plete sterilization. For gas sterilization, the *Bacillis subtilis* spore is used as the bacterial test culture, because it is one of the organisms most resistant to ethylene oxide.

Operating a Gas Sterilizer. The chamber is loaded in the same manner as the autoclave, allowing space between the items for the gas to circulate. However, this is not as critical as in the autoclave, because air pockets do not form in the containers and gas will circulate in all directions. Heat damage is not a problem in gas sterilization, as the heat needed is only slightly higher than room temperature.

Exposure times are dependent upon the type of sterilizer, the gas concentration, the temperature, and the amount of moisture in the chamber. The average exposure time is an hour and forty-five minutes at 130°F, but this varies from manufacturer to manufacturer. Ethylene oxide gas diffuses fairly rapidly in the open air, but many porous wrapping materials absorb the gas and, thus, require longer periods of aeration. These times vary from five to eight hours when a mechanical means of ventilation is used. Under normal room circulation conditions, the period of aeration ranges to seven days. When items are aerated with normal room circulation, personnel should not work in the same area. The storage life of items sterilized by ethylene oxide depends on the type of wrapping used and the place of storage, but items wrapped in plastic wrappers can have a much longer shelf life than items sterilized by the steam autoclave method.

STERILIZATION OF ITEMS USED IN THE MEDICAL OFFICE

Dressings. There are as many different designs of surgical dressings as there are surgical techniques. The American Medical Association has found about 5000 different styles in use. Frequently, the same dressing has several different names.

Some medical offices make their own dressings, but usually the machine-made dressings are less expensive, are more uniform in size and shape, and save considerable time for the medical assistant. These dressings may be purchased in large bulk nonsterile packages and may be rewrapped in smaller packs for autoclaving. Today, many pre-sterilized individual packages can be purchased for a price lower than the cost of the materials and labor. It is recommended that you investigate actual costs on an individual-item basis.

Most dressings and gauze sponges are made of cotton, but some are made of silk, wool, or wood fibers (cellulose). They are folded in various sizes and shapes, with all raw edges carefully placed inside the folds. Ravelings from raw edges could cling to a wound and act as a foreign body. Some dressings have a thin layer of synthetic material that will not adhere to a wound.

Dressings should be sterilized in the autoclave or by dry heat. Wrap them in small packets with a double layer of muslin or with sterilizer paper. Muslin wraps may be reused but must be washed and checked for holes and lint. Muslin will discolor with repeated heating. Each packet should be firm enough to hold together during normal handling but not so tightly packed as to inhibit the flow of steam and heat. The packets are sealed with sterilizer tape, labeled, and dated.

The use of sterilizer tape can serve several purposes: to fasten a package, identify the contents, *and used* and indicate that the pack has been sterilized. Do *initials* not crowd the packs too closely together in the chamber, as this prevents complete circulation of steam and heat. If the office does not have an autoclave and you need sterile dressings, consider presterilized items, or you may be able to make some arrangement with your local hospital for this service.

Remember that a 6-inch pack takes twice as long to penetrate as a 3-inch pack. An indicator should be placed in the thickest part of the pack. It is inadvisable to mix dressings and instruments in the same load because the timing must be set for the longest time that is required for the dressings, and this increased time is hard on the instruments.

Jars, Bottles, and Trays. Jars, bottles, and trays must be wrapped and placed on their sides to be autoclaved. The wraps should be secured with string and not with rubber bands if sterilized by dry heat. If these items are not to be stored sterile, they need not be wrapped. Covers on jars and containers should never be in place, but put to one side or slightly ajar, otherwise steam cannot circulate inside to drive out trapped air. These caps and lids are replaced before being removed from the chamber, taking care not to contaminate them.

Oils and Ointments. The sterilization of oils and ointments presents a different problem. Because steam cannot penetrate oils, it is best to sterilize oily substances by dry heat, usually for two hours at 320°F for a 1-ounce jar. A 4-ounce jar would require 100 minutes for sterilization by dry heat.

The most common item in this group would be gauze dressings impregnated with petroleum jelly (Vaseline). These are sterilized in glass jars or metal instrument boats. Once the container has been opened and some contents removed, it is considered to be contaminated. For this reason, it is best to sterilize small amounts at a time. Use heat-resistant glassware and metals. Do not place the cover directly over the top, but tilt it slightly. Autoclave these items just as you would a fluid (petroleum jelly is the same as mineral oil when heated). Be very careful not to decrease the pressure rapidly, or there will be a boiling over of the oil, which could possibly require a professional service cleaning of the autoclave. Read the manufacturer's instructions. Some guarantees are void if oils and solutions have been processed in the autoclave. The use of dry heat is suggested for these substances.

Several manufacturers sell prewrapped, sterile Vaseline gauze dressings. Because of the difficulty and uncertainty of determining the sterility of oil-based products when attempting to sterilize them in the medical office, purchasing prewrapped materials is the better choice.

Solutions. Some medical offices keep bottles of sterile distilled water or normal saline on hand for rinsing and irrigating purposes. (These solutions are not to be used as injectables.) Sterilization of irrigating and rinsing solutions may be done in an autoclave that has a slow-exhaust cycle; otherwise there will be a boiling over of the solution. To prepare these solutions for autoclaving, use a special Pyrex container that is manufactured for autoclaving liquids (Fig. 23–11A). Either disposable or reusable lids may be purchased that will seal down as they are processed in the autoclave (Fig. 23–11B). Fill the container about two-thirds full, not more, and place a hermetically sealed glass tube indicator, such as a Diack, in the solution. Date and label the contents.

Powders. Powders are best sterilized by dry heat. They are prepared in the same way as are oils. The timing is two hours for a 1-ounce jar at 320°F or one hour at 430°F. Some powders, such as sulfonamides, should be run at the lower temperature of 285°F for three hours. Always check first to make certain a powder may be sterilized by a heat method.

Tubing. Wash and clean well, and rinse with distilled water. Shake out the excess water, leaving a small amount of moisture, which will form steam and drive out the trapped air. Steam pressure sterilization is best for tubing that can withstand the heat; therefore, follow the manufacturer's recommendations. If chemical disinfection is indicated, use 70 percent isopropyl alcohol for 15 minutes, or other recommended agents. Then rinse again with sterile water before use. Nylons have excellent chemical resistance, except for those that are soluble in alcohol and/or phenols. Also, some synthetics absorb chemicals when they are soaked too long.

Rubber Goods. Too much heat, light, moisture, or exposure to certain chemicals destroys many rubbers. These items are sterilized separately not only because they require a different sterilization time, but also because they discolor metals and may stick to them. Improper handling of rubber can destroy it.

Here are general instructions for handling rubber goods. Always rinse rubber in cool running water immediately after use. If necessary, such items should be placed in a basin of disinfectant, then

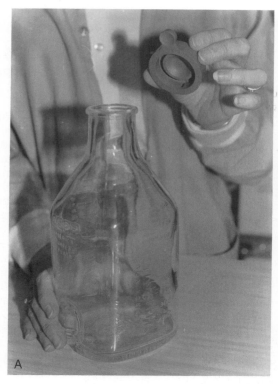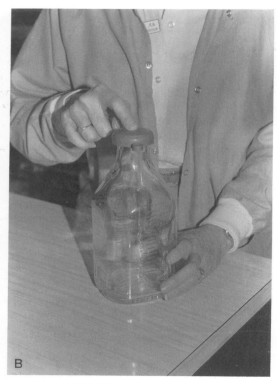

Figure 23–11
Sterilizing solutions. **A**, A heat-resistant glass bottle. **B**, A special rubber stopper.

washed well in warm water and cleansing agents, such as soap. Do not use strong detergents, scouring powders, ammonia compounds, or alcohol on rubber. Open all pockets and folds while cleaning, and remove metal clips. Rinse well in warm water, and towel-dry as thoroughly as possible. Powder with a glove talcum to prevent sticking. Hot water bottles and ice bags should be drained by hanging upside down. When they are dry, they should be inflated and capped. The inside surfaces of rubber should not be allowed to touch. Tubing should be hung over two pegs to prevent sharp turns in rubber, which may crack. Do not soak rubber too long. All rubber goods should be dusted with powder and wrapped if placed in storage.

Methods of sterilization of rubber goods include autoclaving and ethylene oxide gas. Chemicals are used for disinfection. Rubber goods are prepared for chemical disinfection in the same manner as for sterilization, but they will have to be rinsed with sterile water after being removed from the disinfectant solution.

Procedure 23–5

STERILIZING RUBBER GLOVES

PROCEDURAL GOAL

To wash, dry, and wrap rubber gloves for sterilization in the autoclave.

EQUIPMENT AND SUPPLIES

Blood and body-fluid protection barriers (goggles, masks, and aprons or gowns), as necessary (see Appendix C, Recommendations for Prevention of AIDS Transmission)
Household bleach mixed with water 1:10 (10 percent solution)
A low-sudsing detergent
4″ × 4″ gauze
Glove wrappers
Gloves to autoclave
Nonsterile gloves to wear

Procedure continued on opposite page

PROCEDURE

1. Immediately after use, soak soiled gloves in a cool 10 percent bleach solution for at least ten minutes. (Protect yourself by wearing nonsterile gloves.)
   Purpose: To lessen the chance of cross-contamination from blood or body secretions. The cool temperature prevents coagulation of blood and other contaminants.
2. Rinse the gloves in cool water, then sanitize them in a low-sudsing detergent.
3. Inspect for holes and residual contaminants.
   Purpose: Discard torn gloves.
4. Allow the gloves to dry completely on one side and then the other.
   Purpose: Wet glove surfaces will stick together during the autoclave process and will not be usable.
5. Reglove yourself. Place a 4″ × 4″ gauze square into the palm of each glove (below).
   Purpose: The gauze prevents the glove from adhering to itself during the sterilization process. Gauze is now preferred to powdering the glove because it eliminates chemical irritation of the operator's hand.

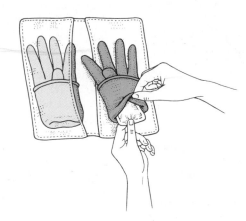

6. Put the gloves into a glove envelope, with the thumbs up and toward the center fold.
   Purpose: Placement of the gloves should be uniform; they should be in a position for easy removal.
7. Close the envelope and wrap it with autoclave paper or cloth.
   Purpose: Double-wrapping is necessary.
8. Label the package with the date, glove size, and your name or initials (below).

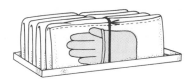

9. Place the package on its edge in the autoclave and steam-sterilize for 15 minutes, being careful to stack the packs vertically and allowing space for circulation.
10. Run the autoclave according to the manufacturer's directions.
11. Store the gloves on dry, covered shelves.
    Purpose: These items may be considered sterile for 28 to 30 days if they are in a double wrap.

Procedure continued on following page

TERMINAL PERFORMANCE OBJECTIVE

Given contaminated gloves, sanitize, dry, wrap, and autoclave them within 30 minutes, completing each step of the procedure correctly and in the correct order, as determined by your evaluator.

STERILIZATION IN SPECIALTY OFFICES

Obstetrics and Gynecology. Routine examination equipment, such as vaginal specula and uterine dressing forceps, is sometimes carelessly cleaned and "flushed through" chemical disinfectants. Any instrument that comes in contact with a patient should be sterilized in an autoclave for 15–20 minutes with 15 lb of pressure at 250°F, or it should be sterilized with a sporicidal chemical before it is used for another patient. If the instrument does not penetrate tissue, it may be stored under clean or medically aseptic conditions. Some physicians prefer to use disposable specula for routine pelvic examinations. Any instrument that penetrates the tissue **must be sterilized and stored sterile.** Some examples include the uterine biopsy punch, uterine tenaculum, cervical dilators and sounds, and any item used for the insertion of an intrauterine device.

Urology. These offices have many problems that are unique to urology. Such problems have lessened with the use of disposable syringes, catheters, and solution bowls. Items used for insertion into the urethra and for bladder instillation must be sterile. Reusable catheters are a major source of contamination and are not recommended. Office-sterilized instillation medications may contain pyogenic substances even if they are sterile. It is best to use reliable commercially prepared solutions.

If cystoscopic examinations are done in the office, extreme care must be taken to maintain sterility. A majority of these procedures are now done in the hospital. Office vasectomies must be done with sterile operating room techniques to prevent contamination.

Ophthalmology. The major concern here is in the careless use of eyedrops and careless handling of the medicine dropper. The use of stock solutions has been discouraged because of the dangers of the solution becoming a culture for pathogenic bacteria. Eye ointments present a similar problem. Only sterile solutions should be used if there is a laceration or ulceration of the eye. Instruments used for the removal of a foreign body should be sterile. It is advisable to reserve a medication for the patient for whom it is prescribed and not to use it on other patients.

Ear, Nose, and Throat. Routine examination instruments are sterilized after use and stored in a clean area. The main danger here is in the changing of dressings, placing of packs, and performing of minor surgery. Dressing forceps are often sanitized and returned to a sterilant solution and used again before the time lapse required to sterilize. There is frequently some carelessness in handling such items as tracheotomy tubes.

Neurology. Most neurologic offices do not use many items that puncture the skin, so sterilization technique may become lax or may never be practiced. The most crucial technique done in the neurologic office may be a spinal puncture, but this is rare nowadays, since most physicians prefer to use the hospital for this procedure. Surveys have shown that on rare occasions spinal needles that have been carefully cleaned and autoclaved have caused aseptic meningitis as a result of pyogens in the distilled water. This can be avoided by using disposable needles that have been sterilized by dry heat or gas sterilization.

Pediatrics. It has been known for many years that the main source of cross-infection in pediatrics has been the thermometer. Because it is used so frequently, there is some carelessness in sanitizing the thermometer before chemical sterilization. The chemical sterilant may not be changed or the container sterilized as frequently as it should be. Sometimes, alcohol alone is used, and this solution is not a sporocide or virucide, especially for hepatitis virus. Thermometers used by patients with hepatitis should be discarded and should not be used again. Disposable thermometers prevent cross-infection. Single-use thermometer sheaths are available in both oral and rectal types and are easy to use.

There is also carelessness involved in removing small foreign objects from the skin, such as splinters. Sterile procedures and sterile instruments must always be used when entering the skin, regardless of how uncooperative the patient may be.

Thoracic Medicine. The most common source of contamination here is in the use of the pulmonary function test equipment. These machines are difficult to sterilize, and asepsis is frequently ignored. The interior of the apparatus is not accessible and cannot be sterilized except by gas sterilization. The parts that are nearest the patient should be autoclaved or carefully sterilized in a chemical sterilant. Disposable parts such as mouthpieces and tubes are available.

REFERENCES AND READINGS

Bates, B.: *A Guide to Physician Examination*, 2nd ed. Philadelphia, J. B. Lippincott Co., 1983.

Bonewit, K.: *Clinical Procedures for the Medical Office*, 2nd ed. Philadelphia, W. B. Saunders Co., 1984.

Coates, H. W.: *Care and Handling of Surgical Instruments*. Chicago, V. Mueller Division, American Hospital Supply Corp., 1977.

Fuerst, R.: *Microbiology in Health and Disease*, 15th ed. Philadelphia, W. B. Saunders Co., 1983.

Fuller, J. R.: *Surgical Technology: Principles and Practice*, 2nd ed. Philadelphia, W. B. Saunders Co., 1986.

Nealon, T. F.: *Fundamental Skills in Surgery*, 3rd ed. Philadelphia, W. B. Saunders Co., 1979.

Perkins, J. J.: *Principles and Methods of Sterilization in Health Sciences*, 2nd ed. Springfield, IL, Charles C Thomas, 1983.

23

CHAPTER OUTLINE

VOCABULARY

See Glossary at end of book for definitions.

abscess
biopsy
cannula
cerumen
curettage
cyst

dilatation
dissect
fistula
glaucoma
lumen

obturator
patency
polyps
stylus
suppuration

24

Instruments for Minor Surgery and Clinical Procedures

OBJECTIVES

Upon successful completion of this chapter you should be able to

1. Define the terms in the Vocabulary for this chapter.
2. Differentiate between ring-handled and thumb-grasp, straight and curved, plain-tipped and toothed, serrated and plain-jawed, and ratchet and box-locked instruments.
3. Describe the uses and characteristics of each of the four classifications of instruments.
4. Identify scissors by function and using the appropriate sharp-sharp, blunt-blunt, or blunt-sharp category.
5. Differentiate between a hemostat and a needle holder.
6. Describe the usage(s) for each of the seven types of forceps.
7. Name two instruments used in each of the following specialties: gynecology, ophthalmology, otolaryngology, and urology.
8. Name two instruments used during each of the following: biopsy and wound repair.
9. Name and state the use of each of the instruments mentioned for the routine physical examination and neurologic testing.
10. Recall three rules regarding the care of surgical instruments.

Upon successful completion of this chapter you should be able to perform the following activity:

1. Correctly identify, spell the names of, and determine the uses of standard office instruments.

Instruments are fundamental to the performance of diagnostic procedures and patient treatments. With the growth of urgent care centers and an increase in outpatient surgery, the medical assistant now must care for and use a greater variety of surgical instruments. The administrative medical assistant must properly spell the names of instruments when transcribing medical dictation, as well as purchase and inventory them by name. The clinical medical assistant must know which instruments are used for each procedure in order to package them for sterilization and setup, and to assist the physician during surgery or an examination. Chapter 23 covers the care and cleaning of instruments. This chapter describes the names and classifications of the instruments frequently found in the medical office and their use.

IDENTIFYING THE PARTS OF SURGICAL INSTRUMENTS

Instruments have clearly identifiable parts and can be visually differentiated from one another. The basic components are the handle, the closing mechanism, and the part that comes into contact with the patient, commonly called the jaws. Many instruments may be ordered straight (str) or curved (cvd), depending on the operator's preference.

Instruments have either ring handles (finger-rings) or spring handles (sometimes called thumb-handled or thumb grasp). Included in the instruments with a ring handle are scissors, and tweezers are listed under spring-handled instruments. A ring-handled forceps is shown in Figure 24–1A; a spring-handled thumb forceps is pictured in Figure 24–1B.

Ratchets resemble gears and are located just below the ring handles. Ratchets are used to lock an instrument into position. Most ratchets can be closed at three or more positions, depending on the thickness of the material being grasped. An example of an instrument with a ratchet closing mechanism is shown in Figure 24–1C. Another type of locking mechanism is the box lock (Fig. 24–1D).

The inner surfaces of the jaws on some instruments have saw-like teeth called serrations, and both ring-handled and thumb-type instruments may have them. These serrations may be crisscross, horizontal, or lengthwise (Fig. 24–1E). Serrations prevent small blood vessels and tissue from slipping out of the jaws of the instrument.

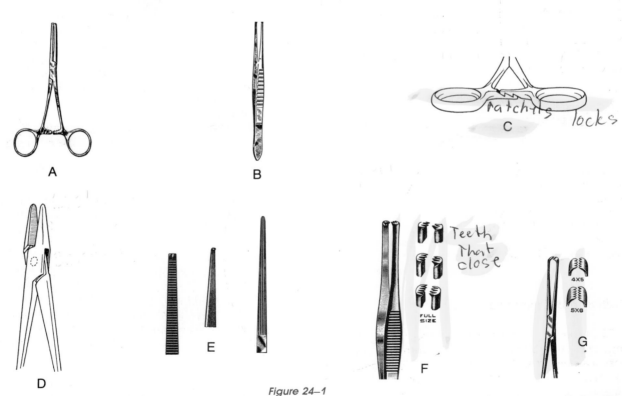

Figure 24–1

Identifying parts of an instrument. **A**, Ring handle. **B**, Thumb-type or spring-type handle. **C**, Ratchets. **D**, Box-lock. **E**, Serrations (horizontal, crisscross, longitudinal). **F**, Mouse-toothed (rat-toothed). **G**, Allis tissue forceps.

Jaws may be plain-tipped or mouse-toothed (Fig. 24–1F). If the tooth is large, the tip may be called rat-toothed rather than mouse-toothed. Toothed instruments are usually called tissue forceps and are identified by the number of intermeshing teeth (e.g., 1 × 2, 2 × 3, 3 × 4). Figure 24–1G shows part of an *Allis tissue forceps*. Because this forceps is used to grasp delicate soft tissues, the teeth are finer, shallow, and more rounded; others may be sharper and deeper. Still others have sharp hook-like single or double teeth, such as the *tenaculum* and *vulsellum*. Usually, the *tenaculum* has a single sharp hook on each jaw (see Fig. 24–9D). However, the *vulsellum* (Fig. 24–9C) has a double hook that resembles the fangs of a snake. Toothed instruments commonly have ratchets for locking into towels or human tissues.

An instrument is usually named for its use (*splinter forceps*, for removing splinters) or after the person(s) who developed it (*Mayo-Hegar needle holder*). Many general instruments are identified by the part of the body where they are used, such as the *rectal speculum* and the *nasal speculum*.

There are thousands of surgical instruments, and there are great variations in their names. The same instrument may carry two or three different names, depending on the physician or the part of the country. A physician may ask for a clamp or a forceps when a *Kelly hemostat* is wanted, and you will need to know what a clamp or forceps means in each case. As in building words from word parts, if you train yourself to recognize the distinctive parts of instruments and the reasons for each part, you will quickly build a working knowledge of hundreds of instruments.

CLASSIFICATIONS OF SURGICAL INSTRUMENTS

Surgical instruments are generally classified according to their use, and most belong to one of four groups:
1. Cutting and dissecting.
2. Grasping and clamping.
3. Retracting.
4. Probing and dilating.

Cutting and Dissecting Instruments

These are the cutting, incising, scraping, punching, and puncturing instruments. Included are scissors, scalpels, chisels, curettes, punches, drills, and needles. Instruments with a sharp blade or surface can cut, scrape, or **dissect**.

Surgical Scissors. Figure 24–2 shows the many different types of scissors found in a medical office. A pair of scissors is composed of two parts joined together by a screw and a screw joint. When a pair of scissors is completely closed and held to the light, the two blades seem to touch only at the tips. As the instrument is closed, this meeting place travels from the joint to the tip, giving the shearing action. Scissors are identified as straight or curved. The blade points are characterized as sharp or blunt. Thus, a pair of scissors is described as sharp-sharp (s/s), sharp-blunt (s/b), or blunt-blunt (b/b).

All-purpose *operating scissors* (Fig. 24–2A through C) are also called *surgical scissors*. The most frequently used are 5½-in long. They may be ordered in ½-in lengths, from 4½ to 5½ in. There are some other specialty scissors that are longer. As the name implies, these scissors are used to cut tissue or lengths of fine suture.

The blunt *dissecting scissors* (Fig. 24–2D) are used for dissecting or exposing growths or vessels from the surrounding tissue. The *Mayo* style shown in the figure has a beveled blade. The blades of *dissecting scissors* usually are narrower than those of the blunt-blunt *surgical scissors*. Both tips of a *dissecting scissors* are blunt, and some *dissecting scissors* have blades on the inside and outside edges, allowing the scissors to shear and separate subcutaneous tissues as the scissors are opened as well as closed.

The *Lister bandage scissors* (Fig. 24–2E) are used to remove bandages and dressings. The probe tip is blunt and can be easily inserted under bandages, with relative safety and little discomfort to the patient. Also, the tip is less likely to probe into the skin, as a sharp-tipped scissors may do. The *Burnham finger bandage scissors* (Fig. 24–2F) are useful when a tip smaller than that of the *Lister* is needed, as on a finger bandage. The *gauze shears* (Fig. 24–2G) are used to cut to size not only gauze but also such things as rubber sheeting, tubing, and adhesive strips.

The *Littauer stitch*, or *suture*, *scissors* (Fig. 24–2H) are among the several popular types of scissors employing a break or hook to get under a suture. When an incision has sufficiently healed, the suture is cut with these scissors, and the end pulled with a *thumb dressing forceps*.

The *iris scissors* (Fig. 24–2I) were originally used in eye surgery. Many physicians, however, prefer it to suture scissors or, in some cases, to general operating scissors. The usual length of *iris scissors* is 4 in; however, longer or shorter patterns are manufactured. The tips may vary, as with the *operating scissors* (e.g., straight or curved, blunt or sharp).

Scalpels. Scalpels are used to make incisions. Most scalpels are disposable or have disposable

Scalpels

blades furnished in different shapes and sizes (Fig. 24–3). The three standard handles are No. 3, No. 3L (long), and No. 7. No. 3 handle is most commonly used, and No. 3L is the same except for its increased length. No. 7 handle is more delicate and is used in narrower places. Combinations of disposable blades and handles are available in various blade sizes. The most commonly used blade is No. 11. Depending on the area to be incised, Nos. 10, 12, and 15 are also popular. Only blades with numbers between 10 and 15 will fit on No. 3, No. 3L, and No. 7 handles.

Grasping and Clamping Instruments

Clamping instruments are used for many different tasks. Many have a sharp tooth or teeth and are used to retract, hold, and manipulate human tissue. The most common clamping instruments are the hemostats, which were originally designed to stop bleeding or to clamp severed blood vessels. Other clamping instruments are used to grasp other instruments or sterilized materials. Sometimes hemostats and the other clamping instruments are used interchangeably.

Forceps. There are several hundred different types of forceps. Used alone, the term is extremely broad and does not identify any particular instrument.

Hemostatic Forceps. Figure 24–4*A* through *C* shows three commonly used hemostats. These instruments are employed to clamp off small blood vessels and to hold tissue. In hospitals, a wide variety of hemostats is used, whereas in the medical

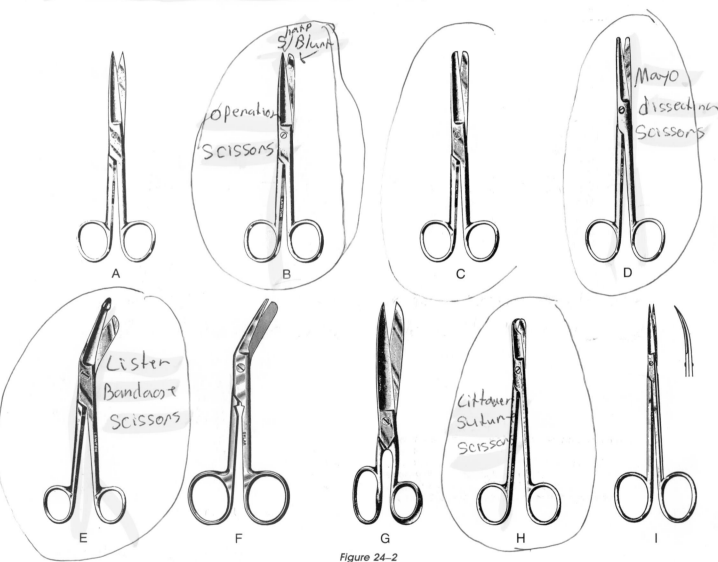

Figure 24–2

*Scissors. **A,** Operating scissors, straight or curved, sharp-sharp. **B,** Operating scissors, blunt-sharp. **C,** Operating scissors, blunt-blunt. **D,** Mayo dissecting scissors, straight or curved, 6¾ in. **E,** Lister bandage scissors, 5½ in. **F,** Burnham finger bandage scissors. **G,** Gauze shears, army-type, 7½ in. **H,** Littauer stitch (or suture) scissors, 5½ in. **I,** Iris (eye) scissors, straight or curved, 4⅛ in.*

24

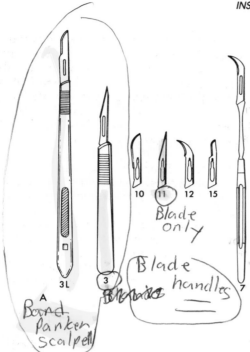

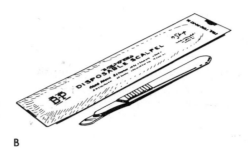

10 11 12 15

Blade only

Blade handles

3L 3 7

A

Board Panker scalpell

Figure 24–3
*Scalpels and blades. **A**, Bard-Parker operating scalpels (handles with various disposable blades). **B**, Packaged, disposable sterile blade and reusable handle.*

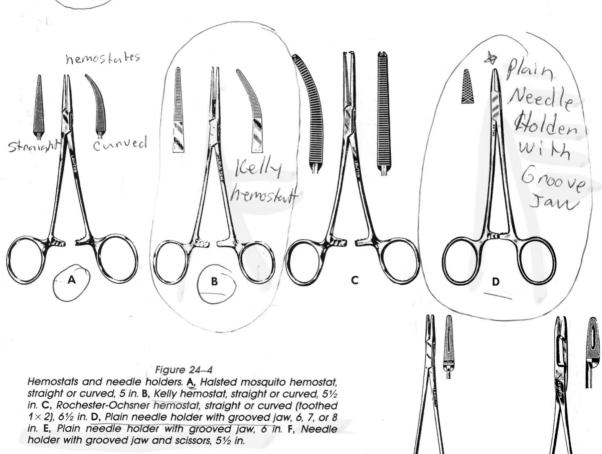

hemostates

Straight *curved*

Kelly hemostatt

Plain Needle Holden with Groove Jaw

A B C D

E F

Figure 24–4
*Hemostats and needle holders. **A**, Halsted mosquito hemostat, straight or curved, 5 in. **B**, Kelly hemostat, straight or curved, 5½ in. **C**, Rochester-Ochsner hemostat, straight or curved (toothed 1 × 2), 6½ in. **D**, Plain needle holder with grooved jaw, 6, 7, or 8 in. **E**, Plain needle holder with grooved jaw, 6 in. **F**, Needle holder with grooved jaw and scissors, 5½ in.*

office, most hemostats have jaws that are fully serrated or serrated halfway and do not have teeth. The size and length of the hemostat vary according to the size of the vessels being clamped. Hemostatic forceps may be straight or curved, plain-tipped or rat-toothed. The *Halsted mosquito hemostat* (Fig. 24–4A) and the *Kelly hemostat* (Fig. 24–4B) are the most commonly used in minor surgical procedures. The *Rochester-Ochsner hemostat* (Fig. 24–4C) may be used for larger clamping jobs.

for small blood vessels

Needle Holders. Figure 24–4D through F shows some commonly used needle holders. The jaw of a needle holder firmly grasps a suture needle as it is passed through the skin flap adjoining an incision. A needle holder with thin jaws may be advantageous for holding the fine needles used in plastic surgery or eye surgery. The jaws of needle holders are shorter and look stronger than those of hemostats of the same size. The jaws are always serrated, and some popular needle holders contain a groove down the length of the jaw.

Splinter Forceps. The four types of splinter forceps shown in Figure 24–5A through D are quite different in construction. However, they all are used to grasp foreign bodies embedded in the skin or under fingernails. The fine tips lend themselves

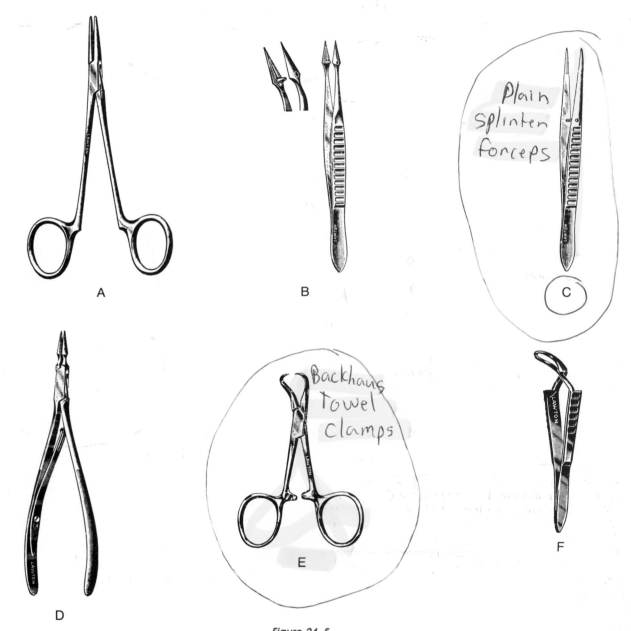

Plain splinter forceps

Backhaus towel clamps

Figure 24–5
Splinter forceps and towel clamps. **A,** *Physician's splinter forceps (ring handle).* **B,** *Hunter splinter forceps (thumb or spring handle).* **C,** *Plain splinter forceps.* **D,** *Virtus splinter forceps.* **E,** *Backhaus towel clamp.* **F,** *Jones towel clamp (spring handle).*

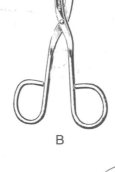

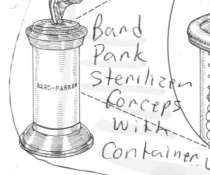

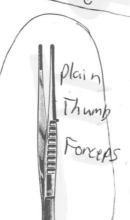

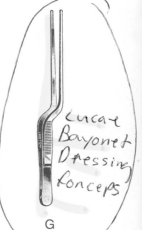

24

Figure 24–6

Sterilizer, tissue, and dressing forceps. A, Sterilizer forceps (tongs), three-pronged, 8 in. B, Sterilizer forceps, 8 in. C, Bard-Parker sterilizer forceps and container. D, Allis tissue forceps. E, Plain tissue forceps, 5½ in. F, Plain thumb forceps, 5½ in. G, Lucae bayonet dressing forceps, 5½ in.

particularly to the retrieval of splinters and other foreign objects.

Towel Forceps. The two most popular styles of towel clamps, or towel forceps (Fig. 24–5*E* and *F*), are used to place sterile drapes around the site of the operation, thus creating a sterile field. The towel clamps hold the various layers of draping or towels in place. All towel clamps have sharp hooks, which are used occasionally to hold the drape to the edge of the incision. A towel clamp may be used to encircle and lift a tubular structure such as a vessel or the *vas deferens* during a surgical procedure. The curved tips allow them to hang freely without interfering with the line of vision. Towel clamps come in various lengths from 3 to 6½ in. The use

of fenestrated drapes (disposable, plastic-backed paper towels with an opening in the middle) for minor office surgery has decreased the popularity of autoclaved cloth towels and towel clamps.

Sterilizer Forceps. The illustrated types of sterilizer forceps (Fig. 24–6*A* and *B*) are used to retrieve sterilized items such as instruments, syringes, and needles from the autoclave. Both types shown have curved jaw surfaces, which facilitate holding the items. Many types are available. The *Bard-Parker sterilizer forceps and container unit* may be preferred because a spring-operated, metal float-basket rises as the forceps is withdrawn, thus helping the forceps not to touch the sides of the container and break sterile technique. When the forceps is at rest in the container, the attached lid provides a seal from the environment (Fig. 24–6C).

Tissue Forceps. The *Allis tissue forceps* (Fig. 24–6D) is used to grasp tissue such as muscle or skin flaps surrounding the surgical wound. The same function is served by the *plain tissue forceps* (Fig. 24–6E), but the Allis tissue forceps has a much more gentle grip because the teeth are less sharp.

Dressing Forceps. The *plain thumb forceps* (Fig. 24–6F) is primarily a dressing instrument designed to handle with a "no-touch technique" surgical dressings. It is manufactured in lengths of 4 to 12 in, with varying serrated jaws, and does not have teeth. The *Lucae bayonet forceps* (Fig. 24–6G) is a simple, angled thumb forceps. It is used to best advantage in the nose and ear to insert packing or remove foreign objects. The bayonet shape provides better vision. Bayonet forceps are manufactured in lengths up to 8½ in. Occasionally, they are toothed.

Retracting Instruments

Retracting instruments hold tissue away from the surgical wound (incision), so their use in minor surgery is limited. By physician preference, the *Allis* tissue forceps and the *Kelly hemostat* are used to retract during most minor surgical procedures. A retractor may be hand held (in which case an assistant is required to hold it in place) or self-retaining (holding itself in place by means of a ratchet).

Probing and Dilating Instruments

These instruments are used for both surgery and examinations. Probes may be used to search for a foreign body in a wound or to enter a **fistula.** Dilators are used to stretch a cavity or opening for examination or before inserting another instrument to obtain a tissue specimen.

Probes. The *grooved director* (Fig. 24–7A and B) is used to guide a cutting instrument, such as the scalpel, as an artist's stick is used against the canvas to steady the paintbrush. Notice that the director may have a probe tip (Fig. 24–7B), which makes it easier to explore the direction of a fistula. Probes and directors come in lengths ranging from 4 to 12 in, and with or without bulbous tips. The slender construction of the *Larry probe* (Fig. 24–7C) makes it suitable for rectal examinations. Probes also are

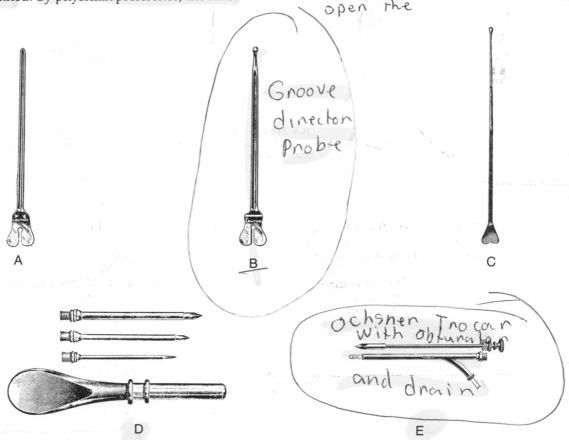

Figure 24–7

Probes and trocars. **A,** *Grooved director, plain tip.* **B,** *Grooved director, probe tip.* **C,** *Larry probe, bulbous tip.* **D,** *Nested trocar, three sizes.* **E,** *Ochsner trocar with obturator and drain.*

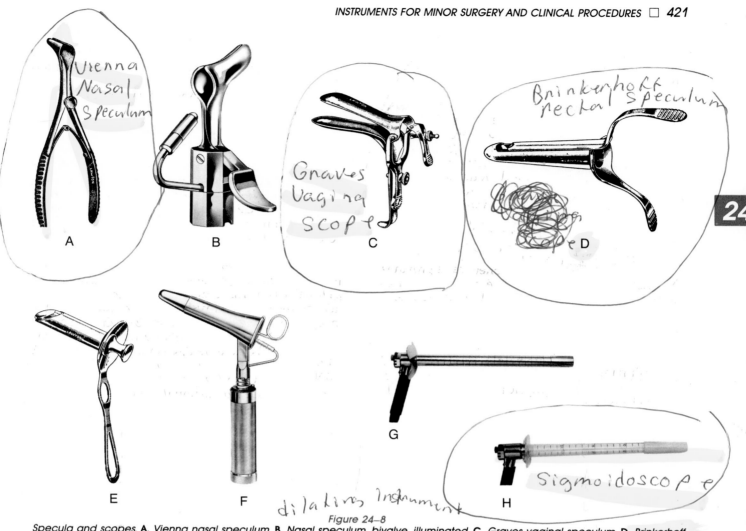

Figure 24–8

Specula and scopes. **A,** *Vienna nasal speculum.* **B,** *Nasal speculum, bivalve, illuminated.* **C,** *Graves vaginal speculum.* **D,** *Brinkerhoff rectal speculum.* **E,** *Hirschman anoscope.* **F,** *Illuminated anoscope with removable obturator.* **G,** *Sigmoidoscope, reusable, illuminated, 25 cm (obturator not shown).* **H,** *Sigmoidoscope, disposable, fiberoptic.*

useful for exploring foreign bodies embedded in subcutaneous tissues.

Trocars and Obturators. A trocar consists of a sharply pointed **stylus** (**obturator**) contained in a **cannula** (outer tube). The trocar is inserted into the body as a unit. The stylet (obturator) is necessary to gain entry into the body. The cannula is used to hold the cavity open after entry. Once the trocar is inserted, the stylet (obturator) is withdrawn, allowing other instruments to pass through. Figure 24–7D shows a nested trocar (three sizes). The *Ochsner trocar* (Fig. 24–7E) has a drain attached. Trocars come in various sizes and are used to withdraw fluids from cavities or for draining and irrigating with a catheter.

Specula. The most common dilator is the speculum (Fig. 24–8). A speculum is an instrument for opening or distending a body orifice or cavity to permit visual inspection. A *bivalve speculum* (Fig. 24–8A through C) is one with two valves or parts,

sometimes referred to as blades or bills. The valves are spread apart, thus dilating the opening. The *Brinkerhoff rectal speculum* (Fig. 24–8D), used to examine the rectal wall, has no blades or bills.

Scopes. Scopes are viewing instruments equipped with a light source. Generally, the dilating scopes do not have blades or bills that would increase dilation after the instrument has been inserted. The *anoscope* (Fig. 24–8E and F) is approximately 3½ in (8.9 cm) in length and enables examination of the anal area and lower rectum. Because of its limited length, the *anoscope* is usually not illuminated. The *proctoscope* (not shown) is approximately 6 in (15 cm) in length and facilitates examination of the rectum above the limits of the *anoscope*. The *sigmoidoscope* (Fig. 24–8G and H) is approximately 10 in (25 cm) in length and permits examination of the sigmoid bowel area. Both the *proctoscope* and the *sigmoidoscope* must be illuminated.

An obturator may also be a part of a scope. The

obturator for the *rectal scope* (Fig. 24–8E) is smooth and rounded to ease insertion of the instrument through the anal sphincter muscle.

SPECIALTY INSTRUMENTS

Although all instruments fall under the same four categories as the surgical instruments just discussed, the remaining instruments are organized into specialty groupings. Presenting the instruments in this manner makes it easy to see how the instruments relate to particular examinations. In addition to recognizing the name and usage of each instrument, you must organize and set out the instruments needed for each particular examination on what is called a *tray setup.*

Instruments for Gynecology

The *vaginal speculum* (see Fig. 24–8C), used in the vaginal examination, is manufactured in different sizes.

The *Sims uterine curette* (Fig. 24–9A) is one of six sizes frequently used. Curettes are spoon-shaped scraping instruments used to remove minor polyps, secretions, and bits of afterbirth (placental matter) and to obtain specimens from the uterine cavity. Identical sizes with dull blades also are available.

The *Bozeman uterine dressing forceps* (Fig. 24–9B) and the *Foerster sponge forceps* (Fig. 24–9E) are used to reach the cervix, uterus, and vagina. Designed to hold sponges or dressings, they are used to swab the area or apply medications.

The *Schroeder uterine vulsellum forceps* (Fig. 24–9C)

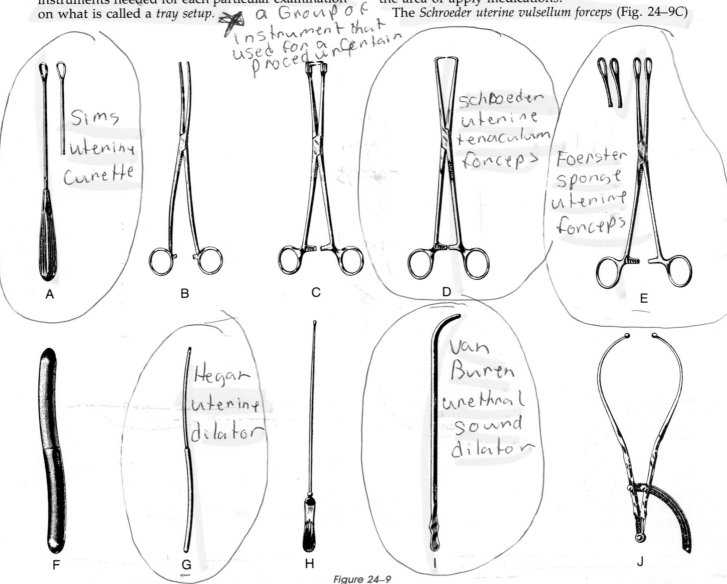

Figure 24–9

Instruments for gynecology. **A,** *Sims uterine curette, sharp or blunt, 12 in.* **B,** *Bozeman uterine dressing forceps.* **C,** *Schroeder uterine vulsellum forceps, straight, 9 in.* **D,** *Schroeder uterine tenaculum forceps, 9 in.* **E,** *Foerster sponge forceps (uterine sponge forceps), straight or curved, 9½ in.* **F,** *Hegar uterine dilator, double-ended, largest.* **G,** *Hegar uterine dilator, double-ended, smallest.* **H,** *Sims uterine sound.* **I,** *Van Buren urethral sound.* **J,** *Martin pelvimeter.*

24

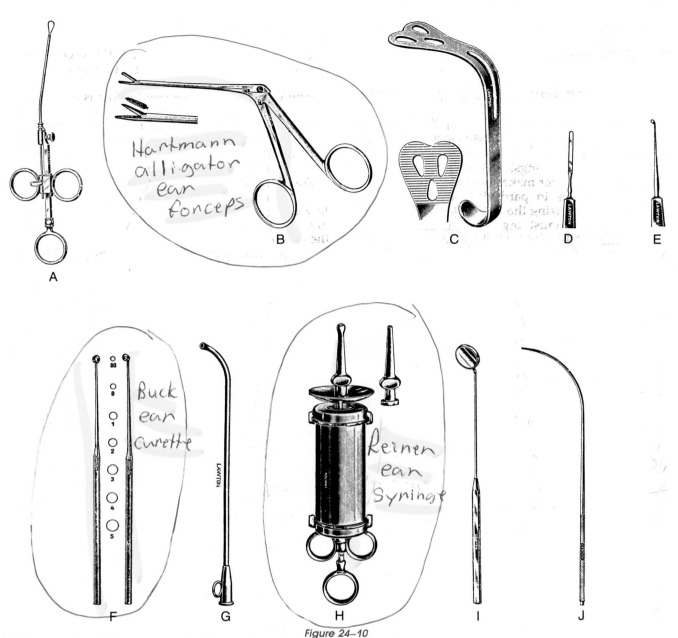

Hartmann alligator ear forceps

Buck ear curette

Reiner ear Syringe

Figure 24-10

*Instruments for ophthalmology and otolaryngology. **A,** Krause nasal snare. **B,** Hartmann "alligator" ear forceps, plain or toothed. **C,** Weider "metal" tongue depressor. **D,** Dix eye foreign body spud, flat end. **E,** Laforce eye foreign body spud ("golf-club" eye spud). **F,** Buck ear curette. **G,** Hartmann eustachian-tube catheter. **H,** Reiner ear syringe with shield and control handle, plain tip and bulbous tip. **I,** Laryngeal mirror. **J,** Ivan laryngeal metal applicator.*

and the *Schroeder uterine tenaculum forceps* (Fig. 24–9D) are used to hold tissue, such as the cervix, while obtaining a tissue specimen or for lifting the cervix to view the fornix.

The *Hegar uterine dilators* (Fig. 24–9F and G) come in sets of eight sizes. They are double-ended, so there are actually 16 different sizes. Uterine dilators are used to dilate the cervix for examination and for **dilatation** and **curettage** (D & C).

The *Sims uterine sound* (Fig. 24–9H) is used to check the **patency** of the cervical os. The *Martin pelvimeter* (Fig. 24–9J) is used to measure the female

pelvis to determine whether or not it is possible to deliver the fetus through the birth canal.

Instruments for Ophthalmology and Otolaryngology

The *Vienna nasal speculum* (Fig. 24–8A) and the *illuminated nasal speculum* (Fig. 24–8B) are used to spread the nostrils for examination of the nasal cavity. By spreading the valves, the physician can examine for nasal **polyps** or sources of irritation or can introduce an applicator or snare into the naris.

The *Krause nasal snare* (Fig. 24–10A) has a wire loop that, when tightened, may be used to remove polyps from the nasal cavity. A similar snare, smaller in size, is available for use in the ear.

The *Hartmann "alligator" ear forceps* (Fig. 24–10B) has a 3½-in shaft. It is so called because the jaw moves with an action similar to that of an alligator's jaw. It is inserted through either the nasal or the ear speculum and is used for grasping and removing foreign objects. The alligator jaw is made in a variety of styles (for example, cup jaw or with teeth) so that it can remove foreign bodies or polyps of different shapes.

The *Wieder "metal" tongue depressor* (Fig. 24–10C) retracts the tongue during throat, postnasal and oral examinations.

The physician is frequently called upon to remove foreign bodies from the eye. Deeply embedded foreign objects are, of course, handled by a specialist; however, the *Dix eye foreign body spud* (Fig. 24–10D) is helpful in office procedures, as is the *Laforce "golf club" eye foreign body spud* (Fig 24–10E).

Buck ear curettes (Fig. 24–10F) are used to remove foreign matter from the ear canals. They are made with sharp or blunt scraper ends and are manufactured in various sizes.

The *Hartmann eustachian tube catheter* (Fig 24–10G) is used to blow air into the eustachian canal, which connects the nasopharynx to the cavity of the middle ear.

The *Reiner ear syringe* (Fig. 24–10H) is used for removal of **cerumen** (wax) and for irrigations. All types are fitted with a piston, by means of which a stream of fluid is forcibly injected into the ear or cavity. A small splash shield is mounted behind the tip to collect the wash-back into a basin held beneath the ear. The three-ringed handle facilitates a firm grip. It is supplied with a plain catheter or a bulbous tip.

The *laryngeal mirror* (Fig. 24–10I) is used for examination of the larynx and postnasal areas. Laryngeal mirrors also are made in various sizes and may be purchased with mirror surfaces that do not fog.

The *Ivan laryngeal metal applicator* (Fig. 24–10J) holds cotton in place with its scored or roughened end. It has a length of 9 in and a curve that lends itself to use in the throat and postnasal areas. Other metal applicators vary in size and may be either straight or curved.

The *tonometer* (Fig. 24–11) is an instrument used for measuring intraocular tension (pressure) caused by a disease known as **glaucoma.** This instrument is expensive and extremely delicate and requires special care. Figure 24–11A shows the standard *Schiotz tonometer.* This instrument is kept in a special stand and is sterilized for each patient. Figure 24–11B shows the *Digiton electronic tonometer (Schiotz).*

Instruments for Biopsy

Figure 24–12 shows a number of styles of instruments used for obtaining specimens for **biopsy,** which is most commonly done to ascertain the presence of cancer cells.

The *rectal biopsy punch* (forceps) (Fig. 24–12A) is used through a *proctoscope* or *sigmoidoscope* and is made with stems that may be interchanged. These

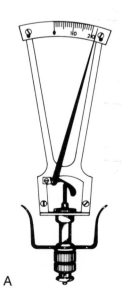
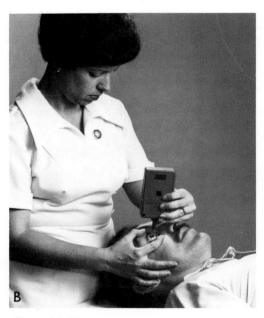

Figure 24–11
Tonometers. **A,** Standard tonometer, Schiotz. **B,** Electronic Digiton tonometer, Schiotz.

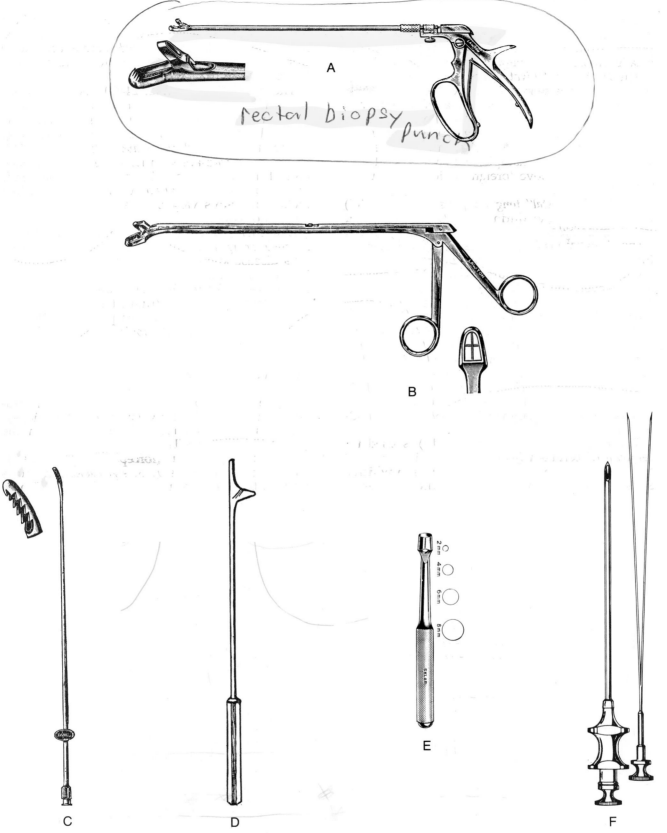

rectal biopsy punch

24

Figure 24–12

Instruments for biopsy. **A,** *Rectal biopsy punch (forceps).* **B,** *Wittner uterine (cervical) biopsy forceps.* **C,** *Novak biopsy curette.* **D,** *Cervical spatula.* **E,** *Cutaneous punch (skin biopsy punch).* **F,** *Silverman biopsy needle with stylus (inserted) and biopsy cannula.*

have different lengths and are made with cupped, basket-type, straight, or angled jaws. The toothed style (not shown) affords a better grip on the tissue during the taking of the specimen. The ring-handled *uterine (cervical) biopsy forceps* (Fig. 24–12B) is one of several styles used for cervical biopsies.

Different techniques for obtaining cervical cells for examination may involve the use of the *Novak biopsy curette* (Fig. 24–12C) or the scraping of cells by using a *cervical spatula* (Fig. 24–12D). Many of these techniques now are done using disposable kits.

The *cutaneous punch* (*skin biopsy punch*) is sometimes called a *dermal punch* (Fig. 24–12E). This is used to biopsy a small piece of skin for diagnostic examination.

The *Silverman biopsy needle* (Fig. 24–12F) has a stylus that works on the same principle as the obturator. When the needle is inserted into the tissue, the stylus is kept in place inside the needle. As the needle reaches the area for biopsy, the stylus is removed, and a split cannula is inserted to pick up the specimen. The needle biopsy can eliminate the necessity for a surgical incision.

Instruments for Wounds

The *Senn retractor and skin hook* (Fig. 24–13A) is a double-ended instrument. The three-pronged end is used as the skin hook. The flat end is a retractor, which is used to hold open small incisions or lacerations for viewing, or to secure a skin edge for suturing. The *Freer dissector and elevator* (Fig. 24–13B) is one type of elevator used to lift the connective tissues from bone during orthopedic surgery. A fingernail drill is used to cut an opening into the fingernail (Fig. 24–13C). The opening releases pressure and allows the drainage of blood that accumulates following certain injuries to the nail. The comedo extractor removes blackheads, which are plugged hair follicles (Fig. 24–13D).

The *abscess needle* (Fig. 24–13E) is attached to a syringe and is used to withdraw fluids or **suppuration** (pus) from a **cyst** or **abscess**. The needles must be sterilized and the points protected while they are stored.

Instruments for Urology

The glass *Asepto irrigation syringe* (Fig. 24–14A) varies in capacity from 1 to 4 oz and comes equipped with a blunt cone tip, a fine pipette tip, or (as shown) a catheter tip. Disposable plastic irrigation syringes are available in disposable irrigation kits (Fig. 24–14B).

The irrigation syringe has a bulb plunger and a glass barrel and is used for irrigating tubing or a body cavity. This type of tip is used to irrigate a catheter.

The *Robinson catheter* (Fig. 24–14C) is a soft rubber urethral catheter, in sizes French 12 to 30. The higher the number, the smaller the **lumen** (open-

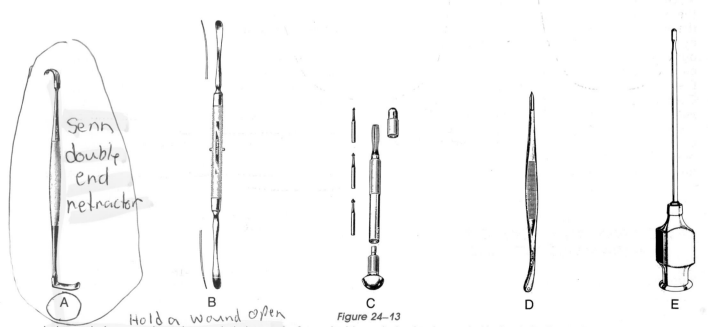

Figure 24–13

Instruments for wounds and wound drainage. **A,** *Senn* double-ended retractor and skin hook. **B,** Freer dissector and elevator. **C,** Fingernail drill with attachments. **D,** Comedo extractor, double-ended. **E,** Abscess needle. (Courtesy of Becton-Dickinson & Co.)

24

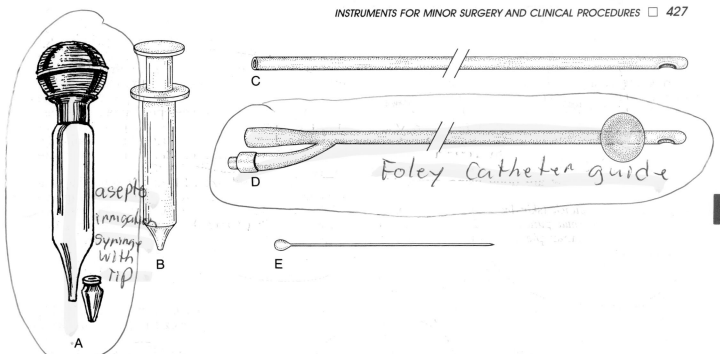

asepto irrigation Syringe with Tip

Foley Catheter guide

Figure 24–14
Instruments for urology. **A,** *Asepto irrigation syringe with tip.* **B,** *Disposable catheter syringe.* **C,** *Robinson catheter.* **D,** *Foley catheter.* **E,** *Catheter guide.*

ing). It is frequently inserted into the bladder to obtain a sterile specimen. Since the urinary tract is sterile, catheterization is always performed using sterile technique.

left in place

The *Foley catheter* (Fig. 24–14D) is an indwelling catheter. It is manufactured with a double rubber lining. After the catheter is inserted into the bladder, a sterile solution is injected into the inner lining. At the end of the inner lining is a balloon, which inflates with the sterile solution and keeps the catheter from slipping out of the bladder until the balloon is deflated. Deflation is accomplished by reversing the technique: the fluid is aspirated out of the balloon with a syringe. Indwelling catheters must be irrigated frequently to make certain that the outer lumen is open for urinary drainage. Catheters may be left in place for two to four weeks. Foley catheters are available in sizes French 8 to 30.

A *catheter guide* (Fig. 24–14E) is a metal device used only when it is impossible to insert a catheter normally. Great caution must be used with the guide so as not to damage tissue in the urethra. No one except the physician should use a guide.

INSTRUMENTS FOR ROUTINE PHYSICAL EXAMINATIONS AND DIAGNOSIS

Auscultation Instruments

Stethoscopes (Fig. 24–15) are used to transmit to the examiner's ears the sounds produced within the body, especially the sounds of the heart, lungs, and bowel. Stethoscopes have two earpieces with flexible tubes leading to the end that is placed on the patient. The flat, disc-shaped endpiece is the *Bowles stethoscope* (Fig. 24–15A). The bell-shaped endpiece is the *Ford stethoscope* (Fig. 24–15B). Many examiners prefer the double endpiece with both disc- and bell-shaped attachments. The *obstetric stethoscope* (Fig. 24–15C) leaves the examiner's hands free to palpate and manipulate the fetus. Some stethoscopes are electronic and amplify sounds.

Illuminated Diagnostic Sets

The sets in Figure 24–16 illustrate several different attachments for the battery-handled (*A*), wall-mounted (*D*), or table-top unit (*E*) that act as the source of power for the lightbulb or fiberoptic filament in the attachment. Attachments and power sources are often interchangeable and include *anoscopes*, *proctoscopes* and *sigmoidoscopes*.

The *diagnostic otoscope attachment* (Fig. 24–16B) provides a hinged magnifying lens that can be pivoted to the right or left side to pass an applicator or other instrument through the speculum. Specula of different sizes may be interchanged on these otoscopes. Each size has a number and specific use. Disposable specula are available and may be economical if only a few sizes are used. The *operating otoscope attachment* (Fig. 24–16C), sometimes called a *therapeutic otoscope*, has a smaller magnifying lens and provides greater access into the ear canal. The *fiberoptic pneumatic otoscope* (Fig. 24–16D) gives an increased level of illumination (owing to the fiber-optic filament) and allows for the injection of air into the ear canal (the pneumatic feature).

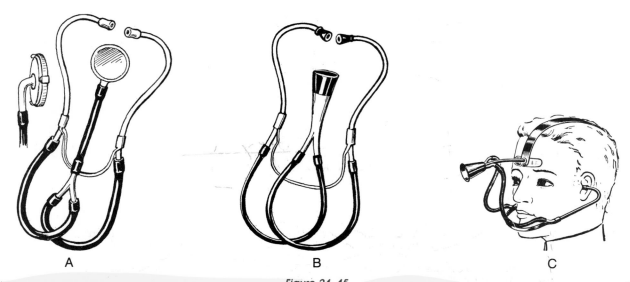

Figure 24–15

*Stethoscopes. **A**, Bowles stethoscope with disk-shaped chest endpiece. **B**, Ford stethoscope with bell-shaped endpiece. **C**, Obstetric stethoscope with headpiece.*

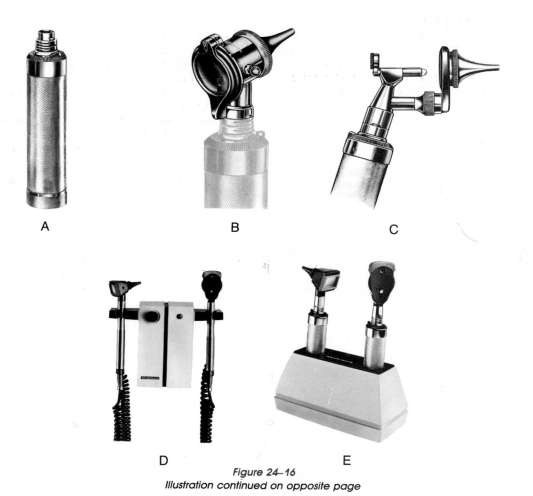

Figure 24–16

Illustration continued on opposite page

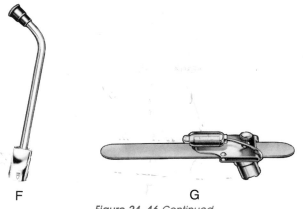

F   G

Figure 24–16 Continued

Illuminating instruments. **A,** *Battery handle for attachments.* **B,** *Diagnostic otoscope (removable speculum).* **C,** *Operating otoscope (removable speculum).* **D,** *Wall-hung transformer unit and handles for fiberoptic pneumatic otoscope and ophthalmoscope.* **E,** *Desk model with rechargeable handles for otoscope and ophthalmoscope.* **F,** *Transilluminator, curved.* **G,** *Tongue depressor holder, illuminating.* (**D,** **E,** *and* **G,** *courtesy of Welch Allyn, Inc., Skaneateles Falls, New York.*)

The *ophthalmoscopes* (Fig. 24–16D, right side, and E, right side) are used to examine the optic nerve, retina, and blood vessels of the interior of the eye. This scope is also used to determine pupillary reaction to light.

The *transilluminator attachment* (Fig 24–16F) is used to pass light through an area such as the sinuses, teeth, or breasts. Because it is flexible and curved, it often is used to examine the throat. A wooden tongue depressor may be inserted into an *illuminated tongue depressor holder* (Fig. 24–16G) for viewing the oral cavity.

Neurologic Instruments

Figure 24–17A shows a *percussion hammer* for testing the patient's reflexes. The *Neurotone-5* (Fig. 24–17B) is a percussion hammer that includes most of the other objects necessary for neurologic testing. The unit includes a tuning fork and brush, needle, and pinwheel attachments.

Tuning forks (Fig. 24–17C) are used to test the perception of sound. They are held by the single stem and gently tapped on the examiner's knuckle, or they may be plucked between the thumb and index finger. It is not advisable to rap it on a hard surface, since this damages the instrument. Tuning forks also help to determine whether the patient is suffering from conduction (sound conduction from the external ear to the cochlea) deafness or from deafness due to damage of the acoustic nerve. The fork is struck sharply to produce sound vibrations and then is held against the patient's mastoid bone or forehead by the examiner. Tuning forks are available in varying tone ranges from low to high.

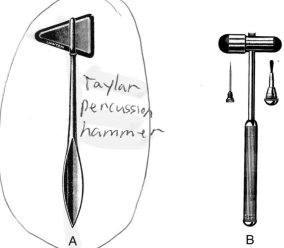

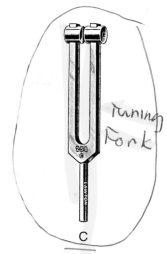

A   B   C

Figure 24–17

Neurologic instruments. **A,** *Taylor percussion hammer.* **B,** *Neurologic hammer with pin and brush.* **C,** *Tuning fork.*

Table 24–1
A Quick Reference Guide to Instruments

Instrument	Function	Use	Frequently Used Example	Frequently Used Size
Scissors	Cutting, dissecting	Cutting away or through tissues or materials	Mayo dissecting Lister bandage Littauer stitch Iris (eye)	6 3/4 in 5 1/2 in 5 1/2 in 4 1/8 in
Scalpel handles Scalpel blades	Cutting, dissecting	Incising or excising tissues or growths	Bard-Parker disposable Bard-Parker disposable	Nos. 3, 3L, 7 Nos. 10–15
Curettes	Cutting, dissecting	Scraping away tissues	Sims uterine Buck ear Krause nasal snare Cervical spatula	10 in 8 in
Biopsy punches	Cutting, dissecting	Excising growths or tissues	Rectal Cervical Cutaneous	13 in 9 1/2 in 2–7-mm set
Hemostats	Clamping	Clamping blood vessels	Rochester-Ochsner Rochester-Péan Kelly Halsted mosquito	6 1/4 in 6 1/4 in 5 1/2 in 3 1/2 in
Splinter forceps	Grasping	Removing foreign bodies	Hunter Physician's Plain Virtus Hartmann "alligator"	5 1/2 in 5 1/2 in 5 1/2 in 5 1/2 in 3 1/2 in
Spuds	Grasping	Removing foreign bodies	Dix eye Laforce "golf club" eye	No size No size
Tissue forceps	Grasping	Grasping soft tissues	Allis Toothed Plain thumb Schroeder uterine vulsellum Schroeder uterine tenaculum	5 1/2 in 5 1/2 in 5 1/2 in 10 in 10 in
Dressing forceps	Grasping	Applying dressings	Plain thumb Lucae bayonet Bozeman uterine Foerster uterine	5 1/2 in 5 1/2 in 10 in 10 in
Needle holders	Grasping	Grasping suture needles	Mayo-Hegar	6 in

Table continued on opposite page

Table 24–1
A Quick Reference Guide to Instruments Continued

24

Instrument	Function	Use	Frequently Used Example	Frequently Used Size
Towel clamps	Grasping	Holding sterile drapes in place	Backhaus Jones	3 in 3 in
Sterilizer forceps	Grasping	Grasping and transferring sterile items	Bard-Parker Transfer Tongs	No size 8 in 8 in
Probes	Probing	Entering and exploring	Grooved director Larry probe Ochsner trocar	4 1/2 in 4 1/2 in Varies
Specula and scopes	Dilating	Viewing and exploring	Vienna nasal Graves vaginal Brinkerhoff rectal Hirschman anoscope Sigmoidoscope Diagnostic otoscope Operating otoscope Fiberoptic otoscope	5 1/2 in S, M, L S, M, L S, M, L 10 in No size No size No size
Dilators	Dilating	Opening or stretching	Hegar uterine Sims uterine sound Van Buren urethral sound	3–4 mm to 17–18 mm Varies Varies
Retractors	Retracting	Holding open wounds or cavities	Senn Wieder tongue depressor	Varies No size
Catheters	Irrigating, drainage	Exchanging fluids or air	Hartmann eustachian Robinson urinary Foley urinary	Nos. 00–4 French 14–18 French 14–20
Syringes	Irrigating	Cleansing, medicating	Reiner ear Asepto Catheter	No size 30–50 cc 30–50 cc
Mirrors, lights	Inspecting	Viewing	Laryngeal Transilluminator	9 in Varies
Applicators	Applying	Applying medications	Buck ear/nasal Brown ear/nasal	6 in 6 in
Hammers	Percussing	Testing reflexes	Taylor percussion Neurotone-5	No size No size
Tuning forks	Percussing	Testing hearing	Hartmann	No size
Stethoscopes	Auscultating	Listening to body sounds	Bowles Ford Obstetric	No size No size No size
Meters	Measuring	Testing size, pressure	Tonometer Pelvimeter	No size No size

Procedure 24–1

PROCEDURAL GOAL

To identify, correctly spell the names of, and determine the usage of standard office instruments or those selected by your instructor.

EQUIPMENT AND SUPPLIES

Bard-Parker transfer forceps
Curved hemostat
Straight hemostat
Dressing forceps (thumb)
Allis tissue forceps
Towel clamp
Scalpel and blade
Vaginal speculum
Dissecting scissors
Bandage scissors
Ophthalmoscope
Paper and pencil

PROCEDURE

1. Look for the following parts that determine usage: box-lock, serrations, finger rings, cutting edge, noncutting edge, thumb type, teeth, ratchets, and electric attachments.
   Purpose: To determine the combination of features and parts for each instrument.
2. Consider the general classification of the instrument: cutting and dissection, grasping and clamping, retracting, or probing and dilating.
   Purpose: The clue to the name of the instrument may be found by determining the classification.
3. Carefully examine its teeth and serrations.
   Purpose: The clue to the name of the instrument may be found by determining its distinctive parts.
4. Look at the length of the instrument to determine the area of the body for which it is used.
   Purpose: The clue to the name of the instrument may be found by determining where it can reach.
5. Try to remember whether the instrument was named for a famous physician, university, or clinic.
   Purpose: Many instruments are named for the inventor.
6. If the instrument is a pair of scissors, look at the points and determine whether they are sharp-sharp, sharp-blunt, or blunt-blunt.
   Purpose: The clue to the name of a pair of scissors may be found by determining the combination of points.
7. Carefully compare the instrument with similar instruments that you know, to determine if it is in the same category or has the same name.
   Purpose: The clue to the name of an instrument may be found with the knowledge you already have.
8. Write, with correct spelling, the complete name of each instrument, including its category and usage.

TERMINAL PERFORMANCE OBJECTIVE

Given the instruments listed, or those chosen by your evaluator, correctly identify and spell the names of nine of 10 instruments (minimum performance of 90 percent), including each instrument's category and usage, within ten minutes, as determined by your evaluator.

CARE AND HANDLING OF INSTRUMENTS

Since instruments are expensive and the physician's skill is dependent upon the quality of the instruments, the medical assistant must properly care for each instrument to maximize the life of the instrument and ensure that every part is in safe, working order.

Most instruments are made of fine-grade stainless steel. The term stainless is usually taken too literally. Although stainless steel does resist rust and keeps a fine edge and tip longer, even the best stainless steel may develop water spots and stains, especially if water with a high mineral content is used. Proper hardness and flexibility are important. Inexpensive instruments may be too brittle or too soft. Mistreatment of chrome-plated instruments can cause minute breaks in the finish, which may become a source of contamination or may tear the surgeon's gloves.

Instruments should be carefully examined when they are purchased. Scissors should be tested to see if they shear the full length of the blades, completely to the tip. This can be checked by cutting a piece of cotton. If the scissors cut cleanly and do not chew at any point, even at the tip, they are functioning correctly. Teeth and serrations should be checked to see if they intermesh completely and if the jaws are even on the sides and tip. Each instrument should be felt over its entire surface for any rough areas that may tear or snag the surgeon's gloves. Box-locks and hinges must work freely but should not be too loose. Thumb- and spring-handled instruments must have the correct tension and meet evenly at the tips.

Under no circumstances should instruments be bunched together or allowed to become entangled. Avoid mixing stainless steel instruments with ones of aluminum, copper, or brass. This may cause electrolysis and may result in etching. Even mixing stainless steel with chrome-plated instruments is best avoided. If an instrument is accidentally dropped, it may be permanently damaged. If scissors are dropped with the blades partially open, there will be a nick at the point at which the blades cross. Do not leave ratchets closed. Do not leave an instrument clamped onto material such as a drape or gauze.

Reserve a special place during the surgical procedure to receive contaminated instruments. This is usually a basin of disinfectant solution placed in the sink or within reach of the assistant. If a metal basin is used, it is advisable to place a small towel on the bottom of the basin to prevent damage to the instruments as they are dropped into the solution. Never allow blood or other coagulable substances to dry on an instrument. If immediate cleaning is not possible, they should be rinsed well and placed in a cold water solution of a blood solvent and a mild detergent. The detergent increases the wetting ability of the water, allowing the instrument surfaces to be better exposed to the solution. It is best to use a detergent that has a neutral pH. It should be low-sudsing and easy to rinse off. Each manufacturer of the various disinfectants and blood solvents recommends the correct dilution and time of immersion for its product. Read the label.

Upon completion of the surgical procedure, the receiving basin for the instruments is transferred from the area to the cleaning and sterilization room. It is important to remove used instruments from the patient's view as soon as possible.

Separate the various types of instruments. Sharp instruments should be carefully handled to prevent damage to cutting edges or possible injury to the person sanitizing them. Rubber and plastic items are easily punctured and often discolor metals. Some plastic and rubber goods should not be soaked too long because they will discolor. Plastics may become porous and lose their glossy surface. Sanitize and sterilize surgical packs without delay. The instruments must be ready for the next scheduled procedure or any emergency. Surgical packs should be processed daily at a designated time.

REFERENCES AND READINGS

Bates, B.: *A Guide to Physical Examination*, 3rd ed. Philadelphia, J. B. Lippincott, 1983.

Coates, H. W. (ed.): *Care and Handling of Surgical Instruments*. Chicago, V. Miller Division, American Hospital Supply Corp., 1977.

Fuller, J. R.: *Surgical Technology: Principles and Practice*, 2nd ed. Philadelphia, W. B. Saunders Co., 1986.

Nealon, T. F., Jr.: *Fundamental Skills in Surgery*, 3rd ed. Philadelphia, W. B. Saunders Co., 1979.

24

CHAPTER OUTLINE

VOCABULARY

See Glossary at end of book for definitions.

arrhythmia	pulses
arteriosclerosis	bounding
atherosclerosis	elastic
congestive heart failure	intermittent
hyperventilation	irregular
meniscus	thready
	unequal

25

Vital Signs

OBJECTIVES

Upon successful completion of this chapter you should be able to

1. Define and spell the words in the Vocabulary for this chapter.
2. Cite the average, normal values for body temperatures measured orally, rectally, and by the axillary method.
3. List five circumstances that will cause the body temperature to increase or decrease.
4. List four types of fevers.
5. Cite the normal ranges for pulse rate, rate of respiration, and blood pressure.
6. Locate seven pulse sites.
7. Describe each of the following pulses: thready, elastic, intermittent, irregular, bounding, and unequal.
8. Cite two reasons for obtaining the pulse rate at the apical site.
9. List four circumstances that cause the pulse rate to increase or decrease.
10. Describe each of the following types of respiration: apnea, dyspnea, bradypnea, tachypnea, orthopnea, hyperventilation.
11. List the five physiologic factors affecting the blood pressure.
12. Differentiate between essential hypertension and secondary hypertension.
13. Describe the sounds of each of the Korotkoff phases.
14. List the common causes of errors when obtaining a blood pressure measurement.

Upon successful completion of this chapter you should be able to perform the following activities:

1. Measure orally, rectally, or by the axillary method, the body temperatures of adults and children.
2. Determine pulse rates and respiration rates of adults and children.
3. Determine a patient's blood pressure using an aneroid and mercury sphygmomanometer.
4. Measure a patient's height and weight.

Measuring and recording the patient's vital signs is an important preface to every physical examination and is usually the responsibility of the medical assistant. The vital signs are the patient's temperature, pulse, respiration, and blood pressure. These four signs are abbreviated *TPR* and *BP* and may be referred to as *cardinal signs*. It is essential to understand the significance of the vital signs in health and disease and to be able to accurately measure and record them. The patient's height and weight are not considered vital signs but are obtained at the same time as the vital signs. Therefore, the procedure for measuring height and weight is included in this chapter.

The vital signs are influenced by many factors, both physical and emotional. A patient may have rushed to arrive at the office on time or may have consumed a hot or cold beverage just before the examination. A patient may be angry or afraid of what the doctor may find. Most patients, for one reason or another, are apprehensive during an office visit. These emotions may alter the vital signs, and it is necessary for the medical assistant to help the patient relax before taking any readings. It sometimes is necessary to obtain some measurements a second time, after the patient is calmer or more comfortable. To obtain a better picture of the patient's vital signs, you may be asked to record the vital signs three times: at the beginning of the visit, during the visit, and just before the patient leaves the office.

Physicians realize that, in the past, some patients were treated for false high blood pressure caused by the temporary emotions or conditions that were a reaction to the medical environment. Cardiologists recognize high blood pressure (hypertension) as a medical diagnosis only when it can be established that the blood pressure is persistently elevated. The hypertensive patient or the patient suspected of having hypertension may be taught to take his or her own pulse and blood pressure in the relaxed atmosphere of the home to obtain average readings and to help the physician establish a definite diagnosis.

Accuracy is essential. A change in one or more of the patient's vital signs may indicate a change in general health. Variations may indicate the presence or disappearance of a disease process and, therefore, a change in the treatment plan. Although you will obtain vital signs routinely, it is not a routine task. These findings are crucial to a correct diagnosis, and you should never perform them with indifference or casualness. In addition to accurate measurement, you must use extreme care when charting your findings on the patient's medical record.

TEMPERATURE

A patient's temperature is an important part of the physical diagnosis. The Fahrenheit (F) scale has been used most frequently in the United States, but many doctors and hospitals now are using the centigrade (or Celsius) scale. In the home, however, most patients continue to use the Fahrenheit scale. Most temperature readings are obtained orally. When obtained rectally, the body's temperature registers more quickly and slightly higher (99.2° to 99.6°F, 37.3° to 37.5°C) than if the oral method is used. This is because the rectum provides a tighter closure around the thermometer (with less air circulating and cooling the area) and is near the abdominal organs, which are naturally warmer than the oral cavity. The patient's body temperature is more accurately measured by the rectal method, but it is not as convenient to obtain. Occasionally, it may be necessary to place the thermometer under the arm. This reading is called the *axillary* temperature. Because this area is cooler than the mouth, the thermometer will register the body temperature one degree lower than when the oral method is used.

When obtaining temperatures orally is the routine method of measurement, you do not have to indicate this method when recording the reading; however, you do record an "R" for rectal and an "A" for axillary readings. In pediatrics, it is assumed that the temperature reading is obtained by the rectal method. Therefore, indicate "O" for oral and "A" for axillary. Some medical facilities may require the methods to be recorded for all three.

In both health and disease, the body's temperature varies during a 24-hour period. It is influenced by many external and internal conditions. Higher temperatures occur in the late afternoon hours (following food ingestion and activity), during exercise, and in extreme emotional states such as anxiety or anger. Increased metabolism and the presence of bacterial infection raise the body's temperature. Lower temperatures occur in the early morning hours (after long hours of sleep), during starvation, and after exposure to extreme cold. A slowed metabolism, shock, and **congestive heart failure** lower the body temperature (Table 25–1).

The accepted normal temperature is 98.6°F (37°C) when measured orally. When the body's temperature is elevated, it is frequently said that the person "has a temperature." However, this expression should be avoided, since a person always has a temperature, whether normal, subnormal, or elevated. Normal temperature might be better called the average temperature since some individuals have a temperature that is slightly lower or higher than 98.6°F in the normal state. A persistently elevated temperature is called a *fever* and warrants thorough investigation. The are several classifications for fevers.

In a *continuous fever* (Fig. 25–1A), the temperature is elevated and remains at the elevated level with no, or very little, fluctuation within a 24-hour period. In an *intermittent fever* (Fig. 25–1B), the temperature is elevated at certain times within a 24-

Table 25–1

Causes of Changes in Body Temperature*

Increase in Body Temperature	
CONDITION	CAUSE
Illness	Bacterial infection, producing fever
Activity	Increased muscular activity, leading to increased body temperature
Food intake	Increased metabolism, resulting in increased body temperature
Emotions	Stress and strong emotional reactions, causing increased body temperature
Exposure to heat	Increase in heat, producing increased body temperature
Pregnancy	Increased metabolism, leading to increased body temperature
Drugs	Some drugs increase body temperature by increasing metabolism or muscular activity
Age	Infants have body temperatures 1–2°F higher than those of adults
Decrease in Body Temperature	
CONDITION	CAUSE
Illness	Viral infection, resulting in subnormal body temperature
Activity	Decreased muscular activity, causing decreased body temperature
Fasting	Decreased metabolism, producing decreased body temperature
Emotions	Depression and shock, leading to decreased body temperature
Exposure to cold	Decrease in heat, resulting in decreased body temperature
Drugs	Some drugs decrease body temperature by decreasing metabolism or muscular activity
Age	Elderly have decreased metabolisms

*Average temperature = 98.6°F (37°C). Normal variations from 97° to 99.6°F (36.1° to 37.5°C).

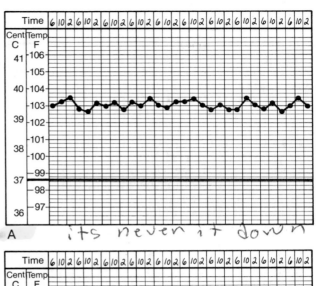

A   *its never it down*

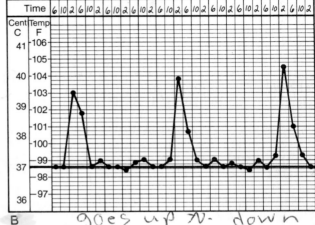

B   *goes up N down*

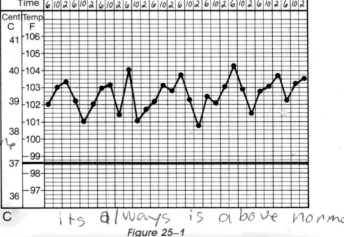

C   *its always is above normal*

Figure 25–1

Temperature charts illustrating specific fevers. **A,** Continuous fever. **B,** Intermittent fever. **C,** Remittent fever.

coming N going temperature

hour period but falls to normal or even subnormal during this period. In a *remittent fever* (Fig. 25–1C), the temperature fluctuates greatly but never falls to the normal level. A fever is said to be *relapsing* when it recurs after one or more days of normal temperature. *infections.*

Fevers resolve or disappear by *lysis* or *crisis*. Lysis occurs when a fever gradually falls over a period of several days. If a fever falls abruptly within a 36-hour period, it does so by crisis. Frequently, a fever crisis is accompanied by profuse sweating (diaphoresis). Diaphoresis also occurs in night sweats, extreme weakness, and nervousness. Chills and rigor (shivering) are frequently found in patients who are having a fever crisis.

when the fever goes down

Thermometers

Three types of clinical thermometers are used: rectal, oral, and security-tipped (Fig. 25–2). The differences in these three types are the bulb shapes.

25

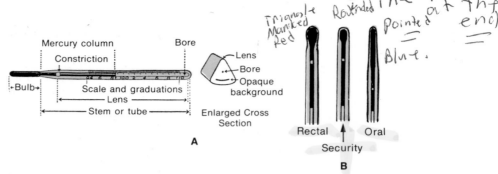

Figure 25–2
A, *The cross section of the clinical thermometer is triangular-shaped. The lens must be held at eye level to see and read the level of mercury.* **B,** *Illustration of the construction of the bulbs. The rectal thermometer is stubby. The security thermometer is often used for axillary temperatures. The oral thermometer has a longer, more slender bulb.*

The different shapes identify which thermometer to use for a particular area of the body. The rectal and security-tipped types are constructed so as not to puncture the mucous membranes of the rectum, and both may be used for axillary temperatures.

Thermometers should be stored in separate, clean containers, either dry or soaking in 70 percent isopropyl alcohol or other suitable disinfectant solution. The choice of a solution should be based on its disinfecting effectiveness and safety for use on human tissues. After use, a thermometer should not be returned to its container until it has been sanitized, then separately disinfected. At least once each week, the containers should be thoroughly cleaned and the solutions, if any, changed. Label the container as to the thermometer type, that is, oral or rectal. Patients are very alert to and apprehensive about the type of thermometer being used, where it was used last, and its cleanliness. Even though your thermometers are disinfected, you can add more protection by using a disposable sheath that slips over the entire length of the thermometer. Patients feel more at ease knowing that the thermometers do not come into contact with their bodies.

Thermometers are manufactured in two scales: Fahrenheit and Celsius. Figure 25–3 compares these two thermometers. Table 25–2 is the conversion table and includes a list of converted temperatures. The thermometer works on the principle that mercury expands with heat. Inside the thermometer is a column of mercury that rises in reaction to the amount of heat produced at the bulb when it is placed in the patient's mouth or rectum, or under the patient's arm.

Preparing the Thermometer. Hold your fingers under running water to check that the water temperature is cool. Warm water will cause the mercury to rise, and you will need to shake down the mercury before using the thermometer. Hot water will break the thermometer. Rinse the thermometer clean before use. Lower the mercury column to below 95°F (35°C) by shaking with a snap of the wrist. Be sure to hold the thermometer tightly between your thumb and forefinger at the end opposite the bulb. Be careful not to strike the thermometer against a hard object, as the glass will break and the mercury will spill. Such spills require special handling as mercury is a poisonous substance.

TIPS FOR OBTAINING TEMPERATURES

- *Do not take an oral temperature within 30 minutes after the patient has eaten, drunk, or smoked.*
- *Label containers to differentiate thermometers that are contaminated or soaking from those that are clean.*
- *Label rectal thermometers carefully. If you are not using the different bulb types for identification, mark the stem ends of the rectal thermometers with red nail polish.*
- *Keep rectal thermometers in solutions separate from the oral and axillary thermometers.*
- *Use separate security-tipped bulbs for obtaining axillary temperatures.*

Obtaining Temperatures Rectally

The rectal method is usually required for the very young patient, patients with breathing difficulties, or patients who are uncooperative or unconscious. The procedure is the same as for the oral method, except the bulb must be lubricated with jelly. The patient's temperature will register on the thermometer within two minutes. Stay with the patient or have the parent stay with the patient. Adults should be kept in the prone or Sims position until the thermometer is removed. Place an infant in the supine position. Hold the legs straight up with one hand, and hold the thermometer in place with the other. Alternatively, restrain the small child in the prone position with one hand at the buttocks, and

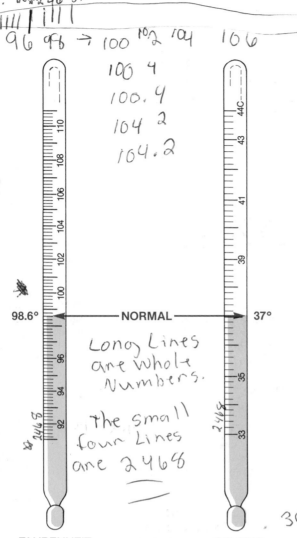

Handwritten annotations near figure:
96 98 → 100 102 104 106

100 4
100.4
104 2
104.2

Long Lines
are whole
Numbers.

the small
four lines
are 2468

98.6° — NORMAL — 37°

FAHRENHEIT — *Higher Number*
A

CELSIUS — *is Lower*
B

305.

Figure 25–3

The Fahrenheit and Celsius clinical thermometers compared to show the difference in scales and normal body temperature, which is about 98.6°F or 37°C when measured orally.

Using the Electronic Thermometer

Electronic thermometers record rapidly, usually within five seconds, and claim an accuracy of ±0.2°F (Fig. 25–4). They have color-coded disposable tips for both oral and rectal use. The temperature reading on the dial remains displayed until it is released, which allows ample time to read and record the findings. Electronic thermometers require adjustment, and care must be taken to have the dial at eye level while adjusting it. Many models are available, and some require additional fine adjustments. Be certain to follow the manufacturer's instructions to ensure accuracy.

PULSE RATE

The pulse rate is such a routine part of the physical examination that it is often taken in a mechanical way, and some of the finer aspects are neglected. The pulse rate is a method of counting the heartbeat by feeling the pulsing of an artery. What is felt is the expansion and relaxation of the artery in response to the pressure changes of each heart beat. When the heart contracts, pressure throughout the arteries increases, and the arteries expand. When the heart relaxes, arterial pressure decreases, and the arteries relax. Each constriction

hold the thermometer in place with the other. You must never leave a thermometer in an infant or child without you or the parent holding onto it.

Obtaining Temperatures by the Axillary Method

Recent studies reveal that the axillary temperature may be as accurate as the other methods. For example, the presence of feces in the bowel may cause a falsely elevated rectal temperature, and the rectal method is not the best choice for patients with hemorrhagic diseases such as leukemia. The axillary method is gaining in popularity in geriatrics. Axillary temperatures take more time to register the correct body temperature, but the method is safe, simple, and easily accessible.

Table 25–2
Temperature Conversion Scale:
Fahrenheit to Celsius*

F	C	F	C	F	C
95.0	35.0	100.2	37.9	105.4	40.8
95.2	35.1	100.4	38.0	105.6	40.9
95.4	35.2	100.6	38.1	105.8	41.0
95.6	35.3	100.8	38.2	106.0	41.1
95.8	35.4	101.0	38.3	106.2	41.2
96.0	35.5	101.2	38.4	106.4	41.3
96.2	35.6	101.4	38.5	106.6	41.4
96.4	35.7	101.6	38.6	106.8	41.5
96.6	35.9	101.8	38.7	107.0	41.6
96.8	36.0	102.0	38.8	107.2	41.8
97.0	36.1	102.2	39.0	107.4	41.9
97.2	36.2	102.4	39.2	107.6	42.0
97.4	36.3	102.6	39.3	107.8	42.1
97.6	36.4	102.8	39.4	108.0	42.2
97.8	36.5	103.0	39.5	108.2	42.3
98.0	36.6	103.2	39.6	108.4	42.4
98.2	36.8	103.4	39.7	108.6	42.5
98.4	36.9	103.6	39.8	108.8	42.6
98.6	37.0	103.8	39.9	109.0	42.7
98.8	37.1	104.0	40.0	109.2	42.9
99.0	37.2	104.2	40.1	109.4	43.0
99.2	37.3	104.4	40.2	109.6	43.1
99.4	37.4	104.6	40.3	109.8	43.2
99.6	37.5	104.8	40.4	110.0	43.3
99.8	37.6	105.0	40.5		
100.0	37.7	105.2	40.6		

*To convert degrees F to degrees C, subtract 32, then multiply by 5/9. To convert degrees C to degrees F, multiply by 9/5, then add 32.

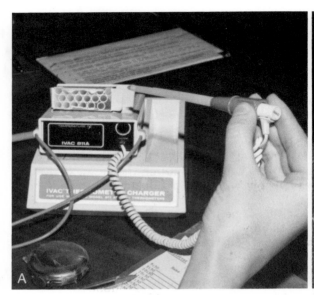
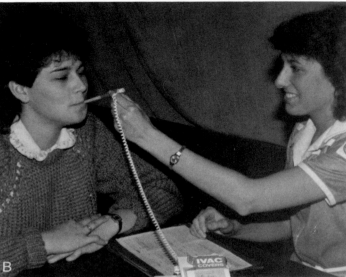

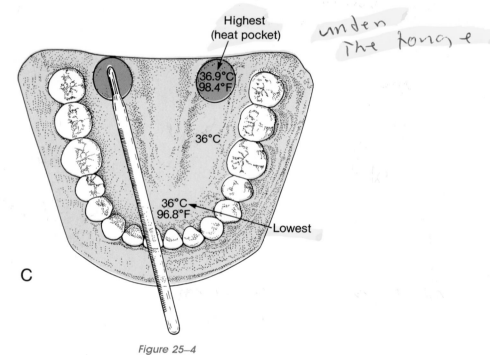

under the tongue

Figure 25-4

A, *The electronic thermometer will register a patient's temperature within five seconds.* **B,** *Special care is taken so that the probe is inserted* not *under the tongue.* **C,** *Areas of the mouth that give the highest and lowest readings.*

and relaxation of the heart muscle is a heartbeat, and each resulting expansion and relaxation of the arteries is the pulse rate. Normally, heartbeat (rate) and pulse rate are the same. The pulse rate varies from person to person. It is affected by the individual's activities and illnesses. The average adult pulse rate is from 60 to 90 pulsations, or beats, per minute. During resting periods, the pulse rate is usually 60 to 70 beats per minute. During activity,

it may be from 70 to 90. The pulse rate of a young athlete at rest may be as slow as 50 beats per minute. Since the body must balance heat loss by increasing circulation (a faster heart rate), the pulse rate is proportionate to the size of the body. The smaller the body, the greater the heat loss and the faster the heart must pump to compensate. Therefore, infants and children normally have faster pulse rates of 90 to 120 beats per minute.

Pulse Sites

A pulse rate may be counted anyplace where an artery is near the surface of the body. This rhythmic throbbing may be felt at the following arteries: radial, brachial, carotid, temporal, femoral, popliteal, and dorsalis pedis (Fig. 25–5).

The radial artery is the most frequently used site for counting the pulse rate. It is best found on the thumb side of the wrist, just above the wrist bones.

The brachial pulse is felt at the inner (antecubital) aspect of the elbow. It is the artery heard and felt when taking a blood pressure. It is also felt in the groove between the biceps and triceps muscles on the inner surface of the arm, just above the elbow.

The apical heart rate (Fig. 25–6), or the heartbeat at the apex of the heart, is heard with a stethoscope. It is frequently the method of choice for infants and young children. An apical count may be requested if the patient is taking cardiac drugs or has bradycardia (slow heartbeat) or a rapid, irregular pulse at one of the other pulse sites. The physician may listen to the apical beat while you count the pulse at another site. This is to determine equal pulse between the heartbeat and the artery. The stethoscope is placed just below the left breast. Count for one minute, and note the method by placing an "AP" beside the recorded count.

The carotid artery is located between the larynx and the sternocleidomastoid muscle in the front and to the side of the neck. It is most frequently used in emergencies and during cardiopulmonary resuscitation (CPR). It can be felt by pushing the muscle to the side and pressing against the larynx.

The femoral pulse is located at the site where the femoral artery passes through the groin. One must press deeply below the inguinal ligament. The popliteal pulse is found at the back of the knee. The patient must be in a recumbent position, with the knee slightly flexed. The popliteal artery is deep and difficult to feel. This artery is palpated and listened to with the stethoscope when a leg blood pressure reading is necessary. The dorsalis pedis artery is felt on the top of the foot, just slightly lateral to the midline, beside the extensor tendon of the great toe. This pulse may be congenitally absent in some patients. A good pulse rate at this site is an indicator of normal lower limb circulation and arterial sufficiency.

25

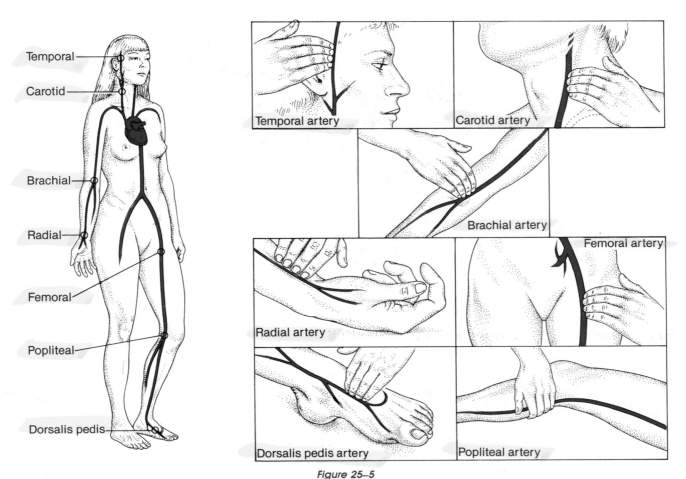

Figure 25–5
The pulse sites. Although the radial artery is the most frequently used, it is important for the medical assistant to be able to obtain a pulse rate from any of the alternative sites.

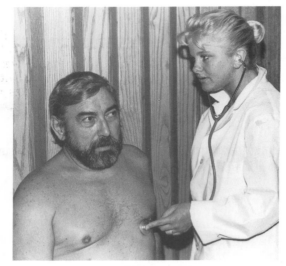

Figure 25–6
The stethoscope is placed at the apex of the heart for the apical heart rate. The specific anatomic location is the left intercostal space, between the fifth and sixth ribs, at the midpoint of the left clavicle.

Determining the Pulse Rate

The patient should be in a comfortable position, with the artery to be used at the same level or lower than the heart. The limb should be well supported and relaxed. The patient may be lying down or sitting. As with all pulse readings, the pads of your first three fingers are placed over the artery with slight pressure. The pulse is counted for one minute, and any irregularities or variations from the normal quality, such as **arrhythmias** or **pulses** that are **thready**, **elastic**, **intermittent**, **irregular**, **bounding**, or **unequal** are noted and recorded. Some pulses are more difficult to feel than are others, and the correct pressures to be used for each patient and site require practice and experience. Both you and your patient should be in relaxed positions. The sensitivity in your counting fingers is greatly reduced if you are in an awkward position. Too much pressure obliterates the patient's pulse and too little pressure prevents detection of irregularities or all of the beats. Record the number of beats counted in one minute. If the pulse rate is counted at any site other than the radius, the site should be recorded.

RESPIRATION RATE

One complete inhalation and exhalation is called a respiration. The normal adult respiration rate is 16 to 20 respirations per minute. The respiration rate is usually in proportion to the pulse rate, at the ratio 1:4. It is somewhat slower in older persons and faster in infants and children. The respiration rate generally increases as the body temperature rises. Examples of the respiration, pulse, and temperature ratios follow.

Respiration	Pulse	Temperature
16	64	98.6°F
20	80	99.0°F
24	96	101.0°F
28	112	104.0°F

Variations occur in the respiratory rate (fast or slow), volume (deep or shallow), and rhythm (regular or irregular) (Fig. 25–7). There are specific medical terms to describe the character of a person's breathing. Dyspnea, meaning difficult breathing, occurs in patients with pneumonia or asthma. It also occurs after physical exertion or at very high altitudes. Other alterations in breathing are bradypnea (abnormally slow respiration), apnea (temporary cessation of respiration), tachypnea (excessively rapid breathing), and hyperpnea (increased depth of breathing). Hyperpnea is usually accompanied by **hyperventilation** and is frequently found in emotional conditions. Orthopnea is difficulty in breathing while lying down, as found in patients with congestive heart failure.

Counting Respirations

Because the respiration rate is easily controlled and patients self-consciously alter their breathing rates when they are being watched, it is best to count the respirations while appearing to count the pulse. Keep your eyes alternately on the patient's

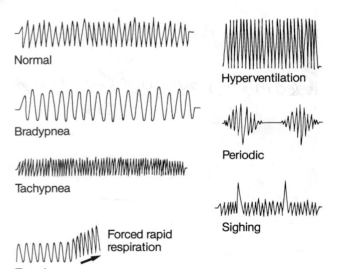

Figure 25–7
Various breathing patterns called spirograms, which are recorded by a spirometer.

chest and your watch while you are counting the pulse rate, and then, without removing your fingers from the pulse site, determine the respiration rate. It may be easier to count the respirations first, as that number is not as hard to remember. If the patient is lying down, the arm may be crossed over the chest so the respirations can be felt with the rise and fall of the chest. Count the respirations for one minute, noting any variation or irregularity in the rate. Record both the pulse and respiration counts on the medical record at the same time.

The pulse and respiration rates are usually counted while an oral temperature is being obtained. Doing the three procedures together is very efficient, and the patient cannot distract you with conversation. After recording the pulse and respiration counts, remove the thermometer and record that reading.

Procedure 25–1

DETERMINING ORAL TEMPERATURE, PULSE RATE, AND RATE OF RESPIRATION

25

PROCEDURAL GOAL

5 minutes

To determine and record a patient's temperature, pulse rate, and rate of respiration, as part of the assessment of the patient's general physical condition.

EQUIPMENT AND SUPPLIES

An oral thermometer with a Fahrenheit scale
A supply of tissues
A watch with a second hand
Nonsterile gloves

PROCEDURE

1. Wash your hands. Follow universal blood and body-fluid precautions (see Appendix C). Glove yourself with nonsterile gloves.
2. Introduce yourself and correctly identify the patient (below left).
   Purpose: To make sure you have the right patient.

ORAL TEMPERATURE
3. Rinse a clinical thermometer under cool running water, letting the water run from the bulb to the stem (below right).
   Purpose: To remove antiseptic solution, which may produce a bitter taste.

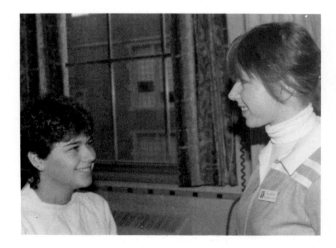
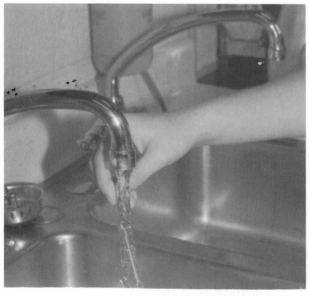

Procedure continued on following page

4. Shake down the thermometer, allowing yourself enough room so that you do not strike it on an object and break it (below left).
   Purpose: To allow the column of mercury to fall to 95°F or lower.
5. If you are not gloved, ask the patient to open the mouth and to place the thermometer under their own tongue. Then ask the patient to keep the lips firmly closed and to breathe through the nose (below right).
   Purpose: Air seeping into the mouth will interfere with an accurate body temperature reading.

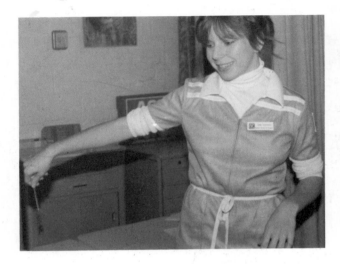 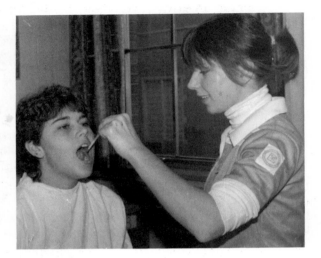

6. Advise the patient that the thermometer needs to be held in place for at least five minutes (below left).
   Purpose: The mouth is an area where air may enter, so it is necessary to extend the time for an accurate reading.

count fast

PULSE

It is advisable to count the patient's pulse and respirations while the thermometer is in the patient's mouth. You may wish to reverse the steps of this procedure and count the patient's respirations before the pulse, as the respiration number is easier to remember.

7. Turn the patient's palm downward in a relaxed position.
   Purpose: The patient's radial artery is more easily palpated when the patient is relaxed and in this position.
8. Gently grasp the palm side of the patient's wrist with your first three fingertips, just over the radius (below right).
   Purpose: If you press too hard, your patient's artery will be occluded, and you will feel no pulse.

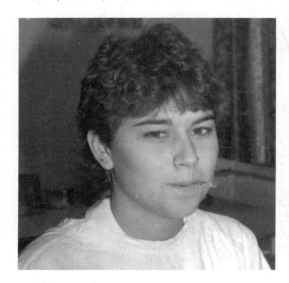 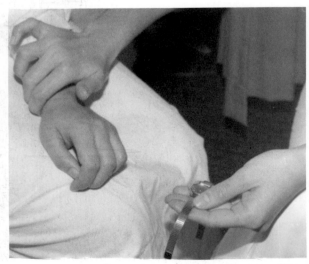

Procedure continued on opposite page

9. Count the beats for one full minute, using a watch with a second hand.
   Purpose: Counting for the full minute allows you to obtain an accurate count, including any irregularities in rhythm and volume.
10. Remember the count and any irregularities so that you can note it later, on the patient's medical record. Leave your fingers on the patient's pulse site and proceed to the respirations count.
    Purpose: Patients should not know that you are counting their respirations.

RESPIRATIONS

If you have not counted the patient's respirations before the pulse count, the respirations count should be taken immediately following the pulse count and while the thermometer is still in the patient's mouth.

11. Count the respirations for one full minute, using a watch with a second hand.
    Purpose: Counting for the full minute allows you to obtain an accurate count, including any irregularities in rhythm or depth or unusual breathing such as apnea or dyspnea.
12. Release the patient's wrist, and record the pulse and respirations findings on the patient's medical record.
13. Follow universal blood and body fluid precautions. Apply gloves, remove the thermometer, and wipe it dry from stem to bulb with a tissue (below top).
    Purpose: Wiping with a tissue cleans the surface for visibility and prevents cross-contamination.
14. Read the thermometer, making certain that you hold it at eye level. Look for the silver column of mercury, and follow it until it ends. Align the end of the column to the scale marked in degrees (below bottom).
    Purpose: Holding the thermometer at eye level facilitates an easier and more accurate reading.

25

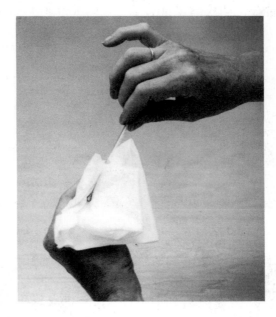

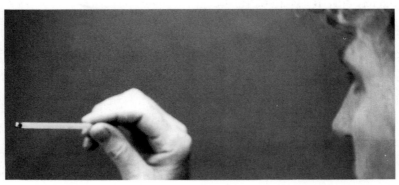

Procedure continued on following page

15. Shake down the mercury column to 95°F.

16. Rinse the thermometer in cool running water, then soak it in a separate soap solution. Later, you will sanitize and rinse the thermometer, and then sterilize it by soaking it in a chemical sterilant for an amount of time prescribed by the manufacturer. After complete sterilization, dried thermometers may be stored in a dry container or in containers of antiseptic solution (below).
Purpose: Thermometers must be thoroughly sterilized and dried before being returned to their containers for use with another patient.

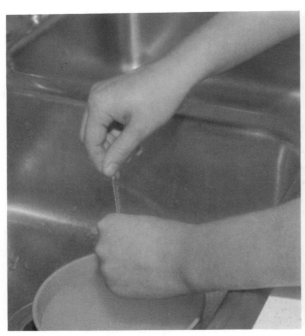 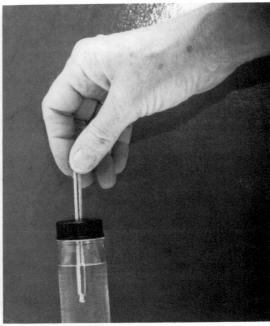

17. Discard gloves, and record the temperature reading on the patient's medical record. Remember to include the method if it is part of the accepted procedure.

18. Unless otherwise instructed, record the temperature first, then the pulse, then the respirations, for example, T—98.6 (degrees), P—72, R—16. It may be abbreviated: 98.6—72—16.

TERMINAL PERFORMANCE OBJECTIVE

Given a patient and the necessary equipment, obtain and record a patient's oral temperature within ±0.2°F of your evaluator's reading, a pulse rate within ±2 beats of your evaluator's count, and a respirations rate within ±1 count of your evaluator's count, within seven minutes, while observing the principles of medical asepsis, patient safety, and good communication.

Procedure 25-2

DETERMINING AN ADULT'S TEMPERATURE RECTALLY

2 minutes

PROCEDURAL GOAL

To determine a patient's temperature rectally when requested by the physician.

EQUIPMENT AND SUPPLIES

A rectal thermometer with a Fahrenheit or centigrade scale
A supply of tissues or gauze squares
A tube of lubricant
Nonsterile gloves

PROCEDURE

1. Wash your hands. Follow universal blood and body-fluid precautions (see Appendix C). Glove yourself with nonsterile gloves.
2. Introduce yourself and correctly identify the patient.
   Purpose: To make sure you have the right patient.
3. Rinse a rectal clinical thermometer under cool running water, letting the water run from the bulb to the stem.
   Purpose: To remove antiseptic solution, which may be irritating to the rectal mucosa.
4. Shake down the thermometer, allowing yourself enough room so that you do not strike it on an object and break it.
   Purpose: To allow the column of mercury to fall to 95°F (35°C) or lower.
5. Squeeze a small amount of a water-soluble lubricant or oil-based jelly onto the tissue or gauze.
   Purpose: Putting the thermometer directly into the lubricant container will contaminate the rest of the lubricant.
6. Lubricate the bulb end of the rectal thermometer.
   Purpose: Lubrication removes some of the danger of injuring the mucous membrane of the patient's rectum.
7. Position the patient prone or in the Sims position, and drape appropriately.
8. Gently lift or push aside the buttock, and insert the thermometer into the rectum to about 1 to 1½ in.
   Purpose: Careful and correct placement avoids injury to the mucosa of the bowel.
9. Hold the thermometer in place for two minutes, being certain to keep your hand on the thermometer.
   Purpose: To protect the patient from being injured by the thermometer.
10. Remove the thermometer, and wipe dry from stem to bulb with a tissue.
    Purpose: Wiping with a tissue cleans the surface for visibility and prevents cross-contamination.
11. Read the thermometer, making certain that you hold it at eye level. Look for the silver column of mercury, and follow it until it ends. Align the end of the column to the scale marked in degrees.
    Purpose: Holding the thermometer at eye level facilitates an easier and more accurate reading.
12. Read and record the rectal temperature on the patient's medical record, for example, 99.6 (R) or 37.5 (R).
13. Shake down the mercury column to 95°F (35°C).
14. Rinse the thermometer in cool running water, then soak it in a separate soap solution. Later, you will sanitize and rinse the thermometer, and then sterilize it by soaking it in a chemical sterilant for an amount of time prescribed by the manufacturer. After complete sterilization, dried thermometers may be stored in a dry container or in containers of antiseptic solution.
    Purpose: Thermometers must be thoroughly sterilized and dried before being returned to their containers for use with another patient.

TERMINAL PERFORMANCE OBJECTIVE

Given a patient and the necessary supplies, determine and record the patient's rectal temperature, within three minutes, adhering to acceptable principles of medical asepsis, patient safety, and good communication, within ±0.2°F or ±0.1°C of your evaluator's reading.

Procedure 25-3

DETERMINING AN ADULT'S TEMPERATURE BY THE AXILLARY METHOD

10 minutes

PROCEDURAL GOAL

To determine a patient's temperature using the axillary method when requested by the physician.

EQUIPMENT AND SUPPLIES

A clinical thermometer with a Fahrenheit or centigrade scale (security-tipped or rectal bulb type is recommended)
A supply of tissues or gauze squares
Soap, water, and a towel to wash and dry the axilla
An alcohol sponge
Nonsterile gloves

PROCEDURE

1. Wash your hands. Follow universal blood and body-fluid precautions (see Appendix C). Glove yourself with nonsterile gloves.
2. Introduce yourself and correctly identify the patient.
   Purpose: To make sure you have the right patient.
3. Rinse a short-bulbed clinical thermometer under cool running water, letting the water run from the bulb to the stem.
   Purpose: To remove antiseptic solution, which may be irritating to the patient's skin.
4. Shake down the thermometer, allowing yourself enough room so that you do not strike it on an object and break it.
   Purpose: To allow the column of mercury to fall to 95°F (35°C) or lower.
5. Set the thermometer in a safe place on tissue or a gauze square.
6. Wash the patient's axilla.
7. Wipe with an alcohol sponge.
   Purpose: Alcohol quickens drying by evaporation.
8. Place the bulb of the thermometer into the center of the armpit, pointing the stem to the upper chest.
9. Instruct the patient to hold the arm tightly against the ribs with the other hand.
10. Advise the patient that the thermometer needs to be held in place for at least ten minutes.
    Purpose: The axilla is an area where air may enter, so it is necessary to extend the time for an accurate reading.
11. Remove the thermometer, and wipe dry from stem to bulb with a tissue.
    Purpose: Wiping with a tissue cleans the surface for visibility and prevents cross-contamination.
12. Read the thermometer, making certain that you hold it at eye level. Look for the silver column of mercury, and follow it until it ends. Align the end of the column to the scale marked in degrees.
    Purpose: Holding the thermometer at eye level facilitates an easier and more accurate reading.
13. Read and record the axillary temperature on the patient's medical record; for example, 99.6 (A) or 37.5 (A).
14. Shake down the mercury column to 95°F (35°C).
15. Rinse the thermometer in cool running water, then soak it in a separate soap solution. Later, you will sanitize and rinse the thermometer, and then sterilize it by soaking it in a chemical solution for an amount of time prescribed by the manufacturer. After complete sterilization, dried thermometers may be stored in a dry container or in containers of antiseptic solution.
    Purpose: Thermometers must be thoroughly sterilized and dried before being returned to their containers for use with another patient.

TERMINAL PERFORMANCE OBJECTIVE

Given a patient and the necessary supplies, determine and record the patient's axillary temperature, within 11 minutes, adhering to acceptable principles of medical asepsis, patient safety, and good communication, within ±0.2°F or ±0.1°C of your evaluator's reading.

Procedure 25–4

DETERMINING A CHILD'S TEMPERATURE RECTALLY

PROCEDURAL GOAL

To determine a child's temperature rectally when requested by the physician.

EQUIPMENT AND SUPPLIES

A rectal thermometer with a Fahrenheit or centigrade scale
A supply of tissues or gauze squares
A tube of lubricant
Nonsterile gloves

PROCEDURE

1. Wash your hands. Follow universal blood and body-fluid precautions (see Appendix C). Glove yourself with nonsterile gloves.
2. Introduce yourself to the parents and correctly identify the child-patient.
   Purpose: To make sure you have the right patient.
3. Rinse a rectal clinical thermometer under cool running water, letting the water run from the bulb to the stem.
   Purpose: To remove antiseptic solution, which may be irritating to the rectal mucosa.
4. Shake down the thermometer, away from the child and allowing yourself enough room so that you do not strike it on an object and break it.
   Purpose: To protect the child from injury and the equipment from possible breakage.
5. Squeeze a small amount of a water-soluble lubricant or oil-based jelly onto the tissue or gauze.
   Purpose: Putting the thermometer directly into the lubricant container will contaminate the rest of the lubricant.
6. Lubricate the bulb end of the rectal thermometer.
   Purpose: Lubrication removes some of the danger of injuring the mucous membrane of the patient's rectum.
7. Position the child on the back with the legs up in the air, and hold the thermometer in place with your hand (bottom left).

Or

Position the child in the prone position, with one hand at the buttocks and the other hand holding the thermometer in place (bottom right).

25

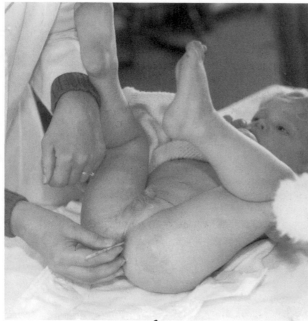

infants

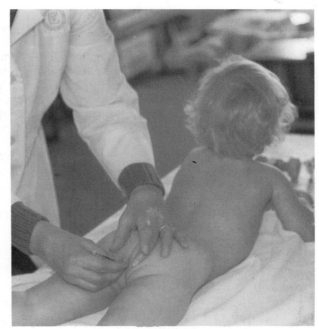

child

Procedure continued on following page

8. Gently push aside the buttock and insert the thermometer into the rectum to about 1 to 1½ in.
   Purpose: Careful and correct placement avoids injury to the mucosa of the bowel.
9. Hold the thermometer in place for two minutes, being certain to keep your hand on the thermometer.
   Purpose: To protect the patient from being injured by the thermometer.
10. Remove the thermometer, and wipe dry from stem to bulb with a tissue.
    Purpose: Wiping with a tissue cleans the surface for visibility and prevents cross-contamination.
11. Read the thermometer, making certain that you hold it at eye level. Look for the silver column of mercury, and follow it until it ends. Align the end of the column to the scale marked in degrees.
    Purpose: Holding the thermometer at eye level facilitates an easier and more accurate reading.
12. Read and record the rectal temperature on the patient's medical record; for example, 99.6 (R), or 37.5 (R).
13. Shake down the mercury column to 95°F (35°C).
14. Rinse the thermometer in cool running water, then soak in a separate soap solution. Later, you will sanitize and rinse the thermometer, and then sterilize it by soaking it in a chemical sterilant for an amount of time prescribed by the manufacturer. After complete sterilization, dried thermometers may be stored in a dry container, or in containers of antiseptic solution.
    Purpose: Thermometers must be thoroughly sterilized and dried before being returned to their containers for use with another patient.

TERMINAL PERFORMANCE OBJECTIVE

Given a child-patient and the necessary supplies, determine and record the patient's rectal temperature, within three minutes, adhering to acceptable principles of medical asepsis, patient safety, and good communication, within ±0.2°F or ±0.1°C of your evaluator's reading.

BLOOD PRESSURE

Blood pressure is the pressure of the blood against the walls of the arteries. This pressure is determined by the pumping action of the heart, the resistance of the blood's flow through the arteries, the elasticity of the arterial walls, the amount of blood in the vessels, and the blood's viscosity (thickness). Because of these influencing factors, there are actually two blood pressure readings. The *systolic* pressure is the highest pressure level that occurs when the heart is contracting and the pulse beat is felt. The diastolic pressure is the lowest pressure level when the heart is relaxed and no pulse beat is felt. *Systole* (heart contraction) and *diastole* (heart relaxation) together make up the *cardiac cycle*.

Blood pressure is read in millimeters of mercury, abbreviated mm Hg. However, the abbreviations are not necessary when recording the reading on the patient's medical record. Blood pressure is recorded as a fraction, with the systolic reading the numerator (top) and the diastolic reading the denominator (bottom), for example, 130/80. The average normal blood pressures follow.

The male adult may have a reading slightly higher than that of the female adult. A child's reading is usually lower than an adult's. Older persons may have a slightly higher reading. A reading of 150/90 mm Hg may be considered a normal reading for a patient 60 years of age. The numeric difference between the systolic reading and the diastolic reading is called the *pulse pressure*. Blood pressure during quiet rest or basal conditions is called *basic*, or *basal*, blood pressure.

When tracking a patient's blood pressure, frequent readings should be taken about the same time of day and by the same person. *Normotension* is the term for normal blood pressure. A person is said to have *hypertension* (elevated blood pressure) if the pressure is persistently above normal. Hypertension may have no known cause (essential hypertension), or it may be associated with some other disease (secondary hypertension). Essential hypertension is common among Americans. Secondary hypertension often accompanies renal diseases, pregnancy, endocrine imbalances, obesity, **arteriosclerosis**, **atherosclerosis**, and brain injuries. Temporary hypertension may occur with stress, pain and exercise.

Hypertension has been called the silent disease because it has no symptoms, and persons may go for long periods of time without knowing that they have a problem. Often, hypertension is discovered by accident during the medical or dental treatment of another problem. Long-term, untreated hypertension is suspected to be a major cause of strokes.

		Adults Over 18 Years of Age		
	Children	NORMAL	HIGH NORMAL	HYPERTENSION
Systolic	Not established	Up to 140	130–139	Over 140
Diastolic	Not established	Up to 90	80–89	Over 90

Hypotension is abnormally low blood pressure and may be caused by shock, both emotional and traumatic; hemorrhage; central nervous system disorders; and chronic wasting diseases. Persistent readings of 90/60 mm Hg or below are usually considered hypotensive. *Orthostatic*, or *postural*, hypotension is the temporary fall in blood pressure that occurs when a person rapidly changes from a recumbent position to a standing position or when a person stands motionless in a fixed position, such as standing at attention. Some medications can cause orthostatic hypotension. The patient may feel suddenly dizzy and have blurred vision or may actually faint.

Measuring Blood Pressure

The instrument used to measure blood pressure is called the sphygmomanometer. The term manometer refers to an instrument used to measure the pressure of a liquid or a gas. Sphygmo means pulse. Thus, sphygmomanometer means an instrument used for measuring blood pressure in the arteries. The instrument consists of an inflatable cuff, an inflatable bulb with a control valve, and a pressure gauge. There are two common types of pressure gauges: the mercury column (Fig. 25–8*A*) and the aneroid dial (Fig. 25–8*B*). Sphygmomanometers are delicately calibrated instruments and must be handled carefully. They should be re-calibrated regularly, either by you or a medical supply dealer. Check your sphygmomanometers for accuracy. The recording needle on the aneroid dial sphygmomanometer should rest within the small square at the bottom of the dial. The **meniscus** of mercury on the mercury column sphygmomanometer should rest at zero (0). Inexpensive models are available in drug stores and retail stores for patients to use to measure their own blood pressure at home. More sophisticated electronic and computerized sphygmomanometers are also available for home use.

The sphygmomanometer must be used with a stethoscope. The objective of the procedure is to use the inflatable cuff to obliterate (cause to disappear) circulation through an artery, similar to using a tourniquet. The stethoscope is placed over the artery just under the cuff, and then the cuff is slowly deflated to allow the blood to flow again. As blood flow is resumed, the cardiac cycle sounds may be heard again through the stethoscope, and gauge readings are taken when the first and last sounds are heard.

25

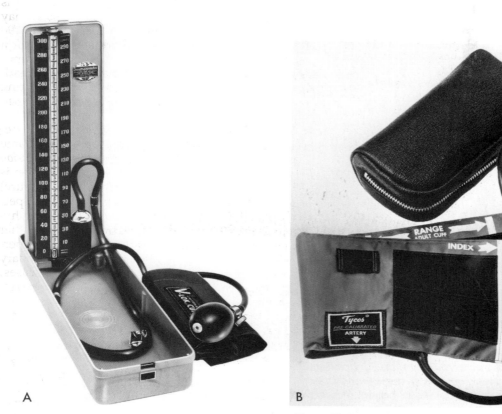

A

B

Figure 25–8

A, *Baum mercury manometer. (Courtesy of Baum Co.)* **B**, *Tycos aneroid manometer. (Courtesy of Tycos Co.)*

Heart Sounds. These are the two basic sounds produced by the functioning of the heart during the cardiac cycle. The first sound produced at systole (contraction) is dull, firm, and prolonged and is heard as a "lubb" sound. The second sound, produced at diastole (relaxation) when the heart valves close, is shorter and sharper and is heard as a "dupp" sound. The "lubb–dupp" is the sound of one heartbeat.

Korotkoff Sounds. The Korotkoff sounds are the sounds heard during the measurement of blood pressure. These sounds are thought to be produced by the vibrations of the arterial wall as the wall suddenly distends when compressed by the blood pressure cuff. However, it has not been determined whether the sounds come from within the wall itself or from the blood passing through the vessel. The sounds were first discovered and classified into five distinct phases by Nicolai Sergeevich Korotkoff, a Russian neurologist.

Phase I. This is the first sound heard as the cuff deflates. The blood is resurging into the patient's artery and can be heard quite clearly as a sharp, tapping sound. Note the gauge reading when this first sound is heard. Record this as the *systolic pressure.*

Phase II. As the cuff deflates, even more blood flows through the artery. The movement of the blood makes a swishing sound. If proper procedure is not followed in inflating the cuff, these sounds may not be heard because of their soft quality. Occasionally, blood pressure sounds completely disappear during this phase. The loss of the sounds and their reappearance later is called the *auscultatory gap.* The silence may continue as the needle or the column of mercury falls another 30 mm Hg. Auscultatory gaps occur particularly in hypertension and certain heart diseases. So, if you notice such a gap, be certain to report it to the physician.

Phase III. A great deal of blood is now pushing down into the artery. The distinct, sharp tapping sounds return and continue rhythmically. If you do not inflate the cuff enough, you will miss the first two phases completely, and you will incorrectly interpret the beginning of phase III as the systolic blood pressure (phase I).

Phase IV. At this point, the blood is flowing easily. The sound changes to a soft tapping, which becomes muffled and begins to grow fainter. Occasionally, these sounds continue to zero (0). This may occur in children, after exercise, with a fever, or in pregnancy if anemia is present. The American Heart Association recommends that the beginning of phase IV be recorded as the diastolic reading for a child. Some physicians call the change at phase IV the "fading sound" and want it recorded between the systolic and the diastolic recordings (for example, 120/84/70, with the "84" representing the gauge reading when the sounds of phase III have ended and those of phase IV are beginning. Other physicians consider phase IV the true diastolic pressure.

Phase V. All sounds disappear in this phase. Note the gauge reading when the last sound is heard. Record this as the *diastolic pressure.*

Procedure 25–5

DETERMINING A PATIENT'S BLOOD PRESSURE

PROCEDURAL GOAL

To perform a blood pressure measurement that is correct in technique, accurate, and not uncomfortable to the patient.

EQUIPMENT AND SUPPLIES

Sphygmomanometer
Stethoscope
Antiseptic sponges

PROCEDURE

1. Wash your hands.
2. Clean the ear pieces and diaphragm of the stethoscope with the antiseptic sponges (facing page, top left).
3. Introduce yourself and correctly identify the patient.
   Purpose: To make sure you have the right patient.
4. Observe the patient for signs of anxiety or distress.
   Purpose: An anxious or distressed patient may have a falsely high blood pressure reading.
5. Explain what you are about to do (facing page, top right).
   Purpose: Your manner and approach may relax the patient.

Procedure continued on opposite page

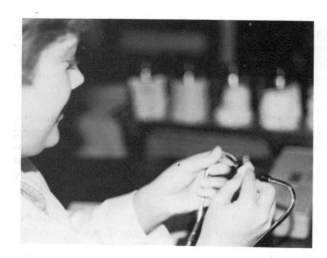
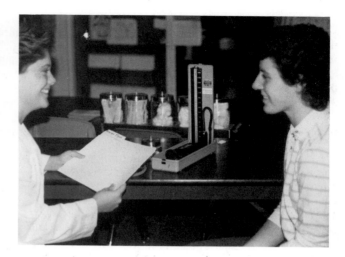

25

6. Seat the patient for at least five minutes, legs uncrossed and feet flat on the floor. The patient may be placed in the supine position.

7. Palpate the brachial and radial arteries simultaneously. Palpate both right and left arms. If one arm has a stronger pulse, use that arm. If the pulse is equal, select the right arm.
   Purpose: A stronger pulse will be easier to measure. If both are equal, selecting the right arm is the universal method.

8. Determine the correct cuff size.
   Purpose: An incorrect cuff size will prevent accurate measurement of the blood pressure.

9. Support the patient's arm at heart level or lower and roll the sleeve to about 5 in above the elbow. If the sleeve is too tight, remove the clothing.
   Purpose: Tight clothing will constrict the brachial artery and interfere with an accurate reading.

10. Center the cuff bladder over the brachial artery, with the connecting tube away from the patient's body and the tube to the bulb close to the body.

11. Place the lower edge of the cuff with the tubing connections about 1 in above the natural crease of the inner elbow.

12. Wrap the cuff snugly and smoothly.

13. Attach the sphygmomanometer tubes to the cuff (below).

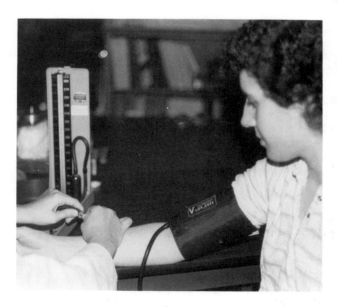

14. Position the gauge of the sphygmomanometer so that it is at eye level.
    Purpose: Instruments can be read accurately only at eye level.

Procedure continued on following page

15. While palpating the radial pulse, observe the gauge and inflate the cuff until you can no longer feel the pulse. Then deflate the cuff, and mentally add 30 mm to the reading where you lost the pulse.
    Purpose: This is to determine the maximum inflation level needed to find phase I of the Korotkoff sounds.

16. Check the pulse rate for one minute.
    Purpose: You will need to wait one to two minutes between any inflations of the cuff. Take the time to determine the patient's pulse rate.

17. Insert the ear pieces, turned down and forward, into your ears.

18. Straighten all tubing.
    Purpose: Knocking the tubings together can produce sounds that will interfere with hearing the Korotkoff sounds.

19. Palpate the brachial artery, and place the stethoscope diaphragm over the artery firmly enough to obtain a seal but not so tight that the artery is constricted. The diaphragm should be just below, but not touching, the cuff or tubing (below left).

20. Close the valve, and squeeze the bulb to inflate the cuff at a rapid but smooth rate to the maximum inflation level that was previously determined. This process should take seven to ten seconds.

21. Open the valve slightly, and deflate the cuff at the constant rate of 2 mm Hg per second (below right).
    Purpose: Careful, slow release will allow you to listen to all the sounds.

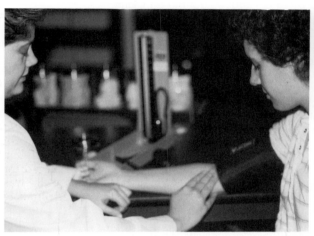 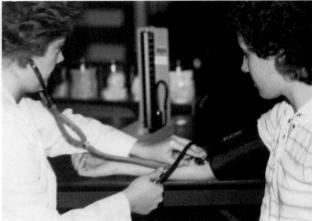

22. Listen throughout the entire range of deflation until the sounds have stopped for at least 10 mm Hg.

23. Remove the stethoscope from your ears, and record the systolic and diastolic readings as BP 120/80.

24. If you are uncertain of your reading, release the air from the cuff. Wait one to two minutes, then repeat the process.
    Purpose: You must wait this time to allow the circulatory congestion to dissipate.

25. Remove the cuff from the patient's arm. Disconnect the tubes from the cuff, and place the equipment back in the sphygmomanometer box (below).

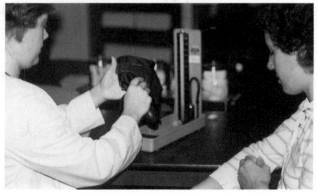

Procedure continued on opposite page

26. Sanitize the ear pieces of the stethoscope.
27. Help the patient with any clothing adjustment.
28. Alert the physician to any unusually high or low readings or any other unusual findings.

TERMINAL PERFORMANCE OBJECTIVE

Given a patient and the supplies listed, determine a patient's blood pressure within ±4 mm Hg of your evaluator's reading, within five minutes, and record the reading on the patient's medical history with 100 percent accuracy.

COMMON CAUSES OF ERRORS

1. The limb being used is not at the same level as the heart. (It is not necessary for the manometer to be at the same level as the heart.)
2. The rubber bladder in the cuff has not been completely deflated before starting or retaking a reading.
3. The mercury column is allowed to drop too rapidly, resulting in an inaccurate reading.
4. The patient is nervous, uncomfortable, or too anxious, which may cause a reading higher than the patient's actual blood pressure.
5. The cuff is improperly applied:
   a. The cuff is too large or too small (Fig. 25–9)
   b. The cuff is not around the arm smoothly.
   c. The cuff is too loose or too tight.
   d. The bladder is not centered over the artery.
   e. The rubber bladder bulges out from the cover.
6. Failing to wait one to two minutes between measurements.
7. Defective instruments:
   a. Air leaks in the valve.
   b. Air leaks in the bladder.
   c. Dirty mercury column.
   d. Mercury column or aneroid needle that is not calibrated to zero.

Palpatory Method. The systolic pressure may be checked by feeling the radial pulse rather than hearing (auscultatory method) it with the stethoscope. Place the cuff in the usual position and palpate the radial pulse, noting the rate and rhythm. Now inflate the cuff until the pulse disappears, and then add 30 mm more of inflation to get above the systolic pressure. Do not remove your fingers from the pulse or change the pressure of your fingers. Now, slowly release the pressure in the cuff, and wait for the pulse to be felt again. Note the reading on the gauge, and record the first pulse felt as the systolic pressure. The diastolic and the Korotkoff phases cannot be determined by this

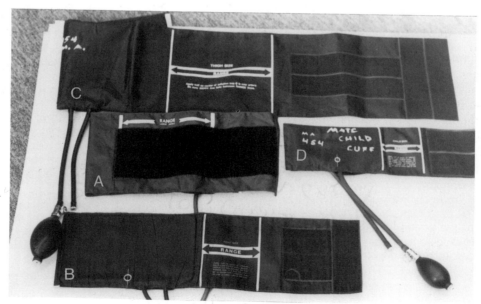

Figure 25–9
*Several sizes of blood pressure cuffs. **A,** Regular-sized adult cuff. **B,** Large-sized adult cuff, for the muscular or obese arm. **C,** Thigh-sized cuff, which may be used on the upper leg or the muscular or obese arm. **D,** Child-sized cuff, for small children and adults with very thin arms.*

method, and its use, other than in combination with the auscultatory method, is not recommended.

MEASURING HEIGHT AND WEIGHT

The patient's height and weight are often helpful in diagnosis, and the medical assistant must determine these readings with accuracy and empathy. Some patients are sensitive or secretive about their body weight. Your manner and approach are very important in keeping many patients from feeling embarrassed or shy.

The location of the scale should be considered. Whether your patients are obese, petite persons who do not want their weight known to others, or handicapped with appliances that must be removed, make certain that your office scale is placed in an area of privacy.

It is not necessary to remove shoes and clothing if patients are consistently weighed and measured with them on. Although the exact weight and height may not be determined, changes in the patient's weight and height can be detected and analyzed.

Do not comment on a patient's progress in a weight program; this is the physician's or counselor's responsibility. When the physician prescribes weight measurement at home, make certain that the patient understands the importance of weighing himself or herself each day at the same time in clothing of similar weight. Body weight may vary considerably from early morning to late afternoon. Teach the patient how to record the weight on a graphic record and how to make any other important notations. (For a chart of suggested normal weights, see Chapter 21).

Procedure 25–6

MEASURING A PATIENT'S HEIGHT AND WEIGHT

PROCEDURAL GOAL

To accurately weigh and measure a patient as part of the pre-examination process.

EQUIPMENT AND SUPPLIES

A balance scale with a measuring bar
Paper towels

PROCEDURE

1. Wash your hands.
2. Introduce yourself and correctly identify the patient.
3. Explain what you are about to do.
   Purpose: Your manner and approach may relax the patient.

WEIGHT

4. Place a paper towel on the scale.
   Purpose: To prevent cross-contamination.
5. If the scale is not at zero (0), return all weights of the scale to zero (0), and check to see that the balance bar pointer floats in the middle of the balance frame (facing page top).
   Purpose: A floating pointer indicates that the scale is properly adjusted and in balance.
6. Help the patient onto the scale on the paper towel. The patient's weight on the scale will now throw the balance bar off balance. The pointer will tilt to the top of the balance frame (facing page bottom).
7. Move the large lower weight into the groove closest to the estimated weight of the patient. The grooves are calibrated in 50-lb increments. If you choose a groove that is more than the patient's weight, the pointer will immediately tilt to the bottom of the balance frame. You have gone too far. Go back one groove.
   Purpose: To adjust the weights until the pointer floats in the middle of the frame.

Procedure continued on opposite page

25

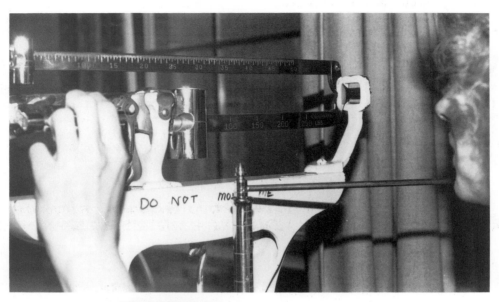

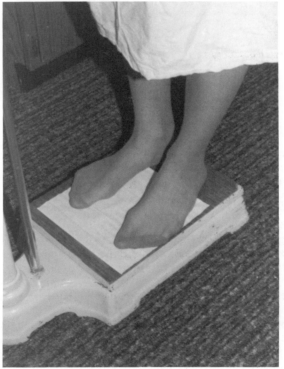

Procedure continued on following page

8. Ask the patient to stand still, and slide the small upper weight to the right along the ¼-lb markers until the pointer balances in the middle of the balance frame.
   Purpose: The pointer will float between the bottom and the top of the frame when both the lower and the upper scale weights together balance the scale with the patient's weight. Leave the weights in their places.

Add two Number Together

HEIGHT
9. Ask the patient to stand tall and to look straight ahead.
10. Adjust the height bar so that it just touches the top of the patient's head. Leave the bar as set.

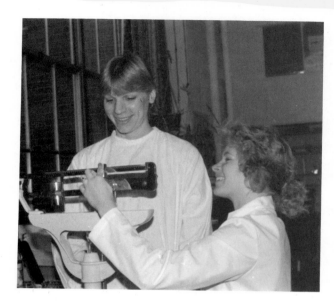

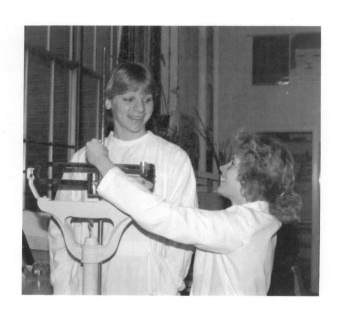

11. Assist the patient off the scale and with dressing, if necessary.
12. Read the weight scale. Add the numbers at the markers of the large and small weights, and record the total, to the nearest ¼ lb, on the patient's medical record (for example, Wt 102¾).
13. Record the height. Read the marker at the movable point of the ruler, and record the measurement, to the nearest quarter inch, on the patient's medical record (for example, Ht 64¼).
14. Return the weights to zero (0), and return the measuring bar to zero (0).

TERMINAL PERFORMANCE OBJECTIVE

Given a patient and the equipment and supplies listed, determine the weight and height of the patient, within two minutes, and within ±¼ lb and ¼ in of your evaluator's measurements.

Divide 64¼ by 12

Height

6 Ft = 72 inches

$$\frac{5 \ R4 \ \times \frac{1}{4} \ inches}{12 \overline{|64|}}$$
$$\frac{60}{4}$$

REFERENCES AND READINGS

Bates, B.: *A Guide to Physical Examination*, 2nd ed. Philadelphia, J. B. Lippincott Co., 1981.

Bonewit, K.: *Clinical Procedures for Medical Assistants*, 2nd ed. Philadelphia, W. B. Saunders Co., 1984.

Diekelmann, N. et al.: *Fundamentals of Nursing*. New York, McGraw-Hill, 1980.

DuGas, B. W.: *Introduction to Patient Care: A Comprehensive Approach to Nursing*, 4th ed. Philadelphia, W. B. Saunders Co., 1983.

Jarvis, C. M.: Vital signs: how to take them more accurately and understand them more fully. *Nursing '76*, April, pp. 31–37, 1976.

Kirkendall, W. M.: *Recommendations for Human Blood Pressure Determination by Sphygmomanometers*, Report of a Subcommittee of the Postgraduate Education Committee of AHA. Dallas, American Heart Association, 1980.

Lancour, J.: How to avoid pitfalls in measuring blood pressure. *American Journal of Nursing* 76:773, 1976.

Macleod, J. (ed.): *Clinical Examination: A Textbook for Students and Doctors by Teachers of the Edinburgh Medical School*, 4th ed. Edinburgh/London, Churchill Livingstone, 1976.

Sorensen, K. C., and Luckmann, J.: *Basic Nursing: A Psychophysiologic Approach*, 2nd ed. Philadelphia, W. B. Saunders Co., 1986.

Wood, L. A., and Rambo, B. J.: *Nursing Skills for Allied Health Services*, Vol. 2, 2nd ed. Philadelphia, W. B. Saunders Co., 1977.

25

CHAPTER OUTLINE

History and Background
- Drug Sources
- Drug Names
- Drug Regulation

Drug Interactions With the Body
- Uses of Drugs
- Fate of Drugs
- Factors That Influence the Effect of a Drug
- Classifications of Drug Actions

Approaches to Studying Pharmacology
- Reference Materials
- Learning About Drugs

Calculating Drug Dosages for Administration
- Mathematical Equivalents
- Ratio and Proportion
- Calculating Dosages
- Systems of Measurement
- Pediatric Dose Calculations
  - Procedure 26–1: Calculating the Correct Dosage For Administration
  - Procedure 26–2: Calculating the Correct Dosage For Administration Using Two Systems of Measurement
  - Procedure 26–3: Calculating the Correct Dosage For a Child When Only an Adult Medication is Available

VOCABULARY

See Glossary at end of book for definitions.

angina pectoris
cardiotonic
ion
nomogram
permeability

26

Introduction to Clinical Pharmacology

OBJECTIVES

Upon successful completion of this chapter you should be able to

1. Spell and define the words listed in the Vocabulary for this chapter.
2. List the six ethical and legal responsibilities in administering medications.
3. Differentiate between a drug's generic name and trade name.
4. Cite three dangers of using over-the-counter drugs.
5. List the information needed in each of the four parts of a prescription.
6. Cite the DEA regulations for prescription drugs under each of the five Schedules of the 1970 Controlled Substances Act.
7. Define three types of drug dependency.
8. Cite five clinical uses of drugs.
9. List, in order, the five steps that describe the fate of a drug in the human body.
10. Cite ten factors that influence the effect a drug may have on the body.
11. Recall at least ten terms that classify drugs according to their actions on the body.
12. Describe the use of the Physicians' Desk Reference.

Upon successful completion of this chapter you should be able to perform the following activity:

1. Given various medication orders and available medications packaged in different strengths, apply standard dosage calculation formulas to calculate correct dosages to be administered to patients.

This chapter provides an overview and an introduction to the basic concepts of clinical pharmacology. *Pharmacology* is the broad science that deals with the origin, nature, chemistry, effects, and uses of drugs. *Clinical pharmacology* deals with the biologic effects a drug has on the patient when used as a medical treatment. It covers the actions of a drug in the body over a period of time, including the rate at which body tissues absorb a drug, where a drug is distributed or localizes in the tissues, the chemical changes of the drug that occur in the body, the specific effects a drug has on the body, the route by which a drug is excreted, and, finally, *toxicity*, which is a drug's poisonous effect.

As a result of the rapid, technical advances in drug therapy and biochemistry, the importance of how the body deals with a drug is now emphasized more than the specific effects that a drug has on the body. As a medical assistant, you should have a general understanding of the types of drugs that are available. For every drug that you administer, you should know the functional changes that particular drug brings about in the body. That is, you should know the drug's *effect*, and how the body absorbs, utilizes and eliminates the drug, which is the *fate* of a drug. With the advent of new drugs and with information on what happens to drugs once they are in the human body being discovered almost daily, you will continually need to update your knowledge of the specific drugs used in your particular practice. Your role as the person responsible for administering medications and instructing patients on drug administration may change from time to time, but you must always assist the physician, and sometimes the pharmacist, in providing safe drug therapy for the patients. Despite differences in the duties of drug administration assigned to you by your individual physician or region, the following ethical and legal considerations are your responsibility:

- To be informed about the drugs that you administer.
- To ensure that a drug being used is correct in its order, dosage, route, time, and use.
- To pre-assess the patient for any adverse effects, such as allergy or drug-to-drug or drug-to-food interactions.
- To administer a drug appropriately.
- To be alert to any adverse effects that might occur immediately following the administration of a medication.
- To provide comfort, encouragement, and teaching to patients to ensure patient understanding, safety, and cooperation while they are on drug therapy.

HISTORY AND BACKGROUND

Drug Sources

Some drugs have been with us since ancient times. Written recipes using opium, castor oil, al-

cohol, and iron have been found on Egyptian papyrus and Sumerian clay tablets dating back to 2000 BC. In medieval times, drugs derived from plants included belladonna (used to treat gastrointestinal disorders), ipecac (used to induce vomiting and now in many cough medicines), and digitalis (used in the treatment of cardiac disorders). The South American Indians have used quinine for reducing fevers and curare, a skeletal muscle relaxant, as an arrow poison for centuries.

Today, pharmacology has become a science, and the drug industry is able to isolate the chemical components of natural drugs and manufacture them synthetically, in a form purer than the plant counterpart. The development of pure drugs enables the administration of drugs to be exact, establishing dose-response relationships, that is, knowing exactly how much of a particular drug is needed to bring about a desired effect.

Natural Sources. Drugs can be obtained from the leaf, seed, sap, stem, or root of certain plants. For example, digitalis is an extract from the leaf of the purple foxglove (*Digitalis purpurea*); opium comes from the unripe capsules of the opium poppy (*Papaver somniferum*); ipecac, from roots of the *Cephaelis ipecacuanha*; and quinine, from the bark of the cinchona tree. As far back as the Stone Age, humans prepared extracts, fluid extracts, and tinctures from plants. *Alkaloids* are the nitrogenous chemicals extracted from plants and, in pure medicinal form, are quite potent. Although there are exceptions, drugs whose names end in "ine" are alkaloids. Morphine and atropine are examples. *Glycosides* are the sugars, such as glucose, extracted from plants, and their names usually end in "in" (for example, digoxin and digitoxin). Other products of plants include oils, such as castor oil; volatile oils, such as peppermint and clove; gums, used as soothing lotions or suspending agents; resins, such as pine; and tannins, used as protective coatings over burns.

Animals are another natural drug source and often supply replacement hormones for human therapy. Animal fats are used as bases for ointments. Insulin is a hormone extracted from the cells of the beef or sheep pancreas, and thyroid extract is obtained from the thyroid glands of some animals that are slaughtered for food. Some antibiotics come from substances that are excreted or secreted by bacteria, yeasts, and molds.

Minerals also supply a wide variety of natural drugs, such as sodium chloride and potassium, dietary replacements, and mineral oil.

Synthetic Sources. Early in the 19th century, chemists began isolating and extracting the pure principles from crude plant extracts. The first extraction of a pure form of a plant principle was morphine, discovered in 1805. This advance made dosage control possible. Further advances resulted in synthetic drugs, which are chemicals that duplicate the physical properties of natural substances. Synthetic drugs often can eliminate the many side effects that occur with natural substances, and have increased potency (power). Oral insulin is one example of a synthetic replacement of a natural substance. Another is aspirin. In the late 19th century, a chemist experimenting with synthetic quinine discovered, by accident, salicylates. A later chemist discovered that coating salicylates with acetic acid made a safer form of salicylate. Thus, acetylsalicylic acid, or aspirin, was invented. Most drugs manufactured today are the controlled, more potent, synthesized substances that duplicate or replace the outdated, less reliable natural sources.

Drug Names

A single drug may have up to four different names:

- An organic name.
- A chemical name.
- A generic name.
- A trade name.

Some drugs have the same name in more than one of these categories. As an example, the various names of the **cardiotonic** drug digitalis follow.

Organic Name. This is the species name for a natural substance. *Digitalis purpurea* is a genus of herbs commonly called the purple foxglove whose leaves furnish digitalis.

Chemical Name. The chemical name of a drug represents its exact formula and is frequently difficult to understand. The chemical formula for digitalin, the digitalis glycoside extracted from the leaves, is $C_{36}H_{56}O_{14}$, with a hexose sugar name of *6-desoxy*-D-allose, $CH_3(CHOH_3)CH$ $(O\text{-}CH_3)$-CHO. Chemical names are used by chemists and manufacturers. You will not need to know the formulas for drugs.

Generic Name. The generic name is the common name of the chemical or drug, and it is usually descriptive of a drug's chemical structure. This name is not owned by any particular company. It is nonproprietary, that is, not protected by a trademark. In this example, *digitalis* is the generic name. Consumer group efforts have resulted in legislation in several states requiring pharmacists to fill prescriptions with generic forms of prescribed drugs rather than with the more expensive brand names, unless the physician specifically states a substitute is not acceptable. These groups claim that the less expensive generic products are the same as the more well-known brand names. Studies now show that generic substitutes may not always be chemically equivalent to certain name brands and that some generic drugs may not be as reliable as their name brand counterparts. Further testing and studies are being performed to resolve some of the controversy concerning equivalent formulations of products among various manufacturers and the high costs of name brand medications.

Trade (Brand) Name. The trade name is the name by which a particular manufacturer identifies the drug. A drug will have a different trade name with each pharmaceutical company that manufactures it. The trade names for digitalis include *Crystodigin* and *Purodigin*.

Drug Regulation

Drugs are regulated and controlled in their manufacture and distribution by the federal government. Basically, these regulations govern the following four areas of drug production:
1. Drug development and evaluation before release for human use.
2. Drug quality and standardization.
3. Dispensing and administering drugs.
4. Drug use.

Drug Development and Evaluation. The Food and Drug Administration (FDA) is an agency of the United States Department of Health and Human Services and makes mandatory the testing of all drugs before release to the public. Testing includes toxicity tests in laboratory animals, then clinical studies in a controlled group of voluntary patients. A manufacturer must prove not only the safety of a drug but also its effectiveness. A drug that is safe but cannot be proved to have an advantageous effect on the human body will not be approved by the FDA. When all the phases of the preclinical and clinical studies pass investigation, the FDA will approve a new drug for marketing. Only one of ten new drugs ever reaches the clinical testing phase. Very few new drugs reach the consumer. After approval, a manufacturer must continue to demonstrate a drug's effectiveness and safety and must submit reports whenever unexpected adverse reactions are discovered. If there is evidence that an approved drug no longer appears safe or effective, the FDA may suspend or withdraw the drug from manufacture and distribution at any time.

Drug Quality and Standardization. Manufacturing standards are established by the FDA to ensure the proper identity, strength, purity, and quality of drugs shipped in interstate commerce, which includes nearly all the drugs that we encounter in the medical office. Every manufacturer must consistently do the following:

- Identify every drug by a particular color, form, shape, size, and label.

- Produce every dose at the same tested strength.
- Produce the exact formula approved by the FDA.
- Use ingredients that are free from contaminants and of the highest quality.

Dispensing and Administering Drugs. There are two methods of dispensing drugs: over the counter (OTC) and by prescription. Over-the-counter drugs are available to the public for self-medication. These drugs have been approved by the FDA and are considered safe for patients to use without the physician's advice. Most are very low in dosage and have more of a placebo effect than a therapeutic effect. The real dangers of OTC drugs are

1. Patients may self-medicate and avoid professional medical care when it is needed.

2. OTC drugs may mask signs and symptoms that are necessary to making correct medical diagnoses.

3. Multiple-drug interactions can lead to adverse reactions or toxicity.

Federal law makes drugs that are dangerous, powerful, or habit-forming illegal to use except under a physician's order. A *prescription* is an order written by the physician for the compounding or dispensing and administration of drugs to a particular patient. Sometimes, an order may be written for the medical assistant on the patient's medical record, or to a nurse on the patient's chart. However, a prescription most often needs a written order on a prescription blank for the pharmacist to fill. A prescription must be given, and signed, by the physician, or the order cannot be carried out. There are four parts to a prescription, as follows:

- *Superscription*: Patient's name and address, the date, and the symbol R$_x$ (Latin for recipe, meaning "take").
- *Inscription*: Names and quantities of the ingredients.
- *Subscription*: Directions for compounding. Prescription writing is not as complicated for the physician as in earlier times, because pharmaceutical manufacturers now prepare most medications ready for dispensing or administration. Rarely will a pharmacist have to compound or mix a medication.
- *Signature*: Directions for the patient. It is usually preceded by the symbol S (Latin for signa, meaning "mark"). This is where the physician indicates what instructions are to be put on the label to tell the patient how, when, and in what quantities to use the medication.

Prescription directions may be in English or Latin. There are set terms and abbreviations, a medical shorthand of sorts. It is easier to write "tab. 1 t.i.d. c. aq. p.c." than "one tablet three times each day with water after meals." A typical prescription is shown in Figure 26–1.

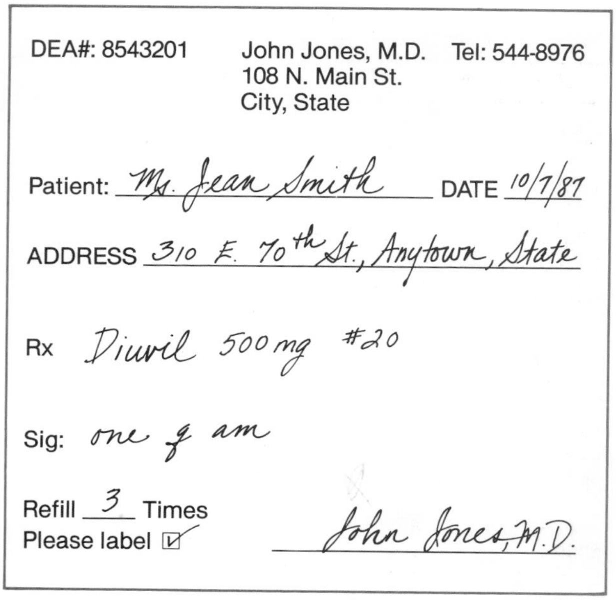

DEA#: 8543201   John Jones, M.D.   Tel: 544-8976
108 N. Main St.
City, State

Patient: *Ms. Jean Smith*   DATE *10/7/87*

ADDRESS *310 E. 70th St., Anytown, State*

Rx   *Diuvil 500 mg   #20*

Sig: *one q am*

Refill *3* Times
Please label ☑   *John Jones, M.D.*

Figure 26–1
A sample prescription.

The medical assistant does not write prescriptions but must know prescription terms and abbreviations to communicate with the physician and the pharmacist and to administer medications by written order. The more common terms and abbreviations are listed in Table 26–1. Keep all prescription pads safe and out of view of the public.

Drug Use. Before the first law regulating the sale of foods and drugs in the United States was enacted in 1906, the consumer did not know the actual ingredients of food and drugs. Cough medications contained excessive amounts of codeine. Vitamin and mineral supplements contained high levels of alcohol. A popular soft drink contained cocaine as its active ingredient. Over the years, more than 50 pieces of legislation have been enacted to control the dispensing and administration of drugs. See Table 26–2 for a brief history of drug legislation.

Today, narcotics and various other substances are controlled and regulated by the Drug Enforcement Agency (DEA), a branch of the Justice Department. The DEA regulates drugs under five schedules of controlled substances, known as Schedules I, II, III, IV, and V. Drugs are listed under a particular schedule, based on their abuse potential and medical usefulness. These schedules not only list the drugs regulated by each category, but also address regulations concerning the writing, telephoning, and refilling of prescriptions, and the storage and maintenance of drugs. Every medical practice should have a copy of the controlled substances regulations. The medical assistant may secure this list from a regional office of the DEA. It is also important to be on the DEA's mailing list to receive

Table 26–1
Common Prescription Abbreviations

Abbreviation	Latin	Translation
aa	ana	of each
a.c.	ante cibum	before meals
ad	ad	up to
ad lib.	ad libitum	as much as needed
a.m.	ante meridiem	morning
ante	ante	before
aq.	aqua	water
b.i.d.	bis in die	two times a day
c̄	cum	with
capsul.	capsula	capsule
contra	contra	against
elix.	elixir	elixir
emul.	emulsum	emulsion
et	et	and
ext.	extractum	extract
f., or ft.	Fac or fiat	make
fl.	fluidus	fluid
gm.	gramma	gram
gr.	granum	grain
gt.	gutta	drop
gtt.	guttae	drops
h	hora	hour
h.s.	hora somni	hour of sleep (bedtime)
inj.		injection (to be injected)
kg.		kilogram
M.	misce	mix
mcgm.		microgram
noct.	nocte	at night
o		other
o	omnis	every
O.D.	oculus dexter	right eye
O.S.	oculus sinister	left eye
p.c.	post cibum	after meals
p.r.n.	pro re nata	whenever necessary
pil.	pilula	pill
pulv.	pulvis	powder
q.	quaque	every
q.d.	quaque die	every day
q.h.	quaque hora	every hour
q.i.d.	quater in die	four times a day
q.n.	quaque nocte	every night
q.n.s.	quantum non satis	quantity not sufficient
qo		every other
q.s.	quantum satis	quantity sufficient
q.2h.	quaque secunda hora	every two hours
q.4h.	quaque quarta hora	every four hours
Rₓ	recipe	take
S, or Sig	signa, signetur	write (on the label)
s̄	sine	without
sat.		saturated
sol.	solutio	solution
s.o.s.	si opus sit	if needed
sp.	spiritus	spirit
ss.	semis	one half
stat.	statim	immediately
suppos., supp.	suppository	suppository
syr.	syrupus	syrup
tab.	tabella	tablet
t.i.d.	ter in die	three times a day
tr. (tinct.)	tinctura	tincture
troc.	troche	lozenge
U.		unit
ung.	unguentum	ointment
ut dict.	ut dictum	as directed

Table 26–2
Brief History of Drug Legislation

Date	Legislation	Purpose
1906	Pure Food and Drug Act	To regulate the sale of drugs
1914	Harrison Narcotic Act	To regulate the manufacture, sale, dispensing, and prescribing of narcotics by the Treasury Department
1938	Food, Drug, and Cosmetic Act	To regulate the quality of drugs through interstate commerce by the Food and Drug Administration, a branch of the Department of Health and Social Services
1951	Durham-Humphrey Act	To provide stricter enforcement of the dispensing of habit-forming hypnotic drugs
1965	Drug Abuse Control Amendment	To provide stricter enforcement of the dispensing of dangerous drugs, including stimulants
1970	Controlled Substances Act	To combine the 50 former federal laws into one piece of legislation. Bureau of Narcotics and Dangerous Drugs (BNDD) established
1973	Drug Enforcement Act	To replace the BNDD (see above) with the Drug Enforcement Agency (DEA)

26

updates as drugs are added or deleted, or moved from one schedule to another.

Schedule I. Includes substances that have no accepted medicinal use and a high potential for abuse. The possession of these drugs is illegal. Drugs included in this schedule are heroin, LSD (lysergic acid diethylamide), marijuana, mescaline, and peyote.

Schedule II. Includes various narcotics such as opium, the opium derivatives (e.g., morphine), and the synthetic opium derivatives (e.g., synthetic morphine and methadone); stimulants, such as cocaine and amphetamines; and the commonly abused depressant barbiturates. To write these prescriptions, a physician must have a special license (DEA number). The prescription must be entirely handwritten by the physician on Federal Triplicate Order Forms imprinted with the DEA number or with the DEA number written in by the physician. These prescriptions must be filled within 72 hours and may not be refilled. In an emergency, a physician may telephone a Schedule II order to the pharmacist. However, the amount of the drug must be limited, and the physician must furnish to the pharmacy, within 72 hours, a written, signed prescription for the drug prescribed. If these drugs are kept in the medical office, they must be stored under lock and key and routinely counted and inventoried. The law requires that a dispensing record be kept on file for two years (or as otherwise specified by state law) and be subject to inspection by the DEA. The record must include the following:

- Full name and address of the patient.
- Date of order.

- Name, dosage form, and quantity of the drug.
- Method (administered or dispensed).

Schedule III. Includes the lesser abused combination drugs that contain limited quantities of codeine, narcotic substances, or amphetamine-like substances. The physician must handwrite the prescription, but a DEA number is not required. Refills, up to five in any six-month period, are allowed, but they must be indicated on the original prescription order. When changes or additions are made by telephone, the physician must directly communicate with the pharmacist, and a written prescription order confirming the telephone request should be forwarded to the pharmacist as soon as possible.

Schedule IV. Includes the minor tranquilizers and hypnotics that have a lesser potential for abuse. Prescriptions may be handwritten by the medical assistant under the physician's direction, but the physician must sign them. Up to five refills are allowed within a six-month period. Requests for refills may be telephoned to the pharmacist by the medical assistant under order of the physician, but the physician should record the order on the patient's medical record. Schedule IV drugs include meprobamate (Equanil), chlordiazepoxide (Librium), diazepam (Valium), flurazepam (Dalmane), chloral hydrate, and the non-narcotic analgesic propoxyphene (Darvon).

Schedule V. Includes miscellaneous mixtures containing limited amounts of narcotic drugs. Prescription orders and refills are the same as for Schedule IV drugs. Examples are most cough medications containing codeine and some drugs used for gastrointestinal disorders, such as Donnagel and diphenoxylate (Lomotil).

Drug Abuse. Any drug from aspirin to alcohol may be misused or abused. Today, there is a tremendous increase in the use of illegal and legal drugs. Nationally, treatment programs are available everywhere for people in all walks of life. Programs include detoxification, rehabilitation, and long-term rehabilitation maintenance. The AMA recognizes the problem of drug and alcohol abuse among physicians and other health professionals and has initiated therapy programs for its members. Medical assistants may frequently encounter patients who are misusing or abusing drugs. It is important for you to be alert to the symptoms of drug dependence and to notify the physician when you suspect a patient, or co-worker, of having a problem with drug or alcohol dependency.

Drug misuse is the improper use of common drugs that can lead to dependence or toxicity. Examples of persons with chronic dependencies include people who cannot have a bowel movement unless they take a laxative, those who have used nasal decongestants for so long that they cannot breathe without the use of nasal sprays, or those who take so many antacids that they suffer systemic metabolic alkalosis. Alcoholic beverages are used by an estimated 75 million Americans. Even the controlled, social drinker can misuse alcohol and experience nausea, vomiting, a hangover, or dangerous accidents.

Drug abuse is taking too much of a drug continually or periodically, in a manner that is considered not acceptable behavior by society. Drinking alcohol socially is acceptable. Drinking on the job is considered abusive. Cigarette smoking is a example of a once-accepted use of nicotine that is more and more being considered a form of drug abuse.

Drug dependency is the advanced stage of drug abuse. Dependency is the inability to function unless under the influence of a substance. *Psychological dependency* is the compulsive craving for the effects of a substance. *Habituation* is a milder form of psychological dependence. In this case, a person forms a habit of using a substance even to the detriment of physical health and well-being. Drinking coffee and soft drinks that contain caffeine and smoking cigarettes are common examples of habituation. *Physical dependence* is a person's need for a substance to avoid physical discomfort. This type of dependence occurs when abused substances produce biochemical changes, usually in the nervous system tissues. Discontinuing a substance that causes physical dependency creates the withdrawal syndrome. *Addiction* is a term that is now too broad to have any real meaning, and is being replaced by the term *dependence*.

The following five types of drugs are the most commonly abused:

1. The potent narcotic analgesics, such as heroin and morphine.
2. Depressant drugs, such as the barbiturates, sedatives, hypnotics, and anti-anxiety agents.
3. Psychomotor stimulants, such as cocaine and amphetamines.
4. Hallucinogens and psychosis-imitating drugs, such as LSD, mescaline, and peyote.
5. *Cannabis* derivatives, such as marijuana and hashish.

Regardless of the type of drug abused, it will have two effects on the person: acute and chronic. The acute effect is what the person feels when *intoxicated*, or directly under the influence of a particular substance. The chronic effects include the temporary or permanent physical and mental changes that result from long-term abuse.

The medical assistant often is called upon to answer patient questions concerning drug abuse and problems. You should read and keep up to date on the drug-related issues of our society. You should also have available for patients pamphlets and agency referral names for each of the five types of commonly abused drug previously listed.

DRUG INTERACTIONS WITH THE BODY

The study of pharmacology used to focus on the *desired effect* a drug has on the human body, that is, the so-called end result. Now, knowledge of what happens to a drug while it is in the body (that is, the *fate* of the drug) is more important than the drug's effect, which we also now know is often far from the drug's "end result." This shift has more value because we know that different patients react to the same dose of a drug in very different ways and that the same patient may react to the same dose of a drug differently at various times. Simply knowing the effect of a drug does not ensure the safety of the patient.

Uses of Drugs

Drugs may be called pharmaceuticals, medicines, or medications. As a form of therapy (that is, the treatment of disease by medicines) drugs occupy a prominent position. However, drugs also are used for other than therapeutic purposes. The uses of drugs include

- Therapeutic: Used to cure a disease, such as antibiotics used to cure bacterial infections.
- Palliative: Used to relieve the symptoms of a disease, such as pain relievers.
- Preventive: Used to prevent a condition, such as Dramamine for motion sickness.
- Replacement: Used to replace or supplement what the body is not producing, such as insulin for the diabetic or vitamins and minerals.
- Diagnostic: Used to aid in the diagnosis of a disease or condition, such as dyes used in radiography examinations.

Generally, therapeutic drugs either eradicate foreign substances from the body, such as antibiotics destroying pathogens, or interfere with the functioning of the patient's own cells, tissues, or organs. This interference always has the potential to be poisonous to the body. However, the object of *rational drug therapy* is to control the degree of interference and to bring about the desired effect without any adverse, or *untoward*, effects.

Most drugs that affect the body tissues either bring about stimulation (increased activity) or depression (decreased activity). Some drug reactions are much more complicated: a drug may increase activity at the cellular level, which in turn decreases the activity of a particular organ, or vice versa. For example, a drug may decrease the nerve impulse transmission of certain cells in the heart, resulting in an increased heart rate. Some drugs stimulate one area of the body while depressing another. Morphine depresses the cough mechanism yet increases the mechanism that causes vomiting. Epinephrine (Adrenalin) decreases (constricts) the openings of the blood vessels yet increases (dilates) the opening of the bronchial tubes.

Although most drugs can ultimately be classified as stimulants or depressants of some area of the body (especially the central nervous system), it is important to know how and where a drug affects the body as well as what the drug does. Many drugs bring about the same effect, but in different ways from different parts of the body. For example, many drugs reduce blood pressure. Some act by depressing or stimulating central nervous system sites; some by relaxing the smooth muscle in the vessels in the heart; and others by decreasing the total fluid volume in the tissues. The end result, or effect, of all these methods is the same, a decreased blood pressure. However, each method is very different. Pain can be relieved by drugs acting in different ways at different sites. Some pain relievers act by relaxing smooth muscle spasms (antispasmodics); others block sensory nerve impulses to an area (local anesthesia); and still others dull the general senses of a patient so that an awareness of pain is lost (analgesics or general anesthesia).

People differ greatly in their reactions to drugs. Knowledge of how and where a drug produces its effect helps the physician to know which type of drug to use and when two or more drugs may be used for a more advantageous effect (*synergistic effect*). For example, treating a hypertensive patient with two drugs may be of more value than therapy with just one drug.

The Fate of Drugs

By knowing how the body handles a drug and what happens to the drug in the body, we can know the *onset* of a drug's activity (beginning), when its *intensity* is likely to peak, the *critical concentration* (the minimum amount of chemical necessary in the fluids that bathe the tissues for the tissues to respond to the drug), and the *duration* of a particular drug's activity. All these facts help to determine the dosage form, dosage amount, route, and frequency of administration of medications. The fate of a drug includes the following:

- *Absorption*: How a drug is absorbed into the body's circulating fluids, known as the *routes*.
- *Distribution*: How a drug is transported from the site of administration to the various points in the body.
- *Action*: What changes the drug causes once it has reached its destination.
- *Biotransformation*: How the drug is inactivated, including the time it takes for a drug to be *detoxified* and broken down into by-products.
- *Excretion*: The route by which a drug is excreted, or eliminated, and the amount of time such a process requires.

Drug Absorption. What happens to a drug from the time it is administered until it reaches the bloodstream is the first factor in determining the route of drug administration. An important point to remember is that no matter where a drug is absorbed, it can have one of two actions on the

No drug remains truly localized

body: *local* (restricted to one spot or part; not general) or *systemic* (affecting the body as a whole). However, most drugs are used for their systemic effects. Even when drugs are used for local purposes, we know that none remain truly localized in the body. Any chemical that comes into contact with even the most superficial surface, such as the skin, has the potential to be absorbed into the bloodstream and to circulate to other tissues and organs. When we decide whether a drug is local or systemic, we should be thinking more of its intended use rather than its effect on the human organism.

Oral Route. Oral medications are convenient, safe, and inexpensive. However, drugs that can be destroyed in any way by the digestive tract must be given by injection. Injections are rapid but increase the danger of overdose or possible infection. The majority of oral medications are absorbed by the small intestine, but a few are absorbed more rapidly in the stomach. After absorption into the bloodstream from the small intestine, drugs are carried to the liver. In this organ, much of the drug's potency is inactivated before it circulates to the tissues. This inactivation by the liver often makes it necessary to administer higher dosages orally than when given by injection.

Food slows the absorption of drugs. Therefore, many medications are best prescribed one hour before or two hours after the ingestion of food. Food may also bind the drugs to them or in some other way destroy a drug. Tetracyclines, for example, are destroyed by milk products and antacids containing calcium salts. Patients on tetracycline should be advised not to eat dairy products or take liquid or solid forms of antacids.

The stomach acids present during digestion alone may destroy certain drugs. Because some drugs are destroyed by the components of the digestive tract or irritate the empty lining of the stomach, many oral drugs are *enteric-coated* to keep them intact for passage into the small intestine or to prevent gastric irritation or vomiting.

Some drugs are not affected by the digestive processes but cannot be absorbed through the intestinal walls into the bloodstream. For example, neomycin has no effect when taken orally (unless it is used to "sterilize" the bowel itself prior to bowel surgery). Other drugs may be unable to cross the bowel mucosa because of their poor solubility in lipids (fats), or they are inactivated by the pH of the gastrointestinal (GI) tract.

It is important to remember these absorption factors when administering medication by the oral route. If a patient has responded to a drug previously but now is not, it may be important to question the patient's food-medication cycle. It could be that the patient is no longer taking the medication on an empty stomach as directed.

Parenteral Route. Parenteral means "beside the digestive tract" and is the term for administering drugs by injection (hypodermically, under the skin). The parenteral route is the surest and fastest one, but there are several factors that determine its effectiveness.

The first is the amount of blood supply to the site of injection. The absorption of a drug in an aqueous (water) solution is faster in an area with more blood vessels. Therefore, drugs deposited in the muscle will be absorbed faster than drugs deposited in the upper layers of the subcutaneous tissues. The *intramuscular route* (IM) is chosen in an emergency for fast action or when larger amounts of the medication must be absorbed. The *subcutaneous route* (SC, or sub-cu) is chosen when a slower, prolonged effect is desired.

A second way that parenteral drug absorption may be controlled is physically. A drug's absorption may be quickened by hand massage after injection. Absorption may be slowed by injecting the drug in a physical form that slows absorption. One way of slowing the absorption of a drug and, therefore, increasing the duration of its effect is to suspend the drug in a solution that prolongs absorption, such as colloidal substances, fatty substances (oil), insoluble salts or esters, and epinephrine (Adrenalin), which acts by constricting the blood vessels, thus retarding circulation and absorption. Insulin is suspended in protamine, which is a water-soluble protein extracted from the sperm of certain fish. Heparin is suspended in gelatin. Penicillin G is suspended with procaine (hydrochloride) salts. Aqueous drugs suspended in these substances slowly dissolve in the tissues over a long period of time, and the patient can be spared costly, frequent, and sometimes painful injections. Local anesthetics are sometimes mixed with epinephrine to keep the anesthetics and their effects in an area longer.

The third parenteral route is *intravenous* (IV), which is directly into the vein. This route is instantaneous and can be dangerously irreversible. Because of the dangers of intravenous administration, only those members of the medical team who are licensed to do so may inject medication intravenously. **The medical assistant is not licensed to perform the intravenous administration of medications to patients.** Because IV administration is so dangerous, medications given by IV are usually administered in small doses through an intravenous infusion (IV drip) to prevent toxic effects in the brain or the heart. Sometimes, an accidental overdose can be slowed by the application of a tourniquet between the injection site and the heart or the application of ice packs to the site. Both methods can constrict the blood vessels and retard the flow of the drug through the circulatory system.

Other forms of parenteral routes include the *intradermal* injection, which is below the skin but superficial to the subcutaneous tissues. This route is used mostly for allergy testing and skin testing.

(See Chapter 31, section on allergy testing.) *Intrathecal*, or *intraspinal*, injections are used for spinal anesthesia and administering certain antibiotics into the spine for the treatment of meningitis. *Intraarticular* or *intralesional* injections are used for administering steroids into joints and lesions, or anticancer drugs into cancerous tumors.

Mucous Membrane Absorption. Drugs may be absorbed by the mucous membranes of the mouth, throat, nose, eyes, rectum, vagina, and the respiratory and urinary tracts. Some applications have a local effect, such as nasal sprays, eye drops, and a rectal suppository for constipation. Others have a systemic effect, such as a rectal suppository to control vomiting or a nitroglycerin tablet dissolved under the tongue (sublingual) to dilate the blood vessels and relieve the pain of **angina pectoris.** *Inhalation* is used to concentrate locally drugs in the lower respiratory passages or to produce systemic effects such as general anesthesia.

Topical Absorption. These routes include the application of medications to the skin, eyes and ears. Most drugs are not absorbed by the outer layers of the skin. However, drugs in ointments, creams, lotions, and aerosols can be applied for the treatment of skin itching, inflammation, or other discomforts and for the treatment of skin infections with antibiotics. Nitroglycerin (for angina) and dimenhydrinate (Dramamine, for motion sickness) are two drugs that can be absorbed through the skin for systemic effects. *Dermal patches* containing these medications can be taped to the body for a slow, prolonged time-release of the drugs.

Drug Distribution. Once a drug is absorbed, it must be transported by the circulatory system to the area where it will have its effect. In the bloodstream, drugs can attach to plasma proteins and then be freed to pass from the blood into the site of action. Drugs are then carried through the fluids bathing the cells into the cells of the tissues and organs. The amount of blood supply to a part affects the speed with which drugs reach certain tissues. The high degree of blood circulating through the brain, heart, liver, and kidneys ensures that drugs will be concentrated in these areas rapidly. Drugs accumulate much more slowly in muscle, fat, and bone tissues.

The blood-brain barrier is a functional barrier between the brain cells and the capillaries circulating blood through the brain. This barrier determines which substances can cross. For the substances that can, it regulates the degree and rate of their absorption into the brain tissue. The general anesthetic thiopental sodium (Pentothal Sodium) is able to cross the blood-brain barrier immediately and produces sleep within seconds, whereas other sleep-producing drugs, such as the barbiturates, cross slowly and may take as long as 30 minutes to an hour to produce the same effect. While these drugs remain in the body, they may cross the blood-brain barrier several times, being redistributed to the rest of the body's tissues, then returning to the brain tissue. This is why some patients go back and forth between sleep and wakefulness.

Drugs can be distributed to the fetus of a pregnant woman by blood circulation exchange. Therefore, drugs of all types should be avoided during pregnancy. Some drugs may attach to and accumulate in bone tissue, which may interfere with normal growth and development. Tetracycline is an example. Distribution of this drug to the unborn fetus or a young infant may lead to its accumulation on the teeth and later discoloration of the tooth enamel. For the most part, this is a problem of the deciduous teeth (first set); however, administering tetracyclines to older children can cause a brownish discoloration of the permanent teeth.

Drug Action. No one theory explains why drugs act the way they do. The following is a general summary of the various theories of drug action:

1. Drugs are believed to combine with body chemicals on the cell surface or within the cell itself. Correct cells are chosen because a particular drug has a *specific affinity* for a particular cell. The specific cell recipient is called a *receptor,* and the drug that has the affinity for it and produces a function change in the cell is called the *agonist.*

2. Not all drugs that bind to specific cells cause a functional change in the cell. These drugs act as an *antagonist* to the natural process, and work by *blocking* a sequence of biochemical events.

3. Some drugs are believed to act by affecting the enzyme functions of the body. Drugs attach to enzyme substances and rob the enzymes from cells. As a result, the enzyme products needed for normal cellular function are not supplied, and the cell fails to function properly.

4. Certain anti-infective drugs have a *selected toxicity* for pathogens or parasites that have invaded the body. Penicillin and sulfonamides work because they poison, or interfere with the life processes of, bacteria without affecting the life processes of normal human cells. Research scientists continue to look for differences between cancer cells and normal cells to enable them to apply the principle of selected toxicity in cancer treatment. Most of the anticancer drugs in use today are not selectively toxic, and normal human cells are also poisoned by the cancer drugs.

5. Both drugs that have a selective affinity for cells and those that bind with enzymes can be counteracted by administering large amounts of the natural substances with which the drugs compete. This process is known as administering an *antidote* to a drug that may be acting as a poison.

6. Some drugs alter the function of cells by affecting the physical properties of the cell membrane rather than altering the biochemical processes

26

within the cell itself. This is especially true of drugs that affect nerve cells, such as anesthetics and alcohol. A change in the cell membrane changes the **permeability** of the membrane, which in turn changes the flow of **ions** in and out of the cells. This change in ion flow changes the polarity (opposite effects at two extremities, the two extremities being inside and outside the cell membrane) on which nerve pulses are conducted and produces general sleep or stupor.

Biotransformation of Drugs. This is the process by which drugs are converted into harmless byproducts. These by-products are then more easily eliminated by the kidneys. Most drugs are broken down by the enzyme activity of the liver. The ability to break down the chemical components of a drug varies among individuals. Factors that determine this ability include age, the presence of other drugs, and liver disease. In some patients on long-term drug therapy, a drug may overstimulate the enzyme activity of the liver. This results in a too rapid destruction of the drug, and the patient has to take larger and larger doses for the drug to be effective. This situation is called *tolerance*.

Excretion of Drugs. The kidneys are the most important route for the elimination of drugs. Most drugs are filtered out of the circulation, broken down into harmless particles, and then excreted in the urine. Because the kidneys are so important in the elimination of drugs from the body, drug therapy must be carefully monitored in patients with kidney disease or malfunction. Drugs are also eliminated through the sweat glands and saliva and in bile. Exhalation, another mechanism for drug elimination, is the basis for measuring alcohol concentrations in the blood by the breathalyzer test. Drugs may be eliminated through the milk glands of the lactating mother, which means a woman breastfeeding a child has to be extremely careful about taking medications.

Factors That Influence the Effect of a Drug

As stated earlier, different people react to the same dose of medication in different ways, and the same patient can react to the same dose of the same drug differently on various occasions. The following factors are important in determining the correct medication for a patient.

Body Weight. A person's weight has a direct relationship with the effects of medication. Basically, the same dosage has a greater effect on a person who weighs less, and a lesser effect on a patient who weighs more. Manufacturers of adult medications calculate dosages based on a normal adult weight (approximately 150 pounds). Sometimes, the physician will adjust the dosage to better suit the patient's body size. Pediatric medications are designed for the body weight or body surface area of children. If adult medications are used for children, the correct dosage must be calculated and adjusted for the child's body weight.

Age. In the newborn and the very elderly, age has its greatest effect on the body's response to a drug. This usually has to do with immature or deteriorating body systems. In addition, both groups are particularly sensitive to drugs that affect the central nervous system and to toxicity. Dosage calculations for these two groups must be carefully decided, and therapy usually begins with very small doses.

Sex. Drugs may affect men and women differently. As previously mentioned, the pregnant woman has to be extremely cautious, when taking medications, to avoid damage to the developing fetus. In addition, some drugs have side effects that can stimulate uterine contractions, causing premature labor and delivery. Intramuscular medications are absorbed faster by men. Because women have a higher body fat content and a musculature with less blood supply, intramuscular drugs remain in their tissues longer than in men's tissues. During certain times of the menstrual cycle, the immune response system is suppressed, and antibiotics given at this time may not be as effective as at other times.

Time of Day. *Diurnal* means "during the day" or "time of light." Diurnal body rhythms play an important part in the effects of some drugs. Sedatives given in the morning will not be as effective as when administered before bedtime, because the central nervous system is more stimulated and more resistant to the effects of the drug. Steroid administration is preferred in the morning because it best mimics the body's natural pattern of steroid production and elimination. Diuretics are best administered in the morning to reduce the need for the patient to get up during the night to void.

Pathologic Factors. Patients may adversely respond to drugs in the presence of liver or kidney disease because the body will not be able to detoxify and excrete chemicals properly. In patients with liver or kidney disease, some drugs may cause unconsciousness or death. Patients with other diseases or disorders may react quite differently than expected. Therefore, a thorough medical history is always required before administering medications. Even temporary pain and fever may alter the expected effect of a drug.

Immune Responses. The presence of a drug can stimulate a patient's immune response, and the patient will develop antibodies to a particular chemical. If the same drug is again administered, the patient will have an allergic reaction to the drug, ranging from a mild reaction to a serious respiratory and circulatory emergency.

Psychological Factors. People may respond differently to a drug because of the way they feel about the drug. If a patient believes in the therapy, even a *placebo* (sugar pill or sterile water thought to be a drug) may help or bring about relief. A patient's personality can affect whether or not he or she will be cooperative in following the directions for a particular drug, and a patient's negative mind-set, or mental attitude, can reduce an expected response to a drug.

Tolerance. Tolerance is the phenomenon of reduced responsiveness to a drug. *Congenital tolerance* is an inborn resistance. *Acquired tolerance* occurs after taking a particular drug for a period of time. *Cross tolerance* occurs when a patient acquires a tolerance to one drug and becomes resistant to other similar drugs. *Physical dependence* often accompanies tolerance. The body becomes so adapted to the presence of the drug that it cannot function properly without it. To withdraw the drug is to throw the body out of its equilibrium, causing the well-known withdrawal syndrome.

Cumulation. When a drug is taken too frequently to allow for proper elimination, it accumulates in the tissues. The result is a more intense effect and a longer duration. Cumulation can cause overdose and toxicity. Proper dosage and timing of administration is the best prevention of drug accumulation.

Idiosyncrasy. Occasionally, a person reacts to a drug in a manner that is unexpected and peculiar to that individual only. An idiosyncrasy may manifest itself in many different ways, such as a hypnotic drug keeping a person awake, acting as a stimulant to this person rather than as a depressant. Usually, these reactions cannot be explained.

Classifications of Drug Actions

Clinical pharmacology is a complex subject. To make the subject easier, drugs are classified according to their actions on the body (for example, chemotherapeutics or emetics). Drugs also may be classified according to the body system that they affect (for example, drugs acting on the cardiovascular system). The following is a glossary of terms describing some basic drug actions. As you read some of the examples, remember that a drug classified as one type of agent may have other uses and actions on other systems of the body. For example, a drug classified as a diuretic may also be an antihypertensive drug, and a vasodilator may also be a respiratory antispasmodic. It takes time to understand not only the basic classification of a particular drug but also the many secondary uses and effects it has on the human body.

Adrenergic. A drug that acts like epinephrine, a hormone produced by the medulla of the adrenal glands (called adrenaline in Great Britain). It can be administered parenterally, topically, or by inhalation and acts as a vasoconstrictor, antispasmodic, or mimic of any of the effects that natural epinephrine has on the body. Adrenergics are used as emergency heart stimulants and to counteract allergic conditions such as hives and asthma. They are the most effective drug for counteracting the effects of anaphylactic shock. Adrenergic drugs are called *sympathomimetic* because their actions resemble the natural functions of the sympathetic nervous system.

Analgesic. A drug to relieve pain by lessening the sensory function of the brain. Analgesics vary greatly in their ability to relieve pain and range from aspirin to the opium derivatives. For narcotic analgesic examples, see Narcotic.

Analgesic–Antipyretic–Anti-inflammatory. A drug that relieves pain (usually originating in the joints, muscles, teeth, head, skin, and connective tissue), reduces fever (antipyretic), or acts as an anti-inflammatory or antirheumatic. Examples include acetaminophen (Tylenol), aspirin (acetylsalicylic acid), phenylbutazone (Butazolidin), ibuprofen (Advil, Motrin, Nuprin), naproxen (Naprosyn), piroxicam (Feldene), and indomethacin (Indocin).

Anesthetic. A drug used to produce insensibility to pain or the sensation of pain, local or general. *Topical anesthetics* are applied to the surfaces of the skin and mucous membranes and have a local action. *Local anesthetics* are infiltrated (injected into the tissues or nerves), intraspinal, or caudal (injected into the base of the spine). Their effects are local. *General anesthesia* is systemic and produces sleep.

Antibiotic. Agents that are produced both by living organisms and synthetically and are effective against bacterial infections. Some antibiotics are selective and have a *narrow spectrum*. Others have effects on a wide range of microorganisms and are called *broad-spectrum* antibiotics. There are four groups of antibiotics:

1. Those that result in the death of the bacterial cell (bacteriolytic). Examples include the penicillins (Pentids, Bicillin, Amoxil, and Ampicillin), cephalosporins (Keflin, Keflex), and bacitracin.
2. Those that interfere with the genetic production and reproduction of bacteria (bacteriostatic). Examples include the tetracyclines, streptomycin, gentamicin, erythromycin, chloramphenicol, and griseofulvin.

26

3. Those that dissolve the bacterial cell membranes (bacteriostatic or bacteriocidal). Examples include amphotericin and nystatin.

4. Those that interrupt the bacterial metabolic processes (bacteriostatic). Examples include the sulfonamides, aminosalicylic acid (PAS), and isoniazid (INH).

Antidepressant. Several drug groups are used to treat depression, including antidepressants, antipsychotics, antianxiety agents, psychomotor stimulants, and lithium. Antidepressants include amitriptyline HCl (Elavil) and imipramine pamoate (Tofranil).

Antifungal. Preparations to treat systemic or local fungal infections (mycoses), which include

1. Those that treat the serious systemic fungal infections that spread to various vital organs via the bloodstream. One example is amphotericin B (Fungizone).

2. Those that are taken orally to treat ringworm-type infections of the skin, hair, and nails. An example is griseofulvin (Fulvicin-U/F).

3. Those that are used to treat the yeast-like fungal infections, such as **Candida albicans (moniliasis)** of the vagina, mouth (thrush) or skin. Examples include miconazole (Monistat) and nystatin (Mycostatin).

Antiepileptic. Agent used to reduce the number or severity of epileptic attacks. These agents may be called anticonvulsants. However, convulsions do not occur in all types of seizures. Examples include sedatives and hypnotics (see following), phenytoin (Dilantin), methylphenidate HCl (Ritalin), and, sometimes, dextroamphetamine sulfate (Dexedrine).

Antihistamine–Histamine Blocker. An agent used to counteract the effects of histamine. Histamine is a natural substance in the body's tissues that aids in the body's inflammatory response to tissue injury and regulates the secretion of stomach acid. However, when histamine is released, it creates side effects that are the signs and symptoms of allergy, or even anaphylaxis, in certain hypersensitive persons. Antihistamines are used for the relief of allergic disorders, insect-sting reactions, and acute anaphylactic reactions. Because a side-effect of antihistamines is drowsiness, they may also be used for sedation or motion sickness prevention. Examples include brompheniramine maleate (Dimetane), chlorpheniramine maleate (Chlor-Trimeton), diphenhydramine HCl (Benadryl, Benylin), and promethazine HCl (Phenergan).

Histamine blockers may be used to inhibit gastric acid secretions in the treatment of upper gastrointestinal problems and peptic ulcers. Examples are cimetidine (Tagamet) and ranitidine (Zantac).

Antihypertensive. A drug used to treat hypertension. There are many drugs for treating hypertension, including the following: diuretics (see following); sympathetic blocking agents (see following), such as atenolol (Tenormin), Metoprolol tartrate (Lopressor), nadolol (Corgard); centrally acting agents, such as methyldopa (Aldomet); and vasodilators (see following).

Antispasmodic. An agent that relieves or prevents spasms from musculoskeletal injury or inflammation and from neurologic disorders resulting from central nervous system damage, or spasms of the smooth muscles such as the intestines or the uterus. Examples include methocarbamol (Robaxin) and carisoprodol (Soma), and levodopa (L-dopa). *Parkinson disease*

Antitussive (Cough Suppressant). An agent that suppresses the cough reflex and dries up the secretion and normal discharge of a cough. Examples are dextromethorphan HBr (Romilar), codeine, and terpin hydrate with codeine.

Bronchodilator. An agent used to treat chronic bronchitis, bronchial asthma, and emphysema. Oral medications include aminophylline (Theophylline) and theophylline anhydrous (Theo-Dur). Parenteral medications include epinephrine (Adrenalin, Sus-Phrine). Aerosol inhalation medications include albuterol (Ventolin, Proventil) and isoproterenol HCl (Isuprel).

Carminative. A medication that relieves flatulence and aids in the expulsion of gas from the stomach and intestines. It usually contains a volatile oil or carbonated beverage.

Cathartic. An agent that increases and hastens bowel evacuation (defecation). Commonly called a laxative. The types range from mild laxatives to *purgatives*, which are severe cathartics. Some work by increasing the amount of bulk in the bowel. Others work by irritating the intestinal mucosa, which produces movement.

Chemotherapeutic. Now mostly refers to those chemical substances used to treat cancerous conditions and tumors. However, medically, it is the term for any drug that is used as an agent to treat infections.

Cholinergic. Drugs that act like the parasympathetic nervous system. They function to help restore energy and mimic the natural physiological process that occurs when acetylcholine (a natural neurotransmitter) stimulates cholinergic nerves to transmit impulses to certain body structures and organs. Cholinergic drugs decrease the heart rate and act on smooth and skeletal muscle. However, because the site of action is so difficult to localize, or target, these drugs have limited clinical usefulness.

Decongestant. A drug that relieves local congestion in the tissues, usually the mucous membranes. The most popular are the nasal decongestants, such as ephedrine or phenylephrine (Neo-Synephrine). Decongestants are often combined with antihistamines.

Diaphoretic. A drug used to induce or increase perspiration.

Digestant. A drug that promotes the progress of digestion. Enzymes, antacids, and bile salts are included in this group.

Diuretic. A drug that increases the function of the kidneys and stimulates the flow of urine. It increases the water content of the blood through osmosis or salt action, freeing water from the tissues and reducing edema. Examples include hydrochlorothiazide (Diazide, Esidrix, HydroDiuril), furosemide (Lasix).

Emetic. A drug used to induce vomiting. Ipecac syrup is commonly used, and mild mustard and plain tepid water are home remedies used as emetics. _warm salt water_

Expectorant. A drug used to increase the secretions and mucus from the bronchial tubes. It makes a cough more productive (expectoration) and breaks up congestion. Some expectorants are combined with antihistamines. An expectorant has an effect opposite that of a cough suppressant.

Hemostatic. A drug used to control bleeding; a blood coagulant. Absorbable hemostatics are applied directly to a wound, and an artificial clot is formed that is gradually absorbed. Gelfoam and Surgicel are examples.

Hypnotic. A drug that produces sleep and lessens the activity of the brain. A hypnotic has a sedative action when used in smaller doses. The barbiturates, both oral and injectable, are the most common hypnotics: pentobarbital (Nembutal), phenobarbital (Luminal), amobarbital (Amytal), secobarbital (Seconal), and secobarbital and amobarbital (Tuinal).

Hypoglycemic. Drugs used to compensate for a lack of effective insulin activity, such as the prompt-acting and long-acting insulins; or drugs that stimulate the pancreas to release insulin, such as chlorpropamide (Diabinese) and tolbutamide (Orinase). _diabetes_

Miotic. An agent that causes the pupil of the eye to contract.

Mydriatic. An agent used to dilate the pupil of the eye. Used by ophthalmologists in eye examinations.

Narcotic. Any of a group of drugs that depress the central nervous system and cause insensibility or stupor. Natural narcotics include the opium group. Synthetic narcotics include codeine phosphate (methylmorphine), meperidine HCl (Demerol), methadone (Dolophine), morphine sulfate, pentazocine (Talwin), and propoxyphene HCl (Darvon).

Opiate. The habit-forming drugs that are derived from or contain opium, such as morphine, codeine, heroin, papaverine, and tincture of opium (paregoric).

Parasympathetic blocking agent. Drugs that are called anticholinergic or cholinergic blocking agents because they block certain effects of acetylcholine (see Cholinergic). These agents include atropine sulfate, dicyclomine HCl (Bentyl), and methscopolamine (Scopolamine). Parasympathetic blocking agents are effective antidotes to cholinergic overdose and are used as gastrointestinal antispasmodics for the management of peptic ulcer, gastritis, and colitis. They are also used as heart rate stimulants, bronchial dilators and pupil dilators for ophthalmic examinations.

Sedative. A drug that ~~reduces excitement~~; a quieting agent that does not produce sleep as a hypnotic drug does. Antianxiety agents may also be classified as sedatives. Sedatives may be hypnotic drugs given in smaller doses or drugs such as the bromides, paraldehyde, chloral hydrate, or flurazepam (Dalmane). The newer antianxiety agents include alprazolam (Xanax), chlordiazepoxide HCl (Librium), diazepam (Valium), and meprobamate (Equanil and Miltown).

Steroids. Drugs that mimic certain chemicals in the body such as the male and female hormones (testosterone, progesterone, and estrogen) and the hormones of the cortices of the adrenal glands. Agents affecting the female and male reproductive systems are used to treat reproductive system imbalances, for birth control, and in labor and delivery. The adrenocorticosteroids (commonly, cortisone) are widely used as anti-inflammatory, antiallergic, and antistress agents.

Sympathetic Blocking Agent. Drugs that are called adrenergic blocking agents (or _sympatholytic_) because they block certain functions of the adrenergic nerves (see Adrenergic). These agents are mainly useful in treating cardiovascular conditions such as hypertension, angina, and cardiac arrhythmias. Some examples are phenoxybenzamine HCl (Dibenzyline), phentolamine mesylate (Regitine), and propranolol HCl (Inderol).

Tranquilizer. A calming agent that reduces anxiety and tension without acting as a depressant.

26

Tranquilizers are called "psychotherapeutic" drugs. In recent years, this group of drugs has greatly increased in number. The phenothiazine derivatives are often used. These include chlorpromazine (Thorazine), perphenazine (Trilafon), and thioridazine (Mellaril).

Vasoconstrictor. A drug that causes the blood vessels to constrict, narrows the lumen of a vessel, raises blood pressure, and causes the heart to beat more forcefully. Vasoconstrictors may be used to stop superficial bleeding, raise and sustain blood pressure, and relieve nasal congestion.

Vasodilator. The opposite of a vasoconstrictor. A drug that dilates blood vessels, lowers blood pressure by making the blood vessel lumen larger, and causes the heart to pump less forcefully. Used in the treatment of hypertension, angina pectoris, and peripheral vascular diseases. Nitroglycerin placed sublingually gives prompt vasodilation. Non-nitrate vasodilators include propranolol (Inderal) and nadolol (Corgard), both sympathetic blocking agents.

APPROACHES TO STUDYING PHARMACOLOGY

A pharmaceutical glossary could be endless. Many terms are combinations of the condition to be treated with the prefix "anti" (for example, antianginal, antianxiety, antiarrhythmic, anticoagulant, anticonvulsant, antidiarrheal).

Notice how these names emphasize the drug's effect (use) rather than its action in the body. More recent classifications, such as *parasympathomimetic* and *cholinesterase inhibitors*, describe the pharmacologic action rather than the therapeutic use; however, both viewpoints are necessary for a more complete understanding of drugs and what they do once in the human body.

Of course no one can remember all there is to know about clinical pharmacology. Even if you did one day, there would be more to learn the next. The number of new drugs being introduced into use far exceeds the number of older drugs being replaced or discontinued. Thus the number of drugs available for clinical use grows beyond the possible knowledge of one person. Therefore, numerous resources are necessary for study and review of the details concerning particular drugs. Remember, when in doubt, look it up before you use a drug.

Reference Materials

A good pharmacology textbook is handy for studying the principles and concepts of each drug classification. There are several comprehensive editions available in hospital and university bookstores. In addition, reference and cross-reference books that are updated annually or periodically should be available for easy reference. Most references list drug information in the following sequence:

1. *Action*: How the drug acts in the body.
2. *Indication*: The conditions for which the drug is used.
3. *Side Effects*: An effect on the body other than theone(s) for which the drug is given.
4. *Adverse Effects*: An effect on a tissue or organ system other than the one being sought by the administration of a medication.
5. *Precautions*: Actions necessary because of special conditions of the patient, drug, or environment that need to be considered for the drug to be successful or not harmful.
6. *Contraindications*: Conditions that make the administration of a drug improper or undesirable.
7. *Toxic Effects*: The poisonous effects and symptoms of toxicity.
8. *Dosage and Administration*: The usual route, dosage, and timing for administering the drug.

Package Inserts. Every drug package contains an insert describing all the significant aspects of using the drug, including information on the chemical formulation of the drug and clinical studies. The information on the inserts is controlled by the FDA.

Physicians' Desk Reference (PDR). This reference book is published annually by the Medical Economics Company, Inc. For physicians who subscribe to *Medical Economics Magazine*, it is provided free of charge. Copies can be purchased through the publisher or in local bookstores. Supplements are published throughout the year. This reference contains information on approximately 2500 drugs, and the product descriptions are identical to the package inserts. The drug manufacturers pay for this space, so the PDR could be called the "yellow pages" of the drug industry.

The book's sections are color-coded and cross-referenced for easy use. The various sections allow you to begin searching for information concerning a drug from any starting point. You can start with the usage, classification, generic name, manufacturer's name, or trade name of a drug or what the drug looks like. There is a special photographic section for visual product identification. Once you know which drug you want to study, the Product Information Section lists the actual package insert information alphabetically, first by the manufacturer, then by the brand name.

AMA Drug Evaluations. This reference is published by the American Medical Association and replaces a former publication called *New Drugs*. The book provides information on over 1000 drugs, without the bias or endorsement of any particular brand or group of drugs.

The American Hospital Formulary. This reference is published by the American Society of Hospital Pharmacists and is available by subscription. The information is contained in a two-volume set, with four to six supplements added each year. Generic names are listed, and it is divided into sections based on drug actions.

The U.S. Pharmacopeia (USP). This publication was first printed in 1820, and new editions are still published every five years. England and Canada each publish similar volumes. The *Pharmacopeia* is usually not an appropriate reference purchase for the medical office.

The U.S. Pharmacopeia/National Formulary (USP/NF). This reference is the official source of drug standards for the United States. The *Pharmacopeia* was just recently combined with the *National Formulary*, which lists the chemical formulas for all accepted drugs. This new combined reference lists and describes all the approved medications that are considered useful and therapeutic in the practice of medicine. Single drugs rather than combined products (compound mixtures) are listed. If a drug name is the same as the official name in this volume, the drug will have the initials "USP" after it; for example, digitoxin, USP.

Learning About Drugs

The study of pharmacology is difficult, at best. However, there are a few ways you can make it easier.

First, take opportunities to observe the use of drugs in patient care. Studying about epinephrine (Adrenalin) becomes more meaningful when you see how its cardiovascular actions get a patient through an anaphylactic episode. More memorable than any textbook!

Second, concentrate on the most important drugs in each classification. For example, learn about digitalis (cardiovascular), morphine (narcotic analgesic), epinephrine (autonomic nervous system blocker), and atropine (autonomic nervous system mimetic). As you expand your knowledge to other drugs in each classification, you will easily understand new drugs by noting the similarities and differences between them and the basic, important drugs you studied first.

Third, learn about a drug's primary action and use, then expand your knowledge to its other actions and uses. Soon, you will be able to name the drug that is usually indicated for a particular condition. Then, by knowing a drug's secondary effects, you will be able to understand what side effects are likely to occur during the use of the drug. More important, you will be aware of the contraindications for the drug (conditions that make the use of the drug improper or undesirable). Knowledge of the drug's actions will also enable you to predict what toxic reactions could occur from overdose (Table 26–3).

It is hoped that pharmacology will always remain exciting and interesting to you as you work with patients and the other members of your team and that you will continue to assess and evaluate new drugs as their administration becomes your responsibility.

CALCULATING DRUG DOSAGES FOR ADMINISTRATION

The correct dosage of a medication may depend on the patient's age, weight, or state of health or on what other drugs the patient may be taking. Often, the physician will order a medication in a dosage that is different from that of the medications you stock. The difference may be in the system of measurement, the strength, or the form. There are formulas and mathematical tables of conversion for calculating the correct dosage of medication to be administered. Let's look at how you arrive at the correct calculation, one step at a time.

Mathematical Equivalents

You may need to review some basics of arithmetic before you begin to tackle drug calculations. You must thoroughly understand the addition, subtraction, multiplication, and division of fractions and decimals; the relationship of decimals and fractions; and how they are converted from one to the other. In addition, you need to review how decimals and percentages are converted back and forth from one another. Table 26–4 provides some examples of these relationships.

The table shows that a fraction is, in another sense, a ratio. For example, ¼ (a fraction) is the same as the ratio 1:4 (one-to-four). If there is one apple and four oranges, then the number of apples that you have is ¼ the number of oranges, and the ratio of apples to oranges is 1:4. Now, divide the numerator 1 by the denominator 4 (a fraction is also an automatic division problem waiting to be solved):

$$\begin{array}{r} .25 \\ 4\overline{)1.00} \end{array}$$

The act of dividing a fraction results in a decimal number. Decimal numbers can then be converted to percentages by moving the decimal two (2) spaces to the right:

.25 = 25.0%, commonly written 25%.

Table 26–3
Alphabetic Cross-Reference by Brand Name to the Drugs Mentioned in this Chapter

Brand Name	Generic Name	Classification (by first mention)	Brand Name	Generic Name	Classification (by first mention)
Adrenalin	Epinephrine HCl USP	adrenergic	Lasix	Furosemide USP	diuretic
Advil	Ibuprofen	analgesic	L-Dopa	Levodopa	antispasmodic
Aldomet	Methyldopa USP	antihypertensive	Librium	Chlordiazepoxide HCl	antianxiety
Amoxil	Amoxicillin USP	antibiotic	Lithium	Lithium	antidepressant
Ampicillin	Ampicillin USP	antibiotic	Lomotil	Diphenoxylate HCl USP	antidiarrheal
Amytal	Amobarbital	hypnotic	Lopressor	Metoprolol tartrate	antihypertensive
Aspirin	Aspirin USP	analgesic	Luminal	Phenobarbital	hypnotic
Atropine	Atropine sulfate	anticholinergic	Mellaril	Thioridazine	tranquilizer
Benadryl	Diphenhydramine HCl, USP	antihistamine	Miltown	Meprobamate	antianxiety
			Monistat	Miconazole	antifungal
Bentyl	Dicyclomine HCl	anticholinergic	Morphine	Morphine sulfate USP	narcotic
Benylin	Diphenhydramine HCl USP	antihistamine	Motrin	Ibuprofen	analgesic
			Mycostatin	Nystatin	antifungal
Bicillin	Penicillin G benzathine USP	antibiotic	Naprosyn	Naproxen	analgesic
			Nembutal	Pentobarbital	hypnotic
Butazolidin	Phenylbutazone USP	analgesic	Neo-Synephrine	Phenylephrine HCl	decongestant
Chlor-Trimeton	Chlorpheniramine maleate	antihistamine	Nitrostat	Nitroglycerin USP	vasodilator
			Nuprin	Ibuprofen	analgesic
Codeine	Codeine phosphate USP	narcotic	Orinase	Tolbutamide	hypoglycemic
Corgard	Nadolol	antihypertensive	Paregoric	Tincture of opium	opiate
Crystodigin	Digitalis	cardiotonic	Pentids	Potassium penicillin G	antibiotic
Dalmane	Flurazepam	sedative	Phenergan	Promethazine HCl	antihistamine
Darvon	Propoxyphene HCl USP	narcotic	Proventil	Albuterol	bronchodilator
Demerol	Meperidine HCl	narcotic	Purodigin	Digitalis	cardiotonic
Dexedrine	Dextroamphetamine	antiepileptic	Regitine	Phentolamine mesylate	adrenergic blocker
Diabinese	Chlorpropamide	hypoglycemic	Ritalin	Methylphenidate USP	antiepileptic
Diazide	Hydrochlorothiazide USP	diuretic	Robaxin	Methocarbamol	antispasmodic
Dibenzyline	Phenoxybenzamine HCl	adrenergic blocker	Romilar	Dextromethorphan HBr USP	antitussive
Digitoxin	Digitalis	cardiotonic			
Dilantin	Phenytoin	antiepileptic	Scopolamine	Methscopolamine	anticholinergic
Dimetane	Brompheniramine maleate	antihistamine	Seconal	Secobarbital	hypnotic
			Soma	Carisoprodol	antispasmodic
Dolophine	Methadone	narcotic	Tagamet	Cimetidine	histamine blocker
Dramamine	Dimenhydrinate	antiemetic	Talwin	Pentazocrine	narcotic
Elavil	Amitriptyline HCl	antidepressant	Tenormin	Atenolol	antihypertensive
Ephedrine	Ephedrine HCl USP	decongestant	Terpin Hydrate and Codeine	Terpin hydrate with codeine	antitussive
Equanil	Meprobamate	antianxiety			
Esidrix	Hydrochlorothiazide USP	diuretic	Theo-Dur	Anhydrous theophylline	bronchodilator
Feldene	Piroxicam	analgesic	Theophylline	Aminophylline USP	bronchodilator
Fulvicin-U/F	Griseofulvin	antifungal	Thorazine	Chlorpromazine	tranquilizer
Fungizone	Amphotericin B USP	antifungal	Tofranil	Imipramine HCl	antidepressant
HydroDiuril	Hydrochlorothiazide USP	diuretic	Trilafon	Perphenazine	tranquilizer
Inderal	Propranolol HCl	adrenergic blocker	Tuinal	Secobarbital and amobarbital	hypnotic
Indocin	Indomethacin USP	analgesic			
Ipecac	Ipecac	emetic	Tylenol	Acetaminophen USP	analgesic
Isuprel	Isoproterenol HCl	bronchodilator	Valium	Diazepam	antianxiety
Keflex	Cephalexin	antibiotic	Ventolin	Albuterol	bronchodilator
Keflin	Cephalothin sodium USP	antibiotic	Xanax	Alprazolam	antianxiety
			Zantac	Ranitidine	histamine blocker

Now, we can see all the relationships of Table 26–4. Using the example of apples and oranges, you can see that 1 is .25, or 25%, of 4. Therefore the apple is .25, or 25%, the number of oranges. If you need to review any of these concepts, please stop now and practice these steps of arithmetic. To go on without this background could be very frustrating as you attempt to understand problems in dosage calculations.

Ratio and Proportion

We have just reviewed that *ratio* is one way of expressing a fraction, or division problem, and shows the relationship of the numerator to the denominator. The comparison of *two* ratios is called a *proportion*. A proportion is written as follows:

$$\frac{4}{16} = \frac{1}{4} \text{ or } 4{:}16 :: 1{:}4$$

Table 26–4
Mathematical Equivalents

Percentage	Decimal	Fraction	Ratio
25%	.25	1/4	1:4
50%	.5	1/2	1:2
60%	.6	3/5 (6/10)	3:5
.5%	.005	1/200	1:200
.1%	.001	1/1000	1:1000
85%	.85	17/20	17:20
1%	.01	1/100	1:100

This is read as 4 divided by 16 equals 1 divided by 4, or four is to sixteen as one is to four. What we are saying here is that both ratios have the same proportions and are equal to one another even though the numbers are different. This is the key to calculating drug dosages. The physician's order for a medication may be a ratio different from that of the medication we stock, and we will then compare the ordered ratio to the available ratio (what we have in stock) to find the correct proportion to administer. However, before going on, there is more background material that we need to know.

The preceding proportion example has all the answers in it; there is nothing to solve. In calculating dosages, we use mathematical proportions, but with one element unknown. We must solve for that unknown, or "x." For example:

$$\frac{4}{16} = \frac{1}{x}$$

Always in a proportion, we solve the problem by *cross-multiplication*. Do not confuse this with plain multiplication. If you see an equal sign (=) between two fractions, you know this is an *equation* to be *cross-multiplied*.

$$\frac{1}{x} = \frac{4}{16}$$

Now cross-multiply:

$$4 \times x = 16 \times 1$$

Therefore:

$$4x = 16$$

We know what 4x equals, but next we must find what 1x, or x, equals. To find the value of x, we must find a way to leave x (or 1x) alone on one side of the equation. We can change 4x to 1x by dividing the number 4 by itself:

$$4x \div 4 = 1x$$

But what we do on one side of an *equation*, we must do on the other side, or the equation will not be equal anymore. Therefore, we divide 16 by 4:

$$16 \div 4 = 4$$

The answer is x = 4! Let's put it all together now.

$$\frac{1}{x} = \frac{4}{16}$$
$$4 \times x = 16 \times 1$$
$$4x = 16$$
$$\frac{4x}{4} = \frac{16}{4}$$
$$1x = 4$$

We take the answer 4 and replace the "x" with it in the ratio. We have solved for "x."

$$\frac{4}{16} = \frac{1}{4}$$

Calculating Dosages

When calculating dosages, a standard set of formulas is used. These formulas employ certain specific terms. Every drug has a *strength* (potency) and a *dosage unit* (*amount*). The strength is the quantity of the drug held together in a particular form. The amount (volume) is what contains the drug. It may be a solid form, such as a tablet, or a liquid form, such as 1 cubic centimeter (cc) of injectable physiological saline. In liquids, the drug strength is often called the *solute*. The solute is dissolved in an amount called the *solvent*. It is important to understand which measurements pertain to the strength (potency) of a drug and which pertain to the unit of dosage (form, volume, or amount). For example, a vial of injectable material may read "500 mg/cc." This means there are 500 mg (strength) of drug in every cc (amount) of liquid. When an oral medication reads "5 gr," it means that there are 5 grains (strength) in every tablet (amount). Let's use these two examples and the proportion formula previously reviewed to work out two problems: (1) filling a syringe and (2) administering tablets.

1. **Order:** Give 250 mg of a drug.
   Available: A vial marked 500 mg/cc.
   Standard Formula:

   $$\frac{\text{available strength}}{\text{ordered strength}} = \frac{\text{available amount}}{\text{amount to give}}$$

   Problem: Given the strength of the drug needed, the amount of fluid to be withdrawn must be determined.

   We will set up a proportion with the three known quantities: the strength of the drug in the vial, the unit of fluid in which that strength is contained, and the strength of the drug the physician wishes to be administered to the patient.

   Apply the problem to the standard formula:

   $$\frac{500 \text{ mg}}{250 \text{ mg}} = \frac{1 \text{ cc}}{x \text{ cc}}$$
   $$500 \times x = 250 \times 1$$
   $$500x = 250$$
   $$\frac{500x}{500} = \frac{250}{500}$$
   $$1x = \frac{1}{2} \text{ cc} = 0.50 \text{ cc}$$

   Solution: Administer 0.50 cc of the drug.

2. **Order:** Give 10 gr (grains) of a drug.
   Available: A bottle with tablets labeled 5 gr each.
   Standard Formula:

   $$\frac{\text{available strength}}{\text{ordered strength}} = \frac{\text{available amount}}{\text{amount to give}}$$

Problem: Given the strength of the drug needed, the number of tablets to be administered must be determined.

We will set up a proportion with the three known quantities: the strength of the drug in each tablet, the unit amount that is one tablet, and the strength of the drug the physician wishes to be administered to the patient.

Apply the problem to the standard formula:

$$\frac{5 \text{ gr}}{10 \text{ gr}} = \frac{1 \text{ tablet}}{x \text{ (no. of tablets)}}$$

$$5 \times x = 10 \times 1$$

$$5x = 10$$

$$\frac{5x}{5} = \frac{10}{5}$$

$$1x = 2 \text{ tablets}$$

Solution: Administer 2 tablets.

Use the *standard formula* for any type of calculation. You may be using strengths that are measured in International Units (IU), as with insulin or penicillin; grams; milligrams; grains; or percentages. The forms in which drugs may be prepared include cubic centimeters (cc), or milliliters (ml); minims; drops; drams; ounces; pints; gallons (for making up diluted stock solutions from concentrated solutions, such as with alcohol and hydrogen peroxide); or spoonfuls. Follow the steps previously shown, and above all, discipline yourself to write down each step with complete calculations. This is the only way to ensure maximum accuracy and the safety of your patients. If you have difficulty with the calculation, or the answer does not seem quite right, ask the physician to check your calculation. A double check is always preferred.

Systems of Measurement

Sometimes, the physician will order a medication in a strength that is totally different from the one on the label of the vial or bottle. For example, the physician may order one grain of a drug, but the available dosage form is in milligrams. Before you can use the ratio and proportion formulas to arrive at the amount to administer, you first must convert to one system or the other. The best way is to convert to the measurement system that is on the label (what is available). After all, that is the system you will have to use. Dosage calculations would be easier if pharmacology dealt with just one system of measurement. Unfortunately, there are three: the metric system, the apothecary system, and the household system.

The *metric system* of weights and measures is now used throughout the world as the primary system for weight (mass), capacity (volume), and length

(area). In the United States, it is used for scientific work, including most pharmaceuticals. However, some medication forms still use the older apothecary system, which necessitates learning the two systems and the relationships (conversions) between the two. A few hints about each system follow.

The metric system of weights and measures is a decimal system, which means that it uses the base ten (10). Each higher measure is 10 times the measure at hand; each lower, 1/10 the measure. The fraction is always written as a decimal, and the number precedes the letters designating the actual measure. Thus, one and a half liters would be written 1.5 L (Table 26–5). The *cubic centimeter* (cc) and the *milliliter* (ml) are interchangeable. In the metric system, 1 cc is a measurement of area, and an area this size holds exactly 1 ml (1/1000 of a liter) of fluid (volume). In fact, if you were to weigh 1 ml of water contained in 1 cc of area under certain conditions of temperature and barometric pressure, it would also weigh exactly 1 *gram* (gm). In the metric system, these three basic units of measurement are convertible from one to the other.

With the *apothecary system*, the basic unit of weight is the *grain* (gr), and the basic unit of volume is the *minim* (M.). As in the metric system, these two units are related: the grain is based on the weight of a single grain of wheat, and the minim is the volume of water that weighs one grain. Either roman or arabic numerals may be used, but it is not proper to use them together in the same prescription. Either symbols or abbreviations are used; for example, one and a half drams might be written ʒiss or d 1½. The number follows the symbol or abbreviation. Table 26–6 compares the units of weight and volume in the metric and the apothecary systems.

The *household system* is used in most American households. This system of measurement is important for the patient at home who has no knowledge of the metric or apothecary systems. The basic measure of weight is the *pound*; the basic measure of volume, the *drop*. The household drop is equal to the apothecary minim, so these two systems are sometimes easily interchangeable. Both the house-

Table 26–5
Abbreviations and Symbols for Selected Weights and Measures

	Apothecary System			Metric System
	♏	Min. (M.)	minim	gm	gram
	Ə	scr	scruple	L	liter
	ʒ	dr	dram	cc	cubic centimeter
fl	ℨ	f dr	fluid dram	ml	milliliter
	℥	oz	ounce		
fl	℥	fl oz	fluid ounce		
	O	pt	pint		
	C	gal	gallon		
		gr	grain		

Table 26–6
Comparison of Weights and Measurements

Apothecary Table of Weights

APOTHECARY		APPROXIMATE METRIC EQUIVALENT		
60 grains (gr)	= 1 dram (dr ʒ)	60 to 65	milligrams (mg)	= 1 grain
8 drams	= 1 ounce (oz ʒ)	4	grams	= 1 dram
12 ounces	= 1 pound (lb)*	30 to 32	grams	= 1 ounce
		370 to 375	grams	= 1 pound
		0.37 to 0.375	kilograms	= 1 pound

Metric System of Weights

METRIC		APPROXIMATE APOTHECARY EQUIVALENT	
1000 micrograms (mcg)	= 1 milligram (mg)	gr 1/60	= 1 mg
1000 milligrams	= 1 gram (gm)	gr 15–16	= 1 gm
1000 grams	= 1 kilogram (kg)	2.2 lb (avoir.)	= 1 kg

Apothecary Table of Volume

APOTHECARY		APPROXIMATE METRIC EQUIVALENT	
1 minim (m)			= 0.06 ml
60 minims	= 1 fluid dram (fl dr)	4 ml	= 1 fdr (fl dr)
8 fluid drams	= 1 fluid ounce (fl oz)	30 ml	= 1 foz (fl oz)
16 fluid ounces	= 1 pint (pt or O)	500 ml or 0.5 liter	= 1 pint
2 pints	= 1 quart (qt)	1000 ml or 1 liter	= 1 quart
4 quarts	= 1 gallon (gal or C)	4000 ml or 4 liters	= 1 gallon

Metric Table of Volume

METRIC		APPROXIMATE APOTHECARY EQUIVALENT	
1000 milliliters (ml)†	= 1 liter (L)	15 minims	= 1 ml
1000 liters	= 1 kiloliter (kl)	1 quart	= 1 liter or 1000 ml

From Falconer, Mary W., et al.: The Drug, The Nurse, The Patient, 6th ed. Philadelphia, W. B. Saunders Co., 1978, p. 57.
*Note that in the avoirdupois table there are 16 ounces in one pound. In the Troy table there are 12 ounces in one pound as with the apothecary.
†One cubic centimeter (cc) is often used in place of one milliliter (ml). A milliliter of water occupies approximately one cubic centimeter of space.

26

hold and the apothecary systems use the terms dram and ounce as units of measurement, so always be sure of which system you are using. Medications are not measured in household weights, but many prescriptions contain directions using the household measurements of volume. Liquid oral medications are taken by the drop, teaspoon, or tablespoon, and are supplied in bottles labeled in ounces or pints. Table 26–7 shows the household system of measurement (note that there are some apothecary equivalents).

Pediatric Dose Calculations

As noted earlier in the chapter, there is no perfect system for converting adult medications to proper pediatric dosages. In most cases, children are not able to tolerate adult medications, as a child's me-

Table 26–7
Household Measures and Equivalents*

1 minim	= 1 drop
1 teaspoon	= 5 ml or 75 drops
4 teaspoons	= 1 tablespoon (15 cc)
1 dessert spoon	= 2 drams
1 tablespoon	= 4 drams
4 tablespoons	= 1 wineglass
16 tablespoons (liquid)	= 1 cup (liquid)
12 tablespoons (dry)	= 1 cup (dry)
1 cup	= 8 fluid ounces
1 glass	= 8 fluid ounces
1 wineglass	= 2 fluid ounces
1 pint	= 1 pound
1 tablespoon	= 16 cc
1 ounce	= 1 whiskey glass

*These measure and equivalents are approximate because of the great variation in household measuring devices.

tabolism is very unstable compared with that of an adult. When it is necessary to administer an adult medication to a child, the following formulas are accepted. Calculating dosage in this manner is permitted only under the direct order and supervision of the physician.

Fried's Law. This calculation is for children under one year of age and is based on the age of the child in months compared with a child 12½ years old. The calculation assumes that an adult dose would be appropriate for a child aged 12½ years (150 months).

$$\text{Pediatric dose} = \frac{\text{child's age in months}}{150 \text{ months}} \times \text{adult dose.}$$

Young's Rule. For children over one year of age.

$$\text{Pediatric dose} = \frac{\text{child's age in years}}{\text{child's age in years} + 12} \times \text{adult dose.}$$

Clark's Rule. Based on the weight of the child. This system is much more accurate, since children of any age can vary greatly in size and body weight. Clark's rule uses 150 pounds (70 kg) as the average adult weight and assumes that the child's dose is proportionately less. The formula is

$$\text{Pediatric dose} = \frac{\text{child's weight in pounds}}{150 \text{ pounds}} \times \text{adult dose.}$$

West's Nomogram. Calculates the body surface area of infants and young children. Many physicians use the **nomogram**, because even a small miscalculation could be critical, especially when a child is ill, underweight, or overweight (Fig. 26–2).

$$\text{Pediatric dose} = \frac{\begin{array}{c}\text{basic surface area of child}\\ \text{(in square meters)}\end{array}}{1.73 \text{ square meters}} \times \text{adult dose.}$$

You need complete mastery in calculating dosages, whether they be for children or adults. Until you master the arithmetic, the accurate placement of the decimal point, converting equivalents from one system to another, and the use of the ratio and

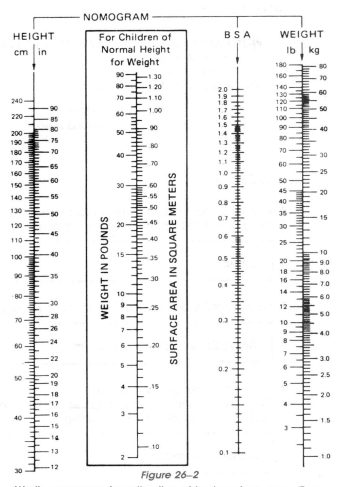

Figure 26–2

West's nomogram for estimation of body surface area. (From Behrman, R. E., and Vaughan, V. C., III: Nelson Textbook of Pediatrics, 13th ed. Philadelphia, W. B. Saunders Co., 1987.)

proportion formula for every type of calculation, you must practice problems in dosages and solutions with someone who can check your work. Mastery of dosage calculations may take some time and much practice, but as with any other skill, you can achieve it if you take the time to understand the basics first, then advance to the concepts of ratio and proportion and, finally, the calculation of specific drugs and solutions.

Procedure 26–1

CALCULATING THE CORRECT DOSAGE FOR ADMINISTRATION

PROCEDURAL GOAL

To calculate the correct dosage amount and choose the correct equipment when the physician orders 2.4 million IU (International Units) of Bicillin (penicillin G benzathine) to be administered to a patient.

Procedure continued on opposite page

EQUIPMENT AND SUPPLIES

Premixed syringes of Bicillin in the following two strengths:
   0.6 million IU/syringe
   1.2 million IU/syringe
Standard mathematical formula:

$$\frac{\text{available strength}}{\text{ordered strength}} = \frac{\text{available amount}}{\text{amount to give}}$$

PROCEDURE

1. Read the order in quiet surroundings to make sure that you fully understand it.
2. Using pencil and paper, write out the order.

> Order:

3. Examine the drug labels to see what strengths and amounts are available.

> Available Strengths and Amounts:

4. Write down the standard formula.
   Purpose: To eliminate the chances of error, orders should never be carried out unless the calculations are completed in writing.

> Standard Formula:

5. Rewrite the formula, replacing the unknown values with the known quantities. The unknown "x" will be the amount of the drug to give ("amount to give").

> Formula with Known Quantities:

6. Work the proportion problem by cross-multiplying to solve for x.

7. State your answer by filling in the blanks, as follows:
   To administer 2.4 million IU of Bicillin, I would select _____ of the premixed syringes labeled _____.

TERMINAL PERFORMANCE OBJECTIVE

Given the necessary physician's order and equipment, calculate the correct dosage with 100 percent accuracy, within three minutes, as determined by your evaluator.

26

Procedure 26–2

*CALCULATING THE CORRECT DOSAGE FOR
ADMINISTRATION USING TWO SYSTEMS OF
MEASUREMENT*

PROCEDURAL GOAL

To choose the correct system of measurement and calculate the correct dosage amount when the physician orders 120 mg (milligrams) of a drug to be administered to a patient.

EQUIPMENT AND SUPPLIES

Tablets labeled 1 gr (grain) each
Standard mathematical formula:

$$\frac{\text{available strength}}{\text{ordered strength}} = \frac{\text{available amount}}{\text{amount to give}}$$

Conversion equivalent:

$$1 \text{ gr} = 60 \text{ mg}$$

PROCEDURE

1. Read the order in quiet surroundings to make sure that you fully understand it.
2. Using pencil and paper, write out the order.

> Order:

3. Examine the drug labels to see what strengths and amounts are available.

> Available Strengths and Amounts:

4. Convert the ordered system of measurement to the system of measurement on the label.

> 120 mg equals how many grains?

5. Write down the standard formula.
   Purpose: To eliminate the chances of error, orders should never be carried out unless the calculations are completed in writing.

> Standard Formula:

6. Rewrite the formula, replacing the unknown values with the known quantities and using the system of measurement on the label. The unknown "x" will be the amount of the drug to give ("amount to give").

> Formula with Known Quantities:

7. Work the proportion problem by cross-multiplying to solve for x.

Procedure continued on opposite page

8. State your answer by filling in the blanks, as follows:
   To administer 120 mg of a drug from tablets labeled 1 gr (grain) each, I would give _____ tablet(s).

TERMINAL PERFORMANCE OBJECTIVE

Given the necessary physician's order and equipment, calculate the correct dosage with 100 percent accuracy, within three minutes, as determined by your evaluator.

Procedure 26–3

CALCULATING THE CORRECT DOSAGE FOR A CHILD WHEN ONLY AN ADULT MEDICATION IS AVAILABLE

26

PROCEDURAL GOAL

To calculate the correct dosage amount for a 90-pound child using Clark's rule.

EQUIPMENT AND SUPPLIES

Adult dosage 250 mg/cc
Clark's rule:

$$\text{Pediatric dose} = \frac{\text{child's weight in pounds}}{150 \text{ pounds}} \times \text{adult dose}$$

Standard mathematical formula:

$$\frac{\text{available strength}}{\text{ordered strength}} = \frac{\text{available amount}}{\text{amount to give}}$$

PROCEDURE

1. Read the order in quiet surroundings to make sure that you fully understand it.
2. Using pencil and paper, write out the order.

   Order:

3. Examine the drug labels to see what strengths and amounts are available.

   Available Strengths and Amounts:

4. Write down Clark's rule.
   Purpose: To eliminate the chances of error, orders should never be carried out unless the calculations are completed in writing.

Procedure continued on following page

Clark's Rule:

5. Using Clark's rule, replace the unknown values with the known quantities. The unknown "x" will be the pediatric strength ordered ("pediatric dose").

Clark's Rule with Known Quantities:

6. Write down the standard formula.
   Purpose: To eliminate the chances of error, orders should never be carried out unless the calculations are completed in writing.

Standard Formula:

7. Rewrite the formula, replacing the unknown values with the available quantities and the pediatric strength just determined. The unknown "x" will be the amount of the drug to give ("amount to give").

Formula with Known Quantities:

8. Work the proportion problem by cross-multiplying to solve for x.

9. State your answer by filling in the blanks, as follows:
   To administer an adult medication labeled 250 mg/cc to a 90-pound child, I will give _____ cc.

TERMINAL PERFORMANCE OBJECTIVE

Given the necessary physician's order and equipment, calculate the correct dosage with 100 percent accuracy, within three minutes, as determined by your evaluator.

Now that you have an introductory understanding of clinical pharmacology, and some guidelines for calculating drug dosages, you are ready to move on to Chapter 27, Administration of Medications. This chapter covers the medical assisting process in drug administration and therapy.

Answers to Procedures 26–1 through 26–3

26–1. To administer 2.4 million IU of Bicillin, I would select 2 of the premixed syringes labeled 1.2 million IU per syringe.

26–2. To administer 120 mg of a drug from tablets labeled 1 gr each, I would give 2 tablets.

26–3. To administer an adult medication labeled 250 mg/cc to a 90-pound child, I would give 0.6 cc.

REFERENCES AND READINGS

Asperheim, M. K.: *The Pharmacologic Basis of Patient Care*, 5th ed. Philadelphia, W. B. Saunders Co., 1985.

Bonewit, K.: *Clinical Procedures for Medical Assistants*, 2nd ed. Philadelphia, W. B. Saunders Co., 1984.

DuGas, B. W.: *Introduction to Patient Care: A Comprehensive Approach to Nursing*, 4th ed. Philadelphia, W. B. Saunders Co., 1983.

Rodman, M. R., and Karch, A. M.: *Pharmacology and Drug Therapy in Nursing*, 3rd ed. Philadelphia, J. B. Lippincott Co., 1985.

Sheridan, E., Patterson, H. R., and Gustafson, E. A.: *Falconer's The Drug, The Nurse, The Patient*, 7th ed. Philadelphia, W. B. Saunders Co., 1985.

Tallarida, R. J.: *Most-Prescribed Drugs (MPD 85)*. Philadelphia, W. B. Saunders Co., 1985.

26

CHAPTER OUTLINE

VOCABULARY

See Glossary at end of book for definitions.

hermetically sealed
radical mastectomy
viscosity
volatile

27

Administration of Medications

OBJECTIVES

Upon successful completion of this chapter you should be able to

1. Spell and define the words listed in the Vocabulary for this chapter.
2. List five factors of patient assessment that may influence whether or not you should continue with an order to administer a drug.
3. State two situations in which it may be your responsibility to further assess an ordered drug before administering it.
4. State two environmental factors that would contraindicate the administration of a medication.
5. Recall the "Three Befores" and the "Five Rights."
6. List the basic solid and liquid oral dosage forms and give an example of each.
7. For each of the five mucous membrane sites, cite the methods for administering medications.
8. Differentiate among the nine types of topical medications.
9. For each parenteral method, list the preferred needle gauge(s) and lengths, and the usual syringe size.
10. State the risks of reusable injectable equipment, and three advantages of disposable injectable equipment.
11. List the contraindications for administering a parenteral drug at any particular site.
12. Locate the anatomic landmarks for each intramuscular injection site.
13. List the special considerations of anatomy when administering injectable medications to infants and small children.

Upon successful completion of this chapter you should be able to perform the following activities:

1. Fill a syringe from an ampule or vial using sterile technique.
2. Administer a medication using the intramuscular method.
3. Administer a medication using the Z-tract intramuscular method.
4. Administer a medication using the subcutaneous method.
5. Administer an allergy test using the intradermal injection technique.

Drug therapy has become one of the most significant aspects of patient care and one of the most significant responsibilities that a physician may delegate to a medical assistant. The medical assistant who is asked to administer medications must have a thorough understanding of the scientific principles of drug therapy and the confidence and assurance to follow through with the physician's request. Chapter 26, Introduction to Clinical Pharmacology, is an introduction to how drugs interact with the body, the basic routes of administration, and the standard formulas for dosage calculation. This chapter, Chapter 27, builds on the last, developing the specific skills of patient assessment and drug administration. Most of the drugs administered in the medical office will be by injection (parenterally). Most oral medications will be filled by prescription and will be started by the patient at home. Occasionally, you may be required to instill drops into a patient's eye, ears, or nose, or you may be called upon to insert a rectal suppository into a pediatric patient.

No matter what type of medication you are to administer, the order must come from the physician. If the physician delegates to you drug administration as part of your job, it must be allowable under state laws. Every state has a medical practice act that will define whether or not a medical assistant can administer drugs under the supervision of a physician. Some states allow medical assistants to administer only certain types of medications, some prohibit medical assistants from giving injections. Information concerning the scope of practice for medical assistants in your particular state should be obtained from your local government or medical society. You should know what the law states and how your duties fit into that law.

DRUG THERAPY ASSESSMENT

Although medications may be given only under the direct order and supervision of the physician, you are a part of the assessment and problem-solving processes in the care of the patient. In medicine, assessment never ends and never is the responsibility of just one person. A physician gives the order to administer medication to a patient based on a medical assessment, but you also must continue to assess the patient and the patient's environment as you follow through with the order. The physician depends on you to be alert to changes or new information that could result in a condition or consequence that would make the use of a drug improper or undesirable. Before giving every medication, you should assess the patient, the drug, and the environment.

Patient Assessment

Assessment of the patient includes the patient's history and current status. As you are about to act

on a physician's order, you too should mentally review the following factors that may influence whether you continue with the order or return to the physician for further clarification.

- Are there any conditions that may contraindicate the use of the drug or the dosage ordered?
- Do you have special knowledge of any other drug use (a dependency, or the use of prescription or over-the-counter drugs) that may contraindicate the completion of the medication order?
- Does the patient have any allergies to drugs of this type or to certain foods or animals that may indicate that this drug will produce a similar allergic effect?
- Are the patient's age, height, and weight correct for the dosage ordered?
- Is there a reason that the route chosen for administration may not be desirable? For example, injections may be ordered for a particular site. However, you notice that at the site there is an injury, a swelling, or a recent change in texture or pigmentation, which would contraindicate the use of the site for injection.

Patient assessment does not end with the administration of the drug. Observe patients carefully for drug reactions that may follow injectable medications. Patients receiving penicillin (a drug with a high incidence of allergic response) or allergy immunotherapy (administering repeated injections of dilute extracts of the substance that causes the allergy; also called desensitization) must remain in the office for 20 to 30 minutes in case of acute anaphylactic reaction. Acute anaphylactic reaction can result in respiratory failure and circulatory collapse within minutes if not reversed with epinephrine. Lesser allergic reactions include hives, swelling, and itching. An antihistamine, such as Benadryl, may need to be administered (see Chapter 22, Basic Concepts of Asepsis, and Chapter 39, First Aid).

Drug Assessment

Drug assessment includes evaluation of the dosage ordered and the drug itself. No medication should be administered without a written order. If you are to administer a medication by verbal order, be sure to have the physician sign or write the order on the patient's medical record as soon as possible. If there is doubt about a particular order, written or verbal, do not give the drug until you are sure that it is what the physician intends. If you still have doubts, confidentially and politely request that the physician personally administer the drug. Remember that you take the responsibility if you do not understand an order but administer it anyway.

You must also evaluate the drug's appropriateness. For example, you have a patient who is a diabetic, and the physician orders Ornade. You know that Ornade is a time-released antihistamine and that Orinase is an oral hypoglycemic. Never hesitate to question a misinterpretation or possible mistake on a drug order. So many drugs sound and are spelled alike that mistakes are possible. If you do not know the details of the drugs that you are administering, you will not be able to assess their appropriateness and, therefore, to support the physician and safeguard the patient.

Know the appropriate dosages. The standard abbreviations for dosages may not be clearly written, and you may need to know whether the order was for a minim (M.) or for a milliliter (ml). Since there are 15 to 16 minims in a milliliter, to guess or not to know the appropriate dosage, in this case, could result in a patient receiving 15 times the desired amount, or 1/15 the necessary amount. Either way, harm may come to a patient from an irresponsible act on your part.

Environment Assessment

The patient's surroundings could determine an order's inappropriateness. The patient may become hysterical or uncooperative about receiving the medication, or the patient's family may protest the use of the drug. A patient may come to the office for a weekly drug treatment, but the physician may not be present. Drugs should not be administered to patients, even on order, if there is not someone present who can not only administer emergency first aid but also reverse acute anaphylactic reactions with injectable epinephrine. The medical assistant cannot inject epinephrine without an order. In the absence of a physician, there would be no one to give that order in an emergency.

The environment must be safe for drug administration. Be sure that the patient is comfortable and protected from further injury. If a patient is to receive an injection, make sure to place the patient in a position that best exposes the site and protects the patient from injury in case he or she faints or has a drug reaction. If the patient is to take an oral medication with water, be sure that he or she is seated in a position that will prevent choking. Because any medication is potentially dangerous to a patient, there also must be emergency drugs, readily available, to counteract any adverse effects that might occur immediately following the administration of a medication. Emergency drugs should be in injectable form for rapid effect. Typically, emergency carts include adrenergics, such as epinephrine; anticholinergics, such as atropine; bronchodilators; and antihistamine-histamine blockers.

A note about your own environment. The entire process of administering medications should be completed in quiet surroundings and with concentration. When you are preparing and administering a medication, do not do anything else, including talking. The process requires organized and concise

movements and involves "The Three Befores" and "The Five Rights."

The "Three Befores"

Before administering any drug, check the label for the correct drug choice and dosage three times:

1. **Before** removing the drug from the shelf. Make sure you start with the right medication and dosage.

2. **Before** pouring or preparing the drug. A double check while you work.

3. **Before** returning the drug to the shelf. A third check. Drugs are returned to the shelf before you leave the medication room to administer the medication to the patient.

The "Five Rights"

Before you leave the medication room, take the time to say "yes" to the following five questions. Do I have the

1. **Right** patient? Check the name on the patient's chart. (Before administering the drug, you will again check, by greeting the patient by name, to be sure that you have the right person.)

2. **Right** drug? Compare the written drug name with the label of the container that you are using. Does it seem appropriate? Know the medications that you are using. Never prepare medications from a bottle with a damaged label. READ THE LABEL THREE TIMES.

Compare the written order with the strength labeled on the container. If the ordered strength is not available, you will have to give more or less, depending on the situation. (Drug calculation formulas are located at the conclusion of Chapter 26.) READ THE LABEL THREE TIMES.

3. **Right** dose? Compare the written dosage order with the amount of drug that you prepare (number of tablets, quantity of solution). (Drug calculation formulas are located at the conclusion of Chapter 26.) READ THE LABEL THREE TIMES.

4. **Right** time? Should the medication be given now? Is it the correct time of day? Is it the correct time in a series of administrations? Is it the correct time in the body cycle?

5. **Right** route? Can the patient receive this medication by the route ordered? Is the particular drug available for the route ordered? Is the route an appropriate one?

If you can say "yes" to all the preceding questions, then and only then are you ready to administer the drug.

DRUG FORMS AND ADMINISTRATION

As discussed in Chapter 26, the chosen route of drug administration determines whether or not the drug will have an effect and, often, the intensity of the effect. A drug prepared for one route but administered by another route may not have any effect at all or may potentially be dangerous. Each route requires different dosage forms.

Solid Oral Dosage Forms

The basic forms are tablets, capsules, powders, and lozenges (troches). Pills are rarely manufactured today, but many people mistakenly call tablets "pills."

Tablets. Tablets are compressed powders or granules that, when wet, break apart in the stomach, or in the mouth if they are not swallowed quickly. Tablets may be *sugar* coated to taste better, or *enteric* coated to resist the acid action of the stomach. *Triturated* tablets are coated with a **volatile** liquid that dissolves in the mouth. An antacid tablet is an example.

Capsules. Capsules are gelatin coated and dissolve in the stomach, or they may be coated with substances that protect them from the acid action of the stomach. Timed- or sustained-release capsules are designed to dissolve at different rates, over a period of time, to reduce the number of times a patient has to take a medication.

Powders. Powders are no longer popular. Effervescent antacids and laxatives are now being manufactured in the form of a large tablet.

Lozenges (troches). Lozenges are flattened discs that are dissolved in the mouth for coating the throat.

Oral Administration. Make sure the patient has enough water to transport the drug to the stomach. Make sure that the patient is able to swallow the medication. It may be helpful to place the medication on the back part of the tongue, or the swallowing reflex can be stimulated by placing ice on the lips or tongue just prior to administering the drug. If a patient has difficulty in swallowing or is very young, you may crush and mix the solid form in a soft food, such as applesauce, provided that the food does not interact with the drug, or the drug is not enteric coated or a timed-release capsule. If your patient has been vomiting or is nauseated, an alternative route might be necessary.

Liquid Oral Dosage Forms

Many types of liquid forms are available. They differ mainly in the type of substance used to dissolve the drug: water, oils, or alcohol.

Syrups. A solution of sugar and water, usually containing flavoring and medicinal substances. Cough syrups are the most common. In diabetic patients, syrups should be used with caution.

Emulsions. Mixtures of oil and water that improve the taste of otherwise distasteful products. Cod liver oil is an example.

Gels and Magmas. Minerals suspended in water. Because minerals settle, these products must be shaken before use. Milk of magnesia is an example.

Aromatic Waters. Aqueous solutions containing volatile oils such as oil of spearmint, peppermint, or clove.

Tinctures. An alcoholic preparation of a soluble drug or chemical substance, usually from plant sources. Examples are tinctures of belladonna and of opium. Less potent examples are camphorated tincture of opium (paregoric) and tincture of benzoin. One nonvegetable tincture is tincture of iodine.

Fluidextracts. Combinations of alcohol and vegetable products that are more potent than tinctures. For example, belladonna fluidextract has a higher percentage of the powdered belladonna leaf than does tincture of belladonna.

Extracts. Very concentrated combinations of vegetable products and alcohol or ether that are evaporated until a syrupy liquid, solid mass, or powder is formed. Extracts are many times stronger than the crude drug itself.

Elixirs. Aromatic, alcoholic, sweetened preparations. Elixir of phenobarbital is one example; the alcoholic cough medicines terpin hydrate with codeine and plain elixir of codeine are two more. Elixirs differ from tinctures in that they are sweetened. They should be used with caution in patients with diabetes or in alcohol abusers.

Oral Administration. If the drug is not intended to coat the oral cavity or throat, liquid medications may be followed by a quantity of water. Use a straw for fluid iron preparations, acids, and certain other minerals to avoid staining the teeth. Then rinse the mouth with water. Liquid medications are not recommended for patients who are too weak to pour the liquid and to hold it steady in the spoon. Liquid medications are ideal for children. Solid drugs should not be administered to children until they reach the age when they can safely swallow a solid drug form without the danger of aspirating the drug.

Mucous Membrane Forms

Some mucous membranes are selected for their ability to absorb medication for a systemic effect. The most commonly used areas are the gums, cheeks (buccal), under the tongue (sublingual), rectum, and the respiratory mucosa (inhalation). Nasal, ophthalmic, rectal, and vaginal preparations may also be applied to these mucous membranes for their localized effects.

Rectal Administration. The rectal mucosa provides a rapid absorption even though the surface of the rectum is small. Drugs are absorbed directly into the bloodstream, without being altered as they would be by the digestive processes, and without irritation to the patient's gastric mucosa. Rectal medications are useful if the patient is nauseated, vomiting, or unconscious. Manufacturers supply rectal medications in the form of gelatin or cocoa butter–based suppositories, which melt in the warmth of the rectum and release the medication, or in the form of enemas. Suppositories and enemas are also used for their local effect, that is, to treat constipation. Rectal suppositories are used to soften the stool or stimulate evacuation of the bowel; enemas, to cleanse and evacuate.

The best time to administer a rectal drug intended for a systemic effect is following a bowel movement or enema. The patient should be cautioned to remain lying down for 20 to 30 minutes to prevent accidental evacuation of the drug by a bowel movement or elimination of the enema. Suppositories intended to treat constipation, of course, are administered to bring about bowel evacuation. The patient should be instructed to insert the suppository about two inches above the rectal sphincter muscles; a little mineral oil or vegetable oil may be used as lubrication. If suppositories are individually wrapped in foil, make sure the patient knows that the foil is the wrapper and is not part of the treatment.

Vaginal Administration. Vaginal suppositories, tablets, creams, and fluid solutions are used to treat local infections. Irrigating solutions (douches) may be used as anti-infectives or to acidify the area. Creams and foams are available as local contraceptives. Vaginal installation is most effective if the patient remains lying down; many preparations are therefore prescribed at bedtime. The patient may need to wear a pad to absorb drainage. Liquid medications can be applied to tampons and inserted for a period of time; then a pad is usually not needed. Solid suppositories and tablets may be lubricated or moistened with water and inserted by hand or with an applicator. Creams are instilled with applicators. Prepackaged, disposable irrigation kits are available for douching.

In addition to prescription douches, many over-the-counter preparations are now marketed. Advise your patients that vaginal secretions have their own wash-effect that is antiseptic in nature. Frequent douching can remove the secretions and change the acidity of the vaginal canal, resulting in infection caused by either normal flora or invading bacteria. When instructing patients, confirm that the patient can differentiate the urinary meatus from the vaginal orifice and the rectum. Mistakes could result in vaginal infections or in damage or infection to the urinary tract. A simple drawing and explanation may be required.

Inhalation. Inhalation drugs are supplied in the form of droplets, vapors, or gas. Because of the large surface area and the rich blood supply of the respiratory membranes, the respiratory tract absorbs medications more rapidly than any other mucous membrane. Inhalation can be used to produce a local effect, such as with medications to liquify bronchial secretions or to dilate the bronchi to bring relief to asthmatic or emphysemic patients. In addition, inhalation may be used for systemic effects, such as with oxygen and general anesthesia. Most inhalant substances do spill over into the bloodstream, however, and caution must be taken not to bring about cardiac irregularities and central nervous system side effects. Hand-held inhalers are very common today. Each brand is different, and the patient needs to carefully read the package insert for proper use of the inhaler.

Oral Administration. Mouth and throat agents come in the form of sprays, swabs, sublingual tablets, and buccal tablets. The mouth and throat membranes may be treated locally with antiseptics for oral hygiene and local infections; with anesthetics for relief of pain; and with astringents that form a protective film over the mucous membranes. The patient may have to gargle, or the area may be painted or sprayed. To paint or spray the throat, first look for the area of inflammation to be treated: otherwise the part needing treatment may be missed entirely. Avoid touching the posterior pharynx (back of the throat); this causes gagging and possibly vomiting.

Sublingual tablets are placed under the tongue, where they are rapidly absorbed into the bloodstream by the rich supply of capillaries. Sublingual absorption is systemic and by-passes the acids in the stomach, which inactivate many medications. Nitroglycerin, used for treating the chest pains of angina pectoris, is one of these medications. Used properly, it can bring relief within minutes. Instruct patients not to chew or swallow the medication, and tell them that a mild tingling will be felt under the tongue as the medication dissolves. The lack of the tingling feeling usually indicates that the medication has expired or, for some other reason, is inactive. The patient should be instructed not to

27

smoke, eat, or drink during administration of the drug.

Buccal tablets are placed between the cheek and the upper molars. The same rules of sublingual administration apply to buccal administration.

Nasal Administration. Nose drops, nasal sprays, and tampons are used for their localized effect, but like the inhalation drugs, they may spill over into the bloodstream, causing a change in the heart rate, an increase in blood pressure, or central nervous system stimulation. Nasal medications are commonly used for blocked nasal passages (decongestants) and nosebleeds (hemostatics). Nose drops should be instilled with the patient's head tilted back. Then the patient should be instructed to tilt the head forward to distribute the medication properly. Short, quick breaths will help spread the solution. Any medication spilling down the throat should be expectorated; swallowing nasal preparations can result in systemic side effects.

Nasal sprays are designed for administration with the patient's head upright. Be sure that the spray tip is centered in the nostril and not against the side of the cavity. Nasal decongestant sprays are often misused by patients. Be sure to teach the patient not to exceed the amount or frequency ordered by the physician. If too much is used, these drugs can dry the mucosa and make congestion worse.

Topical Forms

With a few exceptions, topical drugs are local in their effect. Most drugs applied to the skin cannot be absorbed into the bloodstream (unless there is a break in the skin). However, large amounts of a drug left on the skin for a long period of time can be absorbed and cause systemic poisoning. For example, the previous use of hexachlorophene soaps on hospital infants caused toxic reactions and even infant deaths. Now this drug is banned from use in nonprescription soaps and lotions. Oil-based substances have a better chance of being absorbed through the skin than do substances that are water based. One of the most common causes of poisoning in adults is the absorption of oil-based insecticides.

Skin medication forms include lotions, liniments, ointments, compresses, creams, and patches.

Lotions. Often used to control itching, lotions are applied by dabbing with a soft cloth, cotton ball, or tongue blade. Calamine is an example. Rubbing will increase the itching or irritation. If the condition is contagious, the medical assistant should wear gloves. Some lotions are used to relieve congestion and pain in muscles and joints. In these cases, the application is covered with a thick cloth to retain heat. It is said that these lotions and heat dilate the superficial blood vessels, thus drawing blood to the surface and away from the congested parts. However, this is controversial. Many believe that the effects of these lotions are limited to the skin surface where the medication is applied.

Liniments (emulsions). Liniments have a higher portion of oil than do lotions, and volatile active ingredients may be added. Liniments are often used to protect dried, cracked, or fissured skin.

Ointments. Ointments are semisolid medications containing bases such as petrolatum and lanolin, or nongreasy bases. Ointments are applied to dry, scaly areas with little or no hair and can exert a prolonged effect. Ointments are used in small amounts and are applied with firm strokes to avoid increasing itchiness. Ointments that stain clothing should be covered. An ointment should be removed from a jar or tube with a tongue blade to prevent contamination of the remaining medication.

stays on top

Soaks, Compresses, and Wet Dressings. These aqueous solutions of substances with mild astringent properties have a soothing, cooling, antipyretic effect when applied to blistered and oozing areas. Bandages may be soaked in the solution, then applied to the patient, or the patient's extremity may be immersed in the solution and then wrapped in cloth. Plastic wrap can be applied over the bandage or cloth, or the wet dressing can rest on a plastic-covered surface until the air dries the bandage. If the solution contains a dye, the patient should be advised that the treatment will stain clothing or bedding.

Hot Soaks and Compresses. Hot compresses are used to treat abscesses and cellulitis. Extreme care must be taken to avoid burning the patient. Hot soaks are applied for up to 20 minutes; after this amount of time, circulation to a part reaches maximum flow and dissipates heat as fast as the compress can create it (see Chapter 32, Procedure 32–1).

Creams. Creams contain active ingredients incorporated into emulsions that vanish when they are rubbed into the skin. *rub into the skin*

mixed

The Transdermal Patch. Nitroglycerin and scopolamine (used to treat motion sickness) can be absorbed slowly through the skin to create a constant, timed-release systemic effect. The nitroglycerin patch is particularly useful for patients with frequent attacks of angina. The scopolamine patch is placed behind the ear, and additional amounts of the drug can be released with gentle pressure. With dermal patches, drugs can be administered in a timed-release manner for up to three days. *24 hrs to a week* *apply a NON Hairy area*

Ear Drops and Irrigations. Topical ear medications have a local effect and come in the form of drops and irrigations. Medications are instilled into the ear canal to treat infections, reduce inflammation, and bring about local anesthesia. Drops should be instilled with the patient lying down on the unaffected side. Ear drops are supplied in small bottles, with a dropper attached to the cork or cap. The bottle should be held in the hand for a few minutes to warm the solution to body temperature. Drops that are too cold or too warm can cause pain or dizziness. If the contents need mixing, roll the bottle between the palms; do not shake. The patient should lie still for 15 to 30 minutes to allow the medication to coat the ear canal and to be absorbed. Cotton ear plugs should not be used unless specifically ordered. In addition, ear irrigations are performed with the patient sitting; in infants, the patient should be supine (for procedure, see Chapter 29).

Eye Drops, Ointments, and Irrigations. Drug forms for medicating the eye are sterile. Eye solutions come in dropper bottles; ointments are supplied in small tubes. Drops and ointments should not be applied to the sensitive cornea of the eye. Tips of the dropper and the tube must not touch any portion of the eye or eyelid. Drugs instilled into the eye are generally absorbed slowly and affect only the area in contact. However, some medications can act systemically if improper administration techniques are used. If a medication is allowed to flow into the lacrimal system, it can travel down into the nasal cavity and can be absorbed into the circulatory system. To avoid this, you should apply pressure to the inner angle (inner canthus) of the eye with a tissue immediately following instillation of the medication onto the lower eyelid. Eye drops and ointments are placed between the eyeball and the lower lid. To teach the patient to self-administer eye drops, demonstrate how to hold back the head, open the eye wide, and let the drops fall into the lower portion of the eye. Tell the patient not to worry if the drops run onto the face; the solution is harmless (for procedure, see Chapter 29).

Parenteral Medication Forms

Injectable medications must be sterile and in liquid form. The drug is usually in a solution that is minimally irritating to human tissues, such as physiologic saline or sterile water, and may contain a preservative or a small amount of antibiotic to prevent bacterial growth in the vial. All injectable medications are dated. Before use, check the expiration date, and examine the solution for possible deterioration. A parenteral medication is administered with a sterile syringe and needle.

Ampule. A small **hermetically sealed** glass flask, usually containing a single dose of medication.

Ampules have a neck with a weak point that is broken just before use. To open an ampule,

1. Gently tap the top of the ampule with your fingers to settle all the medication to the bottom portion of the flask.

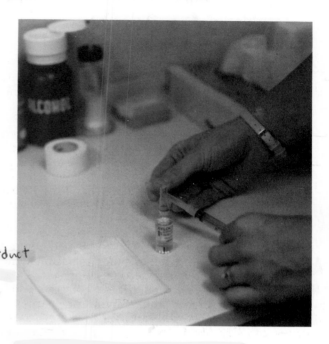

2. Wipe the neck clean with alcohol.

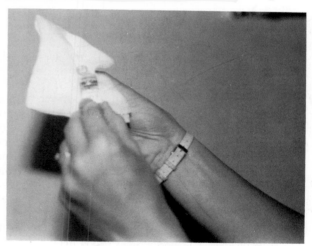

3. It may be necessary to use a small file provided by the manufacturer to score an ampule at the breaking point to facilitate easier breaking.

4. Sharply tap the top so that the top breaks away from you.

5. If the top does not snap off easily, it may be necessary to "bend" it off. Hold each half of the ampule between your thumbs and fingers, in front of you and above waist level.

6. Snap your wrists toward your body to break the neck of the ampule in two. You will hear a pop

because the ampule is vacuum sealed. The glass is designed not to shatter, and the medication will not spill out. Without touching the sides, a syringe and needle unit is inserted into the ampule, and the medication is withdrawn into the syringe.

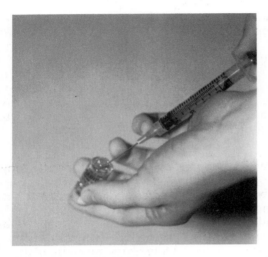

Single-Dose Vial. A small bottle with a rubber stopper through which you insert a sterile needle to withdraw the single dose of medication inside. Before a sterile syringe and needle unit can be introduced into the solution, the rubber stopper must be wiped in a circular motion with alcohol or another suitable disinfectant.

Multi-Dose Vial. A bottle with a rubber stopper that contains enough medication for multiple injections (Fig. 27–1). A vial may contain 30 cc of a drug. If the usual dosage is 0.5 cc, the bottle contains enough medication for 60 injections. Vials vary greatly in size, from 2 cc to 100 or more doses

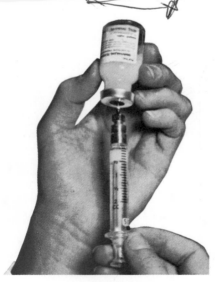

Figure 27–1
Filling a syringe from a multiple-dose vial. Keep the syringe at eye level.

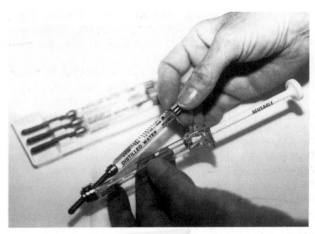

Figure 27–2
The Wyeth Fast-trak tubex system with a prefilled, unit-dose needle and syringe that fits into the metal cartridge for injection. Penicillin is frequently given with this type of syringe.

Because multi-dose vials are entered more than once, extreme caution must be taken every time a needle is inserted into the medication. Contamination could cause very serious infections in future patients. If at any time, you feel that an error has been made or you suspect possible contamination, discard the vial. Never return unused medication to the vial. Learn to withdraw fluids to the correct mark. If you have more medication than you need in the syringe, eject the excess after you remove the unit from the vial. However, remember, your employer will not tolerate excessive waste of drugs due to imprecise withdrawing of medications for injection.

Vials are vacuum sealed. Each time you withdraw medication from a vial, you must first replace the portion of withdrawn medication with the same portion of air. Not enough replaced air will make it difficult to withdraw the medication; too much replaced air will force the medication into the syringe without your pulling on the plunger to withdraw it.

Prefilled Syringe. A sterile disposable syringe and needle unit packaged by the manufacturer with a single dose of medication inside and ready to administer.

Cartridge Injection System. A prefilled syringe and needle that is loaded into a metal cartridge for administration (Fig. 27–2). The prefilled syringes are purchased by the box, and you use the same cartridge-loader over and over.

Parenteral Medication Equipment

Both syringes and needles are manufactured in countless varieties for specific purposes and, sometimes, for specific medications. For example, there is a special syringe for insulin. Also, there is a special syringe unit for diabetics to use for self-injecting.

Hypodermic needles are manufactured in many lengths and widths, depending on the depth needed and the **viscosity** of the medication to be injected. Needles may be purchased separately or as part of a needle-syringe unit. Figure 27–3 shows the construction of a needle and the three common types of needle points. There are some facts to remember about the construction of a hypodermic needle. The following statement was prepared by the Becton-Dickinson Company:

The size of the needle is governed by four factors: safety, rate of flow, comfort of the patient, and depth of penetration. There are three standard dimensions: length, outside diameter of the cannula, and wall thickness. Regular needles are measured for length from where the cannula joins the hub to the tip of the (needle) point.

Needle Gauge. The width of a needle is called its *gauge,* and needle gauges range in size from 14 (the largest) to 28 (the smallest). The smallest gauges (27–28) are used for intradermal injections when a very small opening is desired. These fine needle widths leave a small amount of medication just below the surface of the skin, with a minimum amount of injury. Gauges 25 and 26 are commonly used for subcutaneous injections. With a medication that is in an aqueous solution and is easily injected through a small opening, these two gauges cause minimal tissue damage, and the patient experiences less pain. Larger needles (20 to 23) are usually necessary for intramuscular injections when the medication is thick, such as penicillin, or the length of the needle requires the extra support of a thicker gauge. A patient cannot feel the difference between a 20- and a 22-gauge needle. In fact, the medication is not forced as strongly into the tissues with the larger 20-gauge needle as with the 22-gauge one, and the patient actually experiences less pain. Needles larger than 20 gauge are not used for drug therapy. They are mostly used for venipuncture, blood donations, and blood transfusions.

Needle Length. The choices of needle lengths vary from 3/8 in to 4 in, depending on the area of the body to be injected and the route (depth) used. Intradermal injections require only the short 3/8-in needle. Needles that are 1/2 or 5/8 in long are used for subcutaneous injections. Longer needles are necessary for depositing drugs intramuscularly. The choice of a 1-in, 1 1/2-in, 2-in, 2 1/2-in, or 3-in length depends on both the muscle being used and the size of the patient.

Syringes. Figure 27–4 illustrates the construction of a 2.0-cc and a 10.0-cc syringe. The parts of a

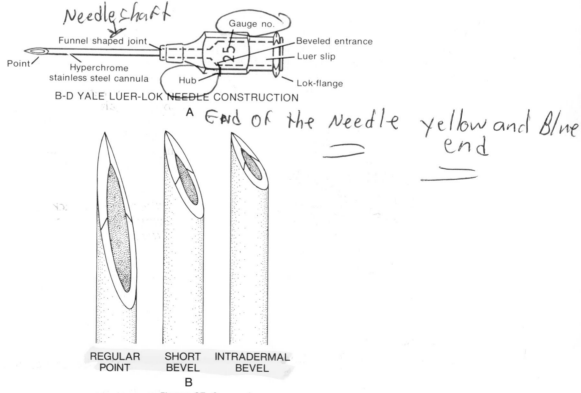

B-D YALE LUER-LOK NEEDLE CONSTRUCTION

A

REGULAR POINT   SHORT BEVEL   INTRADERMAL BEVEL

B

Figure 27–3

A, *The construction of a hypodermic needle.* **B,** *Needle points.*

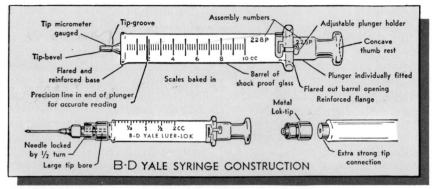

Figure 27–4

The basic construction of syringes, showing the 10-cc syringe and the 2-cc syringe. (Courtesy of Becton-Dickinson Co.)

syringe are its barrel, calibrated scale(s), plunger, and tip (Fig. 27–5). *Regular* syringes that hold up to 3.0 cc (ml) are usually calibrated with two scales: cc (ml) and minims. Larger *regular* syringes are calibrated in cc (ml) only. The *tuberculin* syringe is used for small quantities of drug, as it holds only up to 1.0 cc of injectable material (Fig. 27–6). The *insulin* syringe is calibrated in units specifically for diabetic use (Fig. 27–7).

Most syringes and needles are disposable—the advantages being the prevention of cross-infection, equipment that has not been damaged by use, and freedom from the duties of autoclaving and sterilization. Disposable needles are siliconized and are extremely smooth and sharp. Disposable units are packaged in sealed, rigid plastic containers (Fig. 27–8A) or in peel-apart paper wrappers (Fig. 27–8B). Both have an internal, rigid plastic sheath protecting the needle. Both individual needles and syringe-needle units are color coded for easy identification. Do not attempt to cut expenses by purchasing inferior or unknown brands of needles or syringes. Table 27–1 summarizes the needle and syringe sizes used for injections.

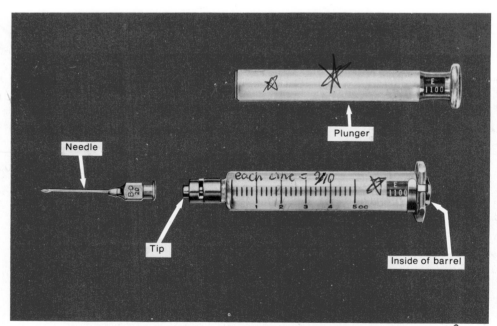

Figure 27–5

The parts of a hypodermic needle and syringe.

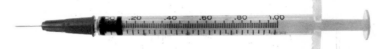

Figure 27–6
The disposable 1.0-cc tuberculin syringe with a detachable needle. This type of syringe is generally used for intradermal injections such as allergy test and for measuring minute amounts of medication subcutaneously.

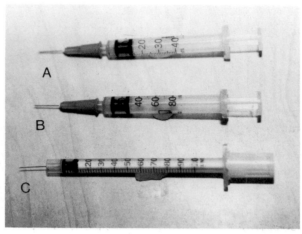

Figure 27–7
*Insulin syringes have special calibrations to accommodate the various strengths of insulin manufactured. The drug is administered by concentration, called Units (U), not by cubic centimeters (cc) or milliliters (ml). The U 100 syringe is becoming the "standard." **A,** Insulin syringe U 40. **B,** Insulin syringe U 80. **C,** Insulin syringe U 100.*

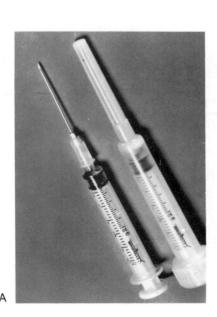

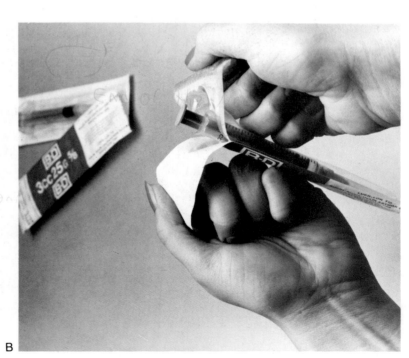

Figure 27–8
***A,** A rigid, disposable plastic package containing a syringe and needle unit. (Courtesy Wyeth Co.) **B,** Sterile paper packaging containing a syringe and needle unit. (Courtesy Becton-Dickinson Co.)*

Table 27–1
Needle and Syringe Sizes for Injections

Route	Gauge	Length	Syringe
Intradermal	27–28	3/8 in	Tuberculin
Subcutaneous	25–26	1/2, 5/8 in	2 cc; tuberculin; insulin
Intramuscular	20–23	1–3 in	2–5 cc

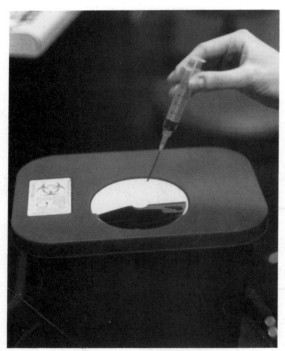

Figure 27–9
A rigid, puncture-resistant, disposable container into which needle-syringe units are placed immediately after use.

Destruction of Used Syringes and Needles. In 1975, the Centers for Disease Control in Atlanta, Georgia, recommended the following:

Because of the impossibility of knowing which patient's blood may be contaminated with hepatitis virus or other organisms, extreme caution must be applied in handling used syringes and needles whether in isolation or not....Used needles need not be recapped; they should be placed in a prominently labeled, impervious, puncture-resistant container designed specifically for this purpose. Needles should not be purposely bent, because an accidental needle puncture may occur.

The U.S. Environmental Protection Agency Office of Solid Waste, in its *Draft Manual for Infectious Waste Management* (September 1982), states that

Because of the potential for physical injury, the EPA believes that it is not prudent to retrieve needles, to handle them or to clip them. The preferable management system for (needles) is placement directly into a puncture-proof container so that subsequent handling (of the container) is without risk of physical injury from the (needles).

After giving an injection, dispose of the syringe and needle by placing them into a closed container immediately (Fig. 27–9). The cap should not be replaced on the needle, and the needle should not be cut or broken.

Reusable Needles and Syringes. Reusable needles and syringes are not recommended; however, there are some medications that must be administered in glass syringes (Fig. 27–10). If you must use reusable needles and syringes, the Centers for Disease Control further states, "Reusable needles and syringes should be rinsed thoroughly in cold water after use; the needle should be placed in a puncture-resistant rigid container; syringes and needles should be wrapped using the double-bag technique and decontaminated and sterilized." This procedure should be used **before** you begin the sanitization and final sterilization process for reuse or before discarding worn-out items. You cannot be too careful when handling contaminated equipment.

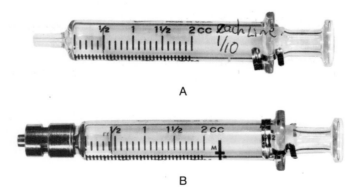

A

B

Figure 27–10
*Reusable 2-cc glass syringes. **A,** Plain tip. **B,** Metal Luer-Lok tip. Glass syringes may be necessary for certain drugs that erode plastic.*

Procedure 27–1

PROCEDURAL GOAL

To fill a syringe with the correct amount of medication, using sterile technique.

EQUIPMENT AND SUPPLIES

A vial or ampule containing the material to be injected
Antiseptic sponges
A sterile needle and syringe unit
A written order, including the drug name, strength, and route

PROCEDURE

1. Read the order and choose a correct vial of medication.
   Purpose: To check the medication the first of three times.

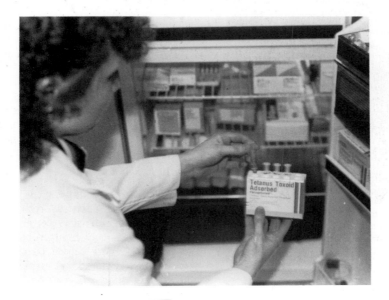

2. Choose the correct syringe and needle size, depending on the site and the quantity of medication to be injected.
3. Wash your hands.
4. Compare the order to both the name of the drug on the vial of medication and the amount to be withdrawn in the syringe.
   Purpose: To check the medication the second of three times.

Procedure continued on following page

27

upside down

5. Gently agitate the medication by rolling the vial between your palms (below left).
   Purpose: To mix any medication that may have settled.
6. Check the quality of the medication and the expiration date.
   Purpose: Medications may become contaminated or outdated.
7. Cleanse the rubber stopper of the vial with the antiseptic sponge, using a circular motion (below right).

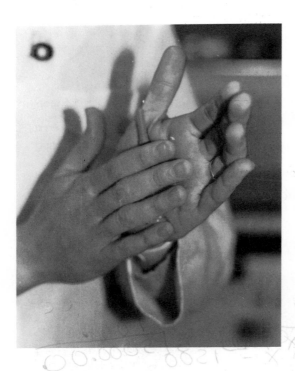

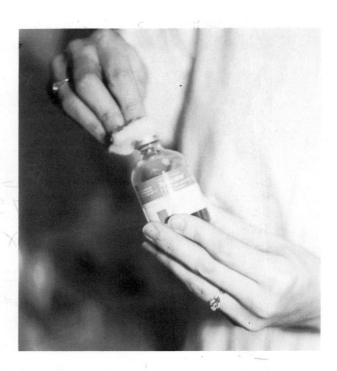

8. Set down the vial. (You may hold the vial in the palm of your minor hand while you continue, if you do not contaminate the rubber stopper.)
9. Take the needle-syringe unit and remove the cap from the plastic protective case, or peel away the protective wrapper.
10. Remove the syringe.
11. Grasp the plunger and draw up an amount of air equal to the amount of medication ordered.
    Purpose: Not enough replaced air will make it difficult to withdraw the medication; too much replaced air will force the medication into the syringe without your pulling on the plunger to withdraw it.
12. Grasp the plastic sheath covering the needle between two fingers on the posterior side of your minor hand, and pull the syringe out of the sheath with your major hand.
    Purpose: To keep the sheath sterile for replacing it on the needle for transportation to the patient. The sheath may not be placed on a nonsterile surface or touched near its opening.
13. If you are not already holding the vial with the sheath in your minor hand, pick up the vial with the same hand that is holding the empty sheath, being careful not to touch the sheath to any nonsterile surface.

Procedure continued on opposite page

14. Turn the vial upside down without touching the rubber stopper (below left).
15. Fully insert the needle into the center of the rubber stopper with your major hand.
16. Inject the air in the syringe into the vial.
17. Slowly pull back on the plunger until the proper amount of medication is withdrawn.
    Purpose: Withdrawing medication rapidly will cause air bubbles to form in the syringe.
18. While the needle is still in the vial, check to see that there are no air bubbles in the syringe.
    Purpose: Air bubbles displace medication, and the patient will not receive the proper amount of medication.
19. If there are air bubbles, slip the fingers holding the vial down to grasp the vial and syringe as a single unit.
    Purpose: This frees your major hand.
20. With your free hand, tap the syringe until the air bubbles dislodge and float into the tip of the syringe.
21. Gently expel these tiny air bubbles through the needle, then continue withdrawing the medication.
22. Withdraw the needle from the vial, and replace the sheath over the needle without the needle touching the sides of the sheath.
23. Return the medication to the shelf or the refrigerator, checking that you have the correct drug and dosage (below right).
    Purpose: This is the third of the "Three Befores" of drug checking.
24. Clean the area.

27

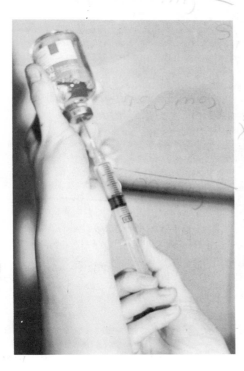
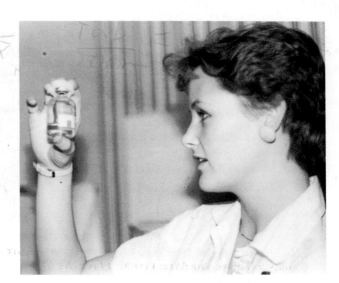

TERMINAL PERFORMANCE OBJECTIVE

Given the necessary equipment and supplies, fill a syringe with a medication, with no break in sterile technique and no errors in any step of this procedure, within two minutes, as determined by your evaluator.

PARENTERAL ADMINISTRATION

With practice, giving medications by injection will become easy and even automatic, but as stated before and stressed often, always follow the physician's orders, the "Three Befores," and the "Five Rights." Develop techniques that provide maximum safety and comfort for the patient. Injections are least painful when the needle is inserted swiftly and the medication injected slowly. Remember that the same aseptic conditions necessary for minor surgery are necessary whenever you penetrate the protective skin barrier (see Chapter 31).

Injections are not given near bones or blood vessels. Injections should never be given in an area where there is scar tissue, a change in skin pigmentation or texture, or excess tissue growth such as a mole or a wart. The point of injection should be as far as possible from any major nerve, and the site selected should be capable of holding the amount of medication that is injected. Never inject into an arm from which the lymph nodes have been removed (as after a **radical mastectomy**), as the medication cannot be absorbed into the bloodstream.

Make certain that all materials are ready for use. Many offices have a central room where medications are prepared. The medication is then taken to the waiting patient in another room. Handling medication administration in this way has many advantages, but care must be taken that the syringe and needle unit are transported with sterile technique. After a syringe is filled, the cap is replaced for transport to the patient. Never wrap a needle in gauze or cotton.

When carrying a syringe and needle, hold it horizontally and parallel to your body. Never transport more than one injection at a time, unless two or more are for the same patient or unless you have a special medication tray that has a named position for each syringe. Never combine two medications in a single syringe unless specifically ordered by the physician. If you are preparing a medication for the physician to give, place the vial or empty ampule beside the filled syringe. This shows what medication is in the syringe and offers a double check. *Never give a medication that someone else prepared*

Use a professional approach and tell the patient what you are going to do. Small talk can keep the patient's mind off the procedure. Never tell a patient that it will not hurt; you may destroy your credibility. Make the patient as comfortable as possible, and allow for privacy. Never allow the patient to stand during the procedure. Keep the equipment out of the patient's sight as much as possible. Wear gloves and other blood and body-fluid protection barriers, as necessary (see Appendix C, Recommendations for Prevention of AIDS Transmission).

Intramuscular Injections

Intramuscular injections are given into the muscle when (1) drugs will irritate the subcutaneous tis-

sues, (2) a more rapid absorption is desired, or (3) the volume of the medication to be injected is large. The angle of insertion is 90 degrees (Fig. 27–11), and the preferred sites are the *gluteus medius, vastus lateralis, deltoid, and ventrogluteal muscles* of the adult (Fig. 27–12). It is believed that some intramuscular injections are not given with a long enough needle, and medications may therefore be deposited into the upper adipose (fatty) tissue by error. Fatty tissue does not absorb medications well, and the medication may remain at the site of the injection. Be certain to select needles that are long enough, especially for obese patients.

When locating a site for an intramuscular injection, expose the site so that you are able to visualize and palpate the landmarks correctly. Table 27–2 lists the sites as well as the criteria for choosing one site over another.

Vastus Lateralis (Thigh) Site. This muscle is part of the *quadriceps group* of the thigh. It is one of the body's largest muscles, and because it is developed at birth, it is considered the safest for infants. Many experts feel that as a site for adult intramuscular (IM) injections, the vastus lateralis is better than either the deltoid or the dorsogluteal sites because there are fewer major nerves and blood vessels in the vastus lateralis. The vastus lateralis muscle fills the midportion of the upper, outer thigh. In the adult, it can be located from one hand's width below the proximal end of the *greater trochanter* to one hand's width above the top of the *patella* (knee cap). Wyeth Laboratories states, "For infants and children, the acceptable position of this region lies below the greater trochanter of the femur and within the upper lateral quadrant of the thigh" (Fig. 27–13). The adult patient may sit or lie supine, but

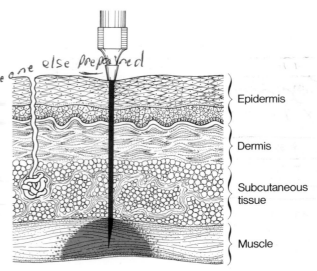

Figure 27–11

An anatomical illustration of the intramuscular injection. Note that the needle is given at a 90-degree angle and deposits the medication into the large central part of the muscle.

Epidermis

Dermis

Subcutaneous tissue

Muscle

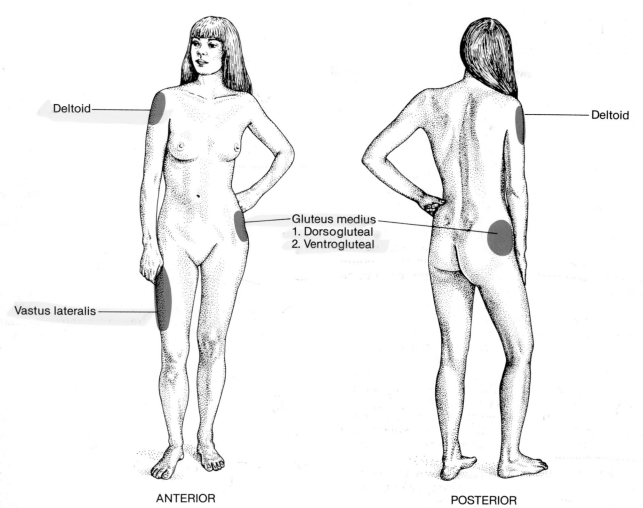

Deltoid

Vastus lateralis

Gluteus medius
1. Dorsogluteal
2. Ventrogluteal

Deltoid

ANTERIOR

POSTERIOR

27

Figure 27–12
The commonly used muscles for intramuscular injection.

Table 27–2
Types of Injections

Method	Drug Amount	Sites	Examples
IM	Adult, 1–2 cc	Deltoid	Adrenalin (epinephrine)
	Adult, 2–5 cc	Vastus lateralis	Penicillin
		Dorsogluteal, ventrogluteal	Demerol (meperidine)
	Child, 1–2 cc	Vastus lateralis, ventrogluteal	Penicillin
IM, Z	As above	Dorsogluteal Ventrogluteal	Irritating drugs
SC	Adult, 0.1–2.0 cc	Deltoid Thigh Abdomen	Insulin Vaccines Toxoids
	Child, 0.5 cc	Deltoid Thigh, abdomen	Vaccines Toxoids
ID	Adult and child, 0.1–0.5 cc	Forearm	Tuberculin test, skin tests

it is easier to locate the vastus lateralis with the patient lying down.

No used for infants

Dorsogluteal (Gluteus Medius) Site. This is the traditional site for deep IM injections. However, complications due to sciatic nerve injury are frequent enough that experts are suggesting that this site be abandoned and replaced with the vastus lateralis and ventrogluteal sites. The dorsogluteal site continues to be popular, and it is still acceptable for adults if care is taken to locate the exact site. It is recommended that this site *not* be used for infants. The patient must lie in the prone position. To relax the muscles, the toes should be pointing inward. To locate the site, draw an imaginary diagonal line starting at the *greater trocanter* of the femur, across the buttocks, to the *posterior spine of the ilium*. Palpate these bony prominences to make certain that you are at the correct site. The injection is made into the gluteus medius muscle several inches below the *iliac crest* (Fig. 27–14).

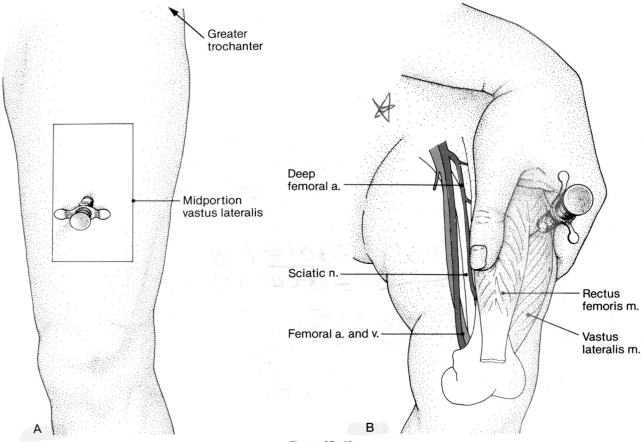

Figure 27–13
The vastus lateralis muscle is the preferred site for intramuscular injections in infants and children. **A,** *Site selection for adults.* **B,** *Site selection for infants and children.*

Children

Ventrogluteal (Gluteus Medius) Site. Although considered safe, this site is not used as frequently as the others. This technique uses a larger mass of the gluteus medius muscle than when using the dorsogluteal site. The area is free of major nerves and blood vessels, and it is considered safe for both infants and adults (Fig. 27–15). All types of IM medications can be injected here, including the thick oily preparations. To locate the site, place your right palm on the patient's *greater trocanter,* then put your index finger on the *anterior iliac spine,* and spread your middle finger back as far as possible from your index finger, trying to touch the *crest of the ilium.* The center of the triangle formed by your index and middle fingers is the site for the injection. Choose the hand that is the opposite of the patient's side, that is, use your left hand to palpate the patient's right ventrogluteal site, and your right hand to palpate the patient's left side. For a child, you will need a 1-in needle, whereas in an obese adult patient, you may need a 2½-in needle to reach the depth of the muscle.

Deltoid Site. The deltoid muscle, the mu cap of the shoulder, is located at the top upper, outer arm. The muscle mass is some limited, so it cannot hold a large volume of n cation. This triangular muscle is located bet the *acromion* and *deltoid tuberosities* and fills an approximately two fingerbreadths below the *mion process* (Fig. 27–16). The major nerv blood vessels located in the posterior portion arm must be avoided. Aqueous medicatic most appropriate here, for example, vitamin frequent injections are ordered, rotate the s alternate the right and left arm. The deltoid acceptable for adults and older children, should not be used when the muscle is sr underdeveloped. For a small arm, you may only a 25-gauge ⅝-in needle; the 23-gauge needle is most often used for the average-sized When injecting, expose the entire shoulder ra than rolling up the sleeve. Grasp the muscle, a stretch the skin before injecting the medication. Th patient may be seated or lying down.

27

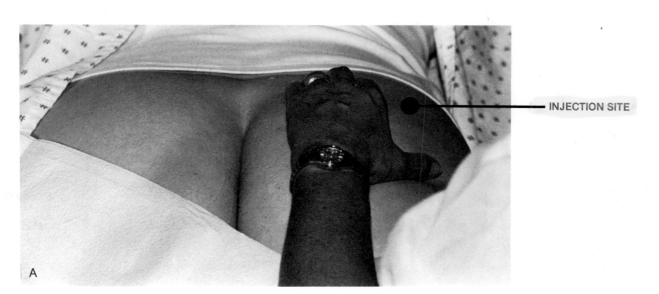

INJECTION SITE

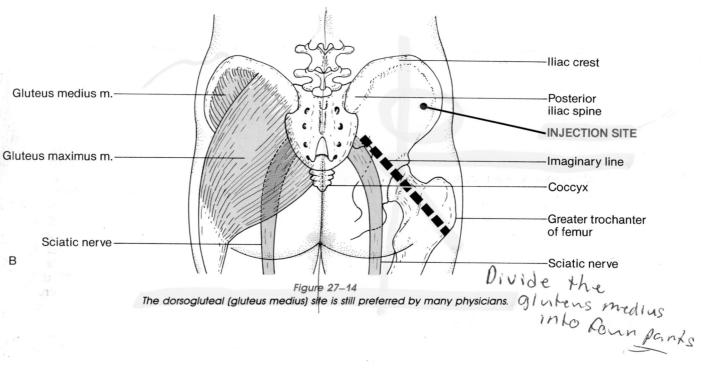

Iliac crest

Gluteus medius m.

Posterior
iliac spine

INJECTION SITE

Gluteus maximus m.

Imaginary line

Coccyx

Greater trochanter
of femur

Sciatic nerve

Sciatic nerve

B

Figure 27–14
The dorsogluteal (gluteus medius) site is still preferred by many physicians.

Divide the
glutens medius
into four parts

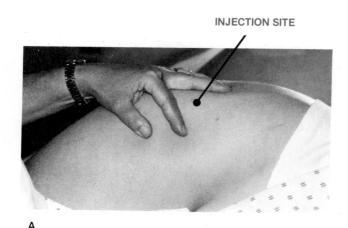

INJECTION SITE

A

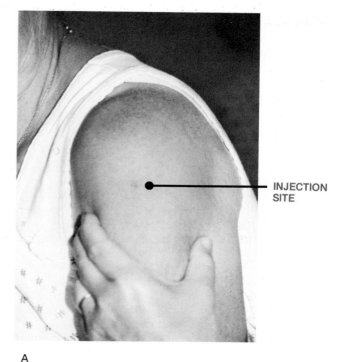

INJECTION SITE

A

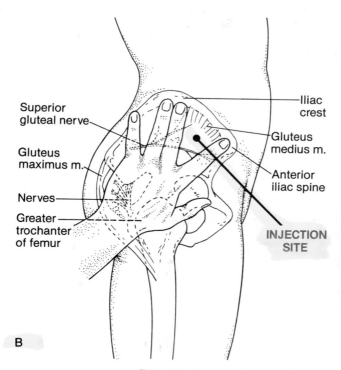

Superior gluteal nerve

Gluteus maximus m.

Nerves

Greater trochanter of femur

Iliac crest

Gluteus medius m.

Anterior iliac spine

INJECTION SITE

B

Figure 27–15
The ventrogluteal site can be used for most intramuscular injections.

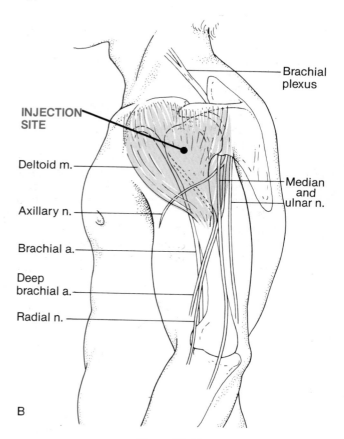

Brachial plexus

INJECTION SITE

Deltoid m.

Axillary n.

Brachial a.

Deep brachial a.

Radial n.

Median and ulnar n.

B

Figure 27–16
The deltoid muscle site is used for both intramuscular and subcutaneous injections. It is not recommended for infants, because the muscle is not developed until later in childhood.

Procedure 27-2

GIVING AN INTRAMUSCULAR INJECTION

PROCEDURAL GOAL

To inject medication into the muscle, using a needle and syringe of the correct size, as directed by the physician.

EQUIPMENT AND SUPPLIES

A vial or ampule containing the material to be injected
Antiseptic sponges
A sterile needle and syringe unit
A written order, including the patient's name, when to give the drug, the route of administration, and the name and strength of the drug
Nonsterile gloves (see Appendix C, Recommendations for Prevention of AIDS Transmission)

PROCEDURE

1. Wash your hands. Follow universal blood and body-fluid precautions (see Appendix C). Glove yourself with nonsterile gloves.
2. Select the correct medication from the shelf or the refrigerator.
   Purpose: Some medications must be refrigerated.
3. Read the label to be sure that you have the RIGHT DRUG and the RIGHT STRENGTH.
   Purpose: One medication may be manufactured and prepackaged in different strengths; for instance, a particular drug may be available in vials of both 250 mg/cc and 500 mg/cc.
4. Warm refrigerated medications by gently rolling between your palms.
5. Prepare the syringe, calculating the RIGHT DOSE.
6. Transport the medication to the patient.
7. Greet and identify the patient by name.
   Purpose: To be sure that you have the RIGHT PATIENT.
8. Position the patient comfortably.
9. Expose the site.
10. Cleanse the patient's skin with the antiseptic sponge, using a circular motion, moving outward from the center (bottom left).
11. Compare the order with the prepared medication, and the patient to the name on the order, to make sure that this is the RIGHT TIME to administer the drug.
    Purpose: This is the last of the five checks to be made before administering a medication. If there is any doubt, do not proceed. Check first with the physician.
12. Remove the sheath from the needle.
13. With the thumb and first two fingers of your minor hand, spread the skin tightly at the site to be injected, or pinch a large portion of the muscle at the site to be injected (bottom right).
    Purpose: Smoothing the skin by stretching or pinching facilitates the insertion of the needle.

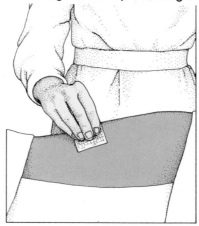 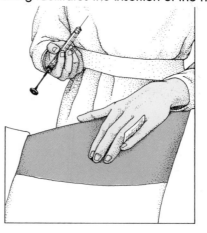

Procedure continued on following page

14. Grasp the syringe as you would a dart, and with one swift movement, insert the entire needle up to the hub, at a 90-degree angle into the muscle (below).
Purpose: The depth of the injection is determined by the choice of needle length, not by how far you insert the needle. Once the needle is at the tissue layer, do not move the needle while injecting the medication. Being in as far as the hub helps to keep the needle in one place.

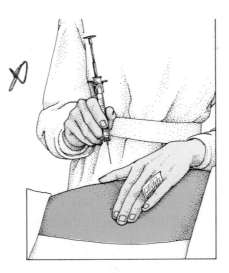 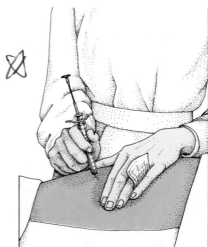

15. Withdraw the plunger slightly to be sure that no blood enters the syringe (bottom left).
Purpose: Blood in the syringe means that the needle is in a blood vessel and is not in the muscle tissue. You may *not* administer an intramuscular medication by the intravenous route.
16. If blood appears, immediately withdraw the syringe, and compress the injection site with the sponge.
17. Begin again with step 1.
Purpose: Blood is now mixed with the medication, and the medication is considered contaminated. Blood may interact with the drug and may be irritating to the intramuscular tissues.
18. If no blood appears in the syringe, push in the plunger slowly and steadily until all medication has been administered (bottom right).
Purpose: A rapid injection may tear the muscle tissue.

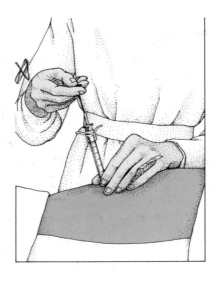 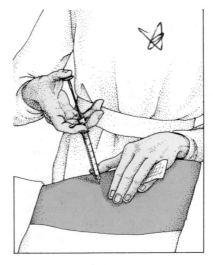

19. ~~Cover the area with the sponge, and withdraw the needle at the same angle of insertion (below~~ left).
20. Gently massage the site with the antiseptic sponge.
    Purpose: Massage helps to increase absorption and to decrease pain (below right).
21. Make sure that your patient is comfortable and safe.
22. Dispose of the needle and syringe.
23. Observe the patient for any adverse reaction. You may need to keep the patient under observation for 20 to 30 minutes.
24. Wash your hands.
25. Record the drug administration on the patient's medical record, and on the required DEA record if the medication is a controlled substance.

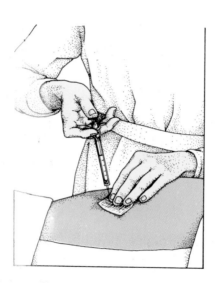 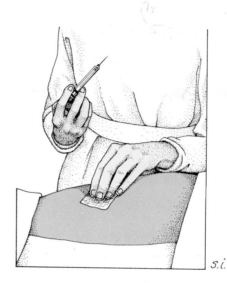

TERMINAL PERFORMANCE OBJECTIVE

Given a patient, an order, and the necessary equipment and supplies, prepare and administer a medication, using the intramuscular route and observing the "Five Rights" and the "Three Befores," and record the administration of the drug on the patient's medical record, within ten minutes, with no break in sterile technique and no omissions or errors in any step of the procedure, as determined by your evaluator.

Z-Tract Intramuscular Injection

Some intramuscular medications are irritating to the skin and subcutaneous tissues. The injection must be given in such a way as to prevent any leakage back from the deep muscle into the upper subcutaneous layers. The Z-tract method displaces the upper tissue laterally before the needle is inserted (Fig. 27–17). The skin is pulled to one side before the tissue is grasped for the injection. After the needle is withdrawn, the tissue is released, with the needle tract to one side of where the medication is deposited in the muscle. The medication cannot leak out. These medications are always injected into the gluteus medius muscle of the buttocks. Because the medication is so irritating to the tissues, the needle should be changed after withdrawing the medication from the vial.

Some medications require the injection of 0.5 cc of air following an injection. This air will clear the needle of the medication and will prevent the medication from flowing back along the tract of the injection. This air can be pulled into the syringe after the medication has been drawn in. Because the syringe is pointed downward during the injection, the air will float to the other end of the syringe and will be the last to enter the tissue. Wait a few seconds before withdrawing the needle. Wait ten seconds before releasing the skin.

Many medications that require the Z-tract method should not be massaged after injection; just hold a sponge over the area for a few seconds. Walking will help the medication absorb. Use alternate sides for multiple or frequent injections.

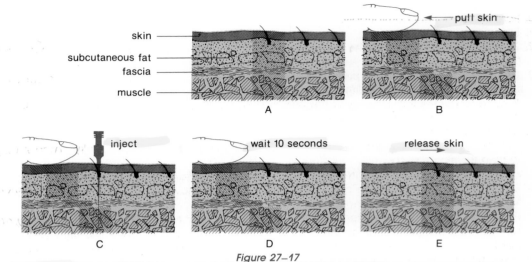

Figure 27–17

The "Z-tract" method of intramuscular injection is used when medications are irritating to subcutaneous tissues. This technique helps prevent the medication from leaking back into the subcutaneous tissues.

Procedure 27–3

GIVING A Z-TRACT INTRAMUSCULAR INJECTION

PROCEDURAL GOAL

To inject a medication into the muscle using a needle and syringe of correct size and the Z-tract method, as directed by the physician.

EQUIPMENT AND SUPPLIES

A vial or ampule containing the material to be injected
Antiseptic sponges
A sterile needle and syringe unit
A written order, including the patient's name, when to give the drug, the route of administration, and the name and strength of the drug
Nonsterile gloves (see Appendix C, Recommendations for Prevention of AIDS Transmission)

PROCEDURE

1. Wash your hands. Follow universal blood and body-fluid precautions (see Appendix C). Glove yourself with nonsterile gloves.
2. Select the correct medication from the shelf or the refrigerator.
   Purpose: Some medications must be refrigerated.
3. Read the label to be sure that you have the RIGHT DRUG and the RIGHT STRENGTH.
   Purpose: One medication may be manufactured and prepackaged in different strengths; for instance, a particular drug may be available in vials of both 250 mg/cc and 500 mg/cc.
4. Warm refrigerated medications by gently rolling the container between your palms.
5. Prepare the syringe, calculating the RIGHT DOSE.
6. If the manufacturer so directs, draw 0.5 cc of air into the syringe.
7. Replace the sheath on the needle, and give a slight turn to loosen the needle. Secure a new needle, still in its sheath, to the tip of the syringe. Discard the contaminated needle.
   Purpose: The needle that was used to withdraw the medication is covered with a substance irritating to the skin and subcutaneous tissues.
8. Transport the medication to the patient.
9. Greet and identify the patient by name.
   Purpose: To be sure that you have the RIGHT PATIENT.

Procedure continued on opposite page

10. Position the patient comfortably.
11. Expose the site.
12. Cleanse the patient's skin with the antiseptic sponge, using a circular motion, moving outward from the center.
13. Compare the order with the prepared medication, and the patient with the name on the order, to make sure that this is the RIGHT TIME to administer the drug.
    Purpose: This is the last of the five checks to be made before administering a medication. If there is any doubt, do not proceed. Check first with the physician.
14. Remove the sheath from the needle.
15. Pull the skin to one side and hold it firmly in place. If the skin is slippery, use a dry gauze sponge to hold the skin in place.
    Purpose: Displacing the skin prevents irritating medications from leaking back to the surface.
16. Grasp the syringe as you would a dart, and with one swift movement, insert the entire needle up to the hub, at a 90-degree angle into the muscle.
    Purpose: The depth of the injection is determined by the choice of needle length, not by how far you insert the needle. Once the needle is at the tissue layer, do not move the needle while injecting the medication. Being in as far as the hub helps to keep the needle in one place.
17. Withdraw the plunger slightly to be sure that no blood enters the syringe.
    Purpose: Blood in the syringe means that the needle is in a blood vessel and not in the muscle tissue. You may *not* administer an intramuscular medication by the intravenous route.
18. If blood appears, immediately withdraw the syringe, and compress the injection site with the sponge.
    Purpose: To minimize bleeding and bruising.
19. Begin again with step 1.
    Purpose: Blood is now mixed with the medication, and the medication is considered contaminated. Blood may interact with the drug and may be irritating to the intramuscular tissues.
20. If no blood appears in the syringe, push in the plunger slowly and steadily until all medication has been administered.
    Purpose: A rapid injection may tear the muscle tissue.
21. Wait a few seconds, then cover the area with the sponge, and withdraw the needle at the same angle of insertion. Wait ten seconds, then release the skin.
22. If the manufacturer recommends it, gently massage the site with the antiseptic sponge.
    Purpose: Massage helps to increase absorption and to decrease pain.
23. Make sure your patient is comfortable and safe.
24. Dispose of the needle and syringe.
25. Observe the patient for any adverse reaction. You may need to keep the patient under observation for 20 to 30 minutes.
26. Wash your hands.
27. Record the drug administration on the patient's medical record, and on the required DEA record if the medication is a controlled substance.

TERMINAL PERFORMANCE OBJECTIVE

Given a patient, an order, and the necessary equipment and supplies, prepare and administer a medication using the Z-tract intramuscular route, observing the "Five Rights" and the "Three Befores," and record the drug administration on the patient's medical record, within ten minutes, with no break in sterile technique and no omissions or errors in any step of the procedure, as determined by your evaluator.

Subcutaneous Injections

Subcutaneous injections are given just under the skin, into the fatty areolar layer called *adipose tissue* (Fig. 27–18). Smaller doses of less irritating drugs are given by this method. The angle of insertion is 45 degrees; however, heparin and insulin are usu-ally administered at a 90-degree angle. The deltoid area is an injection site; however, the abdomen, thigh, and upper back may be used (Fig. 27–19). When multiple or frequent injections are ordered, the sites must be rotated. It is best to keep a rotation record. Most analgesics and immunizations are administered by subcutaneous injection.

when
[Charting the Medication given

give 4-15-91.

area   your
Right Arm   Initials
R A

RA   RUQ = hip
LA   LUQ = hip (IM)
RT (Im)   injection
LT
R Abd (SQ)

Specify
IM
SQ
ID

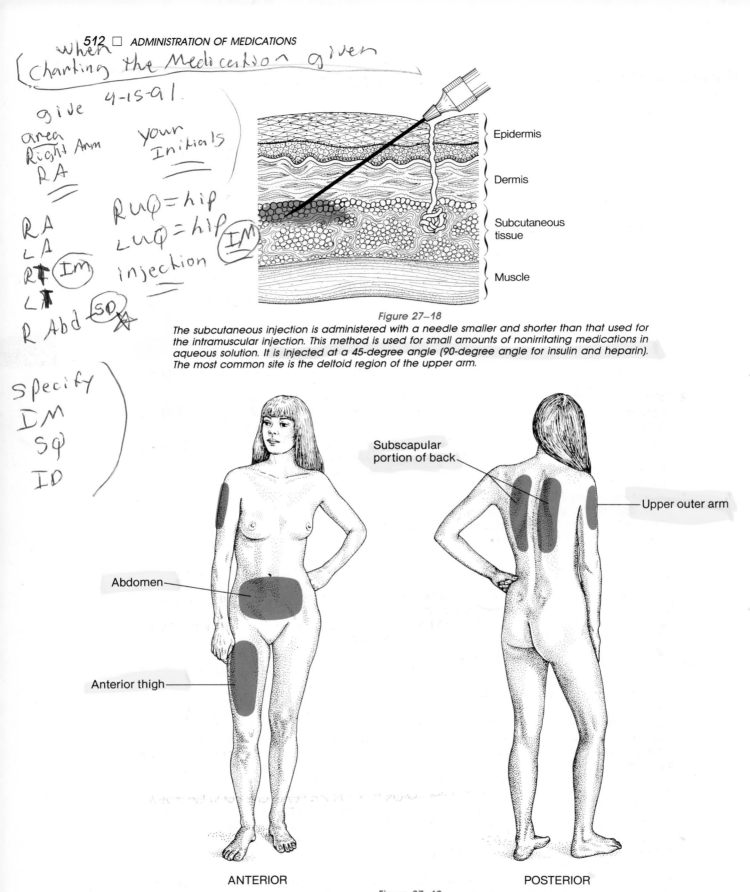

Epidermis

Dermis

Subcutaneous tissue

Muscle

Figure 27-18

The subcutaneous injection is administered with a needle smaller and shorter than that used for the intramuscular injection. This method is used for small amounts of nonirritating medications in aqueous solution. It is injected at a 45-degree angle (90-degree angle for insulin and heparin). The most common site is the deltoid region of the upper arm.

Subscapular portion of back

Upper outer arm

Abdomen

Anterior thigh

ANTERIOR

POSTERIOR

Figure 27-19
Areas of the body commonly used for subcutaneous injections.

Procedure 27–4

PROCEDURAL GOAL

To inject a medication into the subcutaneous tissue using a needle and syringe of correct size, as directed by the physician.

EQUIPMENT AND SUPPLIES

A vial or ampule containing the material to be injected
Antiseptic sponges
A sterile needle and syringe unit
A written order, including the patient's name, when to give the drug, the route of administration, and the name and strength of the drug
Nonsterile gloves (see Appendix C, Recommendations for Prevention of AIDS Transmission)

PROCEDURE

1. Wash your hands. Follow universal blood and body-fluid precautions (see Appendix C). Glove yourself with nonsterile gloves.
2. Select the correct medication from the shelf or the refrigerator.
   Purpose: Some medications must be refrigerated.
3. Read the label to be sure that you have the RIGHT DRUG and the RIGHT STRENGTH.
   Purpose: One medication may be manufactured and prepackaged in different strengths; for instance, a particular drug may be available in vials of both 250 mg/cc and 500 mg/cc.
4. Warm refrigerated medications by gently rolling the container between your palms.
5. Prepare the syringe, withdrawing the RIGHT DOSE.
6. Transport the medication to the patient.
7. Greet and identify the patient by name.
   Purpose: To be sure that you have the RIGHT PATIENT.
8. Position the patient comfortably.
9. Expose the site.
10. Cleanse the patient's skin with the antiseptic sponge, using a circular motion, moving outward from the center.
11. Compare the order with the prepared medication, and the patient with the name on the order, to be sure that this is the RIGHT TIME to administer the drug.
    Purpose: This is the last of the five checks to be made before administering a medication. If there is any doubt, do not proceed. Check first with the physician.
12. Remove the sheath from the needle.
13. With the thumb and first two fingers of your minor hand, form a skin fold by picking up the tissue or by pulling the skin taut.
    Purpose: Smoothing the skin facilitates the insertion of the needle.
14. Grasp the syringe between the thumb and the first two fingers of your major hand with your palm up, and with one swift movement, insert the entire needle up to the hub at a 45-degree angle.
    Purpose: The depth of the injection is determined by the choice of needle length, not by how far you insert the needle. Once the needle is at the tissue layer, do not move the needle while injecting the medication. Being in as far as the hub helps to keep the needle in one place.
15. Withdraw the plunger slightly to be sure that no blood enters the syringe.
    Purpose: Blood in the syringe means that the needle is in a blood vessel and not in the muscle tissue. You may *not* administer a subcutaneous medication by the intravenous route.
16. If blood appears, immediately withdraw the syringe, and compress the injection site with the sponge.
    Purpose: To minimize bleeding and bruising.
17. Begin again with step 1.
    Purpose: Blood is now mixed with the medication, and the medication is considered contaminated. Blood may interact with the drug and may be irritating to the subcutaneous tissues.

Procedure continued on following page

18. If no blood appears in the syringe, push in the plunger slowly and steadily until all medication has been administered.
    Purpose: A rapid injection may damage the tissues.
19. Cover the area with the sponge, and withdraw the needle at the same angle of insertion.
20. Gently massage the site with the antiseptic sponge.
    Purpose: Massage helps to increase absorption and to decrease pain.
21. Make sure that your patient is comfortable and safe.
22. Dispose of the needle and syringe.
23. Observe the patient for any adverse reaction. You may need to keep the patient under observation for 20 to 30 minutes.
24. Wash your hands.
25. Record the drug administration on the patient's medical record, and on the required DEA record if the medication is a controlled substance.

TERMINAL PERFORMANCE OBJECTIVE

Given a patient, an order, and the necessary equipment and supplies, prepare and administer a medication by the subcutaneous route, observing the "Five Rights" and the "Three Befores," and record the drug administration on the patient's medical record, within ten minutes, with no break in sterile technique and no omissions or errors in any step of the procedure, as determined by your evaluator.

Intradermal Injections

Intradermal injections differ from subcutaneous injections in that they are given *within the skin*, not under the skin layer (Fig. 27–20). When correctly administered, a small wheal (elevation) is raised on the skin. A very short needle and a small gauge are used. The angle of insertion is 15 degrees, almost parallel to the skin surface. The best site of injection is the center of the forearm, but the upper chest and back areas are also used (Fig. 27–21). An area with minimum hair is preferred. Most intradermal injections are skin tests for allergies.

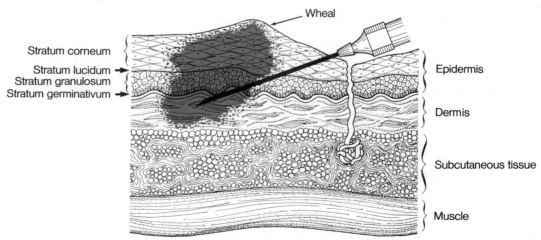

Figure 27–20
The intradermal injection is administered just under the epidermis. The drug is dispersed into an area rich with nerves, so it causes momentary burning or stinging. Minute amounts of medication are injected. This method is used to test for allergies, drug sensitivities, and susceptibility to some diseases.

27

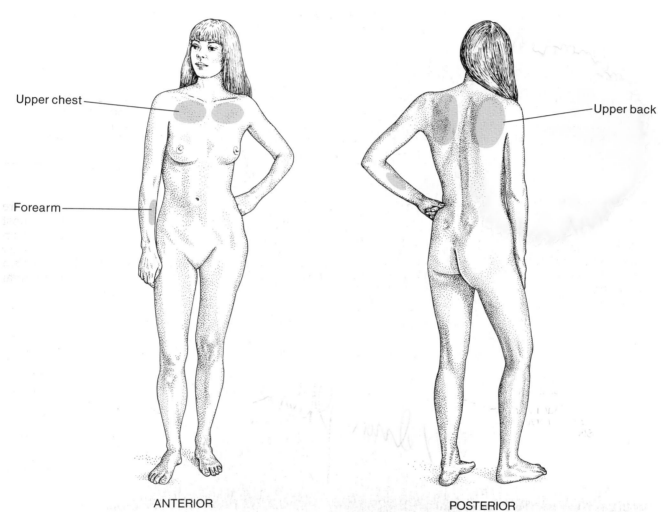

Upper chest

Forearm

Upper back

ANTERIOR

POSTERIOR

Figure 27–21
Sites recommended for intradermal injections.

Procedure 27-5

PROCEDURAL GOAL

To inject a medication into the skin using a needle and syringe of correct size, as directed by the physician.

EQUIPMENT AND SUPPLIES

A vial or ampule containing the material to be injected
Antiseptic sponges
A sterile needle and syringe unit
A written order, including the patient's name, when to give the drug, the route of administration, and the name and strength of the drug
Nonsterile gloves (see Appendix C, Recommendations for Prevention of AIDS Transmission)

PROCEDURE

1. Wash your hands. Follow universal blood and body-fluid precautions (see Appendix C). Glove yourself with nonsterile gloves.
2. Select the correct medication from the shelf or the refrigerator.
   Purpose: Some medications must be refrigerated.
3. Read the label to be sure that you have the RIGHT DRUG and the RIGHT STRENGTH.
   Purpose: One medication may be manufactured and prepackaged in different strengths; for instance, an allergen may be available in 1:000, 1:100, or 1:10 dilutions.
4. Warm refrigerated medications by gently rolling the container between your palms.
5. Prepare the syringe, withdrawing the RIGHT DOSE.
6. Transport the medication to the patient.
7. Greet and identify the patient by name.
   Purpose: To be sure that you have the RIGHT PATIENT.
8. Position the patient comfortably.
9. Locate the antecubital space, then find a site several fingerwidths down the forearm.
10. Cleanse the patient's skin with the antiseptic sponge, using a circular motion, moving outward from the center.
11. Allow the antiseptic to dry.
    Purpose: Because the injected drug is deposited so near the skin surface, the antiseptic could interact with the drug.
12. Compare the order with the prepared medication, and the patient with the name on the order to be sure that this is the RIGHT TIME to administer the drug.
    Purpose: This is the last of the five checks to be made before administering a medication. If there is any doubt, do not proceed. Check first with the physician.
13. Remove the sheath from the needle.
14. With the thumb and first two fingers of your minor hand, stretch the skin taut.
    Purpose: Stretching the skin facilitates the insertion of the needle.
15. Grasp the syringe between the thumb and first two fingers of your major hand, palm down, with the needle bevel upward.
16. At a 15-degree angle, carefully insert the needle through the skin about ⅛ inch, keeping the needle visible through the skin.
17. Turn the syringe 180 degrees to turn the bevel downward.
    Purpose: To prevent the medication from breaking through the skin by the force of the injection.
18. Slowly and steadily inject the medication.
    Purpose: A rapid injection may force the substance through to the surface.
19. When a wheal appears, stop, and withdraw the needle.
20. Do not massage.
    Purpose: Massaging will interfere with the intended results.
21. Make sure that your patient is comfortable and safe.
22. Dispose of the needle and syringe.

Procedure continued on opposite page

23. Observe the patient for any adverse reaction. You may need to keep the patient under observation for 20 to 30 minutes.
24. Wash your hands.
25. Record the drug administration and any reactions that occurred at the site of the injection on the patient's medical record.

[handwritten: Drug Right-celf anm]
[handwritten: A]
[handwritten: 26" 5/8 inch]

TERMINAL PERFORMANCE OBJECTIVE

Given a patient, an order, and the necessary equipment and supplies, prepare and administer a medication by the intradermal route, observing the "Five Rights" and the "Three Befores," and record the drug administration and reactions on the patient's medical record, within ten minutes, with no break in sterile technique and no omissions or errors in any step of the procedure, as determined by your evaluator.

[handwritten: .05   The value of each line is 100th]
[handwritten: 2 | .10]

Infants and Children

Administering injections to infants and small children requires some special considerations. The choice of a site is based upon muscular development as well as the absence of major nerves and blood vessels. The most popular site for intramuscular injection is the vastus lateralis muscle (lateral thigh). Other sites are avoided for the following reasons:

- Babies do not have well-developed deltoid muscles.
- The sciatic nerve is proportionately larger in the infant.
- The gluteus medius is not well developed until the child is walking.

The best policy is to ask the physician to show you just where to inject. Any site selected for infants and children has a greater margin for error because the muscles are smaller than the muscles of the adult.

Babies have to be restrained by another assistant or the parent to avoid injury. If the child is old enough to understand, be honest and explain that the injection may "sting" for a minute, but that it is important to hold very still. Obtain assistance when giving an injection to an uncooperative child. You may keep the fact that the child is to receive an injection from the child until the last minute, but always let the child know. After the injection, praise the child for being helpful; show appreciation and assurance. By doing this, the child will remember more than just the "hurt" of the needle and will trust in you and the process of health care in general. Many children like to have a band-aid applied after the injection as a badge of bravery. Do not give a used syringe to a child for play. It is contaminated and must be disposed of properly.

27

REFERENCES AND READINGS

Asperheim, M.: *The Pharmacologic Basis of Patient Care*, 5th ed. Philadelphia, W. B. Saunders Co., 1985.

Behrman, R., and Vaughan, V. C., III: *Nelson Textbook of Pediatrics*, 13th ed. Philadelphia, W. B. Saunders Co., 1987.

Bonewit, K.: *Clinical Procedures for Medical Assistants*, 2nd ed. Philadelphia, W. B. Saunders Co., 1984.

DuGas, B. W.: *Introduction to Patient Care: A Comprehensive Approach to Nursing*, 4th ed. Philadelphia, W. B. Saunders Co., 1983.

Fuller, J. R.: *Surgical Technology: Principles and Practice*, 2nd ed. Phildadelphia, W. B. Saunders Co., 1986.

Malseed, R. T., et al.: *Pharmacology: Drug Therapy and Nursing Considerations*. Philadelphia, J. B. Lippincott Co., 1982.

Reiss, B. S., and Melick, M. E.: *Pharmacological Aspects of Nursing Care*. Albany, NY, Delmar, 1984.

Rodman, M. J., and Karch, A. M.: *Pharmacology and Drug Therapy in Nursing*, 3rd ed. Philadelphia, J. B. Lippincott Co., 1985.

Sheridan, E., et al.: *Falconer's The Drug, The Nurse, and The Patient*, 7th ed. Philadelphia, W. B. Saunders Co., 1985.

Sorensen, K. C., and Luckmann, J.: *Basic Nursing: A Psychophysiologic Approach*, 2nd ed. Philadelphia, W. B. Saunders Co., 1986.

[handwritten: 28]

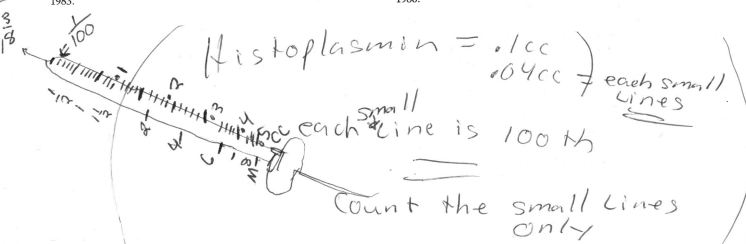

[handwritten: Histoplasmin = .1cc) .04cc each small lines   each small line is 100th   Count the small lines only]

CHAPTER OUTLINE

VOCABULARY

See Glossary at end of book for definitions.

acidosis	exogenous	resonance
atrophy	exophthalmos	symmetry
bilirubin	hydrocele	thrombose
bruit	jaundice	tinnitus
cyanosis	nevi	uremia
emphysema	pallor	vertigo
endogenous	passive	vitiligo
excoriation	postpartum	

28

Assisting with Routine Examinations

OBJECTIVES

Upon successful completion of this chapter you should be able to

1. Define the words listed in the Vocabulary for this chapter.
2. List seven parts of the medical history.
3. Differentiate between signs and symptoms (objective findings and subjective findings).
4. Describe each of the four parts of the Problem-Oriented Medical Record and recall the acronym used for this system.
5. Describe, with an example of each, the six methods of examination.
6. Describe the basic principles of properly draping a patient for examination.
7. List 11 positions for physical examination.
8. Discuss the basics of the routine physical examination.
9. List the sequence of a routine physical examination.

Upon successful completion of this chapter you should be able to perform the following activities:

1. Obtain patient information, and record it in the medical history.
2. Prepare the examination room for the routine physical examination.
3. Assist in the positioning and draping of patients.
4. Assist with a routine physical examination.

Clinical responsibilities vary widely, depending upon the physician's specialty and the extent of reliance upon the medical assistant. Some physicians are reluctant to delegate clinical duties; however, the physician who does utilize the assistant appreciates how time is saved and professional skills can be enhanced. The medical assistant can ease the roles of both the physician and the patient in many office procedures.

To be effective, you must develop the ability to

- Communicate with the patient and the physician easily and professionally.
- Evaluate patient needs and respond to these needs.
- Follow the physician's instructions quickly, accurately, and confidentially.

There is much the medical assistant can do to facilitate the quality of patient care and the physician's schedule. The successful medical assistant orchestrates a routine that is organized yet flexible enough to adjust to the individual problems that may arise.

PREPARING FOR THE PHYSICAL EXAMINATION

Patient care does not start with the physical examination; it begins when the patient makes first contact with the office. Even before the examination, you have the opportunity to react to and interact with the patient to ensure that he or she feels comfortable during the process and that all the necessary information is collected.

Attitude Toward the Patient

More than ever, medicine emphasizes the importance of communicating with the patient and providing a warm and caring environment. Positive reactions and interactions with the patient are essential to providing good patient care. As the patient progresses through the various stages of health care, all members of the medical team must exercise a variety of special skills to enhance the process. These skills are not all technical and medical in nature; many involve the art of caring for the patient as a human being. Because medical care is of an extremely personal nature, the medical assistant must always remember that each patient is an individual with certain anxieties. These anxieties often cause people to act and react in different ways, and effective verbal and nonverbal communication with each patient is essential.

You can do much to put a patient at ease through the tone of your voice and the ease and confidence of your movements and by showing a sincere interest. In other words, give the patient your undivided attention, and let each patient know you *want* to give him or her your attention. The patient is not concerned with the problems of the office staff, nor are you there to impress the patient with your medical knowledge. You are there for one purpose—to give each patient the best possible care.

The Medical Record

When a new patient calls or comes in for an appointment, some medical offices ask the patient to complete a special self-history form (Fig. 28–1). Besides being useful for diagnosing and treating the patient, the self-history allows the patient more participation in the process. The form may be mailed to the patient's home a week before the appointment or may be completed in the office during the first visit.

If you are responsible for taking a portion of the medical history, do it in an area free from outside interference and beyond the hearing range of other patients. Patients will not talk freely where they may be overheard or interrupted. The room should be physically comfortable and conducive to confidential communications.

Listen to the patient. Do not express surprise or displeasure at any of the patient's statements. Remember, you are there not to pass judgment but to gather medical data. Your responses should show interest and concern and should not be judgmental. Do report the information gained to the physician in an organized manner, exactly as given by the patient, without opinion or interpretation.

In some medical offices, the physician takes the medical history, during the patient's initial interview. The physician will correlate the physical findings with the information in the history. Questioning the patient is the usual method of obtaining this vital information. The complete medical history and the physical examination cannot be separated and are the first basic skills of the medical profession.

Terms and Abbreviations. Here are some terms and abbreviations used in writing a patient's medical history.

Chief complaint (CC): Usually the reason for the patient's seeking medical care. Often it is recorded in the patient's own words. It is a list of the patient's current symptoms.

Present illness (PI): An amplification of the chief complaint. It is usually written in chronologic sequence with dates of onset.

Systems review (SR) or review of systems (ROS): A guide to general health; tends to detect conditions other than those covered in the present illness. It is obtained by a logical sequence of questions, beginning with the head and proceeding downward.

Past history (PH) or past medical history (PMH): Covers the dates and questions regarding the pa-

EAST MADISON CLINIC, S.C.
1912 Atwood Avenue
Madison, Wisconsin 53704
608-241-4611

Date _Aug 28, 1986_

☐ Single
☒ Divorced
☐ Married
☐ Widowed

NAME ___Rose Ann Peterson___

S. S. No. ___495-63-2371___   Date of Birth ___11-16-40___

OCCUPATION _Receptionist_   YEARS OF HIGH SCHOOL _12_ COLLEGE _____
POSTGRADUATE _____

DATE OF LAST PHYSICAL ___5-10-85___

ARMED SERVICES? _____ WHEN & WHERE _____

WEIGHT TODAY _121_ 1 YEAR AGO _123_   MAXIMUM WEIGHT _135_ MINIMUM ADULT WEIGHT _116_

Please answer the following questions. Where boxes are provided to check, place a check mark in front of the disease or condition which you have had. If you do not understand the question fully, the nurse will assist you. **This form must be completed and returned to the clinic at least one week prior to your appointment.**

FAMILY HISTORY:

Relative	Living? (Give Present Age)	If Deceased At What Age?	Cause of Death
Father	77		
Mother	76		
Brothers: 1			
2			
3			
4			
5			
or more			
Sisters: 1	50		
2			
3			
4			
5			
or more			

HAS ANY RELATIVE EVER HAD ? (Check Boxes)

WHICH RELATIVE?

☒ Cancer   _aunt_
☐ Tumor
☐ Leukemia
☐ Bleeding problems
☐ Anemia
☐ Diabetes
☐ Gout
☐ Rheumatism or arthritis
☐ High blood pressure
☐ Heart disease
☐ Strokes
☐ Epilepsy

WHICH RELATIVE?

☐ Ulcers
☒ Kidney disease   _self_
☐ Kidney stones
☒ Gall stones   _self_
☒ Lung disease   _Father_
☐ Mental disorders
☐ Suicide
☐ Thyroid disease
☐ Migraine
☐ Tuberculosis
☐ Asthma
☐ Allergies

HAVE YOU HAD A FAMILY HISTORY OF: (Check the ones that apply)
☐ Hay fever   ☐ Asthma   ☐ Emphysema   ☐ Bronchiectasis

EMC-180

28

Figure 28–1

One example of a patient self-history, which may be mailed to the patient the week before the initial visit. The self-history includes a family history as well as the patient's own medical history.

Help with diagnosis + treatment

Illustration continued on following page

PERSONAL HISTORY: *Just your History*

PAST ILLNESSES: (Check the ones you have had)

☒ Measles ☐ Scarlet fever ☐ Typhoid fever
☒ Chicken pox ☐ Rheumatic fever ☐ Asthma
☒ Whooping cough ☐ Diphtheria ☒ Nephritis (Brights Disease)
☐ Poliomyelitis

MEDICAL ILLNESSES OR HOSPITALIZATIONS: (Please describe briefly)

Glomeruli Nephritis - Chronic   What Year *1959*
                                                              & 1961

SURGICAL OPERATIONS: *Gall Stones & Appendix removed*   What Year *1973*
        Tubal Fulgeration   *1983*

BROKEN BONES OR ACCIDENTS: *Broken Rib from coughing*   What Year *1970*

HAVE YOU EVER HAD: ☐ Sweats   ☐ Fevers   ☐ Bleeding

HAVE YOU EVER HAD ANY ALLERGIES AND/OR DRUG REACTIONS?   Yes ☐   No ☒

If yes, to what agent or drug? _____

DRUGS: (Check the ones you have taken or are taking)

☐ Laxatives ☐ Digitalis ☐ Sleeping Pills ☐ Insulin
☐ Sedatives ☐ Thyroid ☐ Aspirin ☐ Hormones
☒ Tranquilizers ☐ Stimulants ☐ Cortisone ☒ Birth control pills

IMMUNIZATIONS: (Shots - check the ones you have had)

☐ Smallpox vaccination in the last 6 years.
☐ Tetanus (not antitoxin) in the last 2 years.
☐ Polio in last 2 years.

EXAMINATIONS: (Check the ones you have had)

☒ Chest x-ray last year
☒ EKG (Heart Tracing)   When *1959*
☒ UGI (X-ray stomach)   When *1973*
☐ Proctoscopic   When _____
☐ Barium enema   When _____
☒ IVP (Kidney X-ray)   When *1959-61-75*
☐ BMR   When _____
☐ Thyroid studies   When _____

HABITS: (Check the ones you have)

☒ Tobacco   ☒ Alcoholic beverages   ☒ Coffee   ☐ Tea   Other_____

GENERAL: Do you have or have you had? (Check those that apply).

☐ Frequent sweats, fevers or chills ☐ Nervousness ☐ Allergies
☐ Night sweats ☐ Recent weight gain ☐ Drug reactions
☐ Recent weight loss ☐ Intolerance to heat or cold

HAVE YOU HAD EXPOSURE TO: (Check the ones that apply)

☐ Dust ☐ Hay ☐ Stonecutting ☐ Foundry Work ☐ Fumes
☐ Mold ☐ Silage ☐ Sandblasting ☐ Metal polishing

REVIEW OF SYSTEMS: (Head, eyes, ears, nose and throat) (Check any that apply to you.)

☐ Headache ☐ Bothered by bright lights ☐ Itching ear canals ☐ Hoarseness
☐ Loss of hair ☐ Blurring of vision ☐ Fullness or popping in the ears ☐ Change of voice
☐ Excessive tearing ☐ Loss of vision ☒ Nasal stuffiness ☐ Difficulty swallowing
☐ Dryness of the eyes ☒ Have you worn glasses ☐ Loss of smell or taste ☐ Bleeding gums
☐ Pain behind the eyes ☐ Painful red eyes ☐ Nosebleeds ☐ Pyorrhea
☐ Pain in the eyes ☒ Ringing in the ears ☐ Sneezing ☐ Trench mouth
☐ See flashing lights ☐ Loss of hearing ☐ Postnasal drip ☐ Sores in mouth
☐ See black spots ☐ Drainage from ears ☒ Sinus infections

Figure 28–1 Continued

Illustration continued on opposite page

LUNGS: (Check the items that apply)
☒ Morning cough   ☒ Cough during the day   ☐ Pleurisy   ☐ Wheezing
☐ Evening cough   ☒ Sputum with cough   ☐ Cough up blood   ☐ Frequent colds
☐ Blood clot to lungs (embolus)

HEART: (Check the items that apply)
☐ Fatigue, (tired feeling) with work   ☐ Pain in chest when working
☐ Shortness of breath with walking   ☐ Rapid beating of the heart
☐ Shortness of breath with work   ☒ Irregular beating of the heart
☐ Shortness of breath lying down   ☐ Nightmares
☐ Awake at night with cough   ☐ Pain or numbness in legs when walking
☐ Cough on lying down   ☐ Pain, or whiteness, of hands in cool weather (or in cool water)
☐ Awake at night short of breath   ☐ Awake at night with tightness in chest
☐ Awake at night with pain in chest   ☐ Swelling of hands
☐ Pain in chest on walking   ☐ Swelling of feet or legs
☐ Pain in chest on running   ☐ Sleep on more than one pillow
☐ Pain in chest after meals

BLOOD, BLOOD VESSELS AND SKIN: (Check the items that apply)
☒ Bruise easily   ☐ Anemia, history of   ☐ History of lymphoma   ☒ Psoriasis
☐ Red spots on hands - feet   ☐ Bleed easily   ☐ History of pernicious anemia   ☐ Hives
☐ Swollen glands   ☐ History of leukemia   ☐ Skin rash   ☐ Fungus infection

STOMACH, INTESTINES AND COLON: (Check the items that apply)
☐ Appetite poor   ☐ "Heartburn" or "Indigestion"   ☐ Intolerance to fried, fatty, greasy foods or milk   ☐ Jaundice   ☒ Gaseousness
☐ Nausea, upset stomach   ☒ Bloating   ☐ Pain in abdomen   ☒ Passage of gas
☐ Vomiting   ☐ Belching   ☐ Hunger pains   ☐ Colic   ☐ Fissure
☐ Fever, recurrent   ☒ Diarrhea   ☐ Mucous in bowel movements   ☐ Grease in bowel movements   ☒ Hemorrhoids
☐ Chills, recurrent   ☐ Constipation   ☐ Blood in bowel movements   ☐ Fistula
☐ Change in bowel habits or stools   ☐ Black bowel movements   ☐ Pain with bowel movements
☐ Vomit blood

BLADDER AND SEX ORGANS: (Fill in the blanks & check the items that apply)
Number of times of urination daily _____ *5 or 6* _____   Number of times of urination nightly _____ *1* _____
☒ Blood in urine   ☐ Colic, kidney   ☐ Loss of urine with cough, laughing, straining, etc.   ☒ Satisfied with sex
☐ Burning on urination   ☐ Pain in flank   ☒ Completely emptying bladder after urination
☐ Discharge   ☐ Pain in side   ☐ Soiling undergarments
☐ Kidney Stone   ☐ Desire to urinate, but unable to pass urine   ☐ Venereal disease

FOR MEN ONLY: (Check the items that apply)
☐ Decreased force of stream   ☐ Straining   ☐ Difficulty with erection   ☐ Difficulty with production of sperm
☐ Small stream   ☐ Stream starts and stops   ☐ Dribbling

FOR WOMEN ONLY: (Check the items that apply & fill in the blanks)
Menses, onset, age _____ *11 yr.* _____   ☐ Bleeding after or pain with intercourse
Menses, stopped, age _____   No. of pregnancies _____ *2* _____
Last period began _____ *Aug 25, 1986* _____   No. of live births _____ *2* _____
Period prior to this one began _____ *July 21, 1986* _____   No. of miscarriages _____
No. of pads or Tampons per period _____ *15* _____   No. of dead births _____
    Light _*1*_ Heavy _____ Soaked _____   ☐ Toxemia with pregnancy
No. of days flow _____ *5* _____   ☒ Family history of cancer of the breast _*aunt*_
No. of days between periods _____ *26* _____   ☐ Mass in the breast
☒ Any discharge between periods   ☐ Discharge from the nipple
☐ Pain with menses
☐ Bleeding between periods

BONES, MUSCLES AND JOINTS: (Check the items that apply)
☐ Aching muscles   ☐ Trick knee   ☐ Infection in the bones   ☒ Sciatica
☐ Aching joints   ☐ Had gout   ☒ Popping in the joints *Knee*   ☐ Lumbago
☐ Swollen joints   ☐ Had rheumatoid arthritis   ☐ Pain in hips, knees, ankles, and with walking   ☐ Rheumatism
☐ Red and swollen joints   ☐ Had lupus erythematosis   ☐ Had other _____
☒ Joint stiffness in the A.M.   ☐ Infection in the joints

BRAIN AND NERVES: (Check the items that apply)
☐ Fits or convulsions   ☐ Weakness of arms or legs   ☐ Memory loss   ☐ Tremors or shaking
☐ Coma or unconsciousness   ☐ Pins and needles sensation   ☐ Poor coordination   ☐ Muscular twitching
☐ Fainting spells   ☐ Inability to feel pain   ☐ Difficulty concentrating   ☐ Head Injury
☐ Dizziness   ☐ Inability to feel cold   ☐ Difficulty buttoning shirts   ☐ Encephalitis (sleeping sickness)
☐ Loss of balance   ☐ Inability to feel heat   ☐ Difficulty tying shoes   ☐ Meningitis
☐ Paralysis (can't move arm or leg)   ☐ Personality change

28

Figure 28-1 Continued

tient's *usual childhood diseases (UCD or UCHD),* major illnesses and operations, allergies, accidents, and immunizations.

Family history (FH): Details regarding the patient's mother and father, their health, and, if deceased, the cause and age of death. Hereditary tendencies are recorded here and may include siblings and offspring.

Social history (SH): Social history includes the patient's eating, drinking, smoking, and sleeping habits; hobbies; interests; and methods of exercise. The physician may wish to inquire about the patient's *occupational history (OH).*

Signs and Symptoms. Many times, you will hear that certain findings and conclusions in a medical history are either objective or subjective. Sometimes, these two terms are confused, as are the terms signs and symptoms, which may be used interchangeably with objective and subjective, respectively.

Subjective findings, or symptoms, are perceptible only to the patient; they are what the patient feels. An ache, pain, or dizziness is felt only by the patient, and only the patient can tell you it exists. The patient tells the physician about these symptoms, and the physician records them as subjective findings or symptoms. Symptoms of the greatest significance in identifying a disease are called cardinal symptoms.

Objective findings, or signs, are perceptible to a person other than the patient, specifically the physician. They are the signs that a physician detects when examining a patient. The physician feels, sees, or hears the signs that are often associated with a certain disease or abnormal condition. Objective findings are dependent upon another person's senses. A mass that a physician feels in the patient's abdomen is an objective finding. It is a sign of an abnormal condition.

Other terms that require understanding are the words functional and physical (organic). When a condition or disease is functional, it means that the disease is without discoverable, or organic, cause, that is, the organ appears normal but its function is not normal. A functional disease is any disease that alters the body functions but is not associated with any apparent organic, or physical, reason. A physical, or organic, disease or condition is one in which the abnormality can be seen or felt.

Problem-Oriented Medical Record (POMR). This method of medical record keeping introduced a logical sequence to recording the information obtained from the patient. It is based on the scientific method and was designed to "solve a problem." The medical history and the physical examination fit into a special format designed to clarify each patient problem. The format includes supporting data that aid in solving the patient's problem. Because the POMR is universally organized, it is clear to anyone who reads the record. It lends to better audit of the medical record. The POMR is said to be the tool that revolutionized communication among the members of the health team caring for the patient. The system is designed for and easily adapted to computerized medical records systems.

Dr. Lawrence L. Weed is credited with bringing this logical system of patient record keeping to the medical profession. The POMR system includes four basic parts:

1. *Data Base.* The record of the patient's history, physical examination, and initial laboratory findings. As new information is added, it becomes a part of this data base.

2. *Problem List.* A list of the identified patient problems kept in the front of the patient's chart. It is the "Table of Contents" or the "Index" of the chart. Each problem entered here is numerically listed and dated and is supported by the data base. If the problem is resolved, the date of problem resolution is entered next to the problem.

3. *Initial Plan.* A written plan for each problem identified on the problem list, outlining further studies, treatments, and patient education.

4. *Progress Notes.* Structured notes that correspond to each problem on the problem list, including (1) subjective data, (2) objective data, (3) assessment of the problem, and (4) plans (diagnostic studies, treatments, and patient education). The first letter of each part of the progress note spells SOAP; therefore, this portion of the POMR system is called "soap notes."

Further information on the POMR system may be found in Chapter 11, Medical Records Management.

Procedure 28-1

PROCEDURAL GOAL

To obtain an acceptable written background from the patient to help the physician determine the etiology and effects of the present illness. This includes the chief complaint, present illness, past history, family history, and social history.

SUPPLIES AND EQUIPMENT

A history form
Two pens, red and black ink
A quiet, private area

PROCEDURE

1. Greet and identify the patient in a pleasant manner. Introduce yourself and explain your role.
   Purpose: To make the patient feel at ease.
2. Find a quiet, private area for the interview, and explain to the patient the need for the requested information.
   Purpose: An informed patient is more cooperative and, thus, more likely to contribute useful information.
3. Complete the history form by asking appropriate questions. A self-history may have been mailed to the patient prior to the visit. If so, review the self-history for completeness.
   Purpose: The self-history is designed to save time and to involve the patient in the process.
4. Speak in a pleasant, distinct manner, remembering to keep eye contact with your patient.
   Purpose: Positive nonverbal behavior creates a friendly atmosphere.
5. Record the following statistical information on the patient information form:
   a. Patient's full name, including middle initial.
   b. Address, including apartment number and zip code.
   c. Marital status.
   d. Sex (gender).
   e. Age and date of birth (DOB).
   f. Telephone number.
   g. Employer's name, address, telephone number.
6. Record the following medical history on the patient history form:
   a. Chief complaint.
   b. Present illness.
   c. Past history.
   d. Family history.
   e. Social history.
   Purpose: This is information that the physician needs to know to make an accurate assessment and diagnosis. The physician usually completes the review of systems during the pre-examination interview.
7. Ask about allergies to drugs and any other substances, and record them in red ink on every page of the history form.
   Purpose: The presence of an allergy may alter medication and treatment procedures.
8. Record all information legibly and neatly, and spell words correctly. Print rather than write in longhand. Do not erase; if you make an error, draw a single line through the error and initial the correction.
   Purpose: To maintain a medical record that is understandable and defensible in a court of law.

Procedure continued on following page

28

9. Check for accuracy by repeating back to the patient the spelling of the name and the address, zip code, and phone number.
10. Thank the patient for cooperating, and direct him or her back to the reception area.
11. Review the record for errors before you hand it to the physician.
12. Use the information on the record to complete the patient's chart as directed by the physician. Keep the information confidential.
    Purpose: All facts and information concerning the patient must remain in the office. This information may be legally and ethically discussed with only the physician.

TERMINAL PERFORMANCE OBJECTIVE

Given a quiet, private area, interview the patient to obtain an accurate and useful patient medical record. The time will vary according to the patient's degree of illness and the openness of the communication, but under normal circumstances, collecting information should be accomplished within 15 minutes. When you are finished, the record should be complete in scope and depth, accurate, and legible, as determined by your evaluator.

ASSISTING WITH THE PHYSICAL EXAMINATION

Methods of Examination

Examinations are performed as both a routine confirmation of the absence of illness and a means of diagnosing disease. There are six methods of examining the human body. All six methods are part of every complete physical examination.

Inspection. This is the art of observation: the ability to detect significant physical features (Fig. 28–2*A*). The focus of this method of examination ranges from the patient's general appearance—the general state of health, including posture, mannerisms, and grooming—to the more detailed observations that may include body contour, **symmetry**, visible injuries and deformities, tremors, rashes, and color changes.

Palpation. This method uses the sense of touch (Fig. 28–2*B*). A part of the body is felt with the hand for the purpose of determining its condition or that of an underlying organ. It may include touching the skin or the more firm feeling of the abdomen for underlying masses. This technique involves a wide range of perceptions: temperature, vibrations, consistency, form, size, rigidity, elasticity, moisture, texture, position, and contour. Palpation is performed with one hand, both hands (bimanual), one finger (digital), the fingertips, or the palmar aspects of the hand. A pelvic examination is done bimanually, whereas an anal examination is performed digitally. Do not confuse palpation with palpitation, which is a throbbing pulsation.

Percussion. This tapping or striking of the body, usually with the fingers or a small hammer to elicit sounds or vibratory sensations, aids in the determination of the position, size, and density of an underlying organ or cavity. The effect of percussion is both heard and felt by the examiner. It is helpful in determining the amount of air or solid matter in an underlying organ or cavity. The two basic methods of percussion are direct and indirect. Direct (immediate) percussion is performed by striking the body with a finger. Indirect (mediate) palpation is used more frequently and is done by the examiner placing his own finger on the area and then striking the placed finger with a finger of the other hand (Fig. 28–2*C*). Both a sound and a sense of vibration are evident here. The examiner will speak of sounds in terms of pitch, quality, duration, and **resonance**.

Auscultation. This is the process of listening to sounds arising from the body—not the sound produced by the examiner as in percussion, but sounds that originate within the patient's body. This is a difficult method of examination because the examiner must distinguish between a normal and an abnormal sound. A stethoscope is usually used to amplify sounds (Fig. 28–2*D*). Auscultation is particularly useful in appraising sounds arising from the lungs, heart, and abdomen and in distinguishing **bruits**, murmurs, rhythms, durations, and quality. Indirect listening is done with the stethoscope, whereas direct auscultation is done by the examiner placing the ear directly on the patient's body.

Mensuration. This is the process of measuring. Measurements are taken of the length and diameter of an extremity, the extent of flexion or extension of an extremity, or the pressure of a grip. The expansion of the chest or the circumference of the head can be measured. The patient's height and weight are measurements. Hearing and vision are measured, and measuring is done for pregnancy. Measurements are taken using tape measures or small rulers and are usually reported in centimeters.

Manipulation. This is the forceful, **passive** movement of a joint to determine the range of extension

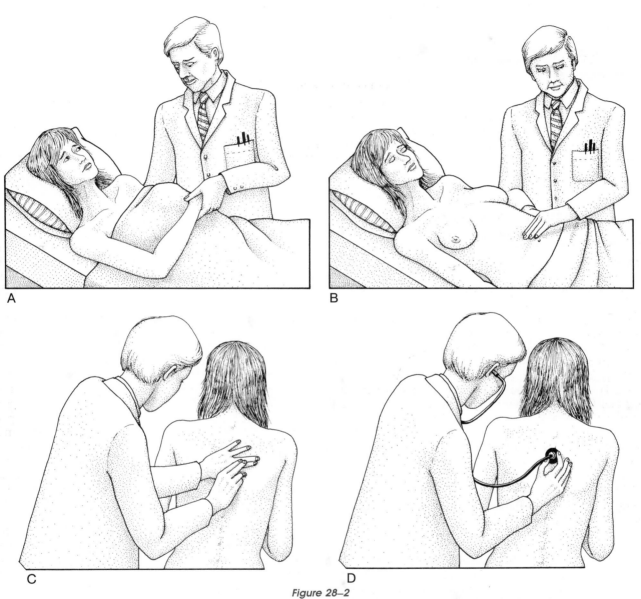

28

Figure 28–2

Four standard methods of physical examination. **A,** *INSPECTION. The art of observation. The physician is inspecting the patient's hand with his eyes for any visible signs of abnormality.* **B,** *PALPATION. The physician may use the sense of touch to determine the size of a part or the presence of abnormal growths. Palpation also may be performed with two hands (bimanually) or the fingers (digitally).* **C,** *PERCUSSION. A part of the body is tapped with the hands or a percussion hammer.* **D,** *AUSCULTATION. The sense of hearing is used to listen to a body sound. The stethoscope amplifies what can be heard.*

or flexion of a part of the body. Manipulation may or may not be grouped with palpation. It is usually considered separate from the four standard methods of examination (inspection, palpation, percussion, and auscultation) and is grouped with mensuration, especially by the orthopedist and the neurologist. Insurance and industrial reports often request this information in detail.

Positioning and Draping for Physical Examinations

There are various positions in which a patient may be placed to facilitate a physical examination. The medical assistant instructs the patient about, and assists the patient into, these positions with as much ease and modesty as possible. The medical assistant helps the patient to maintain a position during the examination with as little discomfort as possible.

Draping with an examination sheet protects the patient from embarrassment and keeps the patient warm, but the sheet must be positioned so that it allows complete visibility for the examiner and does not interfere with the examination. During the general examination, each part of the body is exposed one portion at a time. For gynecologic and rectal examinations, the sheet may be positioned on the diagonal across the patient. The following positions are used for medical examinations.

Horizontal Recumbent (Supine). Recumbent means lying down; supine means lying down with the face upward. Either term is used to describe the patient who is lying flat with the face upward (Fig. 28–3A). These terms are not used when instructing the patient; they are most often used when transcribing surgical and radiological reports.

Dorsal Recumbent. Dorsal refers to the back. The dorsal recumbent position places the patient lying face upward, with the weight distributed primarily to the surface of the back (Fig. 28–3B). This is accomplished by flexing the knees so that the feet are flat on the table. This position relieves muscle tension in the abdomen and is used for examination of the abdomen and for resting. In the *dorsal elevated* position, the patient lies face upward with the head and shoulders slightly elevated, in a somewhat modified Fowler position (see following).

Lithotomy. The word parts of this term do not describe a body position; the name applies to the historical use of this position to perform a lithotomy (incision to remove a stone). The patient is placed on the back, with the knees sharply flexed, the arms placed at the sides or folded over the chest,

and the buttocks to the edge of the table. The feet are supported in table stirrups or are hung in hammock-like knee supports (Fig. 28–3C). The stirrups should be placed wide apart and somewhat away from the table. If the heels are too close to the buttocks, the possibility of leg cramps is increased, and it is more difficult for the patient to relax the abdominal muscles. Make sure that the stirrups are locked in place. A towel is placed under the patient's buttocks, and a drape is placed over the patient's abdomen and knees. The drape should be large enough to cover the breasts if the patient is not wearing a gown. The drape must be long enough to cover the knees and touch the ankles, and wide enough to prevent the sides of the thighs from being exposed. The physician will push the drape away from the pubic area when the examination begins.

Trendelenburg. The patient is supine on a table that has been raised at the lower end about 45 degrees (Fig. 28–3D). This places the patient's head lower than the legs. The patient's legs are then flexed over the end. This position is sometimes used in cases of shock or low blood pressure. Recent studies in emergency care question the value of lowering the patient's head, and experts are suggesting that this position is no longer necessary for shock victims. It is also a position for abdominal surgery because the abdominal viscera gravitate upward and out of the way of the surgical procedure. A sheet is placed over the patient, covering from the underarms to below the knees.

Fowler and Semi-Fowler. These two positions are quite similar (Fig. 28–3E and F). The patient is sitting on the examination table with the head elevated. The head usually is raised to a level of about 90 degrees. This position is useful for examinations and treatments of the head, neck, and chest. In the the semi-Fowler position, the head may be elevated to a lesser angle, which is more comfortable, and the legs are supported at the knees, usually with a pillow or a flexed hospital bed. The semi-Fowler position is used for patients who are having difficulty in breathing. The drape will vary according to the exposure of the patient, but the female breasts should be covered and the drape should extend to the feet.

Jackknife. The patient is placed on the back with the shoulders slightly elevated and the legs flexed sharply up over the abdomen (Fig. 28–3G). This places the thighs at right angles to the abdomen, and the lower leg at right angles to the thighs. This position, also called the *reclining* position, is used for the passing of a urethral sound. Placement of the drape is similar to that for the lithotomy position. (The proctologic position is often incorrectly referred to as the jackknife position.)

28

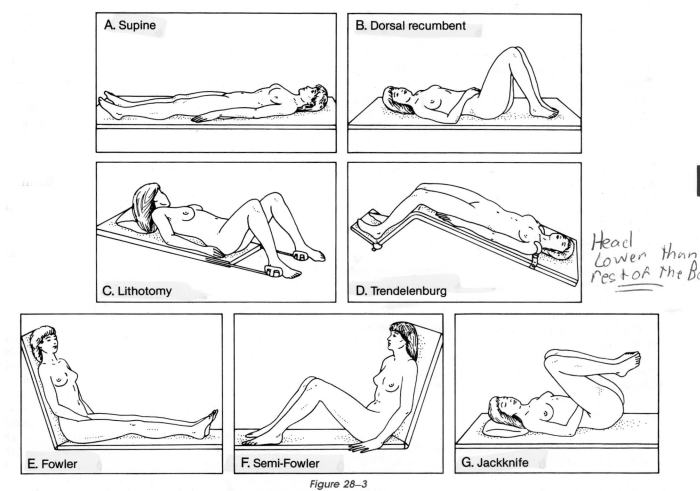

A. Supine

B. Dorsal recumbent

C. Lithotomy

D. Trendelenburg

Head Lower than the rest of The Body

E. Fowler

F. Semi-Fowler

G. Jackknife

Figure 28–3

The basic positions with the patient lying face upward. **A,** The horizontal recumbent (supine) position. **B,** The dorsal recumbent position. **C,** The lithotomy position is preferred for the gynecologic examination. **D,** The Trendelenburg position usually is used for hospital surgery. **E,** Fowler position. **F,** Semi-Fowler position is often used for patients having difficulty in breathing. **G,** The jackknife position has long been confused with the proctologic position. It is used in urologic procedures.

Prone. The patient is lying face down on the table, on the ventral surface of the body (Fig. 28–4A). This is the opposite of the supine position and is another one of the recumbent positions. The patient is covered with a drape large enough to cover from the midback to below the knees. The drape on the female patient should extend high enough to cover the breasts if she is to be turned over to the dorsal recumbent position during the examination.

Sims. This position is sometimes called the *lateral* position. The patient is placed on the left side, with a towel or small pillow under the left cheek. The left arm and shoulder are drawn back behind the body so that the body's weight is predominantly on the chest. The right arm is flexed upward for support. The left leg is slightly flexed, and the buttocks are pulled to the edge of the table. The right leg is sharply flexed upward (Fig. 28–4B). A towel is placed on the upper left thigh, just below the perineal area. A sheet is placed over the patient, extending from under the arms to below the knees. The physician will raise a small portion of the sheet from the back of the patient to sufficiently expose the rectum. The remaining portion of the sheet will cover the patient's chest area and thighs. This position is used for rectal examinations, since the rectal ampulla is dropped down into the abdominal cavity; this facilitates entrance to and examination of the rectum. It is also used for perineal and some pelvic examinations.

Proctologic Position on a Proctologic Table. This position requires an examining table (Fig. 28–5) that can be elevated and tilted in the center and lowered at the head and legs. The patient's head and legs are at an angle lower than the buttocks. It must be stressed that the patient's body is flexed at the hip joint and not at the waist (Fig. 28–4C). If this flexion is not correct, the patient will experience considerable discomfort, and the bowel will not be displaced forward. A fenestrated drape is best, but a single sheet may be draped in a "U" around the anal area. Do not bind the patient's legs together with the drape because it may be necessary to separate the legs during the examination. This position is the superior choice for a sigmoidoscopic examination because it straightens the rectosigmoid area and displaces the lower bowel. It is a convenient position for examining the perineal area, the anus, and hemorrhoids.

Knee-Chest. As the term implies, the patient rests on the knees and the chest (Fig. 28–4D). The head is turned to one side, with one arm flexed under the abdomen and the other hanging over the side of the table, or both arms extended along the sides of the body. The thighs are perpendicular to the table and are slightly separated. The patient's back should not be rounded, but curved inward somewhat to an anterior convexity. The patient will need assistance in order to obtain this position correctly, and it is a difficult position for most patients to maintain. If the correct knee-chest position cannot be obtained, the patient may have to be placed in a knee-elbow position. This position puts less strain on the patient and is easier to maintain. The knee-chest position is also known as the *genupectoral*; the knee-elbow is also called the *genucubital*. These positions are used for the same types of examinations as the proctologic positions. An aperture (opening) drape is used, or a single sheet may be draped in a "U" and pinned over the patient's back at the sacral area. Two smaller sheets may be used, with one sheet over the patient's back and the other from the curve of the buttocks down over the thighs. It will be necessary to join the two sheets together on each side of the examination area with towel clamps. The knee-chest position is sometimes used as therapy for a **postpartum** prolapsed uterus.

Basics of the Routine Physical Examination

It has been said that there is no such thing as a complete physical examination, nor is there a need for one. Examinations vary greatly, depending on the physician's specialty and the reason for the examination. There may also be a variance in the sequence of an examination as individual patient needs are addressed. This chapter reviews an average routine that an examiner might follow. It gives an overview of the process, with some of the terminology and descriptive pathology that is commonly used or seen. Since each physician has individual preferences, only basic instruments are described.

Presenting Appearance (General Appearance). The physical examination really starts as soon as the patient appears before the examiner. Either of the terms *presenting appearance* and *general appearance* may be used on the medical record. These terms note whether or not the patient appears well and in good health. The patient may appear disoriented or in distress. The patient's responses to the opening remarks or questions may show an alertness or dullness.

Gait. The patient's gait, that is, the manner or style of walking, will often give some information. The patient may limp, walk with the feet wide apart, or have difficulty in maintaining his or her balance. The analysis of gait is usually done with the patient walking a straight line or may be done without the patient knowing that he or she is being observed. Some of the terms used are *ataxic* (which describes an unsteady, uncoordinated walk over a wide base), *slapping* or *steppage* (in which the advancing leg is lifted high enough for the toes to clear the ground), *drag-to* (in which the feet are

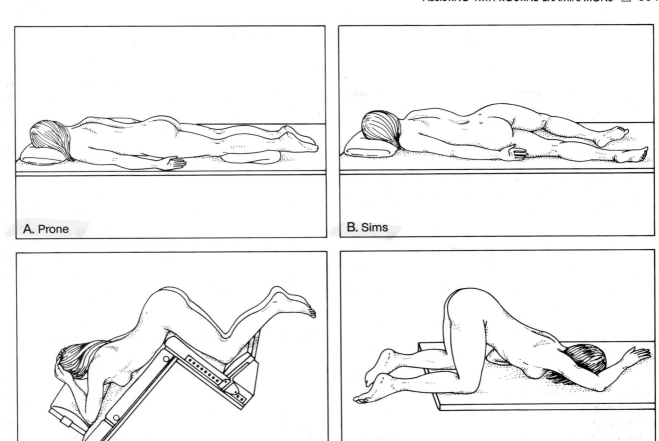

Figure 28–4

The basic positions with the patient lying face down. **A,** *The prone position.* **B,** *The Sims or lateral, position.* **C,** *The proctologic position.* **D,** *The knee-chest position.*

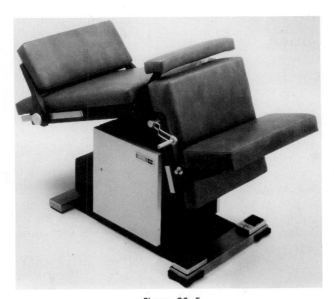

Figure 28–5

A special examination table for proctologic examinations. (Courtesy Ritter, Liebel-Flarsheim, a division of Sybron Corp., Cincinnati, OH.)

dragged rather than lifted), and *spastic* (in which the legs are held together and move in a stiff manner, the toes seeming to drag and catch).

Stature. The patient's height is measured. The physician notes the body build and proportions. Any gross (immediately obvious; taking no account of details, or minutiae) deformities are recorded. Sometimes, abnormalities in height or body proportion may be due to hormonal imbalances.

Posture. A patient's posture may indicate an area of pain. A rigid posture may indicate a fixed spine, and an altered posture may result from an extremity with limited motion. The patient may say that he cannot sleep unless in a sitting position (frequently seen in heart and lung diseases). *Torticollis* (*wryneck*) may be present as a result of a spasm or the shortening of the neck and chest muscles. Examination of the spine may show abnormal curvatures such as *kyphosis* (humpback), *scoliosis* (curvature of the spine), or *lordosis* (abnormal or exaggerated curvature of the lumbosacral area, which causes the buttocks to protrude excessively).

Body Movements. These may be classed as voluntary or involuntary. The voluntary movements are the patient's normal habits and have limited clinical value, unless they are the result of an abnormal condition. Involuntary movements are frequently *tics*, which may be habit spasms (usually found around the eyes, neck, or face) or the result of various conditions. Tics are involuntary, rhythmic movements by a group of muscles that goes into spasm at irregular intervals. A *tremor* is an involuntary trembling or quivering. A tremor may be the beating of the thumb against a flexing finger or a rhythmic oscillation of the head, as may occur in old age.

Speech. In addition to social history, speech may reveal an abnormal condition. Some basic speech defects are *aphonia*, the inability to speak because of a loss of the voice, commonly seen with severe laryngitis or overuse of the voice; *aphasia*, the loss of the power of expression through speech, writing, or sign due to injury or disease of the brain centers; and *dysphasia*, a lack of coordination and failure to arrange words in proper order, usually due to a brain lesion. Other comments concerning speech may include *incoherent*, *jumbled*, or *slurred*.

Breath Odors. These may or may not be diagnostic, although they often are associated with poor oral hygiene or dental care. **Acidosis** will give the strong odor of acetone, which is sweet and fruity. Acidosis may result from diabetes mellitus, starvation, or renal disease. A musty odor is usually associated with liver disease, and the odor of ammonia may be found in cases of **uremia**.

Nutrition. Charts are published containing what is considered normal weight for the age and height of females and males. A patient is generally thought of as being overweight or underweight in comparison with these accepted averages. Obesity may be due to one of two origins: **exogenous**, involving excessive caloric intake in relation to the expenditure of calories, or **endogenous**, involving certain endocrine imbalances.

Edema is the accumulation of fluid in the intercellular tissue spaces of the body and usually refers to the accumulation of fluid in the subcutaneous spaces when commented on in the nutrition section. Edema must be differentiated from fat by the simple test of pressing a finger on the skin over a bony area, such as the ankle, and observing whether or not a pit or depression remains. Edema will leave a whitened pit for a few moments and is recorded as *pitting edema*. Fat does not pit but returns to skin level immediately after the finger is removed.

Skin. Comments on the skin are included as a part of the general appearance, unless the chief complaint involves a condition related to the skin. If so, then the skin is listed as a separate category. In the physical examination, the skin is considered a separate organ of the body. Concerns include abnormal coloring such as redness, **cyanosis**, **pallor**, or excessive brown patches. **Jaundice** may indicate an increase in the level of **bilirubin** in the blood. Decreased pigmentation is found in **vitiligo**, which is the acquired loss of melanin and is characterized by white patches. Lesions, ulcers, and bruises may be the result of pathologic conditions. Skin texture refers to smoothness, roughness, and scaling. Loss of elasticity is when the skin does not return immediately to normal when it has been pulled or stretched. This can occur as an inherited condition or from prolonged injury, such as excessive exposure to the sun.

Fingernails and toenails often give some indication of a person's health. Brittle, grooved, or lined nails may indicate either local infection or systemic disease. *Clubbing* of the fingertips is associated with some congenital heart diseases. *Spooning* of the nail is seen in some severe iron deficiency anemias. *Beau's lines* appear after an acute illness but will grow out and disappear.

Hair Distribution. The distribution or the lack of hair and hair texture are important. Excessive hair, especially facial hair in the female, indicates some bodily change. Heavy abdominal or thigh hair may be an indication of a pathologic condition.

Sequence of the Routine Physical Examination

There is a routine, or sequence, to the physical examination of the patient. The following descriptions of the process will have variations depending on the examiner. Consult your medical dictionary for definitions and further descriptions of the diseases and conditions mentioned. Instruments used in the routine physical examination appear in Chapter 24.

Preparing the Patient. After the physician interviews the patient, you prepare the patient for the physical examination. Usually, you take the patient's height, weight, and vital signs at this time. Give your patient a brief explanation of the type of examination to be done. Patients are more cooperative and less anxious if they understand what is expected of them. Remain with the female patient throughout the examination unless the physician excuses you from the room. A female assistant in the room during the examination of the female patient can avert potential lawsuits. If a patient objects to disrobing, then you must tactfully explain the necessity of adequate exposure in order to facilitate a careful examination. Failure to properly prepare the patient often leads to unnecessary delays and difficulties for the physician. Do not ask the patient to disrobe in an area that is not private, safe for the patient's personal belongings, or warm.

Rapport is accomplished by conversation, but as soon as the physician begins the examination, keep your conversation to a minimum and remain inconspicuous. When the patient is properly positioned and draped, notify the physician that you are ready.

The examination usually starts with the patient seated on the examining table. If the physician uses reflected light, then the light source should be behind the patient's right shoulder. If illuminated instruments are used, then the standard overhead lights are sufficient. Be careful not to shine a light directly into the patient's eyes. Turn on lights while they are directed away from the patient, and then carefully move the light toward the area to be examined.

Head. The patient's head and face are usually the starting place for the examination. The face reflects the patient's state and tells the examiner a great deal. It may appear puffy, especially the eyelids, giving the appearance that the patient has just awakened. The puffiness may be due to myxedema or a medication such as cortisone. With scleroderma, the facial skin is characteristically tight and **atrophied**. *Lipid* or fatty patches that collect in the eyelids, usually near the center, are called *xanthelasma*. These appear as yellowish white, slightly elevated small patches and may or may not be associated with disease.

Neck. The neck is examined for *range of motion* (ROM) by having the patient move the head in various directions. One limitation that may appear is torticollis. *Bounding* is an involuntary slight nodding of the head synchronized with the pulsation of the heart. The thyroid gland is given special attention for symmetry, size, and texture. The examiner manually palpates the thyroid area, and the patient is asked to swallow several times. The medical assistant may help by giving the patient a small amount of water in a paper cup. The examiner palpates the thyroid gland both anteriorly and posteriorly. The carotid artery is palpated and auscultated for possible *bruit* (an abnormal sound or murmur). The lymph nodes are palpated. Swollen lymph nodes usually are present when there is infection in the face, head, or neck.

Eyes. Eyes are checked for reaction to light into the pupils; this is known as *light and accommodation* (L & A). The color of the sclera may be abnormally red or yellow. The movements of the eyes are tested by having the patient follow the examiner's finger. **Exophthalmos** is an important observation that is seen in some cases of hyperthyroidism or of a tumor or fat pad behind the eyeballs. Intraocular pressure is checked using the tonometer in most individuals past the age of 35. Pressure within the eyeball could indicate the presence of glaucoma, which results in pathologic changes in the optic disc, visual defects, and eventual blindness.

Ears. The ears are examined using the otoscope. Symptoms of the ear include deafness, pain, discharge, **vertigo**, and **tinnitus**. The external ear is first checked for redness of the ear canal or the presence of ear wax (cerumen). The tympanic membrane (eardrum) may be seen in most patients and appears pearly gray. Scars appearing on the eardrum are frequently the result of earlier, chronic ear infections or perforations. The color of the eardrum is important to the diagnosis because it may indicate fluids such as blood or pus behind the drum in the middle ear. The patient may be asked to swallow several times in order to observe movement of the tympanic membrane, which occurs on pressure changes in the eustachian tube. The eustachian tube equalizes air pressure between the middle ear and the throat.

Mouth and Throat. The mouth, or oral cavity, is usually thought of in terms of oral hygiene and dental care. A history of sore throats, bleeding gums, tooth extractions, or voice changes requires careful examination. The status of dental hygiene includes the condition of the teeth, how the patient cares for the teeth and gums, and whether or not the teeth of the upper and lower jaws meet properly (occlude) for chewing. Normal gums are pale pink, glossy, and smooth and do not bleed when pressure from a tongue depressor is applied. *Pyorrhea*, the discharge of pus from the dental periosteum, is a progressive condition. It is also called *periodontitis*.

The palatine tonsils are usually visible. Tonsils may be enlarged and pitted. The pharyngeal tonsils (adenoids) are not easily accessible but may be visualized using the mouth mirror. The examiner will use a tongue depressor and a piece of gauze to grasp the tongue for careful examination of it. The floor of the mouth is examined by both inspection and palpation for enlarged lymph nodes, salivary gland function, and ulcerations. The insides of the cheeks are also examined for any abnormal marks or color.

Nose. The nasal cavity and the nasopharynx may reveal the presence of a discharge from the sinuses known as a *postnasal drip* (PND), a common occurrence. Other abnormalities may be obstructions, a deviated septum, polyps, or ulcerations. The nasal cavity basically requires an examination of the color and texture of the mucosa. When a patient has a nosebleed, it is correctly called *epistaxis*. The sinus meatus cannot be seen, but the frontal and maxillary sinuses may be examined by the application of pressure over the area and transillumination.

Chest. While the patient is still in the sitting position, the chest, heart, lungs, and breasts are examined. The chest is examined for symmetric expansion. A tape measure may be used, especially if there is a variation between the upper and lower chest expansion. A patient with a history of **emphysema** may display a chest that is barrel-like. It is necessary to know the landmarks, or *topography*, of the chest in order to know where the underlying organs are located (Fig. 28–6).

With the stethoscope to the patient's back, the examiner listens to the lung sounds. The patient is asked to take deep and regular breaths during this examination. This may produce a slight dizziness, which is not abnormal; the patient may be assured that it is only the result of the deep respirations and will rapidly pass. The types of respiration are noted. Some common variations in respiration can be found in Chapter 25, Vital Signs. Chest sounds heard by the physician may be described as various types or as *rales* (abnormal sounds that vary from coarse musical sounds to the whistling or squeaking sounds frequently heard in asthma or bronchitis). The term *stridor* describes a wheezing sound or a shrill, harsh, or crowing sound. Next, the examiner will tap (percuss) the patient's back at various points to determine the resonance of the chest and diagnose possible tuberculosis. The patient may be asked to take more deep breaths at this time.

Syncope (fainting) and chest pains warrant careful examination. Much of the examination of the cardiovascular system also depends on data gained from the vital signs (Chapter 25). Because it takes considerable concentration to interpret the heart sounds, it is necessary to have complete silence when the examiner is listening to the patient's heart. The heart is examined using a stethoscope from both the anterior and posterior approaches to the patient. Further examination may include auscultation on the left, lateral side. In cases of heart disease, the examiner may spend an extended period of time listening to the heart sounds.

Reflexes. The patient's reflexes are checked with the patient in the sitting and supine positions.

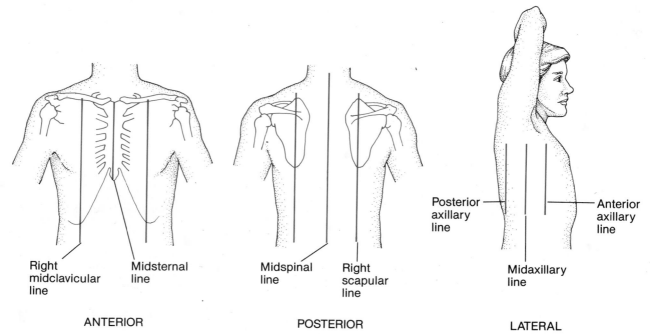

Right midclavicular line   Midsternal line   Midspinal line   Right scapular line   Posterior axillary line   Anterior axillary line   Midaxillary line

ANTERIOR   POSTERIOR   LATERAL

Figure 28–6
Topography of the chest showing the anatomic landmarks.

any joint

While the patient is sitting, the biceps are checked with the patient's arm flexed and supported by the examiner. The knee-jerk (patellar reflex) and the ankle-jerk (Achilles reflex) are checked using tapotement with either the fingers or the reflex hammer. The plantar reflexes (Babinski and Chaddock reflexes) are tested with the patient in either the sitting or the lying position.

Breasts. A careful breast examination is part of the examination of every female, whether or not the patient is symptomatic. The patient is usually examined in the sitting position, but may be examined later in the supine position. Breast cancer is the most common malignancy occurring in women, and early detection is the key to successful treatment. Women should be questioned whether or not they perform self-examination at home and instructed in the proper procedures. The American Cancer Society has excellent pamphlets and films to supplement the physician's instructions (Fig. 28–7).

Abdomen. The patient is lowered to the dorsal recumbent position and the drape is lowered to the pubic hair line. The gown is raised to just under the breasts. A towel should be placed over the female breasts if a gown is not worn. Whether right- or left-handed, the examiner stands to the patient's right side. The patient's arms may be

HOW TO EXAMINE YOUR BREASTS

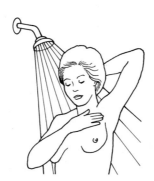

1 In the shower:

Examine your breasts during bath or shower; hands glide easier over wet skin. Fingers flat, move gently over every part of each breast. Use right hand to examine left breast, left hand for right breast. Check for any lump, hard knot or thickening.

2 Before a mirror:

Inspect your breasts with arms at your sides. Next, raise your arms high overhead. Look for any changes in contour of each breast, a swelling, dimpling of skin or changes in the nipple.

Then, rest palms on hips and press down firmly to flex your chest muscles. Left and right breast will not exactly match – few women's breasts do.

Regular inspection shows what is normal for you and will give you confidence in your examination.

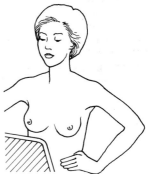

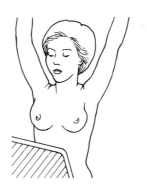

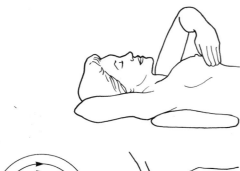

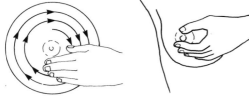

3 Lying down:

To examine your right breast, put a pillow or folded towel under your right shoulder. Place right hand behind your head – this distributes breast tissue more evenly on the chest. With left hand, fingers flat, press gently in small circular motions around an imaginary clock face. Begin at outermost top of your right breast for 12 o'clock, then move to 1 o'clock, and so on around the circle back to 12. A ridge of firm tissue in the lower curve of each breast is normal. Then move in an inch, toward the nipple, keep circling to examine every part of your breast, including nipple. This requires at least three more circles. Now slowly repeat procedure on your left breast with a pillow under your left shoulder and left hand behind head. Notice how your breast structure feels.

Finally, squeeze the nipple of each breast gently between thumb and index finger. Any discharge, clear or bloody, should be reported to your doctor immediately.

Figure 28–7
The Breast Self-Examination (BSE). (Courtesy of the American Cancer Society.)

28

placed at the side, or the hands may be crossed over the chest. If the table is narrow and the patient cannot relax completely, it may help to have the patient tuck the thumbs under the buttocks in order to relax the shoulders. Relaxation of the abdominal muscles is absolutely essential for the abdominal examination. It sometimes helps to place a small pillow under the patient's head or the knees. If the patient exhibits ticklishness, it is best to disregard it and try to continue the examination by changing the routine.

It is important to know the topography of the abdomen and the underlying organs. Mentally divide the abdomen into quadrants (Fig. 28–8A). The vertical line extends from the xiphoid process of the sternum to the symphysis pubis; the horizontal line crosses the abdomen at the level of the umbilicus (navel). Another method of dividing the abdomen is by regions, or sections (Fig. 28–8B). Note that the right and left hypochondriac regions are composed almost entirely of the costal margins. This is because the abdomen extends up under the rib cage to the dome of the diaphragm. The liver and spleen are located in these two regions.

Abdominal symptoms that a patient may give during the history include *dyspepsia* (indigestion), *dysphagia* (difficulty in swallowing), a change in bowel habits, excessive *flatulence* (gas), nausea, and

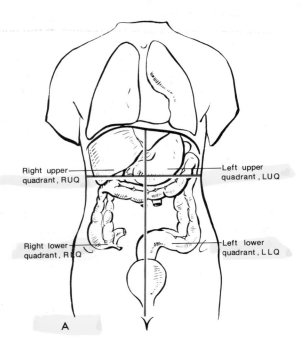

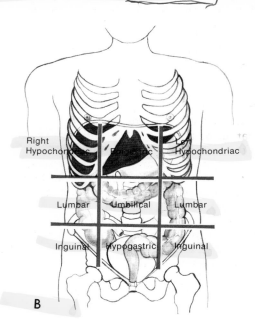

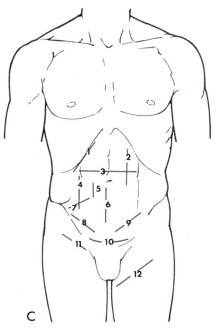

Figure 28–8
A, Quadrants of the abdomen. **B,** Regions of the abdomen. (From Chabner, D.-E.: The Language of Medicine, 2nd ed. Philadelphia, W. B. Saunders Co., 1981.) **C,** Incisions of the abdomen, anterior view: (1) subcostal; (2) paramedial; (3) transverse; (4) upper right rectus; (5) midrectus; (6) midline; (7) lower right rectus; (8) McBurney, or right iliac; (9) left iliac; (10) suprapubic; (11) hernia; (12) femoral. (From Fordney, M. T.: Insurance Handbook for the Medical Office, 2nd ed. Philadelphia, W. B. Saunders Co., 1981.)

vomiting. General abdominal discomfort is common, since abdominal pain is frequently referred pain, that is, pain that is felt in the abdomen but is actually being generated from an organ elsewhere.

The inspection of the abdomen begins with noting any change in skin color such as jaundice. *Striae* (silver stretch marks), *petechiae* (small purple hemorrhagic spots), cutaneous *angiomas* (spider **nevi**), scars, and visible masses may be observed. The contour of the abdomen may be flat, rounded, or bulging in localized areas. A bulging in the right and left lumbar regions (the flanks) may be the result of the presence of free abdominal fluid (*ascites*). Abdominal hernias are examined with the patient in the supine and standing positions. To complete the abdominal examination, the patient may be placed in the knee-elbow position to better determine the presence of free abdominal fluid. The Sims position may also be used for this purpose.

Rectum. The rectal examination usually follows the abdominal examination or may be part of the examination of the male and female genitalia. The patient's comfort and dignity are vital. The examination is limited to an area of within 6 to 8 cm (2.5 to 3.5 in). The examiner needs one to two finger cots or an examining glove and lubricating jelly. A good light must be directed at the perineal area.

The rectum of the male is usually checked when the patient is in a standing position bending over the end of the examining table. This position allows the examiner to check the prostate gland as well. The prostate gland is checked for size, shape, and consistency. The anus and perineal area are inspected for inflammation, rashes, **excoriation**, or external hemorrhoids (Fig. 28–9). The buttocks are spread to facilitate visualization of the anus. If a *fissure* (abnormal crack or cleft) or *fistula* (abnormal tube-like passage) is present, the patient will feel pain. These abnormalities make the digital examination of the rectum difficult to perform. The anal sphincter muscle is palpated; internal hemorrhoids are difficult to palpate unless they are **thrombosed**.

The rectum of the female may be examined while the patient is in the lithotomy position for the pelvic examination. The posterior vaginal wall and the anterior rectal wall are palpated by the examiner by placing the index finger into the vaginal canal and the middle finger into the rectum.

Male Genitalia. Examination of the male reproductive system includes inspection of the penis and the prepuce (foreskin), if present, the glans, and the urethral meatus. The presence or absence of any ulcers, scars, nodules, or discharge from the urethra is noted. The scrotum is examined for enlargement and tenderness, which may be the result of a **hydrocele**, edema, or tumor. The inguinal and femoral areas are inspected and palpated for bulges of possible hernias.

Cancer of the testes is common in males aged from 15 to 34 years and accounts for 12 percent of all cancer deaths. In the early stages, it can be treated effectively. The American Cancer Society recommends a monthly, three-minute self-examination after a warm shower when the skin of the scrotum is loose. The patient should roll and palpate each testicle to locate any hard lumps or nodules (Fig. 28–10). The first sign of testicular cancer usually is an enlargement of one testicle or a change in its consistency.

28

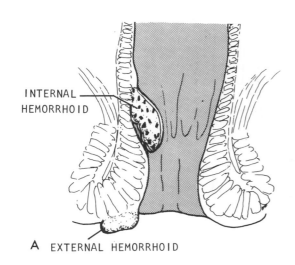 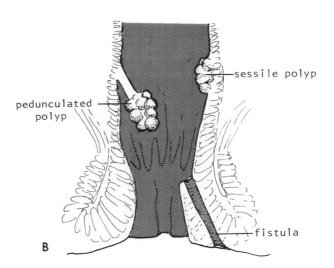

INTERNAL HEMORRHOID

A EXTERNAL HEMORRHOID

pedunculated polyp

sessile polyp

fistula

B

Figure 28–9
Anorectal abnormalities. **A,** Hemorrhoids. **B,** Polyps and fistula. (*From Chabner, D.-E.: The Language of Medicine, 2nd ed. Philadelphia, W. B. Saunders Co., 1981.*)

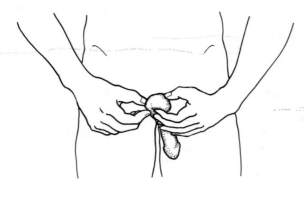

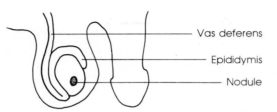

Vas deferens

Epididymis

Nodule

Your best hope for early detection of testicular cancer is a simple three-minute monthly self-examination. The best time is after a warm bath or shower, when the scrotal skin is most relaxed.

Roll each testicle gently between the thumb and fingers of both hands. If you find any hard lumps or nodules, you should see your doctor promptly. They may not be malignant, but only your doctor can make the diagnosis.

Following a thorough physical examination, your doctor may perform certain x-ray studies to make the most accurate diagnosis possible.

Figure 28–10
The Testicular Self-Examination (TSE). (Redrawn from For Men Only, New York, American Cancer Society.)

Procedure 28–2   *ASSISTING WITH A ROUTINE PHYSICAL EXAMINATION*

PROCEDURAL GOAL

To help the physician examine patients by preparing the necessary equipment and ensuring patient safety and comfort during the examination.

EQUIPMENT AND SUPPLIES

Stethoscope	Cotton balls	Examination gloves
Sphygmomanometer	Head mirror	Vaginal speculum
Ophthalmoscope	Examination light	Blood and body-fluid
Otoscope	Pen-light	protection barriers (gog-
Scale	Percussion hammer	gles, masks, and aprons or
Tape measure	Nasal speculum	gowns), as necessary (see
Tongue depressors	Lubricating gel	Appendix C, Recommen-
Gauze sponges	Two finger cots	dations for Prevention of
		AIDS Transmission)

PROCEDURE

1. Prepare the examining room according to acceptable medical aseptic rules. Clean with alcohol or disinfectant the furniture and tray surfaces that will be used. Prepare clean table and pillow paper on the examination table.
   Purpose: There should be no evidence of the previous patient.
2. Wash your hands. Follow universal blood and body-fluid precautions (see Appendix C).
3. Locate the instruments for the procedure. Set them out in the sequence that the examiner will follow.

Procedure continued on opposite page

4. Identify the patient, and determine if the patient understands the procedure. If the patient does not understand, explain what you and the physician will be doing.
   Purpose: To increase patient cooperation during the examination.
5. Measure and record the patient's vital signs, height, and weight. Report any unusual findings to the physician as soon as possible.
   Purpose: To gather data needed before the examination begins.
6. If a specimen is needed, instruct the patient on how to collect the specimen, and hand the patient the proper specimen container, already labeled with the patient's name.
   Purpose: To obtain a specimen that is clearly identifiable as that patient's.
7. Direct the patient to the lavatory, and have the patient empty his or her bladder.
   Purpose: To have the patient's bladder empty for the examination.
8. Hand the patient a gown and sheet. Instruct the patient on how to put the gown on and to use the sheet. Tell the patient to have a seat on the examination table after applying the gown. Help patients with undressing as needed; however, most patients prefer to undress in privacy, if possible.
9. Assist during the examination by handing the physician each instrument as it is needed.
10. If the physician requires a specific position, explain to the patient what you want him or her to do, and assist the patient into that position.
11. If the examination includes a pelvic examination, help the patient into the lithotomy position, and have a warmed speculum ready for the physician.
12. Listen to the patient and help diminish his or her fears. Apply a hand to his or her shoulder, or hold hands if needed.
13. If specimens are taken, label them immediately.
14. When the physician has completed the examination, allow the patient to rest for a moment, then help the patient from the table. Assist with dressing, if necessary.
15. Remove all soiled equipment to the proper area.
16. Change the paper goods or linens with minimal movements to prevent stirring the dust and air.
17. Clean table-top surfaces with disinfectant or alcohol.
18. Prepare specimens for transport or examination.
19. Dispose of blood and body-fluid protection barriers, and wash your hands.
20. Record the necessary notes on the patient's chart and forward it to the physician for further notations.
21. Return to the patient and ask him or her if there are any questions. Give the patient any final instructions, and schedule the next appointment if that is appropriate.
    Purpose: To clarify directions, eliminate any misunderstandings, and allow the patient to discuss any concerns. If there are misunderstandings or concerns beyond your scope of experience or skill, you must arrange for the physician to speak with the patient again.

28

TERMINAL PERFORMANCE OBJECTIVE

Given a patient and the necessary equipment, (1) prepare for and assist in the examination of a patient, (2) care for the examination room, specimens, and the patient's medical record, and (3) conduct an exit interview with the patient, within a period of ten minutes (not including the time of the actual examination), by correctly completing every step of the procedure in the proper order, as determined by your evaluator.

REFERENCES AND READINGS

Bates, B.: *A Guide to Physical Examination*, 2nd ed. Philadelphia, J. B. Lippincott Co., 1983.
Bonewit, K.: *Clinical Procedures for the Medical Office*, 2nd ed. Philadelphia, W. B. Saunders Co., 1984.
DuGas, B. W.: *Introduction to Patient Care: A Comprehensive Approach to Nursing*, 4th ed. Philadelphia, W. B. Saunders Co., 1984.

Fuerst, R.: *Microbiology in Health and Disease*, 15th ed. Philadelphia, W. B. Saunders Co., 1983.
Macleod, J. (ed.): *Clinical Examination: A Textbook for Students and Doctors by Teachers of the Edinburgh Medical School*, 4th ed. Edinburgh/London, Churchill Livingstone, 1976.
Sorensen, K. C., and Luckmann, J.: *Basic Nursing: A Psychophysiologic Approach*, 2nd ed. Philadelphia, W. B. Saunders Co., 1986.
Wood, L. A., and Rambo, B. J.: *Nursing Skills for Allied Health Services*, Vol. 2, 2nd ed. Philadelphia, W. B. Saunders Co., 1977.

CHAPTER OUTLINE

VOCABULARY

See Glossary at end of book for definitions.

amenorrhea	congenital	incontinence	paraplegia
ankylosis	contraindication	induration	presbyopia
arrhythmia	diplopia	leukoderma	pruritus
asthma	eczema	microcephaly	ptosis
bariatrics	erythema	multiparous	rhinitis
cauterization	hydrocephaly	myringotomy	vesiculation
chancre			

Assisting with Specialty Examinations and Treatments

OBJECTIVES

Upon successful completion of this chapter you should be able to

1. Spell and define the words listed in the vocabulary for this chapter.
2. Discuss six disorders of the female reproductive system.
3. Identify the causative organisms of three sexually transmitted infections.
4. Discuss two diagnostic procedures available to the obstetrics-gynecology (OB/GYN) specialist.
5. Define the five-point scale grading of Papanicolaou smear reporting.
6. List nine temporary methods of contraception.
7. Discuss five common disorders of the ear.
8. Describe the Apgar test.
9. Review some special considerations for the pediatric patient.
10. Differentiate between proctoscopy and sigmoidoscopy.
11. Cite two conditions treated by the proctologist.
12. Cite three disorders of the genitourinary tract.

Upon sucessful completion of this chapter you should be able to perform the following activities:

1. Administer, and read and record the results of a tine Tuberculin Test.
2. Test vision using a Snellen Distance Visual Acuity Chart.
3. Assist with a pelvic examination.
4. Irrigate a patient's eye and ear with a sterile solution.
5. Instill sterile drops into a patient's eye.
6. Measure and record the head circumference of an infant.
7. Assist with a proctosigmoidoscopy.

Protocols exist for the various physical examinations performed in the medical office; however, particular methods of examination and treatment vary among physicians, based on individual needs and habits.

In the specialist's office, emphasis is given to a specific area of the body or a particular complaint. Medical assistants perform many specialty procedures and must assist in the specialty examination.

This chapter discusses, in alphabetical order, each specialty and its most commonly used procedures. Specific diseases and diagnostic aids such as x-rays and laboratory tests are also mentioned as they apply to the specialty.

ALLERGOLOGY

This specialty concerns the diagnosis and treatment of allergic conditions. It is difficult to separate allergology and immunology; to understand one, it is necessary to have a degree of understanding of the other. In a normal immune reaction, an antigen unites with an antibody and results in the elimination of the harmful antigen. An allergic reaction is the same, but the interaction of the antigen and the antibody is accompanied by a harmful effect on the body tissue and by excessive release of a substance called histamine. This abnormal immune response is referred to as "hypersensitive reaction," and the diseases arising from it are called "diseases of hypersensitivity." Among such diseases are allergy, hay fever, serum sickness, and transfusion reactions (see Chapter 22).

Symptoms of an allergy can occur for the first time at any age. The substances that produce an allergic response can be eaten, inhaled, injected, or applied topically to the skin. The response to these antigens, or allergens, as the allergists prefer to call them, bears no relationship to the type of material involved. For example, foods may cause **eczema, rhinitis,** or **asthma.** Pollens may also cause any of these conditions. When rhinitis is caused by a pollen, it is given a special name, hay fever, although "hay" is not necessarily the causative agent.

An allergic reaction does not occur on the first contact with the allergen, because the antibodies have not yet been produced by the body. It may occur on the second contact, when the antibodies have been released and are in reserve in the body tissues. The reaction may not occur until later in life, when contact with the allergen suddenly develops into a sensitivity. An allergy is said to be a reaction to a substance that ordinarily is harmless to most people. There are almost as many allergens, such as pollens, foods, plants, animal fur, insect bites, and chemicals, as there are substances. Reactions range from mild sneezing to severe serum sickness, or anaphylactic shock, which can be fatal unless immediate emergency measures are taken.

The diagnosis of an allergy is made by taking a very careful history from the patient, performing a careful and complete physical examination, and following this up with selected laboratory tests, which may include x-ray studies, blood and urine examinations, and skin tests. This history and physical examination are always made by the physician, but the skin tests and laboratory tests are usually the responsibilities of a medical assistant or laboratory technician. Since skin tests are potentially very hazardous to perform, they should always be conducted under supervision of a physician. It should be emphasized that skin tests by themselves are not strictly diagnostic of an allergy, but when combined with a careful history and other factors, they are helpful in establishing the diagnosis. Skin tests are ordinarily performed by one or more of several methods: scratch, intradermal, ophthalmic, or patch.

Scratch Test

The most common and possibly the least satisfactory test is the scratch and puncture test. It is most popular because it is rapid and simple to perform. The tests may be performed on any smooth surface of the skin, but the arm and back are most popular. The arm is safer (either the outer surface of the upper arm or the palmar surface of the lower arm), since a serious reaction may be limited by the application of a tourniquet above the site. However, the back is favored in infants and in young children because of the large area of skin available. It is also easier to immobilize the child in this position.

A reaction usually occurs within 10 to 30 minutes. If the reaction is positive, a wheal (hive) will be formed at the site of the scratch. The interpretation of the test should always be based on a comparison of this reaction with that of the control, which is a scratch with a plain base fluid free from any allergy-producing extract.

The interpretation, or reading, of the skin tests is performed by the physician. However, a few doctors delegate this step to the trained skin tester. Reactions are commonly graded from 2 to 4. No precise definition of a reaction can be given, and indeed the intensity may vary among individuals. However, as a general rule, a 2 reaction implies a wheal that is definitely larger than that of the control. A larger wheal is interpreted as a 3, whereas the presence of pseudopods (finger-like extensions around the periphery of the wheal) may be read as a 4. Carefully wipe off the extract to stop the reaction when a strong reaction is occurring. Erythema, or reddening, around the wheal is usually disregarded in the interpretations. Frequently, the large or significant reactions are accompanied by local itching (Fig. 29–1).

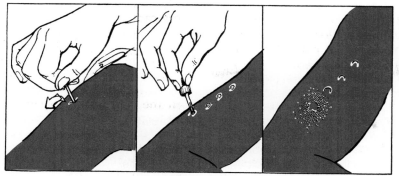

Figure 29–1
Technique for the scratch test. The degree of sensitivity is measured on a numeric scale (shown in color on inside of front cover of this text).

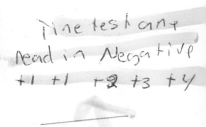

Intradermal (Intracutaneous) Test

This method can be used if a patient has shown a questionable or negative reaction to the scratch method. This test is more sensitive than the scratch test. Extracts are injected into the skin, with the usual sterile technique, in a dose of 0.01 to 0.02 cc. The reaction time is identical to that of the scratch test; however, the antigen is more dilute. Remember that the extract cannot be wiped off as in the scratch method. This method is always done on the patient's arm. This is a safety measure. In a severe reaction, apply a tourniquet immediately above the reaction area in order to retard absorption of the extract. Immediately prepare epinephrine to be administered on the physician's orders.

Tine Test. The tine tuberculin test is administered with a sterile, simple, multiple-puncture, disposable intradermal device for the detection of tuberculosis infection. Each test unit consists of a stainless steel disc attached to a plastic handle. Projecting from the disc are four triangular-shaped prongs (tines) that are 2 mm long and approximately 4 mm apart. The tines have been dipped in a sterile solution containing substances extracted from tuberculosis cultures. The substance on the tines is called old tuberculin (OT).

The preferred site for the tine test is the upper third of the forearm. Avoid areas with excessive hair, scarring, or any other abnormality of the skin surface. Alcohol, acetone, or ether may be used to cleanse the skin. The area must be thoroughly dry before application of the tines.

The results should be read at 42 to 78 hours after the test is given. **Vesiculation** or the extent of **induration** is the determining factor in reading the results: redness without induration is of no significance. The reading should be made in good light, with the forearm slightly flexed. The size of the induration is determined in millimeters by inspection, measuring, and palpation. The tests come with cards for measuring and reading. Interpretation of readings: vesiculation—positive reaction; induration of 2 mm or more—doubtful reaction, further testing needed; induration less than 2 mm—negative. There are no known **contraindications** for this test; however, testing should be done with caution in patients with tuberculosis. Adverse reactions include pain, itching, and discomfort at the test site. Rarely, bleeding may occur at the puncture site, but it is of no significance.

29

Procedure 29–1

PERFORMING A TINE TUBERCULIN TEST

PROCEDURAL GOAL

To perform a tine tuberculin test, read the reaction, and record the results.

EQUIPMENT AND SUPPLIES

Gauze sponge
Antiseptic such as acetone, alcohol, or ether
Blood and body-fluid protection barriers (goggles, masks, and aprons or gowns), as necessary
(see Appendix C)

One tine test unit
Nonsterile gloves

Procedure continued on following page

PROCEDURE

1. Wash your hands. Follow the universal blood and body-fluid precautions. Glove yourself with nonsterile gloves.
2. Assemble the materials needed.
3. Identify the patient and explain the procedure.
   Purpose: Explanations help gain patient cooperation and alleviate apprehension.
4. Expose the forearm, and cleanse the site with antiseptic and sponge, using a circular motion, wiping from the inside to the outside. Allow the site to air-dry.
   Purpose: The preferred site for testing is the volar surface of the upper third of the forearm. The area should be cleaned and dried before application of the tine test.
5. Remove the protective cap while holding the plastic handle.
   Purpose: The cap is removed to expose the four tines.
6. Grasp the patient's forearm firmly, and stretch the skin of the forearm tightly.
   Purpose: The patient may jerk the arm and cause scratching if it is not held firmly.
7. Apply the disc with gentle pressure, and hold it there for at least one second before releasing the tension of the forearm. Withdraw the unit.
   Purpose: Sufficient pressure should be exerted so that the four puncture sites and the circular depression of the skin from the plastic base are visible.
8. Clean the work area.
9. Wash your hands.
10. Observe the reaction on the patient's arm 48 to 72 hours after testing.
11. Record your findings on the patient's chart.

TERMINAL PERFORMANCE OBJECTIVE

Given a patient and the appropriate materials, perform a tine tuberculin test on a patient within five minutes, and read and record the findings within 48 to 72 hours after testing, completing each step correctly and in the proper order, as determined by your evaluator.

Patch Test

This method of testing is of some value in diagnosing dermatitis. In the patch test, the suspected material is placed on the skin (near the original lesion, if possible), covered with a small square of cellophane, and held down with strips of adhesive or transparent tape or even collodion. The reaction is read within one to four days (Fig. 29–2).

RAST (Radioallergosorbent Test)

This laboratory procedure measures minute quantities of specific antibodies against foods by the use of radioisotopes. A venipuncture is performed, and a blood specimen is collected, which is then sent to a specialized laboratory. The RAST generally provides no more information than direct skin testing, which is less expensive and provides immediate results. Thus, skin testing is currently the preferred means for diagnosing allergies.

Environmental Control

Patients with allergies are encouraged to make their surroundings as free as possible from the offending allergens and are instructed in the various methods of doing so. One way is the elimination of animals, feathers, and dust-collecting items within the house. The garden is checked for offending grasses and pollens. Foods that cause problems are best eliminated. Contact allergens such as soaps and cosmetics are avoided.

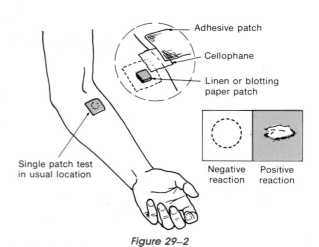

Figure 29–2
Technique for the patch test for skin allergies. (From Miller, B. F., and Keane, C. B.: Encyclopedia and Dictionary of Medicine, Nursing, and Allied Health, 4th ed. Philadelphia, W. B. Saunders Co., 1987.)

ANESTHESIOLOGY

Anesthesiology is the branch of medicine concerned with the administration of anesthetics and the maintenance of the patient while under anesthesia. An anesthesiologist is a specialist in this branch of medicine, and the term is usually reserved for the physician administering the anesthetic. An anesthetist is one who administers anesthetics; this may be a nurse-anesthetist or a physician-anesthetist. The word "anesthetic" was given to medicine by Dr. Oliver Wendell Holmes (1809–1894).

Clinical assisting duties in an anesthesiologist's office are extremely limited and are usually confined to the scheduling of appointments for the doctor to administer an anesthetic at a hospital and to the keeping of accounts. Many anesthesiologists do not maintain an office, as we think of a physician's office, but are hospital based and use the services of a secretary. Even so, medical assistants should be familiar with a few terms and definitions that are applicable to this specialty of medicine.

Anesthetics seem to fall into one of two groups, general or local. There is considerable controversy regarding these two terms, but for convenience, they will be used here. A general anesthetic implies a state of unconsciousness, insusceptibility to pain, and a degree of muscle relaxation. General anesthetics are classified according to the route of administration. The *inhalants* are gases or highly volatile liquids; intravenous and rectal anesthetics are the nonvolatile drugs. The term "local anesthetic" is used when loss of sensation is confined to a limited area. Other terms used for local anesthesia are conduction and regional if the anesthesia creates insensibility by blocking sensory nerve conductivity to a region or part. Other local anesthetics are referred to as *tissue infiltration anesthetics*. This is because the immediately surrounding tissue is injected or infiltrated with a local anesthetic so that each individual nerve ending is blocked. The names of local anesthetics usually end with -*caine*. A *topical anesthetic* is a local anesthetic applied directly to a certain area of the skin or mucous membrane, such as a spray on the nasal mucosa.

DERMATOLOGY

This specialty deals with the diagnosis and treatment of skin diseases. The human skin, also called the integument or integumentary system, is the largest organ of the body. It has many different functions: it aids in controlling body temperature, is a barrier to most bacteria, furnishes a sensory system, and is an insulator against outside elements. Both the term "dermis" (Greek) and the term "cutis" (Latin) are used when referring to the skin. Dermatitis and cutitis are synonymous for inflammations of the skin, but dermatitis is by far the preferred term.

The skin has an outer layer, the epidermis, and an inner layer, the dermis, or corium. Blood vessels and nerves, as well as sweat glands, hair roots, and the nail bed, are located in the dermis (Fig. 29–3). Normality of the skin depends on the person's age, sex, and physical and emotional health. The skin reflects both internal and external contact reactions.

29

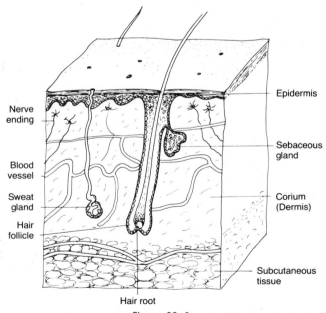

Figure 29–3
The histologic anatomy of the skin and its appendages. (From Chabner, D.-E.: The Language of Medicine, 3rd ed. Philadelphia, W. B. Saunders Co., 1985.)

Examination of the skin is basically inspection followed with detailed examination by palpation, diascopy, and special tests. The *diascope* is a glass plate held against the skin to permit observation of changes produced in the underlying areas by the pressure. The impairments that most frequently bring a patient to the dermatologist's office are the cosmetic disfigurements caused by a skin disease, pain and **pruritus**, and interference with sensations or movements. The possibility that a skin lesion is the result of a systemic condition is sometimes a major concern.

Inspection of the skin may reveal color changes such as **erythema, leukoderma,** jaundice, or vitiligo. Localized red or purple changes may be the result of vascular neoplasms, birthmarks, or subcutaneous hemorrhages (petechiae and ecchymoses). Palpation is used to confirm and amplify findings seen by inspection. Inspection and palpation are interrelated in confirming diagnoses. Palpatory findings may be texture, elasticity, or edema.

One disorder of the skin is *seborrheic dermatitis*, a chronic inflammation of the scalp, commonly called dandruff. It may spread to the face, neck, and body. *Acne vulgaris* is also a disorder of the sebaceous glands and presents as pustules, blackheads (comedones), and cysts. *Furuncles* (boils) and *carbuncles* (clusters of furuncles) are often seen.

Disorders of the skin may be divided into primary and secondary lesions. Primary lesions are those that appear immediately. Macules, papules, plaques, nodules, comedones, cysts, wheals, and pustules are all primary lesions. Secondary lesions never appear originally but are the result of alterations in a primary lesion. Examples of secondary lesions are scales, crusts, fissures, erosions, ulcerations, and scars. A burn gives a blister. The blister is the primary lesion; the blister breaks and an ulceration forms; then healing ends in a scar. The ulceration and the scar are secondary lesions (Fig. 29–4).

Draping a patient for a skin examination depends on the area to be examined. Remember to expose the area adequately but protect the patient's privacy. Try to make the patient as comfortable as possible, and offer support when it is needed.

One dermatology test performed in the dermatologist's office is the *Wood's light examination*. This is a visual examination of the skin made in a darkened room with the ultraviolet lamp. Differences in the ultraviolet light absorption and fluorescence bring out characteristics of some skin diseases, such as *tinea capitis* (ringworm).

ENDOCRINOLOGY

Endocrinology is the study of the function and dysfunction of the glands of internal secretion. Changes due to an endocrine disease may cause alterations in body contour, size, fat distribution, skin texture and pigmentation, and circulation and may have considerable effect on the nervous system. The endocrinologist must be able to distinguish between endocrine dysfunction and the patient's hereditary pattern. This dysfunction in hormone production falls into two categories: deficiency (hypoproduction) and excess (hyperproduction).

Inspection and palpation are the most common methods employed in examining the patient, with inspection being the more prevalent. Of the six endocrine glands in the body, the thyroid and the testes are the most accessible to palpation. The ovaries are palpable to a degree.

Eponyms are used more frequently in endocrinology than in other specialties, but they are slowly being replaced with the true anatomic or pathologic name. Many endocrine disorders are also seen and treated in other specialties. The gynecologist sees the patient with the ovarian changes of **amenorrhea** and menopause. The internist may examine an enlarged thyroid gland that has resulted from an iodine deficiency, or *myxedema* from severe *hypothyroidism*. The ophthalmologist may examine the patient with *exophthalmic goiter*, which gives the appearance of bulging eyes.

Besides the complete physical examination, the physician is aided in diagnosis by a great variety of tests. Some of these tests are x-rays, radioisotopes, and blood chemistry tests.

The medical assistant in an endocrinologist's office will be called upon to participate in the routine physical examination and the collection of blood and urine specimens for diagnostic testing of these glandular disorders. (Some of these tests are discussed in Chapter 33.)

GENERAL SURGERY

A surgeon's practice is what may be called a "referral specialty." That is, patients are usually referred to the surgeon from other specialties or by the family physician. The procedure to be followed in the evaluation of the patient and the comprehensive preoperative examination requires teamwork between the surgeon and the referring physician. An effective working arrangement between these two physicians sometimes depends upon the cooperation of the medical assistant. The referring physician frequently takes care of the initial physical examination and basic preoperative laboratory tests, and then the referring physician's knowledge of the patient's past medical and family history is shared with the surgeon. The surgeon will then have a clear understanding of the objectives of surgery and the patient's preoperative status. The surgeon may offer the patient a simple and understandable description of the operation, its rationale, and possible complications. (This is the basis of "informed consent.")

PRIMARY LESIONS

SECONDARY LESIONS

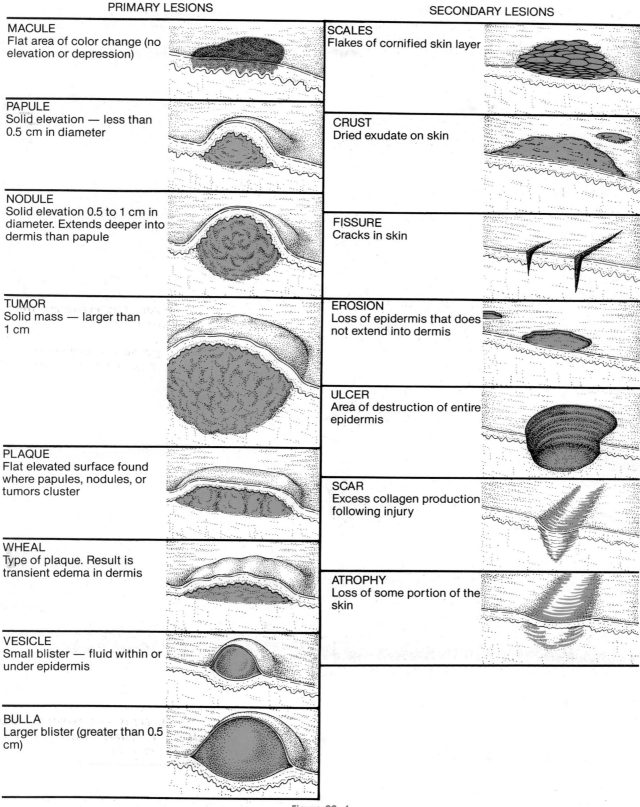

MACULE
Flat area of color change (no elevation or depression)

PAPULE
Solid elevation — less than 0.5 cm in diameter

NODULE
Solid elevation 0.5 to 1 cm in diameter. Extends deeper into dermis than papule

TUMOR
Solid mass — larger than 1 cm

PLAQUE
Flat elevated surface found where papules, nodules, or tumors cluster

WHEAL
Type of plaque. Result is transient edema in dermis

VESICLE
Small blister — fluid within or under epidermis

BULLA
Larger blister (greater than 0.5 cm)

SCALES
Flakes of cornified skin layer

CRUST
Dried exudate on skin

FISSURE
Cracks in skin

EROSION
Loss of epidermis that does not extend into dermis

ULCER
Area of destruction of entire epidermis

SCAR
Excess collagen production following injury

ATROPHY
Loss of some portion of the skin

29

Figure 29–4
Characteristics of common skin lesions.

[handwritten: condition of having gallstones]

The psychologic preparation of the patient is also shared by the referring physician and the surgeon. Anxieties of the patient are normal and inevitable and can be somewhat lessened by the attitude of a good medical assistant. The medical assistant in the surgeon's office can identify the patient with special needs. Families and relatives are anxious about the surgical patient. The medical assistant, with the surgeon's consent, can reduce some of these anxieties with simple explanations and reports.

Assisting the surgeon may include assisting with preoperative examinations and postoperative office visits. Physical examinations would follow the outline given in Chapter 28. The office postoperative care may include dressing changes and suture removal. These are described in Chapter 31.

INTERNAL MEDICINE

Internal medicine is a nonsurgical specialty with several subspecialties, such as gastroenterology, rheumatology, cardiology, pulmonary diseases, and **bariatrics.** Internists are often known as the "diagnosticians of medicine" as well as frequently being considered the "family physicians." The physical examination frequently follows the outline given in Chapter 28.

Gastroenterology

This specialty covers an extremely wide area that includes the stomach, the small intestine, and the bowel down to the rectum. Proctology is concerned with disorders of the rectum and anus.

A patient with a gastrointestinal (GI) problem may complain of such things as nausea, anorexia, or abdominal pain as well as numerous other symptoms. It may be difficult for the medical assistant to organize a patient's complaints when a patient first contacts the office by telephone for an appointment. The patient may say he has a "belly ache" when the discomfort is really in the stomach area; the "belly" is the central portion of the entire abdominal cavity. Or the patient may say he has a stomach ache when the discomfort is in the hypogastric area and not in the epigastric area. Careful questioning will guide the patient to a more precise description of the symptoms.

Emotional factors play an important part in many GI problems, often making the separation of functional disorders and organic disorders difficult. Abdominal pain may be classified as chronic or acute. The "chronic abdomen," or chronic pain, may or may not be abdominal in origin. It may originate in the thoracic cavity or musculoskeletal system. The "acute abdomen" may demand immediate attention, as in acute appendicitis or acute gastritis with possible hemorrhage. Both may demand surgical therapy.

In order to isolate an abdominal problem, it is frequently necessary for the physician to do a sigmoidoscopic examination as well as a pelvic examination on the female patient. The accessory organs of the digestive system also play an important part. These are the liver, the gallbladder, and the pancreas. Jaundice is a sign of liver disease, or obstructive jaundice due to *choledocholithiasis* (a calculus in the common bile duct). *Acute pancreatitis* produces diffuse pain and tenderness in the epigastrium.

Many of the diagnostic tests for GI symptoms are noninvasive in nature. The patient may be asked to have various roentgenograms (x-ray films) of the digestive system. These include barium swallow, upper GI series, and barium enema. The gallbladder is viewed by cholecystography (see Chapter 38). Liver function is checked by various laboratory procedures. The SGOT (serum glutamic-oxaloacetic transaminase) and SGPT (serum glutamic-pyruvic transaminase) are two commonly performed blood tests. The urine is tested for bilirubin and urinary amylase. The stool is tested for occult blood, intestinal parasites and organisms, fat excretion, and color.

[handwritten: Two common Abbreviation COPD — chronic obstructive pulmonary disease]

Pulmonary Medicine

Patients with respiratory problems may present with chronic or acute symptoms. A common complaint seen in this specialty, the upper respiratory infection (URI), may be, like the others, either chronic or acute. Other infections involving the so-called lower respiratory system, the lungs, also present as chronic or acute problems. Many of the infections of the lungs are in the wide group of pneumonias. It is estimated that there are over 50 different causes of pneumonia, ranging from bacteria, viruses, and fungi to chemical irritants. The term pneumonitis is synonymous with pneumonia. The diagnosis of lobar pneumonia refers to an infection involving a segment or lobe of the lung.

Diagnostic aids vary with the possible diagnosis. The most frequently used are x-ray film of the chest, blood count, TB skin tests, and analysis of sputum. Arterial blood tests, pulmonary function tests, and lung scans are also done.

If a patient in the waiting room is coughing very much or if the cough is productive, it would be advisable to have this patient wait for the physician in an examining room. Provide this patient with ample tissues and show him or her where the waste receptacle is located.

[handwritten: Cold — chronic obstructive lung disease. Right = 3 Lobes Left = 2 Lobes (lungs)]

Cardiology

Heart disease is the major cause of death in the United States, as well as the cause of many chronic illnesses. People are concerned and apprehensive about their hearts. No physician would consider examining a patient without checking the patient's heart. Patients seem to derive some therapeutic value from just having a physician "listen to their heart." Auscultation is the primary method of examining the heart.

Examination starts by observing the general appearance of the patient. The physician may notice a degree of cyanosis, facial edema, clubbing of the fingertips, a cough, or shortness of breath. Cardiac disease has many symptoms and many etiologies; hypertension, arteriosclerosis of the coronary arteries, and rheumatic fever are the leading causes. *Congestive heart failure* is the inability of the heart to maintain sufficient circulation to meet the body's needs. **Arrhythmia** may or may not be associated with congestive heart failure. *Angina pectoris* is acute chest pain resulting from a decrease in the blood supply to the heart muscles; it is not a disease but a symptom. The topographic landmarks of the chest (Fig. 29–5) are helpful in describing the heart's location and borders during the examination.

Other diagnostic procedures that aid the physician in the study of the heart include x-ray films; the resting electrocardiogram; and exercise ECGs (stress tests) such as the Master's two-step, treadmill, or bicycle ergometer test (an apparatus for measuring the amount of work done by the patient). The cardiologist also uses such tests as cardiac catheterization and angiocardiogram (see Chapter 37). Cardiac catheterization is accomplished by introducing a small flexible catheter into the vein of the arm, usually the left antecubital, under fluoroscopic guidance, and gently passing it into the right atrium, right ventricle, and on to the pulmonary artery. The pressure of the blood is measured in

these vessels and heart chambers. Samples of the blood are also withdrawn from these areas to determine their oxygen content. The angiocardiogram is a special x-ray procedure using an opaque dye to show the heart and its major blood vessels (see Chapter 38).

To assist in attaining complete relaxation during the cardiac examination, the medical assistant should instruct the patient to void prior to the examination. The room must be warm, since the patient will be disrobed. Silence is a must while the physician is listening to the heart. The assistant should have any available laboratory and x-ray results on hand prior to the examination.

NEUROLOGY

As in other physical examinations, a careful history provides valuable clues in diagnosing neurologic malfunctions. These may be seizures, syncope, **diplopia, incontinence,** and subjective sensations. The patient's general health often complicates a neurologic diagnosis. The purposes of a neurologic examination are to determine whether a nervous system malfunction is present, discover its location, and identify its type and extent. During the history-taking the physician may determine the patient's emotional status, intellectual performance, and general behavior, which may be evident in the patient's grooming and mannerisms. The patient's ability to communicate is also observed at this time.

Each cranial nerve is checked. For example, the first cranial nerve, the olfactory nerve, is examined by the patient's ability to identify familiar odors, such as coffee, tobacco, or cloves. The fifth cranial nerve, the trigeminal nerve, is checked by the patient's differentiating between warm and cold objects held on his or her right and left cheeks.

The motor system is examined by observing the patient's muscular strength and movements. The diameters of the upper arms and the calves of the legs are measured for muscular atrophy. The sensory system is examined by noting the patient's ability to perceive superficial sensations, such as a wisp of cotton brushed on the skin, a light pinprick, or hot and cold touching certain areas. Several reflexes, such as the patellar and Achilles reflexes, are examined. A stroke with a dull instrument on the lateral aspect of the sole of the foot may produce the Babinski sign.

Some other tests include skull x-ray films, angiograms, myelograms, and brain scans. An electroencephalogram (EEG) also is performed. The medical assistant may wish to remind patients to wear some sort of head covering after the EEG, because there may be some contact paste left on the scalp. Conditions such as stroke (cerebral vascular accident, or CVA), cerebral aneurysm, a brain tumor or abscess, Parkinson's disease, or multiple sclerosis (MS) are often seen by the neurologist.

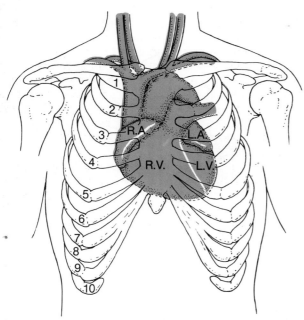

Figure 29–5
Topography of the chest. (R. A., right atrium; R. V., right ventricle; L. A., left atrium; L. V., left ventricle.)

The patient is given a gown and disposable slippers and is asked to disrobe completely, except perhaps for brassiere and underpants. The patient is then seated on the edge of the examining table. The medical assistant hands the physician the various items as they are needed.

OBSTETRICS AND GYNECOLOGY

Examination of the female reproductive system is done to assure normality of the reproductive organs or to diagnose and treat abnormalities of these organs. A gynecologic history includes age at menarche; regularity of the menstrual cycle; amount and duration of the menstrual flow; menstrual disturbances such as dysmenorrhea; intermenstrual or postmenstrual bleeding; and the presence of vaginal discharges. Prenatal care is a major portion of the obstetrics-gynecology (OB/GYN) office's appointments. The first prenatal visit is rather extensive, with a complete history and physical examination and a pelvic examination that includes pelvic measurements, serologic tests, and routine laboratory tests. Follow-up prenatal visits include urinalysis, weight, and blood pressure measurement, and advice on diet and health habits. Any concerns of the patient are alleviated at this time.

The examining room must be adequately equipped, and the surroundings pleasant. A dressing area with an adjacent toilet should be provided. The dressing area should assure privacy and should be equipped with tissues and sanitary protection items. Disposable examination gowns are also placed in this room. Supplies should be checked frequently throughout the day.

The Pelvic Examination

The patient should be instructed to empty the bladder and rectum, completely disrobe, and put on a gown. Unless contraindicated, the patient should be advised at the time the appointment is made not to douche or have sexual intercourse for 24 hours prior to the examination in order to properly evaluate vaginal discharges and to ensure accurate cytologic studies.

The medical assistant should remain in the examining room to provide reassurance to the patient as well as offer legal protection to the physician. Furthermore, the patient should be given assistance in getting on and off the table. The lithotomy position is very awkward to get into unassisted and is embarrassing to the patient.

First, the physician inspects the external genitalia and palpates the perineal body, Bartholin's and Skene's glands, and the urethral meatus. The patient may be asked to ''bear down'' in order to show any muscular weaknesses that may be the result of lacerations of the perineal body during childbirth. A third-degree laceration may have in-

volved the rectal sphincter and may cause rectal incontinence.

Next, the vaginal speculum is inserted for examination of the cervix and the vaginal canal (Fig. 29–6). The normal cervix points posteriorly and is smooth, pink-colored squamous epithelium. The abnormalities most frequently seen are ulcerations (erosions), nabothian cysts, and cervical polyps. Since erosions cannot be palpated, inspection is the only method of knowing their presence. Healed lacerations resulting from childbirth are common in the multiparous patient. Pregnancy increases the size of the cervix, and hormone deficiency causes it to atrophy. The vaginal wall is reddish pink and has a corrugated appearance. Vaginal infections change the appearance of the vaginal mucosa.

After the vaginal speculum has been removed, the physician does a bimanual examination; that is, the minor hand is lubricated and inserted into the vaginal canal and the major hand palpates the abdomen over the pelvic organs (Fig. 29–7). The uterus is examined for shape, size, and consistency. The position of the uterus is noted. The normal uterus is freely movable with limited discomfort (Fig. 29–8). A laterally displaced uterus is usually the result of pelvic adhesions or displacement caused by a pelvic tumor. The uterine adnexa (fallopian tubes and ovaries) are evaluated. The normal tubes and ovaries are difficult to palpate. The physician may now complete the examination by rectovaginal abdominal examination. This is done when the middle finger of the minor hand is inserted into the rectum and the index finger is in the vaginal canal. The rectum is checked by the index finger inserted into the rectum.

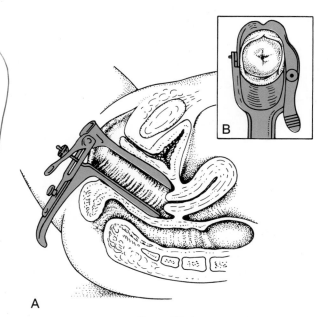

Figure 29–6
A, *Proper position of inserted speculum for examination of the cervix uteri.* **B,** *Normal parous cervix as seen through a speculum.*

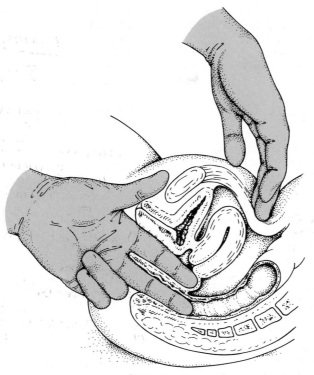

Figure 29–7
Bimanual pelvic examination. The hand on the abdomen brings more of the pelvic contents into contact with the inserted fingers. This technique provides a more adequate palpation of the pelvic viscera than can be accomplished by vaginal examination alone.

29

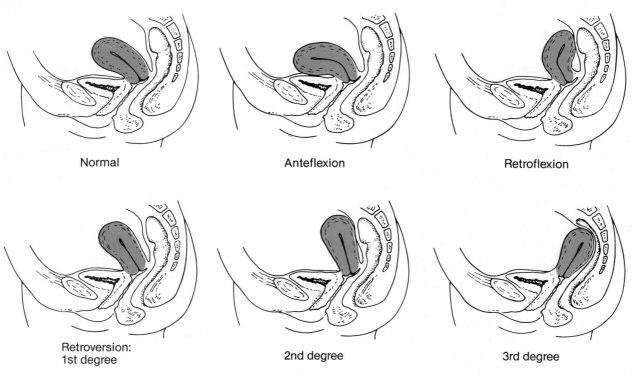

Normal   Anteflexion   Retroflexion

Retroversion: 2nd degree   3rd degree
1st degree

Figure 29–8
Positions of the uterus in sagittal section.

Procedure 29-2

ASSISTING WITH A PELVIC EXAMINATION

[handwritten notes:]
Lubricant
Supplys for a pelvic exam
gloves
Speculum
Vagina
2 Pap swear glass holder
2 glass slides
Request for cytologic examination
form:
Examination Light
Cervical spatula
2 Cervical Brushes
Fixation Spray

PROCEDURAL GOAL

To assist the physician in a routine pelvic examination.

EQUIPMENT AND SUPPLIES

Examination table
Table sheet or table paper
Patient gown
Drape sheet
Vaginal speculum
Lubricant
Examination light
Uterine sponge forceps
Cleansing tissue
Disposable gloves
Cotton applicators
Uterine dressing forceps
Cotton balls
Blood and body-fluid protection barriers (goggles, masks, and aprons or gowns), as necessary
(see Appendix C, Recommendations for Prevention of AIDS Transmission)

PROCEDURE

1. Wash your hands. Follow universal blood and body-fluid precautions (see Appendix C). Glove yourself with nonsterile gloves.
2. Assemble the materials needed, and prepare the room.
3. Identify the patient, and briefly explain the procedure.
   Purpose: Explanations help gain patient cooperation and alleviate apprehension.
4. Instruct the patient to empty the bladder and collect a urine specimen if needed.
   Purpose: Organ palpations are performed on an empty bladder.
5. Instruct the patient to disrobe completely and to put on a gown. Explain proper gown opening (front or back).
6. Assist the patient into the lithotomy position, and apply a drape.
   Purpose: To avoid exposing the patient unnecessarily.
7. Direct the light source into the vaginal speculum.
8. Assist the physician with gloving.
9. Assist the physician with preparation of the smear, labeling, and transportation to the laboratory.
10. Pass the proper instruments to the physician in proper sequence.
11. Apply the lubricant to the physician's fingers.
12. Place the soiled instruments in a basin.
13. Instruct the patient to breathe deeply through the mouth with hands crossed over the chest.
    Purpose: Helps relax muscles.
14. Assist the patient off the table.
15. Instruct the patient to dress.
16. Clean up the room immediately.
17. Wash your hands.

TERMINAL PERFORMANCE OBJECTIVE

Given a patient and appropriate materials, assist in a simulation pelvic examination within 15 minutes, completing each step correctly and in the proper order, as determined by your evaluator.

Disorders of The Female Reproductive System

Spontaneous Abortion. Spontaneous abortion (miscarriage) is the loss of a pregnancy before the twentieth week of fetal development. Common causes are defective development of the embryo, abnormalities of the placenta, endocrine disorders, malnutrition, infection, drug reaction, blood group incompatibilities, severe trauma, and shock. Symptoms include vaginal bleeding of varying degrees of severity and lower abdominal cramping progressing to cervical dilatation with rupture of membranes and complete expulsion of the products of conception. An incomplete abortion results from the partial retention of these products, necessitating a D & C (dilatation and curettage.)

Cervicitis. Cervicitis is an inflammation of the cervix caused by an invading organism. The main symptom is a thick, purulent, whitish discharge with an acrid odor. Dysuria may also be present. Cervicitis is common after vaginal delivery, resulting from infection of cervical lacerations. Treatment consists primarily of antibiotics, although **cauterization**, or electrocoagulation, may be indicated when cervical erosion exists.

Cervical Polyps. Polyps are the second most common lesion of the cervix. They are most prevalent during the reproductive years. The most common symptom is genital bleeding following intercourse, douching, or tampon insertion. Treatment consists of surgical removal of the polyps in the office.

Cystocele. A cystocele is a protrusion of the bladder into the vagina. A diagnosis can be made by requesting the patient to bear down as the vaginal opening is examined. Cystoceles may result from injury during childbirth, obesity, heavy lifting, chronic coughing, and poor musculature due to aging.

Dysmenorrhea. Dysmenorrhea consists of lower abdominal and pelvic pain associated with menstruation. It is one of the most common gynecologic disorders among young females, although it tends to decrease with maturity. The pain is spasmodic. It usually begins 12 to 14 hours prior to the onset of menses and lasts 24 to 48 hours. Dysmenorrhea may be associated with headaches, dizziness, nausea, vomiting, fatigue, low back pain, and diarrhea. The cause of dysmenorrhea is unknown. However, dysmenorrhea may be a symptom of an organic disease, and in this case, must be corrected. Treatment includes analgesics, heat, drugs to decrease uterine contractions, and hormones to suppress ovulation.

Endometriosis. Endometriosis is characterized by the presence of endometrial tissue outside the uterus. It is commonly found in the pelvic area attached to the vulva, urinary bladder, uterus, fallopian tubes, ovaries, intestines, and peritoneum. The cause is unknown, but it is believed to be the result of recent surgery on the uterus, retrograde tubal flow of menstrual fragments, poor nutrition, intercourse during menstruation, or hormonal influences. Use of tampons has also been suggested as a possible cause. Dysmenorrhea and contact pain in the lower abdomen, pelvis, vagina, and back beginning seven days before menses and lasting three days after onset characterize this condition. Other symptoms can include profuse menses, hematuria, rectal bleeding, nausea, vomiting, and abdominal cramps. Treatment includes analgesics, hormonal therapy, and surgery.

Fibrocystic Breast Disease. Fibrocystic breast disease is the presence of multiple, palpable lumps in the breast, usually associated with pain and tenderness that fluctuate with the menstrual cycle. The lumps may be fibrous tumors that have degenerated or sacs filled with fluid. Women with the disease are believed to have a greater risk of developing breast cancer, but this has not been proved.

Fibroid Tumors. Uterine fibroids are benign tumors composed mainly of smooth muscle and some fibrous connective tissue. Fibroids are the common pelvic tumor in women. Their cause is unknown. Menorrhagia (excessive menstruation) is the primary symptom, although the patient may experience bladder or rectal pressure, pelvic pressure, pain, abdominal distortion, and infertility. Treatment consists of surgical removal of small masses, but a hysterectomy (removal of uterus) is indicated when there is greater involvement.

Ovarian Cysts. Ovarian cysts are sacs of fluid or semisolid material located on the ovary. Most cysts are nonmalignant, small, and asymptomatic. They can occur in the follicle or the corpus luteum at any time between puberty and menopause. Large or multiple cysts may cause discomfort, low back pain, nausea, vomiting, and abnormal uterine bleeding. Surgery may be indicated if rupture of the cyst occurs.

Pelvic Inflammatory Disease (PID). PID is any acute or chronic infection of the reproductive system ascending from the vagina (vaginitis), cervix (cervicitis), uterus (endometritis), fallopian tubes (salpingitis), and ovaries (oophoritis). The most common cause of PID is gonorrhea. Uterine infection can also develop following the insertion of an intrauterine device (IUD). Other causative factors include pelvic surgery, tubal examinations, and abortion. Symptoms include a purulent vaginal discharge, fever, malaise, dysuria, lower abdominal pain, bleeding, and nausea and vomiting. PID can be treated with antibiotics, analgesics, and bed rest.

29

Premenstrual Syndrome (PMS). PMS is a number of symptoms that appear one to two weeks before menstruation and that usually subside close to the onset of menses. Symptoms include irritability, nervousness, fatigue, depression, headache, dizziness, numbness of extremities, fainting, asthma, rhinitis, constipation, diarrhea, breast tenderness and enlargement, water retention, backache, palpitations, temporary weight gain, change in appetite, and abdominal bloating. PMS is believed to be a result of salt retention. Treatment consists of diuretics and salt restriction.

Rectocele. A rectocele is a protrusion of the rectum into the vagina. Diagnosis can be made by requesting the patient to bear down as the vaginal opening is examined. Rectoceles are most common in postmenopausal women. Rectoceles may result from pregnancies, instrument deliveries, prolonged labors, obesity, chronic coughing, and lifting heavy objects.

Malignancy of the Reproductive System. The majority of the problems encountered with the female reproductive organs are related to abnormal cell growth. Early screening and preventive intervention are essential. Most malignant tumors require surgical removal. Radiation, chemotherapy, and hormone therapy may be alternative treatment choices. Uterine cancer is the most common reproductive organ cancer, usually affecting women between the ages of 50 and 60. The first signs of uterine cancer include uterine enlargement and unusual bleeding. The only reliable diagnostic procedure is a biopsy. Cervical cancer is asymptomatic until the malignancy has penetrated through the membranes and spread. The earliest symptoms include abnormal vaginal bleeding, persistent discharge, and bleeding and pain during intercourse. Cervical cancer can be detected early by a Papanicolaou (PAP) smear. The American Cancer Society recommends that all women under the age of 40 have a smear performed every three years and that women over 40 have annual smears. Other cancers of the female reproductive organs include endometrial, ovarian, vulvar, and vaginal cancers, and carcinoma of the fallopian tube.

Malignancy of the Breast. Breast cancer is the most common malignancy among females and the leading cause of death among women between 35 and 55 years of age. Although the cause is unknown, other predisposing factors include family history of breast cancer, early menarche and late menopause, first pregnancy after the age of 35 or no pregnancy, high socioeconomic status, obesity, stress, high-fat diet, extensive use of oral contraceptives, and other cancers. The incidence of this cancer is higher in white patients.

Breast cancer appears more commonly in the upper outer quadrant of the left breast. It spreads through the lymphatic and circulatory systems to other parts of the body. Specific signs include

- A lump in the breast.
- Changes in breast shape and size.
- Change in the appearance of the skin.
- Change in skin temperature.
- Drainage or discharge.
- Change in the nipple.

Diagnosis is made through routine monthly breast self-examinations, mammography, ultrasonography, needle aspiration, and surgical biopsy. Treatment consists of

- A lumpectomy (removal of tumor only).
- Simple mastectomy (removal of breast only).
- Modified radical mastectomy (removal of breast and axillary nodes).
- Radical mastectomy (removal of breast, axillary nodes, and muscle of chest wall).

Invasive mammary carcinoma has been classified into four clinical stages:

Stage I: Breast tumors less than 2 cm in diameter.

Stage II: Breast tumors 2 to 5 cm in diameter, or cancers with small mobile axillary lymph node metastases.

Stage III: Breast tumors over 5 cm in diameter with lymph node metastases or skin involvement.

Stage IV: Distant metastases.

Noninvasive mammary carcinomas are classified as Stage TIS (tumor *in situ*).

Sexually Transmitted Infections

Herpes Simplex Virus (HSV). HSV is a virus that is spread by direct skin-to-skin contact with another lesion. There are two strains of the virus, HSV-1 (Type 1) and HSV-2 (Type 2). HSV-1 causes the typical cold sore on the lip or edge of the nose, whereas HSV-2 is the more frequent cause of genital infection. Painful genital fluid-filled vesicles appear on the cervix, labia, vulva, vagina, perineum, or buttocks three to seven days after contact with infected secretions. After the lesions heal, the virus becomes dormant, but additional attacks may recur throughout life. There is some evidence that HSV-2 may cause spontaneous abortion and premature delivery. Newborns can be infected with herpes through active lesions in the birth canal during vaginal deliveries. Brain damage, blindness, or death of the newborn may occur. Most physicians choose to perform a cesarean section when a women has active lesions at the time of birth.

Diagnosis is made by observation of the characteristic vesicles and from patient history. Treatment consists of a combination of antiviral medications such as acyclovir, sulfa-based creams to ease discomfort, and antibacterial agents to combat secondary infections. These herpes lesions are highly contagious, and the medical assistant must avoid contact with all secretions.

Gonorrhea. Gonorrhea is among the most common sexually transmitted diseases. It is widespread throughout the world. It occurs most frequently among lower socioeconomic groups. The causative organism of gonorrhea is bacterium, *Neisseria gonorrhoeae*. The organism is quite fragile and can survive only in a moist, dark, warm area of the body. The most common sites are the vagina, penis, rectum, mouth, and throat. The disease is spread only through direct sexual contact. Infants can become infected during birth if the mother has the disease. Women are usually asymptomatic, but they may develop a greenish-yellow discharge from the cervix. Diagnosis is made by culturing the gonococcus from the discharge of suspected patients. Large doses of penicillin or tetracycline are the recommended treatment.

Syphilis. Syphilis is of unique importance among the sexually transmitted infections because its early lesions heal without treatment and become a major risk to the patient. Since the patient has no symptoms, he or she will think the infection has disappeared. Syphilis is caused by a delicate bacterium called a spirochete, which inhabits the warm moist areas of the genitals and rectum. Syphilis is spread by direct sexual contact or by prenatal transmission to the fetus via the placenta, resulting in an infant with **congenital** syphilis.

The disease progresses through four stages. Symptoms vary according to the stage of involvement. The primary stage (first stage) begins with the organism entering the mucous membranes or the genitals as a result of sexual contact with an infected person. Three or four weeks later, a lesion called a **chancre** appears at the site of organism entrance. Secondary syphilis (second stage) develops six to eight weeks after the chancre. Skin, mucous membranes, and lymph nodes are involved. This stage is characterized by a generalized, painless, nonitching rash. Systemic manifestations include appetite, hair, and weight loss; fever; sore throat; headache; nausea; constipation; and bone, muscle, and joint pain. Without treatment, the disease becomes asymptomatic in two to six weeks. Early latent syphilis (third stage) is asymptomatic and may last for years. The organism is invading the blood vessels, brain, spinal cord, and the bones. After one year, the disease is no longer infectious. Late latent syphilis (fourth stage) is characterized according to the type of involvement, such as internal organs, heart and major blood vessels, and brain and spinal cord.

The diagnosis of syphilis must be confirmed by darkfield examination of the spirochete or by a blood test called VDRL (Venereal Disease Research Laboratory). Penicillin is the treatment for syphilis.

Trichomoniasis. *Trichomonas vaginalis* is the parasitic organism responsible for the infection. The infection can be passed back and forth between sexual partners; therefore, both persons must be treated. The prime and discriminating symptom is a foul, profuse, yellowish, frothy discharge. Diagnosis is made by placing a drop of the secretion on a slide and microscopically identifying the organism. Metronidazole is the drug of choice.

Candidiasis. *Candida albicans* is the yeast-like fungus responsible for this infection. Candida organisms are commonly part of the normal flora of the mouth, skin, intestinal tract, and vagina. Overgrowth of the organism can be caused by long-term antibiotic use, high estrogen levels, diabetes mellitus, and the wearing of tight clothing. Symptoms include itching; dry, bright-red vagina; and vaginal discharge thick with curds. Diagnosis is made by microscopic examination of the discharge mixed with 10 percent potassium hydroxide on a slide. Miconazole cream is the drug treatment of choice.

Diagnostic Testing

Diagnostic testing seen in the medical office includes

Breast Self-Examination. Routine monthly breast self-examinations are the best and most reliable means of detecting breast cancer. Over 90 percent of all initial findings of breast cancer are made by the patient. The American Cancer Society provides excellent pamphlets and films demonstrating the procedure.

Ultrasonogram. Ultrasound is a technique that uses high-frequency sound waves to produce images of solid organs of the body and of accumulations of fluid. Ultrasound can distinguish between cysts and tumors. It is used during pregnancy to determine the number of fetuses, age and sex of the fetus, fetal abnormalities, and position of the placenta.

Mammogram. This is an x-ray film of the breast performed almost exclusively for the detection of breast cancer. The American Cancer Society recommends a single baseline mammogram for all women between 35 and 40 years of age, to be followed by annual mammograms after the age of 50.

Papanicolaou (PAP) Test. A PAP smear is the single most important test performed in the OB/GYN office. A PAP smear is the removal of cells from the cervix and upper vagina to detect the presence of cancer. These cells are scraped from the cervix with a cervical spatula, are spread on a slide, and are sprayed with a commercial fixative of 50

29

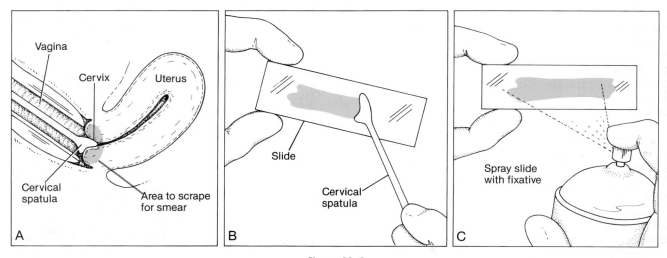

Figure 29–9
Collecting a Papanicolaou smear. **A,** *Scrape a small portion of the mucosa from the cervical os using a wooden cervical spatula.* **B,** *Transfer the specimen onto a slide by moving the spatula over the surface.* **C,** *Fix the slide with an aerosol "fixative" or hair spray.*

percent alcohol and 50 percent ether. The slide is then labeled and sent to the cytology laboratory (Figs. 29–9 and 29–10).

PAP smears are reported on a five-point scale as following:

Grade I: Absence of atypical or abnormal cells.
Grade II: Atypical cytology but no evidence of cancer.
Grade III: Cytology suggestive but not conclusive for cancer.
Grade IV: Strongly suggestive of cancer.
Grade V: Conclusive for cancer.

Pregnancy Testing. Most pregnancy tests are designed to detect the hormone human chorionic gonadotropin (HCG), normally found in the serum and urine of pregnant women about one week after the first missed menses. Urine testing is most commonly performed, and it is more readily available. The test should be conducted on the first urine specimen voided in the morning, because the hormone will be most concentrated.

Pregnancy

The medical assistant should also be knowledgeable about the pregnant female, since many of the OB/GYN patients will be pregnant. Pregnancy is defined as the condition of carrying a developing embryo in the uterus. The duration of pregnancy is approximately 280 days and is divided into first, second, and third trimesters.

The first trimester is the period from the beginning of the last menstrual period through the fourteenth week. It is a period of multiple physical and psychologic changes for the female. For the fetus, it is

a crucial period of organ development. It is during this time that the obstetrician obtains a complete health history of the patient, including family, medical, menstrual, and obstetric histories. The patient also undergoes a complete medical and obstetric examination. Diagnostic testing at this time includes

- Complete blood count.
- Blood type and Rh factor.
- Serologic test for syphilis.
- Rubella titer.
- Sickle cell trait (for black patients).
- Blood glucose (for high-risk patients).
- PAP smear.
- Smears for infections (when indicated).
- Urinalysis.
- Pregnancy test.

The second trimester is the period from the fifteenth through the twenty-eighth week after the last men-

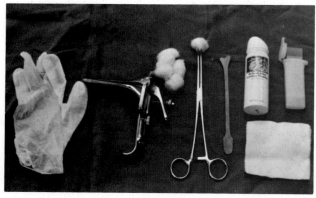

Figure 29–10
Typical set-up for a Papanicolaou smear.

strual period. The uterus has enlarged to above the umbilicus, and the first fetal movements are felt by the patient. In addition to the basic health history and physical examination, assessment by abdominal palpation and fetal heart monitoring are conducted. Diagnostic testing during this period may include amniocentesis, ultrasonography, and x-ray films.

The third trimester is the period from the end of the twenty-eighth week until the time of delivery. This is a period marked by rapid fetal growth. The patient continues to be closely monitored. Childbirth preparation classes usually begin during this time.

Labor is the physiologic process by which the uterus expels the fetus and the placenta. Labor is divided into three stages:

Stage I: Period from onset of labor through complete dilatation of the cervix.
Stage II: Period from complete dilatation of the cervix through the birth of the fetus.
Stage III: Period from the birth of the fetus through the expulsion of the placenta and the membranes.

Family Planning

Family planning refers to the process of deciding whether to have children, how many to have, and when to have them. Choices of whether or not to use a contraceptive method, which to use, and how to use it may be influenced by many external factors and internal feelings.

Permanent methods of contraception include the surgical procedures of vasectomy of the male and tubal ligation of the female. In men, the vas deferens is cut and tied so that sperm will not be ejaculated. In women, sections of the fallopian tubes are cut and cauterized, thus preventing the ovum from reaching the uterus. These two sterilization procedures do not affect physiologic processes or sexual responses.

Temporary methods of contraception include

- Oral contraceptives (Fig. 29–11).
- Minipill.
- Diaphragm (Fig. 29–12).
- Cervical cap (Fig. 29–13).
- Foam, jelly, or cream suppository (Fig. 29–14).
- Sponge (Fig. 29–15).
- Condom (Fig. 29–16).
- Rhythm.
- IUD (intrauterine device) (Fig. 29–17).

OPHTHALMOLOGY

A complete examination of the eye is technical and requires expensive equipment, but the practi-

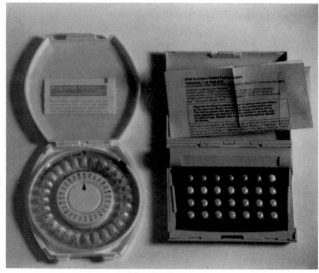

Figure 29–11
The most widely used female contraceptive today is still the pill. Many varieties are available, but the low-dose types are most popular because they have fewer side effects. They are Ortho-Novum 7/7/7 and Triphasil.

29

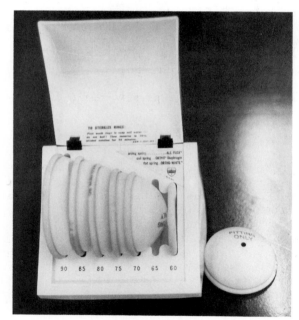

Figure 29–12
Diaphragms come in various sizes and must be fitted by a physician or a specially trained nurse practitioner.

tioner of general medicine does become involved with some examinations and treatments of the eye with the use of basic office equipment. The use of the ophthalmoscope to examine the retina of the eye is an essential part of every complete physical examination. The eye often reflects an individual's general health or may be involved in a systemic disease or injury. The eye may react to a systemic medication the patient is taking.

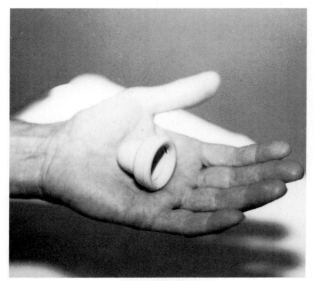

Figure 29–13

The cervical cap has not been released for sale in the United States; however, it is well accepted in Europe. The major advantage is that the cap can hold spermicidal cream and may be left in place for three days.

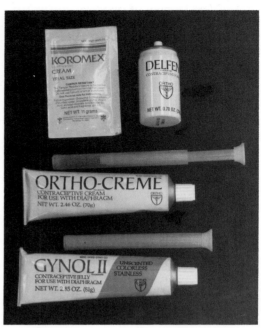

Figure 29–14

Contraceptive foams, jellies, and creams. It is suggested that they be used in conjunction with a barrier-type contraceptive for full effectiveness.

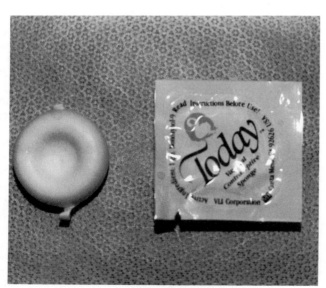

Figure 29–15

The vaginal contraceptive sponge, which is impregnated with a spermicide, must be placed in water before insertion. Caution the patient to keep it in place for ten minutes before intercourse to allow the spermicide to cover the cervix.

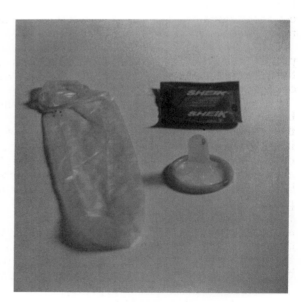

Figure 29–16

The most widely used male contraceptive is the condom. It has the extra advantage of decreasing the danger of infection from sexually transmitted diseases.

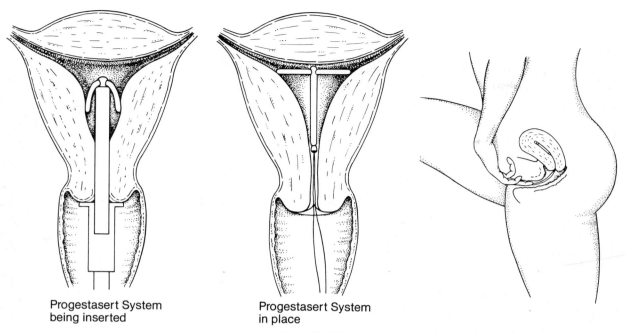

Progestasert System
being inserted

Progestasert System
in place

Figure 29–17
The intrauterine device (IUD) is manufactured as just one product: Progestasert.

29

The most routine eye test, other than the use of the ophthalmoscope, is the distance acuity test, usually given with the *Snellen Chart*. (This test is discussed in more detail later in this section.) This test may be administered by the medical assistant, who may also check the patient's near vision with the *Near Vision Acuity Chart* (Fig. 29–18). This is especially done on the patient past 40 years of age for possible **presbyopia.**

Testing a patient's color vision is important, especially if the patient is in certain occupations. By the age of five, all children should be checked with color vision charts.

The eyelids are examined for edema, which may be the result of nephrosis, heart failure, allergy, or thyroid deficiency. **Ptosis** of the eyelid may be an involvement of the third cranial nerve. Infections of the eyelids are frequently a sty (an infected eyelash follicle), which is painful, or a chalazion (a beady nodule in the eyelid), which is usually not painful unless infected. If the lacrimal ducts are obstructed, the patient has constant tearing, known as epiphora. The conjunctiva of the eye is the delicate membrane covering the eyeball and lining the eyelids. Inflammation of the conjunctiva may be bacterial or viral, and there is a highly contagious conjunctivitis commonly called pinkeye.

The corneal reflex or corneal sensitivity is tested by touching the cornea of the eye quickly with a wisp of cotton. The patient will blink. The pupils of the eyes are normally round and equal in size. Normal pupils constrict rapidly in response to light and during accommodation. This is seen by shining a bright pinpoint light into one eye from the side of the patient's head. The pupil of the illuminated eye constricts, and the pupil of the other eye constricts equally. This test is called light and accommodation (L & A). An older patient's eyes do not accommodate as well as a younger person's. Each eye is checked this way. Then, the patient is asked to look at the physician's finger as it is moved directly toward the patient's nose.

The ophthalmoscope is used for examining the interior of the eye. It projects a bright narrow beam of light that permits the physician to examine the interior parts of the eye and retina through the lens of the eye. It is helpful in detecting disorders of the eyes as well as disorders of other organs, the conditions of which are reflected in the condition of the eyes.

Intraocular pressure has been checked by ophthalmologists for many years, but today many general-practice physicians also check their patients for intraocular pressure. Elevated intraocular pressure, known as glaucoma, causes pressure on the nerve fibers and thus may possibly result in blindness. The tonometer is used to measure this intraocular pressure. The patient is placed in a reclining position or sits with the head resting back on a support. A topical anesthetic is instilled in each eye. After a minute, the patient is instructed to fix his or her vision on a spot on the ceiling. The physician then touches the sterile footplate of the tonometer to the cornea of the eye (Fig. 29–19). The tonometer is an extremely delicate instrument requiring particular care and storage. After each use, it must be sterilized and returned to its stand. Read the manufacturer's instructions and follow them carefully.

60

Nothing can take the place of "the only pair of eyes you will ever have." That is why you are exercising such good judgment in taking care of them as you are now doing.

50

For this reason, you will welcome the suggestion about lenses which are designed and made to give you "greater comfort and better appearance." In man's earliest days he had little use for glasses. He used his eyes chiefly for long distance.

40

He worked by daylight and at tasks with little detail. But now, you use your eyes for much close work—reading, writing, sewing and many other uses which the eyes of primitive man did not know. Now your eyes meet all sorts of lighting conditions, artificial and natural.

30

Many of these conditions produce "overbrightness" or glare. Sometimes it is the direct or reflected glare of sunlight; often it is direct or reflected from artificial light. And very often this glare is uncomfortable—impairs your efficiency. But special lenses, developed by America's leading optical scientists, combat this glare.

25

These lenses give you more comfortable vision and blend harmoniously with your complexion. These lenses are less conspicuous. We are glad to recommend them because they will give you greater comfort and better appearance. Thousands of satisfied wearers testify to their real benefits.

20

You are wise in taking good care of "the only pair of eyes you will ever have." You know how valuable they are, that you can never have another pair. For this reason, you will welcome the suggestion about lenses which are designed and made to give you "greater comfort and better appearance." In man's earliest days he had little use for glasses.

The above letters subtend the visual angle of 5' at the designated distance in inches.

B-858   **BAUSCH & LOMB** ▼   Printed in U.S.A.
                 Mark of Leadership

Figure 29–18
The Near-Vision Acuity Chart for persons older than 40 years who have difficulty with accommodation (adjusting to changes in distance) because the eye muscles no longer respond quickly.

Strabismus, crossed eye, is seen predominantly in a small percentage of young children because it is diagnosed early in life and is treated as early as possible. There are several problems that cause eyes to turn, but most commonly the condition is due to weakness of an extraocular muscle. Evaluation of patients with strabismus includes a cover test, measurement of visual acuity, and a careful ophthalmoscopic examination.

Special techniques employed in the ophthalmologist's office include the use of a *slit-lamp biomicroscope*. This is used to view the fine details in the anterior segments of the eye. It is also used to view a corneal foreign body because it gives a well-illuminated and highly magnified view of the area. The patient with exophthalmia (abnormal protrusion of the eye due possibly to an overactive thyroid or to a tumor behind the eyeball) is checked with the *exophthalmometer*. This instrument is designed to measure the pressure of the central retinal artery. It is helpful in patients with circulatory disease because it measures the blood pressure in the retinal artery.

Distance Visual Acuity

Distance visual acuity is frequently part of a complete physical examination. It is widely used in

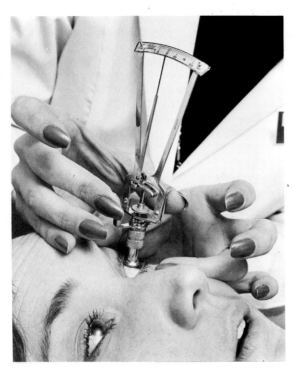

Figure 29–19
Application of a tonometer. (Photograph by Ken Kasper; courtesy of Wills Eye Hospital, Philadelphia, PA.)

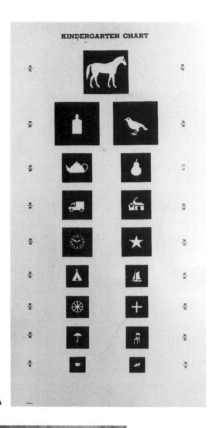

KINDERGARTEN CHART

A

29

schools and industry. To date, it is the best single test available for visual screening. Many cases of myopia, astigmatism, or hyperopia have been detected by this routine test. The most common chart used is the Snellen Alphabetical (Fig. 29–20*B*) chart. This chart has various letters of the alphabet and is for general use. Patients with limited knowledge of the English alphabet can be tested with the "E" chart (Fig. 29–20*C*). In addition, there is a chart available that uses pictures as symbols (Fig. 29–20*A*). This chart is also used for preschool patients, slow learners, or mentally retarded children who have not yet learned the English alphabet. The symbol on the top line of the chart can be read by persons of normal vision at 200 feet. In each of the succeeding rows, from the top down, the size of the symbols is reduced so that a person with normal vision can see them at distances of 100, 70, 50, 40, 30, and 20 feet.

The patient must not be allowed to study the chart before the test. The room or hall should be long enough so that the 20-foot distance can be marked off accurately. The chart should be hung at eye level and illuminated with maximum light, without glare on the chart. The patient may be standing or sitting with the chart at eye level.

Most adults do not need the chart explained, but the assistant must have the patient's cooperation. With the "E" chart, for example, an explanation must be given as to how the E's are to be read. The patient may point up or down, or right or left. The

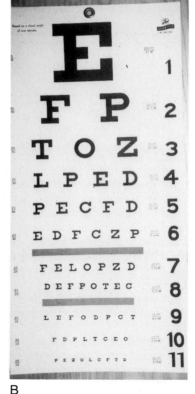

B

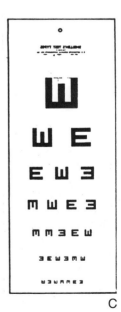

C

Figure 29–20
A, Special chart for children too young to read. B, Testing the patient's eye with the Snellen eye chart. C, The "E" chart, which can be used for children or for persons unable to read English.

patient may prefer to hold three fingers in the same direction that the letter is facing. Use the same routine each time the patient is tested, by starting with the right eye. If the patient is wearing glasses, the physician may want the eyes tested first with the glasses on and then without them. Indicate on the patient's record "with" or "without." Test one eye at a time. Both eyes are to be kept open during the test, but the eye not being tested is to be covered with a paper cup or a piece of cardboard. The paper cup is best because it does not touch the eye. Under no circumstances should the patient use fingers to hold the eye closed.

Allow a moment between changing eyes. The medical assistant should stand beside the chart and point to the line to be read. Start with the line having the larger symbols, then proceed to the lower lines. Record the smallest line that the patient can read without a mistake, and also record any behavioral observations such as squinting, straining, tearing, or turning of the head. Record the responses of each eye separately. The response is recorded as a fraction. The numerator (top number) is the distance of the patient from the chart, the denominator (bottom number) is the lowest line read satisfactorily by the patient. For example, if the patient reads the 20 line at 20 feet, the fraction 20/20 is recorded for that eye. Make certain the record reads "right eye" (O.D.) and "left eye" (O.S.).

Procedure 29-3

MEASURING DISTANCE VISUAL ACUITY USING THE SNELLEN CHART

PROCEDURAL GOAL

To determine the patient's degree of visual clarity at a measured distance, using the Snellen chart.

EQUIPMENT AND SUPPLIES

Snellen eye chart
Eye cover
Patient's chart
Pen or pencil

PROCEDURE

1. Wash your hands.
2. Prepare the examination room. Make sure that (1) the room is well lighted, (2) a distance marker is 20 feet from the chart, (3) the chart is placed at eye level.
3. Assemble the materials needed.
4. Identify the patient, and explain the procedure.
   Purpose: Explanations help gain patient cooperation and alleviate apprehension.
5. Position the patient in a standing or sitting position at the 20-foot marker.
   Purpose: Twenty feet is the standard testing distance.
6. Position the Snellen chart at eye level to the patient.
7. Instruct the patient to cover the left eye.
   Purpose: The right eye is traditionally tested first.
8. Stand beside the chart, and point to each row as the patient orally reads down the chart, starting with the 20/200 row.
   Purpose: Starting with larger letters allows the patient to gain confidence.
9. Record any patient reactions in reading the chart.
   Purpose: Reactions such as squinting, leaning, tearing or blinking may indicate that the patient is experiencing difficulty with the test.
10. Record the smallest line that the patient can read without making a mistake.
11. Repeat the procedure on the other eye.

Procedure continued on opposite page

TERMINAL PERFORMANCE OBJECTIVE

Given a patient and the appropriate supplies, measure and record distance visual acuity of both eyes using the Snellen chart within five minutes, completing each step correctly and in the proper order, as determined by your evaluator.

Eye Irrigation

The purpose of eye irrigation is to relieve inflammation, promote drainage, and wash away chemicals or foreign bodies. Sterile technique and equipment must be used to avoid contamination.

Procedure 29–4

IRRIGATING A PATIENT'S EYES

PROCEDURAL GOAL

To cleanse the eye(s) as ordered by the physician.

EQUIPMENT AND SUPPLIES

Prescribed sterile irrigation solution
Irrigating bulb syringe
Basin for solution
Basin for drainage
Sterile cotton balls
Disposable drape
Towel
Nonsterile gloves
Blood and body-fluid protection barriers (goggles, masks, and aprons or gowns), as necessary
(see Appendix C, Recommendations for Prevention of AIDS Transmission)

PROCEDURE

1. Wash your hands. Follow universal blood and body-fluid precautions (see Appendix C). Glove yourself with nonsterile gloves.
2. Check the physician's orders to determine which eye(s) require irrigation.
   Purpose: To check the abbreviations: O.D. (right eye), O.S. (left eye), O.U. (both eyes).
3. Assemble the materials needed.
4. Read the label of the solution three times.
   Purpose: To follow the rules for administering medications.
5. Identify the patient, and explain the procedure.
   Purpose: Explanations help gain patient cooperation and alleviate apprehension.
6. Assist the patient into a sitting or supine position, making certain that the head is turned toward the affected eye. Place the disposable drape over the patient's neck and shoulder.
   Purpose: This causes the solution to flow away from the unaffected eye so as to reduce the chances for cross-contamination of the healthy eye.
7. Place or have the patient hold a drainage basin next to affected eye to receive the solution from the eye. Position a towel under the basin to avoid getting the solution on the patient (see top, following page).

Procedure continued on following page

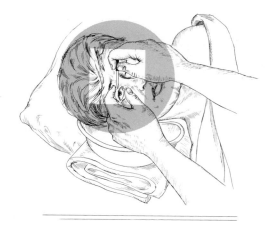

8. Moisten a cotton ball with solution, and cleanse the eyelid and lashes. Start at the inner canthus (near nose) to the outer canthus (farthest from nose) and dispose of the cotton ball.
   Purpose: Debris on the lids or lashes must be cleansed away before exposing the conjunctiva.
9. Pour the required volume of irrigating solution into the basin, and withdraw solution into the bulb syringe.
10. Separate eyelids with the index finger and thumb of one hand, and hold.
11. With the other hand, place the syringe on the bridge of the nose parallel to the eye.
    Purpose: To support and steady the syringe.
12. Squeeze the bulb, directing the solution toward the inner contour of eye and allowing the solution to flow steadily and slowly. Do not allow the syringe to touch the eye or eyelids.
    Purpose: Prevents possible injury to the eye.

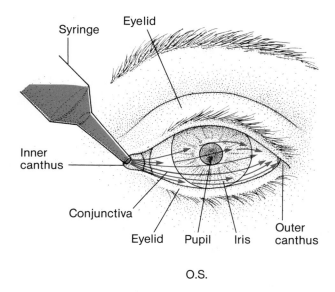

O.S.

13. Dry the eyelid with a cotton ball.
14. Record the procedure on the patient's chart.
15. Clean up the work area.
16. Wash your hands.

TERMINAL PERFORMANCE OBJECTIVE

Given a patient and appropriate supplies, irrigate the patient's eye(s), completing each step correctly and in the proper order, as determined by your evaluator.

Eye Instillation

The purpose of eye instillation is to apply medication. Instillation may also be performed to dilate the pupils prior to examination.

Procedure 29–5

INSTILLING MEDICATION INTO A PATIENT'S EYES

PROCEDURAL GOAL

To apply medication to the eye(s), as ordered by the physician.

EQUIPMENT AND SUPPLIES

Sterile medication with dropper
Disposable drape
Gauze squares
Nonsterile gloves
Blood and body-fluid protection barriers (goggles, masks, and aprons or gowns), as necessary
(see Appendix C, Recommendations for Prevention of AIDS Transmission)

PROCEDURE

1. Wash your hands. Follow universal blood and body-fluid precautions (see Appendix C). Glove yourself with nonsterile gloves.
2. Check the physician's order to determine which eye(s) require medication.
   Purpose: To check the abbreviations.
3. Assemble the materials needed.
4. Read the label of the medication three times.
   Purpose: To follow the rules for administering medications.
5. Identify the patient, and explain the procedure.
   Purpose: Explanations help gain patient cooperation and alleviate apprehension.
6. Assist the patient into a sitting or supine position with the head tilted backward and "looking up."
7. Pull the lower conjunctival sac downward with a gauze square.
   Purpose: Gauze prevents your fingers from slipping.
8. Insert the prescribed number of drops into the eye, directly over the center of the lower conjunctival sac while holding the dropper parallel to the eye and a half inch away.
   Purpose: Never point dropper toward the eye or touch the eye with the dropper.

29

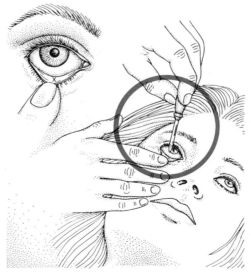

Procedure continued on following page

9. Instruct the patient to close the eye immediately and to rotate the eyeball.
   Purpose: Rotating the eyeball distributes the medication.
10. Dry any excess drainage.
11. Record the procedure on the patient's chart.
12. Clean up the work area.
13. Wash your hands.

TERMINAL PERFORMANCE OBJECTIVE

Given a patient and appropriate supplies, instill drops into the eye(s), completing each step correctly and in the proper order, as determined by your evaluator.

ORTHOPEDIC SURGERY

An orthopedist is concerned with the body's mobility and with diagnosing and treating diseases and abnormalities of the musculoskeletal system. A considerable part of this practice may be caring for fractures, dislocations, strains, sprains, and ruptures.

A common complaint heard in the orthopedist's office is "low back pain." Other diseases seen are rheumatoid arthritis, osteoarthritis, gout, and bursitis.

Besides a careful history, the examination covers basically the back and the extremities. The physical examination of the musculoskeletal system is performed largely by inspection, but palpation and mensuration are also done. The orthopedic physician wants to determine the condition of the muscles, joints, and bones. A large part of the examination is done to determine the direction and the range of active and passive motion in the joints.

The first step is usually inspection of the patient's posture in the standing, sitting, and supine positions. A lateral view of the patient in a standing position shows the position of the head in relation to the trunk of the body. Normal or rigid curves of the cervical, thoracic, and lumbar spine may be seen. Abnormalities such as kyphosis and lordosis are seen in this lateral inspection. Scoliosis is seen from the posterior view. To determine the patient's gait, the physician asks the patient to walk. The physician may observe a limp, possibly due to **ankylosis**, or a scissor gait, as seen in spastic paraplegia.

Each major joint of the body is inspected for range of motion. A goniometer is used for precise measurement of a joint's flexion and extension. Muscles are examined for hypertrophy or atrophy. The measurement of the circumference of an extremity at a given point, such as the calf of the leg or the biceps of the arm, is compared with the opposite side. The tendon reflexes are checked.

The spine, or vertebral column, is referred to in divisions. The first seven vertebrae are the cervical spine, the next twelve are the thoracic spine, and the next five are the lumbar spine. These are the 24 movable vertebrae. Below the lumbar vertebrae are the sacrum and coccyx. When referring to the movable spine, the physician may say C-5, meaning the fifth cervical vertebra, or L-3, meaning the third lumbar vertebra.

Physicians specializing in industrial medicine and worker's compensation cases have special terminology and methods for recording and measuring the musculoskeletal system. The American Academy of Orthopedic Surgeons has published a guide called *Joint Motion: Method of Measuring and Recording*.

The medical assistant must be familiar with such terms as *extension*, which is a movement that increases the angle between the ends of a jointed part, such as a limb straightened. The opposite of this is *flexion*, which is the act of bending or decreasing such an angle. The amount of bending is recorded in degrees (Fig. 29–21). Other terms used are *abduction*, meaning lateral movement away from the middle plane. *Adduction* is movement toward the middle plane.

Radiographs are the most common diagnostic aid used in the orthopedic office. Urinalysis and blood tests are ordered when there is joint involvement or severe pain and swelling. Physical therapy and rehabilitation are also a major part of the therapy.

OTORHINOLARYNGOLOGY

This is the medical specialty that deals with the ear, nose, and throat. It is frequently referred to as otolaryngology or even as a single specialty of otology or laryngology. Usually, the specialty otorhinolaryngology is referred to simply as ear, nose, and throat (ENT). The anatomic point at which the ENT examination begins varies with the physician. Most of the involved area is visible to the physician, with the exception of the nasal accessory sinuses and the middle and inner ear. A large part of this examination consists of the inspection of the mucosa.

If the ears are examined first, the external auditory canal is viewed with an otoscope or a light and

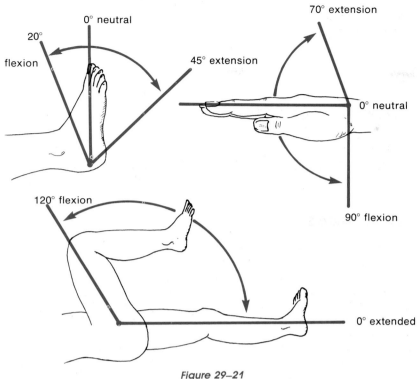

Figure 29–21
Flexion and extension in degrees.

ear speculum. The normal external canal contains a small amount of cerumen (wax). Cerumen is a protective secretion produced to ward off microorganisms. Patients who attempt to remove the wax by using cotton tip applicators often push the wax farther into the canal, which causes the wax to lodge and harden. This impacted wax is uncomfortable and eventually impairs hearing. Patients can have the impacted wax removed to avoid further discomfort or possible ear damage. A softening solution may be instilled into the impacted ear and then followed by irrigation to remove the excess ear wax.

Ear Irrigation

This procedure is performed to remove excessive or impacted cerumen.

Procedure 29–6

IRRIGATING A PATIENT'S EARS

PROCEDURAL GOAL

To remove excessive or impacted cerumen from a patient's ear(s).

EQUIPMENT AND SUPPLIES

Irrigating solution
Basin for irrigating solution
Bulb syringe
Gauze squares
Otoscope
Drainage basin
Disposable drape
Cotton-tip applicators

Procedure continued on following page

PROCEDURE

1. Wash your hands.
2. Assemble the materials needed.
3. Check the physician's orders.
4. Check the label of the solution three times.
5. Prepare the solution as ordered. The solution temperature should be between 95° and 105°F.
   Purpose: Warm solutions are most comfortable to the patient.
6. Identify the patient, and explain the procedure.
7. View the affected ear with an otoscope to locate impaction or a foreign object.
8. Drape the patient.
   Purpose: Draping protects the patient's clothing.
9. Position the patient with the head slightly tilted toward the affected side.
   Purpose: This position allows gravity to help the solution flow from the ear to the basin.
10. Place the drainage basin next to the affected ear.
    Purpose: Prevents solution from running down the patient's neck.
11. Wipe any particles from the outside of the ear with gauze squares.
    Purpose: Prevents the introduction of foreign materials into the ear canal.
12. Fill the syringe.
13. Pull up the auricle of the ear gently with one hand.
14. With the other hand, place the tip of the syringe into the meatus of the ear (below, left).
15. Direct the flow of the solution gently upward (below, right).

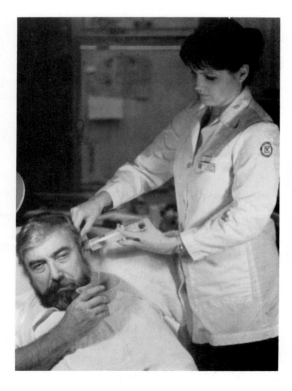

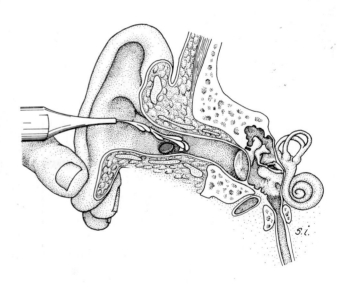

16. Dry the patient's external ear with gauze squares.
17. Dry the ear canal gently with cotton-tip applicators.
18. Inspect the ear with an otoscope to determine the results.
19. Record the procedure on the patient's chart.
20. Clean up the work area.
21. Wash your hands.

Procedure continued on opposite page

TERMINAL PERFORMANCE OBJECTIVE

Given a patient and appropriate supplies, irrigate the ear within five minutes, completing each step correctly and in the proper order, as determined by your evaluator.

Disorders of the Ear

The patient may be given a hearing test with an *audiometer* (Fig. 29–22) to disclose any hearing loss. There are three types of hearing loss: conductive, sensorineural, and central. Conductive hearing loss (external or middle ear disorders) occurs when sound cannot reach the cochlea because of blockage of the ear canal or disorders of the eardrum or ossicles. Factors causing this type of hearing loss include foreign body or cerumen impaction, perforated tympanic membrane, exudate in the middle ear, otosclerosis, and adhesions of the ossicles. Sensorineural hearing loss (perceptive hearing loss) occurs when there is damage to the cochlea or eighth cranial nerve, which conducts sound from the inner ear to the brain. The deafness may be caused by hereditary factors, German measles, trauma, noise, drugs, tumors, aging, and infection. Central hearing loss (brain stem and cerebral hemispheres) is uncommon and usually is characterized by loss of speech rather than of pure tone perception. This type of hearing loss is usually due to lesions or tumors.

The anatomic differences between the adult's and the child's eustachian tube make children far more susceptible to middle ear infections (otitis media). Occasionally, it may be necessary to do a **myringotomy** to drain the exudate from the middle ear.

The inner ear can be invaded by bacteria, especially as a complication of acute otitis media. Vertigo (the sensation of dizziness) may be a symptom of some diseases of the inner ear. Tinnitus (ringing in the ears) is also a subjective symptom. It may be present in labyrinthitis, damage to the eighth cranial nerve, or cerebral arteriosclerosis.

Other disorders of the ear follow.

Otitis externa (swimmer's ear) is a bacterial or fungal infection caused by swimming in contaminated water or heavily chlorinated swimming pools.

External canal blockage is caused by a collection of cerumen or by a foreign body. This may result in reduced hearing, direct tissue damage, or perforation of the eardrum.

Perforation of the eardrum can result from chronic infection, burns, direct blows to the side of the head, insertion of bobby pins and toothpicks, blast injury, and careless use of cotton swabs.

29

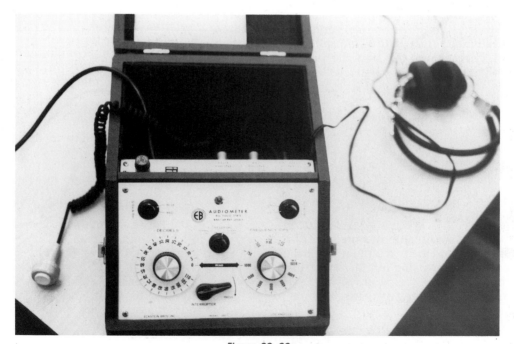

Figure 29–22
The audiometer is used to screen patients who have a possible hearing loss. (Courtesy of Madison Area Technical College, Madison, WI.)

balance

Meniere's syndrome is a dysfunction of the ear labyrinth resulting in swelling and loss of equilibrium. This condition may be caused by infection, allergies, tumors, arteriosclerosis and atherosclerosis, stress, genetic disorders, and poisoning.

Otosclerosis consists of ossification of the stapes against the oval window, resulting in a diminished transmission of sound to the inner ear. The cause is unknown. This condition occurs primarily in females.

Motion sickness is caused by a disturbance within the inner ear. This condition results from any type of motion via transportation (train, car, bus, boat, or plane).

Examination of the Nose and Throat

Examination of the nasal cavity is mainly inspection of the mucous membrane. The common cold and allergies are the main causes of changes in the mucosa. Because the physician cannot see the nasal sinuses, these are examined by palpation and transillumination. If the mucosa is swollen, it may be necessary to spray the area with a vasoconstrictor.

The throat is the area that includes the larynx and pharynx and is viewed with the aid of a mirror and a tongue depressor or piece of gauze to grasp the tongue (Fig. 29–23). In the nasopharynx, the physician looks for enlarged adenoids (pharyngeal tonsils) and for the orifice of the eustachian tube. It may be necessary to grasp the tongue with the aid of a piece of gauze in order to view the laryngopharynx. Spraying the throat with a topical anesthetic helps with the gagging patient.

In the oral cavity, the patient's teeth and gums are carefully examined. The palatine (faucial) tonsils (if present) are checked for size and the presence of crypts. The lingual tonsils are also checked. The salivary glands are palpated.

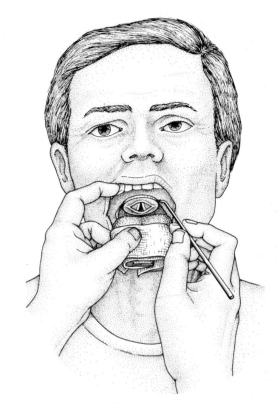

Figure 29–23
Examination of the larynx with a laryngeal mirror and a piece of gauze.

PEDIATRICS

Pediatrics is that branch of medicine dealing with the child and his or her development and care as well as the diseases of children and their treatment. A large percentage of the patients in the pediatric office are "well-baby" or "well-child" care patients. The role of the physician and the medical office staff is to supervise and help maintain the health of these patients. An increasing number of auxiliary health care personnel are being involved in the health services given to young patients. Parents of these young patients must be involved with their care and development. The medical assistant can help a great deal in the communications between the patient, the parents, and the medical staff. The confidence a child develops in the care and the consideration received in the physician's office is the basis of good medical care.

Pediatric care actually starts before the child is born, with the promotion of the mother's good general health before conception and during pregnancy. The confidence and enthusiasm of the parents also affect the infant's physical and emotional well-being.

The newborn's first physical assessment comes at the time of delivery, when the pediatrician assesses the newborn's ability to thrive outside the uterus. The Apgar score is a system of scoring the infant's physical condition at one and five minutes after birth (Table 29–1). The heart rate, respiration, muscle tone, response to stimuli, and color of the infant are each rated 0, 1, or 2. The maximum total score is 10. Those infants with low scores must be given immediate attention.

The frequency of the well-child visits varies with the physician and the community. It may follow this pattern: 2 weeks, 7 weeks, 4 months, 1 year, 2 years, 5 years, 10 years, and 15 years. Immunizations and illnesses significantly increase the frequency of these visits.

As with any other physical examination, the medical history is an essential guide to the pediatric

Table 29-1
The Apgar Scoring System*

Clinical Sign	Assigned Score		
	0	1	2
Heart rate	Absent	Under 100	Over 100
Respiratory effort	Absent	Slow and irregular	Good and crying
Muscle tone	Limp	Some flexion of the arms and legs	Active movement
Reflex irritability	No response	Grimace	Coughing and sneezing
Color	Blue and pale	Body pink, and extremities blue	Pink all over

*The readings are taken by the pediatrician at one-minute and five-minute intervals after birth. At *one minute,* if the score is 7 or less, some nervous system problems are suspected. If the score is below 4, resuscitation is usually necessary. At *five minutes,* if the score is at least 8, the pediatrician can conduct a complete examination. The child is probably reacting normally.

examination. With the infant, the physician is dependent on the parent for the history, but as the child gets older some history may be obtained from the child and clarified or amplified by the parent. Generally, the child is extremely honest regarding the facts of the illness. Close observation also gives the physician considerable information. A wince may indicate tenderness, and the facial expression associated with nausea should alert the physician and the staff.

Explaining what is to be done and showing the child the instruments to be used often contribute to their cooperation. The instruments and the examiner's hands should be warm.

The duties of the medical assistant are to weigh and measure the infant, to record this information on the patient's chart and on the parent's records,

and to check whether immunizations are due (see Chapter 22).

The sequence of the examination varies and is frequently adapted to the cooperation of the child. Leave until last the areas to which the patient may object the most and in which the patient may be the least cooperative. Sometimes, a tongue depressor in each little hand keeps an infant from grabbing the stethoscope.

The physician is concerned with the patient's growth and development. The child's alertness and responses tell the physician a considerable amount. In infancy (birth to two years) and in the young child of preschool age (two to six years), the parent is closely questioned about the child's eating, sleeping, and elimination habits. The school-age child (6 to 12 years or to puberty) is usually a little more cooperative during an examination and can answer most questions without parental assistance. The adolescent (onset of puberty to the cessation of growth, or roughly 12 to 19 years of age) is in a difficult period of life. These patients are usually sensitive, are easily embarrassed, and are concerned about their health and appearance. More physicians are now specializing in adolescent medicine.

Examination of the child during routine well-baby care includes the measurement of the circumference of the infant's head. The head of the infant is measured to determine normal growth and development. If the circumference of the head deviates greatly from normal measurements, **hydrocephaly** or **microcephaly** may be suspected. It is important to discover these conditions as early as possible so that appropriate treatment measures may begin. Measurement of head circumference should be performed during routine office visits until the child is 36 months old. The medical assistant measures the head at the time that the weight and height measurements are determined.

29

Procedure 29-7

MEASURING THE CIRCUMFERENCE OF AN INFANT'S HEAD

PROCEDURAL GOAL

To obtain an accurate measurement of the circumference of an infant's head.

EQUIPMENT AND SUPPLIES

Flexible tape measure
Growth chart
Patient's chart
Pen or pencil

Procedure continued on following page

PROCEDURE

1. Wash your hands.
2. Identify the patient.
3. Gain infant cooperation through conversation.
4. Place the infant in the supine position on the examination table, or the infant may be held by the parent.
5. Hold the tape measure with the zero mark against the infant's forehead, above the eyebrows.
6. Bring the tape measure around the head, just above the ears, to meet at the mid-forehead.

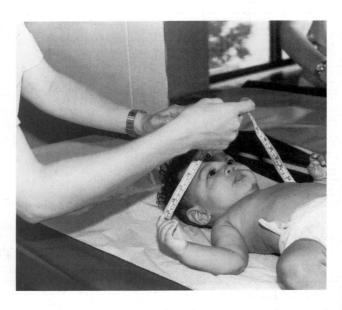

7. Read to nearest 0.01 cm.
8. Record the measurement on the growth chart and patient's chart.
9. Clean the work area.
10. Wash your hands.

TERMINAL PERFORMANCE OBJECTIVE

Given a patient and appropriate supplies, measure and record the head circumference within three minutes, to a minimum performance level of one-eighth inch of the actual reading, as determined by your evaluator.

Ross Laboratories has made growth charts available to physicians for many years (Fig. 29–24). These charts use the *National Center For Health Statistics* (NCHS) system for evaluating and comparing young children's growth rates with similar children of similar ages. Slowed growth patterns and nutritional variances are easily detected. Because boys and girls differ in normal growth rates, separate charts are used. There are charts for two age groups: birth to 36 months, and ages 2 to 18 years. Frequently, medical assistants are asked to plot a growth pattern (Table 29–2).

Many medical offices evaluate young children's

Table 29–2
How to Use the NCHS Growth Charts

1. Look at the vertical column to find *stature, length,* or *weight.*
2. In the horizontal column find your patient's age.
3. Mark an "X" at the spot on the graph where the items in number 1 meet.
4. Next find the percentile in which your patient places as compared with children of the same age.
   a. Trace the percentile line up to the value listed on the right side of the chart.
   b. Remember to alter the percentile if it is not located exactly on the line.
5. Report the results to your physician immediately if the result is above or below the normal range.

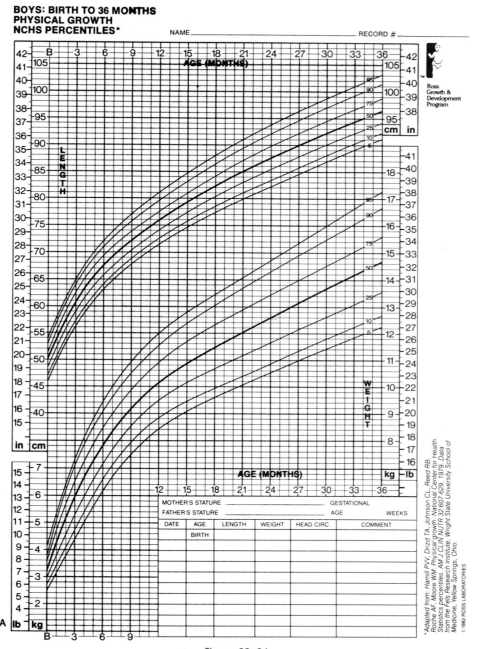

Figure 29–24
National Center for Health Statistics (NCHS) Physical Growth Percentile Charts. **A,** Chart for boys.

Illustration continued on following page

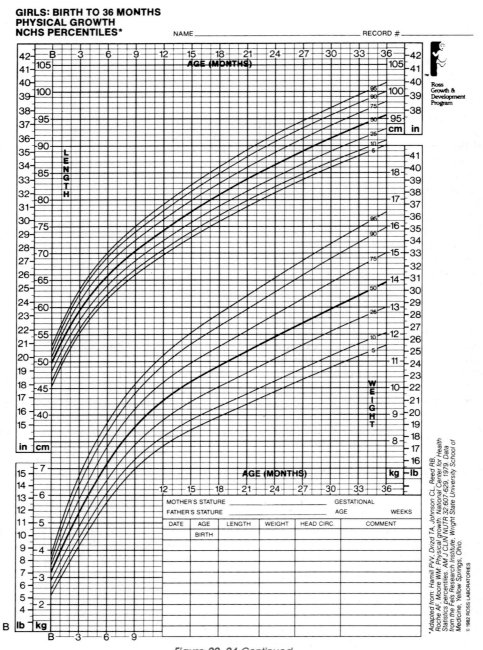

Figure 29–24 Continued
B, *Chart for girls. (Courtesy of Ross Laboratories, Columbus, OH.)*

rates of growth and development with the *Denver Developmental Screening Test*. This test helps detect delays in development and documents normal development in the preschool child. It is a simple screening test and is easy to use. The directions for screening and the scoring system are published with the test. It does not test intelligence but rather focuses on four basic categories: gross motor, fine motor-adaptive, language, and personal-social development. If unusual or unexplained delays are detected, the child can be referred for more detailed diagnosis by a specialist (Fig. 29–25).

Restraints for Children. For routine examinations, it is usually not advisable to use strong restraints. A small child may be held on an adult's lap, with the child's right arm tucked under the adult's left arm. The child's left arm may be held in place by the adult's right hand. The adult's left hand is then free to support the child's head.

For examination and treatment of the ears, eyes, nose, or throat, place the child on the examination table. Immobilize the head as gently as possible (Fig. 29–26). Try to gain the child's cooperation. Ask the parent to assist. The parent can frequently help restrain the child. A familiar face and voice can help to calm children's anxieties and fears.

When restraining a crying child, check your own position and that of the child. Sometimes a child cries from the pain of too tight a hold rather than from the pain of the examination. For example, when holding an infant's legs to expose the buttocks, place your index finger between the ankles to reduce pressure.

When more extensive examinations are necessary, place the child on a large sheet that has been folded lengthwise, keeping the top of the sheet even with the shoulders and the bottom just below the feet. Leave a greater portion of the sheet on the left side of the child. Now bring this longer side back over the left arm and under the body and right arm. Next, bring the sheet back over the right arm and under the body again. The two arms will be completely restrained, leaving the abdomen exposed. When restraining the entire body, bring the right portion of the sheet over the abdomen, and tuck it securely under the entire back and out again on the right side.

Another method of restraint is the mummy style (Fig. 29–27). Fold the sheet into a triangle, and place it on the examining table. The distance from the fold to the lower corner of the sheet should be twice the length of the child. Place the child on the sheet, with the fold slightly above the shoulders. Loosen tight clothing and straighten the child's arms and legs. Bring the lower corner of the sheet up over the child's body. The left corner is brought over the body and tucked under the body snugly, leaving the arm exposed. Bring the opposite corner over the exposed arm and under the child's body.

This restraint can be quickly and easily made and can be used to leave either arm exposed while securing the opposite arm and also the legs and body. It may be pinned if necessary. Elbow restraints may be made by using a blood pressure cuff or a towel wrapped around the elbow several times.

To prevent a small child or infant from rolling the head from side to side, stand at the head of the table and support the child's head between the hands, making certain not to press on the ears or on the anterior or posterior fontanel (see Fig. 29–25A). The reverse of this may be restraining a child with your body by taking the place of the physician (Fig. 29–25B), and the physician's working from above the child's head. This may be used for an examination of the child's eyes. A small infant may be placed crosswise on the table that has both the head and base raised slightly, forming a large V in the table. This prevents the infant from rolling, as might happen on a flat surface.

It is not necessary to drape an infant, but the older child's modesty should be respected. Sincere respect and friendly conversation at the child's level accomplishes a great deal. Always be patient with children. Be certain that they understand what is expected. Always involve the parents as much as possible.

PROCTOLOGY

Proctology is the branch of medicine concerned with the disorders of the rectum and anus. Proctoscopy is an examination of the lower rectum and anal canal through a three-inch-long proctoscope. The proctoscope permits detection of hemorrhoids, polyps, fissures, fistulae, and abscesses (Fig. 29–4). The patient may need an enema for this procedure. Sigmoidoscopy is an examination used to view the lower portion of the sigmoid and rectum through a 10- to 12-inch-long sigmoidoscope. The patient is examined in a knee-chest position or on a special jackknife table. The sigmoidoscope aids in the diagnosis of infection, inflammation, and ulcerative conditions and permits actual viewing of tumors and polyps. The patient must have an enema prior to the examination.

Other diagnostic aids used in the diagnosis of colon and rectum disorders include gastrointestinal series (x-ray films), stool cultures, and tests for occult blood in feces.

Disorders and Diseases

Rectocolonic cancer comprises 15 percent of all cancer and accounts for 20 percent of cancer deaths. It usually occurs after the age of 55. In younger patients, it is often associated with ulcerative colitis.

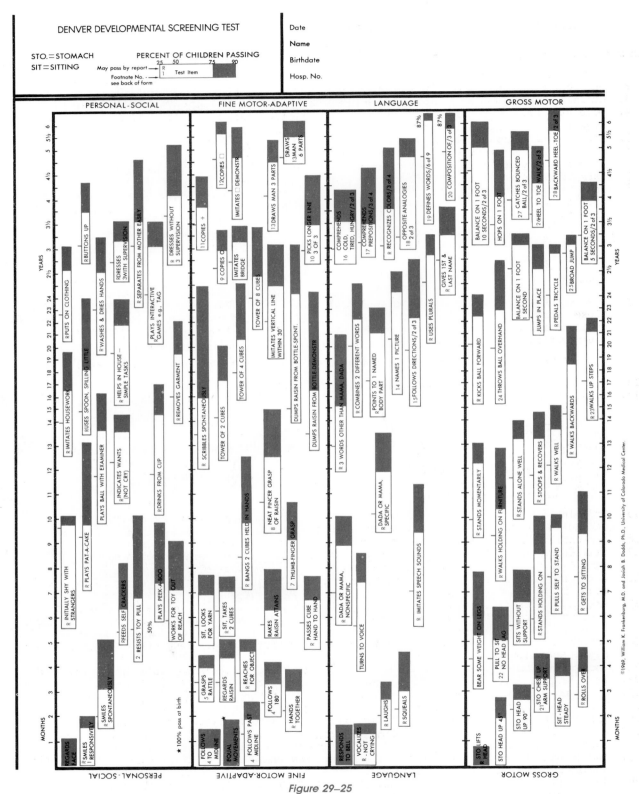

Figure 29–25

The Denver Developmental Screening Test, which is used in most medical offices. (Reprinted with permission, ©1969, William K. Frankenburg, M.D., and Josiah B. Dodds, Ph.D., University of Colorado Medical Center.)

Illustration continued on opposite page

DATE

NAME

DIRECTIONS   BIRTHDATE

HOSP. NO.

1. Try to get child to smile by smiling, talking or waving to him. Do not touch him.
2. When child is playing with toy, pull it away from him. Pass if he resists.
3. Child does not have to be able to tie shoes or button in the back.
4. Move yarn slowly in an arc from one side to the other, about 6" above child's face. Pass if eyes follow 90° to midline. (Past midline; 180°)
5. Pass if child grasps rattle when it is touched to the backs or tips of fingers.
6. Pass if child continues to look where yarn disappeared or tries to see where it went. Yarn should be dropped quickly from sight from tester's hand without arm movement.
7. Pass if child picks up raisin with any part of thumb and a finger.
8. Pass if child picks up raisin with the ends of thumb and index finger using an over hand approach.

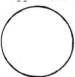

9. Pass any en-closed form. Fail continuous round motions.
10. Which line is longer? (Not bigger.) Turn paper upside down and repeat. (3/3 or 5/6)
11. Pass any crossing lines.
12. Have child copy first. If failed, demonstrate

When giving items 9, 11 and 12, do not name the forms. Do not demonstrate 9 and 11.

29

13. When scoring, each pair (2 arms, 2 legs, etc.) counts as one part.
14. Point to picture and have child name it. (No credit is given for sounds only.)

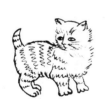   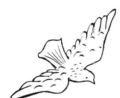   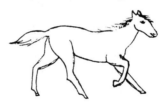   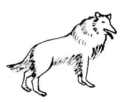   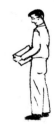

15. Tell child to: Give block to Mommie; put block on table; put block on floor. Pass 2 of 3. (Do not help child by pointing, moving head or eyes.)
16. Ask child: What do you do when you are cold? ..hungry? ..tired? Pass 2 of 3.
17. Tell child to: Put block <u>on</u> table; <u>under</u> table; <u>in front</u> of chair, <u>behind</u> chair. Pass 3 of 4. (Do not help child by <u>pointing, moving head or eyes</u>.)
18. Ask child: If fire is hot, ice is ?; Mother is a woman, Dad is a ?; a horse is big, a mouse is ?. Pass 2 of 3.
19. Ask child: What is a ball? ..lake? ..desk? ..house? ..banana? ..curtain? ..ceiling? ..hedge? ..pavement? Pass if defined in terms of use, shape, what it is made of or general category (such as banana is fruit, not just yellow). Pass 6 of 9.
20. Ask child: What is a spoon made of? ..a shoe made of? ..a door made of? (No other objects may be substituted.) Pass 3 of 3.
21. When placed on stomach, child lifts chest off table with support of forearms and/or hands.
22. When child is on back, grasp his hands and pull him to sitting. Pass if head does not hang back.
23. Child may use wall or rail only, not person. May not crawl.
24. Child must throw ball overhand 3 feet to within arm's reach of tester.
25. Child must perform standing broad jump over width of test sheet. (8-1/2 inches)
26. Tell child to walk forward, 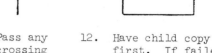 heel within 1 inch of toe. Tester may demonstrate. Child must walk 4 consecutive steps, 2 out of 3 trials.
27. Bounce ball to child who should stand 3 feet away from tester. Child must catch ball with hands, not arms, 2 out of 3 trials.
28. Tell child to walk backward, ◄━◠◠◠◠━ toe within 1 inch of heel. Tester may demonstrate. Child must walk 4 consecutive steps, 2 out of 3 trials.

<u>DATE AND BEHAVIORAL OBSERVATIONS</u> (how child feels at time of test, relation to tester, attention span, verbal behavior, self-confidence, etc,):

Figure 29–25 *Continued*

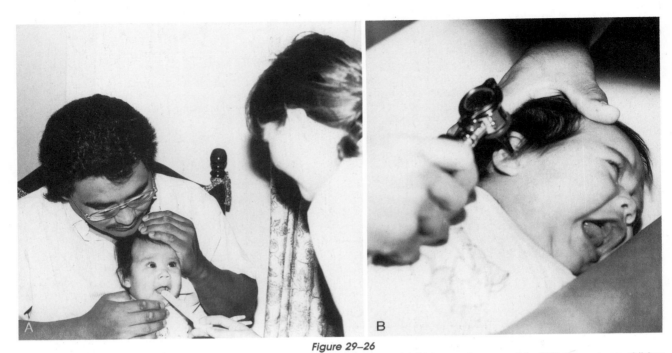

Figure 29–26

A, *Proper method of holding a child for an oral examination. Enlist the child's aid as much as possible. With very young children, parents can be extremely helpful by holding and comforting the child.* **B,** *An acceptable method of immobilizing the head during an ear examination.*

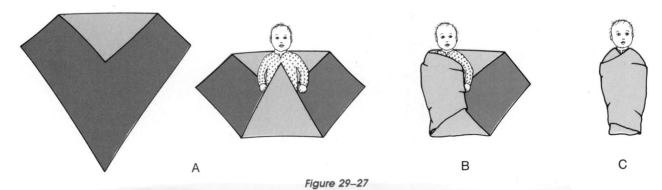

Figure 29–27

A very safe method of restraining an infant. The baby's blanket can serve as the restraining device. **A, B** *and* **C,** *show how to wrap it around the child.*

Rectal cancer is more common in men, while colon cancer is more common in women. Its incidence appears to be associated with low-fiber diets, high-carbohydrate diets, high-fat diets, and genetic factors. At least 70 percent of rectocolonic cancers are anatomically within reach of the sigmoidoscope (ten inches) and approximately 13 percent are found within digital reach (3.2 inches). The American Cancer Society recommends proctoscopy every three years for all persons over the age of 40 and provides an excellent film showing this procedure.

Both the lower portion of the rectum and the anal canal contain vertical folds of mucous membrane called rectal and anal columns. The veins in the mucosa of these folds frequently become dilated, resulting in *hemorrhoids*. They have been associated with standing for long periods, diarrhea, pregnancy, constipation, vomiting, coughing, loss of muscle tone, anorectal infections, hepatitis, and alcoholism.

Polyps are growths protruding from the mucous membrane of the GI tract. There are several varieties, of which most are benign. Most types develop in adults over 45 years of age. Predisposing factors include age, heredity, diet, and infection. Polyps are difficult to diagnose because they are usually asymptomatic and are discovered during sigmoidoscopy or on lower GI x-ray films. The most common symptom is rectal bleeding.

Pruritus ani is associated with itching around the anus, associated with irritation and burning. Contributing factors include excessive rubbing with soap and cloth, poor hygiene, excessive perspiration, spicy foods, diabetes, perfumed toilet paper or colored paper, coffee, alcohol, food preservatives, fungal and parasitic infections, anorectal disease, and certain skin diseases.

Colorectal Examination

Many patients are apprehensive about colorectal examinations. The patient's feelings and concerns must be considered. Most patients suffer from a great deal of anxiety from the moment they enter the examining room. It is important that the assistant create an atmosphere of confidence and calm.

In an attempt to alleviate apprehension, the patient needs to know exactly what to do before the examination begins and may need to be reminded as the examination continues. Let the patient know that the examination is not usually painful, but some discomfort such as cramping can be experienced. Furthermore, the sensations of expelling flatus or of an impending bowel movement may be present. Explain that these sensations are caused by the instruments.

29

Procedure 29–8

ASSISTING WITH PROCTOSIGMOIDOSCOPY

PROCEDURAL GOAL

To assist the physician with the examination of the rectum and colon, to collect specimens as requested, and to promote patient comfort and safety.

EQUIPMENT AND SUPPLIES

Examination table	Basin of water
Sigmoidoscope	Biopsy forceps
Anoscope	Drape sheet
Light source	Patient gown
Suction pump	Towel
Insufflator	Cotton balls
Rectal dressing forceps	Gauze squares
Finger cots	Tissues
Gloves	Specimen bottle with preservative
Lubricating jelly	

Blood and body-fluid protection barriers (goggles, masks, and aprons or gowns), as necessary (see Appendix C, Recommendations for Prevention of AIDS Transmission)

Procedure continued on following page

PROCEDURE

1. Wash your hands. Follow universal blood and body-fluid precautions (see Appendix C). Glove yourself with nonsterile gloves.
2. Assemble the materials in proper order.
   Purpose: To position the instruments according to the physician's preferred order.
3. Test the equipment for proper functioning.
   Purpose: To make certain that the suction device is functioning properly.
4. Identify the patient, and explain the procedure.
5. Instruct the patient to empty his or her bladder.
6. Give the patient a gown, and instruct him or her to remove all clothing from the waist down and to put the gown on with the opening in the back.
7. Assist the patient into the desired position.
   Purpose: Proper positioning is very important for the comfort of the patient and for the accessibility of the rectum and sigmoid colon. The best position can be attained with an adjustable table constructed for this purpose. Special proctologic tables allow the contents of the abdomen to drop forward. The "S" curve of the sigmoid colon is thus allowed to straighten out somewhat, which better accommodates the insertion of the sigmoidoscope.
8. Cover the patient with a drape immediately.
   Purpose: To avoid exposing the patient unnecessarily.
9. Assist the physician as needed. Hand the physician the various instruments and equipment.
   a. Lubricate the physician's gloved finger and instruments.
   b. Attach the inflation bulb to the scope.
   c. Attach the light source to the scope.
   d. Adjust the light source.
   e. Turn on the suction machine.
   f. Hand the biopsy forceps to the physician.
   g. Label the specimen bottle.
10. Observe the patient during the procedure for any undue reactions such as fatigue or fainting, and be ready to offer assistance.
11. Wipe the anal area with tissue at the completion of the examination.
12. Assist the patient into a supine position.
13. Instruct the patient to get dressed.
14. Send the specimen to the laboratory, if collected.
15. Clean the work area.
16. Wash your hands.

TERMINAL PERFORMANCE OBJECTIVE

Given a patient and appropriate supplies, assist in a simulation proctosigmoidoscopy, completing each step correctly and in the correct order, as determined by your evaluator.

UROLOGY

The urologist treats diseases of the genitourinary tract of the male and the urinary tract of the female. Frequently, the urologist works with the gynecologist to treat the female patient. The upper urinary system (kidneys and ureters) is assessed mainly by abdominal palpation. The urinary bladder is palpable when distended, but this is very painful. Much of the urinary survey is dependent on the patient's history, such as frequency or urgency of urination, dysuria, or incontinence. Cystitis is the most common disorder of the bladder, especially in the female. The presence of renal calculi is the most painful. *kidney stones*

A major part of the urologic examination is the urinalysis. The medical assistant must be able to instruct the patient, especially the female, in the collection of a clean-catch urine specimen (see Chapter 35). It is best to have the patient void in the physician's office so that the specimen can be examined immediately. Most urologists prefer to examine a catheterized specimen.

Major complaints presented to the urologist involve changes in the frequency of urination. This is the symptom of several conditions, including *cystitis*, *diabetes mellitus*, and *diabetes insipidus*. This symptom may or may not be accompanied by painful or difficult urination (dysuria). Urgency is another very annoying symptom, since it is the inability to control the release of urine after the desire to urinate occurs. Similar to this is incontinence, the involuntary loss of urine. Stress incontinence is the loss of urine during physical stress, such as during coughing, sneezing, or laughing. This is commonly seen in the **multiparous** woman with a *cystocele* or *urethrocele*.

There are many diagnostic aids in urology, and a complete urinalysis is probably the most common. Renal function tests include determination of serum creatinine and blood urea nitrogen levels. An excretory test is the phenosulfonphthalein test. Frequently employed radiographic studies are the *intravenous pyelogram* and the *retrograde pyelogram*. For the detection of calculi, an x-ray film of the abdomen may show the kidneys, ureters, and bladder. Radioisotopic studies as well as sonography are useful.

Cystoscopy is the examination of the bladder by means of a cystoscope passed through the urethra and into the bladder. The cystoscope illuminates the bladder interior. By means of special lenses and mirrors, the bladder mucosa is examined for inflammation, tumors, and calculi. A catheter can be passed through the cystoscope and on into the ureters and kidneys to obtain samples of urine or to introduce an opaque substance for x-ray films.

There is no special instrument setup for a routine urologic examination unless a special procedure, such as obtaining a catheterized urine specimen, is done. Most offices use prepackaged disposable units for catheterization and for bladder irrigation.

Both male and female patients are disrobed and given a gown. The female is placed in the lithotomy position. The male patient is seated on the examining table, and the physician instructs the patient to do what is needed.

REFERENCES AND READINGS

Bates, B.: *A Guide to Physical Examination,* 2nd ed. Philadelphia, J. B. Lippincott, 1979.

Bonewit, K.: *Clinical Procedures for Medical Assistants,* 2nd ed. Philadelphia, W. B. Saunders Co., 1984.

Cave, J., Hill, J., and Schrader, P. (eds.): *Catalog of Performance Objectives, Criterion-Referenced Measures and Performance Guides for the Medical Assistant.* Kentucky, Vocational-Technical Education Consortium of States, 1978.

Du Gas, B. W.: *Introduction to Patient Care: A Comprehensive Approach to Nursing,* 4th ed. Philadelphia, W. B. Saunders Co., 1983.

Fuller, J. R.: *Surgical Technology: Principles and Practice,* 2nd ed. Philadelphia, W. B. Saunders Co., 1986.

Sherman, J. L., and Fields, S.: *Guide to Patient Evaluation,* 3rd ed. Garden City, NY, Medical Examination Publishing Co., Inc., 1978.

Sorensen, K. C., and Luckmann, J.: *Basic Nursing: A Psychophysiologic Approach,* 2nd ed. Philadelphia, W. B. Saunders Co., 1986.

Wood, L., and Ramber, B. J. (eds.): *Nursing Skills for Allied Health Services.* Philadelphia, W. B. Saunders Co., 1980.

Wyngaarden, J. B., and Smith, L. H., Jr.: *Cecil's Textbook of Medicine,* 16th ed. Philadelphia, W. B. Saunders Co., 1982.

29

CHAPTER OUTLINE

VOCABULARY

See Glossary at end of book for definitions.

abrasion
approximation
caustic
débridement
desquamation

diluent
fascia
lesion
microsurgery
paroxysm

30

Preparing to Assist with Basic Minor Surgery

OBJECTIVES

Upon successful completion of this chapter you should be able to

1. Define and spell the words in the Vocabulary for this chapter.
2. Name and list the usage of ten solutions and medications employed in minor surgery.
3. Identify the types and sizes of suture strands and surgical needles.
4. List all the rules of sterile technique for personnel, the sterile field, and handling equipment.
5. Name five common fears the patient may have when faced with either elective or emergency surgery.
6. State two techniques just prior to minor surgery that may help relieve a patient's fears.
7. Recall at least five preoperative instructions for minor surgery.
8. Name three considerations when choosing the correct patient position for a minor surgical procedure.

Upon successful completion of this chapter you should be able to perform the following activities:

1. Use transfer forceps to move sterile items.
2. Open autoclaved packs to prepare a sterile field for minor surgery.
3. Add sterile items to a sterile field.
4. Remove items from covered, sterile containers.
5. Pour sterile solutions into sterile containers on a sterile field.
6. Glove, using the open-gloving method.
7. Prepare a patient's skin for surgery.

Minor surgery is surgery that is restricted to the management of minor problems and injuries. Almost all medical assistants are expected to glove and assist with the preparation of the sterile field and the patient. A few are expected to assist with outpatient surgical procedures that were once performed in the hospital. Although these more difficult operations may involve complete gowning and gloving with surgical masks and caps, the next two chapters limit discussion and descriptions to the routines necessary to prepare for and assist in minor surgery only. This chapter includes surgical supplies, how to prepare for minor surgery, the difference between a circulating and scrubbed medical assistant, aseptic techniques, and the preoperative preparation of the patient. It prepares you for Chapter 31, in which specific minor surgical procedures and the postoperative care of the patient are presented.

A complete understanding of minor surgery procedures includes material presented in preceding chapters, specifically: Chapter 22, Basic Concepts of Asepsis, in which the principles of microbiology and surgical asepsis can be found; Chapter 23, Sanitization, Disinfection, and Sterilization, in which the processes that do or do not achieve sterility are discussed; and Chapter 24, Instruments for Clinical Procedures and Surgery, which presents the types of instruments used in surgery, their care, and their use. You are urged to refer to these previous chapters frequently while reading these next two.

The following are composites of acceptable procedures and techniques for preparing for minor surgical procedures in the medical office, clinic, and urgent-care center. However, individual practices and preferences may modify some of these procedures as described.

SURGICAL SUPPLIES

When minor surgery is routinely performed, the medical office is usually designed to include a changing room and a recovery area for the patient and a minor surgery room that is separate from the other examining rooms. The minor surgery room should be near a workroom with a sink and an autoclave, if the room does not have its own. It should be easy to clean or decontaminate and uncluttered, to allow easy movement and minimal dust collection. In addition to the operating table, equipment should include a clock with a second sweep, an operating light, sitting stools, and a Mayo-stand. Cabinets with counter tops are necessary to serve as a side or back table during the surgery. All surgical supplies are stored in these cabinets. Supplies used in this room should not be used elsewhere; supplies used elsewhere should not be brought into this room.

Surgical Solutions and Medications

Treatment room supplies include standard solutions and medications that are used in minor surgery and dressing changes. Although the solutions and medications listed here are basic, every practice will have preferred items and methods of applying them. Many of these items are used by the medical assistant. Others are used by the physician only, but the medical assistant is responsible for their care and supply.

Sterile distilled water is kept in two forms. Multiple-dose vials are used for injectable distilled water and as a **diluent** for medications. Larger containers of sterile distilled water are used for rinsing instruments that have been in a chemical disinfectant solution. These containers of sterile rinsing water may be prepared in the office. If you sterilize distilled water in the office, have it periodically tested in a laboratory to confirm sterility.

Sterile physiologic saline solution (0.85 percent sodium chloride) is also stocked in two sizes. The smaller multiple-dose vials are used for injection. The larger containers of physiologic saline are used for rinsing and irrigating wounds. Do not prepare these items in your office; purchase high-quality commercially prepared products.

Povidone-iodine (Betadine) is currently the preferred skin antiseptic. Isopropyl alcohol 70 percent was the antiseptic of choice in the past. Neither of these products is sporicidal. Betadine does not cause the problems of the earlier tincture of iodine and is used in several different ways: as a skin preparation for surgery, as a surgical hand scrub, for saturating dressings, and as a topical ointment.

Surgical soap such as Betadine Scrub, Hibiclens, pHisoHex, Septisol, and Gamophen is used for hand washing, for the patient's skin preparation before surgery, and before the application of an antiseptic.

Hydrogen peroxide (H_2O_2) in a 3 percent solution is used as a mild antiseptic. It kills by its oxidizing power. The oxidizing action creates minute bubbles when applied to a skin **abrasion** or wound and has cleansing action. It is used in irrigations and **débridement** and is nonirritating.

Procaine and lidocaine (Xylocaine) are local anesthetics, and there are many others. They are usually purchased in multiple-dose vials of 30 to 50 cc (ml). When highly vascular areas are involved, anesthetics with epinephrine may be used. Epinephrine causes vasoconstriction at the site, which keeps the anesthetic in the tissues longer, prolonging its effect, and minimizes local bleeding. On the other hand, epinephrine tends to maximize swelling at the site and to distort a close **approximation** of the wound edges. Epinephrine must be used with caution in patients with a history of heart disease.

Tincture of benzoin is applied as a protective coating over ulcers and abrasions. It is used under adhesive tape to increase holding power and to decrease skin sensitivity to the tape. Tincture of benzoin is supplied in spray cans as well as in solution for painting on the skin with an applicator.

Ethyl chloride is used as a skin anesthetic (topical). It is a highly volatile liquid that is sprayed on the skin and evaporates so quickly that the tissue is immediately cooled and numbed. It has a very short duration and is sometimes called "freezing."

Epinephrine,1:1000 (Adrenalin) is a vasoconstrictor used to control hemorrhage, asthmatic **paroxysms**, and shock. It is also used to reverse allergic reactions. Administration can be topical, by inhalation, or parenteral.

Formalin, 10 percent solution, is used to preserve excised tissue for specimens, such as those taken in biopsy or for histologic studies.

Aromatic spirits of ammonia is supplied in bottles or in small glass ampules covered with cotton gauze to prevent injury when they are crushed to open. It is most commonly used for fainting, although recent studies have shown that its dangers may far outweigh any advantages for certain patients.

Vaseline (petroleum jelly, or petrolatum) is used to impregnate gauze squares or strips. It is packaged and sterilized by commercial manufacturers.

Iodoform gauze strips are slender strips of gauze, ¼ to ½ in wide, impregnated with iodoform (96 percent iodine). They are used to pack an abscess, acting as a wick to draw out the infection and as a local antibacterial (Fig. 30–1).

Silver nitrate (AgNO₃) is available in solution or coated on applicator sticks. It is a **caustic** and is

applied topically. It must be kept in light-proof brown containers. The most commonly used solution is 20 percent, but 10 percent and 50 percent solutions are frequently employed. The applicator sticks are convenient for touching oral and nasal **lesions.** Silver nitrate may be used to promote the healing process after surgery.

Instruments

See Chapter 24, Instruments for Clinical Procedures and Minor Surgery.

Accessory Supplies

In addition to surgical instruments, there are other pieces of equipment frequently used in minor surgery.

An *electrosurgical unit* is used to cauterize blood vessels and incise tissue with an electric current.

Fiberoptic lights and headlights supply an intense light in a small area.

Wound drains are rubber drains introduced into wounds at the end of a surgical procedure, if the wound is filled with fluid or is oozing (Fig. 30–2).

Surgical sponges are used to absorb blood and protect tissues during surgery. They also may be used to wipe blood or other debris from the instruments. The 4 × 4 gauze square is used in most minor surgery.

30

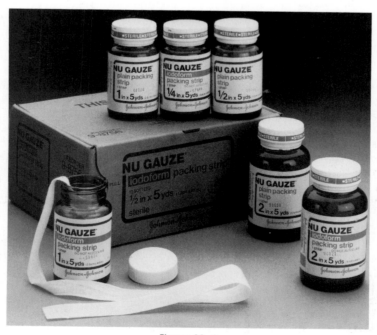

Figure 30–1

Commercially prepared iodoform gauze (Nu Gauze) for packing an abscess and to facilitate drainage. (Courtesy of Johnson and Johnson Products, Inc., New Brunswick, NJ.)

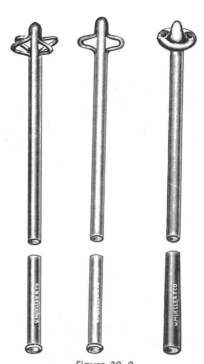

Figure 30–2

Rubber wound drains. (Courtesy of V. Mueller.) (From Fuller, J. R.: Surgical Technology, 2nd ed. Philadelphia, W. B. Saunders Co., 1986.)

Syringes and needles are used to inject local anesthetics, to aspirate fluids from a wound, and to irrigate wounds.

Commercially prepared *disposable packs* are available for most minor surgical procedures. They are time-savers and convenient because they can eliminate linen laundering and supply autoclaving. Their disadvantages include high cost and their lack of custom-designed contents to suit regional prac-

tices and preferences. Available packs include towel packs, skin prep packs, irrigation sets, suture sets, suture removal sets, catheterization sets, biopsy sets, and shave prep packs (Fig. 30–3).

Disposable Drapes

Commercially prepared, paper drapes have a plastic coating on the underside that is nonabsorbent. This barrier reduces the risk of contamination by capillary attraction (see Chapter 22). Disposable drapes are available in several different materials and sizes and may contain an opening (fenestration) for the operative site. A special incisional drape has an adhesive backing around the opening to prevent slippage (Fig. 30–4). This clear incisional drape adheres to the patient's cleansed skin and remains taped to the area throughout the procedure. The skin incision is made with the scalpel through the adhesive drape. In minor surgery in the medical office, disposable drapes are rapidly replacing the use of autoclaved linen towels and towel clamps (Fig. 30–5).

Suture Materials

The word *suture* is used as both a noun and a verb. As a noun, it refers to a surgical stitch or to the material used; as a verb, it refers to the act of stitching. Sutures were used as long ago as 2000 BC. History does not record the first surgical operations and the use of sutures, but ancient medical writings do make reference to using sinews and strings to tie off blood vessels and control bleeding. Hippocrates wrote of his use of sutures, and Aesculapius was said to have used sutures during the

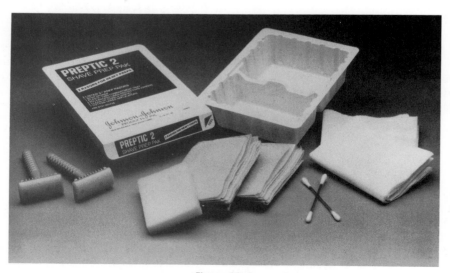

Figure 30–3

This disposable shaving prep kit (Preptic) contains all the necessary items except water. (Courtesy of Johnson and Johnson Products, Inc., New Brunswick, NJ.)

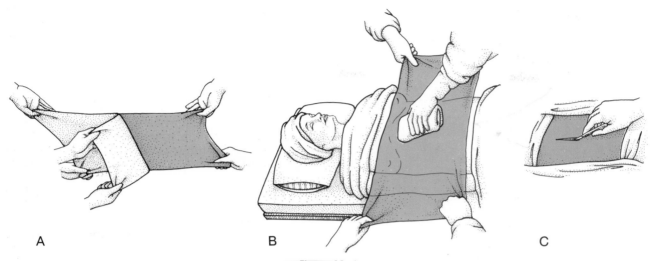

A   B   C

Figure 30–4
Application of the adhesive-backed incisional drape.

Trojan War. Before Joseph Lister, infection and suppuration were inevitable when a wound was closed by sutures. Modern surgery and the use of sutures began in 1865, when Lister developed antisepsis and the disinfection of suture materials. Many kinds of materials have been used over the centuries, including precious metals, horsehair, animal tendons, and cotton and linen cord. Most of the improvements in suture materials and techniques have occurred in the last 50 years.

A suture may also be used as a *ligature*. This is a strand of suture material used to tie off a blood vessel or to strangulate tissue. A ligature may be tied around a skin growth and left there until the growth is strangulated and falls off. If a ligature is used to tie off an internal tubular structure, it must last permanently or long enough for the structure itself to disintegrate. To *ligate* means to apply a ligature.

Types of Sutures

Sutures may be classified as either absorbable or nonabsorbable (Fig. 30–6). The absorbable suture is one that is dissolved and absorbed by the body's enzymes during the process of wound healing; therefore, these sutures do not have to be removed. It is often referred to as surgical gut, and sometimes incorrectly called "catgut." The name came from the use of sheep intestines as fiddle strings by the Arabs. The Arabic word for fiddle is "kit," and these "kitgut" strings were used by surgeons for suturing.

Surgical gut is still made from sheep or beef intestines. Surgical gut that is untreated is called *plain* catgut and is absorbed by the body in five to seven days. Plain catgut is used mostly in tissues that heal rapidly, such as the mucous membrane and subcutaneous tissue.

Chromic catgut is treated with chromic salts, which slows its absorption rate in the tissues. Chromic catgut can last 20 to 40 days before absorption. It causes less inflammation than does plain catgut and is widely used in gynecologic and urologic surgery. Surgical gut must be dipped (not soaked) in a sterile saline solution just before use to soften it. To straighten the strand, grasp each end and pull with a gentle, continuous motion. Never jerk the strand, and handle the material at a minimum to avoid fraying of the suture.

Nonabsorbable sutures are more frequently used

30

used
inside

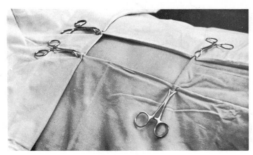

Figure 30–5
Four towels secured with towel clamps mark the boundary of the operative site. (From Nealon, T. F.: Fundamental Skills in Surgery, 3rd ed. Philadelphia, W. B. Saunders Co., 1979.)

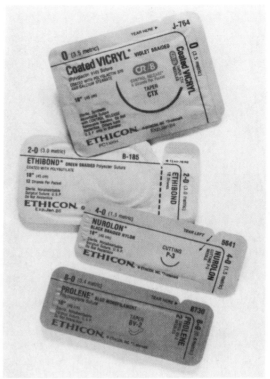

Figure 30–6
Suture packets labeled according to size, type, and length of suture material, type of needle point, and shape of the needle. Note: The second packet from the top contains sutures but no needle. (Courtesy of Ethicon, Inc.)

in the medical office because the majority of suturing is superficial and in areas where the sutures are removed after healing has taken place. These removable sutures are made of many different materials.

Silk is used in a wide variety of tissues because it is easy to tie yet strong. It is treated with Teflon or a similar coating to prevent snagging of the tissue and flaking. *Dermal silk* has an additional coating to allow it to last a little longer in the body.

Surgical cotton is tough and resistant but not as strong as silk. It is used in the same applications as silk but is not as popular. Cotton may be strengthened by dipping the strands in sterile saline before use. Like silk, it is a multifilament (braided) natural fiber and has a tendency to flake.

Stainless steel is the strongest of all sutures and is very well tolerated by the body, but it has distinct disadvantages. Surgical steel is difficult to handle: it can puncture the glove and cause injury to the person handling it. It is easily contaminated during the procedure, and it tends to have a sawing effect on the tissue. Steel is used mostly in orthopedic surgery and on the abdominal **fascia** when great strength is needed. *Surgical staples* are made of stainless steel.

Polyester suture is the second strongest of all the suture materials. It is a multifilament strand coated with Teflon and is used in facial, ophthalmic, and cardiovascular surgery.

Nylon suture is strong, with a high degree of elasticity, and is relatively nonirritating to the tissue. It is supplied in braided or monofilament strands. Because it is so elastic and yet stiff, nylon necessitates placing many knots, and the knots tend to untie if not placed correctly. Nylon is used mostly for skin closure and **microsurgical** procedures.

The sizes of suture material are standard, as set by the *United States Pharmacopeia*. The size is determined by the diameter of the strand. Sutures range from 11–0 (the smallest) to 1–0 (the largest). The higher the number, the smaller the diameter. The 2–0 to 6–0 is used most frequently in the medical office. Another method of writing the suture size is 000 instead of 3–0, 0000 instead of 4–0, and so forth.

Needles

Surgical needles are chosen according to the area in which they are to be used and the depth and width of the desired stitch. They are classified according to shape and by the type of point, shaft, and eye (Fig. 30–7). The shape of a needle may be straight or curved. Straight needles are not easily manipulated and are restricted to use on the surface tissue. A curved needle allows the surgeon to swing the needle beneath the surface and then back up again on the other side. The sharper the curve of the needle, the deeper the surgeon can pass the needle. The point of a needle can be a taper or a cutting edge. A taper is used on delicate tissues; the cutting edge lacerates the skin as the needle is passed through, which is advantageous on the tougher tissues, such as the skin and connective tissue. The head of the needle can have an eye or can be eyeless. Eyeless needles are also called *atraumatic* because they cause the least amount of tissue trauma as the needle is pulled through. Manufacturers supply the suture strands with the suture needle attached in peel-apart packages, or separate needle packs and continuous reels of suture that will need to be autoclaved as used. The majority of suture materials used in the medical office are prepackaged, with the suture strand and needle attached. The most common needle type for minor skin repair is the curved, cutting-edged, atraumatic needle.

PREPARATION FOR SURGERY

Procedure File

Keep a card file for each procedure, listing the preferences of each physician in the office. This is

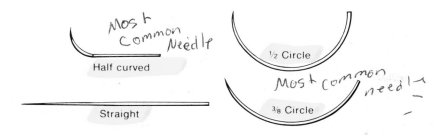

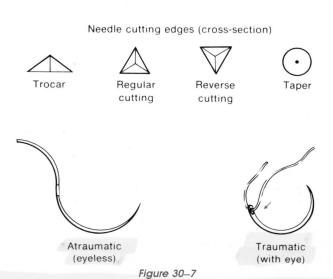

Figure 30–7

Needle shapes and the types of needle points and eyes. Most needles used in the medical office are the atraumatic type.

particularly helpful for complicated procedures and procedures that are seldom performed. Color-code the 5 × 8 cards for each physician, and keep the information current. The cards usually contain information on the following:

- Preoperative instructions
- Preoperative and operative medications
- Universal blood and body-fluid precautions, listing specific protection barriers (goggles, masks, gowns, aprons, and gloves) to be worn by the surgeon and the assistants (see Appendix C, Recommendations for Prevention of AIDS Transmission)
- Instruments used
- Syringe and needle sizes
- Glove sizes
- Postoperative instructions
- The number of days to the scheduled follow-up appointment

A more detailed procedures manual should be developed by you and the physicians. These procedures should be reviewed at regular intervals for revision and development. See Chapter 19 for directions on how to write a procedures manual.

Preparing Sterile Packs

Surgical packs must be prepared the day before the procedure or at least in enough time for the pack to be dry and cool for the procedure. (See Chapter 23, Sanitization, Disinfection, and Sterilization.)

- Before closing the pack to be autoclaved, take a count, on at least two separate occasions, of the items required for the procedure. Use your procedure file card for guidance.
- If the items are numerous, label the pack with the name of the procedure rather than the individual contents.
- Sterilize transfer forceps in a separate pack. If you are not gloved, use the sterile transfer forceps to arrange the instruments on the sterile field in their sequence of use.
- If disposable, sterile towels and drapes are not used, you may autoclave linen towels, one or two to a package. Fanfold the towels so they may be unfolded easily with the transfer forceps.
- In many cases, an entire setup may be autoclaved in one pack (instruments, sponges,

dressings, suture materials, syringes, and needles), but you must be certain that the pack is not so thick that it prevents steam circulation to all the parts of the pack.

- Sterility indicators should be placed in the very middle of large packs to indicate whether or not there is proper sterilization throughout the pack.
- In case of contamination, it is always best to have more than one pack ready for every procedure.

ASEPTIC TECHNIQUE

There is no mystery about aseptic technique. Handling sterile items requires a degree of dexterity and vigilance, but it is really a matter of concentration, with planned movements and steps.

Although the procedures outlined in this chapter and the next are for minor surgery, all the sterile techniques of major surgery must be observed. To have a sound knowledge of sterility and sterile technique, start with the analogy: **Everything sterile is white, everything that is not sterile is black, and there is no gray**.

Sterile surfaces must not come into contact with nonsterile surfaces. Honesty is important; an incomplete or incorrect step may lead to serious wound contamination and postoperative infection.

Personnel

Hands and hair are the two greatest sources of contamination. With practice, you will learn to know what may be touched with the hands and what must be touched only with sterile forceps or sterile gloved hands. Hair that is allowed to fall free over the shoulders and forward will give off a cloud of bacteria; it must be contained back and off the shoulders. In addition, the following rules are fundamental:

- Remember that air currents carry bacteria, so body motions and talking over a sterile field should be kept to a minimum.
- Sterile team members face each other.
- If you lose the sterile field from your line of vision, you can no longer assume the field is sterile; therefore, never turn your back on a sterile field or wander away from the sterile field.
- Nonsterile persons do not reach over a sterile field.

The Sterile Field

A sterile field is any sterile surface, usually containing sterile items. In surgery, a sterile field is created by draping sterile towels, prepackaged or from autoclaved packs, over a Mayo stand or table. A sterile field is also the draped surgical site after the patient's skin has been prepped and draped for surgery. The following rules demonstrate correct field techniques:

- Sterile field towels and sterile table drapes are fanfolded so that they may be unfolded easily by lifting one edge.
- If an entire setup is in a single package and is double-wrapped, the wrappings can be left underneath as the sterile table drape.
- Sterile tables are sterile only at table height.
- Any item below your waist level must be considered contaminated.
- A 1-in edge around the entire sterile field is considered not sterile.
- The edges of all wrappers, packs, and towels are considered not sterile.
- The sides of containers are considered not sterile.
- Sterile goods must not be allowed to come into contact with the 1-in edge around the sterile field, the edges of wrappers, or the sides of containers.
- If the sterility of an item is questionable, consider the item contaminated.

Moisture

Moisture carries bacteria from a nonsterile surface to a sterile surface, therefore:

- A sterile field placed on a drop of moisture results in the contamination of the field.
- Spills contaminate a sterile field.
- A sterile field remains sterile only as long as it is dry.

Handling Equipment

When two medical assistants work with the surgeon, one serves as the circulating assistant and the other serves as the scrub assistant. The scrub assistant washes with the surgical scrub, may perform the patient skin prep, and gloves for the procedure. During the procedure, the scrubbed assistant receives only sterile items, cares for the open sterile field, and passes instruments and supplies to the surgeon. The circulating assistant wears nonsterile gloves, opens sterile supplies before and during the procedure, helps position the patient for the procedure, may perform the scrub prep of the patient, and handles all nonsterile equipment in the room during the procedure. Before every surgery, the team members review which universal blood and body-fluid precautions (such as goggles, masks, aprons, and special procedures) are necessary for the procedure.

If you are the single assistant, you must do all of these functions. The order in which you do things is vital. If you do not do things in the proper order, you might find yourself gloved and sterile with no packs open or with a nonsterile item to retrieve, or you may find that the surgeon is waiting and you cannot work because you do not have on your gloves. Not only is it important to learn aseptic technique, but it is important to learn, step-by-step, how to get from the beginning to the end. Table 30–1 outlines the chronologic steps for the single assistant who must function as both the circulating and the scrub assistants, and Table 30–2 outlines the same steps for the two-assistant team during a minor surgical procedure.

Transfer Forceps. The first sterile procedure that you must master is the use of transfer forceps. If you are the circulating assistant and your hands are not gloved, you must use sterile transfer forceps to touch sterile items or to pass sterile items to the scrub assistant's or surgeon's hand. Even if you are not working with surgical patients, there is rarely a day that you will not need to transfer some sterile item from the autoclave or a sterile package. Sterile transfer forceps may be autoclaved and kept dry in a pack or may be submersed in a sterile solution. The solution must be fresh and the container filled. At the time you change the solution, re-autoclave the transfer forceps and the container. The Bard-Parker transfer forceps, with its closed container system and spring-loaded inner lining, is sometimes preferred over the traditional open container. The closed system may prevent contamination from the air and dust, and the forceps are designed so that they cannot touch the sides of the container. This system must be changed, cleaned, and autoclaved as often as the open systems.

Table 30–1
Preparation for Minor Surgery: Single-Assistant Preparation

1. Wash your hands; gather all supplies STERILE SIDE (Mayo tray): two towel packs; skin-prep pack; patient drape pack; instrument pack; miscellaneous pack(s); three glove packs; masks; goggles; aprons or gowns NONSTERILE SIDE (side counter): syringes; suture material; anesthesia; solutions; additional sponges; dressings; bandages; transfer forceps; waste basin; waste receptacle; nonsterile gloves; masks; goggles; aprons or gowns 2. Escort patient into the room 3. Greet and converse with patient 4. Position patient on table 5. Wash your hands 6. Open first towel pack 7. Open skin prep pack 8. Pour soap and antiseptic solutions 9. Expose the site to be prepped 10. Scrub with the surgical hand wash 11. Glove and arrange sterile field 12. Place sterile towels at skin scrub boundaries 13. Prep the patient's skin 14. Discard skin prep materials 15. Discard gloves; wash your hands 16. Open table drape pack on Mayo stand to create sterile field 17. Open instrument pack(s), and transfer instruments to sterile field. Add sterile syringe unit 18. Add sterile items as requested	19. PHYSICIAN JOINS YOU AND CONVERSES WITH THE PATIENT 20. Open physician's glove pack (PHYSICIAN NOW GLOVES) 21. Open patient drape pack (PHYSICIAN NOW DRAPES THE SURGICAL SITE) 22. Cleanse and hold up anesthesia vial for physician to withdraw anesthesia with sterile syringe (PHYSICIAN WILL NOW ADMINISTER THE ANESTHESIA) 23. Repeat surgical hand wash; reglove with a new glove pack 24. Arrange sterile field instruments and other materials for safety and in sequence; check instrument condition 25. Unwind suture materials, load the first suture into the needle holder 26. Place two gauze sponges at the site 27. Assist the procedure* For PHYSICIAN—instrument pass; maintain field; anticipate needs; cut sutures For PATIENT—retract tissue; sponge blood from wound; specimen care 28. Remove gloves 29. Escort patient to recovery area; reglove 30. Record and prepare specimens 31. Clean the room; clear materials; discard gloves 32. Chart the procedure on the medical record 33. Help the patient to prepare to leave the office 34. Disinfect and sterilize equipment at first available time

*By law, the assistant may not clamp tissue, place sutures, or alter body tissues in any way.

30

Table 30–2

Preparation for Minor Surgery: Two-Assistant Team Preparation

Circulating Assistant	Scrub Assistant
1. Wash your hands; gather all supplies STERILE SIDE (Mayo tray): two towel packs; skin prep pack; patient drape pack; instrument pack; miscellaneous pack(s); three glove packs; masks; goggles; aprons or gowns NONSTERILE SIDE (side counter): syringes; suture material; anesthesia; solutions; additional sponges; dressings; bandages; transfer forceps; waste basin; waste receptacle; nonsterile gloves; masks; goggles; aprons or gowns 2. Escort patient into the room 3. Wash your hands; glove if necessary 4. Position patient on table 5. Expose the site to be prepped; discard gloves 6. Rewash your hands 7. Open one glove pack for your team member 8. Open first towel pack 9. Open skin-prep pack 10. Pour soap and antiseptic solutions 11. Open glove pack for team member 12. Open table-drape pack on Mayo stand to create sterile field 13. Open instrument pack(s), and transfer instruments to sterile field. Add sterile syringe unit 14. Add sterile items as requested	1. Scrub with the surgical hand wash, in preparation for the procedure 2. Greet and converse with the patient 3. Glove 4. Place sterile towels at skin-scrub boundaries 5. Arrange skin-prep sterile field 6. Prep the patient's skin; discard skin prep materials 7. Discard gloves; repeat surgical hand wash 8. Reglove with new glove pack 9. Arrange sterile field instruments for safety and in sequence; check instrument condition 10. Arrange additional items as needed
PHYSICIAN JOINS THE TEAM NOW AND CONVERSES WITH THE PATIENT	
15. Open physician's glove pack 16. Open patient drape pack 17. Cleanse and hold up anesthesia vial for scrub assistant to withdraw anesthesia 18. Open additional items during the procedure 19. Escort patient to recovery area 20. Remove clean items to work area; reglove 21. Clean room 22. Disinfect and sterilize equipment; discard gloves 23. Help the patient prepare to leave the office; schedule next appointment	11. Unwind suture materials, load the first suture into needle holder 12. Assist physician in draping patient 13. Insert syringe and needle into the vial, and draw out desired amount of anesthesia 14. Pass anesthesia to physician 15. Place two gauze sponges at the site 16. Assist with the procedure* For SURGEON—instrument pass; maintain field; anticipate needs; cut sutures For PATIENT—retract tissue; sponge blood from wound; specimen care 17. Record and prepare specimens 18. Clear contaminated supplies 19. Sanitize equipment 20. Remove gloves 21. Chart the procedure on the medical record

*By law, the scrub assistant may not clamp tissue, place sutures, or alter body tissues in any way.

Procedure 30-1

PROCEDURAL GOAL

As a circulating assistant, use transfer forceps to move sterile items on a sterile field or to transfer sterile items to a gloved team member.

EQUIPMENT AND SUPPLIES

A sterile transfer forceps in a sterile forceps container or a Bard-Parker container
A sterile item to move or transfer
A Mayo stand set up with a sterile field and sterile instruments
A sterile gauze sponge in an individual wrapper

PROCEDURE

1. Wash your hands, and dry them carefully.
   Purpose: Water on your hands could run down the forceps and contaminate the forceps and the sterile solution.
2. Peel open the sterile 4 × 4 or 3 × 3 gauze package, and set it down on the counter with the gauze sponge exposed and laying on the inside of the wrapper.
3. Remove the forceps by pulling it straight up and out of the solution, without touching the sides of the container.
   Purpose: If you turn the tips upward, the solution will run onto the nonsterile area and then back down over the sterile end when you turn the tips down again, thus contaminating the forceps and the solution when you return the forceps to the container.
4. Dry the forceps by touching them, points down, to the piece of dry, sterile gauze.
   Purpose: Wet forceps will contaminate a sterile field.
5. Grasp an item on the field with the forceps, points down, and move it to its proper position for the procedure (below, left).
6. Or, transfer an instrument to the surgeon's gloved hand (below, right).
7. Return the forceps, points down, into the forceps container, without touching the container sides.

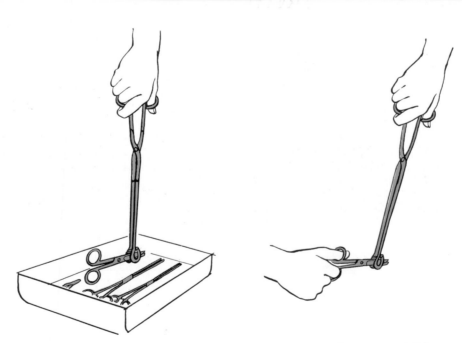

Procedure continued on following page

TERMINAL PERFORMANCE OBJECTIVE

Given the necessary supplies and equipment, move a sterile item into proper position on the sterile field, or transfer the sterile item to the surgeon's hand, within 15 seconds, without a break in sterile technique, as determined by your evaluator.

Procedure 30–2

OPENING AN AUTOCLAVED LINEN PACK THAT WILL SERVE AS THE STERILE TABLE DRAPE

PROCEDURAL GOAL

As a circulating assistant, open an autoclaved pack that contains a linen table drape, using correct aseptic technique.

EQUIPMENT AND SUPPLIES

An autoclaved pack that contains an inner linen towel that will serve as the sterile table drape
A Mayo stand
Disinfectant and gauze sponges

PROCEDURE

1. Check to see that the Mayo stand is dust free and clean. If it is not, clean it with 70% alcohol, or another disinfectant, and gauze sponges.
   Purpose: Although some areas cannot be sterile, steps must be taken to keep contamination to a minimum.
2. Wash your hands, and dry them carefully.
   Purpose: Moisture on your hands contaminates the pack.
3. Place the autoclaved pack on the Mayo stand, and read the label.
   Purpose: Most medical offices have a limited supply of surgical packs; to open a wrong package could mean not having enough instruments for a different procedure.
4. Check the expiration date.
   Purpose: An expired pack is not considered sterile.
5. Position the package so that the outer envelope-flap is face up and at the top as you look at the package (below, left).
   Purpose: This positions the pack for correct opening, using aseptic technique.
6. Open the first flap away from you (below, right).
   Purpose: Otherwise, you will be reaching over a sterile field for the other three flaps.

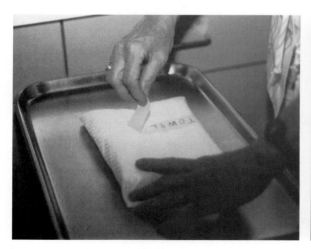
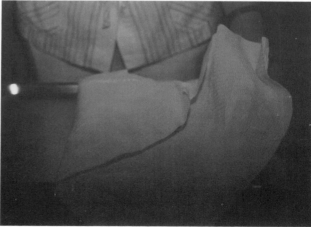

Procedure continued on opposite page

7. Next, pull away the two side flaps. Be careful to lift each flap by reaching under the small folded-back tab and without touching the inner surface of the pack or its contents (below, left).
Purpose: The tab and the outside surface are considered touchable and not sterile. Inside the 1-in tab, the inner surface is considered sterile and not touchable.
8. The last flap is pulled toward you by its tab, exposing the towel (below, right).

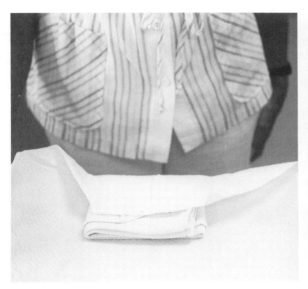 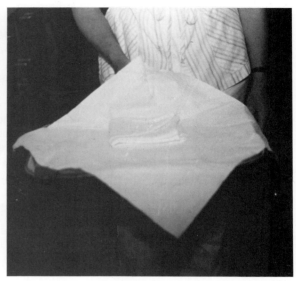

9. Using sterile forceps (or a gloved hand) open the four-folded inside linen in the same manner as steps 6 through 8 previously listed.
10. You now have a sterile table drape as a sterile field to work from and for the distribution of additional sterile supplies and instruments.

TERMINAL PERFORMANCE OBJECTIVE

Given the necessary supplies and equipment, open a sterile linen pack, within 30 seconds and without a break in sterile technique, as determined by your evaluator.

Procedure 30–3

OPENING AN AUTOCLAVED PACK (SETUP) THAT WILL SERVE AS THE STERILE FIELD

PROCEDURAL GOAL

As a circulating assistant, open an autoclaved pack that contains a complete setup, using correct aseptic technique.

EQUIPMENT AND SUPPLIES

An autoclaved pack that contains an entire setup
A Mayo stand
Disinfectant and gauze sponges

PROCEDURE

1. Check to see that the mayo stand is dust free and clean. If it is not, clean it with 70% alcohol, or another disinfectant, and gauze sponges.

Procedure continued on following page

30

Purpose: Although some areas cannot be sterile, steps must be taken to keep contamination to a minimum.

2. Wash your hands, and dry them carefully.
   Purpose: Moisture on your hands contaminates the pack.
3. Place the autoclaved pack on the Mayo stand, and read the label.
   Purpose: Most medical offices have a limited supply of surgical packs; to open a wrong package could mean not having enough instruments for a different procedure.
4. Check the expiration date.
   Purpose: An expired pack is not considered sterile.
5. Position the package so that the outer envelope-flap is face up and at the top as you look at the package.
   Purpose: This positions the pack for correct opening, using aseptic technique.
6. Open the first flap away from you.
   Purpose: Otherwise, you will be reaching over a sterile field for the other three flaps.
7. Next, pull away the two side flaps. Be careful to lift each flap by reaching under the small folded-back tab and without touching the inner surface of the pack or its contents.
   Purpose: The tab and the outside surface are considered touchable and not sterile. Inside the 1-in tab, the inner surface is considered sterile and not touchable.
8. The last flap is pulled toward you by its tab, exposing the contents.

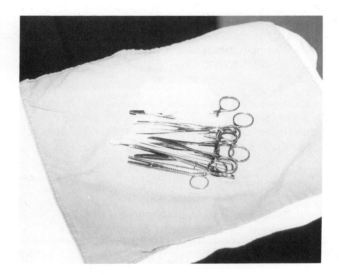

TERMINAL PERFORMANCE OBJECTIVE

Given the necessary supplies and equipment, open a sterile setup pack, within 30 seconds and without a break in sterile technique, as determined by your evaluator.

Procedure 30–4

OPENING A STERILE PACK TO ADD ITS CONTENTS TO A STERILE FIELD

PROCEDURAL GOAL

As a circulating assistant, add instruments from a sterile pack to a sterile field, using correct aseptic technique.

EQUIPMENT AND SUPPLIES

An autoclaved pack that contains at least three instruments or other sterile items
A Mayo stand set up with a sterile field

PROCEDURE

1. Wash your hands, and dry them carefully.
   Purpose: Moisture on your hands contaminates the pack.
2. Position the pack on the palm of your minor hand so that the outer envelope-flap is face up and at the top as you look at the package (below, left).
   Purpose: This positions the pack for correct opening, using aseptic technique.
3. Open the first flap away from you (below, right).
   Purpose: Otherwise, you will be reaching over a sterile field for the other three flaps.

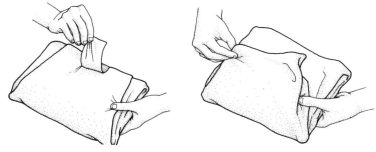

4. Next, pull away the two side flaps. Be careful to lift each flap by reaching under the small folded-back tab and without touching the inner surface of the pack or its contents (below, left).
   Purpose: The tab and the outside surface are considered touchable and not sterile. Inside the 1-in tab, the inner surface is considered sterile and not touchable.
5. The last flap is pulled toward you by its tab, exposing the contents (below, center).
6. By closing your open palm, grasp the items through the cloth at the tip ends (below, right).
   Note: To make this possible, all items must be autoclaved in the same direction.

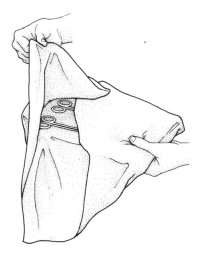
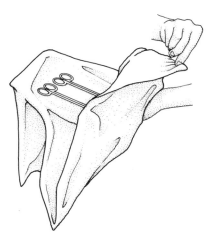
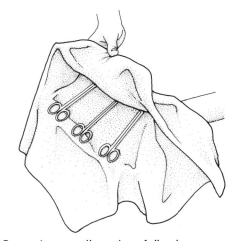

Procedure continued on following page

7. Hold the four flaps back around your wrist with your major hand (below, left).
   Purpose: All parts of the four flaps are now considered not sterile, and you do not want them to touch any part of the instruments or the sterile field.
8. Slide the items, handles first, onto the field.
   Purpose: To avoid damaging the fine tips.
9. Do not reach over the field, yet place the instruments inside the perimeter of the 1-in barrier.
   Purpose: The 1-in perimeter around the sterile field is considered not sterile.
10. Or, hand the items to a gloved team member (below, right).

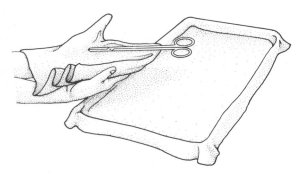 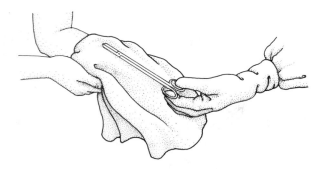

TERMINAL PERFORMANCE OBJECTIVE

Given the necessary supplies and equipment, open a sterile pack and add its contents to a sterile field, within 30 seconds and without a break in sterile technique, as determined by your evaluator.

Procedure 30–5   *ADDING STERILE ITEMS IN A PEEL-BACK WRAPPER TO A STERILE FIELD*

PROCEDURAL GOAL

As a circulating assistant, add the contents of a sterile pack, such as syringes, needles, and suture materials, to the sterile field, using correct sterile technique.

EQUIPMENT AND SUPPLIES

A package containing suture material
A package containing a disposable syringe and needle
A Mayo stand set up with a sterile field

PROCEDURE

1. Wash your hands, and dry them carefully.
   Purpose: Moisture on your hands contaminates the pack.
2. Off to the side of the sterile field, hold the pack in your hand and read the label.
   Purpose: Most medical offices have a limited supply of items; to open a wrong package could mean not having enough supplies for a different procedure.

Procedure continued on opposite page

3. Hold the pack, and grab a peel-away edge in each hand.
4. Open by peeling the two flaps apart. Keep the flaps away from the sterile item by holding them outward. The item should be sticking straight out from between the peel-back sides (below, left). *Purpose:* The edges of a sterile pack are considered not sterile.
5. Continue to peel with a snap of the hands to "pop" the items out of the package and onto the field from a distance of about 8 to 12 in. Do not reach over the field, yet place the item inside the perimeter of the 1-in barrier (below, right).

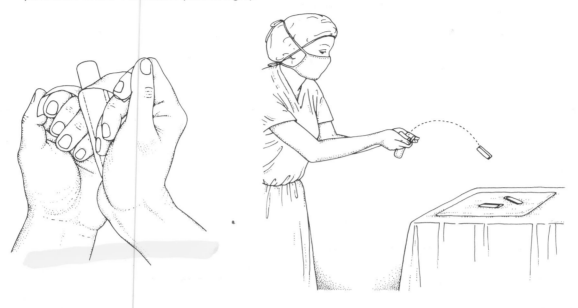

TERMINAL PERFORMANCE OBJECTIVE

Given the necessary supplies and equipment, add sterile prepackaged items to a sterile field, within 30 seconds, without a break in sterile technique, as determined by your evaluator.

Procedure 30–6

REMOVING ITEMS FROM A COVERED, STERILE CONTAINER

PROCEDURAL GOAL

As a circulating assistant, remove items from a covered, sterile jar.

EQUIPMENT AND SUPPLIES

Sterile items in a covered, sterile jar
Sterile transfer forceps
A Mayo stand set up with a sterile field

PROCEDURE

1. Wash your hands, and dry them carefully.
   Purpose: Water on your hands could run down the forceps and contaminate the forceps and the sterile solution.
2. Lift the lid straight up, then slightly to one side. Hold the lid in your hand with it facing downward.
   Purpose: Air currents carry contaminants that could settle on the inside of the lid.

Procedure continued on following page

3. Remove the item from the container with the transfer forceps by pulling the item straight up, without touching the sides of the container.
Purpose: The sides of containers are considered not sterile.

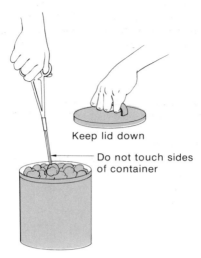

Keep lid down

Do not touch sides of container

4. While still holding the item with the transfer forceps, replace the lid.
Purpose: Sterile jars should be exposed to the air as little as possible.
5. Add the item to the sterile field with the transfer forceps.
6. If the lid must be placed on the side counter, then place it inside up, taking care not to touch the inside surface.
Purpose: The counter top contaminates the sterile, inner surface if the lid is placed inside down.
7. Replace the lid as soon as possible.
Purpose: Sterile jars should be exposed to the air as little as possible.

TERMINAL PERFORMANCE OBJECTIVE

Given the necessary supplies and equipment, transfer a sterile item from a covered container to a sterile field, within 30 seconds, without a break in sterile technique, as determined by your evaluator.

Procedure 30-7

POURING A STERILE SOLUTION INTO A CONTAINER ON A STERILE FIELD

PROCEDURAL GOAL

As a circulating assistant, pour a sterile solution into a stainless steel bowl or medicine glass that is sitting at the edge of a sterile field.

EQUIPMENT AND SUPPLIES

A sterile bottle of solution
A stainless steel bowl or medicine glass
A sterile field
A sink or waste receptacle
Note: A medicine glass or bowl on the sterile field should be near one edge of the field but inside the perimeter of the 1-in barrier.

Procedure continued on opposite page

PROCEDURE

1. Wash your hands, and dry them carefully.
   Purpose: Moisture on your hand may cause the bottle to slip from your hand.
2. Place your hand over the label, and lift the bottle. Note: If the container has a double cap, set the outer cap on the counter inside up (see Procedure 30–5, Step 6), then proceed with Step 3.
3. Lift the lid of the bottle straight up, and then slightly to one side, and hold the lid in your minor hand facing downward.
   Purpose: Air currents carry contaminants that could settle on the inside of the lid.
4. Pour away from the label.
   Purpose: Spills down the side of the bottle stain or make the label unreadable.
5. If the container does not have a double cap, pour off a small amount of the solution into a waste receptacle.
   Purpose: To rinse any contaminants off the bottle lip.
   Note: If the container has a double cap, skip this step and proceed to Step 6.
6. Pour, away from the label, the desired amount into the glass or bowl, without allowing any part of the bottle to touch the glass or bowl.
   Purpose: The bottle exterior is not sterile.

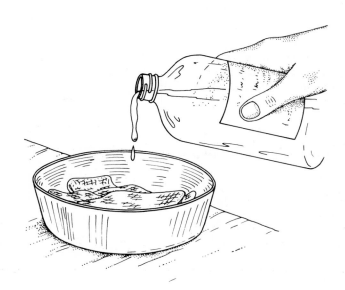

7. Tilt the bottle up to stop the pouring while it is still over the bowl or glass.
   Purpose: Solutions spilled on a sterile field contaminate the field.
8. Remove the bottle from over the sterile field.
   Purpose: Motion over a sterile field should be kept to a minimum.
9. Replace the cap(s) off to the side, away from the sterile field.

TERMINAL PERFORMANCE OBJECTIVE

Given the necessary supplies and equipment, pour a sterile solution into a bowl or glass that is sitting at the outer perimeter of a sterile field, within 15 seconds and without a break in sterile technique or spillage, as determined by your evaluator.

PREOPERATIVE PREPARATION AND CARE OF THE PATIENT

Whether minor surgery is the result of an unforeseen accident or a planned, elective procedure, the patient needs psychologic care as well as physical care. The patient facing any surgical procedure suffers from fear of pain, disfigurement, and often the fear of cancer being discovered. An injured patient may feel anxious about the medical bills or loss of employment. Because surgery is a frightening and dehumanizing experience, you must take the time, both preoperatively and at the time of surgery, to help the patient through these fears and anxieties. The best method is to help the patient talk about the procedure or voice any concerns or misgivings. Questions should be answered directly, but answer only those questions that are within your scope of experience and the policies of the office. If you cannot answer a question, assure the patient that you will relay the question to the physician prior to the procedure. Don't forget to relay the message. What may seem to be a minor or unimportant question to you may be very frightening to the patient. A good technique is to write down the question in front of the patient, then give it to the physician. The minor surgery room can look very frightening to the patient, so, unless the patient is sedated, try to make conversation with the patient while you prepare for the physician's arrival.

The physical preparation may involve obtaining blood and urine for tests the day before surgery, completing forms and permissions, and gathering a current history concerning any recent illnesses or medications. Before the day of surgery, preoperative instructions may include a shave prep, cleansing enemas, food intake restrictions, special bathing, and a sedative medication.

On the day of surgery, the patient's vital signs are recorded, and the patient is assisted in undressing, if necessary, and then is asked to empty the bladder. Keep the patient on schedule but never appear to rush the process.

Preoperative Instructions

When planning office surgery, complete the following procedures before the time of the appointment:

- Have the necessary consent forms ready to sign.
- Give the patient all the necessary preoperative instructions, such as medications to be used and special skin cleansing.
- Instruct patients to bring a relative or friend to drive them home after the surgery.
- When appropriate, instruct the patient to wear special clothing that is easily removed and can be worn over bulky dressings or a cast.
- Instruct the patient to leave jewelry and other valuables at home.
- Call the patient the day before the surgery and confirm any special instructions.

Positioning the Patient

Have the patient disrobe sufficiently to completely expose the surgical area. There is too much risk of contamination in doing the procedure while either you or the patient is holding back clothing that may slide into the area where the physician is working. Clothing may also act as a tourniquet or may make it difficult to apply a proper dressing or bandage. The patient's clothing may also be stained with the skin disinfecting solution or may prevent a large area from being treated properly.

It is equally important to position the patient as comfortably as possible. An uncomfortable position can be held for only a limited time, and the patient will have to move, often in the middle of a procedure. If not comfortable, the patient's muscles may stiffen or ache after the surgery. If bandaging is applied to an area with the patient in an awkward position, the bandage may bind or improperly fit when the patient assumes a normal position. When deciding on the correct patient position, consider where you and the physician will stand or sit, where the instruments will be placed, and the position of the light source. If the patient has an open wound or is bleeding, wear nonsterile gloves to assist the patient into position for the procedure. If the bleeding is profuse, you should wear an apron or gown. If there is danger of blood or body-fluid contamination to your face, wear goggles and a mask.

Preparing the Patient's Skin

The human skin is a reservoir of bacteria (see Chapter 22, Basic Concepts of Asepsis). Resident organisms cannot be removed or completely destroyed; therefore, the skin cannot be sterilized. Transit bacteria, however, can be harmful, and all care must be given to cleanse the patient's skin of transit bacteria as much as possible. Cleansing the patient's skin prior to surgery is called a skin prep. A good skin prep eliminates, as much as possible, the transference of harmful organisms to the incision site. Sometimes, the patient may be instructed to repeatedly cleanse the surgical area with bacteriostatic or antiseptic soap several days before the surgery. A patient may need to shave the surgical area immediately before coming to the office. Disposable skin prep trays are available. A patient skin prep is performed by a gloved assistant.

Procedure 30–8

GLOVING USING THE OPEN-GLOVING (WITHOUT A GOWN) METHOD

PROCEDURAL GOAL

To apply your own sterile gloves to perform sterile procedures.

EQUIPMENT AND SUPPLIES

A pair of packaged surgical gloves in your size

PROCEDURE

1. Perform the surgical hand scrub according to Procedure 22–2.
2. Dry your hands well.
   Purpose: Gloves will not slide easily over moist hands.
3. Open your glove pack. Remember a 1-in area around the perimeter of the glove pack is considered not sterile.
   Purpose: The open glove pack is a sterile field.
4. Glove your major hand first. ~~Right hand~~
   Purpose: This will set up your major hand to do the more difficult step, which is to apply the second glove (below, left).
5. With your minor hand, pick up the glove for your major hand, with your thumb and forefinger grabbing the top of the folded cuff, which is the inside of the glove (below, left).
   Purpose: The inside of the glove will be next to your skin and is considered not sterile.
6. Lift the glove up and away from the sterile pack.
   Purpose: Movement over a sterile field must be kept to a minimum.
7. Hold your hands away from you, and slide your major hand into the glove.
8. Leave the cuff folded (below, right).
   Purpose: You will unfold the cuff later.

30

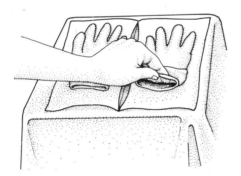

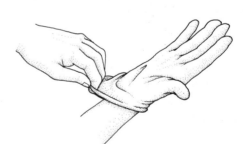

Procedure continued on following page

9. With your gloved major hand, pick up the second glove by slipping your gloved fingers under the cuff so that your gloved hand only touches the outside of the second glove (below, left).
Purpose: Sterile surfaces must always touch sterile surfaces.

10. Slide your second hand into the glove, without touching the exterior of the glove or any part of your other hand (below, center).

11. Still holding your hands away from you, unroll the cuff by slipping the fingers up and out. Stay away from your bare arm (below, right).

12. Now, slip your gloved fingers up under the first cuff and unroll it, using the same technique.

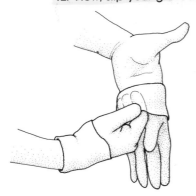 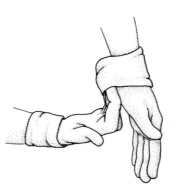 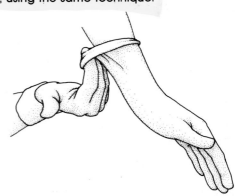

TERMINAL PERFORMANCE OBJECTIVE

Given the necessary supplies, apply a pair of sterile gloves within one minute and without a break in sterile technique, as determined by your evaluator.

Procedure 30-9

PREPARING A PATIENT'S SKIN FOR SURGERY

PROCEDURAL GOAL

To prepare the patient's skin for a surgical procedure to reduce the risk of wound contamination.

EQUIPMENT AND SUPPLIES

Sterile gloves
An autoclaved skin prep pack containing:
    Four tri-folded sterile towels
    12 to 24 4 × 4 gauze sponges
    Eight cotton-tipped applicators
    Two small stainless steel bowls
Antiseptic soap
Antiseptic
Waste receptacle on the side counter
Cotton balls, nail picks, and scrub brushes may also be needed
Blood and body-fluid protection in barriers (goggles, masks, and aprons or gowns), as necessary
(see Appendix C, Recommendations for Prevention of AIDS Transmission)

PROCEDURE

1. Wash your hands, and dry them carefully. Follow universal blood and body-fluid precaution (see Appendix C).
   Purpose: Moisture on your hands contaminates the pack.
2. Open your skin prep pack, following Procedure 30–2.
3. Arrange the items with the transfer forceps.
   Purpose: The skin prep field is a sterile field.
4. Add the soap and antiseptic solutions to the two bowls as described in Procedure 30–7.
5. Expose the site. Use a light if necessary.

Procedure continued on opposite page

6. Glove yourself.
Purpose: To protect the patient from your resident bacteria.
7. Place two sterile towels at the edges of the area to be scrubbed.
Purpose: The area must be scrubbed up to the sterile towels, which will be beyond the opening of the surgical drape when the drape is applied.
8. Start at the incision site, and begin washing with the antiseptic soap on a gauze sponge in a circular motion, moving from the center to the edges of the area to be scrubbed.
Purpose: Circular motion from inside to outside drags contaminants away from the incision site.

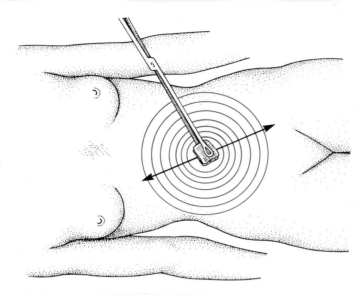

9. After one wipe, discard the sponge, and begin again with a new sponge soaked in the antiseptic solution.
Purpose: After one circular sweep, the sponge is now contaminated with skin bacteria and debris. When you return to the incision site for the next circular sweep, it must be with sterile material.
10. Repeat the process, using sufficient friction for five minutes (or whatever is the policy for the length of time required for the skin prep).
Purpose: Friction aids in the removal of **desquamated cells**.
11. Dry the area, using the same circular technique with dry sponges. The area may be dried by blotting with the third sterile towel.
12. Check to see that no solutions are pooling under the patient.
Purpose: The solution will irritate or burn the skin.
13. Paint on the antiseptic with the cotton-tipped applicators, using the same circular technique and never returning to an area that has already been painted.
14. If the surgeon is not ready to begin the procedure, cover the site with the last sterile towel.

TERMINAL PERFORMANCE OBJECTIVE

Given a patient and the necessary supplies, drape and prep the skin for a surgical procedure, within **seven minutes**, adhering to the principles of surgical asepsis, patient safety, and patient comfort, with no break in sterile technique, as determined by your evaluator.

REFERENCES AND READINGS

Anderson, R. M., and Romfh, R. F.: *Technique in the Use of Surgical Tools.* New York, Appleton-Century-Crofts, 1980.
Bonewit, K.: *Clinical Procedures for Medical Assistants,* 2nd ed. Philadelphia, W. B. Saunders Co., 1984.
DuGas, B. W.: *Introduction to Patient Care: A Comprehensive Approach to Nursing,* 4th ed. Philadelphia, W. B. Saunders Co., 1984.

Fuller, J. R.: *Surgical Technology: Principles and Practice,* 2nd ed. Philadelphia, W. B. Saunders Co., 1986.
Nealon, T. F.: *Fundamental Skills in Surgery,* 3rd ed. Philadelphia, W. B. Saunders Co., 1979.
Sabiston, D. C.: *Textbook of Surgery,* 13th ed. Philadelphia, W. B. Saunders Co., 1986.
Steichen, F. M., and Ravitch, M. M.: *Stapling in Surgery.* Chicago, Year Book Medical Publishers, Inc., 1984.
Vander Salm, T. J. (ed.): *Atlas of Bedside Procedures.* Boston, Little, Brown and Co., 1979.
Wood, L. A., and Rambo, B. J.: *Nursing Skills for Allied Health Services,* Vol. 3. Philadelphia, W. B. Saunders Co., 1980.

30

CHAPTER OUTLINE

VOCABULARY

See Glossary at end of book for definitions.

approximate	in situ	planing
coagulum	irrigation	senile
condylomata	keratosis	slough
hemangioma	pedunculated	untoward
hematoma	photocoagulation	

31

Assisting With Minor Surgery

OBJECTIVES

Upon successful completion of this chapter you should be able to

1. Define and spell the words in the Vocabulary for this chapter.
2. Describe at least six types of wounds.
3. Apply wound management to the three stages of the healing process.
4. Distinguish between the roles of the scrub assistant and the circulating assistant during and after minor surgery.
5. List the routines of minor surgery in correct sequence.
6. Choose the correct type of dressing or bandage to use.
7. List postsurgical routines in correct sequence.
8. Care for and instruct the patient postoperatively.
9. List the safety precautions necessary for electrosurgery.
10. List the safety precautions necessary for laser surgery.

Upon successful completion of this chapter you should be able to perform the following activities:

1. Assist in minor surgery.
2. Assist in wound closure (suturing).
3. Remove a bandage.
4. Change a dressing.
5. Remove sutures.
6. Prepare a patient for electrosurgery.

Because there are so many different minor surgical procedures and setups and because each physician–medical assistant team has individual preferences, we cannot cover all minor surgical procedures or even list all the specific items that may be used for a specific technique. The following procedures are merely composites of acceptable practices in minor surgical techniques. Once you know these basics, with a little bit of background information, you will be able to assist in any minor surgical procedure.

If you have not yet read Chapter 30, you should do so now. Please note in the introduction to Chapter 30 that other chapters in the book should be studied either before or concurrent with this one. Chapter 30 covers, step by step, aseptic techniques and the care of the patient up to the time of surgery. This chapter continues the process at the surgery itself and proceeds to the postoperative care of the patient.

THE HEALING PROCESS

Before you can effectively assist in surgery and wound management, you must have an understanding of wound repair and the healing process. Whether a wound occurs accidentally or as the result of surgery, the repair process is the same. A firm understanding of wound management assists you in understanding the principles of surgical closure techniques and in instructing the patient in postoperative home care.

Terminology of Wounds

A wound is an interruption in the continuity of the internal or external body tissues. A wound may be *intentional* (such as in surgery) or *accidental*, and *open* or *closed* (Table 31–1). An open wound is one with an outward opening where the skin is broken, and the underlying tissues are exposed. A closed, or *nonpenetrating* wound does not have an outward opening, but the underlying tissues are damaged, as in a **hematoma** or contusion (bruise). Closed wounds are usually the result of a blow or a violent jar or shock (concussion) to the body. An aseptic (clean) wound is not infected with pathogens; septic wounds are infected with pathogens.

Open wounds may be classified according to the appearance of their openings. An *incised* wound has a clean edge and is made with a cutting instrument. An incised wound may be the result of intentional surgery or a criminal knife wound. A *lacerated* wound has torn or mangled tissues and is made by a dull or blunt instrument. The *penetrating*, or *puncture*, wound is caused by a sharp, slender object such as a needle or ice pick and passes through the skin into the underlying tissues. A *perforating* wound is a penetrating wound that passes through to a body organ or cavity.

Wound Healing

All wounds go through a healing, or repair, process that has three phases.

The *first phase* (lag) is the period when the blood vessels contract to control hemorrhage, and blood platelets form a network in the wound that acts like glue to plug the wound. Following a complex series of chemical reactions, a substance called fibrin is released into the wound that begins clotting. The fibrin continues to collect red blood cells, more platelets, and white blood cells, and the clot becomes a scab. About 12 hours later, special white blood cells arrive at the site to clear away debris and bacteria. Within one to four days, the fibrin threads contract and pull the edges of the wound together under the clot or scab.

The *second phase* (proliferation) is the wound healing and new growth period and lasts from 5 to 20 days. It is during this phase that the tissues repair themselves. New cells form, and the wound continues to contract and seal. If the wound is a clean surgical incision, complete contraction usually takes place during this phase, and there is no scarring or permanent fibrous tissue (cicatrix) formation.

The *third phase* (remodeling) occurs from the twenty-first day on. Whereas the clean, shallow wound may contract in the first two phases, large or mangled wounds require the time and cellular activity of this third phase to build a bridge of new tissue to close the gap of the wound. The cells produce a fibrous protein substance called collagen (connective tissue) that gives the wounded tissues strength and forms scar tissue. Scar tissue is not true skin; it is usually very strong, but it cannot stand the tension of the normal skin because it lacks elasticity. Scar tissue is also devoid of normal blood supply and nerves.

Wounds are classified by the way they repair themselves. The clean, surgical wound that has been sutured closed and heals quickly without scarring does so by *first intention*. Tissues that are severely damaged, are purposely kept open, or fail to close are said to heal by granulation (healing from the bottom up) which is called *second intention*.

Several factors influence the healing process. People who are young and in good general health and have adequate nutrition heal more rapidly. Adequate protection and resting to the injured area also enhances the healing process. Destruction or re-injury during the second phase can delay healing and increase scarring.

Wounds are susceptible to infection because the normal skin barrier is broken. If there is debris in a wound as a result of the breakdown of the various cellular components, this dead (necrotic) tissue acts

Table 31–1
Types of Wounds

Type	Description
Intentional (performed under surgical asepsis)	
1. Surgical Incision	A neat, clean cut, performed with scapel
2. Hypodermic puncture	Injection under the skin for the purpose of drug administration or fluid withdrawal

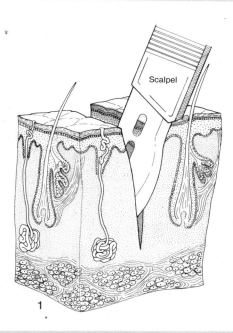

Scalpel

1

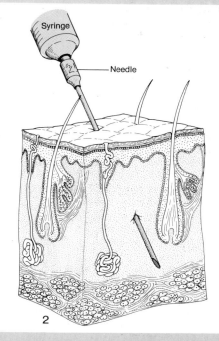

Syringe

Needle

2

Type	Description
Accidental (septic, may cause infection)	
1. Contusion (hematoma)	Closed (nonpenetrating) wound in which blood from broken vessels accumulates in tissues
2. Incision	Neat, clean cut from sharp blade objects, such as glass, knives, or metal

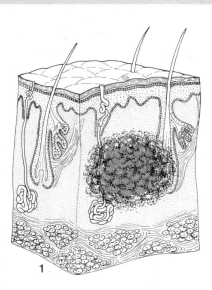

1

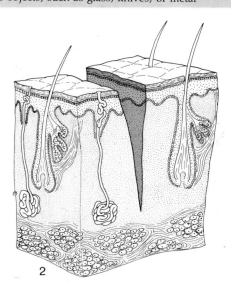

2

Table continued on following page

31

Table 31–1
Types of Wounds Continued

Type	Description
3. Laceration	Jagged, irregular breaking or tearing of tissues, usually caused by a sharp blow to the body
4. Puncture	Skin is pierced by pointed objects, such as pins, nails, splinters, or a bullet

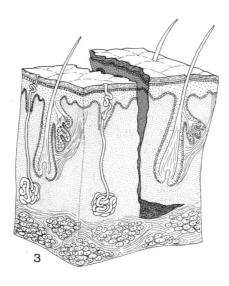

3

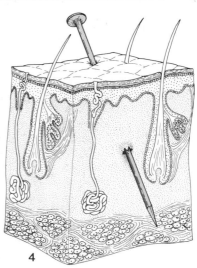

4

| 5. Abrasion | Superficial wound; scraping of the skin |
| 6. Avulsion (sometimes amputation) | Tissue forcibly torn or separated from the body; may be jagged or mutilated, from automobile accidents, gunshot wounds, or animal bites |

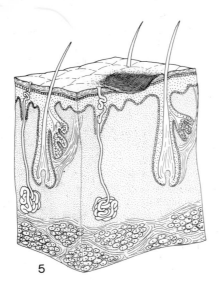

5

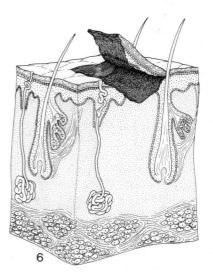

6

as a culture medium for bacterial growth. Suppuration (pus) is necrotic tissue with bacteria, dead leukocytes, and other products of tissue breakdown. Necrotic tissue must be removed. Removal of debris is called **débridement**, which may be natural or a surgical procedure.

Open Wound Healing. Sometimes the physician may prefer no dressing or bandage on small wounds. There are definite advantages to open wound healing:

- There are strong arguments for allowing air to freely circulate in the wound.
- The wound is not irritated or rubbed by a dressing or bandage.
- The wound stays dry, which inhibits bacterial growth, resulting in less chance of infection.
- Sutures stay dry and hold together better.
- In the patient who is shaved prior to surgery, dry shaving nicks heal faster than moist nicks.
- Any pre-existing infection remains localized and is not spread by the dressing or bandage.

ASSISTING IN MINOR SURGICAL PROCEDURES

The physician is ultimately responsible for the surgical patient, but you are ultimately responsible for ensuring that everything you and your physician use in the care of the surgical patient is accounted for, ready for use, and prepared in a safe manner. A surgical conscience is the practice of good aseptic technique and demands that breaks in aseptic technique be reported immediately without regard to delays or embarrassment.

Every team has preferences regarding the sequence in which the team goes about the routines of minor surgery. Once a routine is established, it should be followed in every case. (Sample sequences can be found in Tables 30–1 and 30–2.) Sample set-ups for various types of minor surgery are provided in Table 31–2.

Surgery Routines

After receiving an assignment to assist in a minor surgical procedure (Fig. 31–1), study the physician preference card (see Chapter 30) to review the procedure and note the materials that will be needed. Next, prepare the room and pull the supplies that will be used. Supplies are opened just prior to the procedure; if there is a delay of longer than one hour, however, opened materials must be considered no longer sterile. Supplies should not be placed where they can be knocked over or dropped; wrapped supplies that fall to the floor must not be used. Once supplies are opened, a team member should stay in the room. The circulating assistant opens the packs, beginning with the pack that provides the sterile surface for the remaining sterile items. The Mayo tray is usually prepared as soon as the scrub assistant is gloved and ready to manage the sterile field. Drapes, towel packs, additional sponge packs, and other sterile packages are stacked on the side or back table. Items from this table may be added if needed during the procedure. A basin or trash bucket for waste is placed nearby during the surgery.

The scrub assistant sorts and places the scalpels, hemostats, scissors, tissue forceps, and retractors on the field according to their sequence and frequency of use (Fig. 31–2). Scalpels and sharp instruments should be conspicuously placed so that they do not accidentally harm a team member. If the scrub assistant has not previously prepped the patient, the circulating assistant now performs the patient skin prep. The circulating assistant opens the drape pack. The physician enters the room, gloves, and begins draping the patient with towels or a fenestrated drape. The scrub assistant hands the drapes to the physician, one at a time. In many offices, the scrub assistant alone drapes the site. Once the site is draped, the Mayo stand is positioned below the site, and the scrub assistant stands opposite the physician, over the patient. The circulating assistant cleans the vial of anesthesia with alcohol and holds the vial (with the label up and visible to read) for the scrub assistant or the physician. The scrub assistant or physician lifts the syringe from the sterile field and withdraws the appropriate amount of anesthesia into the syringe. The physician administers the anesthesia, and the scrub assistant immediately places two sponges on the patient, next to the wound site, for sponging blood at the time of the first incision or to sponge an open injury as the first step of the procedure. Local anesthesia is administered either directly into the open wound or into the tissues surrounding the site to be incised. After the anesthesia has taken effect, the physician begins the procedure.

During the procedure, the scrub assistant must protect the sterile field from contamination, notify the physician if there is a break in sterile technique, dispose of soiled sponges into waste receptacles, and anticipate the surgeon's needs for instruments. The physician may verbally request instruments or may use hand signals (Fig. 31–3). As the team works together over time, the physician may not need to give any signals.

Instrumentation is logical: if the physician requests a suture, then scissors will be needed to cut the suture tie; if there is a sudden hemorrhage from a bleeder, the physician will need a hemostat. In gaining experience, the assistant watches, listens, and learns to judge what will be needed or performed next. Pass instruments with a firm and purposeful motion so that the physician will not have to look up. Wait until you feel the physician

Table 31–2
Sample Minor Surgery Set-Ups

Procedure	Side Counter	Sterile Field	Comments	Postoperative Care
Suture repair	Local anesthetic; dressings and bandages; splints or guards; tape; drape; gloves; sterile physiologic saline	Syringe and needle; hemostats (3); scissors; sponges; suture material and needle; tissue forceps or skin hook; needle holder	If an emergency patient arrives in the office with a pressure dressing over a laceration, do not remove the pressure dressing until the physician is ready to suture. If the patient's pressure cloth *must* be removed, have ample sterile dressings ready to apply immediately. Ask the patient the possible length, depth, and exact location of the laceration. Usually there is limited cleansing of a wound because of the bleeding. If not, let the physician instruct you on the necessary cleansing.	Frequently, clean lacerations in a moderately protected area will not be dressed but left open. The patient will be instructed to keep the area clean and dry. Some lacerations may be closed with adhesive strips. These are becoming increasingly popular, since they reduce the chance of infection and do not leave suture scars.
Needle biopsy	Specimen bottle with sufficient fixative or preserving solution; laboratory form and label; local anesthetic; gloves	Biopsy needle; syringe and needle; sponges	A biopsy is the examination of tissue removed from the living body. Biopsies are usually done to determine whether a growth or swelling is malignant or benign; however, it may be done as a diagnostic aid in other diseases or infections. A needle biopsy may be done by aspiration with a needle and syringe or by a special biopsy needle. The specimen is then sent to a pathologist for either a cytologic or histologic examination.	Usually there is no special dressing required after a needle biopsy. A Band-Aid is often sufficient.
Cyst removal	Local anesthetic; disinfectant (skin prep); laboratory form; dressing, size depends on site; gloves; drape; specific bottle with sufficient fixative or preserving solution	Kelly hemostats: 2 str. and 2 cvd.; dressing forceps (2); suture and needle; scissors s/s or s/b; dissector (physician's choice); skin hook; syringe and needle; knife handle with blade # 11 or # 15; tissue forceps (2); Allis forceps; needle holder; sponges; coagulant gel	A sebaceous cyst is a benign retention cyst of a sebaceous gland containing fatty substance of the gland. It is also called a wen. They may occur any place on the body, with the exception of the palms of the hands and the soles of the feet. They are more common on the neck and shoulder, and because they are frequently the source of irritation, they are removed. Ordinarily, the cyst is attached only to the skin and moves freely over the underlying tissue. For cosmetic reasons the physician will make the incision on the natural skin crease lines.	See Suture repair above.
Incision and Drainage (I & D)	Wax or plastic bag for contaminants; extra sponges; medications; skin antiseptic; bandages; ethyl chloride spray; extra applicators; gloves	Hemostats (2); probe; scissors; abscess needle; gauze stripping, iodoform; knife handle with blade # 15; dressing forceps (2); sponges; dressing	An abscess is a localized collection of pus in a cavity formed by the disintegration of tissue. Abscesses may appear on any part of the body. "Furuncle," "boil," and "carbuncle" are names	When dressing the area, several layers of gauze sponges should be placed over the abscess opening, especially if a drain has been inserted, and the gauze anchored with

Table continued on opposite page

612

Table 31–2
Sample Minor Surgery Set-Ups Continued

Procedure	Side Counter	Sterile Field	Comments	Postoperative Care
			applied to different types of abscesses. In most abscesses, pyogenic cocci, usually staphylococci, are found, but it is not uncommon to find secondary organisms. The treatment for abscesses, other than those on the face, is usually incision and drainage. Because of the infectious organisms, extreme caution should be taken in handling the contaminated materials and instruments. The physician may choose to inject a local anesthetic if the abscess is deep rather than to use the ethyl chloride to "freeze" the area. The medical assistant may cut the length of gauze stripping for packing at the physician's request.	bandage. Frequently, a patient is instructed to apply warm moist packs for a couple of days. Daily dressing changes may also be indicated because of the copious drainage.
Cervical biopsy	Specimen bottle 10% formalin; laboratory form; skin antiseptic solution; gloves	Vaginal speculum; uterine dressing forceps (2); cervical biopsy punch; coagulant foam or gel; sponges; uterine tenaculum; vaginal tampon or packing	This is the examination of the tissue removed from the cervical area of the uterus. A biopsy is usually done to determine whether there is a malignancy present. It is also a diagnostic aid in diagnosing other diseases. If the Papanicolaou smear test is positive, it is usually confirmed by a cervical biopsy. The patient is placed in the lithotomy position, with a towel under the buttocks. Since the cervix is devoid of nerve endings that would respond to cutting and burning stimuli, there is very little discomfort. Postbiopsy bleeding may be controlled by the application of a coagulant gel or foam, or the physician may choose to lightly cauterize the area. The physician may also choose to remove a piece of tissue by means of electric conization.	Usually there are no special dressings or packing after a cervical biopsy. The patient is instructed to care for any discharge and to abstain from douching or sexual intercourse for a few days.
Nasal pack	Head mirror and light; emesis basin; medication; laryngeal mirror; tongue depressor; topical anesthetic; gloves	Nasal speculum; cotton applicators; scissors; metal applicator, str. and cvd.; nasal packing with string (4"); dressing forceps (bayonet); hemostatic forceps, str.; medicine glass; nasal pack, 1 in, plain or iodoform	A nasal pack is inserted into the nasal cavity, usually for the purpose of stopping hemorrhage or for the application of medication. The patient is placed in a sitting position, with the back well supported. Drape the front of the patient and give him or her some paper tissues.	The patient is instructed not to remove the pack, and a return visit is scheduled; or the patient is instructed how and when to remove the packing.

31

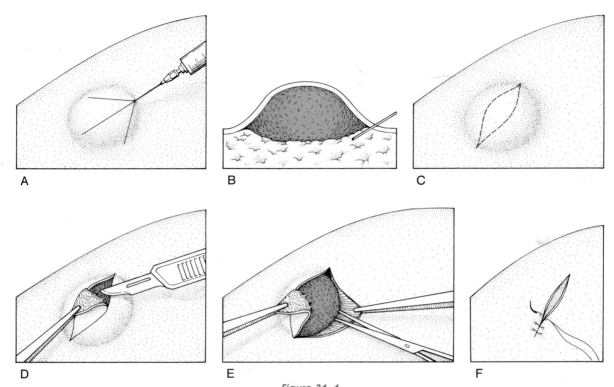

A

B

C

D

E

F

Figure 31–1

Technique of excision of sebaceous cyst, or wen. **A** *and* **B,** *Infiltration of the tissues surrounding the cyst is performed with procaine hydrochloride, 0.5 percent solution.* **C** *and* **D,** *An elliptic incision is made over the cyst to remove a small segment of skin including the puncta.* **E,** *Using the attached ellipse of skin for traction purposes, the cyst is removed intact if possible.* **F,** *Bleeding points are controlled with fine catgut ligatures, and the skin incision is closed with nonabsorbable sutures.*

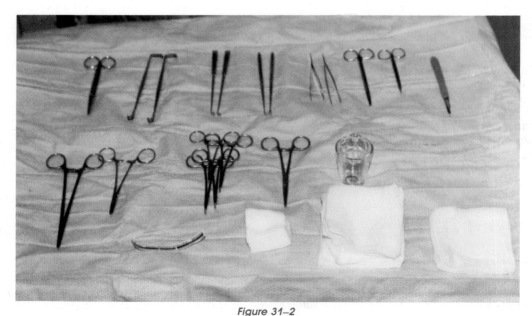

Figure 31–2

Sterile instruments and supplies on a sterile field in preparation for assisting with the minor surgical procedure.

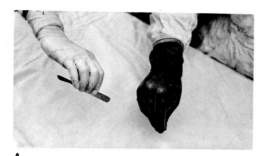

A

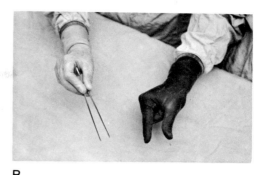

B

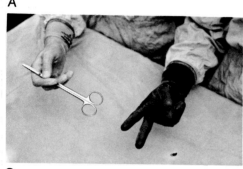

C

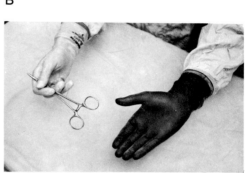

D

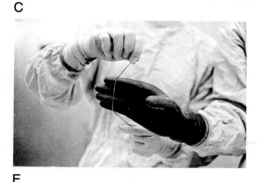

E

Figure 31–3
*Passing instruments. **A,** Hand signal for scalpel. **B,** Hand signal for forceps. **C,** Hand signal for scissors. **D,** Hand signal for hemostat. **E,** Hand signal for suture strand without a needle (free tie). (From Nealon, T. F.: Fundamental Skills in Surgery, 3rd ed. Philadelphia, W. B. Saunders Co., 1979.)*

31

grasp the instrument, so it will not drop onto the patient or to the floor. Pass instruments so that the physician is protected from injury. Pass scalpels blade down. Hold all instruments by their tips, and pass the handle ends into the physician's palm or fingers. Avoid painful slapping of the instruments into the surgeon's hand. Correct passing produces a faint, gentle "snap" as it contacts the gloved hand.

If a specimen is collected during the procedure, it is placed in a sterile glass or basin. Do not remove the specimen from the sterile field until the physician gives the order. The physician may want to examine it again during the procedure.

Procedure 31–1

ASSISTING DURING THE MINOR SURGICAL PROCEDURE

PROCEDURAL GOAL

To maintain the sterile field and to pass instruments in a prescribed sequence during a surgical procedure that involves the making of a surgical incision and the removal of a growth.

EQUIPMENT AND SUPPLIES

Blood and body-fluid protection barriers (goggles, masks, and aprons or gowns), as necessary (see Appendix C, Recommendations for Prevention of AIDS Transmission)
An open patient drape pack on the side counter

Procedure continued on following page

A Mayo stand
A sterile field containing the following:
> A needle and syringe for the anesthesia
> A supply of gauze sponges
> A scalpel handle and a no. 11 blade
> One Allis tissue forceps
> One skin retractor
> Three hemostats
> One medicine glass or bowl (specimen container)

A waste receptacle
A vial of anesthesia
Sterile gloves (at least two pairs)

PROCEDURE

SETUP
1. Scrub with the surgical hand wash; follow universal blood and body-fluid precautions (see Appendix C).
2. Position the Mayo stand over the patient and below the site.
3. Invert the vial of anesthesia, and hold it for the gloved physician to withdraw the prescribed amount of anesthesia into the syringe.
   Purpose: The vial of anesthesia cannot be held after both team members are gloved.
4. Glove.

DRAPE THE PATIENT
5. Grasp the patient drape in the open drape pack by holding one edge or corner in each hand.
6. Lift the drape from the pack without touching the drape to any of the pack edges.
   Purpose: A 1-in barrier around any sterile field is considered not sterile.
7. Drape the surgical site without touching any part of the patient or the operating table with your gloved hands. The physician injects the local anesthesia.
   Note: The physician may drape the patient, while you glove.

ASSIST WITH THE PROCEDURE
8. Position yourself across from the physician. Arrange the sterile field. Check instrument condition.
9. Place two sponges on the patient, next to the wound site.
10. Grasp an Allis tissue forceps by the tips, and pass it to the physician to grasp a piece of tissue to be excised. Pass the handles into the surgeon's open palm with a firm and purposeful motion so that a gentle "snap" is heard as it contacts the surgeon's gloved hand.
    Purpose: The physician will not have to look up to receive the instrument.
11. Grasp the scalpel blade with a hemostat, and mount the scalpel blade onto the scalpel handle. Keep all sharp equipment conspicuously placed on the sterile field.
    Purpose: Sharp instruments that are not clearly visible may injure a team member.
12. Pass the scalpel, blade down, to the physician. The physician will take the scalpel with the thumb and forefinger in the position ready for use.
    Purpose: To protect the physician from injury.
13. Dispose of soiled sponges, using the waste receptacle.
14. Hold clean sponges in your minor hand, to pass as needed.
15. Hold out the specimen container to receive the specimen.
16. If there is a bleeder, or if a hemostat is requested, pass the hemostat in the manner described in Steps 9 and 10.
17. Receive instruments, and put them in the field.
18. Continue to sponge blood from the wound site.
19. Retract the wound edge with a skin retractor if so requested.

TERMINAL PERFORMANCE OBJECTIVE

Given the necessary equipment and supplies, maintain a sterile field, pass instruments to the physician, and sponge blood from the surgical site without a break in sterile technique, injury to the physician, or delays in the flow of the procedure, as determined by your evaluator.

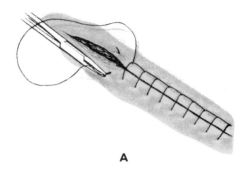 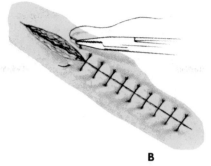

A   **B**

Figure 31–4
Types of skin closures. **A,** *Continuous technique.* **B,** *Interrupted technique. (Courtesy of Ethicon, Inc.)*

Completion of the Surgical Procedure

At the conclusion of the procedure, the physician will begin the wound closure. The techniques and methods of tissue closure vary greatly, and it would be impossible to describe or illustrate all of them. There are two basic methods of suturing: the *continuous* (running) placement of a single strand; and the *interrupted* suture, in which each knot is placed and tied independently so that if one breaks, the others keep the wound closure intact (Fig. 31–4). The majority of skin closures in the medical office are limited to the interrupted technique.

The scrub assistant mounts the suture and needle in the needle holder and passes the unit to the physician. As the physician closes the wound, the scrub assistant assists by cutting the suture and sponging the site. The physician places the first interrupted suture at the midpoint of the incision. Then, each side of the first suture is mentally divided in half again, and the next two sutures are placed at each of these midpoints. The rest of the sutures are placed by the same technique of mentally dividing the remaining suture line in half until the length of the wound edge is totally **approximated.**

Procedure 31–2

ASSISTING WITH SUTURING   **31**

PROCEDURAL GOAL

To assist the physician in wound closure, without a break in sterile technique or injury to other team members.

EQUIPMENT AND SUPPLIES

Blood and body-fluid protection barriers (goggles, masks, and aprons or gowns), as necessary (see Appendix C, Recommendations for Prevention of AIDS Transmission)
Sterile gloves
A sterile field on a Mayo stand
Mayo-Hegar needle holder
Strands of atraumatic suture material
Surgical scissors
Gauze sponges

PROCEDURE

1. Four to five inches over the sterile field, hold the curved needle point up in your minor hand (following page, top left).
Purpose: Keeping the suture material close to the surface prevents the strands from wandering onto a nonsterile area.

2. With the needle holder in your major hand, clamp the needle at the upper third of the total length (near the eyeless connection) with the needle holder (following page, top right).
Purpose: Clamping in the middle weakens or distorts the shape of the needle. Clamping too near

Procedure continued on following page

the thread may cause the suture to detach from the needle. Clamping at the lower third of the needle damages the needle point.

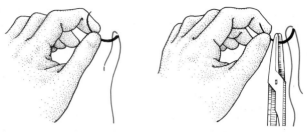

3. With your major hand, hold the needle holder halfway down its shaft, at the box-lock, with the suture needle point up.
    Purpose: To prevent injury to the physician.
4. With your minor hand, hold the suture strand, and pass the needle holder into the surgeon's hand (below).
    Purpose: Holding the strand prevents it from touching anything else as it is being passed.

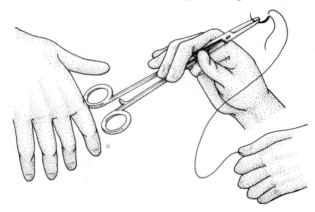

5. Pick up the surgical scissors with your major hand and a gauze sponge with your minor hand.
6. After the physician has placed a closure and holds the two strands taut, cut both suture strands in one motion, between the knot and the physician, at the length requested (about ⅛ in) (below).
    Purpose: Too long a suture may irritate the patient during recovery; too short a suture may untie during recovery.

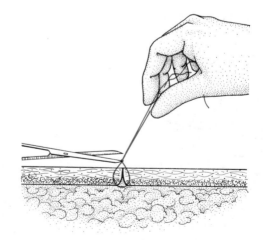

7. Gently blot the closure once with the gauze sponge in your minor hand.
    Purpose: Rubbing or friction may damage the wound edges, and once a gauze sponge has been used, it must be discarded.
8. If additional strands of suture are needed, repeat the process.

Procedure continued on opposite page

TERMINAL PERFORMANCE OBJECTIVE

Given the necessary equipment and supplies, assist in the passing of suture materials and skin closure, without delay to the physician and without a break in sterile technique, as determined by your evaluator.

After skin closure, the wound site is cleaned with wet and dry sponges. This may be done by the surgeon or the scrub assistant. Care must be taken not to disturb the wound edges or the sutures. Next, sterile dressings are placed over the incision, and the drapes are removed. Lift the drapes directly off the patient with minimum movement so as not to disturb the dressing or stir up the air currents. The circulating assistant or the surgeon then applies nonsterile bandage and tape to the dressing. Do not break down your Mayo stand until the patient has left the room. If there is an unexpected contamination of the wound site during the dressing, more materials will be needed from the sterile field.

DRESSINGS AND BANDAGES

Dressings

A dressing (Fig. 31–5A) is a sterile covering placed over a wound to

- Protect the wound from injury and contamination
- Maintain a constant pressure
- Hold the wound edges together
- Control bleeding
- Absorb drainage and secretions
- Hide temporary disfigurement

A dressing usually consists of a strip of lubricated mesh or a nonstick Telfa pad placed over a sutured wound. It is important to use dressings that do not adhere to the wound itself. Gauze squares are usually placed over the nonadhering material. Body cavities or wounds that need to remain open for a time are dressed with long, thin packing material that is often impregnated with an antiseptic or lubricant. This is sometimes called *packing*. Regardless of the type of material, a good dressing must be effective and comfortable and must remain in place. If the dressing covers a hairless area, it may be anchored with tape only, but no tape may touch the wound.

Frequently, small, clean lacerations may be closed with special adhesive strips called Steri-Strips. These strips reduce the chance of infection and do not leave suture scars. Steri-Strips are used on areas of the body that are well protected from movement and stress: they are often used on the face. They should never be used on a knee or an elbow. Since Steri-Strips are a suture replacement, only the physician should place them. The physician places the strips onto the wound in the same sequence and at the same intervals as in interrupted sutures (Fig. 31–5B).

31

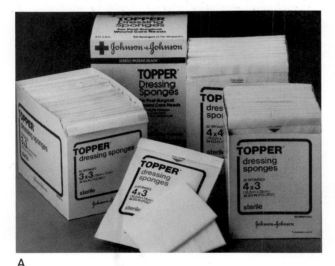

A

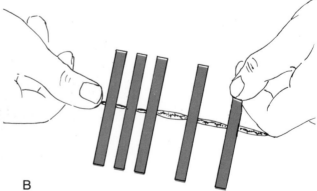

B

Figure 31–5

A, *Probably the most commonly used dressing, this gauze square is manufactured in various sizes to accommodate wound sizes. It may be referred to as a sponge or a flat, but it is manufactured under the name "Topper." Each dressing is packaged individually in pull-apart sterile packages. (Courtesy of Johnson and Johnson Products, Inc., New Brunswick, NJ.)* **B,** *Sterile strip skin closures may be preferred for small lacerations. Sterile strips are applied in the same manner as sutures.*

Bandages

Dressings are usually held in place by bandages, which further help to maintain even pressure, support the affected part, and keep the wound free from injury or contamination. Bandages can be gauze, cloth, or elastic cloth rolls and are bound by tape or tying. Dressings and bandages frequently appear easy and simple to apply, but special skill is required to apply a functional dressing that serves the purpose for which it is intended. Bandages that are too loose fall off. Bandages that are too tight may further harm the patient. Patients do not feel that good medical care has been given them if bandages are messy or uncomfortable. Swelling may occur after a dressing and bandage is applied, and the patient may need a dressing change sooner than scheduled.

Plain gauze roller bandage is almost a thing of the past. It is difficult to handle because it must be applied with reverse spiral turns if the area is uneven. Plain gauze roller bandage has no elasticity and tends to bind. Because it does not adhere to itself, it is also more likely to slip. *Wrinkled crepe–type bandages*, such as Kling, are preferred because they adhere to the various shapes of the body as well as to themselves (Fig. 31–6). Roller bandages are not applied without a dressing.

Plain elastic cloth bandage (Ace) or *elastic roller cloth with adhesive backing* makes a flexible and secure cover (Fig. 31–7). When applying Ace elastic roller bandage as a pressure bandage, especially to the lower limbs, it is absolutely essential to keep the bandage consistent in spacing and tension to assure even pressure. Even and gentle pressure stimulates circulation and healing; but uneven pressure causes constriction points that can create pressure sores or ulcers. All roller bandages are applied from the distal to the proximal part of the area. Bandaging can only remain even and snug if it is wrapped from a smaller to a larger circumference. Elevate the limb while you are bandaging, and work with the roller facing upward, close to the patient's skin. This technique is more likely to keep the tension consistent, and you will be less likely to drop the roll (Fig. 31–8*A*). Common bandaging techniques are shown in Figure 31–8*B* through *H*.

Adhesive bandages are commercially prepared elastic bandages, commonly called Band-Aids. They are available in various shapes to fit the various body parts. Small circular bandages are called "spots" (Fig. 31–9).

Seamless tubular gauze bandage, with or without elastic, is superior material for covering round surfaces, such as the arms, legs, fingers, and toes. It can be used as either a dressing or a bandage. Tubular bandage is applied with a cage-like applicator. Work with the cutting channel of the applicator facing toward the patient. You may start in the middle of the area to be dressed and anchor the dressing, if there is one, with a small piece of tape. Hold the applicator in both hands, and control the tension flow with your fingers as the applicator is gradually rotated and the material slides off. Tubular dressings may be applied with or without slight pressure. Beyond the tip of the bandaged part, give the applicator a full half-turn, place the applicator again over the part, and repeat the process. Be very careful not to create a tourniquet effect when you reverse the applicator. When the desired thickness of the bandage is reached, cut the gauze, and anchor the final dressing with tape (Figs. 31–10 through 31–13). This lightweight gauze should not be used as a stockinette under a cast. Patients should be advised to call the physician's office if there is any problem with the dressing.

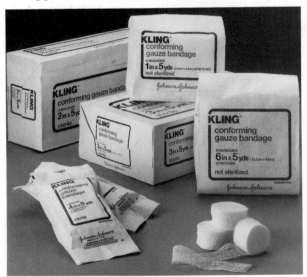

Figure 31–6
A wrinkled-crepe cotton bandage that adheres to itself and conforms to cover the body part. (Courtesy of Johnson and Johnson Products, Inc., New Brunswick, NJ.)

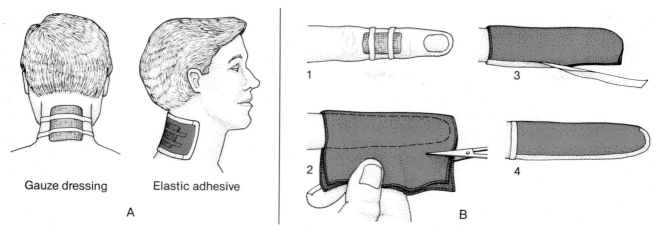

Gauze dressing   Elastic adhesive

A

B

Figure 31–7
Elastic adhesive bandage used on (A) *the neck and* (B) *the finger.*

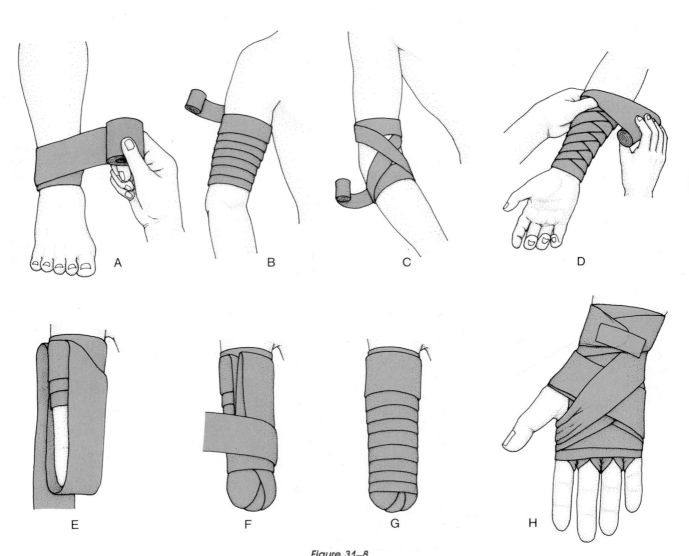

Figure 31–8
A, *Applying a roller bandage. Start at the distal point. Keep the roll close to the patient with the roll upward. Keep tension and spacing consistently even.* **B,** *Circular bandage.* **C,** *Figure-of-eight bandage.* **D,** *Reverse spiral bandage.* **E,** *Recurrent bandage for fingers.* **F,** *Circular turns for fingers.* **G,** *Reverse spiral for fingers.* **H,** *Combination recurrent and figure-of-eight turns for the hand.*

31

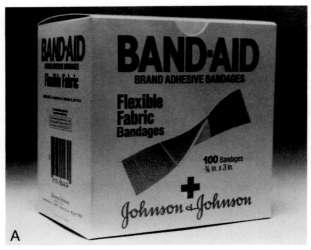

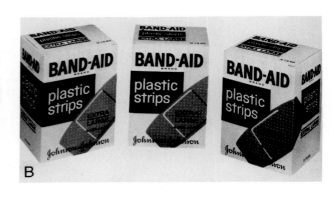

Figure 31–9
Commercially prepared fabric bandages. (Courtesy of Johnson and Johnson Products, Inc., New Brunswick, NJ.)

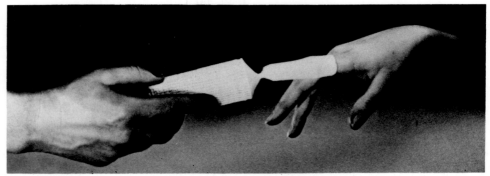

Figure 31–10
Tubegauz applied to a finger. (Courtesy of Scholl, Inc., Hospital Products Division.)

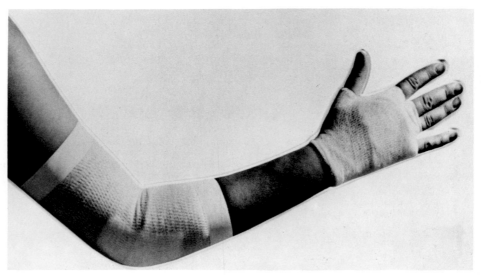

Figure 31–11
Tubegauz applied to elbow and hand. (Courtesy of Scholl, Inc., Hospital Products Division.)

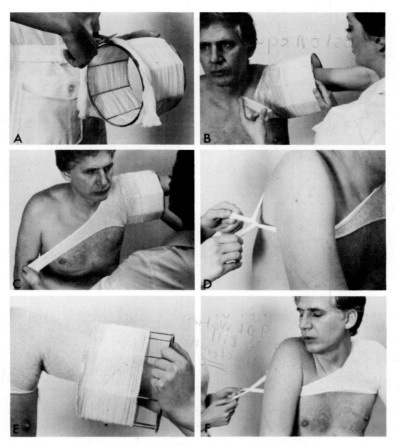

Figure 31-12
Shoulder bandaging with Tubegauz. **A,** With a loaded applicator, make two slits in the Tubegauz, one slit at the top and another at the bottom of the applicator. You will need to make a longer slit at the bottom. **B,** Place the arm through the applicator up to the shoulder. **C,** Pull one tail of the Tubegauz across the chest, the other across the back. **D,** Pulling the pieces taut, tie the two tails under the other arm. **E,** Bring the applicator slightly down the arm, and anchor, then move the applicator to the shoulder. **F,** Cutting from the smooth rim end, make two slits as before, bring tails across back and chest, and tie under the arm. (Courtesy of Scholl, Inc., Hospital Products Division.)

31

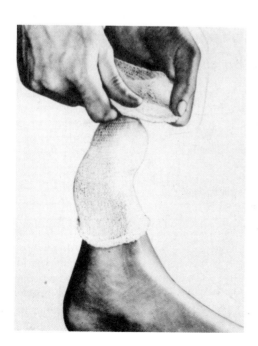

Figure 31-13
Tubegauz applied to toes. (Courtesy of Scholl, Inc., Hospital Products Division.)

POSTSURGICAL ROUTINES

Cleaning the Operatory ~~post on equipment~~

While the circulating assistant escorts the patient from the room, the scrub assistant clears away the sterile field. Follow the universal blood and body-fluid precautions. The scrub assistant should not remove the sterile gloves until all contaminated materials are removed and cared for. Sharp items are placed in separate basins, instruments are taken to the work area, disposable items are properly placed in trash cans, and the linen is removed to the linen hamper. The room should be checked for any blood, spills, or other contamination. Decontaminate the room with soap and disinfectant as necessary. Label any specimens, and prepare them for transportation to the laboratory. Chart the procedure on the patient's medical record, and place the chart on the physician's desk for any additional entries or comments. As soon as there is time, clean and reprocess the instruments and packs. *1 pt Bleach 9 pt water to kill Bacteria*

Postoperative Instructions and Care

Give the patient time to rest after the surgery. If a sedative was administered, make certain that the patient is sufficiently recovered to avoid injury during the journey home. If the patient has been given a topical or local anesthetic, explain to the patient that the anesthesia will soon be wearing off and that there may be discomfort at the site. Check with the physician if a pain medication has not been prescribed. If the physician has prescribed a pain medication, review with the patient the purpose of the medication and the directions for its use. Before the patient leaves the office, set the follow-up appointment.

Postoperative care extends for the total recovery period, not just for the time of immediate care before the patient leaves the office. Most medical assistants are responsible for teaching patients to care for themselves at home following the surgical experience. Since it is a known fact that the concentrative powers of the postoperative patient are diminished following the stress of surgery, instructions should be in writing that is simple in style and easily understood by the patient at home. These instructions can be preprinted forms for each type of surgery or a general form with boxes checked for whichever postoperative instructions apply to a particular patient. Printed instructions should include

- How to apply a hot or a cold compress *and Verbale*
- Whether or not to elevate a limb
- Whether or not to bathe
- Limitations of food intake or exercise
- When to return to work or school
- How to recognize and care for drainage if there is a wound drain in place
- What type of complications necessitate the patient calling the office
- Whether or not to change dressings
- The medications prescribed and their purposes
- The time the next day the patient should call to report in
- The date of the next appointment

Explain to the patient the importance of calling the office if there are any questions or **untoward** changes. If the patient does not call within the next 24 hours, you should call the patient. Many patients tend to "ride it out" or say they didn't want to bother you. Never allow the postoperative patient to leave the office without the physician's knowledge and approval.

Postoperative Return Visits

If the healing process is a long one or if the wound becomes infected, the patient may return for a dressing change. Check the patient's medical record, and follow the physician's instructions carefully. Follow the universal blood and body-fluid precautions. Glove, and wear other protection barriers as appropriate. Place the patient in a comfortable position, and adequately expose the area to be re-dressed. Try to obscure the wound site from the patient's vision, and do not reveal any unpleasant reactions, by either comment or facial expression. If at any time you determine that the wound may be infected, stop and notify the physician.

Reusable Ace bandage is rerolled in your hand as it is taken off the patient. Because microorganisms are carried by the air currents, keep the bandage close to the patient; do not let it fly around as you work.

Tape applied directly to the patient's skin is not the ideal dressing immobilizer. If tape has been used, it is hoped that it has been kept to a minimum. If there is tape holding a dressing in place, cut the tape next to the dressing. Always remove tape by pulling it toward the wound. If tape is adhering to a hairy area of the body, lift the outer tape edge with one hand and slowly and gently separate the underlying hair and skin from the tape with the thumb of your other hand. In other words, peel the skin from the bandage, not the bandage from the skin. Never rapidly "rip" tape from the body. If the tape is not irritating to the patient, it may be advisable to leave the tape on the skin until total healing has taken place. *Both ends*

After the physician examines the wound, you will either apply a new dressing or remove the patient's sutures.

Procedure 31–3

PROCEDURAL GOAL

To remove a wound covering, using sterile technique and without pain or injury to the patient.

EQUIPMENT AND SUPPLIES

Blood and body-fluid protection barriers (goggles, masks, and aprons or gowns), as necessary (see Appendix C, Recommendations for Prevention of AIDS Transmission)
Nonsterile gloves (sterile gloves may be preferred)
Clean towels
Waste receptacle
Bandage scissors
Sterile pack with a thumb dressing forceps and gauze sponges
Hydrogen peroxide or sterile physiologic saline
Surgical soap (optional)

PROCEDURE

1. Wash and dry your hands. Follow the universal blood and body-fluid precautions (see Appendix C). Glove yourself with nonsterile or sterile gloves.
2. Open the forceps pack.
3. Inspect the bandaged area, and ask the patient where the wound is.
   Purpose: To correctly identify the wound site.
4. Position and support the bandaged area.
5. Cut through the entire bandage on the side opposite the wound.
   Purpose: To avoid injuring or contaminating the wound with the scissors.
6. Gently lift each side of the bandage material toward the wound.
   Purpose: Pulling bandage material away from the wound may reopen the edges of the wound.
7. Place the bandage in the waste receptacle.
8. Place toweling under the unbandaged area.
   Purpose: To catch spills and to keep the patient dry.
9. Lift one corner of the dressing with the thumb dressing forceps, toward the wound.
10. If the dressing is not adhering to the wound, lift the other side toward the wound and off.
11. Place the dressing in the waste receptacle away from the patient, but leave it for the physician to examine.
    Purpose: Dressings are examined for the amount of blood lost, drainage, and infection. Occasionally, the physician may smell the dressing if infection is suspected. (Infected wounds have distinct odors.)
12. If the dressing adheres to the wound, pour a small amount of hydrogen peroxide or sterile saline solution onto the dressing, and allow it to soak for a few seconds.
    Purpose: Pulling a dressing that adheres to a wound may reopen the edges of the wound or may remove the scab that has formed.
13. Gently blot the area with a sterile gauze sponge.
14. Lift and hold the gauze sponge by two corners and never touch the surface that touches the wound.
    Purpose: To protect the wound from contamination and to protect you from the wound excretions.
15. If it is necessary to cleanse the area, hold a dry gauze sponge over the suture line or scab with your minor hand.
    Purpose: To protect the wound edges and sutures from injury.
16. Gently scrub the surrounding area with gauze sponges soaked in hydrogen peroxide, sterile saline solution or surgical soap.
17. Rinse by pouring sterile water or saline solution over the site.
18. Cover the area, and call for the physician to examine the wound and the healing process.

31

Procedure continued on following page

TERMINAL PERFORMANCE OBJECTIVE

Given the necessary equipment and supplies, remove a roller bandage and dressing from a patient and clean the area, within five minutes and without discomfort to the patient or a break in sterile technique, as determined by your evaluator.

Procedure 31–4

APPLYING A NEW DRESSING

PROCEDURAL GOAL

To apply a fresh, sterile dressing to a wound.

EQUIPMENT AND SUPPLIES

Blood and body-fluid protection barriers (goggles, masks, and aprons or gowns), as necessary (see Appendix C, Recommendations for Prevention of AIDS Transmission)
Nonsterile gloves (sterile gloves may be preferred)
Mayo stand
Clean towels
Bandage scissors
Sterile dressing pack with two thumb dressing forceps, gauze sponges, cotton-tipped applicators, and a tongue depressor
Local medication or skin antiseptic
Dressing materials
Bandage
Tape
Waste receptacle

PROCEDURE

1. Wash and dry your hands. Follow the universal blood and body-fluid precautions (see Appendix C). Glove yourself with nonsterile or sterile gloves.
2. Open the dressing pack.
3. Place dry toweling under the area to be dressed.
   Purpose: To catch spills and to keep the patient dry.
4. Position and support the area to be dressed.
5. Over the waste receptacle pour the skin antiseptic onto two cotton-tipped applicators.
6. Paint the wound site with the skin antiseptic in a circular motion, from the inside out.
7. Avoid the wound edges.
   Purpose: Cotton adheres to granulation tissue.
8. If the medication is in a spray container, spray in short spurts holding the container 8 to 12 in from the wound, until the medication evenly covers the area.
9. If the medication is an ointment, spread the ointment onto a sterile tongue depressor, then spread the ointment on the new sterile dressing with the tongue depressor.
   Purpose: Spreading ointment directly onto the wound may cause injury to the wound edges or may disturb the sutures.
10. Make sure that both the medication and the dressing cover an area larger than the wound.
11. Secure the dressing with bandage or tape.
12. Give the patient any new instructions.
13. Record the dressing change on the patient's medical history, including how much bleeding or discharge there was on the dressing, the condition of the wound, what medication was applied, and when the patient is to return.

[handwritten notes: chart swelling, Pain Heat, amount of, Redness, Drainage, Color, Odor]

TERMINAL PERFORMANCE OBJECTIVE

Given the necessary equipment and supplies, apply a sterile dressing, within five minutes, without discomfort to the patient or a break in sterile technique, as determined by your evaluator.

Procedure 31–5

PROCEDURAL GOAL

To remove sutures from a healed incision, using sterile technique and without injury to the closed wound.

EQUIPMENT AND SUPPLIES

Blood and body-fluid protection barriers (goggles, masks, and aprons or gowns), as necessary (see Appendix C, Recommendations for Prevention of AIDS Transmission)
Nonsterile gloves (sterile gloves may be preferred)
Suture-removal pack containing
       One suture-removal scissors
       One thumb dressing forceps
       Gauze sponges
Skin antiseptic
Steri-Strips or Butterfly Bandages (optional)

PROCEDURE

1. Wash and dry your hands. Follow the universal blood and body-fluid precautions (see Appendix C). Glove yourself with nonsterile or sterile gloves.
2. Open the suture-removal pack.

31

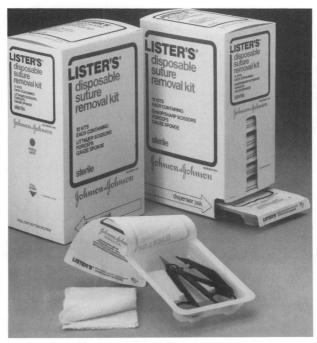

Courtesy of Johnson and Johnson Products, Inc., New Brunswick, NJ.

Procedure continued on following page

3. Place dry toweling under the area.
   Purpose: To catch spills and to keep the patient dry.
4. Position and support the area.
5. If the area has not yet been cleaned, clean and blot dry with a sterile gauze sponge.
6. Place a gauze sponge next to the wound site.
   Purpose: To place the removed sutures.
7. Without pulling, grasp the knot of the suture with the dressing forceps.
8. Cut the suture at skin level (below, left and right).

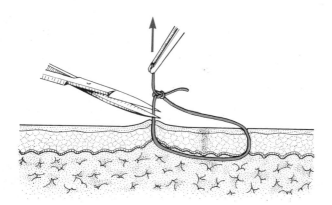
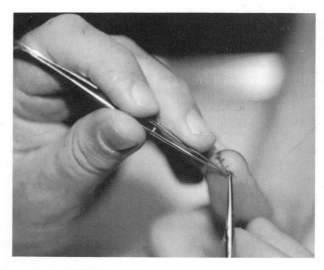

9. Lift (do not pull) the suture toward the incision and out with the dressing forceps (below, left and right).

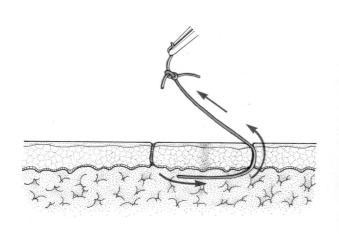
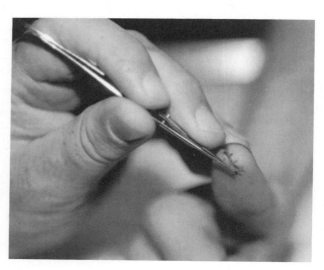

10. Place the suture on the gauze sponge, and check that the entire suture strand has been removed.
    Purpose: Suture fragments left in a wound may cause infection and may prolong the healing process.
11. If there is any bleeding, blot the area with a new gauze sponge before continuing.
12. Continue in the same manner until all the other sutures have been removed.
13. Remove the gauze sponge with the sutures on it, and count the sutures.
    Purpose: To compare the count with the suture placement count on the patient's medical record, to ensure that all sutures are accounted for.
14. The physician may choose to apply Steri-Strips or Butterfly Bandages for added support and strength.
15. Instruct the patient to keep the wound edges clean and dry and not to place excessive strain on the area.

Procedure continued on opposite page

TERMINAL PERFORMANCE OBJECTIVE

Given the necessary equipment and supplies, remove sutures from a healed incision within five minutes, without injury to the patient or a break in sterile technique, as determined by your evaluator.

ELECTROSURGERY

The electrosurgical unit incises, excises, or destroys tissue by using an electric current instead of a scalpel or curette. Electrosurgery is accomplished in minutes, and the shape and size of a surgical site can be well controlled by the surgeon. The electric current works on a minute scale, exploding the cells, which produces carbon and steam by-products. This process also seals the cells and any blood vessels in the area, and cellular oozing and vascular bleeding can be kept to a minimum. In addition, the area is automatically sterilized by the heat generated by the current. Thus, electrosurgery is advantageous because (1) it is swift, (2) it controls bleeding by simultaneously cauterizing the surrounding blood vessels, and (3) it is aseptic in technique.

The dermatologist uses electrosurgery for the removal of warts, moles, skin tags, and various skin blemishes. Some skin cancers, **senile keratoses**, seborrheic keratoses, spider nevi, and **hemangiomas** are also treated. An otolaryngologist may use electrosurgery for the treatment of tonsil tags and nasal polyps and for the control of epistaxis. Proctologic techniques include coagulation of **condylomata**, polyp removal, and the control of bleeding after a biopsy. A gynecologist frequently uses electrosurgery for cervical coagulation and the removal of cervical polyps.

Four separate items are required for electrosurgery: the power unit, the patient grounding pad, the grounding cable (See Fig. 31–14A), and the electrosurgical (electrocautery) needle or pencil (Fig. 31–14B). The grounding cable connects the machine

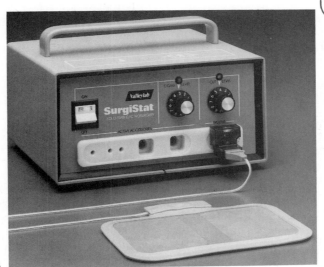

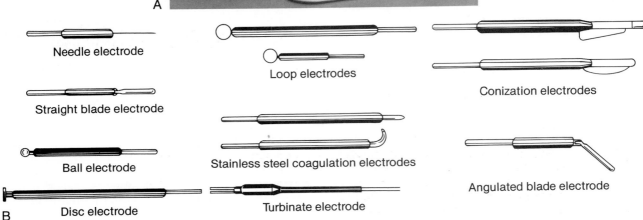

Figure 31–14 **A,** An electrosurgical power unit, which generates the electric currents necessary for electrosurgery. (Courtesy of Valleylab Inc., Boulder, CO.) **B,** Types of electrode pencils and tips used for electrosurgery.

Needle electrode

Straight blade electrode

Ball electrode

Disc electrode

Loop electrodes

Stainless steel coagulation electrodes

Turbinate electrode

Conization electrodes

Angulated blade electrode

to the grounding pad, which is placed on the patient as the electric ground. The pencil attaches to the machine by a long cord and is held by the surgeon. When the surgeon touches the tissue with the pencil, the electric current is activated by a foot pedal or a switch on the pencil, and proceeds from the machine through the cord and pencil into the tissues.

2 Types of Currents

An electric current needs two terminals (biterminal, or bipolar) to complete a circuit. In the *monopolar unit*, the tip of the pencil is the first terminal and becomes the active electrode. The current continues through the patient's body, seeking an exit route that offers the least resistance to its flow back to the power unit. The grounding cable and grounding pad (sometimes called the dispersing plate, or indifferent plate) that is placed on the patient's body is the *ground* acting as the second terminal and provides the path back to the machine to complete the electric circuit. Because the electric current flows through the patient's body, the patient must be grounded with the grounding pad for the current to pass through. If the patient is not grounded, the electric current may burn or lacerate the patient.

If a *biterminal* (bipolar) *coagulation forceps* and unit is used, this dual-tipped forceps passes the electric current from one tip to the other. The two tips are the only two terminals needed to complete the circuit, and a grounding pad is not used.

Types of Current. Two types of current are generated by the electrosurgical unit: *undamped* and *damped*. Undamped current is a steady, unrestricted current and actually cuts tissue when guided through the tissue by an ordinary wire or the point of the pencil. An electrosurgical unit, when set in an undamped or "pure-cut" mode, produces a steady, uninterrupted high-frequency current, and the tissue is divided cleanly, with little or no bleeding.

Damped current is electricity that is restricted and diminished. It is used to coagulate tissue and to stop bleeding. In surgery, *coagulation* is the "clotting" of normal tissue, by physical means, to form a shapeless residual mass. Electrocoagulation is only one method of coagulation, but it is superior to the others, which include thermal coagulation, carbon dioxide coagulation, and coagulation by injection of sclerosing chemicals.

Types of Electrosurgical Techniques. There are four types of electrosurgical techniques: electrocoagulation, electrodesiccation, electrofulguration, and electrosection.

Electrocoagulation coagulates tissues and controls hemorrhage. An active electrode, which may be a needle, disk, knife blade, or ball, is brought into contact with or is inserted into the lesion to be destroyed. A grounding pad may be placed in contact with or near the operative site. The amount of tissue destruction depends on the type of current and the length of time it is applied. This technique uses a moderately damped or modulated undamped current. This procedure may produce a great amount of necrosis, but it is advantageous in the treatment of larger or deeper growths. If bipolar coagulation forceps are used, coagulation takes place only between and immediately around the tips of the bipolar (biterminal) forceps. The destruction causes the tissue to turn grayish white. The tissue **sloughs** between 5 and 15 days, depending on the depth and the size of the area treated. When the slough has completely separated, healthy tissue appears underneath. Patients undergoing coagulation should be instructed that there will be a slight grayish discharge from the site. A topical antibiotic may be given, but it is usually not necessary because the electric current itself creates a sterile area.

Electrodesiccation destroys cells and tissues by means of a short electric spark gap that produces a highly or moderately damped current. The active electrode (usually a needle or ball) is inserted into or applied directly to the lesion. It produces coagulation of the tissue immediately surrounding the site of application or insertion and usually results in less necrosis than does coagulation. Electrodesiccation may be used to destroy granulations and small polyps. It is sometimes used to destroy the stem of a **pedunculated** growth, after the growth has been removed by an instrument, to provide hemostasis and to minimize regrowth.

Electrofulguration is from the Latin "fulgur," meaning lightning or spark. Like electrodesiccation, it also destroys tissue by means of an electric spark, but the needle tip is not inserted into the tissue. It is held about 1 or 2 mm away from the surface of the site, allowing the current to produce a superficial desiccation. A grayish-white **coagulum** is formed on the surface and, depending on the mass, sloughs in a few hours to a few days. Small superficial growths carbonize when sparked and may be lifted off immediately, with no surface evidence.

Electrosection uses slightly damped, modulated undamped, or undamped currents. The active electrode is a knife blade, wire loop, or a needle, and a large conductive metal plate is used as the grounding pad. This technique is used to incise or excise lesions and growths or for superficial **planing**.

Hazards of Electrosurgery. Safety precautions need to be taken with electrosurgery. If not, serious harm could come to the patient. Electric current should not be used around metal; therefore, the patient should be asked to remove all metal items and should be questioned whether or not there are any metal implants. Other implants that may pose a problem are those that may be disturbed by high-frequency voltage, such as pacemakers.

When a grounding pad is used, proper placement is important. The pad should be placed as close as possible to the wound site. Remember that all power concentrates and surges through the small tip of the active electrode and then seeks the grounding pad as the easiest exit pathway or ground. For the current to complete its circuit, there must be solid contact between the patient and the grounding pad; therefore, the grounding pad should not be placed over hair, scar tissue, body protuberances, or highly irregular contours that would make it difficult to maintain an even contact between the pad and the body part. If the grounding pad is bent or wrinkled or has been applied unevenly, the current concentrates in the problem *Needs to be smooth and flat* area, and "hot spots" or "cuts" can occur. A conductive medium (coupling gel) may be used to provide better contact between the patient and the grounding pad, but it must be applied uniformly to the pad and to the patient, covering the entire surface of each. Missed spots may cause burns, and areas coated too thinly may dry out during a lengthy procedure, resulting in hot spots. Pre-gelled electrodes make application easier, but care still must be taken in their application. Also, be careful that the patient is not placed in a position where contact may be made with metal of any type. The area to be treated must be dry and sufficiently exposed, and the patient should be in a comfortable position to limit movement during the procedure.

Procedure 31–6

PREPARING A PATIENT FOR ELECTROSURGERY

PROCEDURAL GOAL

To prepare a patient site for treatment by electrosurgery.

EQUIPMENT AND SUPPLIES

Blood and body-fluid protection barriers (goggles, masks, and aprons or gowns), as necessary (see Appendix C, Recommendations for Prevention of AIDS Transmission)
Nonsterile gloves (sterile gloves may be preferred)
Surgical soap
Distilled water
Skin antiseptic
Skin prep pack
Patient drape pack
Razor (optional)
Electrosurgical unit
An autoclaved pack containing tissue dressing forceps, surgical scissors, and gauze sponges

PROCEDURE

1. Wash and dry your hands. Follow universal blood and body-fluid precautions (see Appendix C). Glove yourself with nonsterile or sterile gloves.
2. Open and set up the skin-prep pack.
3. Drape the area to be treated.
4. If the area must be shaved, lather with surgical soap, and shave the area.
5. Rinse with sterile water.
6. Recleanse the area to be treated with surgical soap, and rinse with sterile water.
7. Paint the skin with an appropriate skin antiseptic.
8. If the antiseptic is alcohol-based, allow the antiseptic to dry thoroughly.
   Purpose: Alcohol is flammable and may form a spark.
9. Cover the area until the procedure is about to begin.
10. Prepare the electrosurgical equipment.
11. Open the instrument pack.
    Purpose: The surgeon may need forceps to hold a growth steady during the procedure and surgical scissors to trim away carbonized tissue.

Procedure continued on following page

TERMINAL PERFORMANCE OBJECTIVE

Given the necessary equipment and supplies, prepare a patient for electrosurgery within five minutes and without a break in sterile technique, as determined by your evaluator.

Anesthesia With Electrosurgery. Local anesthetics may or may not be used, depending on the method of the electrosurgery and the age and sensitivity of the patient. If a local anesthetic is injected into the patient, the surgeon may use a limited amount of anesthetic so as not to place too much liquid in the tissue that could heat with the passing current. Topical skin freezing with ethyl chloride is sometimes done, but care should be taken in using this flammable substance near an electric spark.

Postoperative Care. The crust resulting from electrosurgery is sterile. Thus, the postoperative application of an antiseptic solution is not necessary, nor is a dressing required if the treatment area is small and superficial. A small, dry gauze dressing or Band-Aid may be applied to protect the area from trauma or for cosmetic reasons. Dressings usually are not advisable, since the crust **in situ** should be kept dry, and a dressing may become moist. The patient should be instructed to keep the area dry, protected from trauma, and clean to prevent infection. A follow-up appointment should be scheduled for three to five days, so the area may be examined. Further treatment may be required in two to six weeks.

Care of Electrosurgical Equipment. If there is a break in an electric circuit, electricity will find another path back to the power unit. Breaks in the electric circuit can occur in damaged grounding cables or in the power unit. The grounding cable should be inspected after each surgical procedure. The power unit should be inspected regularly by a qualified engineer, and damaged parts must be replaced immediately. The electrode tips and needles sterilize themselves by means of the electric current, but you will need to keep them clean and polished. Fine steel wool or emery paper may be used for polishing them. The handles and cables may be wiped with alcohol or other germicide. As with all equipment that you must maintain, thoroughly read the manufacturer's instructions.

LASER SURGERY

LASER is the acronym for Light Amplification by Stimulated Emission of Radiation. The first application of these light waves in medicine was in the treatment of diseases of the retina. Later, its application was expanded to **photocoagulation** therapy, and then to thermal vaporization and coagulation at a microscopic level. Today, laser surgery is used on the most delicate human tissues: the eyes, brain, spinal cord, gastrointestinal tract, and fallopian tubes.

Laser equipment is very expensive and, therefore, is mostly found in hospitals, but medical offices are beginning to purchase the equipment. There are many types of laser machines, but all are similar in design. They all have an optical tube, a laser medium, reflective mirrors, and an energy source. The principle behind the laser is that light waves stimulate molecules to generate more light waves until an intense beam of light is created that begins to act like matter. This light beam of "matter" exits from the machine and, when it reaches the human tissues, heats the cells to extremely high temperatures. The cells explode and change to carbon and steam. This coagulation and vaporization process can destroy tumors, abnormal cells, strictures, and ulcers.

Safety Precautions. The laser can be as dangerous as it is powerful. A special set of safety precautions is necessary for all personnel operating laser equipment.

- Safety glasses are required for the operators and the patient.
- Do not use flammable, alcohol-based products to prep the patient.
- Keep sterile saline solution available in case the beam accidentally ignites towels or linens.
- Post warning signs on entry doors.

The dangers of the laser include burns, the inhalation of carbon or steam when tissue is subjected to laser beams, and the electric hazards related to high-wattage equipment. Laser light destroys tissue and, improperly handled, can harm not only the patient but also you and the physician. A full laser safety program should be completed before assisting in laser procedures.

REFERENCES AND READINGS

Anderson, R. M., and Romfh, R. F.: *Technique in the Use of Surgical Tools.* New York, Appleton-Century-Crofts, 1980.
Bonewit, K.: *Clinical Procedures for Medical Assistants*, 2nd ed. Philadelphia, W. B. Saunders Co., 1984.
DuGas, B. W.: *Introduction to Patient Care*, 4th ed. Philadelphia, W. B. Saunders Co., 1983.
Fuller, J. R.: *Surgical Technology: Principles and Practice*, 2nd ed. Philadelphia, W. B. Saunders Co., 1986.

Glass, R. H.: *Office Gynecology*, 2nd ed. Baltimore, Williams & Wilkins, 1978.

Grewe, H. E., and Kremer, K.: *Atlas of Surgical Operations*. Philadelphia, W. B. Saunders Co., 1980.

Nealon, T. F.: *Fundamental Skills in Surgery*, 3rd ed. Philadelphia, W. B. Saunders Co., 1979.

Sabiston, D. C., Jr.: *Textbook of Surgery*, 13th ed. Philadelphia, W. B. Saunders Co., 1986.

Vander Salm, T. J. (ed.): *Atlas of Bedside Procedures*. Boston, Little, Brown and Co., 1979.

Wood, L. A., and Rambo, B. J.: *Nursing Skills for Allied Health Services*, Vol. 3. Philadelphia, W. B. Saunders Co., 1980.

31

CHAPTER OUTLINE

VOCABULARY

See Glossary at end of book for definitions.

arthritis	erythema	quackery
atrophy	extravasation	sprain
bursitis	osteoarthritis	strain
denervated	osteoporosis	tone

32

Assisting With Modalities in Patient Treatment

OBJECTIVES

Upon successful completion of this chapter you should be able to

1. Recall the effects of heat on the body and why heat is an important treatment modality.
2. Identify ten conditions that contraindicate the use of heat in treatment.
3. Differentiate between heat hydrotherapy and dry heat.
4. Recall the effects of cold on the body and why cold is an important treatment modality.
5. Identify at least five applications of moist or dry cold.
6. Explain the importance of physical therapy in the treatment of physical disability occurring from injury or disease.
7. Explain the importance of range-of-motion exercises.
8. Recall three theories of pain control and how physical therapy can help alleviate pain due to either bodily or mental conditions.
9. Create patient-teaching activities for the various applications of heat and cold, crutch walking, and the use of a wheelchair.

Upon successful completion of this chapter you should be able to perform the following activities:

1. Apply, and instruct a patient to apply, a hot moist compress.
2. Apply, and instruct a patient to apply, a hot water bottle.
3. Assist the physician or physical therapist with the administration of ultrasound therapy.
4. Apply, and instruct a patient to apply, an ice bag.

2
Physical
Measures

This chapter describes some of the more common applications of physical agents used in therapy. These physical agents are called *modalities* and include heat and cold therapy with water, the use of electric currents as a form of physical therapy, and therapeutic exercise.

Heat or cold applications to injured or painful body parts have been utilized throughout history. Heat and cold therapies are two well-practiced, commonsense home treatments easily applied with or without the direction of a physician. It is most likely that you have had the occasion to apply heat to a swollen, sore body part, or ice to a burn or bruise. You have been applying the principles we are about to discuss, even though you may not have understood the underlying reasons that these therapies are so useful. These two physical measures, along with some other of the more complicated devices we will discuss in this chapter, are used primarily to improve circulation, minimize pain, and correct or alleviate muscular and joint malfunction.

Physical therapy and therapeutic exercise is the scientific use of physical measures, devices, and body movement to restore normal function to injured tissues. Physical therapy is a separate allied health profession practiced by physical therapists and physical therapy assistants and aides. The Association of Physical Therapists states that "physical therapy treatments should be administered by a trained physical therapist or the treatment should be supervised by a registered physical therapist." Registered physical therapists work mainly in hospitals or in specialized private practices.

Your role may be limited to referring the patient to a physical therapist and explaining pre-appoint-ment instructions, or, if it is permitted in your area of the United States, you may be able to administer limited physical therapy under the supervision of a physician or a registered physical therapist. Before participating in the physical treatment of patients, it is important for you to know which procedures are permitted by state law to be performed by someone other than a licensed physical therapist.

GENERAL PRINCIPLES OF HEAT APPLICATION

Heat produces local vasodilation and increases circulation. It speeds up the inflammatory process, promotes local drainage, relaxes muscles, and repairs tissue cells. Heat can be applied to relax and relieve pain in a **strained** muscle; to promote drainage from an abscess or infected area; to relieve tissue congestion and swelling, such as nasal congestion or a localized collection of **extravasated** blood in the tissues; or to improve the repair time of a **sprained** joint (Fig. 32–1). However, the effects of external heat applications also depend on the following conditions:

- The type of heat used
- The length of time the heat is applied
- The general condition of the patient
- The size of the area needing treatment

Heat can be harmful. Prolonged application of heat increases the secretions of the skin, softening it and lowering its resistance to injury. Extreme heat works adversely by constricting the blood vessels and causing burns. Heat applied too often may increase a patient's tolerance to heat so that the

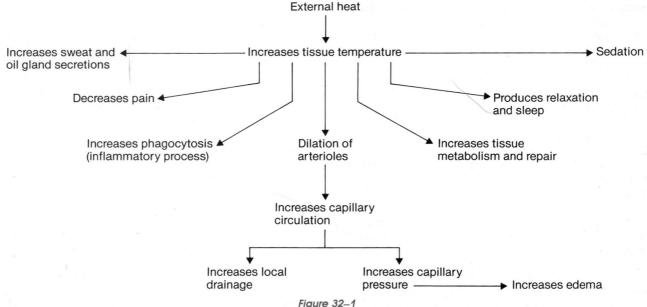

Figure 32–1
Body responses to local heat application. (Adapted from St. Mary's Hospital, Inc., Russelville, AR.)

patient may be burned without knowing it. Infants and the elderly are particularly susceptible to burns, so extreme caution must be used when treating them. Infants and patients who cannot report a burning sensation should be evaluated and watched carefully, as should persons with diseases of the cardiovascular, renal, and respiratory system, and with **osteoporosis**. In addition, special precautions must be taken with patients with impaired circulation, such as those with diabetes. Because heat can increase the inflammatory process, it should never be applied to the abdomen if appendicitis is suspected. In this instance, heat can rupture the inflamed appendix.

When deciding whether or not to treat a body part with heat, the following conditions all are generally contraindications. Of course, there may be special conditions, or directions given by the physician, to treat with heat even though one or more of these conditions exist. However, *do not* treat a patient having any of the following conditions until you have specifically discussed the condition with the physician:

1. Acute inflammatory conditions. Heat should not be used in most acute inflammatory processes for the first 48 hours.

2. Severe circulatory problems, such as blockage and bleeding. Heat can increase the blockage and cause hemorrhaging.

3. The lack of sensation in a body part. There is danger that the patient cannot report burning. A lack of sensation may indicate a lack of circulation in the body part.

4. Pregnancy or menstruation. Heat can cause uterine contractions and increase menstrual flow.

5. Areas containing encapsulated pus and having no drainage. Heat increases the inflammatory process, and the encapsulated area could rupture.

6. Blisters from hot water bottles, heating pads, skin ointments, or salves previously applied by the patient. Heat should not be applied over newly burned skin.

7. Scar tissue does not have a normal supply of blood vessels; therefore, heat is not carried away by blood circulation, and burns could occur.

8. Body areas that may contain malignant tumors. Malignant tumor activity may be stimulated by heat.

9. Erythema, redness of the skin, may indicate a blood clot, which could break loose with an increase in circulation caused by application of heat.

10. Metal materials. Heat concentrates in metal materials, such as metal implants, prostheses, and certain IUDs. Therefore, patients with internal metal devices should not have those areas treated. To avoid burns, metal objects such as jewelry, watches, hearing aids, hairpins, and metal clips must be removed before treatment. Treatment must be administered on nonmetal tables and chairs.

Body parts may be heated to 110°F (44°C) without damage to the tissues. Redness appears because the capillaries become congested with blood at the skin's surface. Continuous heat for more than 20 minutes usually results in the increased circulation carrying away the heat as rapidly as it is applied, and the therapy may lose its effectiveness. Heat applied for more than one hour causes the blood vessels to constrict, thereby decreasing the blood supply to the area and adversely affecting the effectiveness of the treatment.

Moist heat penetrates better than dry heat. Moist heat (heat hydrotherapy) may be applied with hot packs and compresses, soaks, or baths. Dry heat may be applied in the form of hot water bottles or electric heating pads and lamps, or by the use of electric current when we need to treat the deeper tissues. Let's look at some of the more common methods of treatment by heat.

Heat Hydrotherapy

Soaks. With heat hydrotherapy, a body part is immersed gradually into medicated or plain water for approximately 15 minutes at a temperature no greater than 110°F (44°C). The extremities are often treated by this method. Patients can take their own soaks at home, but special instructions in aseptic techniques must be given to the patient if the area being treated is an open wound (see Chapter 31).

Whirlpool Treatment. This method uses a tank with special equipment that agitates the water to provide gentle massage (Fig. 32–2). It is useful for exercise or to cleanse wounds. The temperature is the same as for any method of heat hydrotherapy.

Paraffin Bath. This is especially useful in treating chronic joint disease. A mixture of seven (7) parts paraffin and one (1) part mineral oil is heated to melting at about 127°F. The patient's body part is dipped into the warm paraffin mixture and removed, and then this is repeated until a thick coat is formed on the body part (Fig. 32–3). The paraffin is left on for about 30 minutes and then is peeled off. It leaves the skin soft, warm, and pliable, with a slight erythema.

Hot Moist Compresses. These are used to increase blood flow to small areas of the body, such as the hands. Compresses may be made at home with soft cloths or a clean washcloth. If hot moist compresses are applied to an open wound in the office, use sterile gauze sponges, a sterile solution, and surgically aseptic conditions. Follow the universal blood and body-fluid precautions (see Appendix C, Recommendations for Prevention of AIDS Transmission). Dispose of used materials in a closed container so that personnel and other

32

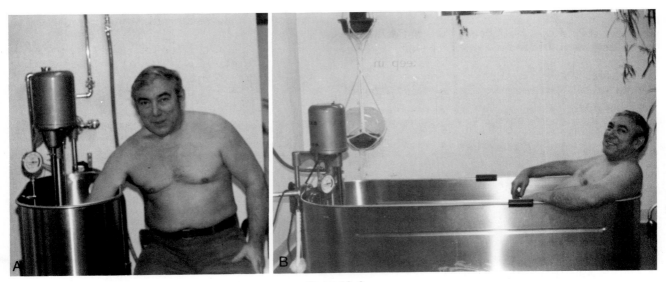

Figure 32–2
*Hydrotherapy tanks are equipped with whirlpools. **A,** The tank provides therapy for the patient's extremities. **B,** A larger tank is used for full-body therapy. (Courtesy of DeanCare, Madison, WI.)*

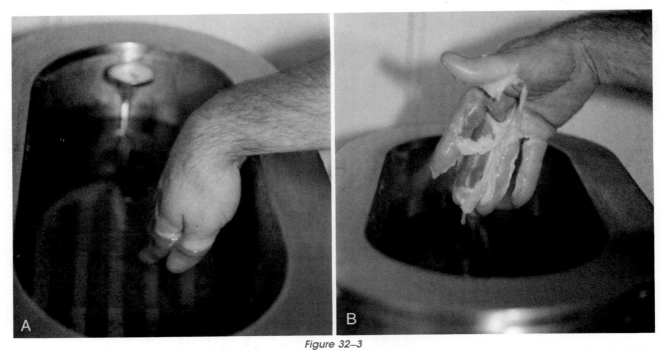

Figure 32–3
*The paraffin bath is especially helpful for pain relief in patients with arthritis. **A,** The hand is dipped into warm paraffin. If a thicker coating of wax is desired, the hand is dipped again. **B,** The warm paraffin is left on the hand for about 30 minutes and then is peeled off.*

patients are not in danger of contact with the contaminated materials (see Chapter 31).

Often, you will be asked to instruct patients on how to apply hot moist compresses at home. Patient instructions for home care should be explicit and simple. The patient should remove all jewelry and should be instructed *not* to apply a hot moist compress if a rash appears or the skin is broken. A plastic covering will help keep in the moisture. A hot water bottle may be used to keep the compress hot. If you are speaking to the patient over the telephone, be sure that the patient writes down the instructions as you read each step. Never assume that the patient knows the correct method. When instructing patients in person, it is best to have preprinted instructions for you to review and give to the patient to take home. The following list of steps may be used in preparing patient instructions for applying hot compresses at home:

1. Moisten a clean hand towel with warm water.

2. Wring it out.

3. The compress should be warm, not hot.

4. Place the towel directly onto the skin.

5. Cover the towel with plastic to keep in the moist heat.

6. Continue the therapy for the prescribed length of time and the prescribed number of times each day.

Commercially prepared hot moist compresses are packs made of canvas containing a silicon gel, which retains heat. They may be purchased for home use and may be heated in warm water.

Procedure 32–1

APPLYING A HOT MOIST PACK (COMMERCIALLY PREPARED COMPRESS)

PROCEDURAL GOAL

To apply a hot moist pack to a patient's arm for the treatment of pain or discomfort, as directed by the physician.

EQUIPMENT AND SUPPLIES

Commercially prepared hot moist packs
Heating tank or vessel
Towels
Forceps

PROCEDURE

1. Using forceps, remove the commercially prepared pack from the hot water tank or vessel.
   Purpose: This type of pack contains a gel substance that retains heat and can burn your hand.

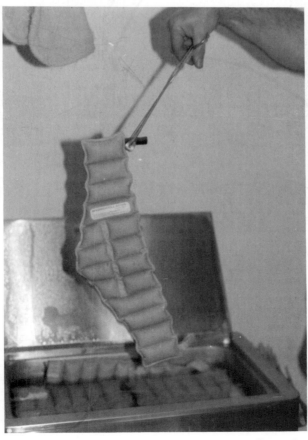

Procedure continued on following page

2. Wrap the pack in six to eight layers of toweling.
   Purpose: The towels hold in the heat and prevent skin burns.
3. Place the patient's arm on an arm board covered with foam rubber, if one is available.
   Purpose: Supporting the arm with padding decreases patient discomfort.

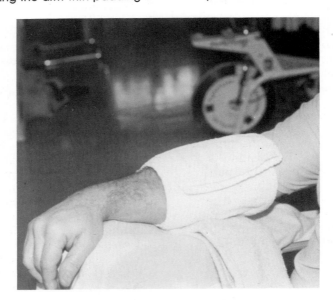

4. Apply the pack to the affected area, and cover it with a towel.
5. Secure the pack with another towel that has fasteners (especially when packing arms or legs).
   Purpose: To keep the pack in place.

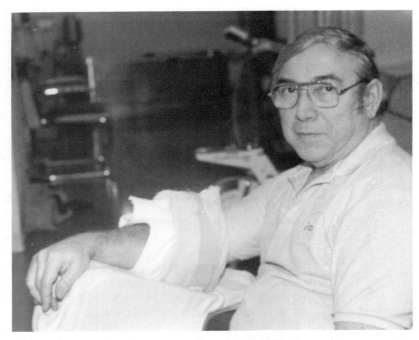

6. Keep the pack in place as ordered by the physician. Times will vary from 15 to 30 minutes.

TERMINAL PERFORMANCE OBJECTIVE

Given a patient, the appropriate equipment and supplies, and a specific order by the physician, apply a hot moist pack to a patient, explaining the procedure while completing each step in the correct order, as determined by your evaluator.

Dry Heat

Methods of dry heat can produce heat on the superficial skin surfaces or penetrate to the deeper muscle tissues. Heating pads, infrared radiation (heat lamps and hot water bottles), and ultraviolet rays generate heat that can penetrate to a depth of 10 mm. Deeper penetration of heat, produced with high-frequency electric current, is called *diathermy*. Diathermy is derived from the Greek words meaning "heating through."

Heating Pads. The least complicated method of applying dry heat, heating pads are often used by the patient at home. When giving instructions for use at home, caution the patient that heating pads must not be used near moisture. Instruct the patient to turn the heat control to low or medium (never the high setting) and to keep the pad on the body part only for a prescribed length of time. Heating pads with automatic thermostats are preferred over the older models that do not control the temperature evenly.

Infrared Radiation Lamps. These generate heat within a metal coil element or a special heat-producing electric bulb. This source of energy produces very shallow heat penetration. The penetration is about 3 to 5 mm, or 0.1 to 0.2 in, and depends on the principle of conduction to warm the deeper tissues (Fig. 32–4). This treatment produces an approximate 1°F temperature increase at the site being treated.

Before treatment, the skin is cleansed to remove any ointments and skin oils. The treatment extends for usually 20 to 45 minutes, according to the physician's instructions. During the course of the treatment, the patient's skin becomes flushed, but a "sunburn" does not occur. However, if used

improperly, the infrared lamp is capable of producing skin burns in exactly the same manner as touching a hot stove or oven. In addition to dry heat treatments, the infrared lamp can be placed above a moist dressing to extend the time of a moist heat treatment.

Maintenance of the infrared lamp is simple. The heating element should be kept in a down position when not in use, to prevent dust from accumulating on the element. The electric connections should be checked and kept in good working condition.

Ultraviolet Radiation. Ultraviolet radiation is produced by the sun or by lamps, sometimes called sun lamps. Ultraviolet radiation is more penetrating than infrared radiation and can cause skin burns or pigmentation changes resulting in tanning. Ultraviolet rays are also capable of killing bacteria. It is this bactericidal action that makes ultraviolet radiation so useful in therapy. It is effective in treating skin diseases caused by bacteria, such as acne, psoriasis, and ulcerations.

Ultraviolet rays are generated by different types of lamps. One type discharges a current of electricity through certain gases in a quartz tube. The process produces ultraviolet rays with very little heat generation. This lamp is called the *cold quartz lamp* and is most frequently used in the physician's office.

There are two types of cold quartz ultraviolet lamps. One type is used for general body radiation. This energy is very potent, and precautions must be taken to avoid tissue damage from over-exposure. The physician must give an exact order in seconds or minutes for the length of exposure and the exact distance between the patient and the lamp. At a distance of 36 in from the unit to the patient, a first-degree burn can be produced in 30 seconds to one minute, a second-degree burn in one to two minutes, and a third-degree burn in two to four minutes.

Test the lamp on the patient's forearm for a few seconds before you begin treatment to determine the presence of skin sensitivity. Some patients cannot tolerate any ultraviolet radiation. A history of sun exposure may help you determine this. Ultraviolet rays are considered carcinogenic if their use is prolonged. Certain drugs, especially the sulfonamides, increase the sensitivity of the skin to ultraviolet rays, and treatments should be postponed or the dosage reduced accordingly. Additional precautions include covering the genitalia and other areas of the patient's body not being treated with a towel. Both the operator and the patient should wear ultraviolet–filtered glasses.

The size of the dose is usually governed by the erythematous response of the patient's skin. Treatments are generally given every other day because 24 hours is not enough time to evaluate the maximum erythematous response of the skin. The penetration of the rays is less than 0.1 mm, and there

32

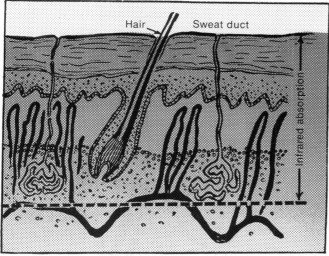

Figure 32–4
The broken line indicates the depth of penetration of the infrared rays into the skin.

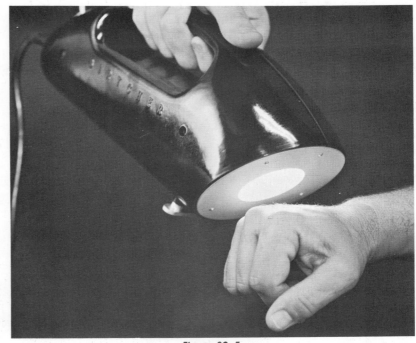

Figure 32–5
The Spot-Quartz is a portable, cold quartz lamp. (Courtesy of the Bircher Corporation.)

may be some tanning of the skin. The intensity of the radiation is greatest when the rays strike the skin at right angles (90 degrees). At an angle of 30 degrees, the intensity decreases to 80 percent (Lambert's cosine law). If the distance from the patient to the lamp is decreased by one half, the strength of the radiation is increased four times (inverse square law). Because of these two factors, it is important that the distance and the angle of the ultraviolet rays are correct and the same for each treatment.

The *portable Spot-Quartz lamp* is useful when treating small areas (Fig. 32–5). The portable lamp is placed near or in contact with the area to be treated. Practically no heat is generated in the lamp coils, thus skins burns do not occur. The treatment time extends from a few seconds to minutes, depending

on the skin condition and the distance between the patient and the lamp. A masking adapter for small areas attaches to the face of the lamp, and a filter (Wood's filter) eliminates the visible light. The glass coils of the lamp must be protected from breakage and must be kept free of dust and soil. They may be cleaned with alcohol.

Hot Water Bottles. These are often used at home without any thought to correct technique. When teaching patients how to use this method at home, caution them to keep the water temperature at or below 125°F (52°C). If the patient is a child, keep the temperature below 115°F (46°C) to prevent burns. A hot water bottle that is less than one-half full conforms better to the body and is more comfortable.

Procedure 32–2

APPLYING A HOT WATER BOTTLE

PROCEDURAL GOAL

To administer dry heat using a hot water bottle.

EQUIPMENT AND SUPPLIES

Hot water bottle
Thermometer
Pitcher
Towel

Procedure continued on opposite page

PROCEDURE

1. Wash your hands.
2. Identify the patient.
3. Explain the procedure, and answer any questions that the patient may ask about home care.
4. Specifically, ask the patient if he or she has any questions about how to perform the treatment.
5. If the patient is not sure how to do the procedure, demonstrate as follows:
6. Fill the pitcher with hot water from the faucet.
7. Check the temperature with a thermometer, to avoid skin burns.
8. Fill the hot water bottle about one-half full.
9. Lay the bottle on a counter, turn the neck upward, and push out excess air.
   Purpose: To eliminate air, which is a poor conductor of heat.
10. Seal the bottle.

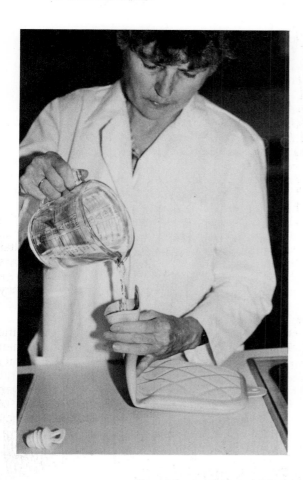 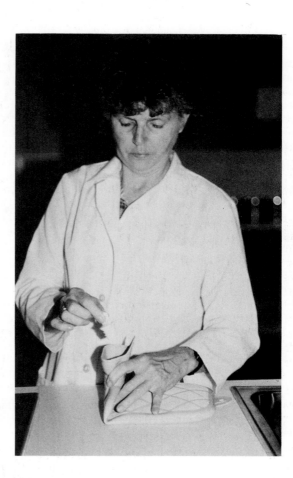

TERMINAL PERFORMANCE OBJECTIVE

Given a patient, the appropriate equipment and supplies, and a specific order by the physician, apply a hot water bottle to a patient, explaining the procedure while completing each step in the correct order, as determined by your evaluator.

Heat Application to Deeper Tissues

Three methods of heat application to the deeper tissues are short-wave, microwave, and ultrasound diathermy. All three forms are applied to increase blood flow and speed up metabolism and electrolyte flow across the cell membranes. Treatment is used to stretch and repair tendons, joint capsules and scars. Treatments usually relieve stiffness of joints, relax muscles, and decrease muscle spasm.

Short-wave Diathermy. This method produces energy similar to that emitted by a radio station transmission. This energy penetrates deep into the body tissues and creates heat. The use of short-wave diathermy may be indicated for all types of inflammatory processes (acute, subacute, and chronic). Many patients report pain relief within 36 to 48 hours. Treatments may be prescribed as often as three times a week, for 20 to 30 minutes.

Two condenser plates are placed on either side of the body part to be treated. As these high-frequency waves are transmitted through the body from one plate to the other, heat is generated in the tissues. Most short-wave diathermy plates are placed one inch from the skin. The dosage panel should be adjusted until a mild heat is felt by the patient. Some patients may believe that if a little warmth produces good results, more heat will be even better. This is not true with short-wave diathermy. Do not increase the volume of energy above the amount ordered by the physician, and carefully explain to the patient that only a gentle warmth is appropriate for effective treatment. Conversely, notify the physician that you need to lower the volume of energy if the amount ordered is too much for the patient. Position the machine so that the patient cannot adjust the controls. If necessary, place a towel on the patient to collect perspiration.

The short-wave diathermy machine must be wiped down after use on each patient. Do not permit the electric cords to tangle. Do not move the machine in any position that will pull the electric cord at any of the connections. The cables leading to the patient electrode plates should not cross one another or touch the patient. Electricity follows the path of least resistance and may flow from one cord to another, thus rerouting the energy away from the area being treated. Almost all machines have "spacers" on the cables to prevent this. Some machines may require a warm-up period before they can be used in treatment.

Microwave Diathermy. This method uses radar waves. It works on the same principle as microwave ovens used for cooking. Microwaves have a higher frequency and shorter wavelength than radio waves. This mode is the easiest to use (one electrode is placed above the body part to be treated), but it has less penetration than does short-wave diathermy. Microwaves cannot be used over moist dressings or near persons with implanted electronic cardiac pacemakers.

Ultrasound Diathermy. Ultrasound energy is sound energy. The basic principle of ultrasonography is the same as that of sonar, used in oceanography. Ultrasonic waves are concentrated into a narrow beam and are transmitted through a medium in the form of vibrations. The customary sounds that we hear are produced by sound waves vibrating at a rate of 100 to 12,000 cycles per second (hertz). Ultrasound waves vibrate at the rate of one million times per second. In therapeutic ultrasound machines, this frequency is created by an electric current passing through an applicator (transducer). In the applicator is a quartz crystal. The current passes through the quartz, causing the quartz to vibrate at an extremely high frequency. When the applicator containing the quartz is brought into contact with the body, the vibrations are transferred and continue through the tissues.

Though the frequency of this vibration is high, the total energy transmitted to the patient is very low. It is normally indicated on an output meter on the machine, in total watts or watts per square centimeter of the applicator element area (Fig. 32–6). Ultrahigh-frequency sound waves do not travel through air. The applicator must be held in contact with the body surface and aided with a *coupling agent*. A coupling agent may be either water or a gel. If the area of the body to be treated can be immersed in a basin or tank, treatment may be administered under water. For areas of the body that cannot be immersed, gel is applied to the applicator and to the body part to be treated. The gel should be water-soluble and nonstaining to clothing or skin.

Ultrahigh-frequency sound waves cause the tissues to vibrate, which in turn vibrates the circulatory system and speeds up circulation. The increased blood flow creates a chemical action in the tissues that has a favorable effect on the body's healing process. All this takes place with little or no heat, and the patient feels no sensation except a little warmth. Because ultrasound waves travel best through water, they penetrate the deep body tissues that have a high water content, such as the muscles. However, because ultrasound waves cannot penetrate and "move" along tissues that have a low water content, such as bone, the waves are capable of concentrating and "bombarding" bone and causing damage. Ultrasound treatment must be used very carefully where bones are near the surface of the skin.

Most acute ailments, such as strains, sprains, and torn muscles and tendons, are treated with ultrasound power as low as 0.5 to 1.0 watt per square centimeter. Ultrasound treatment is not recommended within the first 48 hours for these acute conditions. During this first 48-hour period, the best treatment is application of cold compresses. Chronic conditions, such as **arthritis** and **osteoarthritis,** may be treated at a higher power, 1.5 to 2.5 watts per square centimeter. The duration of any treatment varies from 5 to 15 minutes, depending on the physician's instructions.

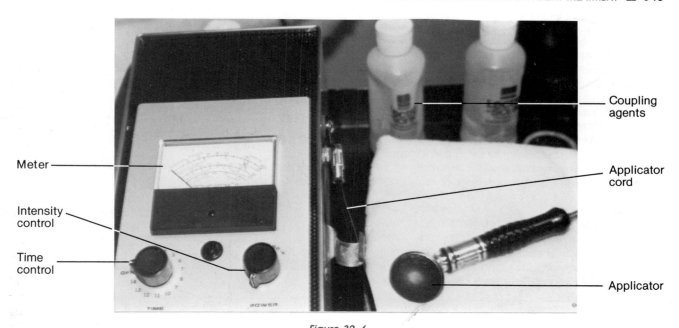

Figure 32–6
The ultrasound machine and its parts are shown here. Notice that the intensity control is at zero. The bottles contain coupling gel.

Procedure 32-3

ASSISTING WITH ULTRASOUND THERAPY

Note: The medical assistant should perform ultrasound therapy only under the supervision of the physician or a registered physical therapist.

PROCEDURAL GOAL

To apply ultrahigh-frequency sound waves to the patient's deep tissues for therapy.

EQUIPMENT AND SUPPLIES

Ultrasound machine
Coupling agent

PROCEDURE

1. Wash your hands.
2. Confirm the patient's identity.
3. Explain the procedure, and ask the patient to indicate if there is any discomfort.
   Purpose: To ensure that the patient does not experience any pain or injury.
4. Question the patient for the presence of any internal or external metal objects.
5. Position the patient comfortably, with the area to be treated exposed.
6. Apply a warmed coupling agent liberally over the area to be treated and to the applicator.
   Purpose: To transmit the sound waves through water or a water-soluble substance.
7. Begin treatment with the intensity control at the lowest setting.
8. Set the timer on the machine.
   Purpose: The timer starts the machine.
9. Increase the intensity control to the ordered amount.
10. Hold the applicator at a 90-degree angle against the patient's skin.
    Purpose: To ensure close contact.

Procedure continued on following page

11. Work the applicator over the area to be treated in a circular fashion, within a radius of two inches per second.
   Purpose: Constant motion prevents "hot spots" from occurring from excessive ultrasonic waves to one area.
12. If the alternative method of "stroking" is ordered, move the applicator in short one-inch strokes so that each stroke overlaps the last stroke about one-half inch.
13. Keep the applicator moving until the timer sounds. The timer shuts off the machine automatically.
14. Return the intensity control to zero.
15. Remove the coupling agent from the patient and from the applicator with a paper wipe.
16. Assist the patient to the dressing room.
17. Record on the patient's medical record the treatment date, area treated, intensity, duration, and any unusual occurrences or reaction(s) that may have occurred during the treatment.

TERMINAL PERFORMANCE OBJECTIVE

Given a patient, the appropriate equipment and supplies, and a specific order by the physician, assist with an ultrasound treatment, completing each step of the procedure in the correct order, as determined by your evaluator.

GENERAL PRINCIPLES OF COLD APPLICATION

closes the vessels

Cold applications such as ice packs and cold compresses act as vasoconstrictors and cause contraction of the involuntary muscles of the skin. These two actions cause a reduced blood supply to the skin and numbing of the sensory nerve endings. Cold applications are used to control bleeding or to slow down inflammatory reactions. Cold reduces swelling and relieves pain. Occasionally, it is used to slow down the activity of living cells, thereby controlling infection. It is important to understand that while cold applications prevent further swelling, they do not reverse any swelling that is already present in the tissues. Such swelling is later treated with heat.

Cold applications may be used in an emergency to treat burns and to control internal bleeding and edema. Cool sponge baths, using cool water and alcohol, are employed to reduce fevers. A generalized lowering of the body's temperature depresses the activity of the body, slowing the heart and the pulse rate and decreasing cellular activity.

Pressure

Cold Compresses

Cold compresses are applied to small areas such as the face and the head. Gauze sponges or wash cloths are most often used. The first cloth should be applied gently so that the patient gets used to the cold. Compresses should be changed every three minutes, and the total treatment is ordered usually for 20 minutes at a time. Advise patients to check the skin for signs of redness and swelling at the application site. Applications should be stopped if the cold causes pain.

Ice Packs

Ice packs can be applied to the head to treat headache, fever, delirium, and minor head injuries; to the abdomen to slow down inflammation within the abdominal or pelvic cavity; or to the eyes to control swelling and inflammation. Ice packs may be prescribed following some surgical procedures to control swelling and bleeding and may be used to relieve the symptoms of hemorrhoids.

Usually, an ice pack is applied up to one hour or until the patient complains of pain from the cold or numbness, whichever occurs first. Ice packs should be covered with a cloth or towel to keep the patient dry. Ice packs without a covering may be too cold for the patient to tolerate.

Do not assume that a patient knows the correct technique of applying an ice pack. Instruct the patient on how to care for and apply ice packs at home. Ice packs may be made from items around the home such as plastic bags and towels. Commercially prepared dry ice packs may be purchased, but they are effective only for a few minutes. The best method for applying an ice pack is with the purchased ice bag.

Treatment

THERAPEUTIC EXERCISE

A therapeutic exercise program is designed to correct specific disabilities of the patient. An exercise program may restore mobility, coordination, and strength to a part or may result in relaxation and relief of tension or pain. Extensive evaluation of the patient's actual physical condition is necessary when exercise therapy is prescribed. This is also a time when a great amount of patient education and encouragement is required. The physical therapist and the physician work together in eval-

Procedure 32-4

PROCEDURAL GOAL

To instruct a patient on how to apply dry cold to a body area to prevent swelling.

EQUIPMENT AND SUPPLIES

Ice bag
Small cubes or chips of ice
Towel
Blood and body-fluid protection barriers (goggles, masks, and aprons or gowns), as necessary (see Appendix C, Recommendations for Prevention of AIDS Transmission)
Nonsterile gloves

PROCEDURE

1. Wash your hands. Follow the universal blood and body-fluid precautions (see Appendix C).
2. Identify the patient.
3. Explain the procedure, and answer any questions that the patient may ask about home care.
4. Specifically ask the patient if he or she has any questions about how to perform the treatment.
5. If the patient is not sure how to do the procedure, demonstrate as follows:
6. Check the bag for possible leaks.
7. Fill the bag with small cubes or chips of ice until it is about two-thirds full.
   Purpose: Small chips conform better to the body part.
8. Push down on the top of the bag to expel excess air, and apply the cap.
   Purpose: To remove air, which is a poor conductor of cold.
9. Dry and cover the bag.
10. Help the patient position the ice bag on the affected area.
11. Advise the patient that the damaged tissues will benefit from the cold even though the treatment may feel uncomfortable.
12. Advise the patient to leave the ice bag in place for about one-half hour or until the area feels numb.
13. Check the skin for color, feeling, and pain.
    Purpose: If the area being treated becomes very painful, remains numb, or is pale or blue, the ice bag should be removed and the physician notified.
14. Clean the ice bag by emptying the water, rinsing it, and allowing it to dry in the air without the cap on.
15. Chart the procedure and the patient teaching session.

TERMINAL PERFORMANCE OBJECTIVE

Given the necessary equipment, teach a patient to fill, apply, and care for an ice bag, completing each step of the procedure in the correct order, as determined by your evaluator.

---

uating the best type of treatment. Often, therapeutic exercise is combined with the heat and heat hydrotherapy treatments already mentioned in this chapter.

Joint Mobility

If motion is restricted even for a short period of time, the joint tissues become dense, hard, and shortened. These changes occur even in normal joints in as short a time as four days. It is important to institute joint exercise as soon as possible during therapy. Treatment of joint immobility or disability is accomplished either actively or passively by exercising a joint to its highest degree of possible motion.

Active Exercise. Active exercise is body movement voluntarily initiated and controlled by the patient, although the patient may be assisted by the physical therapist or physical therapist assistant.

Active exercise may require specialized equipment, similar to gymnasium equipment. Some devices that are prescribed are stationary bicycles and free weights.

Passive Exercise. Passive exercise is moving a body part without the voluntary action of the patient. The movement is performed by someone other than the patient or by the force of a machine.

Range-of-Motion (ROM) Exercises. ROM exercises are specially designed exercises that move each joint of the body through its full range of motion (Fig. 32–7). After an injury to a joint, it is recom-

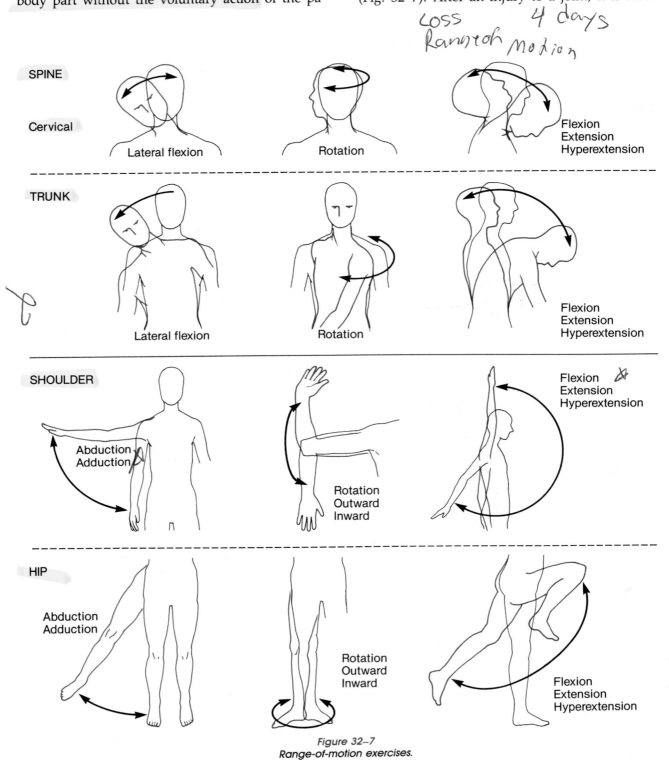

Figure 32–7
Range-of-motion exercises.

Illustration continued on opposite page

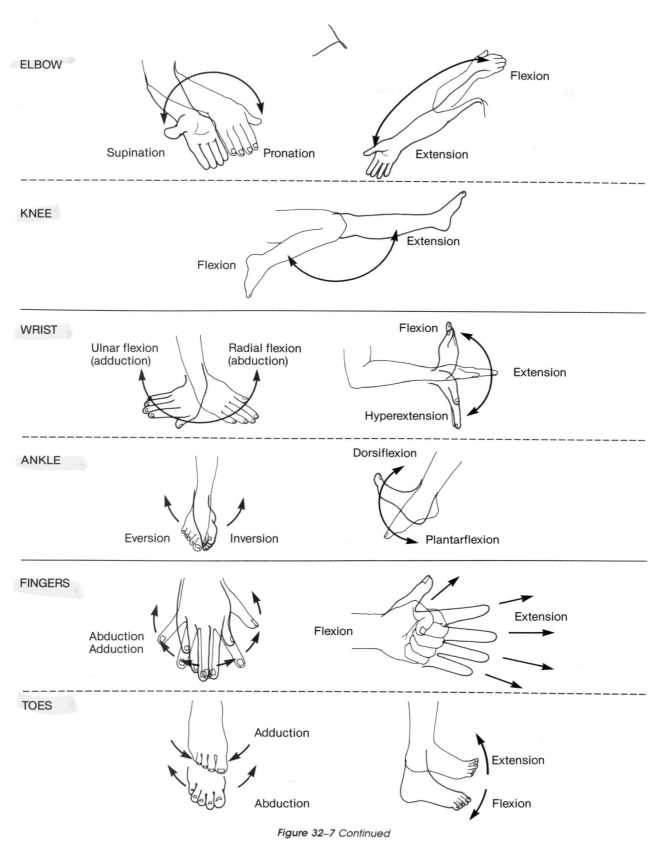

ELBOW
Supination — Pronation
Flexion
Extension

KNEE
Flexion
Extension

WRIST
Ulnar flexion (adduction)
Radial flexion (abduction)
Flexion
Extension
Hyperextension

ANKLE
Eversion — Inversion
Dorsiflexion
Plantarflexion

FINGERS
Abduction
Adduction
Flexion
Extension

TOES
Adduction
Abduction
Extension
Flexion

Figure 32–7 Continued

32

mended that the patient exercise the injured part to its full range of motion three times, at least twice daily. If the patient cannot exercise actively, another individual can exercise the part passively. Range-of-motion exercises should be done slowly and gently, and only after the patient has been specifically instructed in correct techniques by a physical therapist. If the exercises are done too early or improperly, pain and even fracture or bleeding within the joint can occur.

Muscle Training and Strength

Muscle training is used to teach patients to gain or regain use of their muscles. This training can involve rehabilitation of muscle control lost as a result of physical trauma or diseases, such as poliomyelitis or cerebral palsy, or learning to use crutches or a wheelchair. Endurance exercises are used in the rehabilitation of the patient whose goal is to return to an active life after a long and debilitating illness or injury.

Electromuscle Stimulators. These are low-voltage machines that create a controlled electric current similar to that coming from an ordinary wall outlet. These low-voltage currents are useful for stimulating the motor and sensory nerves supplying the muscles. Such stimulation provides a passive means of exercising a muscle when a patient cannot activate the muscle voluntarily because of nerve damage. The purpose of the treatment is to revitalize a muscle or prevent **atrophy** of normal muscle.

Small electrode pads are moistened with tap water to increase their contact with the patient's skin. The pads are held by the technician until they are strapped into place. The machine is then operated by passing electric currents into the patient's muscles. The path of the electric current varies, depending on the exact placement of the two pads. As the current is applied to the muscles, the various waves act like the body's own nerves, causing the muscles to contract and relax.

One type of therapeutic current can stimulate and exercise **denervated** muscles and, if applied often enough, maintain a nearly normal muscle **tone.** Stimulation is also beneficial in retraining a patient to use injured muscles. The current artificially contracts and relaxes the muscles, and the patient is able to remember the feel of moving the body part. This often produces spectacular results and demonstrates to the patient that a muscle is not "dead" but can be revitalized.

Crutches. Crutches are used for mobility in cases of leg injury. You may be asked to help the patient select and adjust the proper size of crutches. Have the patient stand tall, with the head and back straight. If extra support is needed to maintain posture while measuring the crutches, have the patient stand straight against a wall. Adhere to the following steps to ensure a comfortable fit:

flat shoes

1. Crutch tips should be placed about 6 in away from and parallel to the toes. (A thin person should move the tips slightly forward; a heavy person, with wide hips, should allow more space between the crutches and the toes.)
2. Adjust the length of the crutches so that two or three fingers fit between the armpit and the crutch top (about 2 in). You may measure from the anterior axillary fold to the heel and then add 2 in more.
3. Have the patient bend the elbow about 20 to 30 degrees when holding the hand grip.
4. Ask the patient to push down on the crutches and lift the body slightly. Now the arms should be nearly straight.
5. The hands and the arms should hold all the body weight with each stride. (Remember that weight borne by the axillary region may cause permanent nerve damage.)
6. Ask the patient to walk a few steps to be sure that the weight is distributed properly (Fig. 32–8).
7. As crutch-walking skills improve, so will posture. Instruct the patient to make adjustments at regular intervals. (Young children outgrow crutches rapidly. Check for fit frequently.)

Here are some tips that you can preprint for distribution to patients who are using crutches:

- Check to be sure that all wing nuts are tight.
- Check your crutch tips for wear. Crutch tips may be purchased at any drugstore or hardware store.
- Foam pads at the armpits and around the hand grips are more comfortable.
- Wear a sturdy low-heeled shoe on your unaffected foot.
- Keep the injured leg as relaxed as possible, and bend the knee to ensure that it clears the floor.
- Avoid scatter rugs, spills on the floor, extension cords, pets, and walking in the dark.
- Special safety equipment for the kitchen and bathroom is available for purchase or rental.

Wheelchairs. Wheelchairs use arm muscles rather than leg muscles for mobility. The folding wheelchair is very popular because it is lightweight and folds easily for travel.

The following suggestions can help patients to maneuver safely in and out of wheelchairs:

- Lock the chair so that it cannot move.
- Fold back the foot rests.
- Back into the chair, and support yourself on the arm rests as you lower your body into the seat.
- To leave the chair, first lock the chair and then fold back the foot rests.
- Lift your body, supporting yourself on the arm rests.
- Place your unaffected foot flat on the floor, just slightly under the seat.
- Push into an upright position, using your thigh muscles along with your arm and shoulder muscles.

always have a wheelchair next to their good side

32

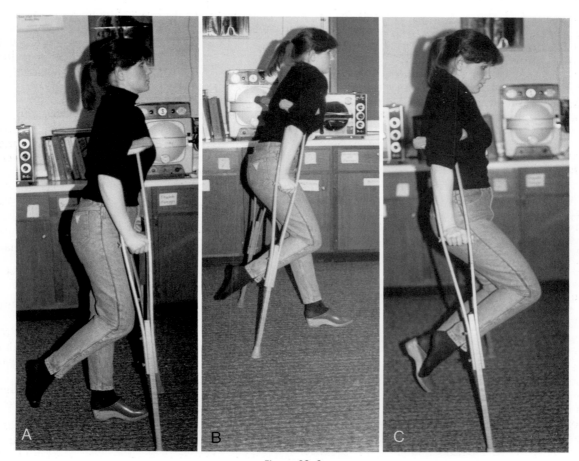

Figure 32–8
One type of crutch walking, the swing-through gait, is shown here. It is used when the affected foot can bear no weight. **A,** *The unaffected foot bears the body weight, both crutches are advanced together.* **B,** *The arm muscles bear the body weight as the body swings through.* **C,** *Completion of one step. With weight back on the unaffected foot, both crutches will be advanced again to get ready for the next step.*

Relief of Tension and Pain

A growing branch of medicine and physical therapy employs exercise to relax the muscles and to provide relief from tension and pain resulting from stress or a wide variety of physical disorders.

Pain Control. This includes such techniques as relaxation, massage, the application of heat and liniments, mechanical electric stimulation, acupuncture, and hypnosis. Mechanical electric stimulation was introduced one hundred years ago as an analgesic. It was regarded as **quackery** at that time, even though some patients reported pain relief. Acupuncture, adapted from ancient Chinese techniques, has received wide acceptance during the last few decades. Along with acupuncture, hypnosis has proved helpful in pain relief for many patients. During the last ten years, the effectiveness of relaxation exercises, heat, and massage for pain relief have been explained scientifically.

There are several theories about pain and its control. The "gate theory" offers one possible explanation. In 1937, Ronald Melzack and Patrick Wall hypothesized that pain signals can be modified by a hypothetic gate in the spinal cord that opens and closes. Gentle stimulation causes impulses to travel so fast that they rush ahead and close the gate, which keeps the pain signals from reaching the brain.

Since this theory was first proposed, we have learned that our bodies contain morphine-like substances called *cephalins* and *endorphins*. These two analgesic substances are found naturally in the brain and spinal cord and appear to block the transmission of pain signals upward along the spinal cord to the brain. Another discovery is that certain thick sensory fibers extending from tactile receptors in the skin can compete with and suppress the transmission of pain to the brain from the thinner nerve fibers.

The most significant number of chronic pain sufferers seen in the medical office are those with muscle or joint pain such as arthritis, **bursitis**, and low back pain. All the physical pain control techniques previously mentioned have been useful in treating these conditions. *Intractable pain* is defined as that which cannot be relieved except through the use of addicting drugs or incapacitating sedation. The patient with chronic, prolonged, unrelenting pain becomes a slave to the torment. Indeed, pain may destroy a person's personality or life productivity. Until the last decade, intractable pain was managed by surgical excision of the sensory nerve pathways (pain receptors) to the brain.

For the patient with intractable pain, the electric muscle stimulator can increase blood flow through the area and relieve pain. The TENS-PAC is one type that transmits electric stimulation to the patient's nerves by touching the skin (Fig. 32–9) and is called a "transcutaneous electric nerve stimulator." Patients can be taught to use this device at home.

Massage. Massage is a form of passive exercise that relieves tension and pain. Massage activates the thicker tactile receptors in the skin, which compete with the pain signals. The systematic, therapeutic stroking or kneading of the body or a body part can effectively relieve localized pain as well as pain at a distant site.

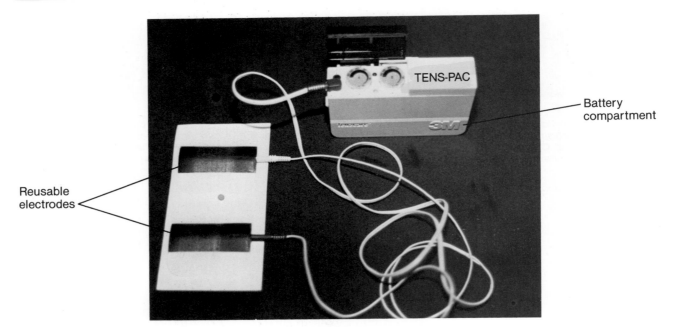

Figure 32–9
The small, portable Tens-Pac is prescribed by physicians to help control acute pain.

The medical assistant is usually not asked to apply therapeutic massages to patients, but you should be familiar with the terminology used:

- *Effleurage* is a stroking movement. In natural childbirth, a light circular stroke of the lower abdomen is done in a rhythm with controlled breathing to aid in the relaxation of the abdominal muscles.
- *Friction* is deep stroking or rubbing that involves deeper tissues. The traditional back rub uses friction.
- *Pétrissage* is a kneading or rolling type of massage with pressing of the muscles. It is also called *foulage*.
- *Tapotement* is a rapidly repeated, light percussion or tapping done with the sides of the hands. It may be called vibratory if it is done with a vibratory instrument or a sound.

The emphasis of this chapter has been on the basic physical techniques that are used to treat and promote the repair of diseased or injured tissues and to relieve pain. Many of these treatments will be performed by you under the supervision of the physician or the physical therapist. If you are interested in the numerous other therapies that are performed in hospitals or physical therapy practices, you should consider visiting one of these institutions to observe firsthand how these modalities are further integrated into the restoration and rehabilitation of the patient to normal health and functioning.

REFERENCES AND READINGS

Bonewit, K.: *Clinical Procedures for Medical Assistants*, 2nd ed. Philadelphia, W. B. Saunders Co., 1984.

Miller, B. F., and Keane, C. B.: *Encyclopedia and Dictionary of Medicine, Nursing, and Allied Health*, 4th ed. Philadelphia, W. B. Saunders Co., 1987.

Swanson, M. A.: *Crutches on the Go*. Issaquah, WA, Medic Publishing Co., 1984.

Taylor, R.: *Physical Therapy: Improving Movement and Function*. Daly City, CA, Krames Communications, 1984.

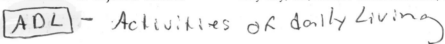

ADL – Activities of daily Living

32

CHAPTER OUTLINE

VOCABULARY

See Glossary at end of book for definitions.

accuracy	hematoma	quality control
aliquot	hemolyzed	reference laboratory
antibody	occult	requisition
anticoagulant	photometer	specimen
cerebrospinal fluid (CSF)	preservative	stat.
fast		

Introduction to the Laboratory and Specimen Collection

Upon successful completion of this chapter you should be able to

1. Define and spell the terms listed in the Vocabulary for this chapter.
2. Discuss the medical assistant's role in coordinating laboratory tests and results.
3. List the 11 departments found in most laboratories.
4. State at least 15 rules for laboratory safety.
5. Define the objective of quality control in the laboratory.
6. Identify the parts of a microscope.
7. Name at least five reasons physicians order laboratory tests.
8. List the information required on a laboratory requisition.
9. Cite the chemistry tests commonly ordered by physicians.

Upon successful completion of this chapter you should be able to perform the following activities:

1. Focus the microscope under low power, high power, and oil immersion.
2. Collect a throat culture for either immediate testing or transportation to a laboratory.
3. Collect a contaminant-free urine specimen, using clean-catch, midstream technique.
4. Perform an occult blood test on a stool specimen.
5. Perform a glucose level determination on a whole-blood specimen.

THE ROLE OF THE MEDICAL ASSISTANT

Laboratory tests are an essential part of a medical diagnosis, an aid to treatment, and frequently a control of medication. Only a physician may request laboratory testing for a patient. The medical assistant is responsible for a number of these laboratory testing procedures. The assistant must know the normal range of these tests, proper patient preparation, and the procedure for each. The assistant must carefully follow all laboratory instructions in obtaining the specimens, labeling, and sending them to the laboratory. There must be good communication between the patient, the office staff, and the laboratory personnel. The assistant should make patients feel more at ease with these procedures and, thus, elicit more cooperation.

It is the medical assistant's responsibility to alert the physician to any abnormal results or findings. This is accomplished by either circling or underlining the abnormality in red. Laboratory results are not filed until they are reviewed by the physician. Usually, the assistant contacts the patient concerning reports, follow-up procedures, and office visits.

INTRODUCTION TO THE LABORATORY

The laboratory is the place where specimens are tested, analyzed, and evaluated. Precise measurements are made, and the results are then calculated and interpreted. Tests are performed manually (by hand) or through automation (by using specialized instruments). These tests are performed by professionally trained medical technologists, medical laboratory technicians, and other allied health personnel. The *medical technologist (MT)* has a bachelor's degree and one year of clinical training. The *medical laboratory technician (MLT)* has one year of college and one year of clinical training. Both become certified by the successful completion of a national certifying examination. In addition to certification, many states regulate laboratory personnel by requiring state licensure.

Medical laboratories are located in either hospitals or nonhospital facilities. Nonhospital facilities include physician's offices, clinics, public health departments, HMO's (health maintenance organizations), and private **reference laboratories.** The head of a laboratory is the *pathologist,* a physician specially trained in the nature and cause of disease. The laboratory is divided into various departments, which may include (1) hematology, (2) chemistry, (3) microbiology, (4) specimen collection and processing, (5) blood bank, (6) coagulation, (7) serology, (8) bacteriology, (9) parasitology, (10) urinalysis, and (11) special chemistry. The laboratory in the physician's office usually performs procedures in hematology, chemistry, microbiology, and urinalysis.

Hematology. Whole blood is the specimen used for the majority of the tests performed. The numbers of *leukocytes* (white blood cells), *erythrocytes* (red blood cells), and *thrombocytes* (platelets) are actually counted. Observation is also made of the size, shape, and maturity level of these blood components. The results of these tests are used to diagnose anemias, leukemias, and clotting disorders.

Chemistry. Tests are usually performed on *serum,* the liquid part of blood left after a clot has formed. Urine and other body fluids may also be tested. The most common procedures performed measure levels of glucose (to determine blood sugar levels), enzymes (to determine heart damage), and electrolytes (to determine sodium, chloride, potassium, and bicarbonate levels).

Microbiology. Organisms are grown and identified from blood, urine, sputum, and wound specimens. Susceptibility testing is then performed on these organisms to determine proper antibiotic therapy. Microbiology deals with the study of bacteria, fungi, yeasts, parasites, and viruses.

Urinalysis. Urinalysis includes the physical, chemical, and microscopic examination of urine. In the physical examination, the color, transparency, and odor of the urine are noted. Chemical analysis is performed to measure levels of glucose, protein, ketones, blood, bilirubin, urobilinogen, and pH. Microscopically, the urine is examined for the presence of red, white, and epithelial cells, casts, crystals, yeasts, parasites, and bacteria.

Laboratory Safety

Basic safety rules must be observed at all times in the laboratory to avoid personal injury and to prevent equipment damage. Any accident must be reported to the physician or supervisor. Hazards in the laboratory can be classified as either physical, chemical, or biologic.

Physical hazards include fires resulting from electric malfunction or open flames from Bunsen burners or alcohol lamps. All laboratory personnel must be familiar with the location of fire extinguishers and fire escape routes. Keep all electric equipment in proper repair, and always follow manufacturers' instructions.

Chemical hazards may be caused by burns, poisons, or carcinogenic substances. Caution should be taken in handling all chemicals and specimens to avoid spills, splashes, or accidental mouth aspiration from pipetting. Skin or eyes that come into contact with any chemicals must be immediately washed with water for at least five minutes. Pipetting should be performed only with safety bulbs or filters.

Biologic hazards can result from the use of specimens and reagents capable of transmitting disease. The laboratory work area must be disinfected before and after each use when dealing with biologicals. Eating, drinking, smoking, or mouth pipetting is not allowed. Gloves should be worn. Laboratory aprons or coats should be worn. Specimens and any contaminated materials must be disposed of through sterilization or incineration. Hands must be washed before and after every procedure. Extreme caution and common sense are essential at all times in the laboratory.

LABORATORY RULES

1. Avoid eating, drinking, or smoking.
2. Keep pens, pencils, and fingers away from mouth and face.
3. Pull long hair back and up.
4. Avoid mouth pipetting.
5. Report all accidents to physician or supervisor.
6. Wear laboratory coat or apron.
7. Wipe spills and splashes immediately.
8. Wash hands before and after every procedure.
9. Follow manufacturer's instructions for equipment operation.
10. Know the location of all safety equipment and supplies and fire escape routes.
11. Wear protective gloves.
12. Avoid wearing chains, rings, bracelets, and other loose hanging jewelry.
13. Clean work area before and after every procedure.
14. Disinfect or sterilize specimens and materials contaminated with blood or microorganisms.
15. Avoid storage of food and beverages in laboratory refrigerator.
16. Repair malfunctioning equipment immediately.
17. Be familiar with appropriate first aid procedures.
18. Properly ground all electric equipment.
19. Clearly label all reagents and solutions.
20. Be a professional at all times.

Quality Control

The objective of **quality control** in the laboratory is to ensure the **accuracy** of test results while detecting and eliminating error. Quality control is a major part of the routine in most medical laboratories. Mandated by law, quality-control programs monitor all aspects of laboratory activity, from specimen collection through the processing, testing, and reporting steps. Programs check supplies, reagents, machinery, personnel, and actual test performance. Equipment performance and maintenance are also monitored. Specially prepared quality-control samples are tested along with patient samples. The results of testing performed on the quality control samples must be within a pre-established range before the patient results can be reported. The quality-control samples, called controls, are usually supplied with pre-packaged kits intended for use in the small laboratory. The controls should be analyzed at specified intervals. For example, positive and negative controls supplied with pregnancy test kits should be performed with each patient specimen. Urinalysis dipsticks (used for chemical examination of urine) should be checked daily and each time a new container is opened. Controls for automated chemistry analyses should be performed at specified intervals during the day. Consistent results of controls ensure constant conditions throughout the testing sequence.

THE MICROSCOPE

Every medical laboratory is equipped with a microscope. This indispensable instrument is used to view objects too small to be seen with the naked eye. The microscope is helpful in identifying microorganisms in urine sediment and other body fluids. The microscope is employed to evaluate stained blood, urine, and throat smears and to determine blood cell counts. Since the microscope is an expensive and technical instrument, special care must be taken in its operation, care, and storage (Fig. 33–1).

Microscopes are either *monocular* or *binocular*. A monocular microscope has one eyepiece for viewing, and a binocular has two. The *eyepiece*, or *ocular*, is located at the top of the microscope and contains a lens to magnify what is being seen. The usual magnification is ten times ($\times$ 10). The ocular is attached to a barrel or tube that is connected to the microscope *arm*. Under the arm is the *revolving nosepiece*, to which are attached the *objectives*. Most microscopes have three objectives, and each has a different magnifying power. The shortest objective has the lowest power ($\times$ 10). Low power is used to scan the field of interest and then focus on a particular object. Greater detail is observed with the next longest objective, which is high power ($\times$ 40). The longest objective, oil immersion ($\times$ 100), allows for the finest focusing of the object.

The arm of the microscope connects the objectives

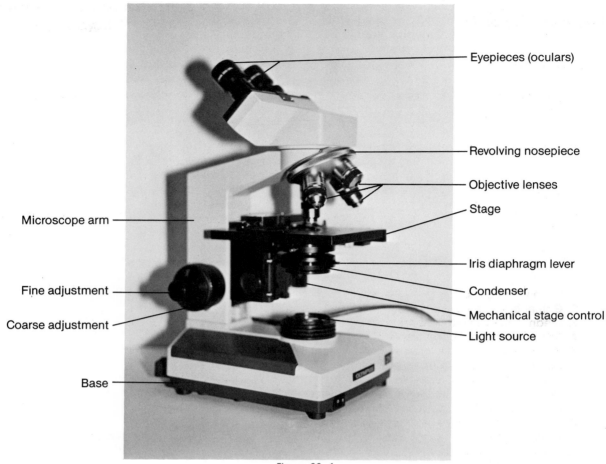

Eyepieces (oculars)

Revolving nosepiece

Objective lenses

Stage

Iris diaphragm lever

Condenser

Mechanical stage control

Light source

Microscope arm

Fine adjustment

Coarse adjustment

Base

Figure 33–1
Parts of a microscope.

and oculars to the *base,* which both supports the microscope and contains its light source. Together, the *condenser* and the *iris diaphragm* direct and regulate the light up through the objective. Just above the base are the focusing knobs. The *coarse adjustment* is used only with low power, and the *fine adjustment* is used with high power and oil immersion. The *stage* of the microscope holds the slide to be viewed.

Microscopes are very precise and expensive instruments that require careful handling. The amount of routine maintenance depends on the amount of daily use. Dirt is the enemy of the microscope, which must be kept scrupulously clean at all times. The microscope should always be stored in a plastic dust cover when not in use. Lenses should be cleaned before and after each use with lens paper and lens cleaner. Any other type of tissue scratches the lenses or leaves lint residue behind. The use of solvent cleaners such as xylene is not recommended on a routine basis because it may loosen lenses. Xylene can be used to remove oil that has dried on the lenses. Oil, makeup, dust, and eye secretions all can obstruct vision through the lens as well as cause the possible transmission

of infection. Finally, the body of the microscope should be dusted with a soft cloth.

Microscopes should be placed in a permanent location in the laboratory, on a sturdy table in an area where they cannot be bumped. If a microscope must be moved, it should be carried securely, with one hand supporting the base and the other holding the arm. When storing the microscope, it should be left with the low power objective in the lowest position. The stage should be centered.

SPECIMEN COLLECTION

The medical assistant is responsible for the collection of many different types of **specimens.** The most common specimens are blood, urine, and swabs for culture. Less often, feces, gastric contents, **cerebrospinal fluid (CSF),** tissue samples, semen, and aspirates such as synovial fluid or amniotic fluid are submitted for testing. These specimens are analyzed for levels of many chemicals and drugs, types and numbers of cells present, and the presence of microorganisms.

Procedure 33-1

PROCEDURAL GOAL

To focus properly the microscope, using a prepared slide, under low power, high power, and oil immersion.

EQUIPMENT AND SUPPLIES

Microscope
Lens tissue
Lens cleaner
Slide containing specimen

PROCEDURE

1. Wash your hands.
2. Gather the materials needed.
3. Clean the lenses with lens tissue and lens cleaner.
4. Adjust seating to a comfortable height.
5. Plug the microscope into an electric outlet, and turn on the light switch.
6. Place the slide specimen on the stage, and secure it.
7. Turn the revolving nosepiece to low power.
8. Carefully raise the stage while observing with the naked eye from the side.
9. Focus the specimen, using the coarse-adjustment knob.
10. Switch to fine adjustment, and focus the specimen in detail.
11. Adjust the amount of light by closing the iris diaphragm and lowering the condenser.
12. Turn the revolving nosepiece between the high power objective and oil immersion.
13. Place a small drop of oil on the slide.
14. Carefully swing the oil immersion objective into place.
15. Adjust the focus with the fine-adjustment knob.
16. Increase the light by opening the iris diaphragm and raising the condenser.
17. Identify the specimen.
18. Return to low power.
19. Lower the stage.
20. Center the stage.
21. Remove the slide.
22. Switch off the light and unplug the microscope.
23. Clean the lenses with lens tissue, and remove oil with lens cleaner.
24. Wipe the microscope with a cloth.
25. Cover the microscope.
26. Clean the work area.
27. Wash your hands.

33

TERMINAL PERFORMANCE OBJECTIVE

Given the necessary equipment and supplies, focus the microscope on a prepared slide, progressing from low power to high power and, then, to oil immersion within five minutes, using proper techniques so as not to damage the slide or the microscope. Correctly complete each step of the procedure in the correct order, as determined by your evaluator.

The results of these tests, along with other diagnostic testing, patient history, and physical examination, lead the physician to a diagnosis or rule out a particular disease. Management of the patient's condition may require repeated testing, such as routine glucose level determinations in the diabetic patient. If a patient is receiving medication, the physician may request therapeutic drug monitoring, to be certain that the patient is actually taking the medication and to detect possible toxic levels. Patients being given diuretics for the treatment of high blood pressure may need to have their potassium levels checked on a routine basis. Occasionally, the physician may request a test to determine the patient's baseline level, for comparison with the results of future tests.

Screening tests, such as routine urinalysis, are performed in order to detect hidden disease in otherwise apparently healthy individuals. A urinalysis may reveal the presence of diabetes, liver disease, or pathology of the urinary tract. Some screening tests are required by law in certain states. Persons applying for a marriage license may be required to have a VDRL (Venereal Disease Research Laboratory) test to detect syphilis. Some states require screening of newborns for hereditary metabolic defects such as phenylketonuria and hypothyroidism. Tests may reveal the extent of disease or degree of damage done to an organ or body system. For example, the measurement of the rise of certain enzymes after a heart attack can indicate the amount of heart damage. Repeated testing can allow the physician to follow the course of a disease and assess the effectiveness of the treatment. A person diagnosed as having leukemia will have daily white blood cell counts performed before receiving chemotherapy.

The importance of accurate specimen collection cannot be overemphasized. If not performed correctly, it can easily lead to inaccurate results. If the tests are to be accurate indicators of the patient's state of health, it is imperative that the concepts of specimen collection be understood and followed exactly.

The correct specimen must be collected in the correct container, for example, blood may be collected using a vacuum tube system (Fig. 33–2). These tubes are available in a variety of sizes with and without **preservatives** and **anticoagulants.** The tubes are color-coded so that the color of the stopper denotes which, if any, additive is present (Table 33–1).

The medical assistant should always check the laboratory's specimen requirements manual for any unfamiliar tests. The manual lists all specimen collection information. Any unanswered questions should be resolved by calling the laboratory before collection of the specimen.

Care must be taken to avoid contamination of the specimen or the assistant. The correct collection and handling of the specimens used in various micro-

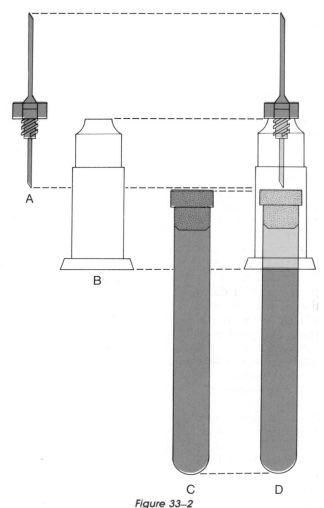

Figure 33–2
*Vacuum tube blood-collecting system. **A**, Needle; **B**, holder; **C**, vacuum tube; **D**, assembled unit.*

biologic procedures are absolutely essential if the results are to be of any value in the diagnosis of the disease and the treatment of the patient. Expiration dates on swabs, tubes, transport media, and other collection containers should be checked before these items are used.

An improperly handled specimen may become contaminated or may contaminate the surrounding

Table 33–1
Vacuum Tube Blood-Collecting System

Stopper Color	Anticoagulant in Tube	Uses of Tube
Red	None	For clotting blood and obtaining serum
Purple	EDTA	For most hematology studies
Blue	Sodium citrate	For coagulation studies
Green	Heparin	For special hematology tests

environment. Follow the universal blood and body-fluid precautions. All blood and other body fluids from *all* patients should be considered infective. See Appendix C, Recommendations for Prevention of AIDS Transmission.

Sufficient samples should be collected for the tests requested by the physician. Amounts may vary based on the methods used. If a report is returned from the laboratory with the term *"insufficient sample,"* it indicates a request for additional specimen. Be certain to clarify any questions concerning the previous specimen by calling the laboratory before collecting a new one.

Many testing procedures require that patients be given a specific set of instructions to follow. For example, patients may be required to **fast** 8 to 12 hours prior to the collection of blood and urine. They may need to follow a high-carbohydrate diet for several days prior to a *glucose tolerance test*. Some foods and medication must be discontinued. The physician will discuss medication alterations with the patient. Sometimes, it might not be medically advisable to discontinue the medication, and this must be noted on the laboratory **requisition.** The laboratory will then be alerted to the possible drug interferences, and it may be able to use an alternative test method.

The specimen collected must be a true representative sample. A swab for a wound culture collected from the surface of the wound will generally not yield the same results as one taken from the depths of the wound. A **hemolyzed** blood specimen, or one taken from an atypical area such as a **hematoma** or the area above an intravenous (I.V.) hookup, will show marked differences in many tests. If a large volume of specimen is collected, such as a 24-hour urine or fecal fat specimen, the total volume or weight must be carefully measured and recorded. The specimen must be well mixed before an **aliquot** is removed and submitted for testing.

The specimen must be handled, processed, and stored according to the instructions, to avoid causing any alterations that would affect test results. Check whether the specimen needs to be kept warm or cool. Specimens such as urine require chilling if the testing is not going to be done immediately. Some cultures or specimens need to be kept at body temperature after collection. Gonococcal cultures and semen tests are two such examples, since cooling kills the gonococci and sperm. **Cerebrospinal fluid (CSF)** should be incubated if culturing cannot be performed immediately. When required, serum must be separated from the cells as soon as possible after the specimen has clotted, to prevent alterations caused by the metabolism of the cells. Specimens for bilirubin testing must be protected from light. Some specimens need to be frozen to prevent chemical constituents from changing. Consult the laboratory specimen requirements to be certain that each specimen is handled and processed properly.

A completed requisition must accompany each specimen sent to the laboratory. The information must be carefully printed in ink. All copies must be legible. Be sure to complete all necessary items on the requisition. The following information in usually required when specimens are sent to the laboratory:

1. Physician's name, account number, address, and phone number.
2. Patient's full name, surname first.
3. Patient's address.
4. Patient's insurance number.
5. Patient's age, birthday, and sex.
6. Source of specimen.
7. Date and time of collection.
8. Specific test requested.
9. Medications the patient is taking.
10. Possible diagnosis.
11. Indication of whether test is **STAT** (needed immediately).

If the specimen is to be mailed, it must be carefully packaged to prevent breakage, damage, or contamination of all persons handling it. See Appendix C, Recommendations for Prevention of AIDS Transmission. Containers of liquid specimens may be wrapped in absorbent material and inserted in unbreakable tubes with safe-top lids. The lids are taped shut so that no leakage occurs if the specimen container breaks. Place all specimens in a second container, such as an impervious bag, for transport. The completed requisition goes inside the outermost wrap. Usually, Styrofoam mailers (Fig. 33–3)

33

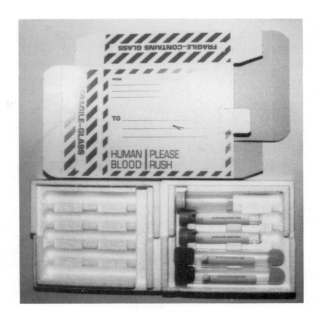

Figure 33–3
Example of a good mailing package for specimens. It is made of plastic foam for protection of the contents.

are used because they cushion the sample and also provide insulation. Styrofoam inserts can be shaped to fit around the specimen containers. A warning label specifying the etiologic agent or biological specimen is affixed to the outside of the container. The specimen should be given to the laboratory courier or mailed at a post office immediately so that it is not exposed to temperature extremes.

Collection of Microbiology Specimens

Medical assistants are often called upon to collect specimens for the identification of possible microorganisms. A microbiology specimen must contain as few contaminants as possible and must be composed of material from the actual site of the infection. Contaminants lead to confusing culture results. For example, if urine for culture is not collected using clean-catch technique, the contaminants present will increase the colony count and confuse the results. The test will have to be repeated, and this leads to greater cost and time delay in treating the patient. Wound swabs should be taken from the depths of the wound; surface organisms may not be the true cause of the infection.

Knowledge of the optimal collection times is necessary for the best chance of recovery of the causative organisms or collection of positive serologic specimens. Urinary tract infections are best diagnosed from the first specimen voided in the morning since the specimen has been incubating in the bladder overnight. In addition, this specimen is most likely to have a high number of microorganisms. Blood for serologic testing is usually collected during the acute stage of the disease, and again during the convalescent stage. The results of the two are compared; a rise in antibody titer is usually diagnostic.

A sufficient sample must be obtained to perform all tests requested. For example, in cases of suspected tuberculosis (TB), the physician may order a Gram stain, acid-fast stain, and cultures for TB, aerobes, and anaerobes. The patient must be instructed to collect at least 10 ml of a first morning sputum specimen.

The proper collection containers, media, and procedures must be used. These include sterile, nonbreakable containers with tight-fitting lids (Fig. 33–4); polyester (not cotton) swabs (Fig. 33–5); appropriate transport media for aerobic and anaerobic cultures; and the immediate inoculation of swabs for gonococcus cultures onto pre-warmed modified Thayer-Martin agar. If possible, obtain specimens for culture before antibiotics are given. This is particularly important for throat and gonococcus cultures. If an antibiotic has been given, note it on the requisition, and send the specimen to the laboratory immediately for inoculation onto the media.

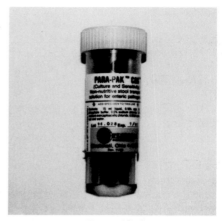

Figure 33–4
Sterile nonbreakable collection container with tight-fitting lid.

Even small amounts of the antibiotic interfere with the culture.

Throat and urine specimens are frequently collected in the physician's office to assist in the diagnosis of "strep throat" and urinary tract infections. "Strep throat" is caused by an organism called *Streptococci* and, if left untreated, can cause serious complications such as rheumatic fever, rheumatic endocarditis, and glomerulonephritis. The organism most commonly isolated in the urine is *Escherichia coli*. The medical assistant collects the throat culture specimen and instructs the patient to collect a clean-catch urine specimen.

Throat cultures are collected by gently swabbing the back of the throat and the surfaces of the tonsils with a sterile swab. The mouth and tongue should not be touched. This prevents contamination of the swab with the normal flora of the mouth. This procedure can be accomplished best by depressing the tongue and instructing the patient to say "ah."

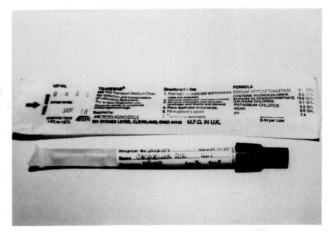

Figure 33–5
Sterile swab collection tube.

Procedure 33–2

COLLECTING A SPECIMEN BY SWAB FOR THROAT CULTURE AND FOR DIRECT SLIDE TESTING

PROCEDURAL GOAL

To collect a throat culture, using sterile technique, for either immediate testing or transportation to the laboratory.

EQUIPMENT AND SUPPLIES

Blood and body-fluid protection barriers (goggles, masks and aprons or gowns), as necessary (see Appendix C, Recommendations for Prevention of AIDS Transmission)
Nonsterile gloves (sterile gloves may be preferred)
For on-site testing:
    Sterile swab
    Sterile tongue depressor
For transport:
    Sterile swab
    Sterile tongue depressor
    Transport medium

PROCEDURE

1. Wash and dry your hands. Follow universal blood and body-fluid precautions (see Appendix C). Glove yourself with nonsterile or sterile gloves.
   Purpose: To reduce the spread of infection.
2. Gather the materials needed.
3. Position the patient so that the light shines into the mouth.
   Purpose: Visualization of the area to be swabbed.
4. Remove the sterile swab from the sterile wrap with your dominant hand, and grasp the sterile tongue depressor with your nondominant hand.
   Purpose: Better control of the swabbing process.
5. Instruct the patient to open the mouth and to say "ah." Depress the tongue with the depressor.
   Purpose: Saying "ah" helps elevate the uvula and reduces the tendency to gag. The tongue is depressed so that you can see the back of the throat.
6. Swab the back of the throat between the tonsillar pillars and especially the reddened, patchy areas of the throat and the tonsils.
   Purpose: Pathogenic organisms are found in the back of the throat and on the tonsils.

33

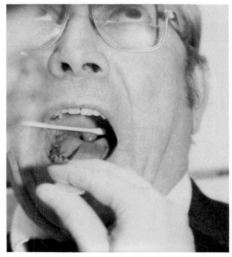

Procedure continued on following page

7. Place the swab into the transport medium, label it, and send it to the laboratory. If testing is performed in the office, inoculate a blood agar plate and label it. If direct slide testing is requested, return the labeled swab to the laboratory.
   Purpose: Transport media prevents the swab from drying. Labeling immediately after collection prevents mixing up specimens.
8. Dispose of contaminated supplies.
   Purpose: Prevents the spread of infection.
9. Disinfect the work area.
10. Wash your hands.

TERMINAL PERFORMANCE OBJECTIVE

Given the appropriate equipment and supplies, and using sterile technique, swab a throat and transfer the specimen into a transport medium or onto a glass slide within three minutes. Correctly complete each step of the procedure in the proper order, as determined by your evaluator.

Urine specimens must be collected, by the clean-catch method, directly into a sterile container. Urine cultures are performed whenever the patient reports to the physician with symptoms that might indicate infection.

Procedure 33-3

COLLECTING A CLEAN-CATCH URINE SPECIMEN FOR CULTURE OR ANALYSIS

PROCEDURAL GOAL

To collect a contaminant-free urine sample for culture or analysis, using midstream, clean-catch technique.

EQUIPMENT AND SUPPLIES

Sterile container with lid
Antiseptic towelettes
Set of written instructions

PROCEDURE

1. Label the container and give the patient the supplies.
   Purpose: Labeling the container avoids possible mixing up of specimens.

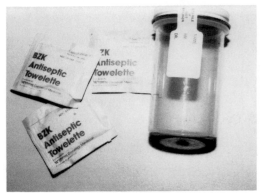

Procedure continued on opposite page

2. Explain the instructions to adult patients or to the guardians of child patients.
   Purpose: Instructions must be understood if they are to be followed. By talking to the patient, you can determine if the patient understands.

   Female. Ask the patient to remove underclothing and to sit on the toilet, with one knee to the side as far as possible. Loosen the cap so that it can be removed from the container with one hand. Use fingers to spread the labia apart. Continue to hold the labia in this position throughout the entire procedure. Use three separate towelettes to clean the area from front to back three times—once down each side, and then once down the middle. Place the lid of the specimen cup, top side down, on a clean surface. Do not touch the rim or the inside of the lid or cup. Begin to urinate into the toilet, then hold the cup in the stream and collect a portion of the urine. Finish urinating into the toilet. Replace the lid on the container, and if needed, wipe the container with towels. For specimens collected at home, note the time on the container, and refrigerate until transporting to the laboratory. For specimens collected in the office, note the time on the container and process immediately or refrigerate.

   Male. Loosen cap on the container. Retract the foreskin (if present), and use an antiseptic towelette to cleanse the glans and the urethral opening. Place the lid of the specimen cup, top side down, on a clean surface. Do not touch the rim or the inside of the lid or cup. Begin to urinate into the toilet, then hold the cup in the stream and collect a portion of the urine. Finish urinating into the toilet. Replace the lid on the container, and if needed, wipe the container with towels.

   Infants. Obtain a sterile urine pouch. Using antiseptic towelettes, carefully cleanse the perineum and genital area. Tape the pouch in place over the penis or on the labia. Hold the infant so that the pouch is in position and urine flows into the pouch without touching the skin. Stimulate urination by placing the infant's feet in cold water, if necessary. Remove the pouch as soon as the specimen has been collected. Transfer the specimen to a sterile container.

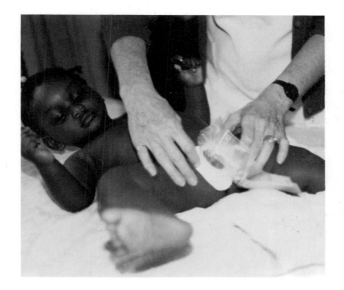

33

TERMINAL PERFORMANCE OBJECTIVE

Given the necessary supplies, explain the collection of a mid-stream, clean-catch urine sample to a patient within one minute, and correctly complete each step of the procedure in the proper order, as determined by your evaluator.

Occult Blood

Screening tests for **occult** blood in the stool are routinely performed to detect bleeding in the intestinal tract, which may indicate cancer, polyps, or other lesions of the colon or rectum. The test can be performed in the office during a rectal examination, or the patient may be instructed to collect a sample at home. Most test procedures use a paper impregnated with a gum resin called guaiac, which turns blue when a developer is added and blood is present. Home tests are also available. The test paper impregnated with the reagents is dropped into the toilet bowl after a bowel movement. The patient then watches for the color change, as explained in the instructions.

The guaiac tests are subject to interferences. Vitamin C in large doses causes false negatives. Iron, red meats, and certain raw, leafy vegetables can cause false positives. Contamination with menstrual blood or collection of the specimen when hemor-

rhoids are present results in a positive test result. If patients are collecting specimens at home, they must be given supplies and instructions. *Hemoccult* slides (Smithkline Diagnostics) come in packets of three, for collection on three consecutive bowel movements. The patient should be free of vitamin C and be on a nonmeat diet for two days prior to the beginning of collection. The stool should be passed into a clean container, and then a small sample should be smeared on the paper in the appropriate windows of the slide with the wooden applicator provided. Oxidizing cleaning agents present in the toilet bowl can cause false positives if the sample is retrieved from the bowl. It is convenient to place the labeled slides, applicators, and instructions in an envelope addressed to the office. After the specimens have been collected, the slides may be mailed back to the office. The testing of specimens collected in the office is often done using rolls of guaiac paper. A sample from the glove following a rectal examination is also sufficient for testing.

Procedure 33–4

PERFORMING AN OCCULT BLOOD TEST

PROCEDURAL GOAL

To explain the collection of a stool specimen and to perform an occult blood test on the specimen obtained.

EQUIPMENT AND SUPPLIES

Blood and body-fluid protection barriers (goggles, masks, and aprons or gowns), as necessary (see Appendix C, Recommendations for Prevention of AIDS Transmission)
Nonsterile gloves (sterile gloves may be preferred)
Collection slides
Applicator sticks
Developer
Written instructions

PROCEDURE

1. Supply the patient with an addressed envelope containing slides, applicator sticks, and written instructions including diet restrictions. Have the patient return the slides to the office.
   Purpose: Most screening for occult blood is done on samples collected at home.

Procedure continued on opposite page

2. Wash and dry your hands. Follow universal blood and body-fluid precautions (see Appendix C). Glove yourself with nonsterile or sterile gloves.
3. Open test window on the back of the slide, and add two drops of developer to each test area. Look for the development of a blue color, which indicates a positive test for hidden blood.
4. Add developer to the on-slide performance monitor at the bottom of the slide window. Look for correct reactions in the positive and negative control circles. If the on-slide monitor does not perform as expected, the results of the patient test are invalid. Do not report them. If the on-slide monitor shows the developer is reacting as expected, the patient results may be reported.
   Purpose: The monitors are a form of quality control of the procedure to ensure that the guaiac paper and developer react as expected.
5. Record the results of the patient and the on-slide monitor.

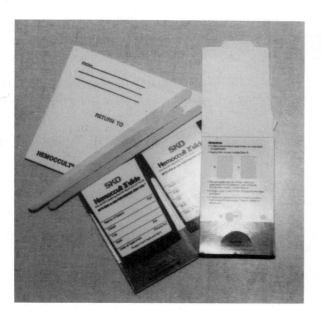
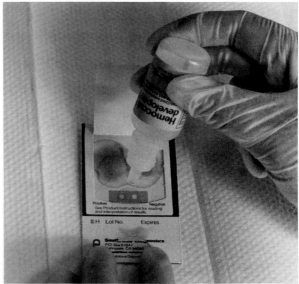

TERMINAL PERFORMANCE OBJECTIVE

Given the necessary supplies, explain the collection of a stool sample to a patient. Test the sample according to the instructions in the test kit, within three minutes and correctly complete each step of the procedure in the proper order, and obtain the correct reading, as determined by your evaluator.

33

Collection of Semen

Semen analysis is usually performed for fertility studies, especially after vasectomies in order to establish the effectiveness of the *vasectomy*. The patient is advised to refrain from intercourse for two to four days before the sample is collected. Instruct the patient to collect the total specimen in an opaque glass container. Masturbation or coitus interruptus may be employed as methods of obtaining the specimen, but if the latter is used, great care must be taken to collect the entire ejaculate. Condoms should never be employed, as the latex has definite spermicidal qualities. The cap of the container must be tightly closed, with the patient's name, the date, and the time of ejaculation written on the label. The specimen must be kept at body temperature and must be delivered to the laboratory within three hours after collection.

BLOOD CHEMISTRY TESTS

Blood Glucose. The most common blood chemistry test performed in the laboratory of the physician's office is the blood glucose level. It is used in the diagnosis of diabetes and as an aid in the control of the diabetic patient. It may also be requested in screening for hypoglycemia (low blood sugar). If the laboratory does not perform other chemistry tests, the enzymatic glucose stick methods produced by Bio-Dynamics (Chemstrip bG) and Ames (Glucostix and Visidex) will probably be the method used because the sticks can be read with the naked eye and require no additional instruments for testing. However, if the physician chooses, a portable meter can be purchased to mechanically determine the reading. The meter gives a more accurate reading than can be obtained by visual comparison of the colors. This **photometer** measures the amount of light reflected off the reacted reagent pad and converts the measurement into a digital readout of the blood glucose level. The photometers are designed for use with one particular reagent manufacturer's strips and are not interchangeable.

Procedure 33–5

**BLOOD GLUCOSE LEVEL DETERMINATION BY
CHEMSTRIP bG**

PROCEDURAL GOAL

To perform a blood glucose level determination by Chemstrip bG on whole blood.

EQUIPMENT AND SUPPLIES

Blood and body-fluid protection barriers (goggles, masks, and aprons or gowns), as necessary (see Appendix C, Recommendations for Prevention of AIDS Transmission)
Nonsterile gloves (sterile gloves may be preferred)
Whole-blood specimen
Gauze
Chemstrip bG
Accu-Chek II

PROCEDURE

1. Wash and dry your hands. Follow universal blood and body-fluid precautions (see Appendix C). Glove yourself with nonsterile or sterile gloves.
2. Assemble the materials needed.
3. Mix the blood specimen.
4. Remove the test strip from the container and recap tightly.
   Purpose: Test strips are affected by moisture and must be carefully stored to maintain their reactivity.
5. Deposit a large drop of blood on the test pad, covering the pad completely (facing page, top and center).
   Purpose: The pad must be completely covered for accurate reading by the machine.
6. Wait exactly 60 seconds.
   Purpose: Timing is critical.
7. Wipe the drop of blood off the pad with gauze.
8. Wait exactly 60 seconds.
9. Compare the color-reacted pad with the color chart, or use the Accu-Chek II photometer to determine the reading. Follow the manufacturer's instructions (facing page, bottom).
10. Record the reading.
11. Clean the work area.
12. Wash your hands.

TERMINAL PERFORMANCE OBJECTIVE

Given a whole blood specimen and the appropriate supplies, perform a blood glucose level determination within five minutes and to a minimum performance level of ½ color block of the known reading, as determined by your evaluator.

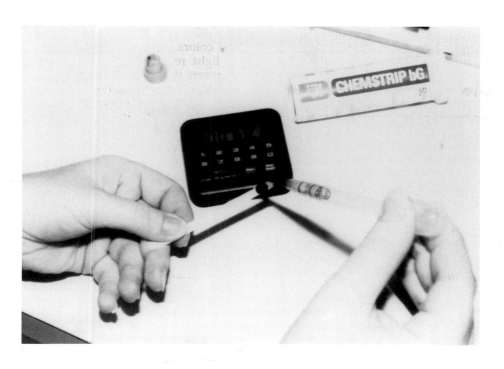

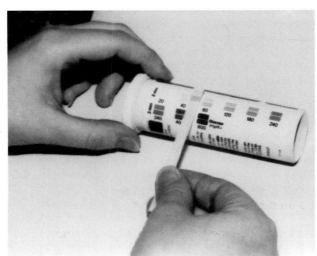

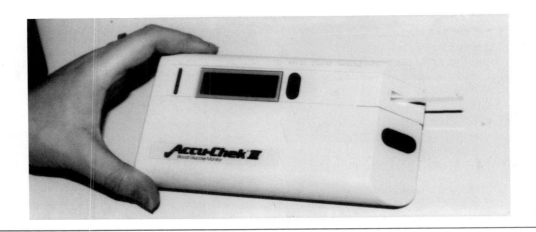

33

Table 33–2

Panels and Profiles

Panel/Profile	Tests Included	Requirement	Expected Range MALE (16–65)	UNITS
Chemistry panel	Glucose	2 ml serum: 1 serum- separation tube	75–125	mg/dl
	BUN (blood urea nitrogen)		6–25	mg/dl
	Creatinine		0.6–1.5	mg/dl
	Uric acid		4.0–8.5	mg/dl
	SGOT (ASG) (aspartate aminotransferase)		0–50	mU/ml*
	Cholesterol		135–300	mg/dl
	Triglycerides		30–175	mg/dl
	LDH (LD) (lactate dehydrogenase)		100–225	mU/ml
	Total bilirubin		0.1–1.1	mg/dl
	Albumin		3.2–5.2	g/dl
	GGT (gamma glutamyltransferase)		0–60	mU/ml
	Alkaline phosphate		15–100	mU/ml
	Calcium		8.2–10.5	mg/dl
	Phosphorus		2.1–5.0	mg/dl
	Iron		30–180	µg/dl
	Sodium Na$^+$		136–145	mmol/L
	Potassium (K$^+$) ⎫ Electrolytes		3.2–5.5	mmol/L
	Chloride (Cl$^-$) ⎬		98–108	mmol/L
	Bicarbonate (HCO$_3^-$) ⎭		22–32	mmol/L
Electrolyte panel	Sodium (Na$^+$)	1 ml serum: 1 serum- separation tube, no hemolysis	136–145	mmol/L
	Potassium (K$^+$)		3.2–5.5	mmol/L
	Chloride (Cl$^-$)		98–108	mmol/L
	Bicarbonate (HCO$_3^-$)		22–32	mmol/L
Lipid profile	Triglycerides	3 ml serum: 1 serum- separation tube. Cannot be done on lipemic serum because of triglyceride interference with HDL. Fasting specimen required.	30–175	mg/dl
	Cholesterol		130–300	mg/dl
	HDL (high-density lipoprotein) Cholesterol		30–70	mg/dl (M)
			40–90	mg/dl (F)
	LDL (low-density lipoprotein) Cholesterol		60–180	mg/dl
Thyroid panel	Triiodothyronine (T$_3$) uptake	1 ml serum: 1 serum- separation tube	35–49% (M)	
			33–46% (F)	
	Thyroxine (T$_4$) radioimmunoassay (RIA)		4.0–11.0	µg/dl
	T$_7$ (calculated)		1.4–5.4 (M)	
			1.3–5.1 (F)	
OB Profile	ABO	2 red top tubes: spin unopened and send intact. Positive RPR results in additional tests and cost.		
	Rh factor			
	Antibody screen		Negative	
	Rubella			
	RPR (rapid plasma reagent)		Negative	

*U stands for units. Enzymes are measured in terms of reactivity, which is expressed in units.
Courtesy General Medical Laboratories, Madison, WI.

Other blood chemistry tests commonly ordered by the physician include tests for serum calcium, uric acid, blood urea nitrogen, and cholesterol.

Serum Calcium. Calcium is essential in the formation of bone tissue, in muscular activity, and in blood coagulation. When there is a deficiency of calcium, tetany occurs. This condition is characterized by a twitching of muscle fibers and tetanic convulsions. An increase of serum calcium is found in hyperparathyroidism, multiple myeloma, and some respiratory diseases.

Uric Acid. This test is used basically to aid in the diagnosis of gout, a metabolic disease marked by acute arthritis and inflammation of the joints. An increase in uric acid levels is also seen in severe kidney damage and toxemias of pregnancy.

Blood Urea Nitrogen (BUN). This is a kidney function test. Normally, the kidneys excrete urea. This major product of the kidneys is the end product of protein metabolism. In some kidney diseases, the kidneys do not excrete urea sufficiently, so the urea nitrogen in the blood increases.

Cholesterol. Cholesterol is normally found in the blood, but in some disease states, the cholesterol concentration is increased or decreased. An elevated reading may aid in the diagnosis of liver malfunction, hypothyroidism, and a possibility of atherosclerosis. A decrease is found in hyperthyroidism, anemias, cachexia, and acute infections.

Many times, the physician may order a *panel* or *profile* on a patient. This is a group of tests relating to a particular organ or system. Cardiac, liver, and thyroid profiles are common. Panels may include as many as 20 or more tests relating to a number of different body systems. Panels are performed on sophisticated automated machinery and provide maximum information with minimum sample and cost (Table 33–2).

Many tests run on a small sample of specimen

REFERENCES AND READINGS

Bauer, J. D.: *Clinical Laboratory Methods*, 9th ed. St. Louis, C. V. Mosby Co., 1982.

Graff, Sister L.,: *A Handbook of Routine Urinalysis*. Philadelphia, J. B. Lippincott, 1983.

Slockbower, J. M., and Blumenfeld, T. A.: *Collection and Handling of Laboratory Specimens*. Philadelphia, J. B. Lippincott, 1983.

33

CHAPTER OUTLINE

VOCABULARY

See Glossary at end of book for definitions.

agglutination	hemolysis	sensitivity disk
colony	inoculate	screening test
endotoxin	mordant	toxin

Microbiology for the Physician's Office

OBJECTIVES

Upon successful completion of this chapter you should be able to

1. Define and spell the words in the Vocabulary for this chapter.
2. List three diseases caused by viruses.
3. Describe the appearance of a Gram-positive and a Gram-negative bacterium on a stained smear.
4. Cite the morphologic differences of bacteria.
5. List the equipment needed to perform microbiologic testing in the physician's office.
6. Differentiate between aerobic and anaerobic bacteria.
7. Describe the performance of sensitivity testing.
8. Differentiate between selective and nonselective media.
9. Explain the importance of colony counts for urine cultures.
10. Describe the procedure for identifying group A streptococci in throat cultures.

Upon successful completion of this chapter you should be able to perform the following activities:

1. Inoculate media for cultures.
2. Prepare direct smears and smears from culture.
3. Stain smears using Gram stain.
4. Examine stained smears for the presence of microorganisms.
5. Recognize the morphologic differences of bacteria on stained smears.
6. Perform slide agglutination testing for infectious mononucleosis.

INTRODUCTION TO MICROBIOLOGY

Microbiology is the study of microorganisms, including bacteria, fungi, viruses, rickettsiae, and protozoa. The main objective of microbiologic procedures is to identify the organisms responsible for illness so that the physician can properly treat the patient. These procedures are performed either in the physician's office or in the microbiology department of a medical laboratory.

Bacteria

The study of bacteria is called *bacteriology*. Bacteria are one-celled plant microorganisms. There are numerous ways of identifying bacteria, including their morphology (form and structure), their ability to retain certain dyes, their growth in different physical environments, and the results of certain biochemical reactions.

Bacteria exist in three main forms: round-shaped *cocci*, rod-shaped *bacilli*, and spiral-shaped *spirilla*. They can occur singly, in pairs, in clusters, or in long chains and are widely distributed in the air, soil, water, living animals and plants, and dead organic matter. The *Gram stain* is a method of staining that differentiates bacteria according to the chemical composition of their cell walls. *Gram-positive* bacteria stain purple, and *Gram-negative* bacteria stain red. Bacteria that must have oxygen to survive are known as *aerobic*; others, called *anaerobic*, can live only in the absence of oxygen. The most important classification of bacteria pertains to the toxic effects they have on the body. *Pathogenic* bacteria (disease-causing) attack the body by secreting **toxins** while they are growing, or they release **endotoxins** when they die. After a period of incubation, these poisons cause the symptoms of the disease.

The skin, respiratory tract, and gastrointestinal tract are inhabited by a variety of harmless, normal flora. An infection occurs when bacteria occurring naturally in one part of the body invade another part of the body and become harmful. A common example is the bacterium *Escherichia coli* (normal flora of the intestinal tract) causing a urinary tract infection. Pathogenic bacteria can be transmitted from person to person by many mechanisms, including direct contact (by means of airborne infections, contact with animals, or transmission by insects) and indirect contact (through drinking water or food products or on inanimate objects). Another example is the bacterium *Staphylococcus epidermidis*, normally found on the surface of the skin. When bacteria of this type invade the body, as with a cut, they usually produce an infection.

Fungi

Mycology is the study of fungi and the diseases they cause. Fungi are larger than bacteria and have rigid cell walls. Fungal infections are resistant to antibiotics used in the treatment of bacterial infec-

tions and must be treated with drugs active against the unusual cell walls of this organism. Fungi are present in the soil, air, and water, but only a few produce disease. These infections may be quite superficial, affecting only the skin, hair, or nails. However, some fungi can penetrate the tissues of the internal body structures and produce serious diseases of the mucous membranes, heart, lungs, and other organs. Among the fungal diseases are *ringworm*, *athlete's foot* (tinea pedis), *thrush* (oral candidiasis), *histoplasmosis*, *coccidioidomycosis*, and *blastomycosis*.

Viruses

Viruses, the smallest infectious microorganisms, can be seen only with the aid of an electron microscope. Study of viruses and their diseases is known as *virology*. Viruses cannot be grown on artificial culture media and cannot be destroyed by antibiotic drugs. Viral diseases are transmitted by direct contact, insects, blood transfusion, contamination of food or water, and inhalation of droplets expelled by coughing or sneezing. Some of the more than fifty known viral diseases include the *common cold*, *smallpox*, *chickenpox*, *influenza*, *poliomyelitis*, *measles*, *mumps*, *German measles*, *cold sores*, *shingles*, *viral hepatitis*, *rabies*, *infectious mononucleosis*, *croup*, *viral encephalitis*, and *yellow fever*.

Rickettsiae

Rickettsiae are microorganisms found in the tissue cells of lice, fleas, ticks, and mites and are transmitted to humans by the bite of these insects. Rickettsial diseases include *Rocky Mountain spotted fever*, *typhus*, *Q fever*, and *trench fever*. These diseases are not common in communities with good sanitary conditions, and they can be prevented by insecticides, vaccines, and antibiotics.

Protozoa

In contrast to the previously mentioned microorganisms, the protozoa are animals, not plants. Depending on the protozoon, transmission can occur through insect bites, blood transfusion, sexual contact, and fecal contamination. Pathogenic protozoa include *Plasmodium* (malaria), *Trichomonas* (vaginitis), *Entamoeba histolytica* (dysentery), and *Toxoplasma gondii* (encephalitis).

MICROBIOLOGY PROCEDURES COMMONLY PERFORMED IN THE PHYSICIAN'S OFFICE

Some physicians prefer to perform some of the simple screening procedures in their offices and refer the more complex tests to special laboratories. Others collect specimens in the office and send all of them to larger laboratories for analysis. The basic microbiology procedures most frequently encountered in the small physician laboratory include preparation of direct smears; staining; microscopic examination of smears, wet preps, and potassium hydroxide (KOH) preps; **screening tests** for strep throat and infectious mononucleosis; and screening for urinary tract infections. Many types of tests are available in kit form. The kits supply all needed reagents and most equipment. Directions for the entire test procedure are contained in the kits and must be followed carefully. Known controls are also included to ensure accurate testing. In order to perform microbiologic procedures in the office, the following equipment is needed: a microscope, incubator, staining rack and materials, slides, culture media, inoculation loops, a Bunsen burner, and sterile supplies for specimen collection.

Preparation of Smears

A smear is made on a glass slide that will then be stained and examined under the microscope. A direct smear is made from a swab of the infected area (see Chapter 33); a culture smear is taken from a single cluster of organisms (**colony**) growing on a plate of solid media or in a tube of liquid broth, using a loop. The material must be applied thinly or the resulting smear will be too thick to study under the microscope. Slides should be labeled before the infectious material is applied. This prevents possible incorrect labeling and contamination of hands with infectious organisms. Smears are dried, heat-fixed, and stained.

Staining

Most bacteria are so small and possess so little color that they are difficult to observe. Staining allows the microorganisms to be clearly seen under the microscope. The Gram stain is used most often. This staining procedure consists of applying a sequence of dye, **mordant**, decolorizer, and counterstain to the bacteria. The dyes are taken up differently according to the chemical composition of the cell walls. This serves to classify organisms according to their reactions to the stain and separates them into Gram-positive (which stain purple) and Gram-negative (which stain red).

Types of Media

A variety of growth media is available to promote the optimum growth of microorganisms. A growth medium may be liquid, semisolid, or solid. Liquid broth can be solidified by adding *agar* (a seaweed extract). The agar broth may come in tubes or plates (also called *Petri dishes*). Media can be *selective or nonselective*. Selective media allow the growth of specific bacteria while inhibiting the growth of others. *Eosin–methylene blue (EMB)*, *MacConkey*, and *Thayer-Martin* are examples of selective media. Nonselective media support the growth of most bacteria.

Generally, this medium is blood agar. This contains *sheep blood* and *tryptic soy broth (TSB)*. These media have undergone extensive quality control testing for both sterility and appropriate reactions with certain organisms. An expiration date appears on each tube or plate. The used containers are autoclaved and then disposed.

Blood agar is used for performing throat cultures. The organism that causes strep throat (*Streptococcus*) is able to utilize the red blood cells in the agar for growth. This growth results in a detectable change in the medium called **hemolysis.** For urine cultures, two types of media are used: EMB or MacConkey and blood agar. The organism *Escherichia coli* is commonly isolated from urine.

Cultures

A culture is **inoculated** by passing a swab or loop lightly over the surface of an agar medium in a zigzag pattern. Broths are inoculated by swirling the swab or loop in them. The inoculated tubes or plates are incubated at 37°C for 24 hours and are then examined for growth.

Some organisms require a high concentration of carbon dioxide (CO_2) for growth. Transport plates of chocolate agar or Thayer-Martin agar have a CO_2-generating tablet that is placed in a well in the plate immediately after inoculation (Fig. 34–1). Without this special atmosphere, organisms such as the *Neisseria gonorrhoeae* (which causes gonorrhea) would die. Alternatively, the plate is placed in a

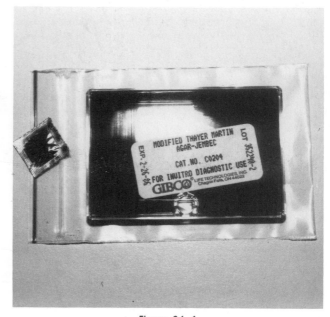

Figure 34–1
Transport plate of modified Thayer-Martin agar for growth of the organism that causes gonorrhea. The plate is inoculated with a swab and labeled, and the CO_2-generating tablet contained in the foil packet is placed in a well in the plate. The plate is sealed in the plastic pouch and kept in the incubator until picked up by the courier.

34

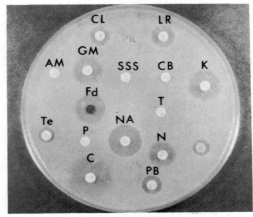

Figure 34–2

Chemotherapy and antibiotics. Testing sensitivity of a bacterium to antibiotics or other chemo-therapeutic agents by the "disk method." (Courtesy of Linda Kaye Hickey; from Fuerst, R.: Frobisher and Fuerst's Microbiology in Health and Disease, 15th ed. Philadelphia, W. B. Saunders Co., 1983.) CL, Coly-Mycin (colistin sulfate); AM, ampicillin; Te, Terramycin (oxytetracycline); P, penicillin; C, chloramphenicol; PB, polymyxin B; N, neomycin; Fd, nitrofurantoin; T, tetracycline; K, kanamycin; LR, cephaloridine; GM, Garamycin (gentamicin sulfate); SSS, triple sulfa (sulfadiazine/sulfameth-azine/sulfamerazine); Cb, carbenicillin; NA, nalidixic acid.

sealed jar with a lighted candle. The burning of the candle generates CO_2.

Sensitivity Tests

Antibiotic susceptibility is used to determine which antibiotics inhibit the growth of organisms and which are most effective in treating the infection. In this test, the bacteria are subjected to a variety of antibiotic-impregnated paper disks. These **sensitivity disks** are placed on a plate of *Mueller-Hinton* agar that has been inoculated with a pure culture of the organism being tested. After incubation, the plate is examined for growth around each disk. A zone of clear medium around the disk indicates that the organism cannot grow in the presence of that antibiotic, and the organism is said to be *sensitive* to the antibiotic. If the organism grows up to the disk, it is *resistant* to that antibiotic, and that antibiotic would not be an effective treatment. The size of the zone around the disk is important. Zone size is affected by the number of organisms present. For this reason, sensitivity testing must always be done using a standardized inoculum of a pure culture (Fig. 34–2).

Procedures for Inoculating Specimens and Preparing and Examining Smears

Aseptic techniques must be strictly observed in the following procedures to ensure safety and good results.

Procedure 34–1

INOCULATING A BLOOD AGAR PLATE FOR CULTURE OF STREP THROAT

PROCEDURAL GOAL

To inoculate a blood agar plate for culture of strep throat.

EQUIPMENT AND SUPPLIES

Blood and body-fluid protection barriers (goggles, masks, and aprons or gowns), as necessary (see Appendix C, Recommendations for Prevention of AIDS Transmission)
Nonsterile gloves
Blood agar plate
Bacitracin disk or strep A disk
Bunsen burner
Inoculating loop
Wax pencil
Swab from patient's throat
Forceps

Procedure continued on opposite page

PROCEDURE

1. Wash and dry your hands. Follow the universal blood and body-fluid precautions (see Appendix C). Glove yourself with nonsterile gloves.
2. Remove the swab from the container. Grasp the plate by the bottom (media side), and lift the cover, or lift the cover while the plate is on the table.
   Purpose: To make handling the plate easier and to prevent contamination of the plate.
3. Roll the swab down the middle of the top half of the plate, then use the swab to streak the same half of the plate. Dispose of the swab properly (below, left).
   Purpose: Rolling the swab ensures contact with the surface of the agar.
4. Sterilize the loop in the Bunsen burner, and allow it to cool.
   Purpose: Loops must be sterilized before and after use, to prevent cross-contamination of specimens.
5. Streak for isolation of colonies in the third and fourth quadrants, using the loop. Use the loop to make three slices in the agar in the area of heavy inoculum. Sterilize the loop (below, right).
   Purpose: Isolated colonies are needed for observation of colony morphology. The agar is sliced where the disk is to be placed, to allow for detection of subsurface hemolysis.

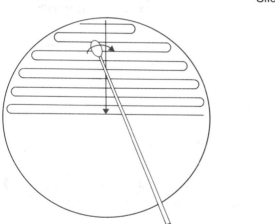

Slice media

Bacitracin disk

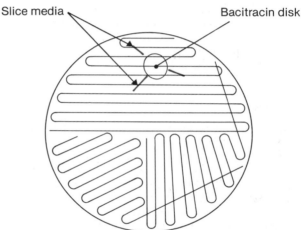

6. Sterilize the forceps and remove one disk from the vial. Place the disk on the agar between the cuts. Sterilize the forceps.
   Purpose: Group A beta-hemolytic streptococci are presumptively identified by their sensitivity to the disk.
7. Label the agar side of the plate with the patient's name and identification number and the date.
   Purpose: Labeling the agar side of dish prevents mixing up specimens.
8. Place the plate in the incubator, with the agar side of the plate on the top.
   Purpose: Placing the plate with the agar side up prevents accumulation of moisture on the surface of the agar.
9. Record all information in the laboratory log and on the patient's chart.
   Purpose: Laboratories must keep records of all tests performed, and these tests are assigned an identifying accession number.
10. Incubate for 24 hours and then examine. Incubate negative cultures for an additional 24 hours.
    Purpose: Some hemolysis patterns are not well-defined after 24 hours of growth.
11. Clean the work area.
12. Wash your hands.

TERMINAL PERFORMANCE OBJECTIVE

Given a specimen and the necessary materials, properly inoculate a blood agar plate within five minutes, and correctly complete each step of the procedure in the proper order, as determined by your evaluator.

34

Procedure 34–2

STREAKING PLATES FOR QUANTITATIVE CULTURES

PROCEDURAL GOAL

To inoculate two plates with urine, using quantitative streaking methods.

EQUIPMENT AND SUPPLIES

Blood and body-fluid protection barriers (goggles, masks, and aprons or gowns), as necessary (see Appendix C, Recommendations for Prevention of AIDS Transmission)
Nonsterile gloves
Urine specimen
Bunsen burner
Inoculating loop
Blood agar plate
EMB plate

PROCEDURE

1. Wash and dry your hands. Follow the universal blood and body-fluid precautions (see Appendix C). Glove yourself with nonsterile gloves.
2. Mix the urine specimen thoroughly by swirling.
   Purpose: Microorganisms settle to the bottom of the specimen when the specimen is allowed to stand.
3. Sterilize the loop, cool, and dip the tip into the specimen.
   Purpose: The loop must be allowed to cool, or the heat will destroy the microorganisms as the loop comes into contact with the urine specimen, resulting in falsely low colony counts on the culture. Urine on the shaft of the loop will run down the shaft and increase the size of the specimen deposited on the plate, resulting in a falsely elevated colony count on the culture.
4. Deposit the specimen on the plate, as indicated in the following diagrams. Use the loop to streak according to one of the following patterns.
   Purpose: Careful streaking of the plates is necessary for an accurate estimate of the organisms present.

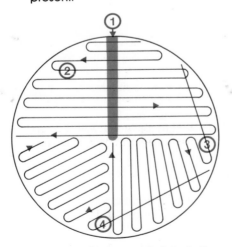
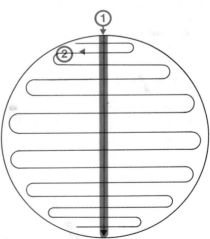

5. Inoculate the second plate in the same manner.
6. Label the bottom of the plates with the patient's name and identification number, and the date.
   Purpose: Labeling the bottom of the plates prevents mixing up of the specimens.
7. Record all information in the laboratory log and on the patient's chart.
8. Place the plates in the incubator, with the agar sides of the plates facing up.
9. Incubate for 24 hours, then identify organisms.
10. Clean the work area.
11. Wash your hands.

Procedure continued on opposite page

TERMINAL PERFORMANCE OBJECTIVE

Given a specimen and the necessary materials, inoculate two plates for culture within five minutes, and correctly complete each step of the procedure in the proper order, as determined by your evaluator.

Procedure 34–3

PREPARING A DIRECT SMEAR OR CULTURE SMEAR FOR STAINING

PROCEDURAL GOAL

To prepare a smear for staining from a clinical specimen or from a culture medium.

EQUIPMENT AND SUPPLIES

Blood and body-fluid protection barriers (goggles, masks, and aprons or gowns), as necessary (see Appendix C, Recommendations for Prevention of AIDS Transmission)
Nonsterile gloves
Clean glass slides
Diamond-tip pen
Wax pencil
Bunsen burner
Saline solution
Specimen

PROCEDURE FOR A DIRECT SMEAR

1. Wash and dry your hands. Follow the universal blood and body-fluid precautions (see Appendix C). Glove yourself with nonsterile gloves.
2. Label the slide with a diamond-tip pen.
   Purpose: Other labels are destroyed in the staining process.
3. Prepare a thin smear by rolling the swab on the slide. Make certain that all areas of the swab touch the slide.
   Purpose: Rolling the swab ensures that all parts of the swab come in contact with the slide so that the organisms that are collected are deposited on the slide. Thin smears are needed for evaluation.

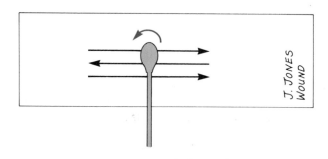

4. Allow the smear to air-dry. Do not wave it or heat-dry it.
   Purpose: Waving the slide spreads pathogens. Overheating organisms distorts them.

34

5. Hold the slide with the smear up. Pass rapidly through the flame of the Bunsen burner. Check the heating process by touching the slide to the back of the hand. The slide should feel warm, not hot. Check it often by touching the back of the slide to the back of the hand. Cool the slide. An alternative method is to use a Bacticinerator (below).
Purpose: Heat-fixing causes materials to adhere to the slide.

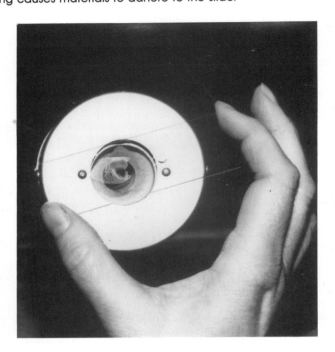

PROCEDURE FOR A CULTURE SMEAR

1. Wash and dry your hands. Follow the universal blood and body-fluid precautions (see Appendix C). Glove yourself with nonsterile gloves.
2. Identify the colonies to be stained by circling them on the back of the plate and numbering them with a wax pencil. Label the slide accordingly (below, left).
   Purpose: This allows accurate identification of colonies.
3. Apply a small drop of saline solution to the slide, using a loop.
   Purpose: Liquid is needed to emulsify the colony. Large drops require a longer drying time.
4. Touch, with a sterile loop, only the top of the colony chosen. Transfer the material picked up to the appropriate area of the slide, and spread it in a circular motion to the size of a dime. Repeat for each colony chosen (below, right).
   Purpose: Only a small amount of colony is needed for staining.

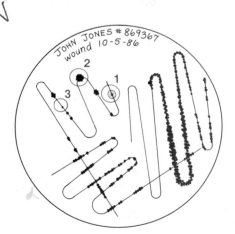

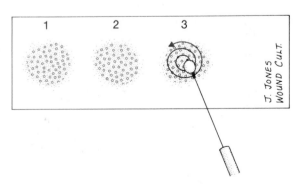

Procedure continued on opposite page

5. Allow the smear to air-dry.
6. Heat-fix the smear.
7. Clean the work area.
8. Wash your hands.

TERMINAL PERFORMANCE OBJECTIVE

Given a specimen swab or culture plate and the necessary materials, prepare a smear for staining within ten minutes, and correctly complete each step of the procedure in the proper order, as determined by your evaluator.

Procedure 34–4

STAINING A SMEAR WITH GRAM STAIN

PROCEDURAL GOAL

To stain a slide, using Gram stain, so that the organisms present are colored appropriately (neither overcolorized nor too strongly decolorized).

EQUIPMENT AND SUPPLIES

Blood and body-fluid protection barriers (goggles, masks, and aprons or gowns), as necessary (see Appendix C, Recommendations for Prevention of AIDS Transmission)
Nonsterile gloves
Gram stain reagents
Staining rack
Forceps
Wash bottle of water
Prepared smear for staining
Absorbent paper

34

PROCEDURE

1. Wash and dry your hands. Follow the universal blood and body-fluid precautions (see Appendix C). Glove yourself with nonsterile gloves.
2. Place the slide face up on a level staining rack.
   Purpose: If the slide is face down, the organisms will not be stained. If the rack is uneven, the stain will run off the slide surface.
3. Flood the slide with *crystal violet.* Time for 30 seconds.
   Purpose: Crystal violet is the primary stain and colors everything purple.
4. Flood the stain off with a sharp stream of water from the wash bottle. With forceps, tip the slide to remove the water.
   Purpose: Using forceps keeps your fingers clean.
5. Flood the slide with *Gram's iodine* (mordant). Time for 30 seconds.
   Purpose: Gram's iodine causes the stain to set in the organisms that are Gram-positive.
6. Flood the iodine off with water. Grasp the slide with forceps, and hold it nearly vertical.
7. Decolorize by running the *decolorizer* (alcohol) down the slide until the smear stops giving off purple stain in all but the thickest portions (about ten seconds).
   Purpose: This is the critical step. The decolorizer removes stain from the organisms that are Gram-negative.

Procedure continued on following page

8. Rinse the slide with water, and return it to the staining rack.
9. Flood the slide with *safranin*, and time for 30 seconds.
   Purpose: Safranin is the counterstain and stains red everything that decolorized.
10. Rinse the slide well with water.
11. Wipe off the back of the slide with an alcohol tissue.
    Purpose: The back of the slide is cleaned to remove traces of stain, which make examination of the smear difficult.
12. Blot the slide dry between sheets of absorbent paper.
13. Clean the work area.
14. Wash your hands.

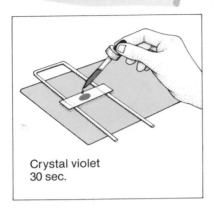

Crystal violet
30 sec.

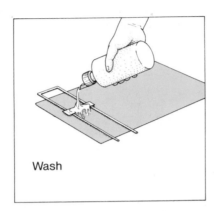

Wash

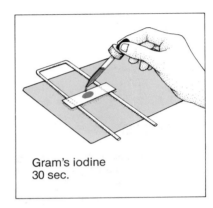

Gram's iodine
30 sec.

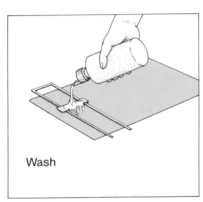

Wash

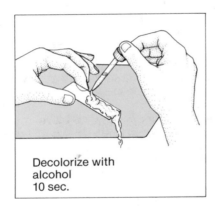

Decolorize with
alcohol
10 sec.

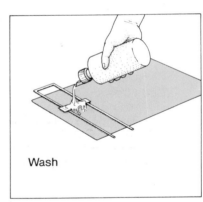

Wash

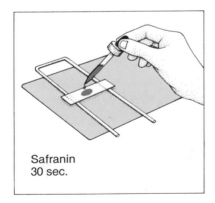

Safranin
30 sec.

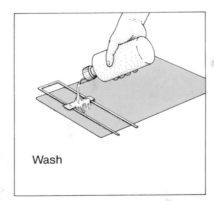

Wash

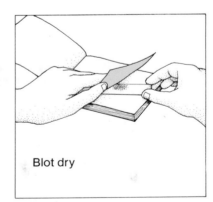

Blot dry

TERMINAL PERFORMANCE OBJECTIVE

Given the necessary materials, stain a smear within five minutes, and correctly complete each step of the procedure in the proper order, as determined by your evaluator.

Procedure 34-5

EXAMINING A SMEAR STAINED WITH GRAM STAIN

PROCEDURAL GOAL

To focus a stained slide under oil immersion, locate an appropriate area for evaluation, and give a morphologic description of the organism seen.

EQUIPMENT AND SUPPLIES

Blood and body-fluid protection barriers (goggles, masks, and aprons or gowns), as necessary (see Appendix C, Recommendations for Prevention of AIDS Transmission)
Nonsterile gloves
Stained slide
Microscope
Immersion oil
Lens paper

PROCEDURE

1. Wash and dry your hands. Follow the universal blood and body-fluid precautions (see Appendix C). Glove yourself with nonsterile gloves.
2. Place the slide right side up, on the center of the stage, over the condenser lens. Focus it under the low-power objective and then under the high-power objective. Place a drop of immersion oil on the slide, and switch to the oil-immersion objective.
   Purpose: If the slide is not right side up, you will be able to focus under the low-power objective but not under the oil-immersion objective.
3. Clear the image, using the fine-adjustment knob. Add light as needed.
4. Scan the slide to locate the thin area where cells are spread out.
   Purpose: Examination of thick areas yields poor results, since staining is not accurate and single organisms are hard to see.
5. Identify the microorganisms seen.
   a. Gram stain: Purple is Gram-positive; red is Gram-negative.
   b. Shape: Cocci are round. Bacilli are rod shaped. Spirilla are curved.
   c. Arrangement: Singly, in pairs, tetrads, chains, or clusters.
   d. Other cells seen: Yeasts, epithelial cells, and WBC's.

34

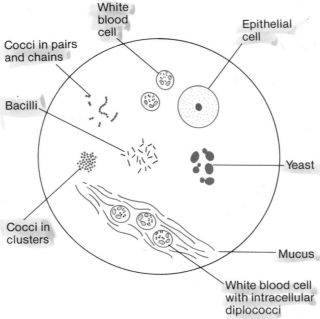

White blood cell

Epithelial cell

Cocci in pairs and chains

Bacilli

Yeast

Cocci in clusters

Mucus

White blood cell with intracellular diplococci

Procedure continued on following page

6. Record the findings.
7. Clean the work area.
8. Wash your hands.

TERMINAL PERFORMANCE OBJECTIVE

Given the necessary materials, examine a smear stained with Gram stain, identify the microorganisms present within 15 minutes, and correctly complete each step of the procedure in the proper order, as determined by your evaluator.

Slide Agglutination Test

The procedure for performing the *Mono-Test* (Wampole Laboratories, Cranberry, NJ) for infectious mononucleosis is included here because it is performed routinely in many small laboratories. The kit contains all the supplies and reagents needed (Fig. 34–3).

The test is an example of **agglutination** reactions found in many testing procedures. In agglutination tests, antigen-coated red cells (or latex particles) and antibodies are combined in a test tube or on slides. The test suspension is rocked for a specified amount of time and is observed for the presence of clumping. The visible clumps indicate a positive test. Known positive and negative controls are run at the same time as the patient's sample. Procedure 34–6 is an example of a slide agglutination test.

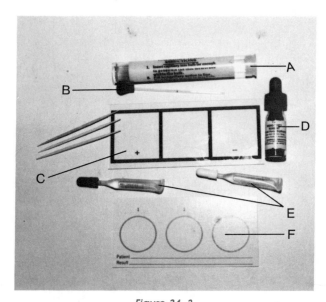

Figure 34–3
Materials contained in a Mono-Test kit (Wampole Laboratories). **A,** *Disposable capillary pipettes;* **B,** *reusable bulb;* **C,** *reusable glass slide;* **D,** *Mono-Test reagent;* **E,** *positive and negative controls;* **F,** *disposable cardboard slide. (Trademark of Wampole Laboratories, Division of Carter Wallace, Inc.)*

Procedure 34–6

MONO-TEST FOR INFECTIOUS MONONUCLEOSIS

PROCEDURAL GOAL

To perform and interpret a slide test for infectious mononucleosis.

EQUIPMENT AND SUPPLIES

Blood and body-fluid protection barriers (goggles, masks, and aprons or gowns), as necessary (see Appendix C, Recommendations for Prevention of AIDS Transmission)
Nonsterile gloves
Mono-Test kit
Blood specimen (serum or plasma)

PROCEDURE

1. Wash and dry your hands. Follow the universal blood and body-fluid precautions (see Appendix C). Glove yourself with nonsterile gloves.
2. Remove the test kit from the refrigerator, and allow the reagents to warm to room temperature. Check the expiration date of the kit.
   Purpose: Outdated or cold reagents do not react as expected.
3. Fill a disposable capillary tube to the calibration mark with serum or plasma (see Chapter 36 for collection of blood). Using the rubber bulb included in the kit, deposit the specimen in the middle circle of the clean glass slide also provided in the kit.
   Purpose: The capillary tube measures the exact amount of sample for accurate testing.

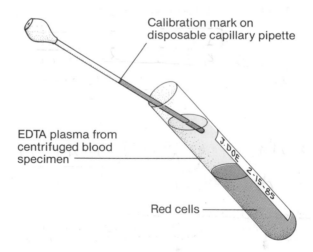

Calibration mark on disposable capillary pipette

EDTA plasma from centrifuged blood specimen

Red cells

4. Place one drop of negative control in the right circle and one drop of positive control in the left circle.
   Purpose: Known controls ensure that reagents are functioning properly.
5. Mix thoroughly the Mono-Test reagent by rolling the bottle gently between the palms of the hands. Squeeze the enclosed dropper to mix all the contents of the bottle.
   Purpose: Reagent red blood cells settle on standing and must be mixed before use.
6. Hold the dropper in a vertical position, and add one drop of Mono-Test reagent to each area of the slide. Do not touch the dropper to the slide.
   Purpose: Holding a dropper vertically ensures delivery of the same size drop. If the dropper touches other materials, it becomes contaminated, and results will be inaccurate.

Procedure continued on following page

7. Using separate stirrers, quickly and thoroughly mix each area, spreading each area out to one inch in diameter.
   Purpose: Failure to use a clean stirrer for each area would invalidate the test because of cross-contamination.

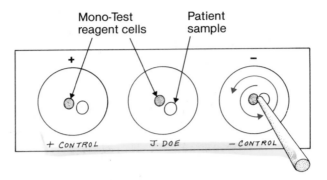

8. Rock the slide gently for exactly two minutes, and observe immediately for agglutination. A dark background is best for viewing.
   Purpose: Timing is always important.
9. Interpret the test results, and record them. Agglutination is positive, and no agglutination is negative.

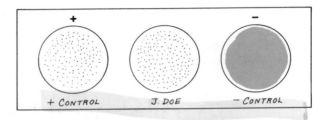

10. Clean the work area.
11. Wash your hands.

TERMINAL PERFORMANCE OBJECTIVE

Given a patient sample and the necessary materials, perform a Mono-Test within ten minutes and correctly complete each step of the procedure in the proper order, as determined by your evaluator.

Rapid Culture Methods

Several companies manufacture rapid culture methods designed for use in small laboratories. The tests selected depend upon the number of tests performed per month and the amount of refrigerator space available for storage. Dry media such as *Microstix-3*, for urine culture plus nitrite testing, and *Biocult GC*, for gonorrhea (both produced by Ames Company), and *Bacturcult*, for urine (Wampole Laboratories), have a long shelf life, do not require refrigeration, and occupy little incubator space (Fig. 34–4*A* and *B*). *Respirastick*, for strep screening, and *Uricult*, for urine culture (both produced by Medical Technology Corporation), are small, screw-top vials containing media on paddles (Fig. 34–4*C*). The vials are self-standing, for growth in any conventional incubator, and do not require refrigeration before use. *Isocult* systems (SmithKline Diagnostics) offer tests for strep screening, urine culture, and yeast, gonococcus, and *Trichomonas* culturing. The long plastic containers can be used in their own incubator or in a conventional incubator. They must be refrigerated before use. The rapid culture methods offer only presumptive identification of most organisms. Further specialization and sensitivity testing require additional materials and procedures.

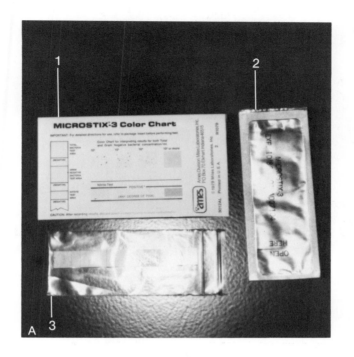

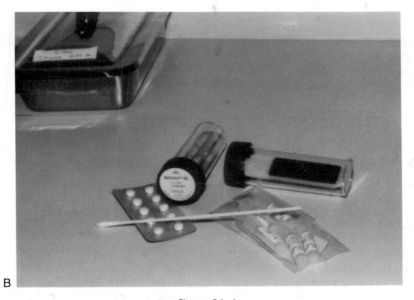

Figure 34–4

A, *Microstix-3 urine culture kit.* **1,** *Color chart for the interpretation of the nitrite test and bacterial colony count;* **2,** *Microstix-3 in foil packet;* **3,** *Microstix-3 in incubation pouch.* **B,** *Biocult GC for the detection of gonorrhea.*

Illustration continued on following page

34

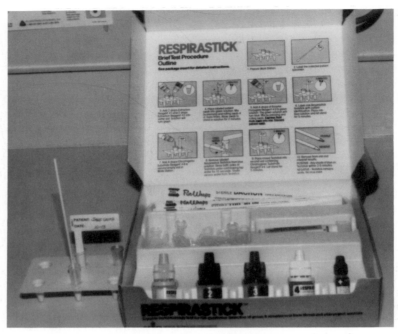

Figure 34–4 Continued
C, Respirastick. This is a culture system used to identify streptococci.

Interpretation of Urine Cultures

Interpretation of urine cultures is performed by estimating the number of colonies and determining if one or more organisms are growing. The number of bacteria present in the urine can be estimated by counting the colonies that grow out after 24 hours of incubation (i.e., colony count) (Fig. 34–5). For example, if 30 colonies are counted on the medium and a 0.001 ml calibrated inoculating loop was used, the bacterial count is 30,000 per ml of urine. The number of colonies is multiplied by 1000, since only 1/1000 ml of urine was cultured. Usually, an infection is indicated when the *colony count* is over 100,000 bacteria per ml of urine.

After the organisms have been counted and isolated from the culture, they can then be identified by various means. Growth characteristics can be observed visually. Agglutination kits and biochemical strip tests are also available for identification of the isolated organisms.

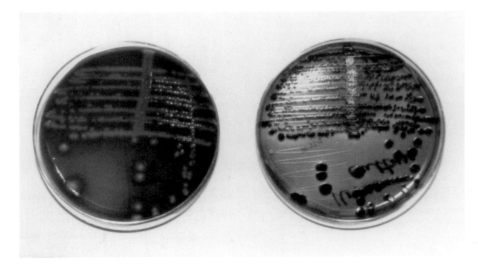

Figure 34–5
A culture showing between 75,000 and 100,000 CFU/ml (colony-forming units/ml). Growth is heavy in the original areas of inoculum and moderate in the third quadrant, and a few colonies are found in the fourth quadrant. The plate on the left is blood agar, and the one on the right is EMB agar (eosin–methylene blue agar). The organism growing is Escherichia coli, *the most common cause of urinary tract infections.*

Interpretation of Throat Culture

Group A beta-hemolytic streptococci (Streptococcus pyogenes) cause septic sore throat and are capable of producing severe complications if not diagnosed and treated. Complications include scarlet fever, rheumatic fever, and glomerulonephritis. Group A beta-hemolytic streptococci may be identified by placing an antibiotic disk, bacitracin, on a streaked plate and observing inhibition of any bacterial growth after 24 hours of incubation (Fig. 34–6). Complete clearing of the agar around the colonies indicates beta-hemolysis.

Several slide and tube tests have been developed for the detection of group A streptococci directly from throat cultures. The tests can be performed while the patient waits. The patient's throat is swabbed, the swab is placed in a tube, reagents are added at timed intervals, and a liquid extract is expressed from the swab onto a slide. Reagents are added and mixed. The slide is gently rocked and then examined for agglutination after a specified time. Agglutination indicates the presence of group A streptococci. The entire procedure can be performed in less than 15 minutes.

A color-change tube test (Ventrescreen, Ventrex Laboratories) for group A streptococci identification directly from a throat swab is also available. The swab is placed in a coated test tube, and extraction reagents are added at timed intervals. The tube is incubated, washed five times with water, and a color reagent is added. Any blue color developing within two minutes is a positive test.

These tests are available in kits that contain all

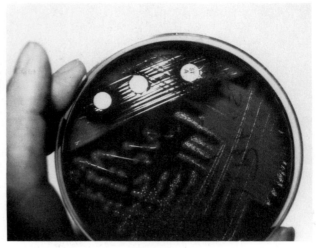

Figure 34–6
Ventrescreen quick tube test for group A streptococci.

the needed supplies. Performance should be checked routinely using known controls.

REFERENCES AND READINGS

Bauer, J. D.: *Clinical Laboratory Methods*, 9th ed. St. Louis, C. V. Mosby Co., 1982.

Feingold, S. M., and Baron, E. J.: *Bailey and Scott's Diagnostic Microbiology*. St. Louis, C. V. Mosby Co., 1986.

Koneman, E. W., et al.: *Clinical Microbiology Educational Series*. Bethesda, MD, Health and Education Resources, 1977.

Koneman, E. W., et al.: *Color Atlas and Textbook of Diagnostic Microbiology*, 2nd ed. Philadelphia, J. B. Lippincott Co., 1983.

Nester, E. W., et al.: *Microbiology*, 3rd ed. Philadelphia, Saunders College Publishing, 1983.

34

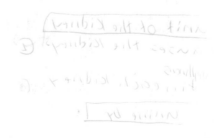

CHAPTER OUTLINE

VOCABULARY

See Glossary at end of book for definitions.

    enzymatic
    ischemia
    myoglobinuria
    phenylalanine

Handwritten notes:

What makes up the urine systems
1. Kidneys = 2   ureter   Bladder   urethra

function of the urine system
1. remove waste from the body
2. Electrolyte Balance.

Normal Adult will urinate
1000 cc – 1500 cc urine Per day

Where are the kidney located
1. above the waist under the muscle in the back.
2. Surrounded by fat to protect the kidneys from Injury.
3. A little over 10% of each heart pump goes into the kidneys.

Functioning unit of the kidney
1. Nephrons causes the kidneys to work   Nephrons
2. over 2 million in each kidney

Kidney will form urine by Three processes
1. Filtration
2. reabsorption
3. Secretion

Ureter - Tubes that comes out the center of the kidey are called urea pelvis. N drain out into the bladder
① about 12-10 inch long ¼ inch wide
② Peristalsis contraction on movement = what pushes the urine out.
③ are lined by Mucous membranes.

Bladder hollow sac that holds fluid
① when its empty it lies in the pelvis behind Pubis Symphysis
② As it fills it come up the lower cavity of the abdominal cavity

Hydronephrosis - condition of water in the kidneys, causes the kidneys to enlarge

Nephropexy - suturing the kidney back into place

the bladder contracts with forces the urine out

Normal Adult bladder will hold
300-400 cc per urine.

Bladder is lined with Mucous membrane and also the urethra

Urethra - The external opening of the bladder
urinary meatus - external opening of urethra
nephritis - inflammation of the kidney.
Pyleonephritis - inflammation of pelvis N kidneys,

Urinalysis

35

kidney
ureter
Bladder
urethra
urinary meatus.

urethra - very narrow 1½ inchs in women
8 inches in a man

Micturation
urination
Voiding
} all mean to empty the Bladder

OBJECTIVES

Upon successful completion of this chapter you should be able to
1. Define and spell the words in the Vocabulary for this chapter.
2. State five types of urine specimens commonly used.
3. Describe the physiology of urine formation.
4. Describe three abnormal colors of urine and the pathologic cause of each.
5. State the importance of performing a specific gravity measurement on urine.
6. Explain the clinical significance of each of the chemical urine tests.
7. Describe how quality control is performed in urinalysis.
8. Describe the appearance of three types of crystals found in urine.
9. Recall the process of performing a complete urinalysis.

Upon successful completion of this chapter you should be able to perform the following activities:
1. Instruct a patient in the collection of a timed urine specimen.
2. Perform a complete urinalysis.
3. Perform a macroscopic quality control on urine.
4. Perform a urinalysis slide test for pregnancy.
5. Demonstrate the performance of a confirmatory test for glucose using the Clinitest method.
6. Demonstrate the performance of the sulfosalicylic acid precipitation test for protein in urine.
7. Demonstrate the proper usage and care of centrifuges, urinometers, and other equipment used in urinalysis.

A routine urinalysis is one of the more common laboratory examinations used in the diagnosis and treatment of disease. It can be easily and quickly performed. The results of a routine urinalysis (abbreviated UA) can reveal diseases of the bladder or kidneys, systemic metabolic or endocrine disorders such as diabetes, and diseases of the liver, such as hepatitis, cirrhosis, or obstruction of the bile ducts. Urinalysis is routinely performed on all patients undergoing physical examinations and on those entering the hospital for treatment.

COLLECTING URINE SPECIMENS

For accurate information, it is important that each urine specimen be properly collected and handled. You should routinely follow the universal blood and body-fluid precautions by using nonsterile gloves and other appropriate barrier precautions when handling urine (see Appendix C, Recommendations for Prevention of AIDS Transmission). Most urine specimens collected in the office are *random specimens*, that is, collected at different times during the day. Because the makeup of urine changes constantly, depending on a person's activity, random specimens are used only for routine screening and initial evaluation.

First morning specimens are preferred because they are usually the most concentrated. They are best for pregnancy testing, culturing, and microscopic examination. *Timed specimens* are submitted when more specific information is needed for proper diagnosis. *Two-hour postprandial urine specimens*, collected two hours after a meal, are used in diabetic screening and for home diabetic-testing programs. *Twenty-four–hour urine specimens* are collected over a period of twenty-four hours to give quantitative chemical analyses, such as hormone levels and creatinine clearance rates (a procedure for evaluating the glomerular filtration rate of the kidneys).

Proper handling of specimens is essential. The chemical and cellular components of urine change if they are allowed to stand at room temperature (Table 35–1). These changes can be avoided by refrigerating the specimen if the analysis cannot be performed within 30 minutes after collection. Occasionally, preservatives must be added.

Routine specimens are collected in nonsterile, disposable containers. For culturing, urine should be collected by catheterization or the clean-catch method into a sterile container. Pediatric specimens are more difficult to collect. A sterile pouch is taped to the cleansed perineum or around the penis (Fig. 35–1). If necessary, the infant may be coaxed into urinating by placing its feet in cool water.

Instructing Patients to Collect Urine

Most patients understand the procedure for collecting a routine urine specimen. However, they

Table 35–1
Changes in Urine at Room Temperature

Constituent	Change
Clarity	Becomes cloudy as crystals precipitate and bacteria multiply
Color	May change if pH becomes alkaline
pH	Becomes alkaline as bacteria form ammonia from urea
Glucose	Decreases as bacteria metabolize it
Ketones	Decrease
Bilirubin and urobilinogen	Undergo degradation in light
Blood	May hemolyze. False-positives possible due to bacterial peroxidase
Nitrite	May become positive as bacteria convert nitrate. Can become negative as bacteria metabolize nitrite.
Casts	Lyse or dissolve in alkaline urine
Cells	Lyse or dissolve in alkaline urine
Bacteria	Multiply twofold every 20 minutes
Yeast	Multiply
Crystals	Precipitate as urine cools. May dissolve if pH changes

will need special instructions for collecting timed specimens. The following set of instructions will help you in your teaching activities with patients who need to collect a 24-hour urine specimen:

CARE OF YOUR SPECIMEN

Do not add anything but your urine into the bottle.
Do not pour out any liquid or powdered preservative from the container.

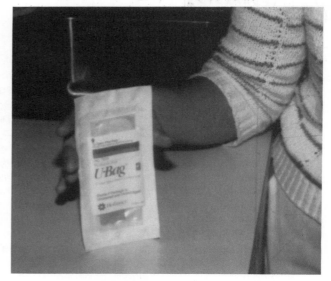

Figure 35–1
Sterile pouch for the collection of pediatric specimens. The pouch is taped to the cleansed genital area. Urination is stimulated by placing the infant's feet in cool water. The sample is emptied into a container by removing a tape plug and allowing the urine to drain. This prevents contamination of the specimen by organisms that may be adhering to the taped opening of the pouch.

If you accidentally spill some of the preservative on you, immediately wash with water and call us.

Always keep the collection bottle refrigerated or cool. Refrigerate or keep in an ice-filled cooler or pail.

Keep the cap on the container.

You may find it more convenient to urinate into the smaller container provided, and then pour the urine into the larger collection bottle.

STEPS FOR OBTAINING YOUR SPECIMEN

1. Upon arising in the morning, urinate into the toilet. Empty your bladder completely.

Do not save this urine. Note exact time, and write it down on the container.

2. Collect all urine voided after this time for exactly 24 hours. Remember that all urine passed at night or during the day in this time period must be saved.

3. Remember to keep the urine cool.

4. At exactly the same time the following morning, urinate completely again. Save this sample. Add it to the collection container. This completes your 24-hour collection.

5. Take all specimens from the 24-hour collection to the medical office, or to the place designated, as soon as possible, maintaining the cool temperature in transit by placing the specimen in a portable cooler or insulated bag.

Procedure 35-1

TEACHING A PATIENT TO COLLECT A TIMED URINE SPECIMEN

PROCEDURAL GOAL

To teach a patient to collect a timed urine specimen.

EQUIPMENT AND SUPPLIES

Small collection container
Large collection container
Set of written instructions

PROCEDURE

1. Add preservative to a large collection container, if required. Determine if the specimen requires a preservative by checking the laboratory specimen requirement manual.
   Purpose: Some constituents undergo degradation if not preserved.
2. Discuss the instruction sheet with the patient. Give the patient a set of written instructions, a transfer container, and the larger labeled specimen container.
   Purpose: Patients may not always understand written instructions, or they may have questions. Labeling of specimen containers prevents the laboratory from receiving unlabeled specimens from patients.
3. Be certain that the patient knows where the collected specimen is to be taken. It may be returned to the office, or it may be taken directly to the reference laboratory. If it is going to be taken to another laboratory, be certain to attach a properly filled out requisition.
   Purpose: Most quantitative urine tests are complicated and are not performed in the physician's office.

TERMINAL PERFORMANCE OBJECTIVE

Given the appropriate equipment and supplies, instruct a patient to collect a timed urine specimen by correctly completing each step of this procedure in the proper order within five minutes, as determined by your evaluator.

35

PHYSIOLOGY OF URINE FORMATION

To understand the meaning of urinalysis results, it is necessary to have a general understanding of the physiology of urine formation and the normal components of urine. Normal body functions and good health depend on homeostasis. Various organ systems supply the body cells with substances such as oxygen and nutrients needed for metabolism and help eliminate the waste products of metabolism such as carbon dioxide. To function normally, body cells need more than a supply of nutrients and the elimination of waste products. Cells need to exist in a stable internal environment, where the composition of the extracellular fluids is constant. The urinary system functions to maintain this composition and, thus, the physiochemical properties of the internal environment.

The urinary tract is composed of paired kidneys located behind the peritoneum, on either side of the lumbar spine. Each drains through a ureter into the bladder. Urine is stored in the bladder until *micturition*, or voiding, when it passes out of the body through the urethra.

Inside each kidney are millions of nephrons, the functional unit of urine formation. In the nephron, blood from the body passes through the afferent arteriole and enters the glomerulus, where the first step of urine formation, filtration, occurs. Water and dissolved chemicals in plasma filter through the glomerulus into Bowman's capsule. Normally, platelets, cells, and larger molecules such as protein and certain drugs do not pass across the glomerular membrane and are not found in the filtrate.

As the filtrate passes through the proximal convoluted tubule, loop of Henle, and distal convoluted tubule, reabsorption of needed chemical substances such as glucose, secretion of excess chemicals, and concentration of the filtrate occur to form urine.

Normally, water constitutes about 95 percent of urine. The other 5 percent includes dissolved chemicals such as urea, uric acid, creatinine, sodium chloride, calcium, sulfates, phosphates, hydrogen ions, and urochrome. The proportion of water and chemicals varies greatly, depending upon the time of day, diet, metabolism, hormones, fluid intake, and nonurine fluid loss. Disease states alter urine volume and change physical, chemical, and microscopic constituents.

PHYSICAL EXAMINATION OF URINE

The first part of a complete urinalysis is the assessment of the physical properties and the measurement of selected chemical constituents of diagnostic importance (Table 35–2).

Table 35–2
Components of the Macroscopic Urinalysis

Physical Property	Chemical Property Measured by Dipsticks
Color	Protein
Clarity	Glucose
Specific gravity	Ketones
Amount*	Bilirubin
Odor*	Blood: intact RBCs, hemoglobin, myoglobin
Foam*	Nitrite
	Urobilinogen
	Leukocyte esterase
	Specific gravity†
	pH†

*Not always assessed.
†Physical properties measured on dipsticks.

Color and Clarity. Normal urine color is a shade of yellow ranging from pale straw to yellow to amber. Color depends on the concentration of the pigment *urochrome* and the amount of water in the specimen. A dilute specimen should be pale, and a more concentrated specimen should be a darker yellow. Variations in color may be caused by diet, medication, and disease. Abnormal colors may be pathologic or nonpathologic (Table 35–3).

Both normal and abnormal urine specimens may range in appearance from clear to very cloudy. Cloudiness may be caused by cells, bacteria, yeast, vaginal contaminants, or crystals. Often, a urine specimen that was clear when voided will become cloudy as it cools when crystals form and precipitate.

Table 35–3
Urine Colors

Color	Pathologic Cause	Nonpathologic Cause
Straw	Diabetes	Diuretics; high fluid intake (coffee, beer)
Amber	Dehydration	Excessive sweating; low fluid intake
Bright yellow		Carotene, vitamins
Red	Blood, porphyrins	Beets, drugs, dyes
Orange-yellow	Bile, hepatitis	Pyridium (phenazopyridine hydrochloride), dyes, drugs
Greenish yellow	Bile, hepatitis	Senna, cascara, rhubarb
Reddish brown	Old blood, methemoglobin	
Brownish black	Methemoglobin, melanin	Levodopa
Salmon pink		Amorphous urates
White (milky)	Fats, pus	Amorphous phosphates
Blue-green	Biliverdin, infection with *Pseudomonas*	Vitamin B, drugs, dyes

Procedure 35–2

PROCEDURAL GOAL

To assess and record the color and clarity of a urine specimen.

EQUIPMENT AND SUPPLIES

Blood and body-fluid protection barriers (goggles, masks, and aprons or gowns), as necessary (see Appendix C, Recommendations for Prevention of AIDS Transmission)
Nonsterile gloves
Urine specimen
Centrifuge tube

PROCEDURE

1. Wash and dry your hands. Follow the universal blood and body-fluid precautions (see Appendix C). Glove yourself with nonsterile gloves.
2. Mix the urine by swirling.
   Purpose: Suspended substances settle when urine stands. If urine is not mixed prior to assessing appearance, the finding will be incorrect.
3. Label a centrifuge tube if a complete urinalysis is being done.
   Purpose: (See Procedure 35–7.) If a complete urinalysis is being done, a portion of the specimen will be centrifuged for microscopic examination. The centrifuged specimen must be labeled to avoid specimen confusion.
4. Pour the specimen into a standard-size centrifuge tube.
   Purpose: Standard-size containers are a better quality control for assessing color and clarity results.
5. Assess and record the color (see Table 35–3):
   Pale straw   *4 colors*
   Yellow
   Dark yellow
   Amber
6. Assess and record clarity:
   Clear—No cloudiness
   Slightly cloudy—Can see light print through tube
   Moderately cloudy—Can see only dark print through tube
   Very cloudy—Cannot see through tube

amount of urine

specific gravity

PH

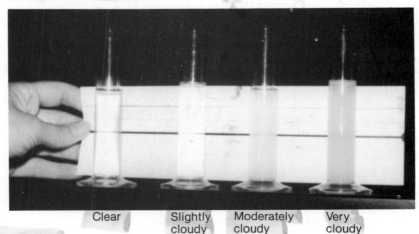

Clear   Slightly   Moderately   Very
         cloudy   cloudy   cloudy

7. Clean the work area.
8. Wash your hands.

Procedure continued on following page

TERMINAL PERFORMANCE OBJECTIVE

Given a urine specimen and the necessary supplies, assess urine color and clarity within one minute and to a ± 1 clarity rating and a ± 1 color rating of your evaluator.

Volume. The amount of urine is rarely measured on a random specimen. With a timed specimen, volume is measured by pouring the entire collection into a large graduated cylinder. Generally, it is not accurate enough to use the markings on the side of the collection container. Once the volume is measured and recorded, a portion of well-mixed specimen called an *aliquot* is removed for testing, and the remainder is discarded or stored, depending on the preference of the laboratory.

The normal volume of urine produced every 24 hours varies according to the age of the individual. Infants and children produce smaller volumes than adults. The normal adult volume is 750–2000 ml in 24 hours, with the average being about 1500 ml. Excessive production of urine is called *polyuria*. It is common in diabetes and certain kidney disorders. *Oliguria* is insufficient production of urine and can be caused by dehydration, decreased fluid intake, shock, or renal disease. The absence of urine production, *anuria*, occurs in renal obstruction and renal failure.

Foam. Normally, the presence of foam is not recorded, but careful observation of this property can be a significant clue to an abnormality. White foam can indicate increased protein. Yellow foam can mean bilirubinuria (see following). Foam is the presence of small bubbles that persist for a long time after the specimen has been shaken; they must not be confused with bubbles that rapidly disperse.

Odor. Like foam, odor is not normally recorded but can be an important clue. Normal urine odor is said to be aromatic. Changes in the odor of urine may be due to disease, the presence of bacteria, or diet. The odor of the urine of a patient with uncontrolled diabetes is described as fruity because of the presence of ketones, which are the products of fat metabolism. An ammonia smell in the urine can be due to an infection. The bacteria break down the urea in the urine to form ammonia. Infection usually imparts a putrid odor. Foods such as asparagus and garlic can also produce an abnormal odor in the urine.

Specific Gravity. Specific gravity (S.G., or sp. gr.) is the weight of a substance compared with the weight of an equal volume of distilled water. In urinalysis, it is the rough measurement of the concentration, or amount, of substances dissolved in urine. The specific gravity of distilled water is 1.000. Normal specific gravity of urine ranges from 1.005 to 1.030, depending on the fluid intake of the patient. Most samples fall between 1.010 and 1.025. Urine specific gravity indicates whether or not the kidneys are able to concentrate the urine and is one of the first indications of kidney disease. The presence of glucose, protein, or x-ray contrast media used in diagnostic studies may also increase the specific gravity of urine. To measure the specific gravity of urine, laboratories use dipstick, urinometer, or refractometer methods.

The *urinometer* is a sealed glass float with a calibrated paper scale in its stem (Fig. 35–2A). With a slight spinning motion, it is placed into a cylinder containing a urine sample, and the value is read at the meniscus of the urine. It requires a quantity of urine sufficient to freely suspend the float, usually around 20–25 ml. If the sample is insufficient to float the urinometer, use a refractometer (see following) or record as QNS (quantity not sufficient).

The urinometer is fragile, and jarring can cause the paper scale in the stem to shift, resulting in erroneous readings. Occasionally, a damaged urinometer loses its calibration. Thus, the calibration of the urinometer should be checked daily with distilled water. The specific gravity of the distilled water should calibrate at 1.000 at 20°C (room temperature). (For example, if the urinometer reads 1.002 in distilled water, 0.002 must be subtracted from the urine readings. However, it is better to replace the instrument.) For each 3°C that the water temperature measures above 20°C, 0.001 must be added to the reading. For each 3°C that the water temperature measures below 20°C, 0.001 must be subtracted from the reading. Use a laboratory thermometer to determine the water temperature.

The *refractometer* measures the refraction of light through solids in a liquid. The result is called the *refractive index*, which, for our purposes, is the same as specific gravity (Fig. 35–2B). The refractometer is both faster and easier to use than the urinometer and requires only a drop of urine. One drop of well-mixed urine is placed under the hinged cover of the instrument, and the value is read directly from a scale viewed through an ocular. The refractometer must be calibrated daily with distilled water.

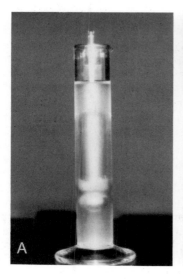
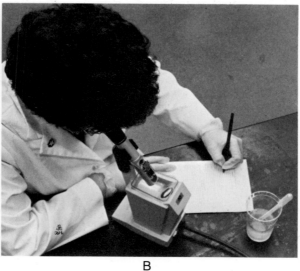

Figure 35–2
A, *A urinometer floating in a clear glass cylinder. The specific gravity reading is taken on the stem of the urinometer as it slowly turns in the specimen.* **B,** *A refractometer is filled with a drop of the urine, the hinged lid is closed, and the specific gravity is read by holding the instrument near a light source and focusing the rotating ring on the eyepiece.*

Procedure 35–3 *MEASURING SPECIFIC GRAVITY USING A URINOMETER*

PROCEDURAL GOAL

To calibrate the urinometer to perform a quality control check and to obtain duplicate specific gravity readings.

EQUIPMENT AND SUPPLIES

Blood and body-fluid protection barriers (goggles, masks, and aprons or gowns), as necessary (see Appendix C, Recommendations for Prevention of AIDS Transmission)
Nonsterile gloves
Urine specimen
Distilled water
Urinometer and cylinder

PROCEDURE

CALIBRATION
1. Wash and dry your hands. Follow the universal blood and body-fluid precautions (see Appendix C). Glove yourself with nonsterile gloves.
2. Fill the glass cylinder two-thirds full with distilled water at 20°C (room temperature).
   Purpose: A quantity of 20 to 25 ml is needed to allow the urinometer to float.
3. Read the specific gravity of the distilled water.
   Purpose: If the urinometer does not read 1.000, a correction factor, or a new urinometer, is necessary.
SPECIMEN
1. Wash and dry your hands. Follow universal blood and body-fluid precautions. Glove yourself with nonsterile gloves.
2. Allow the specimen to come to room temperature if it was refrigerated.
   Purpose: Specific gravity measured by the urinometer is temperature dependent.
3. Mix the specimen well by swirling.
4. Pour the specimen into the clean glass cylinder to two-thirds to three-quarters full.
   Purpose: A sufficient sample must be present to allow the urinometer to float freely.

Procedure continued on following page

35

5. If the sample is insufficient to float the urinometer, record as QNS (quantity not sufficient).
6. With the cylinder on a level surface, gently float the urinometer in the specimen with a spinning motion.
7. While the urinometer is slowly rotating in the specimen, read the lower curve of the meniscus, at eye level.
   Purpose: For accurate results, the urinometer must be read at eye level. Adjust your line of vision to the urinometer: do not hold the cylinder in your hand.

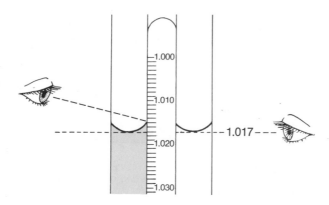

FOR CLOUDY URINE:
1. Read at top of meniscus
2. Add 0.002 to reading

      1.015
    + .002
    ——————
      1.017

FOR CLEAR URINE:
Read at bottom of meniscus at eye level

8. Obtain duplicate readings. (Repeat steps 5 and 6.)
   Purpose: Duplication of test results is a means of quality control of the procedure.
9. Record the results on the laboratory form or on the patient's chart.
10. Clean and dry the equipment, and return it to proper storage.
    Purpose: Urine salts dried on the equipment cause erroneous readings in later tests.
11. Clean the work area.
12. Wash your hands.

TERMINAL PERFORMANCE OBJECTIVE

Given a urine specimen and the necessary supplies, perform calibration and testing for specific gravity within five minutes, to ± 0.002 of the actual specific gravity, as determined by your evaluator.

CHEMICAL EXAMINATION OF URINE

Tests can be performed on urine to detect the presence of certain chemicals that can provide valuable information to the physician. In certain situations, these chemical test results can be critical to the diagnosis.

Reagent strips (dipsticks) are the most widely used technique of detecting chemicals in the urine and are available in a variety of types (Table 35–4). Reagent strips are plastic strips to which one or more pads containing chemicals are attached. Tests are available for pH, specific gravity, vitamin C, leukocytes, protein, ketones, glucose, blood, bilirubin, nitrite, urobilinogen, phenylketones, and others. The presence or absence of these chemicals in the urine provides information on the status of carbohydrate metabolism, liver and kidney function, and the acid-base balance of the patient.

These reagent strips are designed to be used once and then discarded. The directions for each strip are located in the package, and these instructions must be followed exactly to obtain accurate results. A color-comparison chart is located on the label of the container. In addition to reagent strips, various tablet tests are available. Quality controls are also available to ensure reliable test results.

Table 35–4
Urinalysis Reagents

	pH	Protein	Glucose	Ketones	Blood	Bilirubin	Urobilinogen	Nitrite	Leukocytes	Specific Gravity	Phenylketones	Dipstick	Tablet
Multistix 10 SG¹	•	•	•	•	•	•	•	•	•	•		•	
Multistix 9¹	•	•	•	•	•	•	•	•	•			•	
Chemstrip 9²	•	•	•	•	•	•	•	•	•			•	
Multistix 9 SG¹	•	•	•	•	•	•	•	•		•		•	
Chemstrip 8²	•	•	•	•	•	•	•		•			•	
Chemstrip 7	•	•	•	•	•	•	•					•	
Multistix 8¹	•	•	•	•	•			•	•			•	
Multistix 8 SG¹	•	•	•	•	•			•	•	•		•	
Chemstrip 6²	•	•	•	•	•	•						•	
Multistix 7¹	•	•	•	•	•			•	•			•	
Chemstrip 5¹	•	•	•	•	•							•	
Uristix 4¹		•	•					•	•			•	
Chemstrip GP²		•	•									•	
Multistix 2¹								•	•			•	
Chemstrip LN²								•	•			•	
Clinitest¹			•										•
Acetest¹				•									•
Ictotest¹						•							•
Phenistix¹											•	•	

¹Product of Ames Co.
²Product of BMC.

All strips and tablets must be kept in tightly closed containers and should only be removed immediately prior to testing. Reagents should be stored in a cool, dry area. Ames and Bio-Dynamics manufacture the majority of the urinalysis materials used in testing today.

pH. The pH is a measurement of the degree of acidity or alkalinity of the urine. A urine specimen with a pH of 7 is neutral. Less than 7 is acid, and greater than 7 is alkaline. Normal, freshly voided urine may have a pH range of 5.5 to 8.0. Urinary pH varies with an individual's metabolic status, diet, drug therapy, and disease. Colors on the pH reagent pad usually range from yellow-orange for an acid pH to green-blue when the pH is alkaline.

Protein. Protein in the urine in detectable amounts is called *proteinuria* and is one of the first signs of renal disease. We normally excrete a small amount of protein every day, but our testing procedures are designed to detect only pathologic levels in the urine. Proteinuria may be light to heavy, constant, or sporadic. It may be postural (affected by posture) in nature. In orthostatic proteinuria, protein is excreted only when the patient is in an upright position. Generally, first morning specimens from these patients are negative, but protein is found in urine passed throughout the day. Pro-teinuria is a common finding in pregnancy. It is almost always present after heavy exercise. Colors on the protein reagent pad usually range from yellow for negative to yellow-green or green for positive.

Glucose. Glucose is filtered at the glomerulus, but under normal conditions, most of it is reabsorbed by the tubules. The minute quantities normally present are not detected by strips and tablets. Detectable *glycosuria* occurs whenever the renal tubules cannot reabsorb the filtered glucose load. A positive glucose finding is common in urine from diabetic patients and may be the first indication of the disease.

The reagent-strip glucose testing method is **enzymatic.** It detects only glucose; in other words, it is *specific* for glucose. None of the other sugars that can occur in urine are detected by the reagent strips, but *Clinitest* tablets (Ames Company) do detect glucose and many other sugars. Clinitest is a *nonspecific* glucose test. Colors on the reagent strip range from green (low concentration of glucose) to brown (high concentration of glucose).

Ketones. Ketone bodies are the end product of fat metabolism in the body. Acetoacetic acid, acetone, and beta-hydroxybutyric acid are collectively referred to as ketone bodies, or ketones. *Ketonuria*

35

is common in starvation, low-carbohydrate diets, excessive vomiting, and diabetes mellitus. Since ketones evaporate at room temperature, urine should be tested immediately, or it should be tightly covered and refrigerated if not tested promptly. Color reactions on the strip range from pink to maroon when ketones are present. *Acetest* tablets (Ames Company) provide an alternative to strip testing.

Blood. The presence of blood in the urine may indicate infection or trauma to the urinary tract, or bleeding in the kidneys. The blood test pad on the reagent strip reacts with three different blood constituents: intact red blood cells, hemoglobin from red blood cells, and myoglobin, a hemoglobin-like molecule that transports oxygen in muscle tissue.

Hematuria is the presence of intact red blood cells in urine. The color reaction on the reagent strip ranges from orange through green to dark blue when hematuria is present. Hematuria can be due to irritation of the ureters, bladder, or urethra. It is also a common finding in cystitis and in persons passing kidney stones.

Hemoglobinuria is the presence of hemolyzed red blood cells. True hemoglobinuria is rare. It occurs as the result of intravascular red blood cell destruction and can be caused by transfusion reactions, malaria, drug reactions, snake bites, and severe burns. **Myoglobinuria** occurs when muscle tissue

is damaged or injured, such as in crushing injuries, myocardial infarctions, and contact sports. Muscular dystrophy patients often exhibit myoglobinuria. Hemoglobinuria cannot be distinguished from myoglobinuria by strip testing.

Bilirubin and Urobilinogen. *Bilirubin* is a product of the breakdown of hemoglobin (Fig. 35–3). Hemoglobin is released from old red blood cells destroyed in the reticuloendothelial system. It is gradually converted to bilirubin in the liver and then further to urobilinogen in the intestines. Bilirubin is a bile pigment not normally found in urine. Its presence in urine is one of the first signs of liver disease or other disease in which the liver may be involved, such as infectious mononucleosis.

Bilirubinuria can occur even before jaundice or other symptoms of liver disease are evident. It is the result of liver cell damage or obstruction of the common bile duct by stones or neoplasms (tumors). Excessive bilirubin colors the urine yellow-brown to greenish orange. Since direct light causes decomposition of bilirubin, urine samples must be protected from light until testing is complete. *Ictotest* tablets (Ames Company) are more sensitive to bilirubin than are the strips and are often easier to interpret when the urine is highly colored.

Urobilinogen is normally present in urine in small amounts. Increases are seen when there is increased red blood cell destruction and in liver disease. When

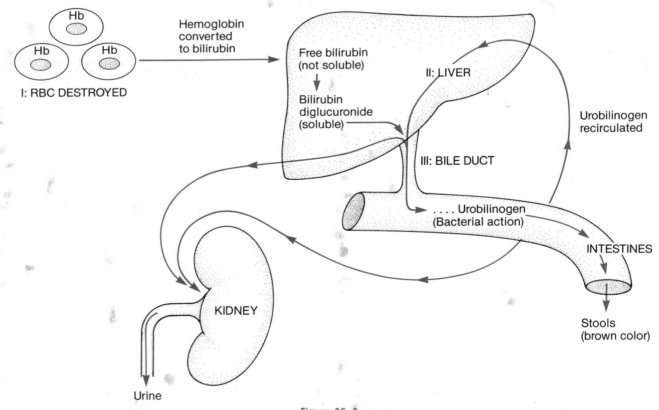

Figure 35–3
Detection of bilirubin and urobilinogen in urine.

there is total obstruction of the bile duct, no urobilinogen is formed in the intestines, none is reabsorbed into the circulation, and hence none is present in the urine. Strip methods cannot detect a decrease in urobilinogen. The reagent strip for positive testing results in color changes from orange through green to dark blue.

Nitrite. Nitrite occurs in urine when bacteria break down nitrate. A positive nitrite test indicates a urinary tract infection. However, not all bacteria are able to reduce nitrate to nitrite. Negative nitrite tests can also occur when there are insufficient bacteria present, or when the urine has not incubated in the bladder long enough for the reaction to occur. *Escherichia coli*, the organism that causes the majority of urinary tract infections, is nitrite positive. False positives can occur if a specimen is allowed to sit at room temperature and contaminating bacteria multiply. False negatives occur if the bacteria further metabolize the nitrite they have produced.

Leukocytes. Leukocytes occur in urine in infections of the urinary tract. They can also be contaminants from the vagina. The *leukocyte esterase test* on reagents strips detects intact and lysed polymorphonuclear white blood cells. However, it does not detect mononuclear white blood cells, which are occasionally present during infections. The test does not react with the small numbers of white blood cells found in normal urine.

Specific Gravity. Reagent strips are available that report specific gravity by the use of colored pads. The individual test pads on the strip give readings every 0.005 on the specific gravity scale from 1.005 to 1.030.

Phenylketones. *Phenistix* (Ames Company) are reagent strips used to detect the presence of phenylketones in the urine. This condition is called *phenylketonuria* (PKU). In this genetically inherited disorder, the body is unable to properly metabolize the nutrient **phenylalanine.**

As high levels of the phenylketones accumulate in the bloodstream, mental retardation occurs. PKU is easily treated by limiting dietary intake of phenylalanine in childhood. Since individuals who are properly treated for the disease do not suffer mental retardation, early detection is very important.

Ascorbic Acid (Vitamin C). Ascorbic acid normally is not found in urine in quantities large enough to interfere with chemical urine tests. However, in persons who habitually consume large quantities of vitamin C, the urine levels of ascorbic acid may affect results of nitrite, glucose, bilirubin, and occult blood tests. STIX reagent strips (Ames Company) or any of the combination strips available detect interfering levels of the drug. If an elevated level is found, the patient should be instructed to discontinue vitamin C intake for 24 hours, and then another urine specimen should be collected for testing.

Procedure 35–4

TESTING URINE WITH CHEMICAL REAGENT STRIPS

PROCEDURAL GOAL

To perform chemical testing on a urine sample.

EQUIPMENT AND SUPPLIES

Blood and body-fluid protection barriers (goggles, masks, and aprons or gowns), as necessary (see Appendix C, Recommendations for Prevention of AIDS Transmission)
 Nonsterile gloves
 Urine specimen
 Reagent strips
 Timer

PROCEDURE

1. Wash and dry your hands. Follow the universal blood and body-fluid precautions (see Appendix C). Glove yourself with nonsterile gloves.
2. Check the time of collection, the container, and the mode of preservation.
 Purpose: Proper specimen identification and screening of specimens for appropriate collection containers and collection procedures prevents testing of inappropriate specimens.

Procedure continued on following page

35

3. If the specimen has been refrigerated, allow it to warm to room temperature.
   Purpose: Certain tests are temperature dependent. Testing of cold specimens may cause false-negative results.
4. Check the reagent strip container for expiration date.
   Purpose: Do not use expired reagents.
5. Remove the reagent strip from the container. Hold it in your hand, or place it on a clean paper towel. Recap the container tightly.
   Purpose: Test strips are sensitive to moisture and must be stored in tightly sealed containers. Contamination from chemical residues on counter tops can affect results.
6. Compare nonreactive test pads with the negative color blocks on the color chart on the container.
   Purpose: Discolored pads have not been properly stored and must not be used for testing.
7. Thoroughly mix the specimen by swirling or inverting.
   Purpose: If settling occurs, certain elements may not be detected.
8. Following manufacturer's directions, note the time, and simultaneously dip the strip into the urine and remove.
   Purpose: Tests are time dependent. Positive tests result in darkening with time.
9. Draw the strip across the lip of the container to remove excess specimen (below, left).
   Purpose: Excess urine on the strip, or prolonged dipping time, affects test results.
10. Hold the strip horizontally. At the exact time, compare the strip with the appropriate color chart on the reagent container.
    Purpose: Holding the strip horizontally prevents runover from one test pad to another and prevents interference from the mixing of chemicals in the test pads.
11. Read the concentration, and record it on the laboratory report form (below, right).
    Purpose: Timing is critical.
12. Clean the work area.
13. Wash your hands.

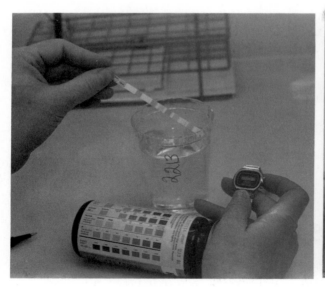 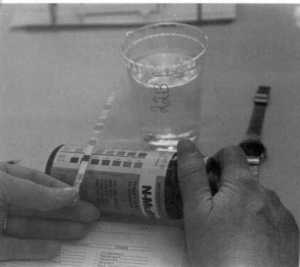

TERMINAL PERFORMANCE OBJECTIVE

Given a urine specimen and appropriate supplies, perform chemical testing of a urine sample within three minutes to a minimum performance level of 100 percent accuracy for negative reactions, and to within ± 1 color block of given test results for positive reactions, as determined by your evaluator.

Confirmatory Testing

Positive reagent strip testing should be confirmed by further testing whenever possible. Verification with a different procedure is preferred over repeating the same procedure to rule out any false reactions that may have been caused by interfering substances on the dipstick.

Positive protein tests should be confirmed by an *acid precipitation test*. Glucose-positive results should be confirmed with Clinitest tablets. Bilirubin-positive results should be confirmed with Ictotest tablets, especially since the dipstick test pad used for bilirubin is often difficult to interpret in highly colored urines. Acetest tablets are used to confirm positive ketone tests.

New tests are constantly being developed and marketed, and existing tests are constantly undergoing improvement. It is important to read the product insert to be aware of changes made in the testing procedure and of product performance.

Procedure 35–5

TESTING URINE FOR GLUCOSE USING CLINITEST TABLETS

[handwritten:] Clinitest 5 drops of urine 10 drop of distilled water

PROCEDURAL GOAL

To perform confirmatory testing for glucose in the urine using the Clinitest procedure for reducing substances.

EQUIPMENT AND SUPPLIES

Blood and body-fluid protection barriers (goggles, masks, and aprons or gowns), as necessary (see Appendix C, Recommendations for Prevention of AIDS Transmission)
Nonsterile gloves
Urine specimen
Clinitest tablet
Clinitest tube
Clinitest dropper
Distilled water
Test tube rack
Color chart
Timer

PROCEDURE

1. Wash and dry your hands. Follow the universal blood and body-fluid precautions (see Appendix C). Glove yourself with nonsterile gloves.
2. Holding a Clinitest dropper vertically, add ten drops of distilled water and then five drops of urine to a Clinitest tube.
   Purpose: Holding the dropper vertically prevents altering the size of the drops.
3. With dry hands, remove a Clinitest tablet from the bottle by pouring the tablet into the bottle cap.
   Purpose: Clinitest tablets react with moisture and become caustic. Handling tablets with moist hands could result in hydroxide burns.
4. Compare the color of the tablet with an unreacted tablet on the color chart.
   Purpose: If the tablet is discolored, it has degenerated and must not be used for testing.

35

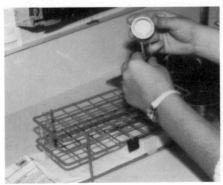

[handwritten:] Centrifuge urine 6 min.

Procedure continued on following page

5. Tap the tablet into the test tube, and recap the container.
6. Hold the test tube at the top.
   Purpose: The tube becomes hot as the reaction progresses.
7. Observe the entire reaction in order to detect the "rapid pass through" phenomenon. (See step no. 10, following).
   Purpose: If "pass through" occurs but is not detected, the reading will be falsely low.
8. When boiling ceases, time exactly 15 seconds, then gently shake the tube to mix the entire contents.
9. Immediately compare the color of the specimen with the "five-drop" color chart, and record your findings.
   Purpose: Color darkens with time. For accurate results, time carefully.

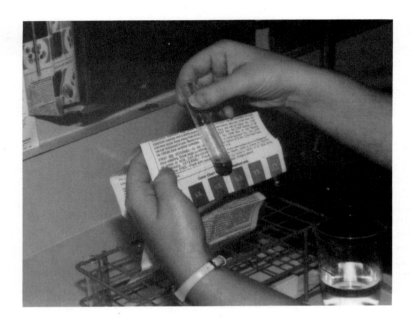

10. If an orange color briefly develops during the reaction, "rapid pass through" has occurred, and the test must be repeated using the "two-drop" color chart.
11. Repeat the test, using ten drops of water and two drops of urine.
12. Compare the specimen color to the "two-drop" color chart.
    Purpose: The five-drop and the two-drop color charts are not interchangeable.
13. Clean the work area.
14. Record the results:
    Negative—Clear
    Trace—Slightly cloudy
    1+—Can see light print through tube
    2+—Can see dark print through tube
    3+—Cannot see through tube
    4+—Large, fluffy precipitate forms and settles, on standing
15. Wash your hands.

TERMINAL PERFORMANCE OBJECTIVE

Given a urine specimen and appropriate supplies, perform the Clinitest procedure for reducing substances in urine within three minutes, and record the results within ± 1 color block of the known value for that specimen, as determined by your evaluator.

Procedure 35-6

PROCEDURAL GOAL

To perform the sulfosalicylic acid (SSA) precipitation test for the presence of protein in the urine.

EQUIPMENT AND SUPPLIES

Blood and body-fluid protection barriers (goggles, masks, and aprons or gowns), as necessary (see Appendix C, Recommendations for Prevention of AIDS Transmission)
Nonsterile gloves
Urine specimen
3 percent sulfosalicylic acid
Centrifuge tube and centrifuge
Test tube and rack
Dropper

PROCEDURE

1. Wash and dry your hands. Follow the universal blood and body-fluid precautions (see Appendix C). Glove yourself with nonsterile gloves.
2. If the urine is cloudy, filter the specimen or use a centrifuged specimen.
   Purpose: If the urine is already turbid (cloudy), the test will be difficult to interpret.
3. In a clear test tube, mix equal volumes of urine and 3 percent SSA.
4. Observe for cloudiness and record:
   Negative—Clear
   Trace—Slightly cloudy
   1+—Can see light print through tube
   2+—Can see dark print through tube
   3+—Cannot see through tube
   4+—Large, fluffy precipitate forms and settles, on standing
   Purpose: This result gives a rough estimation of the protein concentration of the urine.
5. Clean the work area.
6. Wash your hands.

TERMINAL PERFORMANCE OBJECTIVE

Given a urine specimen and appropriate supplies, perform the acid precipitation test within one minute and within ± one grade of the known results as determined by your evaluator.

35

MICROSCOPIC EXAMINATION OF URINE SEDIMENT

The microscopic examination of urine consists of the categorizing and counting of cells, casts, crystals, and miscellaneous constituents of the sediment obtained when a measured portion of urine is centrifuged. The clear upper portion of the specimen is called the supernatant. It is poured off, and a drop of the well-mixed sediment is examined under a microscope. This part of the urinalysis gives the physician information about the course and progress of renal disease as well as detects the presence of infection.

Casts. Casts are formed when protein accumulates and precipitates in the kidney tubules and is washed into the urine. The protein takes on the size and shape of the tubules, hence the term "casts." Casts are cylindric, with flat or rounded ends, and are classified according to the substances observed in them. Certain types of casts are associated with renal pathologic conditions, and others are physiologic, generally being caused by strenuous exercise.

Casts are counted and reported under low-power magnification, but occasionally high-power magnification is needed to identify the type. Since casts tend to migrate to the edges of the coverslip, this area should be examined closely. Casts dissolve in alkaline urine, on standing, so examination of a fresh urine specimen is very important (Fig. 35–4).

Hyaline casts are pale, transparent cylindric structures having rounded ends and parallel sides. Hyaline casts will be missed entirely if subdued light is not used. They are formed when urine flow through individual nephrons is diminished. They can be found in kidney disease but can also be found in urine specimens of normal subjects who have exercised heavily. Occasionally, hyaline casts have granular or cellular inclusions. Cylindroids are hyaline casts with long, thin tails.

Finely and *coarsely granular casts* may be due to exercise but, when present in increased numbers, may indicate renal disease. On close examination, granular casts show a hyaline matrix with coarse or fine granular inclusions. The granules are thought to be due to protein aggregation or degeneration of cellular inclusions.

Red blood cell casts are always pathologic and highly diagnostic. Red blood cell casts occur in glomerulonephritis. They are hyaline casts with embedded red cells, and their presence indicates damage to the glomerular membrane. They may appear brown as a result of the color of the red blood cells present.

White blood cell casts are hyaline casts that contain leukocytes. White blood cells usually have a multi-lobed nucleus, which differentiates them from renal tubular epithelial cells, which have single, round nuclei. White blood cell casts are seen in pyelonephritis.

Renal tubular epithelial cell casts contain embedded renal tubular epithelial cells. These casts are easily confused with white blood cell casts, particularly if the cells have started to degenerate. Renal tubular epithelial cell casts are found when there is excessive damage. Causes are shock, renal **ischemia**, heavy-metal poisoning, certain allergic reactions, and nephrotoxic drugs.

Waxy casts are rarely seen. They appear as glassy, brittle, smooth, homogeneous structures. They are usually yellowish, have cracks or fissures, and have squared or broken ends. They are considered to be degenerated cellular casts and are found in severe renal disease.

Broad casts are from two to six times as wide as other casts. They are formed in the collecting tubules and indicate decreased urine output in several adjacent nephrons.

Occasionally, more than one type of cell will be found in a single cast. Mixed cellular casts have been reported. Absolute identification of the cell types present may be difficult. Be as specific as possible.

Cells. Cells that are found in urine include epithelial cells, which are derived from the lining of the genitourinary tract. Other cells in urine include red blood cells (RBC) and white blood cells (WBC) from the bloodstream. Cells are classified and counted under high-power magnification (Fig. 35–5).

Red blood cells may enter the urinary tract at any point where there is inflammation or injury. They may be found in normal urine in small numbers,

Casts: 100 ×

450 × (to identify cells)

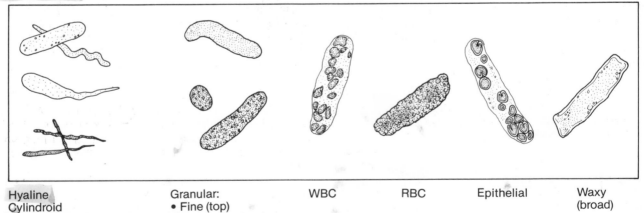

Hyaline
Cylindroid
Mucus (not a cast)

Granular:
• Fine (top)
• Coarse (bottom)

WBC

RBC

Epithelial

Waxy
(broad)

Figure 35–4
Urine casts.

Cells: 450×

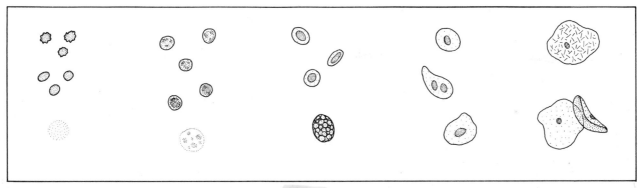

RBC:
• Crenated (top)
• Normal
• Swollen (bottom)

WBC:
• Glitter (bottom)

Round:
• Oval fat body (bottom)

Transitional

Squamous:
• Clue cell (top)
• Folded (bottom)

Figure 35–5
Red and white blood cells in urine.

usually less than 1–2/HPF (high-power field). Persistent hematuria should be investigated. Red blood cells are pale, round, nongranular, and flat or biconcave. They are smaller than white blood cells and have no nucleus. In hypotonic, or dilute, urine, they swell and burst. In hypertonic, or concentrated, urine, they may crenate and wrinkle. When they crenate, they can be mistaken for white blood cells, since the wrinkled surface makes them appear granular. They are often confused with yeast, oil droplets, and droplets of lens cleaner.

White blood cells may occasionally be found in normal urine, but increased numbers, usually greater than 5/HPF, are associated with inflammation or contamination of the specimen during collection. White blood cells are larger than red blood cells, have a granular appearance, and usually contain a multilobed nucleus, although nuclear detail may not be evident.

Renal tubular or *round epithelial cells* are somewhat larger than white blood cells, are round to oval, and have a single, large, oval, and sometimes eccentric nucleus. A few may be found in normal urine specimens, but their presence in increased numbers indicates tubular damage.

Transitional epithelial cells line the urinary tract from the renal pelvis to the upper portion of the urethra. They vary in size from slightly larger than a round epithelial cell to smaller than a squamous epithelial cell. They are round to oval and may have a tail. Occasionally, two nuclei are seen. When transitional cells are present in large numbers, a pathologic condition may exist.

Squamous epithelial cells line the lower portion of the genitourinary tract. When present in large numbers in females, they usually indicate vaginal contamination. Squamous epithelial cells are large, flat, irregular cells and are easily recognized under low-power magnification. They have a single, small, round, centrally located nucleus and often occur in sheets or clumps. Because of their flat nature, the edges of the cells are often rolled or folded.

In identifying epithelial cells, it is helpful to remember the appearance of eggs; round epithelial cells resemble hard-boiled eggs that have been cut in half. Transitional forms resemble poached eggs, and squamous cells resemble fried eggs with large, runny whites.

Crystals. Crystals are common in urine specimens, particularly if they have been allowed to cool. Cooling causes the solid crystals to precipitate out of the urine. The presence of most crystals is not clinically significant unless they are found in large numbers in patients with kidney stones. Occasionally, pathologic crystals are found. Identification of crystals begins with the determination of the pH of the urine. From there, one looks at color, shape, and refractility. Often, a history of drug intake is helpful. Consult Table 35–5 for nonpathologic and pathologic urine crystals. It is not always possible to identify crystals without additional chemical testing.

Miscellaneous Findings. *Oval fat bodies* (Fig. 35–5) are formed when renal tubular epithelial cells or macrophages absorb fats. The fat droplets contained in the cells vary in size and are quite refractile. Oval fat bodies are characteristic of the nephrotic syndrome.

Yeast in urine may indicate vaginal contamination or infection of the urine with yeast. It is common in the urine of diabetic patients. Yeasts are easily confused with red blood cells, are usually oval, may show budding, and are more refractile. To differentiate yeast from red blood cells, a drop of sedi-

35

Table 35–5
Crystals of Urine

Nonpathologic ACID pH	Crystal	Description and Occurrence
	Calcium oxalate	Clear, colorless, bipyramidal or envelope-shaped. Occasionally, shaped like dumbbell or safety pin. Very common
	Uric acid*	Pleomorphic, clear to yellow-brown, flattened, often four-sided, football-shaped, often in rosettes. Quite common
	Hippuric acid	Elongated, six-sided, colorless to yellow-brown, often in clusters
	Amorphous urates	Seen as salmon-pink precipitate in the centrifuge tube. Microscopically: shapeless, sand-like; brownish in color if heavy. Can be dispersed by warming tube prior to centrifugation. Very common
	Sodium urate	Colorless to yellow, long, thin, blunt-ended needles, often in rosettes or clumps
ALKALINE pH		
	Triple phosphate	Colorless "coffin lid" six-sided prisms, often very large. Common in alkaline urines
	Amorphous phosphate	Seen in centrifuge tube as a white precipitate. Microscopically, shapeless, whitish, granular "sand." Can be dispersed by adding acetic acid to the sediment. Fairly common
	Calcium phosphate	Flat plates; long, thin needles or prisms; stars, crosses, or rosettes. Not very common
	Ammonium biurate	Brown "thorn apples" or greasy brown spherules. Rare
Pathologic ALL FOUND AT AN ACID pH		
	Tyrosine needles	Colorless to yellow, fine, silky needles in sheaves, rosettes. Found in severe liver damage, often with leucine
	Leucine spheres	Yellow, radially or concentrically striated spheres. Seen in liver disease
	Bilirubin	Brownish cubes, rhombic plates, or needles in pompom ball arrangement. Free bilirubin stains sediment brown
	Cholesterol plates	Colorless, flat plates with parallel sides and a characteristic notched corner. Seen in some renal diseases
	Cystine	Clear, colorless, hexagonal plates. Seen in the congenital disorder cystinosis
OTHER		
	Radiocontrast dyes	Colorless, long, thin rhombic crystals. Specific gravity may be very high (often greater than 1.050). History will reveal recent x-ray studies
	Sulfa	Clear to brown sheaves of needles with eccentric, central constriction. History of sulfa medication

*May be pathologic.

ment is placed on the blood test pad of a reagent strip. Yeast does not react, but red blood cells do. Red blood cells dissolve when a drop of dilute acetic acid (regular white vinegar) is added to the sediment. The yeast remains intact (Fig. 35–6).

A few *bacteria* may be found in normal urine specimens. Heavy bacterial concentrations in the absence of white blood cells may indicate that the specimen was allowed to sit at room temperature and the bacteria multiplied. Urine specimens with a putrid odor, numerous white blood cells, and bacteria are common in urinary tract infections. Bacteria may be rods or cocci and are identified under high-power magnification.

Sperm are often found in the urine specimens of both males and females. In the latter, their presence represents vaginal contamination of the specimen. Sperm usually have pointed, oval heads and long thread-like tails. They may be motile in fresh urine.

The most commonly encountered parasite in urine is *Trichomonas vaginalis*. It is usually a vaginal contaminant but may also be found in urine specimens from males. When urine is fresh and warm, the trichomonas may be motile. *Trichomonas* organisms are pear-shaped protozoa with four flagella. They are larger than round epithelial cells but smaller than squamous cells. *Trichomonas* organisms die when the specimen is cooled.

Mucous threads can be found in most urine specimens. They appear as pale, irregular, thready structures with tapered ends. Beginners often confuse hyaline casts and mucous threads. Increased numbers are seen in inflammation and when there has been contamination of the specimen with vaginal contents (Fig. 35–4).

Reporting a Microscopic Examination

The slide is first examined under the low-power objective and low light to locate casts. Ten to 15 low-power fields are scanned, and the number of casts is counted and reported. The high-power objective and increased light is used to identify red and white blood cells, epithelial cells, yeasts, bacteria, and crystals. Ten to 15 high-power fields should be scanned, and the number counted, averaged, and reported. The method of counting varies considerably among laboratories. It is important that all workers in the same laboratory use the same counting and reporting systems. Report the results of the microscopic examination as follows (Table 35–6):

1. Separately total the numbers for each element counted, and then average. (Casts, WBC, RBC, and the three categories of epithelial cells are counted, totaled, and averaged.)

2. Casts, WBC, and RBC are reported using numerical ranges based on the average:

0	10–20
0–1	20–30
1–2	30–40
2–5	40–50
5–10	>50

3. Epithelial cells are reported as occasional, few, moderate, or many, according to the following:

0		
0–3	=	occasional
3–6	=	few
6–12	=	moderate
>12	=	many

Each type is calculated individually.

Miscellaneous: 450×

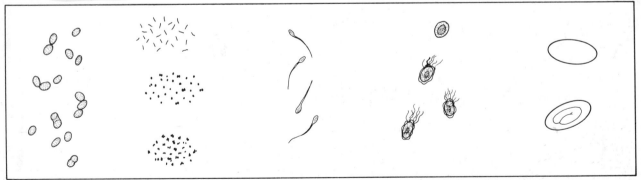

| Yeast | Bacteria:
• Bacilli (top)
• Cocci (middle)
• Amorphous crystals (bottom) | Sperm | Round epithelial cell
Trichomonas | Pin worm eggs:
• Empty shell (top)
• Egg with embryonic worm (bottom) |

Figure 35–6
Miscellaneous findings in urine.

Table 35–6
Calculating a Microscopic Urinalysis

Field	Per Low-Power Field		Per High-Power Field							
	CASTS	MUCUS	WBC	RBC	SQUAMOUS EPITHELIAL	TRANSITIONAL EPITHELIAL	ROUND EPITHELIAL	BACTERIA	CRYSTALS	OTHER
1	0	Few	16	1	1	0	0	Moderate (rods)	Calcium oxalate—few Uric acid—few	—
2	1 hyaline	Few	32	0	3	0	0	Many	Calcium oxalate—few	Yeast
3	1 coarse granular	Moderate	21	2	3	0	0	Many	Calcium oxalate—few	Yeast
4	1 coarse granular	Few	12	1	5	0	1	Moderate	Uric acid—few	—
5	0	Few	25	0	4	0	0	Many	—	—
Total	1 hyaline 2 coarse granular	Few	106	4	16	0	1	Many	Calcium oxalate—few Uric acid—few	Yeast
Average	0.2 hyaline 0.4 coarse granular	Few	21.2	0.8	3.2	0	0.2	Many	Calcium oxalate—few Uric acid—few	Yeast
Report	0–1 hyaline 0–1 coarse granular	Few	20–30	0–1	Few	0	Occasion- ally	Many (rods)	Calcium oxalate—few Uric acid—few	Yeast

4. The remaining elements are estimated as occasional, few, moderate, or many, according to the following:
   Occasional—Not seen in every field
   Few—Covers less than a quarter of the field
   Moderate—Covers approximately half of the field
   Many—Covers the entire field
5. Fibers, hair, talc granules, oil droplets, and other artifacts are not reported (Fig. 35–7).

Artifacts: 100–450×

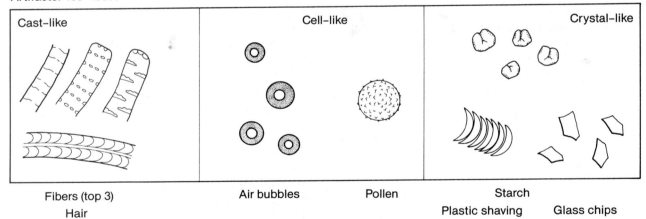

Figure 35–7
Urine artifacts.

Procedure 35-7

ANALYZING URINE MICROSCOPICALLY

PROCEDURAL GOAL

To perform a microscopic examination of urine to determine the presence of normal and abnormal elements.

EQUIPMENT AND SUPPLIES

Blood and body-fluid protection barriers (goggles, masks, and aprons or gowns), as necessary (see Appendix C, Recommendations for Prevention of AIDS Transmission)
Nonsterile gloves
Urine specimen
Centrifuge tube
Centrifuge
Disposable pipette
Microscope slide and coverslip
Microscope
Wax pencil

PROCEDURE

1. Wash and dry your hands. Follow the universal blood and body-fluid precautions (see Appendix C). Glove yourself with nonsterile gloves.
2. Gently mix the urine specimen.
   Purpose: If the urine is not well-mixed, elements that have settled to the bottom of the specimen container will be missed.
3. Pour 10 ml of urine into a labeled centrifuge tube.
4. Place the tube in the centrifuge.
5. Place another tube containing 10 ml of water in the cup opposite.
   Purpose: For proper operation, centrifuges must be carefully balanced. If not properly balanced, damage to the instrument can occur.
6. Secure the lid, and centrifuge for five minutes or for the time specified for your instrument.
   Purpose: Timing varies based upon the speed and the size of the centrifuge head.
7. Remove the tube from the centrifuge after the instrument has come to a full stop.
8. Pour off the clear supernatant from the top of the specimen by inverting the centrifuge tube over the sink drain.
9. Prevent the loss of sediment down the drain.
   Purpose: The sediment is what you will examine under the microscope.

35

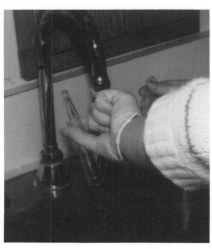

Procedure continued on following page

10. Thoroughly mix the sediment by grasping the tube near the top and rapidly flicking it with the fingers of the other hand until all sediment is thoroughly resuspended.
    Purpose: Elements centrifuge at different rates. Failure to completely mix the entire sediment will cause errors in quantification.

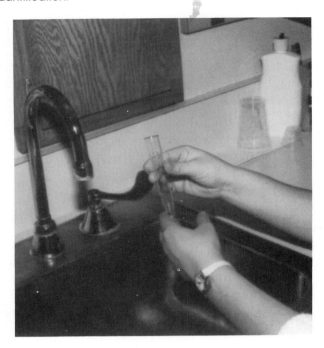

11. Using a disposable pipette, transfer one drop of sediment to a clean, labeled slide.
12. Place a clean coverslip over the drop, and place the slide on the microscope stage.
13. Focus under low power, and reduce the light.
    Purpose: Mucus and casts are easily missed if reduced light is not used. Constant focusing helps locate them.
14. First, scan the entire coverslip for abnormal findings.
    Purpose: Casts tend to migrate to the edges of the coverslip.
15. Examine five low-power fields. Count and classify each type of cast seen, if any, and note mucus if present.
    Purpose: Choose five fields so that one is selected from each corner of the coverslip and the last one is chosen from the middle of the coverslip. If you move to an area and there is nothing there, record a zero.
16. Switch to high-power magnification, and adjust the light.
    Purpose: As magnification increases, more light is needed.
17. In five high-power fields, count the following elements: RBC, WBC, and round, transitional, and squamous epithelial cells.
18. In the same five fields, report the following as few, moderate, or many: crystals (identify and report each type seen separately), bacteria (identify as rods or cocci), sperm, yeast, and parasites.
    Purpose: These three terms are more easily and universally understood than are exact numbers.
19. Average the five fields, and report the results.
20. Clean up the work area.
21. Wash your hands.

TERMINAL PERFORMANCE OBJECTIVE

Given a urine specimen and the necessary supplies, perform a microscopic examination of the urine within 20 minutes to a minimum performance level of $\pm$ 1 reporting range for casts, RBC, WBC, and epithelial cells, and to a minimum performance level of 100 percent for the presence of mucus, crystals, bacteria, yeast, and sperm, as determined by your evaluator.

QUALITY CONTROL

Quality control is a method of checking reagents, procedures, and personnel to ensure that results are accurate. Many commercially prepared products are available for use in both macroscopic and microscopic testing programs. Small laboratories using Ames products often use Chek-Stix for macroscopic quality control. Urintrol (Harleco) and Kovatrol (ICL Scientific) are intended for both macroscopic and microscopic quality control. It is good practice to use these products on a regular basis.

Procedure 35–8

TESTING URINE WITH CHEK-STIX FOR QUALITY CONTROL

PROCEDURAL GOAL

To prepare, test, and record the results of Chek-Stix control product for macroscopic quality control.

EQUIPMENT AND SUPPLIES

Blood and body-fluid protection barriers (goggles, masks, and aprons or gowns), as necessary (see Appendix C, Recommendations for Prevention of AIDS Transmission)
Nonsterile gloves
Chek-Stix
Distilled water
Centrifuge tube
Urinalysis reagent strips and tablets
Parafilm
Timer

PROCEDURE

1. Wash and dry your hands. Follow the universal blood and body-fluid precautions (see Appendix C). Glove yourself with nonsterile gloves.
2. Fill a graduated centrifuge tube with 12 ml of distilled water.
   Purpose: Tap water does not give accurate results because of pH differences.
3. Insert one Chek-Stix reagent strip, and cover the tube with Parafilm. Invert the tube gently for two minutes.
   Purpose: Mixing is required for elution of chemicals from strip.

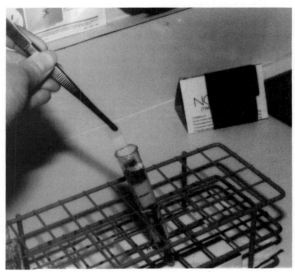

35

Procedure continued on following page

4. After 30 minutes have elapsed, mix again and discard the strip.
5. Test in the same manner as you would do a macroscopic urinalysis. The product may be used as a known, or it may be hidden in a batch of urine specimens and tested as an unknown.
   Purpose: "Blind" testing is often used to eliminate bias when the laboratory personnel know the results in advance.
6. Compare results with those given in the product insert.
   Purpose: Results should be within the range of given values for the procedure to be in control.
7. Record the results in the Quality Control Log.
   Purpose: Values should be monitored over a period of time to check for trends that would indicate deterioration of reagents or problems with any one individual's test procedure. All laboratories must maintain Quality Control logs.
8. If test results show that the procedure is not in control, the following steps should be taken before you report any patient results:
   a. Retest the Chek-Stix with a new test strip, and be sure to time the procedure accurately.
   b. If the procedure is still not in control, prepare a new Chek-Stix and retest with a new reagent strip.
   c. If the procedure is still out of control, open a new bottle of reagent strips, and test with Chek-Stix.
   d. If still out of control, report your findings to your supervisor. Do not report out any patient results until the procedure is in control.
   Purpose: Test results should be an accurate indicator of the patient's condition.
9. Clean up the work area.
10. Wash your hands.

TERMINAL PERFORMANCE OBJECTIVE

Given the necessary supplies, prepare and test the quality control product within 40 minutes, obtaining results that are within the range given for the product, and accurately record the results in the Quality Control Log, as determined by your evaluator.

PREGNANCY TESTING

Medical assistants are often asked about the use of the home pregnancy tests now on the market. These tests are based on the same principles used in the kit methods most often used in laboratories. All the tests detect the presence of human chorionic gonadotropin (HCG) present in urine during pregnancy. The tests vary considerably in their sensitivity. Some of the home tests are able to detect HCG in urine as early as nine days after a missed period. Other tests are more sensitive, but they are not available for home testing. The major drawback to the home test kits is their lack of positive and negative controls, which are supplied with the kits used in the laboratories. However, the home tests do show good agreement with the laboratory methods now in use.

Several types of test kits are now marketed. There are rapid slide agglutination tests, which take only a few minutes to perform, but which generally are not as sensitive as the two-hour tube ring tests. Color-change tube, reagent strip, and flow-through methods offer an easy-to-interpret end point (Fig. 35–8).

Pregnancy tests should be performed on first morning urine specimens, since this is usually the most concentrated specimen of the day and is most likely to give positive results early in the pregnancy. In more advanced pregnancies, random specimens are usually adequate for testing. When done on a routine basis, pregnancy tests give qualitative results. *Qualitative results* give you a yes/no or positive/negative reading. *Quantitative results* require serial dilutions of a timed specimen, using either urine or blood serum.

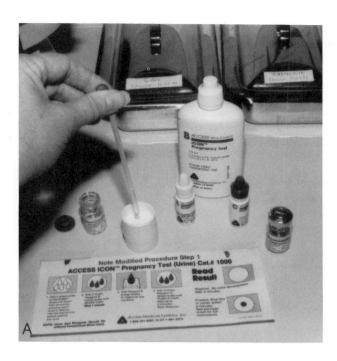

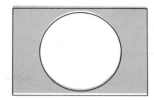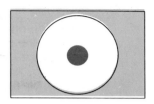

Negative.
No color development
after 2 minutes

Positive.
Blue dot in center
within 2 minutes

B

Figure 35–8
A, *Access Icon pregnancy test. The test is performed in individual disposable cups that have a reagent-impregnated filter paper that develops a blue dot if the test is positive.* **B,** *Access Icon negative and positive tests.*

Procedure 35–9

PERFORMING A SLIDE AGGLUTINATION TEST FOR PREGNANCY

PROCEDURAL GOAL

To perform a slide agglutination test for pregnancy.

EQUIPMENT AND SUPPLIES

Blood and body-fluid protection barriers (goggles, masks, and aprons or gowns), as necessary (see Appendix C, Recommendations for Prevention of AIDS Transmission)
Nonsterile gloves
Urine specimen
Pregnancy test kit
Clean test slide
Disposable mixing sticks
Reagents
Droppers

PROCEDURE

1. Wash and dry your hands. Follow the universal blood and body-fluid precautions (see Appendix C). Glove yourself with nonsterile gloves.
2. Allow reagents to warm to room temperature.
   Purpose: Cold reagents do not react as expected.
3. Clean the slide.
   Purpose: A dirty slide will interfere with testing and make interpretation of results difficult.
4. Hold the dropper vertically, and place one drop of antibody reagent in each of the three circles on the slide, without touching the dropper to the slide.
   Purpose: Drop size changes with the angle of the dropper and can alter the test results. Touching droppers to the slide could contaminate the reagents and alter test results.

Procedure continued on following page

35

5. Place one drop of positive control in the circle labeled + (plus).
6. Place one drop of negative control in the circle labeled − (minus).
   Purpose: The use of positive and negative controls ensures that the reagents are reacting properly and provides end point comparisons.
7. Place one drop of urine in the circle labeled with the patient's name.
8. Mix each well with a separate mixing stick.

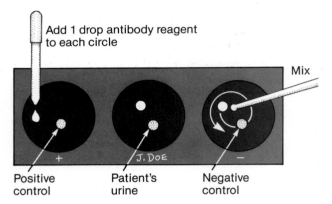

Add 1 drop antibody reagent to each circle

Mix

Positive control Patient's urine Negative control

9. Incubate for 30 seconds without rotation.
   Purpose: Incubation allows the reagents to combine with any HCG present.
10. Mix latex reagent well, including any in dropper.
    Purpose: The latex particles will either agglutinate or not agglutinate. Failure to thoroughly resuspend them before adding them to the slide leads to inaccurate testing.
11. Hold the dropper vertically (or as instructed in the insert), and add one drop of latex reagent to each circle. Do not touch the dropper to the slide.
12. Quickly mix each circle with a separate stick, taking no more than 30 seconds to accomplish mixing.

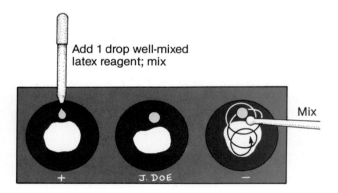

Add 1 drop well-mixed latex reagent; mix

Mix

13. Rotate the slide for two minutes, and observe immediately for agglutination.
    Purpose: Improper timing may allow reagents to dry and cause false results.
14. The controls should react as follows:
    Negative: Agglutination
    Positive: No agglutination

Agglutination of patient's test: Negative test

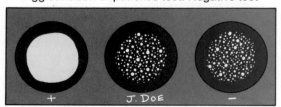

Procedure continued on opposite page

Note: This is an example of agglutination inhibition. In this case, if the test agglutinates, the result is actually negative. In many other test procedures, agglutination would be a positive end point.

15. Clean the work area.
16. Wash your hands.

TERMINAL PERFORMANCE OBJECTIVE

Given a urine specimen and the necessary supplies, perform a slide agglutination test for pregnancy, within five minutes, to a minimum performance level of 100 percent accuracy for positive/negative controls and known specimens, as determined by your evaluator.

CHAPTER OUTLINE

VOCABULARY

See Glossary at end of book for definitions.

anemia	centrifuge	morphology
buffy coat	leukemia	polycythemia vera

Hematology

36

OBJECTIVES

Upon successful completion of this chapter you should be able to

1. Define and spell the terms listed in the Vocabulary for this chapter.
2. List the components of blood and the function of each.
3. Differentiate between plasma and serum.
4. List the blood tests that are performed for a complete blood count and the normal values of each.
5. List body sites used for obtaining capillary and venous blood for testing.
6. Explain the function of a blood-diluting pipette.
7. Identify the parts of a hemacytometer.
8. Name two diluting fluids used for both red and white blood cell counts.
9. Discuss the normal cellular elements that may be observed in a blood smear.
10. State the normal values for the erythrocyte sedimentation rate.

Upon successful completion of this chapter you should be able to perform the following activities:

1. Demonstrate the correct procedure for obtaining a blood sample from a patient by performing a venipuncture.
2. Demonstrate the correct procedure for obtaining a blood sample from a patient by capillary puncture.
3. Perform a microhematocrit on a sample of whole blood.
4. Perform a manual white blood cell count, and calculate the results.
5. Perform a manual red blood cell count, and calculate the results.
6. Demonstrate the proper usage of the Unopette.
7. Prepare and stain a blood smear.
8. Perform a differential cell count on a properly stained blood smear.
9. Evaluate the morphology of red blood cells on a properly stained blood smear.
10. Estimate the number of platelets using a properly stained blood smear.
11. Determine an erythrocyte sedimentation rate.

Hematology is the study of blood. The modern hematology laboratory deals with the *counting* of red blood cells, white blood cells, and platelets; *differentiating* white blood cells on a stained smear; *measuring* the percentage of red blood cells in blood (hematocrit); and *determining* the oxygen-carrying capacity of the blood (hemoglobin).

The *complete blood count* (*CBC*) is the most frequent laboratory procedure ordered on blood. It gives a fairly complete look at the components of blood and can provide a wealth of information concerning a patient's condition. The CBC routinely includes the following:

- Red blood cell count
- White blood cell count
- Hemoglobin determination
- Hematocrit determination
- Differential white blood cell count
- Estimation of platelet numbers
- Red blood cell **morphology** (size and shape)

BLOOD COMPOSITION, FUNCTION, AND FORMATION

Whole blood is composed of formed elements suspended in a clear yellow liquid portion called *plasma*. Plasma makes up about 55 percent of the blood by volume. The remaining 45 percent consists of the formed elements, which are the *erythrocytes* (red blood cells), *leukocytes* (white blood cells), and *thrombocytes* (platelets). The average adult has approximately five to six quarts of blood.

Blood is the vital circulating fluid of the body and has at times been referred to as the "river of life." It is a transportation system bringing numerous substances of nourishment to all the cells of our body for growth, function, and repair and, in turn, carrying waste products away for disposal. In addition, blood functions to maintain the body at a uniform temperature, to keep the other body fluids in a state of equilibrium between alkalinity and acidity, and to carry hormones from the various glands to distant tissues where they are needed.

Plasma is the carrier for the formed elements and other substances such as proteins, carbohydrates, fats, hormones, enzymes, mineral salts, gases, and waste products. Plasma is composed of about 90 percent water, 9 percent protein, and 1 percent of various other chemical substances.

The cellular elements are produced and mature in the bone marrow, spleen, and lymph nodes. Then, they are released into the bloodstream. These cellular elements all have special functions.

The erythrocytes transport oxygen from the lungs to the body cells and carry carbon dioxide away from the cells, back to the lungs to be exhaled. They are disc-like cells that have two concave sides and no nucleus. Their main constituent is the red pigment hemoglobin, which is composed of iron and protein. Hemoglobin actually carries the oxy-

gen and carbon dioxide throughout the body. The life span of an erythrocyte is about 120 days. Then the cell is broken down, and the wastes are stored in the liver. The iron is reused for new red blood cell formation, and the protein is converted into a bile pigment.

The prime function of the leukocyte is to protect the body against infection and disease. The five types of leukocytes are classified into granular and agranular groups. The granular leukocytes are called *polymorphonuclear* leukocytes and include the neutrophils, eosinophils, and basophils. They are characterized by their heavily granulated cytoplasm and segmented nuclei. The *agranular* leukocytes are the lymphocytes and monocytes, which both have clear cytoplasm and a solid nucleus.

Thrombocytes play a vital role in initiating the clotting process of blood. When a small vessel is injured, thrombocytes adhere to each other and the edges of the injury, and form a plug that becomes a blood clot. This blood clot soon retracts and stops the loss of blood.

COLLECTION OF BLOOD SPECIMENS

For most hematology testing, an adequate blood sample can be obtained from capillaries by finger puncture. If a larger sample is required, blood can be obtained from a vein by venipuncture. To perform a CBC, venous blood is collected in a tube containing an *anticoagulant* that prevents clotting. Adding an anticoagulant results in a whole blood sample. When a blood specimen has had anticoagulant added, the liquid portion is called plasma. When a blood specimen is collected without an anticoagulant, it forms a clot and the liquid portion remaining is called *serum*.

Venipuncture

The most common method of obtaining blood for hematology testing is by venipuncture (*phlebotomy*). In a venipuncture, the blood is taken directly from a superficial vein. The vein is punctured with a needle, and the blood is collected in either a syringe or a tube. While a venipuncture is a safe procedure when performed by a trained professional, the procedure must be performed with care. You should routinely use appropriate barrier precautions when handling blood specimens (see Appendix C, Recommendations for Prevention of AIDS Transmission). The good condition of the veins must also be preserved. Much practice is required to become skilled and confident in the art of venipuncture.

Generally, veins in the forearm or the elbow are used for venipunctures (Fig. 36–1). The puncture site should be carefully selected after inspecting both arms. The vein most frequently used is the

720

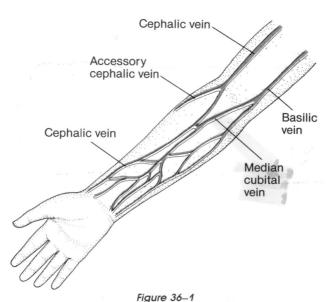

Figure 36–1

Veins of the arm commonly used for venipuncture.

median cephalic vein of the forearm. Alternative sites may be indicated if the area is cyanotic, scarred, bruised, edematous, or burned. You may use veins on the lower forearm, the back of the hand, or the wrist (Fig. 36–2). Use foot or ankle veins only if the patient has good circulation of the legs and you have received permission from your supervisor or the physician.

Performing a venipuncture involves several important steps with which the medical assistant must be thoroughly familiar before attempting the procedure. The first step is to select the proper method

for venipuncture (syringe or Vacutainer). Next, the patient must be prepared for the procedure. Patient preparation is followed by the actual venipuncture and specimen collection. The final step is care of the puncture site before discharging the patient.

Syringe Method. When veins are very small or fragile, the syringe method of venipuncture may be used. The equipment required includes a sterile syringe and hypodermic needle, tourniquet, 70 percent alcohol, sterile gauze, and a blood-collecting tube (Fig. 36–3). Most laboratories today use disposable needles and syringes. The needle and syringe must be assembled carefully to maintain sterility. The tips of both needle and syringe must not be touched, and the needle must not be uncapped until just prior to actual puncture. Needles of 20 to 22 gauge are used for venipunctures. The needle should be inspected to ascertain that it is sharp and smooth. The syringe plunger should be checked for free movement and should be left completely pushed into the barrel so that no air remains in the syringe.

Vacutainer Method. The Vacutainer System (Becton-Dickinson Company) is the most common collection system in use. It consists of evacuated tubes of various sizes with color-coded tops, indicating tube contents (Table 36–1); sterile disposable double-ended needles of different lengths and gauges; and a reusable plastic adapter that holds the needle and guides the tube (Fig. 36–4). Both pediatric- and adult-size adapters and tubes are available. The needle has two sharp ends. The short end is fitted into the adapter, and the longer end is used to puncture the vein. After the vein is entered, the

36

Figure 36–2

Veins on the back of the hand and wrist can be used for venipuncture if veins of the antecubital fossa cannot be used.

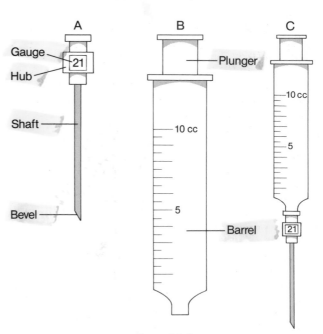

Figure 36–3

*Materials for venipuncture. **A**, Hypodermic; **B**, syringe; and **C**, syringe and needle assembled.*

Table 36–1
Vacutainer Tubes, Contents, and Their Uses

Stopper Color	Contents (Anticoagulant)	Uses*
Red	None	Serum for chemistry, serologic tests, typing, and crossmatching
Royal blue	Chemically clean	Trace metals (iron, lead); serum for chemistry
Black/red mottled (serum separation tube)†	Serum-separator gel	Serum for most chemistries, serologic tests
Black/yellow mottled (chlormerodrin accumulation test) (CAT)†	Clot activator, separator gel	STAT serum collections
Light blue†	Citrate	Coagulation studies, some hematology tests
Lavender†	EDTA	Hematology tests, some chemistries
Black†	Balanced oxalate	Coagulation
Green†	Heparin	Plasma for some chemistries, especially STATs
Gray†	Fluoride	STAT glucose tests, alcohol levels, drug screening

*Specimen requirements vary, depending on the method used in testing. Always check the laboratory specimen requirements manual before collecting a specimen.
†Denotes tubes that must be thoroughly mixed by gentle inversion after the blood is collected.

tube is pushed onto the needle in the adapter, and blood is drawn into the tube by vacuum. When the tube is full, it can be replaced by another tube.

Several tubes of blood can be collected using a variety of color-coded tubes with a single venipuncture. Tubes containing EDTA (ethylenediamine-tetra-acetic acid) anticoagulant additive are recommended for use when doing hematology studies. The white blood cells and platelets are best preserved in this type of tube, and better red blood cell morphology results will be obtained. This ad-

ditive has no adverse effects on the blood sample when a sufficient quantity of blood is obtained. However, problems arise when too little blood is placed in the tube containing the additive. Misleading results and an incorrect diagnosis may occur.

Patient Preparation. Proper patient preparation begins with identification of the patient and a brief explanation of the procedure to minimize anxiety. The patient should be lying down or seated in a chair. Never have the patient standing or sitting on a high stool. Available are special venipuncture chairs with adjustable arm rests and a locking safety mechanism that prevents the patient from falling should fainting occur. (Refer to Chapter 39 for the first aid procedure for fainting.)

All necessary supplies should be within easy reach. When using the Vacutainer method, you should have extra tubes available in case you encounter a bad vacuum. Tourniquets should be flat, broad, and elastic. *Velcro* tourniquets are easy to apply and adjust. They also come in several sizes. Blood pressure cuffs may be used. They can be easily inflated or deflated during the procedure, if necessary.

Alcohol from a dispenser or individual packets is used for most collections. For sterile or aseptic collections, individually packaged *povidone-iodine* swabs are used. Specimens for testing for blood alcohol levels are collected using *benzalkonium chloride* as the antiseptic. Alcohol may not be used for this collection, as it could interfere with the results of the test.

Needle disposal units should be available. Used needles should not be recapped, as this is the most probable cause of accidental needle sticks. Present guidelines for needle disposal recommend that the used needle be removed directly into the needle disposal unit, without cutting or recapping.

Keep your supplies clean and in order. The expiration dates of the evacuated tubes should be checked to be certain that outdated supplies are

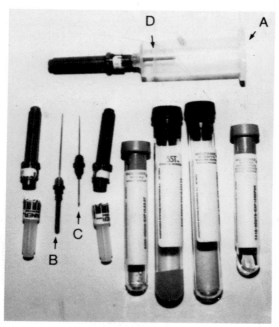

Figure 36–4
The Vacutainer System (Becton-Dickinson Co.) consists of a reusable plastic adapter (A), single-use needles of various lengths and gauges, and color-coded evacuated tubes. A multisample needle (B) is threaded into the adapter. If more than one tube of blood is required, a single-draw needle (C) is used. The first tube is inserted into the adapter and is advanced to the guide line (D) before the venipuncture is performed.

removed from use. Restock supplies as they are used.

Drawing the Blood. The patient's arm is fully extended and supported. A tourniquet is applied to the arm to make the veins more prominent by slowing blood flow. The puncture site is located by gently pressing on the veins with your fingertips. This will determine the direction of the vein and the approximate size and depth. The area around the puncture site is cleansed with alcohol and sterile gauze. The site is then dried also using sterile gauze.

The syringe or assembled Vacutainer system

how to assemble

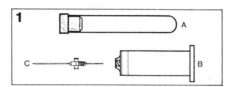

Description of parts:
A. Evacuated Glass Tube with Rubber Stopper
B. Plastic Holder with Guide Line
C. Double-Pointed Needle

A

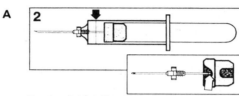

Thread needle into holder...tighten firmly!
Place tube in holder with needle touching stopper.

how to use

1

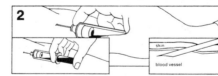

With rear point embedded in stopper, enter tissue—and immediately on tissue entry complete puncture of diaphragm.

B **2**

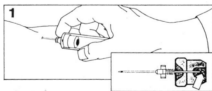

If in vein—blood flows immediately. Note: Technologist with small hands, proceed as you would with a hypodermic syringe. Holder provides finger grip and tube acts as plunger (see inset).

3

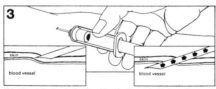

If in tissue instead of vein—blood will not be drawn. Proceed until venipuncture is signaled by intake of blood into VACUTAINER Tube, as shown.

3

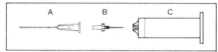

Push tube forward until top of stopper meets guide line. Let go.
Tube stopper will retract below guide line—leave it in that position.
At this stage, the full point of the needle is embedded in the stopper (see cross section) thus avoiding blood leakage upon venipuncture and preventing premature loss of vacuum.

Alternate Method
If needle and adapter are used, follow these instructions in place of steps 1 and 2.

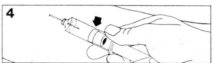

Description of parts:
A. Luer Hub Needle
B. VACUTAINER Adapter
C. Plastic Holder
Thread adapter into holder...tighten firmly!
Attach Luer Needle to Adapter slip as you would needle to a syringe. Place tube in holder with needle touching stopper, then proceed to step 3, above.

4

Where vein cannot be located—to conserve vacuum—remove tube from rear cannula (see arrow) before withdrawing needle from tissue.

5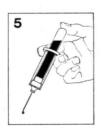

How to obtain blood drops for red and white cell counts, blood smears, etc. After tube is filled —grasp holder as illustrated and press firmly on bottom of tube. After each drop, release pressure and repeat for successive drops.

Additional Information
Incomplete Venipuncture, which may cause the tube to fill slowly or partially, may be corrected by deeper vein entry.
Transfixing of the vein may be corrected by pulling back slowly with needle until flow of blood indicates vein lumen re-entry.
Multiple Specimens (2, 3 or more) may be taken with one venipuncture and without loss of blood by releasing tourniquet while first tube is filling, and switching tubes while needle remains in vein.
Vein occlusion can be minimized by using VACUTAINER Adapter and smaller gauge needles (23, 24 or 25 gauge), thus slowing up flow of blood.
Proper degree of vacuum in each VACUTAINER Tube is doubly assured by the B-D Can Pack.

36

Figure 36–5
B-D Vacutainer method of making a venipuncture. **A,** *How to assemble B–D Vacutainer.* **B,** *How to use B-D Vacutainer. (Courtesy of Becton-Dickinson Co.)*

(Fig. 36–5) is held in one hand, at a 15 to 30 degree angle to the arm. The needle is bevel up and pointing in the same direction as the vein. The skin and vein are entered with one smooth motion until the needle is in the lumen of the vein. The blood is obtained by gently pulling back on the plunger with the other hand while holding the syringe and needle motionless. When using the Vacutainer method, place two fingers at the end of the holder and, with your thumb, push the tube into the adapter. Release the tourniquet as soon as blood begins to fill the tube or to flow into the syringe. When you have obtained the required amount of blood, place a dry sterile gauze pad over the puncture site and remove the needle from the vein.

Care of the Puncture Site. Apply pressure for a few minutes. You may have the patient elevate the arm at this time to prevent oozing of blood. If you have used the syringe method, the blood must be transferred to a tube at this time. Gently insert the needle through the rubber stopper of a vacuum tube. The vacuum inside will draw the required amount of blood into the tube. For tubes that contain additives, gently invert eight to ten times to mix.

Check the puncture site and apply a Band-Aid, if desired. Discard the needle into the designated container, and clean the work area. Complete the laboratory requisition, and forward the blood specimen to the appropriate place. Wash your hands.

Procedure 36–1

COLLECTING A VENOUS BLOOD SPECIMEN

PROCEDURAL GOAL

To collect a venous blood specimen.

EQUIPMENT AND SUPPLIES

Blood and body-fluid protection barriers (goggles, masks, and aprons or gowns), as necessary (see Appendix C, Recommendations for Prevention of AIDS Transmission)
Nonsterile gloves
Needle, syringe and tube or Vacutainer needle, adapter, and tube
70 percent alcohol
Sterile gauze pads
Tourniquet
Band-Aids

PROCEDURE

1. Wash and dry your hands. Follow the universal blood and body-fluid precautions (see Appendix C). Glove yourself with nonsterile gloves.
   Purpose: Prevents the spread of disease.
2. Check requisition for tests ordered and specimen requirements. Gather the materials needed (facing page, top).
   Purpose: Allows for proper specimen collection.
3. Identify the patient and explain the procedure.
   Purpose: Ascertains patient identity, and explanations help gain the patient's cooperation.
4. Instruct the patient to sit with the arm well supported in a downward position (facing page, center).
   Purpose: Veins of the antecubital fossa are more easily located when the elbow is straight.
5. Assemble equipment: Choice of syringe and needle sizes depends upon your inspection of the patient's veins. Attach the needle to the syringe or to the Vacutainer holder. Keep the cover on the needle.
6. Now, label tubes with the patient's name, the date, and time.
7. Apply the tourniquet around the patient's arm three to four inches above the elbow. The tourniquet should never be tied so tightly that it restricts blood flow in the artery (facing page, bottom left).
   Purpose: The tourniquet is used to make the veins more prominent.
8. Select the venipuncture site by palpating the antecubital space, and use your index finger to trace the path of the vein and to judge its depth. The vein most often used is the median cephalic, which lies in the middle of the elbow.
   Purpose: The index finger is most sensitive for palpating. Do not use the thumb, as it has a pulse of its own, which may confuse you (facing page, bottom right).

Procedure continued on opposite page

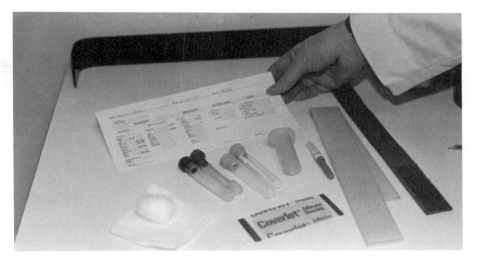

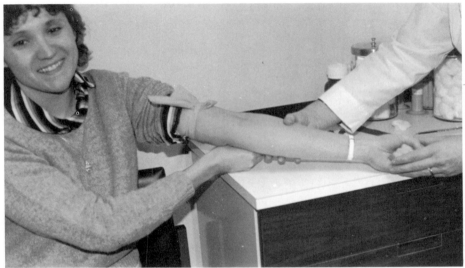

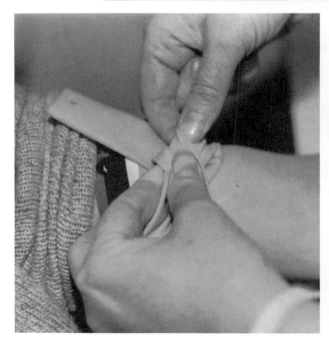

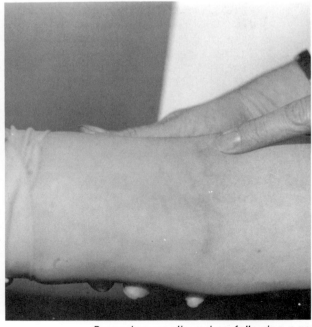

36

Procedure continued on following page

9. Ask the patient to open and close his or her hand several times.
   Purpose: Clenching the fist produces engorgement of the vein.
10. Release the tourniquet after locating the vein.
    Purpose: It should *not* be left in place for more than two minutes. It should be released while the site is cleansed. This prevents hemoconcentration, which can alter test results. ← reapply the tourniquet
11. Cleanse the site, starting in the center of the area and working outward in a circular pattern.
12. Dry the site with a sterile gauze (below, top).
    Purpose: The circular pattern helps avoid recontamination of the area. Puncturing a wet area stings and can cause hemolysis of the sample.
13. Reapply the tourniquet.
14. Remove the needle sheath.
15. Hold the syringe or Vacutainer assembly in your dominant hand. Your thumb should be on top and your fingers underneath.
16. Grasp the patient's arm with the nondominant hand while using your thumb and forefinger to draw the skin taut over the site, to anchor the vein (below, bottom).
    Purpose: Failure to anchor the vein makes puncturing more difficult and painful and may result in a missed vein.

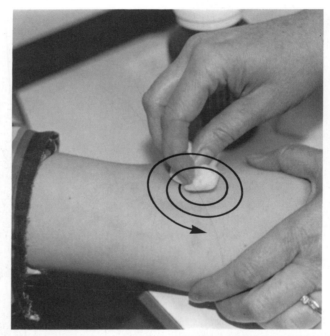

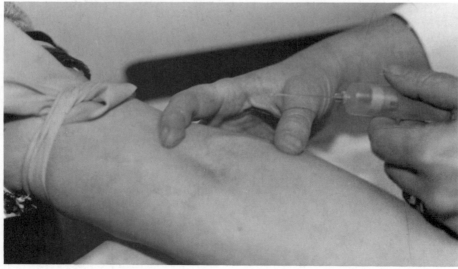

Procedure continued on opposite page

17. Insert the needle through the skin and into the vein with the bevel of the needle up, aligned parallel to the vein, at a 15-degree angle, rapidly, and smoothly (below, top left).
    Purpose: The sharpest point of the needle is inserted first.
18. Slowly pull back the plunger of the syringe with the nondominant hand *or* place two fingers on the flanges of the Vacutainer holder and, with the thumb, push the tube onto the needle inside the holder. Make sure that you do not move the needle after entering the vein. Allow the syringe or tube to fill to optimum capacity.
19. Remove the Vacutainer tube from the adapter prior to removing the needle from the vein.
    Purpose: A nontraumatic venipuncture produces the most reliable results. Proper tube filling ensures the correct ratio of blood to additive. Removal of the tube from the holder prior to removal from the vein prevents any excess blood from dripping from the tip of the needle onto the patient (below, top right, bottom left and right).

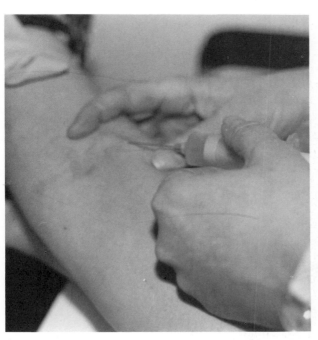

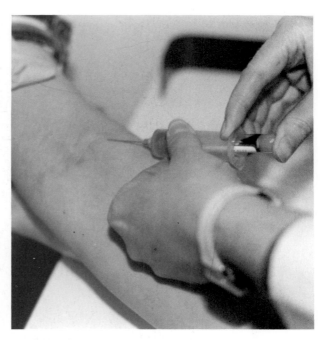

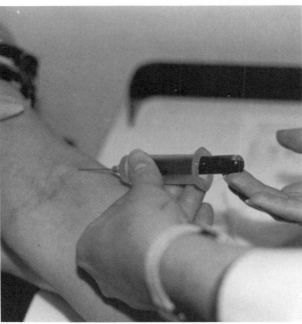

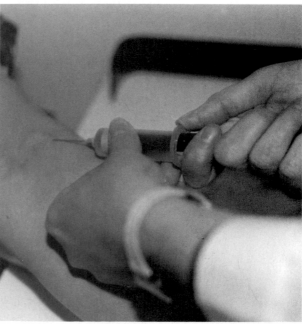

Procedure continued on following page

20. Release the tourniquet as soon as blood starts to flow. It must be released before the needle is removed from the arm.
    Purpose: Removal of the tourniquet releases pressure on the vein and helps prevent blood from getting into adjacent tissues and causing a hematoma.
21. Place a sterile gauze pad over the puncture site and withdraw the needle.
22. Apply direct pressure over the site. The patient may elevate the arm (below, top left and right).
    Purpose: Direct pressure is the best method to stop bleeding. Elevating the arm above the heart also stops bleeding.
23. Transfer the blood to a tube if using a syringe. Gently invert tubes to mix anticoagulants and blood. If tubes were not labeled prior to venipuncture, do so now (below, bottom center).
    Purpose: Prevents clotting of blood. Vigorous mixing may cause hemolysis.
24. Check the puncture site for bleeding.

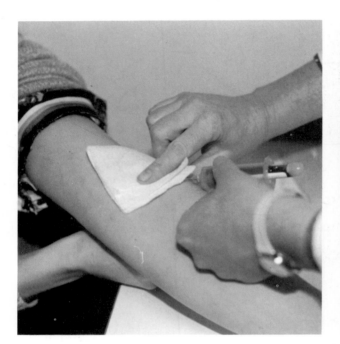

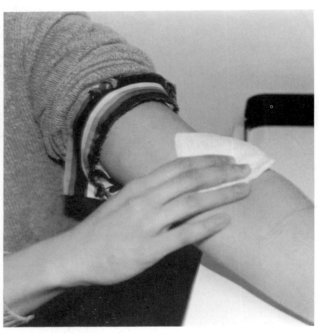

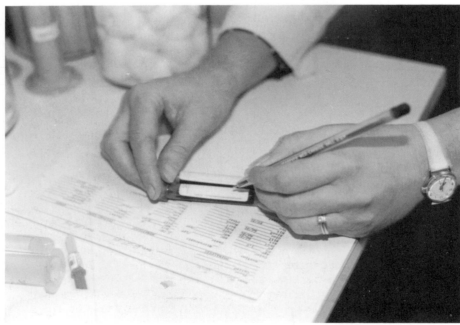

Procedure continued on opposite page

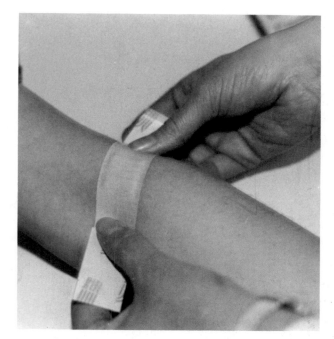

25. Apply a Band-Aid (above).
26. Dispose of the needle safely. Allow it to drop directly into the disposal unit without touching it with your fingers. Do not recap used needles.
    Purpose: Most accidental needle sticks occur when a needle is being recapped. Report any accidents to your supervisor or the physician.
27. Clean the work area. Follow the recommendations for proper disposal of all materials (see Appendix C).
28. Complete the laboratory requisition and route to the proper place.
29. Wash your hands.

TERMINAL PERFORMANCE OBJECTIVE

Given a patient and appropriate supplies, collect a blood specimen by venipuncture using either syringe or Vacutainer method within five minutes and correctly complete each step of the procedure in the proper order, as determined by your evaluator.

Capillary Puncture

Capillaries are small blood vessels connecting the small arterioles to the small venules. The capillary puncture is an efficient means of collecting a blood specimen when only a small amount of blood is required or when a patient's condition makes venipuncture difficult.

Patient Preparation. In adults and children, the usual puncture site is the ring finger, but capillary blood can be obtained from the great finger, the earlobe, toe, or heel (Fig. 36–6). The puncture is made at the tip and slightly to the side of the finger.

The puncture site must be prepared. Gentle massaging or placing the finger in warm water will increase circulation of blood and allow for a good flow of blood. The site is cleansed with 70 percent alcohol and wiped with a dry sterile gauze pad.

Obtaining the Blood. The patient's hand is held in a lateral position, with the skin near the puncture site pulled taut. A sharp-pointed blade called a *lancet* is used. Capillary punctures may also be performed using semiautomated devices such as the *Autolet.* The puncture is performed in one quick, smooth motion. The lancet should puncture the site to a depth of 3 to 4 mm. The first drop of blood is wiped away because it contains tissue liquid and would dilute any results. The second and following

36

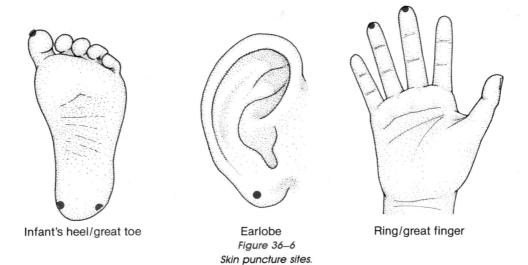

Infant's heel/great toe   Earlobe   Ring/great finger

Figure 36–6
Skin puncture sites.

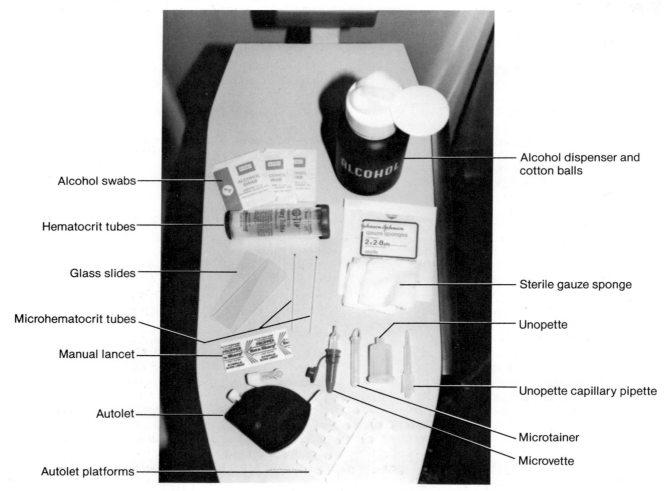

Figure 36–7

Capillary collection devices, clockwise from top: alcohol dispenser with cotton balls, sterile gauze sponges, (left to right) Microvette, Microtainer, Unopette with pipette, Autolet platforms, Autolet, manual lancet, glass slides, microhematocrit tubes, and individually packaged alcohol swabs.

drops are used. The finger is massaged to increase blood flow. Squeezing the finger should be avoided, since this will force tissue fluid to dilute the blood. Samples must be collected quickly to avoid clotting. For this reason, it is important to assemble all equipment needed before performing the capillary puncture (Fig. 36–7).

Pipetting the Blood. Blood must be diluted before blood cells can be counted microscopically because the cellular elements or blood are so concentrated. Blood-diluting pipettes are used to dilute the blood with a diluting fluid, to manually perform leukocyte, erythrocyte, and thrombocyte counts. Blood is collected in glass blood-diluting pipettes, self-filling disposable pipettes, capillary tubes, or on glass slides. Reusable *Thoma*-style pipettes are frequently used for these counts.

Self-filling and self-measuring disposable micropipette systems are also available for counting leukocytes, erythrocytes, and platelets. The *Unopette* system consists of a disposable self-filling diluting pipette and a plastic reservoir prefilled with a precise amount of diluting fluid.

Capillary tubes are available with and without the anticoagulant *heparin*. Tubes with a red ring around one end contain heparin, while those with a blue ring are nonheparinized. The microhematocrit specimen can be collected directly from the finger using the heparinized tubes.

The best specimen for a blood smear is capillary blood smeared directly onto a glass slide. The smear is stained, and the morphology of the cellular components can then be studied.

Procedure 36–2 — COLLECTING A CAPILLARY BLOOD SPECIMEN

PROCEDURAL GOAL

To collect a capillary blood specimen suitable for testing, using fingertip puncture technique.

EQUIPMENT AND SUPPLIES

Blood and body-fluid protection barriers (goggles, masks, and aprons or gowns), as necessary (see Appendix C, Recommendations for Prevention of AIDS Transmission)
Nonsterile gloves
Sterile disposable lancet
70 percent alcohol
Sterile gauze pads
Band-Aids
Supplies for requested test (e.g. pipettes, Unopettes, slides, capillary tubes)

PROCEDURE

1. Wash and dry your hands. Follow the universal blood and body-fluid precautions (see Appendix C). Glove yourself with nonsterile gloves.
2. Greet and identify the patient.
   Purpose: Identification of the patient prior to the collection of the specimen is extremely important.
3. Explain the procedure.
   Purpose: Explanations help gain the patient's cooperation.
4. Assemble the needed materials, based upon the physician's requisition.
   Purpose: Once the skin has been punctured, the collection must proceed as rapidly as possible so the blood does not clot before the entire specimen has been collected.
5. Select a puncture site (side of middle finger of nondominant hand, outer edge of earlobe; medial or lateral curved surface of the heel or the great toe for an infant).
   Purpose: The nondominant hand may have fewer calluses. The side of the finger is less sensitive, and the skin is usually not as thick.
6. "Milk," or very gently rub, the finger along the sides.
   Purpose: This promotes circulation. If the finger is very cold, you may immerse it in warm water or moisten it with warm towels.
7. Clean the site with alcohol, and dry it with sterile gauze.
   Purpose: Puncturing wet skin is painful and can hemolyze the specimen.

Procedure continued on following page

36

8. Grasp the patient's finger on the sides near the puncture site, with your nondominant forefinger and thumb (below, left).
   Purpose: Firmly holding the site allows control of the puncture.
9. Hold the lancet at a right angle to the patient's finger, and make a rapid, deep puncture on the patient's fingertip (below, right).
   Purpose: Lancets are designed to puncture at a depth of 3 to 4 mm which is sufficient to obtain the required drops of blood.
10. Wipe away the first drop of blood.
    Purpose: The first drop of blood contains tissue fluid.
11. Apply gentle pressure to cause the blood to flow freely.
    Purpose: Squeezing liberates tissue that dilutes the blood and causes inaccurate results.
12. Collect blood samples:
    a. Express a large, rounded drop of blood, and fill capillary tubes (bottom, center) (see Procedure 36–3) or pipettes (see Procedure 36–4).

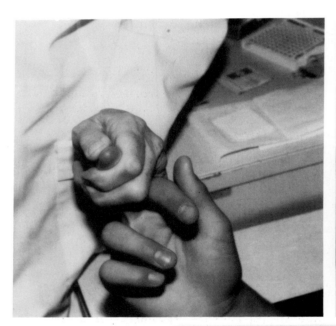
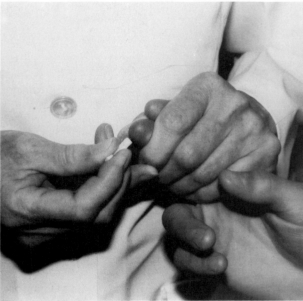

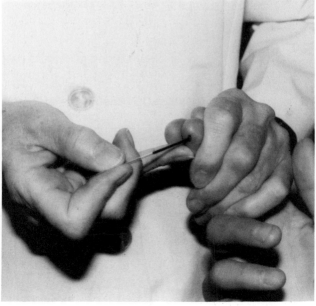

Procedure continued on opposite page

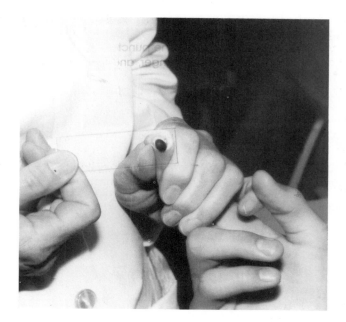

b. Wipe the finger with a clean sterile gauze pad, and place a fresh drop of blood on a slide for a smear (above). Immediately make the smear, using the two-slide method (see Procedure 36–8).

13. Apply pressure to the site with clean sterile gauze.
14. Label all samples and requisitions correctly, and forward to laboratory for testing.
15. Check the patient for bleeding, and apply a Band-Aid if indicated.
16. Dismiss the patient.
17. Dispose of used materials in proper containers.
18. Clean the work area. Follow the recommendations for proper disposal of all materials (see Appendix C).
19. Wash your hands.

TERMINAL PERFORMANCE OBJECTIVE

Given a patient and appropriate supplies, collect a capillary blood specimen suitable for testing, using fingertip puncture technique within three minutes, and correctly complete each step of the procedure in the proper order, as determined by your evaluator.

MICROHEMATOCRIT

The microhematocrit (Hct) is a measurement of the percentage of packed red blood cells in a volume of blood. The test is based on the principle of separating the cellular elements from the plasma. The separation process is speeded up by centrifugation. Two or three drops of blood are collected in two capillary tubes and are placed in a specially designed microhematocrit *centrifuge.*

After centrifugation, the red blood cells will be at the bottom of the tube, the white blood cells and platelets in the center, and the plasma on top. From this separation, the microhematocrit is determined by comparing the concentration of red blood cells with the total volume of the whole blood sample.

The percentage is read by placing the tubes on a special microhematocrit reader. Some microhema-tocrit centrifuges have a built-in reading scale that reads calibrated capillary tubes. Microhematocrits should be performed in duplicate, and the average of the two results reported.

The microhematocrit is a commonly performed test requested by physicians separately or as part of the complete blood count. Since it is a simple procedure requiring only a small amount of blood, it is an ideal test for following the progress of patients.

The normal values vary with the sex and age of the patient (Table 36–2). The values range from a low of 36 percent in women to a high of 52 percent in men. Low microhematocrit readings can indicate **anemia** or the presence of bleeding in a patient, whereas high readings may be caused by dehydration or a condition such as **polycythemia vera.** Values can be influenced by physiologic or pathologic factors as well as collection techniques.

36

Procedure 36–3

PROCEDURAL GOAL

To perform a microhematocrit in duplicate.

EQUIPMENT AND SUPPLIES

Blood and body-fluid protection barriers (goggles, masks, and aprons or gowns), as necessary (see Appendix C, Recommendations for Prevention of AIDS Transmission)
Nonsterile gloves
EDTA anticoagulant blood
Capillary tubes
Sealing clay
Centrifuge
Microhematocrit reader

PROCEDURE

1. Wash and dry your hands. Follow the universal blood and body-fluid precautions (see Appendix C). Glove yourself with nonsterile gloves.
2. Assemble the materials needed.
3. Fill two plain (blue-tip) capillary tubes three-quarters full with well-mixed EDTA anticoagulant blood.
   Purpose: Duplicates should always be done as a means of quality control.
4. Plug the dry end of each tube with a sealing clay.
   Purpose: Sealing the wet end may result in loss of the plug and the sample during centrifugation.
5. Place the tubes opposite each other in the centrifuge, with sealed ends securely against the gasket.
   Purpose: The centrifuge must always be balanced to avoid damage. If the clay ends of the capillary tubes are not outermost against the gasket, the sample will spin out of the tubes. Follow the universal blood and body-fluid precautions (see Appendix C).

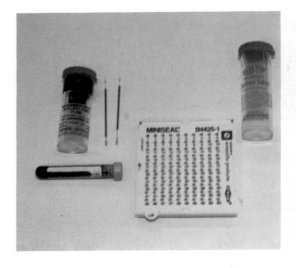 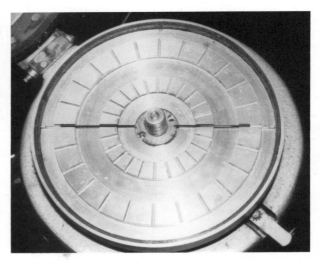

6. Note the numbers on the centrifuge slots and record them.
   Purpose: The sample must be identified throughout the entire procedure.

Procedure continued on opposite page

7. Secure the locking top, fasten the lid down, and lock.
   Purpose: If the locking top is not firmly in place during the spinning cycle, the tubes will come out of their slots and break. The lid is always locked during centrifugation for safety purposes, to avoid aerosols or broken glass from being ejected.
8. Set the timer, and adjust the speed as needed.
   Purpose: The prescribed time is between three and five minutes. Check the manufacturer's instructions for time and speed.
9. Allow the centrifuge to come to a complete stop, and unlock the lids.
10. Remove the tubes immediately.
    Purpose: Tubes left in the centrifuge will show altered results, as the red blood cell layer spreads horizontally.
11. Determine the microhematocrit values, using one of the following methods:
    a. Centrifuge with built-in reader utilizing calibrated capillary tubes.
       (1) Position the tubes as directed by manufacturer's instructions.
       (2) Read both tubes.
       (3) The average of the two results is reported.
       (4) The two values should not vary by more than ± 2 percent.
    b. Centrifuge without built-in reader.
       (1) Carefully remove the tubes from the centrifuge.
       (2) Place a tube on the microhematocrit reader.
       (3) Align the clay–red blood cell junction with the zero line on the reader. Align the plasma meniscus with the 100 percent line. The value is read at the junction of the red cell layer and the **buffy coat**.

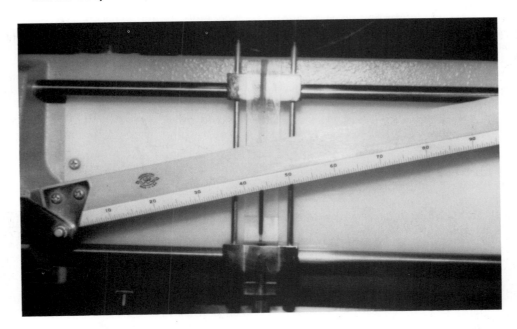

       (4) Read both tubes.
       (5) The average of the two results is reported.
       (6) The two values should not vary by more than ± 2 percent.
12. Dispose of the capillary tubes in a biohazard container.
13. Clean the work area. Follow the recommendations for proper disposal of all materials (see Appendix C).
14. Wash your hands.

TERMINAL PERFORMANCE OBJECTIVE

Given a blood specimen and appropriate supplies, perform a microhematocrit in duplicate within ten minutes, to a minimum performance level of ± 1 percent of your evaluator's results.

36

Table 36–2
Normal Hematology Values

Test	Men	Women
Microhematocrit	42–52%	36–48%
Hemoglobin	13.5–17.5 g/dl	12.5–15.5 g/dl
WBC	4500–11,000 cells/cu mm	4500–11,000 cells/cu mm
RBC	4.5–6.0 million cells/cu mm	4.0–5.5 million cells/cu mm
Platelets	150,000–400,000 cells/cu mm for both	

Differential for Both Men and Women	
Bands	0–7%
Segmented neutrophils	50–65%
Lymphocytes	25–40%
Monocytes	3–9%
Eosinophils	1–3%
Basophils	0–1%

HEMOGLOBIN

The hemoglobin (Hgb) determination is a rough measure of the oxygen-carrying capacity of the blood. Determining hemoglobin concentration can be performed as part of the complete blood count or as an individual test. Many methods of determining hemoglobin concentration have been used throughout the years. Today, the most widely used hemoglobin method is the *cyanmethemoglobin*. A sample of whole blood is diluted in *Drabkin reagent*, which breaks down (lyses) red cells, releasing the hemoglobin into the solution. The chemicals in the reagent react with the released hemoglobin to form the pigment cyanmethemoglobin, which can be measured by using a photometer.

The normal hemoglobin values vary throughout life. Values are normally quite high at birth, decline during childhood, then increase through the teens until the adult levels are reached (Table 36–2). Values range from a low of 12.5 g/dl in women to a high of 17.5 g/dl in men. The various factors that affect the hemoglobin level include age, sex, diet, altitude, and disease.

RED BLOOD CELL COUNT

The red blood cell count is a commonly performed procedure and is part of the complete blood count. The red blood cell count approximates the number of circulating red cells. The function of red blood cells is to transport oxygen to the tissues. The condition in which this oxygen-carrying capacity of the blood is below normal is called anemia. The red blood cell count is usually decreased in anemias.

Increases are found in people with dehydration, polycythemia vera, or severe burns and in people who live at high altitudes, as an adaptation to the lower oxygen content of the air.

The normal values for red blood cell counts range from approximately 4 million cells per cu mm of blood to 6 million cells per cu mm. Red blood cell counts are usually higher in males than females.

WHITE BLOOD CELL COUNT

The white blood cell count is one of the most frequently requested hematology tests. The white blood cell count gives an approximation of the total number of leukocytes in circulating blood. The count is performed to aid the physician in determining if an infection is present. It may also be used to follow the course of a disease and to determine if the patient is responding to treatment.

The normal white blood cell count varies with age, being higher in newborns and decreasing throughout life. The average adult range is between 4500 and 12,000 cells per cu mm. Many factors affect the white blood cell count. Elevation in white blood cells is called *leukocytosis*. Physiologic increases in the white blood cell count are seen in pregnancy, stress, anesthesia, exercise, and exposure to temperature extremes and after treatment with steroids. Pathologic causes of leukocytosis include many bacterial infections, **leukemia**, appendicitis, and pneumonia. A decrease in the white blood cell count is called *leukopenia*. This condition may be caused by viral infections or by exposure to radiation, certain chemicals, and drugs.

METHODS OF COUNTING RED AND WHITE BLOOD CELLS

Manual Counts

Both the red blood cell count and the white blood cell count approximate the number of these circulating cells in the blood. These cellular elements are very concentrated in the blood. Therefore, the blood must be diluted for these cells to be counted microscopically. Blood-diluting pipettes and diluting fluids are used for this purpose. The counts are then performed using the diluted blood, a counting chamber called a *hemacytometer*, a hemacytometer coverslip, and a microscope.

Blood Cell Diluting Pipettes. Blood-diluting pipettes have three basic parts (Fig. 36–8):

- Calibrated stem: Where blood and diluting fluid are aspirated

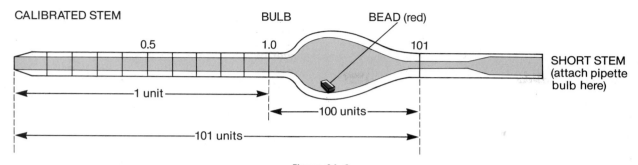

Figure 36–8
Parts of a red cell–diluting pipette.

- Bulb: Where contents are mixed
- Short stem: Where rubber tubing and mouthpiece are attached

The *red-cell diluting pipette* is used to dilute blood for erythrocyte counts. The 0.5 mark on the calibrated stem is the mark to which blood is drawn and the 101 mark on the short stem is the mark to which diluting fluid is drawn. This results in a 1:200 dilution in the bulb (Fig. 36–9). Several commonly used diluting fluids for red cell counts are *normal saline, Hayem,* and *Gower.* Both blood and diluting fluid are aspirated into the pipette by using a pipette bulb (available through Baxter Division, Scientific Products, 1430 Waukegan Road, McGaw Park, IL, 60085-6787) that attaches to the short stem of the pipette.

The *white-cell diluting pipette* is used to dilute blood for leukocyte counts. The pipette is similar to the red-cell pipette, except that it holds less volume and makes a smaller dilution. Blood is drawn to the 0.5 mark and diluting fluid to the 11 mark, resulting in a 1:20 dilution (Fig. 36–9). The diluting fluids used destroy the erythrocytes while preserving the leukocytes. Two common diluting fluids are *0.1 N-hydrochloric acid* and 2 *percent acetic acid.*

Unopettes. Parts of a disposable blood-diluting unit such as Unopette (Becton-Dickinson) consist of a prefilled reservoir containing a premeasured diluting fluid, capillary pipette, and pipette shield (Fig. 36–10). Unopettes are available for counting

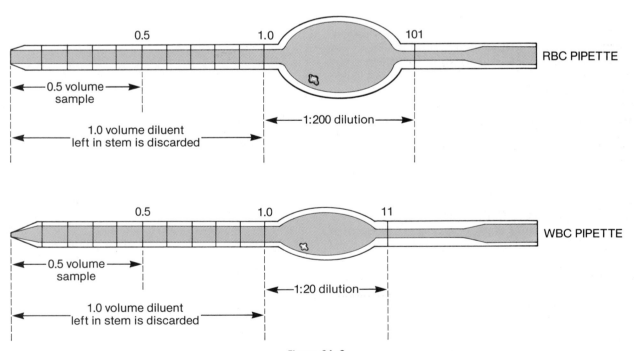

Figure 36–9
Thoma RBC and WBC pipettes. The three major markings on each pipette are shown. The dilution in each pipette is indicated.

36

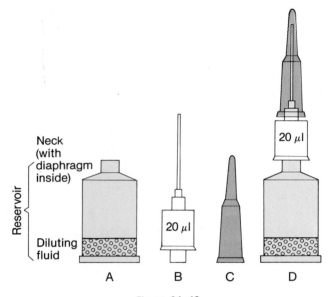

Figure 36-10
*Parts of a disposable blood-diluting unit such as Unopette. **A**, Prefilled reservoir containing premeasured diluting fluid and sealed with diaphragm; **B**, capillary pipette with overflow chamber and capacity marking; **C**, pipette shield; and **D**, assembled unit.*

erythrocytes, leukocytes, and platelets. Package inserts contain detailed instructions that, when correctly followed, result in a more accurate dilution than with the blood-diluting pipettes.

Hemacytometer. The hemacytometer is used to count the cellular elements of the blood. The hemacytometer is a heavy glass slide that, when viewed from the top, has two raised platforms surrounded by depressions on three sides. Each raised surface contains a ruled counting area that is marked off by lines etched into the glass. The depressions surrounding these platforms are called "moats." The raised areas and depressions form an "H." A special hemacytometer coverslip of uniform thickness is used. The coverslip is positioned on the hemacytometer so that it covers the ruled areas, confines the fluid in the chamber, and regulates the depth of the fluid. The depth of the fluid in the most commonly used *Neubauer-type* hemacytometer is 0.1 mm with the coverslip in place (Fig. 36–11).

Each ruled area of the counting chamber consists of a large square, 3 mm × 3 mm. This area, in turn, is divided into nine equal squares, each of which is 1 sq mm. The white blood cell counting area consists of the four large corner squares labeled "W" (Fig. 36–12).

The center squares are used to count the red blood cells. Each center square is subdivided into 25 smaller squares. Only the four corner and center

squares within the large center square are used to count red blood cells (Fig. 36–12).

After the coverslip has been positioned, the hemacytometer is filled, or *charged*. This is accomplished by touching the tip of the diluting pipette or Unopette to the point where the coverslip and the raised platform meet (Fig. 36–13). The fluid will flow by capillary action into one side of the hemacytometer. The opposite side is also filled.

Counting. The hemacytometer is placed on the microscope. White blood cell counts are observed under ×10 objective, and red blood cells are counted under ×40 objective. A counting pattern of left to right and right to left is used to ensure that cells are counted only once. Counts should begin in the upper left corner square. All cells within the squares are counted. Only cells touching top and left boundary lines are counted (Fig. 36–14).

Calculations. Calculations for a red blood cell count are determined by counting both sides of the hemacytometer and obtaining an average. This number is then multiplied by 10,000. For white blood cell counts, the average of the two sides is multiplied by 50.

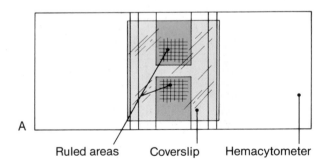

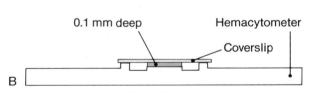

Figure 36-11
*Top (**A**) and side (**B**) views of a hemacytometer. Sample should fill the shaded areas when the chamber is properly filled.*

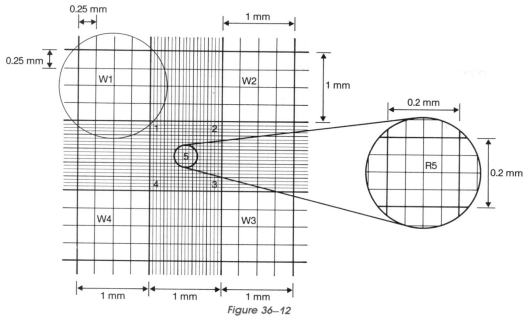

Figure 36–12

Neubauer ruling. The areas labeled "W" are used in counting white cells. Red cells are counted in the five areas in the center square. A blowup of the fifth red cell–counting area is shown as it would appear under the microscope's high-power magnification. Measurements of the ruled areas are shown.

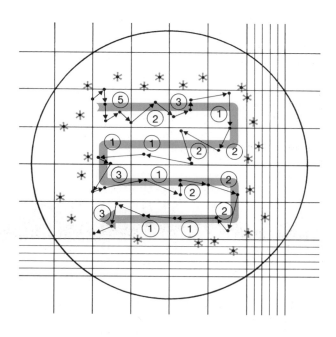

The eye following the field
✳ Not counted into total
◯ Number counted into each square

Figure 36–14

Counting. (1) Begin counting cells in the upper left-hand corner. (2) Proceed across the top row, counting cells, including those that touch the top and left sides of each square. (3) Continue to count the remainder of cells in the same fashion. (4) Count in the direction of the arrows. The number of cells in each square is indicated by a circle.

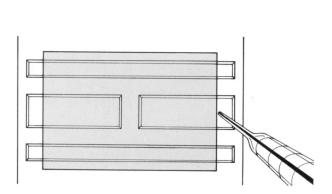

Figure 36–13
Charging the hemacytometer.

36

Procedure 36–4

PROCEDURAL GOAL

To properly fill and dilute Thoma pipettes for use in manual cell counting.

EQUIPMENT AND SUPPLIES

Blood and body-fluid protection barriers (goggles, masks, and aprons or gowns), as necessary (see Appendix C, Recommendations for Prevention of AIDS Transmission)
Nonsterile gloves
Thoma pipettes (red and white blood cell diluting pipettes)
EDTA anticoagulant blood
Diluting fluids
  white-cell diluting fluid—2 percent acetic acid or 0.1 *N*-hydrochloric acid
  red-cell diluting fluid—Hayem normal saline solution
Gauze pads
Pipette bulb
Pipette shaker
Test tube rack

PROCEDURE

1. Wash and dry your hands. Follow the universal blood and body-fluid precautions (see Appendix C). Glove yourself with nonsterile gloves.
2. Assemble the materials needed.
3. Mix the blood well (below, top).
   Purpose: Cells settle when the specimen stands.
4. Attach the pipette bulb to the short stem of the pipette.
5. Hold the pipette between the thumb and the index finger, nearly horizontal with the dominant hand.
6. Hold the well-mixed tube of blood in the nondominant hand, and tilt the tube slightly (below, bottom).

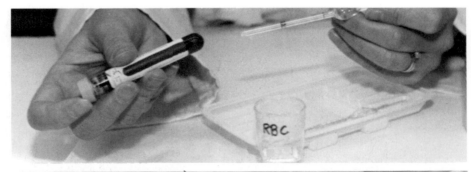

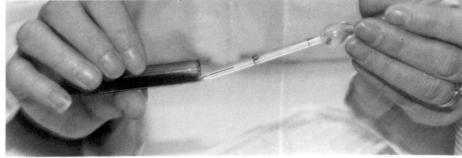

Procedure continued on opposite page

7. Place the tip of the pipette beneath the surface of the blood, and fill to the 0.5 mark, using the pipette bulb. Do not allow any air bubbles, and stop at the mark exactly.
   Purpose: Any error in pipetting will result in an error in the count. Bubbles will cause a falsely lowered count. Drawing blood past the mark will cause a falsely higher count.
8. Wipe the outside of the pipette with a dry gauze pad, and carefully remove any traces of blood. Avoid touching the tip of the pipette to the gauze pad.
   Purpose: Any blood on the outside of the pipette will contaminate the diluting fluid. Touching the pipette tip to the gauze will decrease the volume of blood in the pipette.
9. Tilt the diluting fluid container, and quickly immerse the tip of the pipette beneath the surface of the fluid. Avoid loss of any blood into the diluting fluid.
10. Hold the pipette nearly vertical, and slowly rotate the pipette while filling it with the fluid to the 11 mark on the WBC pipette or the 101 mark on RBC pipette.
    Purpose: Loss of blood into the diluting fluid will lower the count and contaminate the fluid. Mixing while filling causes the bead in the bulb to drop into the fluid and prevents it from trapping any bubbles that would invalidate the test. Holding the pipette in a vertical position while filling prevents entry of air bubbles.

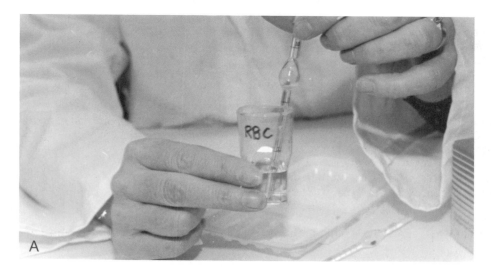

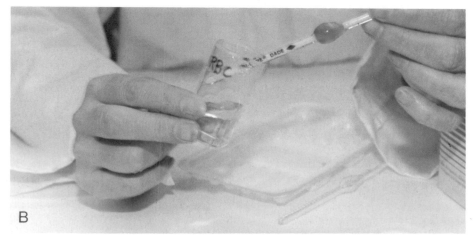

Procedure continued on following page

36

11. Place the tip of the finger over the end of the pipette, and carefully remove the pipette bulb.
    Purpose: Placing the finger over the tip of the pipette prevents the fluid level from moving in the pipette and altering the dilution.

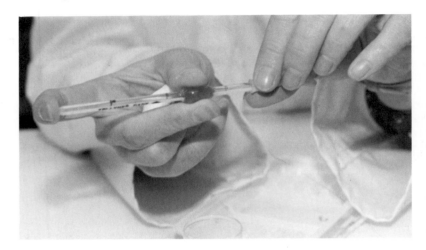

12. Rotate the pipette thoroughly to mix the sample with the finger over the tip.
13. Place the pipette into a tray that has been labeled.
    Purpose: Samples must always be identifiable throughout the entire testing procedure.

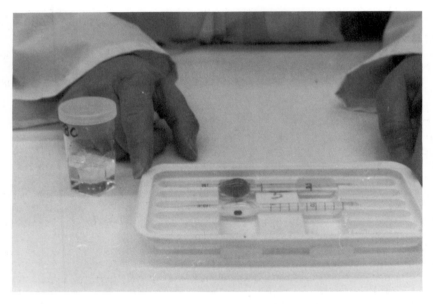

14. Place the pipette on a shaker, and allow it to gently rotate for at least two minutes.
    Purpose: Mixing is necessary to ensure even distribution of cells. Violent bouncing of the pipette will cause the sample to spray out, and insufficient vibration will not adequately mix the sample.
15. Clean the work area. Follow the recommendations for proper disposal of all materials (see Appendix C).
16. Wash your hands.

TERMINAL PERFORMANCE OBJECTIVE

Given a blood specimen and the appropriate supplies, dilute a red and a white blood cell pipette within two minutes and correctly complete each step of the procedure in the proper order, as determined by your evaluator.

Procedure 36-5

PROCEDURAL GOAL

To properly fill a Unopette pipette with blood and to transfer the sample to a Unopette reservoir.

EQUIPMENT AND SUPPLIES

Blood and body-fluid protection barriers (goggles, masks, and aprons or gowns), as necessary (see Appendix C, Recommendations for Prevention of AIDS Transmission)
Nonsterile gloves
Unopette unit
    capillary pipette
    pipette shield
    reservoir
EDTA anticoagulant blood
Gauze pads
Test tube rack

PROCEDURE

1. Wash and dry your hands. Follow the universal blood and body-fluid precautions (see Appendix C). Glove yourself with nonsterile gloves.
2. Remove a Unopette reservoir from the storage container, and recap the container tightly.
   Purpose: The container is humidified. Loss of the humid conditions will allow evaporation, and the remaining Unopettes will give inaccurate results.
3. Use the pipette shield to puncture the diaphragm of the Unopette reservoir. The hole must be large enough to allow the pipette to enter freely.
   Purpose: If the hole is too small, loss of a portion of the sample can occur when the pipette is inserted into the reservoir.
4. Remove the pipette shield.
5. Hold the pipette nearly horizontal.
6. Place the tip of the pipette into a well-mixed tube of blood, and allow the pipette to fill by capillary action until blood reaches the end of the pipette. It will stop by itself.
7. Place a finger over the hole in the end of the pipette to prevent loss of any sample, and carefully wipe the outside of the pipette with gauze to remove all traces of blood.
   Purpose: Blood on the outside of the pipette will enter the reservoir and give inaccurate results.
8. Squeeze the reservoir gently with one hand.
9. While holding your index finger over the hole in the top of the pipette, insert the pipette into the reservoir and seat it firmly in place with a twisting motion.
   Purpose: Squeezing the reservoir before inserting the pipette is necessary. It creates a vacuum, which will draw the sample into the reservoir.
10. Release the pressure on the reservoir, and remove your finger from the top of the pipette. The sample will be drawn into the reservoir.
11. Gently squeeze and release the reservoir several times to rinse all blood from the pipette into the reservoir. Liquid should rise to overflow chamber but should not be forced out of the top of the pipette.
    Purpose: The capillary pipette is calibrated to contain an amount of blood. It must be rinsed several times with the diluting fluid to ensure that all of the sample has been delivered into the reservoir.
12. Mix the contents of the Unopette gently by inversion or by rolling between the palms of your hands.
13. Identify the Unopette.
    Purpose: The sample must be identifiable at all times during the testing procedure.
14. Allow the Unopette to sit for the specified amount of time, as stated in the directions.
15. Place the shield on the top of the prepared Unopette to prevent evaporation.
16. Clean the work area. Follow the recommendations for proper disposal of all materials (see Appendix C).
17. Wash your hands.

36

Procedure continued on following page

TERMINAL PERFORMANCE OBJECTIVE

Given a blood specimen and appropriate supplies, fill a Unopette capillary pipette and transfer to a Unopette reservoir within one minute, correctly completing each step of the procedure in the proper order, as determined by your evaluator.

Procedure 36–6

CHARGING (FILLING) A HEMACYTOMETER

PROCEDURAL GOAL

To fill the hemacytometer for a manual cell count.

EQUIPMENT AND SUPPLIES

Blood and body-fluid protection barriers (goggles, masks, and aprons or gowns), as necessary (see Appendix C, Recommendations for Prevention of AIDS Transmission)
Nonsterile gloves
Neubauer ruled hemacytometer
Hemacytometer coverslip
Lint-free tissue
70 percent alcohol
Blood-diluting pipette or Unopette

PROCEDURE

1. Wash and dry your hands. Follow the universal blood and body-fluid precautions (see Appendix C). Glove yourself with nonsterile gloves.
2. Clean the hemacytometer and coverslip with 70 percent alcohol and lint-free tissue, and thoroughly dry.
   Purpose: Dirt, fingerprints, grease, or lint interferes with filling and counting.
3. Align the coverslip on the chamber.
4. Expel two drops from the well-mixed pipette or Unopette.
   Purpose: Diluent in the calibrated stem contains no cells and must be discarded before filling the chamber of the hemacytometer.
5. Touch the tip of the pipette to the edge of the coverslip in the loading area of the chamber.
6. Controlling the flow with the finger on the pipette or by gentle squeezing of the Unopette, fill the chamber in one smooth motion.
   Purpose: Chamber fills by capillary action. If the pipette is not touching the edge of the coverslip, the chamber will not fill properly.
7. Stop filling when the ruled area is full but do not overfill.
8. Fill both sides of the hemacytometer.
9. Allow the chamber to sit undisturbed for one or two minutes so that the cells settle, but do not allow the sample to dry.
   Purpose: Once the cells have settled in the chamber, the counting procedure is easier. Drying contracts the sample and elevates the count.
10. Clean the work area. Follow the recommendations for proper disposal of all materials (see Appendix C).
11. Wash your hands.

TERMINAL PERFORMANCE OBJECTIVE

Given a properly filled blood-diluting pipette or Unopette and appropriate supplies, fill a hemacytometer chamber within three minutes and correctly complete each step of the procedure in the proper order, as determined by your evaluator.

Procedure 36–7

PROCEDURAL GOAL

To focus properly a hemacytometer, to locate the appropriate areas to count, and to direct your field of vision through the chamber in the proper manner while counting cells.

EQUIPMENT AND SUPPLIES

Blood and body-fluid protection barriers (goggles, masks, and aprons or gowns), as necessary (see Appendix C, Recommendations for Prevention of AIDS Transmission)
Nonsterile gloves
Properly filled hemacytometer (see Procedure 36–6)
Microscope
Hand tally counter

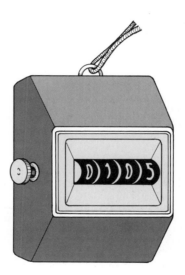

PROCEDURE

1. Wash and dry your hands. Follow the universal blood and body-fluid precautions (see Appendix C). Glove yourself with nonsterile gloves.
2. Place the hemacytometer on the lowered microscope stage under low-power magnification.
   Purpose: The thick chamber will not fit under the objective unless the stage is lowered.
3. Center the ruled area over the opening in the stage.
4. Reduce the light intensity by closing the diaphragm and lowering the condenser.
   Purpose: The unstained cells require reduced light for counting.
5. Raise the stage carefully while watching from the side to be certain that the objective lens does not hit the coverslip.
   Purpose: The chamber or the microscope lens can easily be damaged by improper focusing techniques.
6. Focus and center the correct area (top left large "W" square for counting WBC), using the coarse adjustment and mechanical stage simultaneously.
   Purpose: You will be moving through several planes of focus. When you see the chamber moving through the ocular lens, you will know that you are in approximate focus and will be able to locate the lined area easily.
7. Adjust the light until the cells are easily visible.
   Purpose: Too much light will prevent you from visualizing the cells.
8. Count white cells under low power, by depressing the hand tally once for each cell seen.
   a. Begin in the top row, on the far left.

Procedure continued on following page

36

b. Count the top row, moving visually from left to right.

c. Count all cells within the boundaries of the square, and also cells touching the top and the left-hand lines of the square.

d. Do not count cells touching the right-hand or the bottom lines of the square.

e. When you come to the end of the top row, drop to the second row.

f. Count the second row, moving visually from right to left.

g. Continue counting in this zigzag pattern, ending at the bottom left small square.

   Purpose: Using the same sequence when counting helps you to count all cells that should be counted and to avoid counting cells twice or missing them entirely.

9. When you have finished counting a large square, record the number.

10. Return the tally to zero, move to the next large square, and begin to count.

   Purpose: You need to know the total cells counted in each square individually in order to determine if the chamber was filled correctly. An unevenly filled hemacytometer voids the count.

11. Switch to high power, and focus with the fine adjustment for counting red blood cells (top left "R" square).

12. Locate the remaining squares to be counted, and determine the number of cells in each. For WBC, the counts from each square should vary by no more than ten cells. For RBC, the numbers should vary by no more than 20 cells. Greater variation indicates an unevenly filled hemacytometer. In such cases, the chamber should be cleaned and refilled.

13. Total the cells counted in all four squares for WBC and five squares for RBC.

14. Count the second side of the chamber in the same manner.

15. Average the counts from both sides.

16. Calculate the results.
   RBC—average times 10,000
   WBC—average times 50

17. Record the results.

18. Clean the work area. Follow the recommendations for proper disposal of all materials (see Appendix C).

19. Wash your hands.

TERMINAL PERFORMANCE OBJECTIVE

Given a properly filled hemacytometer and appropriate supplies, count and calculate a manual white or red blood cell count within 15 minutes to a minimum performance level of ± 200 WBC/cu mm and ± 50,000 RBC/cu mm of your evaluator's results.

Automation

Although blood cell counts are usually performed manually in the physician's office, private and hospital laboratories perform them by automation. The many different types of instruments available range from the relatively simple, inexpensive counters to the very complex and expensive machines.

Most of the automated cell counters operate by first diluting the cells in a fluid that conducts an electric current. Then, these diluted cells pass through a special narrow opening in the machine. The passing cells interrupt the flow of current, and each interruption is counted. Some machines use a laser beam instead of an electric current.

Automation has improved the accuracy of cell counting and has resulted in greater efficiency in the laboratory. In addition, automation reduces the frequency of handling the individual blood specimen and decreases the risk of exposure to blood-borne pathogens, such as the hepatitis B virus or HIV (AIDS viruses).

DIFFERENTIAL CELL COUNT

Preparation of Blood Smears

A blood smear enables you to view the cellular components of the blood in as natural a state as possible. The morphology of the leukocytes, erythrocytes, and platelets can be studied. Their size, shape, and maturity can be evaluated. Examining a blood smear is part of a complete blood cell count.

A blood smear is prepared by spreading a drop of blood on a clean glass slide. The slides must be free of dust and grease. The best specimen for a blood smear is capillary blood that has no anticoagulant added. EDTA anticoagulant blood can be used provided the smear is made within two hours of collection.

There are several methods of spreading the drop of blood on the slide that result in a good smear. One method is to place a small drop of blood one-half inch from the right end of a glass slide. The end of a second glass "spreader" slide is placed in

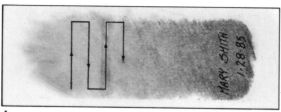

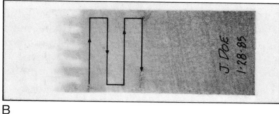

Figure 36–15
Shapes of blood smears. **A** is made by rapidly advancing the spreader slide before the drop of blood extends to the edge of the slide. **B** is made using a special spreader slide with ground edges and corners. Arrows show the pattern for performing a differential in this portion of the smear.

front of the drop of blood at an angle of 30 to 35 degrees. The spreader slide is brought back into the drop until the blood spreads along the edge of the spreader slide. This is done with a quick but smooth gliding motion. The spreader slide is then pushed to the left with a quick, steady motion, spreading the blood across the slide.

A good smear should cover one half to three quarters of the slide. It should show a gradual transition from a thick to a thin end with a feathered edge. It should have a smooth appearance with no ridges, holes, lines, streaks, or clumps (Fig. 36–15). The cells should be distributed evenly, upon microscopic examination.

After the smear has been made, it should be allowed to dry. The slide should be propped up to dry with the thick end down. Do not blow on the slide to dry it. This can cause artifacts in the red blood cells from the moisture in your breath. Once dry, the slide is labeled in the thick portion of the smear by writing the patient's name in the dried blood film. If slides with frosted ends are used, the label can be written on the frosted end.

Following labeling, the slide is fixed in *methanol*, which preserves and prevents changes or deterioration of the cellular components. Many of the quick stains available on the market contain the fixative in the stain.

Staining of Blood Smears

The stains commonly used for examination of blood cells are called *polychromatic* because they contain dyes that will stain various cell components different colors. These stains usually contain *methylene blue*, a blue stain, and *eosin*, a red-orange stain.

These stains are attracted to different parts of the cell. Thus, the cells and their structures are more easily visualized and differentiated. The most commonly used differential blood stain is *Wright stain*.

Wright stain is applied to the slide for approximately one to three minutes. A buffer is added on top of the stain and is mixed by gently blowing until a green metallic sheen appears. This usually takes two to four minutes. The slide is then gently rinsed and is allowed to air-dry. A properly stained smear should appear pinkish to the naked eye.

Identification of Normal Blood Cells

Much useful information can be gathered from the microscopic identification and evaluation of blood cells in a stained smear. A great deal more information can be acquired from the observation of these blood cells than from actual cell counts. Blood smears can impart more knowledge than any other laboratory test.

The features of blood cells that you will observe and evaluate are cell size, nuclear appearance, and cytoplasmic characteristics. The results of observing these three features will allow for cell identification, although much practice is required to be able to recognize and classify all the blood cells that may be seen in various disease states.

Cells are examined under the oil-immersion objective. The light should be bright to facilitate the visualization of colors and small structures. The slide is examined near the feathered end of the smear, where the cells are barely touching each other and are easiest to identify.

Red blood cells are the most numerous of the cellular elements. They are biconcave discs that have no nucleus. The red cells should appear pinkish-tan, as a result of the staining of the hemoglobin within the cells (Fig. 36–16).

Thrombocytes, or *platelets*, are the smallest of the cellular elements. They may be round or oval. No nucleus is present, since the platelet is just a fragment of cytoplasm from a large bone-marrow cell. They stain blue.

Leukocytes are the largest of the normal circulating blood cells. Each of the five types has a characteristic appearance. The granulocytes include neutrophils, eosinophils, and basophils. Granulocytes contain distinctive granules in their cytoplasm and may have segmented nuclei. The agranulocytes include lymphocytes and monocytes. They have few, if any, granules and nonsegmented nuclei. The nuclei of the leukocytes should appear purple, and their cytoplasm may vary from pink to blue or blue-gray.

Neutrophils are known by a variety of names, including *polymorphonuclear neutrophils*, *segmented neutrophils*, *polys*, and *segs*. They are the most numerous white blood cells in circulation in adults. They are produced in the bone marrow, are released into the circulation, and eventually enter tissue to fight off

36

invading microorganisms by engulfing them **(phagocytosis).** Many types of bacterial infections stimulate increased production of neutrophils.

The *segmented neutrophil* nucleus is segmented into two to five lobes that are connected by a strand. The nucleus stains a dark purple. The cytoplasm is pale pink and contains fine pink or lilac granules.

An immature form of the neutrophil is called a *band,* or *stab.* Instead of having a segmented nucleus, where the lobes are separated by a thin filament, the band has an unsegmented nucleus shaped like a horseshoe. The staining is the same as in the segmented neutrophil. An increase in bands is termed a "shift to the left" and is seen in infections such as bacterial meningitis, pneumonia, appendicitis, strep throat, and abscesses and in chronic granulocytic leukemia. The nucleus of the *eosinophil* is divided into two or three lobes that stain purple. The cytoplasm stains pink and contains large round or oval red-orange granules. Eosinophils are phagocytic and are associated closely with allergies such as hay fever and asthma as well as certain parasitic infestations such as trichinosis, amebiasis, and schistosomiasis. The nucleus of the *basophil* is segmented and stains light purple. The large dark blue-black granules contain histamine, which is a part of the allergic response. Little is known about the function of basophils.

Lymphocytes are the second most numerous white cell in adults. In children, they are usually the most numerous. Their nucleus is usually oval or round and smooth. It stains purple. The cytoplasm stains blue. Lymphs, as they are commonly called, are responsible for the recognition of foreign antigens and the production of circulating antibodies for immunity to disease. Increased numbers of lymphocytes are found in most viral diseases; in some bacterial infections such as syphilis, brucellosis, TB, and typhoid and paratyphoid fevers; in leukemias; and in young children who are actively making antibodies. In many viral infections, stimulated or reactive lymphocytes, called *"atypical lymphs,"* are found. These are common in infectious mononucleosis.

Monocytes are the largest white blood cell in the circulation. The nucleus may be oval, indented, or horseshoe-shaped. The cytoplasm stains a dull gray-blue and may contain *vacuoles,* which appear as clear spaces in the cytoplasm filled with fluid or air. Monocytes are called macrophages and ingest bacteria and the debris of cellular breakdown. They are increased in certain viral infections such as hepatitis and mumps; rickettsial infections such as Rocky Mountain spotted fever; and bacterial infections such as brucellosis, TB, and typhoid (Fig. 36–16).

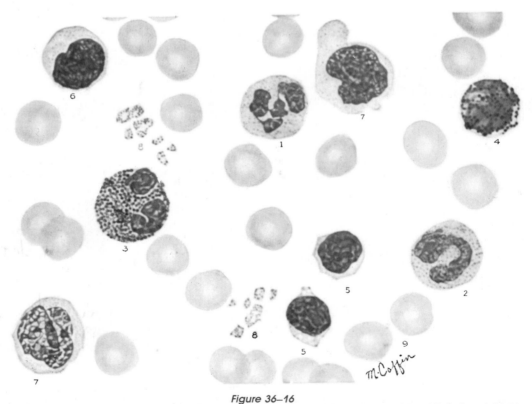

Figure 36–16
Normal cellular constituents of adult human blood. **1,** *Segmented (polymorphonuclear) neutrophil;* **2,** *band (stab) neutrophil;* **3,** *segmented eosinophil;* **4,** *basophil;* **5,** *small lymphocyte;* **6,** *large lymphocyte;* **7,** *monocytes;* **8,** *thrombocytes;* and **9,** *erythrocytes.* (*From Custer, R. P. [ed.]: An Atlas of the Blood and Bone Marrow, 2nd ed. Philadelphia, W. B. Saunders Co., 1974.)*

Differential Examination

A specific area of the stained smear must be examined when doing the differential count. This area must be where the red blood cells are touching but are not clumped, when viewed microscopically. After you have located an appropriate area under low power, focus under oil immersion. The differential examination consists of counting and classifying 100 consecutive white blood cells while moving in a specific winding pattern through the smear. This pattern must be followed to avoid counting the same cells twice. A tally is kept of the cells observed on a *differential cell counter*.

Normal values vary with age (Table 36–2). Many disease states alter the ratios of the different types of leukocytes.

Red Blood Cell Morphology

After determining the differential cell count, the red blood cells are observed and evaluated. Normally, stained red blood cells are the same size and shape and are well filled with hemoglobin. Any variations from the normal state are reported.

Size. Normal-sized red blood cells are known as *normocytic*. If the cells are larger than normal, they are *macrocytic*; if smaller, *microcytic*. The condition in which different sizes of red blood cells are present is called *anisocytosis*.

Shape. Normal red blood cells are round or slightly oval. Cells may be shaped like sickles, targets, crescents, or burrs. *Poikilocytosis* is a significant variation in the shape of the red blood cells.

Content. A red blood cell with the normal amount of hemoglobin is called *normochromic*. Pale-staining cells are *hypochromic* and have less hemoglobin than normal (Fig. 36–17).

Platelet Observation

Platelets, or thrombocytes, are formed in the bone marrow by *megakaryocytes*. As megakaryocytes mature, platelets are shed from the cytoplasm and are

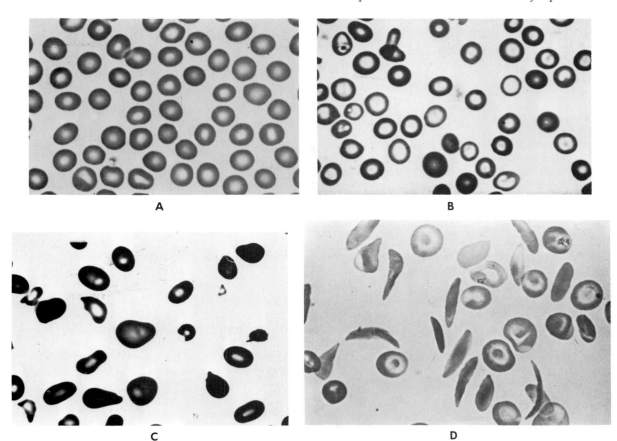

A   B

C   D

Figure 36–17
A comparison of red blood cells. A, Normal blood. B, Iron deficiency anemia. Note lack of color (hypochromia), smaller size (microcythemia), and elliptic cells. C, Megaloblastic anemia. Note varying size of cells (anisocytosis) and large cells (macrocytosis). (All from Henry, J.: Clinical Diagnosis and Management by Laboratory Procedures, 17th ed. Philadelphia, W. B. Saunders Co., 1984.) D, sickle cell anemia, showing sickle-shaped cells and target cells (From Raphael, S. S.: Lynch's Medical Laborarory Techology, 4th ed. Philadelphia, W. B. Saunders Co., 1983.)

36

released into the circulation, where they function in coagulation. When damage to a vessel occurs, platelets form a plug at the site, and eventually a fibrin clot seals the leak. On a stained smear, the morphology of the platelets is observed for any abnormalities. They are small and irregularly shaped and may vary considerably in size. The average number of platelets seen in 10 to 15 fields is reported. The normal platelet count is 150,000 to 400,000 per cu mm. An increase in platelets is called *thrombocytosis*, and a decrease is called *thrombocytopenia*.

Procedure 36–8   *PREPARING A SMEAR STAINED WITH WRIGHT STAIN*

PROCEDURAL GOAL

To prepare and stain a slide that meets the criteria for the performance of a differential examination.

EQUIPMENT AND SUPPLIES

Blood and body-fluid protection barriers (goggles, masks, and aprons or gowns), as necessary (see Appendix C, Recommendations for Prevention of AIDS Transmission)
Nonsterile gloves
Clean glass slides
Transfer pipette or capillary tube
Wright stain materials
EDTA anticoagulant blood specimen

PROCEDURE

1. Wash and dry your hands. Follow the universal blood and body-fluid precautions (see Appendix C). Glove yourself with nonsterile gloves.
2. Assemble the materials needed.
3. Mix the blood specimen.
4. Dispense a small drop of blood onto a slide, about one-half to three-fourths inch from the right end. Use a transfer pipette or capillary tube.
5. Hold the left side of this slide with your nondominant hand.
6. Place the spreader slide in front of the drop of blood at an angle of 30 to 35 degrees. Use your dominant hand.
   Purpose: An angle of 30–35 degrees makes a smear with a good feathered edge.
7. Pull back the spreader slide into the drop of blood, and allow the blood to spread to the edges of the slide.
8. Push the spreader slide forward with a quick smooth motion, maintaining the same angle throughout (facing page, top).
   Purpose: If the motion is not smooth, ridges will occur in the smear.
9. Rapidly but gently wave the slide to accelerate the drying process.
10. Stand the slide with the thick end down, and allow the slide to complete drying.
    Purpose: If the thick end is up, the undried portion of the blood may run down into the dry thin area and ruin the smear.
11. Label the slide when it is dry. Use a pencil, and write the name in the thick end of the smear.
    Purpose: Pencil will scratch the name into the smear and will not wash off in the staining process.
12. Stain according to method used.
    a. Two-step method:
       (1) Place the smear on a staining rack, with the blood side up.
       (2) Flood the smear with Wright stain.
       (3) Time for one to three minutes.
       (4) Add an equal amount of buffer, drop by drop, on top of the Wright stain.
       (5) Blow gently, and mix the two solutions until a green metallic sheen appears. This should appear within two to four minutes.
       (6) Rinse thoroughly with distilled water.
       (7) Drain water from the slide.

Procedure continued on opposite page

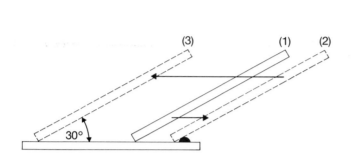

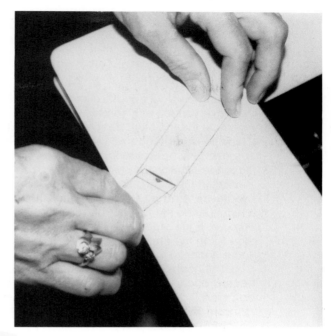

(8) Wipe the back of the smear with gauze.

(9) Stand the smear to dry.

b. Quick stain:

(1) Place the smear into solutions according to the manufacturer's instructions.

(2) Proceed with steps 6 through 9 just listed.

13. Clean the work area. Follow the recommendations for proper disposal of all materials (see Appendix C).

14. Wash your hands.

TERMINAL PERFORMANCE OBJECTIVE

Given a blood sample and appropriate supplies, prepare and stain a blood smear, using Wright stain, within ten minutes and correctly complete each step of the procedure in the proper order, as determined by your evaluator.

Procedure 36–9

PERFORMING A DIFFERENTIAL EXAMINATION OF A SMEAR STAINED WITH WRIGHT STAIN

36

PROCEDURAL GOAL

To perform a differential cell count, evaluate the red blood cell morphology, and estimate the number of platelets.

EQUIPMENT AND SUPPLIES

Blood and body-fluid protection barriers (goggles, masks, and aprons or gowns), as necessary (see Appendix C, Recommendations for Prevention of AIDS Transmission)

Nonsterile gloves

Microscope

Immersion oil

Lens tissue

Lens cleaner

Procedure continued on following page

Differential cell counter
Stained blood smear

PROCEDURE

1. Wash and dry your hands. Follow the universal blood and body-fluid precautions (see Appendix C). Glove yourself with nonsterile gloves.
2. Assemble the materials needed.
3. Clean the microscope with lens tissue and lens cleaner.
   Purpose: Dirty optical surfaces interfere with viewing.
4. Place the slide on the stage, with the smear facing up.
   Purpose: If the slide is face down, you will not be able to focus under oil immersion.
5. Locate an area of the smear where the red blood cells barely touch each other or slightly overlap, using the low-power objective.
   Purpose: If the slide is too thick, the cells will be crowded, small, and difficult to evaluate. If the slide is too thin, the cells will be very far apart and will show the effects of excessive flattening.
6. Focus under oil immersion with the fine-adjustment knob and increased light.
7. Count 100 consecutive white blood cells in a winding pattern, identifying each cell encountered.
8. Record each white cell on the differential cell counter by depressing the appropriate key for each cell.
   Purpose: The differential examination must proceed systematically, to avoid missing cells or counting any cell twice.
9. Evaluate the red blood cells observed in 10 fields.
   a. Record any variations in
      (1) size—microcytosis, macrocytosis, anisocytosis
      (2) shape—poikilocytosis, ovalocytosis, target cells, sickle cells, and so forth
      (3) content—normochromic or hypochromic
   Purpose: The red blood cell evaluation gives the physician important information about the red blood cell population and is an important tool in the assessment of anemias and red blood cell diseases.
10. Count the platelets in ten fields, obtain an average, and multiply that average by 15,000 to give an estimate of the platelet count. The normal platelet count is 150,000 to 400,000 /cu mm. Report the count as normal, decreased, or increased.
    Purpose: Platelet numbers can be a clue to bleeding disorders.
11. Clean the microscope with lens tissue and lens cleaner.
12. Clean the work area. Follow the recommendations for proper disposal of all materials (see Appendix C).
13. Wash your hands.

TERMINAL PERFORMANCE OBJECTIVE

Given a stained blood smear and the appropriate supplies, perform a differential cell count, red blood cell examination, and platelet estimation within 30 minutes to a minimum performance level of 90 percent accuracy as determined by your evaluator.

ERYTHROCYTE SEDIMENTATION RATE

The erythrocyte sedimentation rate (ESR) is a laboratory test that measures the rate at which erythrocytes gradually separate from plasma and settle to the bottom of a specially calibrated tube. The number of these red blood cells that fall in one hour is the ESR. The test is not specific for a particular disease but is used as a general indication of inflammation. Increases are found in such conditions as acute and chronic infections, rheumatoid arthritis, tuberculosis, hepatitis, cancer, multiple myeloma, rheumatic fever, and lupus erythematosus.

Normal values vary slightly with age and sex (Table 36–2). Only increased ESR rates are significant.

Several methods of measuring the erythrocyte sedimentation rate are used, including *Wintrobe*, *Westergren*, and *Landau-Adams*. All these methods are based on the same principle and differ only in the amounts of blood needed and the tube size and calibration used.

The Wintrobe method is commonly used. It consists of a Wintrobe tube that is graduated from 0 to

100 mm and a specially designed Wintrobe rack that holds the tube in a vertical position. A long-tipped *Pasteur pipette* is used to fill the Wintrobe tube with 100 ml of blood, to the zero mark on the tube (Fig. 36–18). The tube is placed in the Wintrobe rack for one hour. At the end of one hour, the level on the tube to which the erythrocytes have fallen is measured. The rate is recorded in mm/hour (Fig. 36–19).

Many factors can affect the sedimentation rate. The tube must be totally filled with blood and must not contain air bubbles. The tube must be allowed to sit in a vertical position undisturbed for a full hour. Minor degrees of tilting may increase the sedimentation rate, and careful timing is important. Jarring or vibrations from nearby machinery will falsely increase the ESR. Testing must be performed within two hours after the blood has been collected.

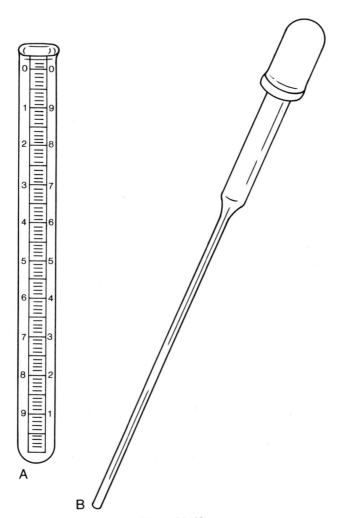

Figure 36–18
Materials for measuring erythrocyte sedimentation rate. **A,** Wintrobe sedimentation rate tube; **B,** long-stemmed Pasteur pipette.

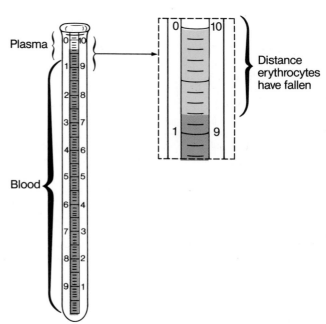

Figure 36–19
Sedimentation rate tube showing the settling of cells. Example shown illustrates a reading of 8 mm.

36

Procedure 36–10

PROCEDURAL GOAL

To properly fill a Wintrobe tube and observe and record the findings of an erythrocyte sedimentation rate, using the Wintrobe method.

EQUIPMENT AND SUPPLIES

Blood and body-fluid protection barriers (goggles, masks, and aprons or gowns), as necessary (see Appendix C, Recommendations for Prevention of AIDS Transmission)
Nonsterile gloves
EDTA anticoagulant blood specimen
Wintrobe tube
Wintrobe rack
Timer
Pasteur pipette
Bulb

PROCEDURE

1. Wash and dry your hands. Follow the universal blood and body-fluid precautions (see Appendix C). Glove yourself with nonsterile gloves.
2. Assemble the materials needed.
3. Check the leveling bubble of the Wintrobe rack.
   Purpose: The rack must be horizontal to ensure that the tube is vertical.
4. Mix the blood well.
   Purpose: Cells settle when the specimen stands, and blood must always be well mixed prior to sampling.
5. Fill the Pasteur pipette with blood, and insert the tip of the pipette to the bottom of the Wintrobe tube.
6. Fill the Wintrobe tube to the "0" mark, by squeezing the bulb of the pipette.
7. Slowly remove the pipette from the tube while keeping the tip of the pipette below the level of the blood.
   Purpose: If the tip of the pipette is above the level of the blood, bubbles will be trapped in the tube and will invalidate the test.
8. Place the tube in a numbered slot in the Wintrobe rack, and set the timer for one hour. The tube must be in a vertical position and free from all vibration.
   Purpose: Jarring will increase the sedimentation rate.
9. Measure the distance the erythrocytes have fallen after one hour. The ESR scale measures from 0 at the top to 100 at the bottom. Each line is one millimeter.
10. Record the findings.
    Purpose: The ESR is reported in mm/hour.
11. Clean the work area. Follow the recommendations for proper disposal of all materials (see Appendix C).
12. Wash your hands.

TERMINAL PERFORMANCE OBJECTIVE

Given an EDTA blood specimen and the appropriate supplies, determine a sedimentation rate, using the Wintrobe method, within 75 minutes to a minimum performance level of ± 1 mm of your evaluator's results.

REFERENCES AND READINGS

Bauer, J.: *Clinical Laboratory Methods*, 9th ed. St. Louis, C. V. Mosby Co., 1982.

Brown, B.: *Hematology: Principles and Procedures*, 4th ed. Philadelphia, Lea & Febiger, 1984.

Diggs, L., Sturm, D., and Bell, A.: *The Morphology of Human Blood Cells*. Abbott Laboratories, 1984.

Miale, J.: *Laboratory Medicine: Hematology*, 5th ed. Philadelphia, Lea & Febiger, 1983.

O'Connor, B.: *A Color Atlas and Instruction Manual of Peripheral Blood Cell Morphology*. Baltimore, Williams and Wilkins, 1984.

Seiverd, C.: *Hematology for Medical Technologists*, 5th ed. Philadelphia, Lea & Febiger, 1983.

Slockbower, J., and Blumenfeld, T.: *Collection and Handling of Laboratory Specimens*. Philadelphia, J. B. Lippincott, 1983.

36

CHAPTER OUTLINE

VOCABULARY

See Glossary at end of book for definitions.

arrhythmia	dyspnea	precordial
cardiac arrest	erythema	vertigo
defibrillator	galvanometer	

Electrocardiography

37

OBJECTIVES

Upon successful completion of this chapter your should be able to

1. Define and spell the terms listed in the Vocabulary for this chapter.
2. Trace the electric conduction system through the heart during depolarization, repolarization, and polarization.
3. Compare the PQRSTU wave pattern traced on ECG paper with the heart's rhythm and other actions.
4. State what the horizontal and vertical lines on the ECG paper indicate.
5. List four types of artifacts commonly seen on an ECG, and list the causes of each.
6. Recall the combination of electrodes used for each lead.
7. State the purpose of using an electrolyte when performing an ECG.
8. List the 12 leads recorded on an ECG; state the electric activity of each; and identify the coding used for each.
9. Discuss the process of standardizing the electrocardiograph.
10. List two heart muscle functions detected by an ECG.

Upon successful completion of this chapter you should be able to perform the following activities:

1. Apply ECG electrodes and lead wires to a patient in preparation for an ECG.
2. Record a 12-lead ECG tracing.
3. Clean up after an ECG procedure and mount the finished ECG tracing.

Electrocardiography is frequently used in the diagnosis of heart disease. It is a painless and safe procedure. To perform electrocardiography, cables with electrodes are attached to the patient. The machine, called an *electrocardiograph*, magnifies many times the natural electric currents generated by the action of the heart. A pattern of the heart waves is traced on heat-sensitive graph paper with a balanced tracing pen, or stylus. This tracing, called an *electrocardiogram* (ECG; or, commonly, EKG), is an exact graphic representation of the heart's rhythm and other heart muscle actions. The tracing is then mounted in a pre-designed folder for the physician to examine and as a permanent record. In many offices, the medical assistant is responsible for both obtaining and mounting the electrocardiogram.

THE HEART'S NATURAL PACEMAKER

The heart is a hollow, muscular organ situated in the chest between the lungs. It weighs approximately 9 oz and is only a little larger than a fist. Its function is to circulate the blood throughout the body.

The heart is really a double pump. On the right side, one pump receives blood that has just come from the body after delivering nutrients and oxygen to the tissues. The right side pumps deoxygenated blood to the lungs, where the carbon dioxide is exchanged for a fresh supply of oxygen. The pump on the left side of the heart receives this fresh oxygenated blood from the lungs and pumps it out through the aorta, to be distributed to all parts of the body.

The heart is divided into four chambers by partitions. The two upper chambers, called the right and left atria, are the receiving chambers. The two lower chambers, called the right and left ventricles, are the pumping chambers. Valves located between each upper and lower chamber open and close in order to permit the flow of blood in one direction. The tricuspid valve is located between the right atrium and ventricle. The bicuspid, or mitral, valve is between the left atrium and ventricle. The wall of the heart possesses three layers: the outer epicardium, the middle myocardium, and the inner endocardium (Fig. 37–1).

A sophisticated electric conduction system, controlled by the autonomic nervous system and located in the myocardium, stimulates the heart muscle contractions, which makes blood move through the chambers of the heart and the rest of the body. Each electric impulse moves through the heart muscle in a twisting, spiral motion. These rhythmic waves cause the heart to "beat."

The cardiac impulse originates in specialized muscle tissue called the *sinoatrial (SA) node*. The SA node is located in the right atrium, just at the junction of the superior vena cava and the atrium.

This wave spreads in concentric circles over the atrial wall, and the atria contract.

The wave then passes through a second area of specialized muscle tissue between the atrium and the ventricle, called the *atrioventricular (AV) node*. In the AV node, the cardiac impulse moves through a band of cardiac muscle that connects the atria with the ventricles. This band, or collection, of tissue is called the *bundle of His*.

From the bundle of His, the transmission of the cardiac wave continues through a mass of cardiac muscle fibers known as the *Purkinje fibers*. The Purkinje fibers end in the muscles of the ventricles, where the cardiac wave causes the ventricles to contract.

This conduction system is so highly organized that transmission is slightly delayed at the AV node, thus allowing time for the atria to first contract and then empty their contents into the ventricles before the ventricles begin to contract.

The transmission of the cardiac impulse from the SA node to the muscles in the ventricles is called *depolarization*. A period of electric *recovery* then occurs and is called *repolarization*. The heart returns to resting (*polarization*), and the entire cycle begins again. The normal cardiac cycle consists of atrial contraction, ventricular contraction, and then recovery and heart rest. This cycle maintains the normal 70 to 90 beats per minute and a normal heart rhythm.

THE CARDIAC CYCLE AND ELECTROCARDIOGRAPHY

The term cardiac cycle refers to one complete heartbeat, which consists of depolarization (contraction), repolarization (recovery), and polarization (relaxation). The cardiac impulse can be transferred to a machine that records this natural electric activity, and this is the physiologic basis of electrocardiography. The electrocardiogram measures the normal conductive mechanism of the heart muscle and detects any disturbances or disruptions of heart rhythm.

The ECG records a series of waves, or deflections, above or below a baseline. Each deflection corresponds to a particular part of the cardiac cycle (Table 37–1). The normal ECG cycle consists of wave forms that have been arbitrarily labeled the *P* wave, *QRS* complex, and *T* wave. The *P wave* reflects contraction of the atria (beginning depolarization). The *P-R interval* reflects the time it takes from the beginning of the atrial contraction to the beginning of the ventricular contraction. The *QRS complex* reflects the contraction of the ventricles (depolarization of both ventricles). The *S-T segment* reflects the time interval from the end of the ventricular contraction to the beginning of ventricular recovery. The *T wave* reflects ventricular recovery (repolarization of the ventricles). After the T wave, there is a period of

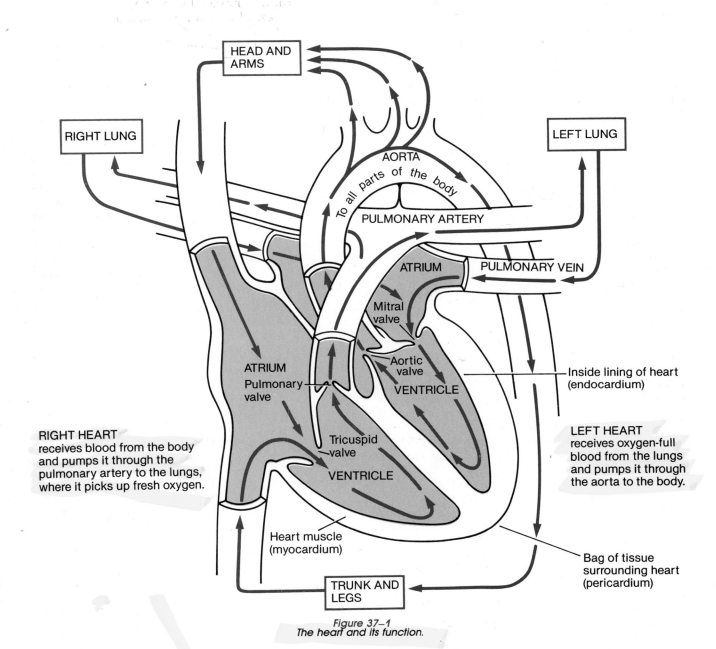

HEAD AND ARMS

RIGHT LUNG

LEFT LUNG

AORTA

To all parts of the body

PULMONARY ARTERY

ATRIUM

PULMONARY VEIN

Mitral valve

ATRIUM

Pulmonary valve

Aortic valve

VENTRICLE

Inside lining of heart (endocardium)

RIGHT HEART
receives blood from the body and pumps it through the pulmonary artery to the lungs, where it picks up fresh oxygen.

Tricuspid valve

VENTRICLE

LEFT HEART
receives oxygen-full blood from the lungs and pumps it through the aorta to the body.

Heart muscle (myocardium)

Bag of tissue surrounding heart (pericardium)

TRUNK AND LEGS

37

Figure 37–1
The heart and its function.

Table 37–1
The Cardiac Cycle

On the electrocardiogram, one complete heartbeat is recorded as PQRSTU.

Waves = The physician Measures and interuped

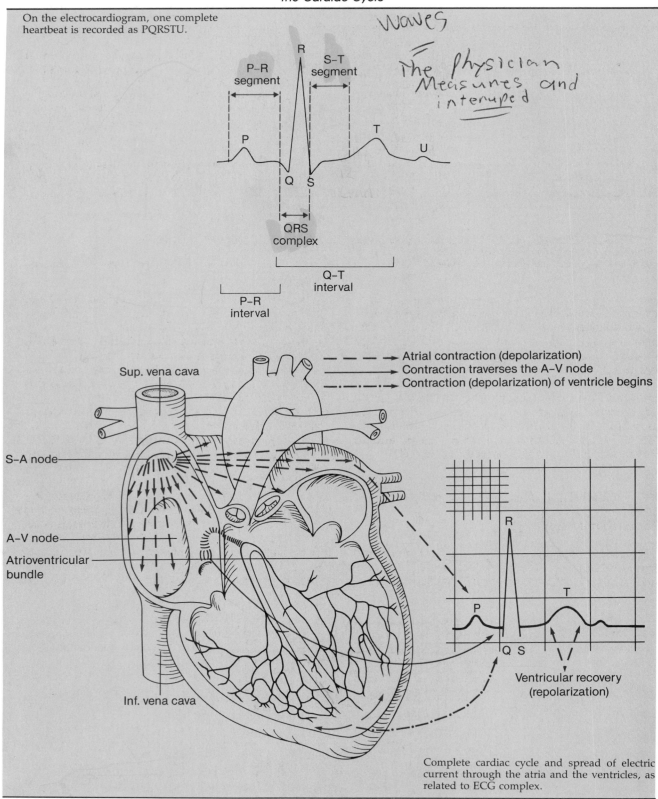

Complete cardiac cycle and spread of electric current through the atria and the ventricles, as related to ECG complex.

Table continued on opposite page

Table 37–1 Continued
The Cardiac Cycle

Stage	Heart Activity	Electric Current
P wave*	Atrial contraction	Atrial depolarization
P-R segment†	Contraction traversing the A-V node	Depolarization traversing the A-V node
QRS complex‡	Ventricular contraction	Ventricular depolarization
S-T segment	Time interval between ventricular contraction and the beginning of ventricular recovery	Time interval between ventricular depolarization and ventricular repolarization
T wave	Ventricular contraction subsides	Ventricular repolarization (electric recovery)
U wave (not always present)	Associated with further ventricular relaxation	Associated with further ventricular repolarization
Baseline§	The heart at rest	Polarization
P-R interval‖	Time interval between atrial contraction and ventricular contraction	Time interval between atrial depolarization and ventricular depolarization
Q-T interval	Time interval between the beginning of ventricular contraction and the subsiding of ventricular contraction	Time interval between the beginning of ventricular depolarization and ventricular repolarization (electric recovery)

*Wave—a uniformly advancing deflection (upward or downward) from a baseline on a recording.
†Segment—a portion of an ECG recording between two consecutive waves. Represents the time needed for an electric current to move on.
‡Complex—the portion of the ECG tracing that represents the sum of three waves (contraction of the ventricles).
§Interval—the lapse of time between two different ECG events.
‖Baseline—a neutral line against which waves are valued as they deflect upward (positive) or downward (negative) from the line.

heart rest (polarization), and the tracing shows a straight line indicating the resting state of the heart. This flat horizontal line is called the baseline. Occasionally, after the T wave, another small *U wave* is seen. It appears in patients who have a low serum potassium level.

By observing and measuring the actual configuration and location of each wave in relation to the other waves and to the baseline, as well as the intervals and segments, the physician is able to detect rhythmic disturbances of the heart and to distinguish different types of cardiac disorders.

THE ELECTROCARDIOGRAM

Electrocardiograph Paper

Electrocardiograph paper is heat-sensitive and pressure-sensitive. The recording, or writing, device of the electrocardiograph is called a *stylus*.

When the machine is on and running, the heated stylus moves along a horizontal line and literally burns the paper. Since the paper is also pressure-sensitive, it must be handled carefully to avoid any markings that would blemish the tracing.

Electrocardiograph paper is graph paper with internationally accepted increments for measuring the cardiac cycle (Fig. 37–2). These universal measurements allow physicians anywhere, anytime to interpret the significance of each person's ECG in the same manner. The medical assistant needs to know the size and the meaning of each square in order to understand its significance.

Each small square measures 1 mm by 1 mm. Every fifth line (both vertical and horizontal) is darker than the other lines and defines a square measuring 5 mm by 5 mm. As the electrocardiograph paper advances, the stylus moves along one horizontal line and intersects with a vertical line every 0.04 second. Therefore, every fifth line intersected represents 0.2 second (0.04 second per line

37

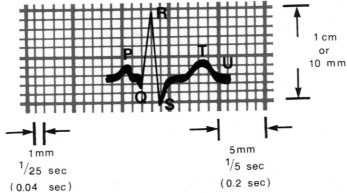

Figure 37–2
Measurements of squares on the ECG paper.

× 5 lines = 0.2 second) in time. Routinely, the electrocardiograph paper advances at a speed of 25 mm per second (5 lines per 0.2 second = 25 lines per second). In one minute, the paper advances 300 5-mm increments.

Electrodes and Electrolytes

Metal *electrodes* are placed on the patient's limbs and chest to pick up the electric activity of the heart. The cardiac impulses are transmitted to the electrocardiograph by metal tips and wires that are attached to the electrodes (Fig. 37–3). The standard 12-lead electrocardiograph has five electrodes. Two electrodes are attached to the fleshy part of the arms and two to the fleshy part of the legs. The fifth electrode is moved to six different positions on the chest.

The cardiac impulses travel from the metal electrodes and wires to an amplifier, where they are magnified (Fig. 37–4). The magnified impulses are then converted into mechanical action by a **galvanometer** and are recorded on the electrocardiograph paper by the stylus.

The skin is a poor conductor of electricity. To aid in the conduction of this electric current, an *electrolyte* is applied to each electrode. Electrolyte products are available in the form of pastes, gels, or pads saturated with electrolyte solution (Fig. 37–5).

Leads

The routine ECG consists of 12 separate *leads*, or recordings, of the electric activity of the heart, from different angles. Each lead must be marked, or coded, in order for the physician to know the angle recorded. New machines automatically mark the 12 leads as the *lead selector switch* is turned. Older models require that the assistant mark, or code, each lead manually. A certain coding system is used to identify each lead recorded. Codes consist of a series of dots and dashes. One standard marking code is illustrated in Table 37–2.

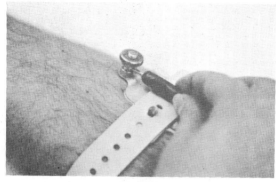

Figure 37–3
Electrode hook-up on a patient's leg. (From Electrocardiography: A Better Way. Milton, WI, The Burdick Corp., 1976.)

Standard, or Bipolar, Leads. The first three leads recorded are called the standard, or bipolar, leads. They are referred to as bipolar because they each use two limb electrodes to record the electric activity. Roman numerals are used to designate these leads (Fig. 37–6).

- Lead I records the electric activity between the right arm and the left arm.
- Lead II records the electric activity between the right arm and the left leg.
- Lead III records the electric activity between the left arm and the left leg.

HELP IN TRACING AN ERROR IN PLACEMENT OF THE BIPOLAR LIMB LEADS

1. If there is interference in limb leads I and II, check the electrode connection on the patient's right arm.
2. If there is interference in limb leads I and III, check the electrode connection on the patient's left arm.
3. If there is interference in limb leads II and III, check the electrode connection on the patient's left leg.

Augmented Leads. The next three leads recorded are the augmented leads. They are AVR, AVL, and AVF. The AV stands for augmented voltage, the R for right arm, the L for left arm, and the F for foot. These leads are unipolar.

- *Lead AVR* records the electric activity from the midpoint between the left arm and the left leg to the right arm (Fig. 37–7A).
- *Lead AVL* records the electric activity from the midpoint between the right arm and the left leg to the left arm (Fig. 37–7B).
- *Lead AVF* records the electric activity from the midpoint between the right arm and the left arm to the left leg (Fig. 37–7C).

Chest, or Precordial, Leads. The last six leads are the chest, or **precordial**, leads. These leads are unipolar and are designated as V1, V2, V3, V4, V5, and V6. Each number signifies the position of the electrode on the chest (Fig. 37–8). Leads V1 through V6 record the electric activity between six points on the chest wall and a point within the heart.

Standardization

Standardization has been determined by an international agreement to ensure that an ECG can be interpreted anywhere in the world. It assumes that the electrocardiograph used has been calibrated

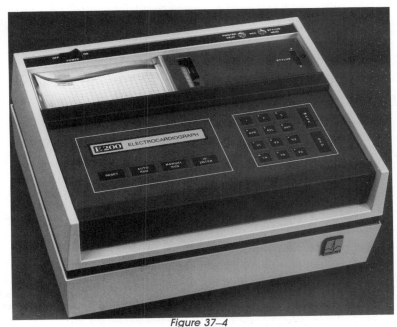

Figure 37–4

Electrocardiograph. (Courtesy of The Burdick Corp., Milton, WI.)

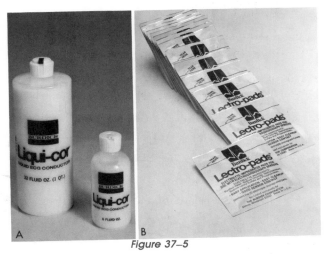

Figure 37–5

Forms of electrolytes. **A**, Electrolyte paste. **B**, Presaturated electrolyte pads. These pads are often preferred because they are not as messy, and they ensure that identical amounts of electrolyte will be at each electrode while eliminating the need for prepping swabs. (Courtesy of The Burdick Corp., Milton, WI.)

Table 37–2

The Standard Marking Codes

	Electrodes Connected	Marking Code
Standard or Bipolar Limb Leads		
Lead 1	LA & RA	•
Lead 2	LL & RA	••
Lead 3	LL & LA	•••
Augmented Unipolar Limb Leads		
AVR	RA & (LA-LL)	—
AVL	LA & (RA-LL)	——
AVF	LL & (RA-LA)	———
Chest or Precordial Leads		
V	C & (LA-RA-LL)	V1 —•
		V2 —••
		V3 —•••
		V4 —••••
		V5 —•••••
		V6 —••••••

(Courtesy of The Burdick Corp., Milton WI.)

[handwritten notes: Count 1 / count / 4 Dashes M / 5 Dashes / 6 dashes / Put it on Pause / Dashes only / count M]

37

according to universal measurements. Before recording a patient's tracing, you must make certain that the machine is correctly standardized.

When a machine is "in standard" (1 STD), 1 millivolt (mV) of electricity causes the stylus to move vertically 10 mm. Thus, it is possible to calculate electric voltages on the vertical axis, by the vertical movement of the stylus on the paper. The stylus should deflect exactly 10 mm when the

standardization button is depressed with a quick pecking motion. The standardization should also be 2 mm wide and rectangular in shape. Each manufacturer's manual explains the method of adjustment to obtain a perfect standardization.

Most machines have three standard (STD) positions that may be used. They are 1/2 STD, 1 STD, and 2 STD. When recording 1/2 STD, 1 mV causes the stylus to deflect 5 mm. If the amplitude (height)

[handwritten note: Must move 10 square up when moving]

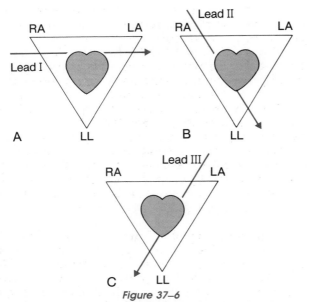

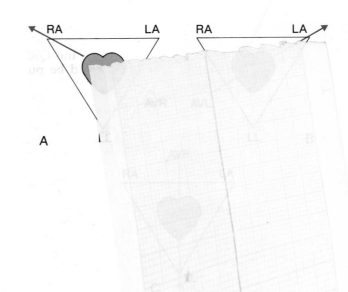

Figure 37-6

The standard limb leads record the electric activity of the heart from three angles. **A,** Limb lead I. The angle recording the heart's voltage between the right arm and the left arm. **B,** Limb lead II. The angle recording the heart's voltage between the right arm and the left leg. **C,** Limb lead III. The angle recording the heart's voltage between the left arm and the left leg.

The augmented lead. When two leads are wired together the machine "thinks" it is recording halfway between the electrodes thus giving a picture of the heart. **A,** AVR is the recording made from the midpoint between LA and LL to RA. **B,** AVL is the recording made from the midpoint between RA and LL to LA. **C,** AVF is the recording made from the midpoint between RA and LA to LL.

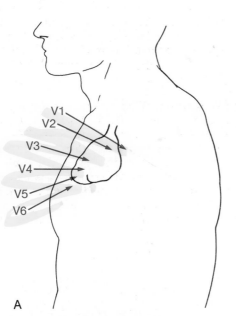

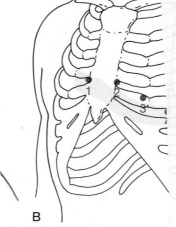

Figure 37-8

A, Chest leads. The chest leads record an additional six views of the heart. From the total of 12 recordings that make up an ECG series—three standard, three augmented, and six chest leads—the physician is able to determine much about the welfare of the heart. **B,** The anatomic placement for each individual chest electrode. V1, Fourth intercostal space at right margin of sternum; V2, fourth intercostal space at left margin of sternum; V3, midway between position 2 and position 4; V4, fifth intercostal space at junction of left midclavicular line; V5, at horizontal level of position 4 at left anterior axillary line; V6, at horizontal level of position 4 at left midaxillary line.

of the QRS complex is too high and is causing the stylus to move off the paper, the machine should be put on 1/2 STD. If the amplitude of the QRS complex is too small, the machine should be put on 2 STD, causing the stylus to deflect 20 mm. Figure 37–9 shows the three standard positions. Make note of any variation from the normal 1 STD. Standardization is usually performed at the beginning of the first lead recording, although some physicians require a standardization within each of the 12 lead recordings.

As mentioned, the universal standard for recording an electrocardiogram is at a speed of 25 mm/second. If the patient's heart rate is very rapid or if certain parts of the complex are too close together, it may be necessary to adjust the paper run to 50 mm/second. This will double the speed of the paper run and extend the recording to twice its normal length (Fig. 37–10). Again, make certain that this is noted on the tracing.

Artifacts

An artifact is unwanted movement of the stylus on the paper produced by outside electric interference. The electrocardiograph is extremely sensitive to any kind of electric activity. Artifacts on the tracing make the interpretation of the recording difficult. The medical assistant should have a thorough understanding of the causes of and remedies for these artifacts. The types of artifacts include wandering baseline, somatic tremor, alternating current, and baseline interruption.

Wandering Baseline. This artifact is a gradual shifting of the stylus away from the center of the paper, usually resulting from unnoticed movement of the patient (Fig. 37–11). If this occurs, remind the patient to remain still. Other causes include electrodes that are corroded or dirty or have been applied too loosely or too tightly; tension on the electrode from a dangling cable; poor-quality electrolyte paste, or too little applied to the electrode; and improper preparation of the patient's skin prior to applying the electrolyte.

Somatic Tremor. Somatic tremor means "muscle movement." Natural electric voltage from muscle movement causes additional stylus movement across the paper. This results in a recording with jagged peaks of irregular height and spacing, and a shifting baseline (Fig. 37–12). Usually, this is because the patient is uncomfortable, apprehensive, moving or talking, or suffering from a disorder that causes body tremors. Explaining the procedure beforehand helps to alleviate apprehension and relaxes the patient. Re-position the patient comfortably, or offer the patient a pillow. Sometimes it helps to place the patient's hands under the buttocks, or ask the patient to take deep breaths. Chills cause somatic tremor. Check the room temperature. The physician may prescribe a sedative for the patient who is having great difficulty in relaxing.

Alternating Current. Commonly known as AC interference, this artifact appears as a series of uniform, small spiked lines on the paper (Fig. 37–13). Alternating current present in nearby equipment or wires can radiate small amounts of energy into the room where the ECG is being performed. Some of this energy can be detected by the sensitive electrocardiograph. Unplug other electric appliances in the room. Move the patient table to another area of the room, or turn the table around. Move the table away from the wall, since the interference may be in the electric wiring in the wall or in an adjoining room. Make certain that your patient is not touching anything off the patient table. If necessary, turn off the overhead fluorescent lights.

If none of the aforementioned procedures eliminates the AC interference, check the machine for proper grounding. You may need to use an external ground wire provided with the machine. Be certain to follow the manufacturer's directions. Check to see that the lead wires are not crossed. Also check the electrodes to be certain they are clean.

Baseline Interruption. This occurs when the electric connection has been interrupted. The stylus moves onto the margin of the paper (Fig. 37–14). The stylus moves violently up and down, or it may record a straight line across the top or the bottom of the paper. Most baseline interruption is caused by noticeable patient movement jarring the electrodes. Other causes can be a broken wire in the patient cable, or cable tips that are attached too loosely to the electrodes.

37

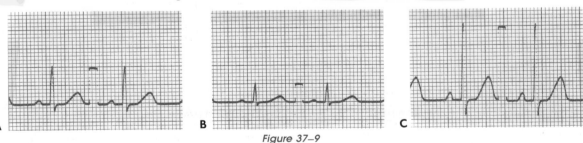

Figure 37–9

Sensitivity control. **A,** Correct standardization of 1 cm (10 mm). **B,** ½ is at half sensitivity of 0.5 cm (5 mm). **C,** 2 is double the sensitivity of 2 cm (20 mm). (From Electrocardiography: A Better Way. Milton, WI, The Burdick Corp., 1976.)

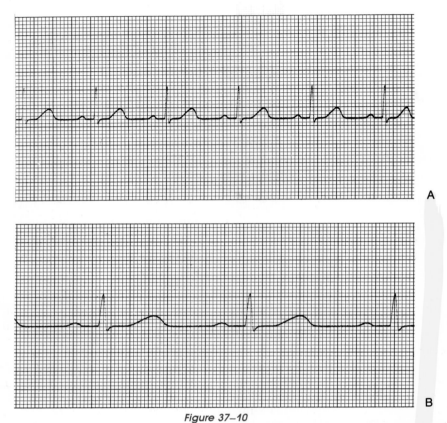

Figure 37–10

Paper run. **A,** *Run 25 is the normal speed for recording, 25 mm per second.* **B,** *Run 50 mm per second. It is used when the heart rate is very rapid, and the complexes are too close together. This extends the complexes twice as far apart.*

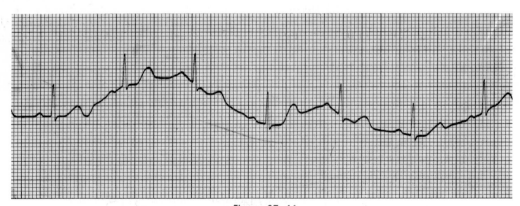

Figure 37–11

Wandering baseline. (Courtesy of The Burdick Corp., Milton, WI.)

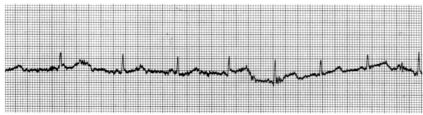

Figure 37–12

Somatic tremor. (Courtesy of The Burdick Corp., Milton, WI.)

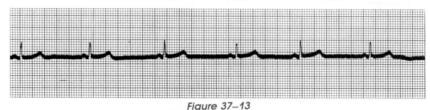

Figure 37–13

AC interference. (Courtesy of The Burdick Corp., Milton, WI.)

OBTAINING THE ELECTROCARDIOGRAM

Preparing the Room and the Patient

The room should be free from interruptions, and the machine should be as far away from other electric equipment as possible. This includes x-ray machines, diathermy equipment, centrifuges, electric fans, refrigerators, and air conditioners. The room should be quiet and warm.

The treatment table should be comfortable and wide enough to avoid muscle movement. The table should be wood or should have some form of insulation between metal legs or surfaces. It is best to position the table so that you are working from the patient's left side.

Small pillows are helpful in relaxing the patient. One pillow may be used under the patient's head, but it should not be pressing down on or elevating the patient's shoulders. A small pillow placed under the patient's knees may also help relax the muscles of the abdomen and the lower extremities.

The patient should be supine, with arms at the sides and the legs not touching one another. If this is not possible, the patient may be placed in a semi-Fowler position or may be seated on a wooden chair. In the sitting position, the patient's feet should be on the floor on a rubber mat or on a wooden footstool or a stack of books. The legs must not hang free, nor should there be any pressure on the back of the lower thighs. If the patient is in a sitting or semi-Fowler position, it is necessary to make a note of this on the patient's recording.

The patient is to disrobe to the waist, and the lower legs are exposed. A patient gown should be put on, with the opening in the front. Shoes and nylons must be removed. Loosen all tight clothing.

It is advisable to have the patient rest for at least ten minutes prior to the recording. Check to determine whether the patient was able to follow the instructions given (Fig. 37–15). Be certain to note on the patient's record any medications that are taken.

Explain the nature and purpose of the electrocardiogram to the patient. Chat with the patient while

37

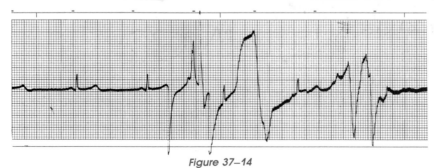

Figure 37–14

Baseline interruption. (Courtesy of The Burdick Corp., Milton, WI.)

INSTRUCTIONS FOR PATIENT BEFORE TAKING AN ELECTROCARDIOGRAM

Name: _____

Your cardiogram appointment is _____, _____ at _____ a.m.
                                     Day   Date   Time   p.m.

These instructions are simple, but it is important you follow them. Please call us if you are unable to follow these instructions or keep your appointment so we may make another appointment.

1. There is no discomfort or sensation in taking an electrocardiogram. No electricity is put into the patient in any way. Small metal plates are placed on the calf of each leg and on each arm, and at different places on the chest. The minute impulse generated by your heart is simply picked up by these plates and recorded by the machine.

2. You will be asked to lie down on a comfortable table while the test is being made by the technician.

3. For your convenience it is best to wear loose clothing, and you will be asked to disrobe to your waist to expose the chest. It will also be necessary to expose your lower legs from the knees down and the upper arms just below the shoulders.

4. The actual test only takes about five minutes, but you will be asked to rest for about half an hour before the test. It is best you do not have a heavy meal for about two hours before the test. There should not be any consumption of cold drinks, ice cream or smoking just before the test. It is also advisable to refrain from excessive exercise just prior to the test. Do not take any medications without the physician's usual instructions and knowledge.

5. During the test you will be asked to lie absolutely still and relax, as the slightest movement interferes with an accurate tracing. Do not talk.

6. The skin on the legs, arms, and chest must be free from skin ointments, oils, and medications.

7. The technician taking the test is especially trained to take the test but is unable to tell you the results of the test, as she is neither trained nor authorized to make any interpretations of the cardiogram. This is the task of the physician.

Figure 37–15

Example of an instruction sheet that is given to the patient at the time the appointment is made for an ECG.

preparing for the procedure. Stress the importance of not moving during the entire procedure, and assure the patient that no electric shock will be felt. Allow time for the patient to ask questions or to express any concerns before you begin the tracing.

Applying the Electrodes and Lead Wires

Expose the patient's arms and legs. Attach an electrode strap to each electrode, then place a small amount of electrolyte on each electrode. Make certain that you have the same amount on each electrode. With the electrode, rub the electrolyte into the skin on the fleshy part of the arms and legs. Rub the skin's surface until a slight **erythema** appears. Wipe off any excess electrolyte. Do not allow your hands to carry the electrolyte from the patient to the equipment. Unequal amounts of electrolyte or the spreading of it to the wires and equipment may cause artifacts.

Position the electrodes with the lead connectors pointing toward the hands and the feet. Place the electrodes on the prepared skin areas. Place each strap around the limb until the hole just meets the hook. Then move the strap one hole tighter, and fasten it. This should provide the correct tension. An accurate tracing cannot be made if the straps are too loose or too tight.

Leave the disc-shaped chest electrode unattached and not directly touching any surface. It will be moved to the six chest points, one lead at a time, during the procedure. A *Welch electrode* is bulb-shaped and may be used for the chest leads. Many multichanneled ECGs use Welch electrodes, which are all connected at the same time. Locate each of the chest lead sites. Squeeze a dab of electrolyte on each electrode site and pinch the bulb slightly. Take care that the bulbs do not touch each other.

Insert the tips of the lead cords into the lead connector holes of the leg and arm electrodes. Check to make certain that you have connected the correct lead terminal into the corresponding electrode. The lead cords are color-coded, but it is still easy to confuse the patient's right and left sides. Rest the patient cable on the patient's abdomen to prevent drag on the cable, which can cause an improper electrode connection. Check to make certain that each lead cord terminal is tight. Plug the patient cable into the patient cable jack on the machine, making certain that it is pushed in all the way.

Procedure 37–1

APPLYING ECG ELECTRODES AND LEAD WIRES

PROCEDURAL GOAL

To create an environment in which your patient is relaxed and at ease, and to properly apply the electrodes and lead wires.

EQUIPMENT AND SUPPLIES

Electrocardiograph
Electrolyte
Electrocardiograph paper
Electrodes
Patient cable
Chest lead strap
Patient gown
Drape sheet
Electrocardiography table
Quiet room
Table paper

PROCEDURE

1. Wash your hands.
2. Gather all the materials needed.
3. Greet and identify the patient.
   Purpose: Identification of the patient is extremely important, to ensure that you have the right patient.
4. Explain the procedure.
   Purpose: Explanations help gain patient cooperation and alleviate apprehension.

Procedure continued on following page

5. Ask the patient to disrobe from the waist up and to remove clothing from the lower legs. Jewelry must be removed.
6. Assist the patient onto the ECG table, and cover the patient with a drape sheet.
   Purpose: To ensure the safety and the modesty of the patient.
7. Make certain that the patient is physically comfortable.
   Purpose: A comfortable and relaxed patient helps reduce somatic tremor.
8. Position the patient so that you are working on the patient's left side, near the heart. Run the power cord away from the patient (below).
   Purpose: These precautions help reduce AC interference.

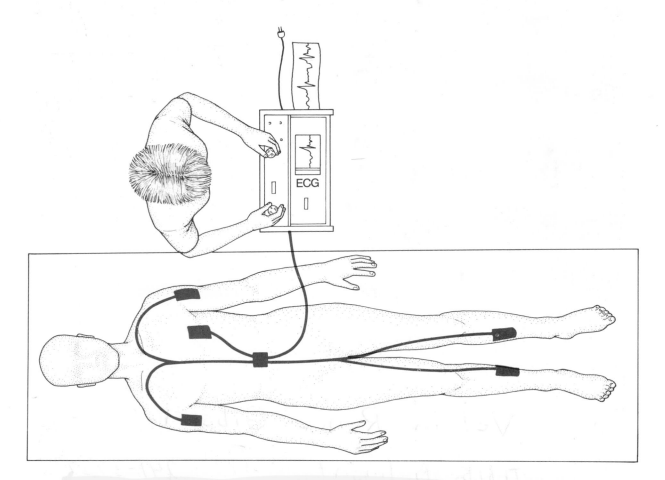

9. Attach the rubber straps to the electrodes and prepare the skin with an electrolyte, using equal amounts at each site. Presaturated electrolyte pads may be used (opposite page, top left).
   Purpose: Unequal amounts of the electrolyte can cause a wandering baseline.
10. Rub the electrolyte briskly into the skin with the electrode (opposite page, top right).
    Purpose: The skin is a poor conductor of electricity, and the electrolyte helps in the conduction of the currents.
11. Place the electrode on the fleshiest portion of the upper arms and lower legs, keeping the lead connectors pointing toward the fingers and the feet (opposite page, bottom left).
    Purpose: The fleshiest parts of the skin minimize chances for somatic tremors.
12. Wrap the rubber straps around each limb until the hole just meets the hook. Then stretch the strap one hole tighter, and fasten it (opposite page, bottom right).
    Purpose: Electrodes that are too tight or too loose could result in artifacts.

Procedure continued on opposite page

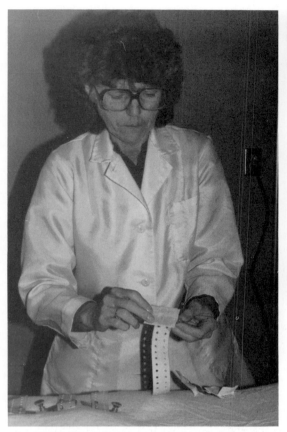

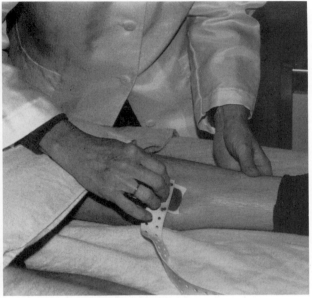

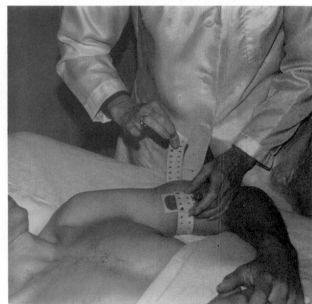

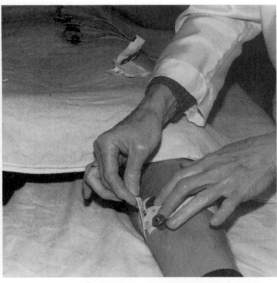

Procedure continued on following page

37

13. Prepare the chest electrode by releasing the rubber ring surrounding the electrode. Lay a folded presaturated electrolyte pad over the metal, and snap the rubber ring in place (below, left).

14. Adjust the chest strap so that the strap weight rests near the right anterior axillary line, and place its plastic anchor plate under the patient's chest, at the level of V4, V5, and V6. The free end of the strap should be placed next to the patient, with the concave side of the weight toward the patient's chest (below, right).

   Purpose: This makes it easier to use the strap when you are running the chest leads.

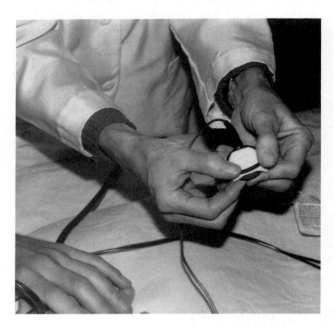
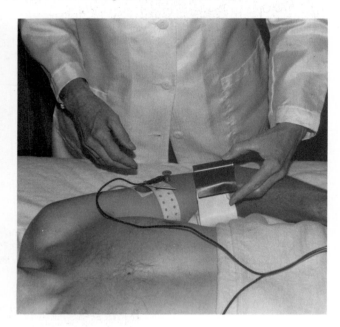

15. Locate V1, place the electrode in V1, and lay the strap over it. Do not stretch the strap. Make certain that the weighted end does not rest on the arm or on the table (below, and following page, top left and right).

   Purpose: These precautions reduce artifacts.

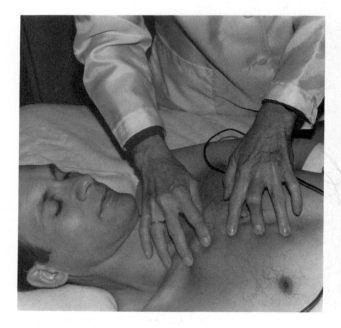
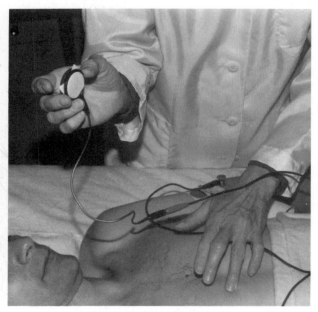

Procedure continued on opposite page

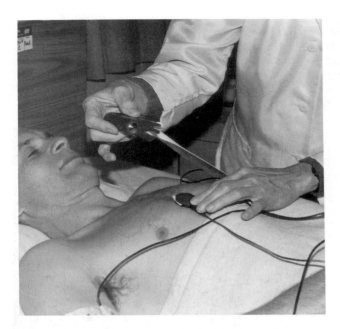 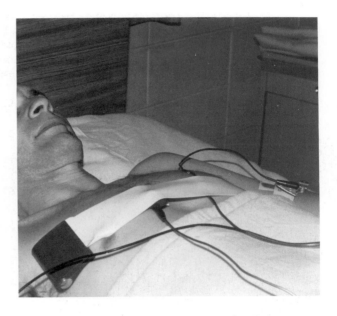

Note: Welch electrodes may be used throughout the chest leads. Locate each of the chest lead sites. Squeeze a dab of electrolyte on each electrode site, and pinch the bulb slightly. Take care that they do not touch each other. Welch electrodes are all connected at the same time (below, and following page, top left and right).

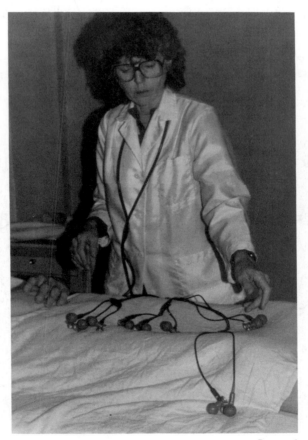

37

Procedure continued on following page

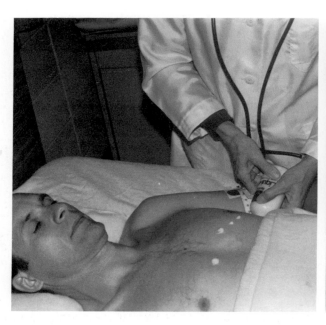
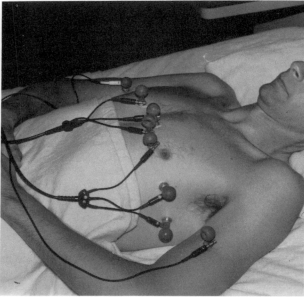

16. Attach the lead wires of the patient cable to the electrodes.
17. Plug the patient cable into the patient cable jack on the machine.
18. Position the lead cable so that it follows the contours of the patient's body and avoids making large loops. To avoid drag, lay the patient cable on the abdomen (below).
    Purpose: Large cable loops produce AC interference, and cable drag causes a wandering baseline.

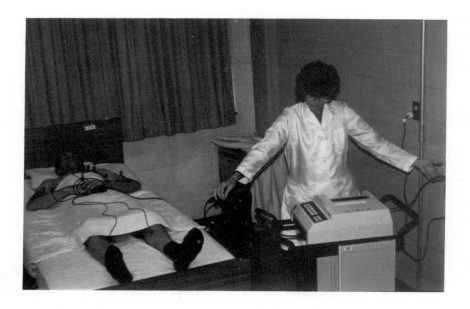

TERMINAL PERFORMANCE OBJECTIVE

Given the appropriate supplies, properly prepare the patient for an electrocardiogram, within ten minutes, by correctly completing each step of the procedure in the proper order, as determined by your evaluator.

Recording the Electrocardiogram

You are now ready to record the patient's electrocardiogram.

Limb Leads. Plug in the electrocardiograph, and allow it to warm up. Check the manufacturer's instructions for the specific amount of warm-up time needed. Set the *lead selector control* to *STD*. Turn the *recorder control* to *ON* and then to *RUN*. Using the *position control knob*, center the *stylus* on the baseline. Check the standardization by pressing the *standardization button* to a height of 10 mm.

After obtaining a proper standardization, turn the *lead selector control* to *lead I*. Code the lead immediately unless the machine does so automatically. Run 8 to 12 inches of the tracing. Switch to *lead II* and *lead III*, and repeat the same steps. Run

[handwritten: il Chicks of the machine]

4 to 6 inches of *AVR*, *AVL*, and *AVF*. Turn the machine to *OFF* while preparing to record the chest leads.

[handwritten: or 7 chicks of the Machine]
[handwritten: Turn Machine on pause]
[handwritten: 7 chick]

Chest Leads. Locate and apply the electrolyte over the six chest locations on the patient. The run begins with the chest electrode over the chest lead V1. Turn the *lead selector control* to either *V* or *V1*, depending on the machine, and the *recorder switch* to *RUN*. Run 4 to 6 inches of recording. Standardize and code the lead. Turn the *recorder switch* to *OFF*. Turning to *OFF* prevents excessive movement of the stylus. Move the chest electrode to V2, V3, V4, V5, and V6, repeating the steps. Having completed all chest leads, slowly turn the *lead selector control* back to *STD*, one lead at a time, in order to avoid possible stripping of the gears in the dial. Run a straight baseline, and turn the *recorder switch* to *OFF*. Unplug the machine.

Procedure 37–2

RECORDING AN ELECTROCARDIOGRAM

PROCEDURAL GOAL

To record a 12-lead ECG tracing of a properly prepared patient.

EQUIPMENT AND SUPPLIES

Electrocardiograph
Electrocardiograph paper
Electrodes
Patient cable
Chest lead strap

PROCEDURE

1. Wash your hands.
2. Greet and identify your patient if you have not already done so while applying the electrodes and lead wires.
3. Plug in the electrocardiograph.
   Purpose: Some machines need a warm-up period.
4. Set the lead selector to STD and the recorder switch to ON.
5. Turn the recorder switch to RUN.
6. Center the baseline, using the position control knob.
7. Check that the standardization is 10 mm.
   Purpose: Universal standard of ECG measurement is ensured.
8. Turn the lead selector control to lead I and record 8 to 10 inches of the lead. Code the lead.
   Purpose: Coding is necessary for identifying the lead.
9. Record leads II, III, AVR, AVL, and AVF, and code them in the same manner by turning the lead selector to the appropriate position. Run the augmented leads 4 to 6 inches only.
10. Turn the machine off.
11. Position the chest electrode for lead V1.
12. Turn the selector control to STD and the recorder switch to RUN, and insert a standardization.
    Purpose: Ensures continued calibration of the machine.
13. Turn the selector control to V and the recorder switch to ON, and obtain a 5- to 6-inch tracing. Code the lead. Turn the recorder switch off.

Procedure continued on following page

37

Purpose: Turning the switch off when changing the chest electrodes keeps the stylus from moving about.

14. Move the chest electrode to the next position, and repeat the previous step for all remaining chest leads.

15. Turn the lead selector to STD slowly, and run out until a baseline only appears. Then turn the recorder switch to OFF, and unplug the machine.

Purpose: Turning the selector rapidly can cause stripping of the gears in the dial.

(handwritten: Metal is a good conductor)

TERMINAL PERFORMANCE OBJECTIVE

Given the appropriate supplies, properly record an electrocardiogram tracing, within ten minutes, by correctly completing each step of the procedure in the proper order, as determined by your evaluator.

POST-TEST PROCEDURES

Equipment Maintenance

Tear off the tracing from the machine. Immediately label the tracing with the patient's name, the date, and your initials. Roll the tracing loosely with the recording on the inside, and place a small paper clip on the very edge. Do not roll tightly, and do not attach the paper clip over any part of the tracing. Tracings scratch easily and should be carefully handled. Set the tracing aside.

Remove the tips of the lead wires from the electrodes, unfasten the rubber straps, and remove the electrodes from the patient. Clean the electrode sites with a warm, wet paper towel, and dry. Assist the patient to a sitting position, but let the patient remain on the table for a few moments. After the patient rests, assist the patient off the table and with dressing, if needed. Change the table paper, and discard any used disposable materials.

Clean the rubber straps with a mild detergent, and dry them. The electrodes must be cleaned with a mild detergent first, then polished with a fine grade of scouring powder. Do not use steel wool or any metal-base polish, as it will interfere with the tracing and cause artifacts. Always rinse the electrodes well, and let them dry before storing them. Use an applicator to clean the connecting holes and the inside of the suction-type chest electrode. Store the machine plug, patient cable, electrodes, rubber straps, and electrolyte near the machine.

Mounting an Electrocardiogram

Today there are many different types of mounts. An office should select the mount that is best adapted to its needs. It is advisable to select a mount that can be easily read in its entirety on one surface. Because tracings are usually a series of records over a period of years, a mount that will last with the passing of time should be selected.

The slotted-type folder best protects the tracings. It can be mounted on one surface and has a longer limb lead, but it is more expensive and takes more filing space. The slotted-folder also takes longer to mount than some of the other styles.

Paper clips and staples should not be used, as they will scratch a tracing. Clear tape can be used, but some tape becomes sticky or yellow with time. Copy machines can be used to make a single-sheet copy of the tracing without damaging the original record. Photocopies take up less filing space.

Regardless of the style of mount used, each ECG should be neatly and carefully mounted, with complete information recorded on each one. The following information must appear on the mount:

- Patient's full name
- Sex
- Age
- Date of ECG
- Medications
- Variation from normal STD and variation from a machine speed of 25 mm/sec

A notation should be made of any variation from the routine, such as a very nervous patient, a different position of the patient, lack of rest before the test, or smoking immediately before the test. If the lead placements were different from the routine, this also should be noted.

Extreme care should be taken when mounting. Do not allow your desk to become cluttered with tracing trimmings. Discard the trimmings into a waste container as you trim them off. Most tracings are easily scratched, so be careful not to damage the tracing with finger rings or sleeve buttons. Do not stack other items on top of the open-faced type of mount.

Do not cut off the lead coding until you are ready to mount that particular lead. Double-check each lead code with the mount placement. Some mounts place the precordial leads horizontally, whereas others place them vertically. Take great care not to mount a lead upside down. If you have been requested to show the STD in a lead, then be careful not to cut it off. Do not cover the tips of the QRS complexes with the sides of the slotted-type mount. Place the mounted ECG tracing on the physician's desk for evaluation with the patient's medical record and any previous ECG tracings.

Procedure 37-3

PROCEDURAL GOAL

To create an appropriate environment for the patient and equipment following an ECG tracing, and to correctly mount the electrocardiogram for the physician to use as an effective and accurate diagnostic tool.

EQUIPMENT AND SUPPLIES

Electrocardiograph
Electrocardiograph paper
Electrodes
Patient cable
Chest lead strap
Cleaning materials
An ECG mount

PROCEDURE

1. Tear off the tracing, and immediately label it with the patient's name, the date, and your initials.
   Purpose: This avoids mix-ups in identification.
2. Disconnect the lead wires from the electrodes, and remove the electrodes from the patient.
3. Wash the electrolyte from the patient's limbs and chest.
   Purpose: Electrolyte solution can cause irritation or can soil clothing.
4. Assist the patient from the table and with dressing, if needed.
   Purpose: Patients may appear weary from the procedure.
5. Clean and dry the electrodes and rubber straps.
6. Discard disposable materials.
7. Store supplies and equipment.
8. Wash your hands.
9. Mount the ECG.
   Purpose: Provides the physician with a easily readable and available form for interpretation.

TERMINAL PERFORMANCE OBJECTIVE

Given the appropriate supplies, properly help the patient after an ECG procedure, clean the work area, and mount the ECG tracing within ten minutes, by correctly completing each step of the procedure in the proper order, as determined by your evaluator.

Interpretation of the Electrocardiogram

Two important heart functions that can be determined by the physician when interpreting the electrocardiogram are heart rate and heart rhythm.

Heart Rate. On the ECG tracing, all heartbeats consist of P waves, QRS complexes, and T waves. It is possible to calculate heart rate on the horizontal axis by measuring the distance between two R waves. To determine the heart rate per minute, divide 300 (the number of 5-mm increments that the ECG paper advances in one minute) by the number of 5-mm increments between the two R waves.

Heart Rhythm. Heart rhythm is determined as being either regular or irregular. The horizontal distance between the P waves is first measured. If the distance is the same, atrial rhythm is regular, and if not, it is irregular. Next, measure the horizontal distance between the R waves. If the distance is the same, ventricular rhythm is regular, and if not, it is irregular.

CARDIAC STRESS TESTING

Cardiac stress testing is conducted to observe and record the patient's cardiovascular response to measured exercise challenges. Stress testing is performed to diagnose cardiac disease that cannot be

37

CARDIAC STRESS TEST

Cardiac stress testing (also known as an exercise tolerance test or treadmill test) is a means of observing, evaluating, and recording your heart's response during a measured exercise test. This test determines your capacity to adapt to physical stress.

There are various reasons that your physician may suggest this test for you:

1. To aid in determining the presence of suspected coronary heart disease.
2. To aid in the selection of therapy.
   a. For angina pectoris (tightness or pain in the chest).
   b. Following a myocardial infarction (heart attack)
   c. Following coronary bypass surgery (open heart surgery).
3. To determine your physical work capacity.
4. To authorize participation in a physical exercise program.

Preparation for the Test

1. Avoid eating a heavy meal within two hours of your appointment.
2. Take your medications as you usually do, unless your doctor advises you not to take them.
3. Wear a shirt or blouse that buttons down the front with slacks, a skirt, jogging pants, or shorts.
4. Do not wear one-piece undergarments, jumpsuits, or dresses.
5. Tennis shoes are ideal if you have them. Otherwise, wear comfortable flat or low-heeled shoes. Do not wear clogs, sling-backs, crepe soles, boots, or high heels, as they make walking on the treadmill more difficult.

The Procedure

When you arrive in the Cardiology Department, areas of your chest may be shaved (men only) to allow the electrodes to adhere lightly to your chest. A blood pressure cuff will be wrapped around your arm, and an electrocardiogram (ECG) is taken while your are at rest. The technician will then demonstrate how to walk on the treadmill and will answer any questions you may have.

You will then perform a graded exercise test on a motor-driven treadmill. You will begin walking very gradually at a rate you can easily accomplish.

Progressively throughout the test, the speed and grade of the treadmill will be increased, you will be walking at a faster pace up a slight incline. At no time will you be asked to jog or run, nor will you be asked to exercise beyond your capabilities.

At all times during the test, trained personnel are in the room with you, monitoring your heart rate and blood pressure and observing you for signs of fatigue or discomfort. We do not wish to exercise you to a level that is medically unsafe or physically distressing.

An ECG is taken again when you finish walking. Your cardiologist will immediately interpret the results of the test and explain his findings to you. If necessary, medications or treatment will be discussed. A letter with the results of the stress test will be sent to your referring physician.

The entire procedure will take 1–1 1/2 hours. If you have any questions regarding the cardiac stress test or any problems with your appointment, please contact us.

detected by the standard resting ECG; to determine an individual's energy performance capacity; or to prescribe a specially designed exercise plan. The stress test is done while the patient is exercising on either a bicycle or a treadmill and under careful supervision.

After you have carefully recorded a patient's history, inform the patient of the details of the procedure. The purpose of the test is to increase physical exertion until a *target heart rate* is reached or signs of deficiency of blood supply to the heart appear. A consent form must be read and signed by the patient. Some offices publish information booklets for their patients (see following).

The chest electrodes are placed on the patient and are connected to the cable wires. One team member demonstrates how to walk on the treadmill. The patient's blood pressure and heart rate are recorded before the test begins. The treadmill is turned on, and a continuous ECG is run during the exercise (Fig. 37–16). The patient's blood pressure and heart rate are also monitored. Immediately after the termination of the test, the blood pressure and heart rate are again recorded. A post-resting ECG is then run on the monitor for five minutes before the patient is discharged.

Stress testing can cause **cardiac arrest.** The medical assistant must be able to recognize symptoms of **dyspnea**, **vertigo**, extreme fatigue, severe **arrhythmia**, and other abnormal ECG readings that may develop during the stress test.

All members of a cardiac stress testing team must be trained in cardiopulmonary resuscitation and must be prepared to terminate testing immediately if the patient is unable to continue or when abnormalities appear on the monitor. It is imperative that the physician be present during this procedure. Besides the monitoring equipment, oxygen and a **defibrillator** must be on hand in the event of cardiac crisis.

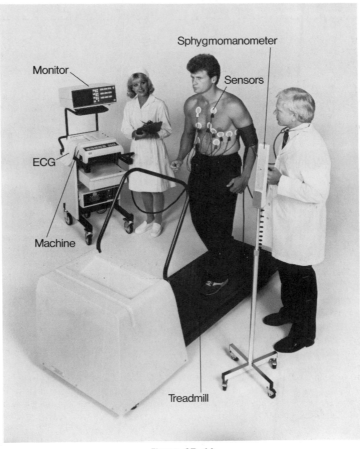

Figure 37–16

Stress test. The medical team in this picture is conducting a stress test. The patient uses the treadmill as directed by the physician, and the patient's heart reaction is displayed on the monitor and is recorded. (Courtesy of The Burdick Corp., Milton, WI.)

REFERENCES AND READINGS

Bonewit, K.: *Clinical Procedures for Medical Assistants*, 2nd ed. Philadelphia, W. B. Saunders Co., 1984.

Burdick ECG Technician Training Program. Minneapolis, MN, presentation by Ronald Korth, Sept. 20, 1984.

Cave, J., Hill, J., and Schrader, P. (eds.): *Catalog of Performance Objectives, Criterion-Referenced Measures, and Performance Guides for the Medical Assistant.* Kentucky. Vocational-Technical Education Consortium of States, 1978.

Electrocardiography—A Better Way. Milton, WI, The Burdick Corp., 1983.

Van Meter, M., and Lavine, P. G.: *Reading ECG's Correctly*, 7th ed. Horsham, PA, Intermed Communications Inc., 1981.

Wyngaarden, J. B., and Smith, L. H., Jr.: *Cecil Textbook of Medicine*, 17th ed., Part VII: Cardiovascular Diseases. Philadelphia, W. B. Saunders Co., 1985.

37

CHAPTER OUTLINE

VOCABULARY

See Glossary at end of book for definitions.

ionizing
rad
radiation
rem
roentgen

38

Assisting With Diagnostic Radiology

OBJECTIVES

Upon successful completion of this chapter you should be able to

1. *Define and spell the words listed in the Vocabulary for this chapter.*
2. *Explain the medical assistant's role related to x-ray procedures.*
3. *List and explain four basic x-ray views.*
4. *Identify the parts of the x-ray machine.*
5. *Discuss the steps involved in x-ray film processing.*
6. *State the purpose of using a contrast medium.*
7. *Identify safety hazards and precautionary measures pertinent to x-ray equipment.*
8. *Discuss the proper care and storage of radiographs in the physician's office.*
9. *Discuss the various special diagnostic procedures, specifically, fluoroscopy, mammography, stereoscopy, thermography, computerized axial tomography, and xeroradiography.*
10. *Recall at least three side effects of radiation overdose.*
11. *Name two things that a patient may be required to do in preparation for an x-ray film.*
12. *Differentiate between diagnostic and therapeutic x-ray procedures.*

Upon successful completion of this chapter you should be able to perform the following activities:

1. *Explain proper preparation of selected radiologic examinations to patients.*
2. *Assist with positioning patients for selected radiologic examinations.*
3. *Assist with the exposing and developing of x-ray films.*
4. *Demonstrate the proper filing of x-ray films and reports.*

Radiology is the specialty of medical science that deals with the study, diagnosis, and treatment of diseases by the use of x-rays, radioactive substances, and other forms of radiant energy. A *radiologist* is a physician who specializes in radiology. *Radiologic technology* is an allied health profession of its own. Technicians spend many years learning to become skilled in this medical specialty. The procedures involved in radiology can be divided into three specialties: diagnostic radiology, radiotherapy, and nuclear medicine. *— Skeletal System*

injected with a radioactive substance — Localize any abnormal Area

The equipment used in radiology is very sophisticated and expensive. It is used primarily by physicians whose specialties require the extensive use of x-ray films, such as orthopedists. Today, patients are usually referred to a radiologist's private practice for any x-ray work-ups.

Medical assistants may schedule the x-ray procedures, record the results, and file the films. Therefore, you must be familiar with radiologic terms and procedures. Physicians who practice general or family medicine may have x-ray equipment available for the occasional chest x-ray film or an x-ray film needed in an emergency. In these situations, the medical assistant may be called upon to expose and develop the film as well as position and prepare the patient for the procedure.

Before proceeding with the main focus of this chapter, a brief introduction is needed about medical assistants and the federal and state regulations that apply in taking and exposing x-rays.

The Consumer-Patient Radiation Health and Safety Act of 1981 directs the Department of Health and Human Services to regulate the training and certification of personnel who administer radiologic procedures in the diagnosis and treatment of injuries and disease in humans. The Act states that

> *Radiographers* perform a comprehensive scope of diagnostic radiologic procedures, and are delegated the responsibility for the operation of radiation-generating equipment. In this law, radiographers are distinguished from personnel whose use of diagnostic procedures is limited to a few specific body sites and/or standard procedures in other clinical specialties, who occasionally may be called upon to assist in diagnostic radiology and whose activities do not, to any significant degree, determine the site or dosage of radiation to which a patient is exposed.

Because medical assistants do not perform a "comprehensive scope of diagnostic radiologic procedures" and because they limit their radiologic procedures to a "few specific body sites" under the direction of a physician, there is considerable question as to whether medical assistants fall within these regulations. Beyond the federal standards, many states also require licensure of any individual who uses equipment that emits **ionizing** radiation. Medical assistants must know their state statutes and must keep informed of any new developments in required credentials.

X-RAYS DEFINED

X-rays, or roentgen rays, were discovered by a physicist, Wilhelm Conrad Roentgen, in 1895. Roentgen received the first Nobel Prize for physics in 1901 for the discovery of these mysterious, or "X," rays. X-rays are a form of **radiation**, similar to light but not visible to the human eye. X-rays have extremely short wavelengths. Their very short wavelength makes them capable of penetrating the body and changing the structure of body cells. Another special property of x-rays is their ability to produce a visible image on film or a fluorescent screen. This visible image produced on special x-ray film is called a *radiograph*.

DIAGNOSTIC RADIOLOGY

Noninvasive procedure — Not opening the body

Diagnostic x-ray procedures allow radiologists to view internal body structures and function. The findings obtained by these procedures help physicians in disease diagnosis and treatment. Today, there are many special diagnostic x-ray procedures available that allow for greater observation inside the body.

A contrast medium is a *radiopaque* substance used *(can be seen)* *(dye)* in diagnostic radiology. It is sometimes used to allow for a more accurate visualization of internal body structures and tissues in contrast to adjacent structures. Contrast media may be gases (air, oxygen, carbon dioxide), heavy metals (barium sulfate, bismuth carbonate), or organic iodines. These can be administered orally, parenterally, or through an enema. Each contrast medium is specific for the examination of a particular organ, body cavity, or passage. The contrast medium makes the area opaque, allowing for both structural and functional visualization as in Figure 38–1. The following is a list of x-ray procedures using a contrast medium and the areas that are visualized:

- angiocardiography—heart and large vessels.
- angiography—blood vessels.
- arteriography—arteries.
- arthrography—joints.
- barium enema—lower intestinal tract. *LGI Large intestine* *(BaE)*
- barium meal—upper intestinal tract (Fig. 38–2). *UGI*
- bronchography—bronchial tree and lungs (Fig. 38–3).
- cholecystography—gallbladder (Fig. 38–4).
- hysterosalpingography—uterus and fallopian tubes (Fig. 38–5).
- intravenous cholangiography—bile ducts.
- intravenous pyelography—renal pelvis, ureters, and bladder (Fig. 38–6). *(IVP)*
- lymphangiography—lymphatic vessels.
- myelography—spinal cord.

Cardiocatheterization — use a dye.

Computed Axial Tomography (CAT Scan). Also known as computed tomography (CT scan), computed axial tomography (CAT scan) was introduced *3D*

M.R.I - Scan has a small opening Magnetic Resonance Imaging, Lay on a table — using the Nonhormal Magnetic of your body no dyes are used.

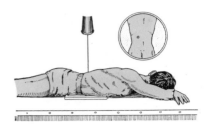

A

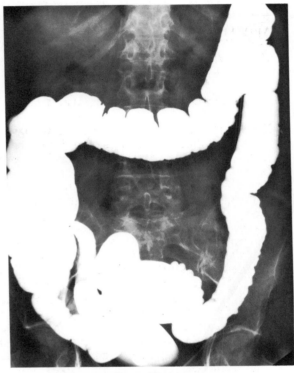

B

Figure 38–1

A, *Positioning the patient for colon x-rays.* **B**, *The radiograph shows the colon distended with barium. (From Meschan, I.: Radiographic Positioning and Related Anatomy, 2nd ed. Philadelphia, W. B. Saunders Co., 1978.)*

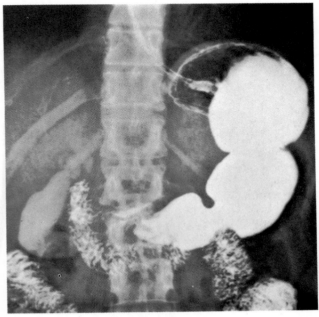

Figure 38–2

Radiograph of the stomach and duodenum (upper GI series). (From Meschan, I., and Ott, D. J.: Introduction to Diagnostic Imaging. Philadelphia, W. B. Saunders Co., 1984.)

ach after a patient swallows a barium mixture. The patient is placed between the x-ray tube and the screen. X-rays pass through the body and project the structures as shadowy images on the screen. The image on the fluoroscope can be recorded on film to produce a permanent record called a photofluorogram.

Mammography. With the advent of new films and exposure techniques, it is now possible to make

in 1972 as another diagnostic x-ray tool. The machine, known as a scanner, examines the body site by rotating a full circle and taking a series of crosssectional x-ray films. Films are made of the structure from all sides. The rates at which the x-rays are absorbed are detected, and a computer calculates the densities into a picture of the body site on a visual screen. The pictures obtained are very detailed and simulate a three-dimensional appearance (Fig. 38–7).

Fluoroscopy. Fluoroscopy, also called radioscopy, is an x-ray examination that permits both structural and functional visualization of internal body structures. Through the use of a contrast medium, motion of a body part can be viewed. Thus, a physician can observe the action of the esophagus and stom-

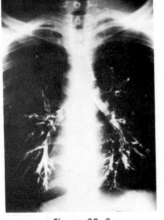

Figure 38–3

Radiograph showing a routine bronchographic film, anteroposterior projection. (From Snopek, A. M.: Fundamentals of Special Radiographic Procedures, 2nd ed., Philadephia, W. B. Saunders Co., 1984.)

38

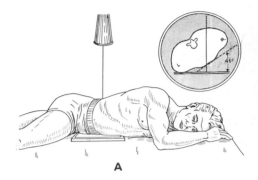

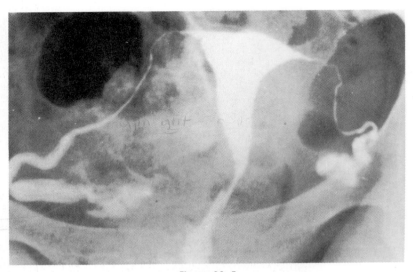

Figure 38–5

A normal hysterosalpingogram using water-soluble media. (From Meschan, I.: Radiographic Positioning and Related Anatomy, 2nd ed. Philadelphia, W. B. Saunders Co., 1978.)

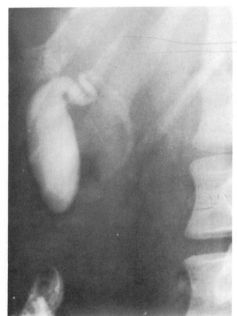

B

Figure 38–4

A, *The proper positioning of the patient for a cholecystogram.* **B,** *Radiograph of the gallbladder. (From Meschan, I.: Radiographic Positioning and Related Anatomy, 2nd ed. Philadelphia, W. B. Saunders Co., 1978.)*

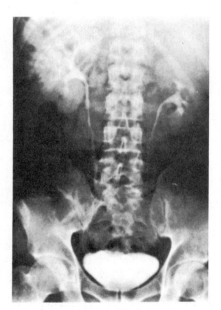

Figure 38–6

An intravenous pyelogram obtained 15 minutes after the intravenous injection of a contrast medium. (From Meschan, I., and Ott, D. J.: Introduction to Diagnostic Imaging. Philadelphia, W. B. Saunders Co., 1984.)

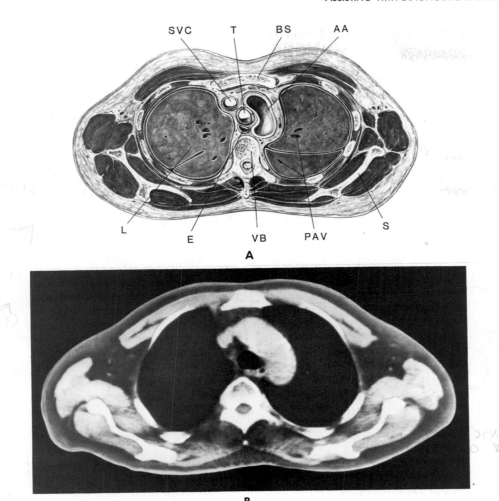

SVC   T   BS   AA

L   E   VB   PAV   S

A

B

Figure 38–7

A computed tomograph through the aortic arch level. Lungs, bone, spine, and blood vessels can be visualized and compared with anatomic drawings. T, trachea; SVC, superior vena cava; L, lungs; E, esophagus; BS, body of sternum; AA, aortic arch; S, scapula; PAV, pulmonary arteries and veins; VB, vertebral body. (From Meschan, I.: Synopsis of Radiologic Anatomy With Computed Tomography. Philadelphia, W. B. Saunders Co., 1980.)

an x-ray visualization of breast tissue to detect tumors and to determine the presence of a malignancy. Lesions too tiny to produce symptoms can also be detected. Mammography is performed without the use of a contrast medium. Mammography should not be considered a substitute for breast biopsy, but it is an effective device for differential diagnosis in fibrocystic disease (Fig. 38–8).

Stereoscopy. This technique, also called stereoscopic radiography or stereoradiography, utilizes a special instrument to view films that have been taken at different angles. This produces a three-dimensional image having depth as well as height and width. Stereoscopy is used primarily for x-ray studies of the skull.

Thermography. This is a technique that reveals internal structures without the use of x-rays but is usually performed by radiographers. Thermography is a heat-sensing technique used primarily in the detection of breast tumors. Using an infrared camera, a photograph is taken that records the variations in skin temperatures. Cool areas appear dark, warm areas light, and intermediate temperatures as various shades of gray. Since inflammatory or malignant areas produce more heat than does surrounding normal tissue, these areas are clearly visible (Fig. 38–9).

38

echography = sonography

Ultrasonography. This procedure is not a radiologic procedure, but it permits visualization of internal structures by the use of high-frequency sound waves that echo off the body. An instrument called a transducer, similar to a microphone, is passed over the body part to be examined. It picks up the echoes, which are then displayed on an oscilloscope. The echoes are produced by the sound waves

Direct sound waves into the body

echo from structure gives a picture.

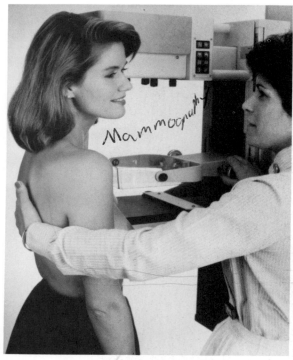

Figure 38–8
The patient is being assisted with the placement of her breast on the film holder in order to get a good image for the mammogram. (Courtesy of Lorad Medical System, Inc., Danbury, CT.)

use To a gel on lotion on the skin

passing through the skin, striking the body part, and bouncing back to the transducer. Since sound waves do not expose the patient to radiation, ultrasound examination is ideal for observing the developing fetus and detecting the presence of multiple fetuses (Fig. 38–10). It is also particularly useful for producing images of soft tissue tumors or lesions in the brain, eyes, abdomen, reproductive organs, and breasts.

Xeroradiography. In xeroradiography, the x-rays are processed on specially treated Xerox paper instead of x-ray film. The process takes only 90 seconds and permits visualization of soft tissues. For this reason, it is most often used to detect lesions or calcifications in the soft tissue of the breast (Fig. 38–11).

upright = a patient stands

Flat Plates. X-rays can also be taken of various body parts without the use of special techniques or the use of a contrast medium. These flat plates are also called plain films. Several x-ray views are usually taken for review by the radiologist. Examples of these diagnostic x-ray films include skull, sinuses, chest, abdomen, and bone.

KUB- Kidney ureten Bladder

X-RAY MACHINE

The x-ray machine consists of tube, table, and control panel (Fig. 38–12). The tube is the part in which the x-rays are produced and then are directed out as an x-ray beam. The entire tube is surrounded by a protective material (lead), except at the point where the rays are emitted. The lead absorbs the radiation like a sponge. The tube is designed to move the entire length of the table. The table is *stationary* where the patient is positioned for the x-ray. It is designed to rotate into different positions, as necessary for specific x-ray films. The control panel contains the knobs for operating the tube and the

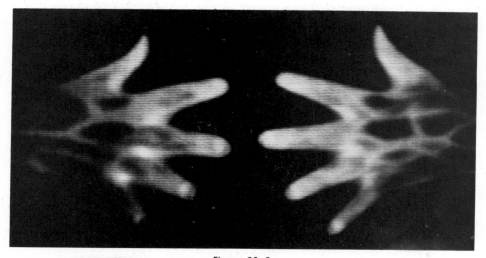

Figure 38–9
A normal hand thermogram. Note that the region of the fingertips is warmer than the remainder of the hand, but the change in warmth is gradual. Vascular structures along the dorsum of the hand are visualized as white streaks. (Courtesy of Dr. W. Reynolds, Henry Ford Hospital, Detroit, MI; from Poznanski, A. K.: The Hand in Radiologic Diagnosis, 2nd ed. Philadelphia, W. B. Saunders Co., 1984.)

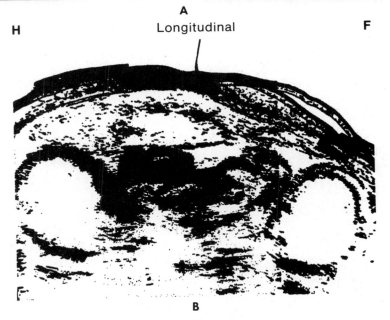

A

H   Longitudinal   F

B

Figure 38–10

A, *Early pregnancy. The fetus is seen in the gestation sac. The crown-rump length (CRL) is 3.3 cm, which is average for 10 weeks gestation. (From Beischer, N. A., and Mackay, E. V.: Obstetrics and the Newborn, 2nd ed. Philadelphia, W. B. Saunders Co., 1986.)* **B,** *The heads of a pair of twins can be seen in this sonograph taken at nine months. Experienced sonographers can determine the infants' positions. (From Gosink, B. B., and Squire, L. F.: Diagnostic Ultrasound, 2nd ed. Philadelphia, W. B. Saunders Co., 1981.)*

38

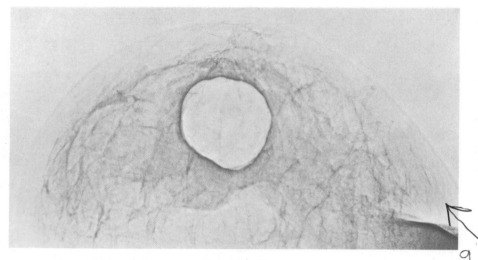

Figure 38–11

A cyst of the breast as seen in a xeroradiograph. (From Schertel L., et al.: Atlas of Xeroradiography. Philadelphia, W. B. Saunders Co., 1977.)

a zerox Machine Takes copies of it

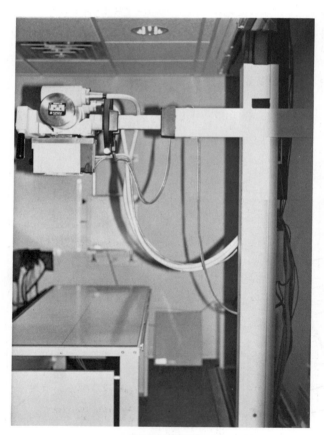

Figure 38–12

A typical office x-ray machine.

table. It is located behind a lead-lined wall, in another area away from the table and the tube.

RADIATION HAZARDS AND SAFEGUARDS

Leadud walls aprons gloves

Excessive exposure to radiation can cause both tissue destruction and a variety of ill effects. Harmful effects include temporary or permanent damage to the skin, eyes, and reproductive and blood-forming organs. X-rays may produce harmful effects on the developing embryo and the fetus, causing malformations or death. Overexposure to x-rays produces a variety of symptoms. These include nausea, fatigue, diarrhea, constipation, bleeding, and loss of appetite.

Signs posted

All radiation exposure is cumulative and adds up to a total radiation dosage that is measured in **rads**, **rems**, or **roentgens.** Monitoring devices called *dosimeters* are worn by persons working near sources of x-rays. These monitors contain special photographic film that is sensitive to radiation and serve as a guide to the amount of radiation to which a person has been exposed. Monitors are submitted periodically for evaluation, and a report of any radiation exposure is maintained on all x-ray personnel.

Radiation exposure can come directly from the x-ray beam or from what is known as scattered radiation. Scattered radiation is the diffusion or deviation of the x-rays that is produced when they pass through a patient or anything in the patient's path. Even though the entire x-ray tube is enclosed in lead, scattered radiation may result from leakage through the tube. To prevent this from happening, all machines must be checked on a regular basis by licensed physicists.

Shielding is of special importance to both patients and personnel. Patients should be protected from unnecessary radiation by using lead aprons to cover the reproductive organs, especially for pregnant patients and all children. Personnel can obtain additional protection by wearing lead aprons and gloves when assisting. The walls of x-ray rooms are also lined with lead, which absorbs the scattered radiation, protecting all others in the area.

In addition to monitors and shielding, all x-ray personnel should have routine periodic blood counts performed to detect the presence of any abnormal or pathologic condition that may result from excessive radiation exposure.

ASSISTING WITH RADIOLOGIC PROCEDURES

As previously stated, there may be occasions when the medical assistant will be called upon to assist in the performance of basic x-ray procedures under the physician's supervision. The medical assistant's x-ray responsibilities may include scheduling examinations; instructing and positioning patients; film processing; and filing and storing films and written reports.

Preparing the Patient

The medical assistant is responsible for preparing the patient for the x-ray procedure. Preparation requires a thorough knowledge of the procedure and the ability to communicate all instructions, both written and oral, to the patient to ensure that these instructions are understood. Written instructions are essential, since oral instructions can be easily forgotten. Most physicians use their own printed material or use product literature provided by pharmaceutical companies detailing step-by-step instructions (Fig. 38–13).

The medical assistant should briefly explain the procedure using proper terminology but should avoid complex descriptions. Encourage the patient to ask questions and discuss any apprehensions. Reinforce the rationale for the x-ray procedure. Many diagnostic x-ray examinations require special preparation by the patient the night before or the morning of the test. Patients may be instructed to eat a low-fat evening meal, not to eat after midnight, to drink plenty of fluids, or take special tablets, laxatives or enemas.

Positioning the Patient

An important responsibility of the medical assistant is the proper positioning of the patient for specific x-ray films. Radiographs are made by directing the x-rays produced by the x-ray tube to-

---

THE COLON X-RAY (BARIUM ENEMA)

Your doctor has requested an x-ray examination of your colon (lower bowel). This is a thorough examination of the colon. A special enema (barium) is given, which allows the colon to be visible on x-rays.

****Please Note:* This preparation is a laxative. It will empty your colon. Expect to have several loose or liquid bowel movements during the night. Do not be alarmed if you experience cramping and feel some weakness.*

The following preparation is necessary to insure a satisfactory examination of the colon.

BEGIN DAY PRIOR TO EXAM DAY

1) Lunch should be a light diet. 1-2 cups soup, 4 Saltines or 1-2 slices bread or toast (butter and jelly ok), 1 serving fruit. May also have: 1 serving cake or up to 3 cookies. Beverage: Any juice, coffee or tea (no milk).

2) Please drink at least one full glass or more of water or clear liquids every 1-2 hours between noon and bedtime. (At least six 8 oz. glasses).

3) 1/2 hr. before evening meal take Fleet Phospho Soda. Pour contents (1 1/2 oz.) into one-half glass cool water. Drink, following immediately with one full glass of water.

4) Eat a liquid evening meal (bouillon, strained fruit juice and plain jello). No solid foods. No dairy products (milk, cream or cheese). No carbonated beverages.

5) At 8 P.M., take four yellow Fleet Bisacodyl tablets, swallowing tablets whole with a full glass of water. Do not chew or dissolve tablets.

6) Drink nothing after taking the tablets.

7) Eat nothing after the evening meal. **(NO BREAKFAST).**

ON THE MORNING OF THE EXAMINATION

1) At least one hour before leaving for your exam use Fleet Bisacodyl Suppository. Remove foil wrap from suppository. Lie on side, insert rounded end of suppository as high as possible in rectum. Wait 15 minutes before evacuating even if urge is strong.

2) On the x-ray table you will be given a barium enema. You will experience a sensation similar to a cleansing enema. It will be only a matter of minutes before you have to go to the bathroom and expel the enema.

3) The radiologist (an x-ray physician specialist) will examine your abdomen by pressing it with his hands and observing the colon with the fluoroscope (television) and x-ray films.

4) When the radiologist has completed his portion of the examination, an x-ray technologist will take some additional films and immediately take you to the bathroom. After you feel you have expelled all of the enema, please have a seat in the hallway and the technologist will take an additional film of your abdomen to visualize your empty bowel.

5) The colon exam will usually require approximately 1/2 hour.

Report to your doctor's receptionist the morning of your examination and you will be given a request slip for your x-rays.

We appreciate your cooperation.

Figure 38–13
Patient instruction sheet for barium enema. (Courtesy of Jackson Clinic, Madison, WI.)

38

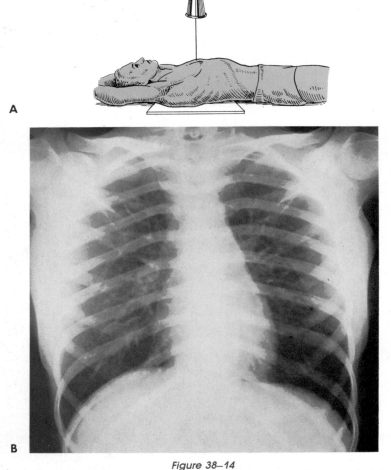

Figure 38–14
A, Patient's position and actual beam of roentgen rays focused on the body, which is positioned in the anterior recumbent position to produce the x-ray image. **B**, Radiograph resulting from the position and exposure in **A**. (From Meschan, I.: Radiographic Positioning and Related Anatomy, 2nd ed. Philadelphia, W. B. Saunders Co., 1978.)

ward a specific body part. The body part must be positioned correctly between the x-ray film and the x-ray tube (Fig. 38–14). The patient's position is determined by the type of examination required and the specific body part to be visualized. Usually, several views are taken in an attempt to achieve a three-dimensional picture for better diagnosis by the radiologist. The basic x-ray views are

- *Anteroposterior (AP) view:* The anterior aspect of the body faces the x-ray tube, and the posterior aspect faces the film. The x-ray beam is directed from front to back (Fig. 38–15).
- *Posteroanterior (PA) view:* The posterior aspect of the body faces the x-ray tube, and the anterior aspect faces the film. The x-ray beam is directed from back to front (Fig. 38–16).
- *Lateral view:* The body part is placed on its side. The x-ray beam is directed from one side (Fig. 38–17).
- *Right lateral (RL) view:* The right side of the body faces the film.

- *Left lateral (LL) view:* The left side of the body faces the film.
- *Oblique view:* The body is placed on a angle. The x-ray beam is directed at an angle (Fig. 38–18).

The basic x-ray positions are

- *Supine position:* The patient lies on his or her back.
- *Prone position:* The patient lies on his or her abdomen.

Terms to describe the direction of the x-ray beam are

- *Axillary:* The beam is directed toward the axilla (underarm).
- *Craniocaudal:* The x-ray beam is directed downward from head to toe.
- *Mediolateral:* The x-ray beam is directed from the midline toward the side of the body part of which a film is being made.

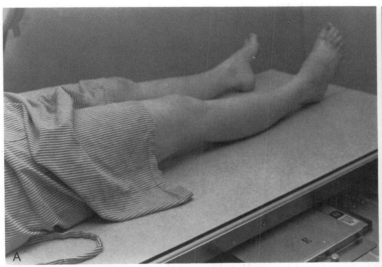
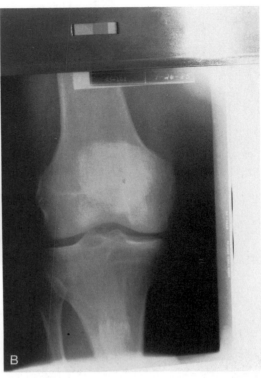

Figure 38–15
A, Anteroposterior view. The beam enters the anterior surface, as in the knee pictured. **B**, Resulting x-ray.

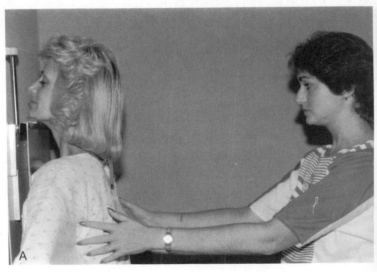
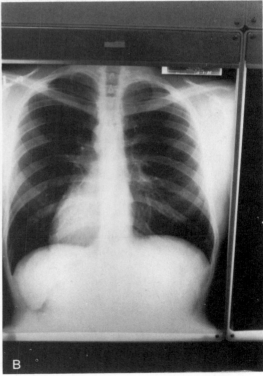

Figure 38–16
A, Posteroanterior view. The beam enters the posterior surface and emerges from the anterior surface, as in the chest example.
B, Resulting x-ray.

38

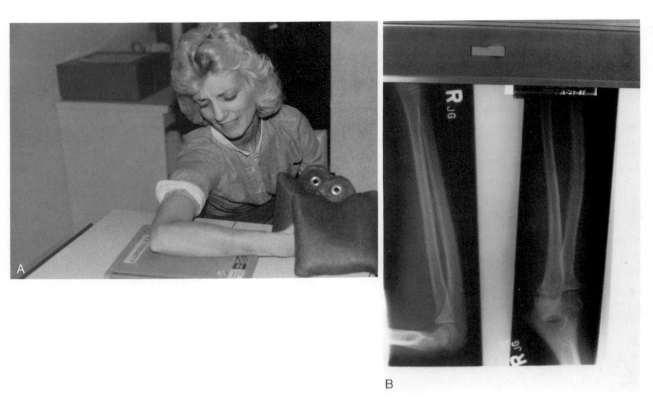

Figure 38–17
A, *Lateral view. A side projection of the right arm.* **B,** *Resulting x-ray.*

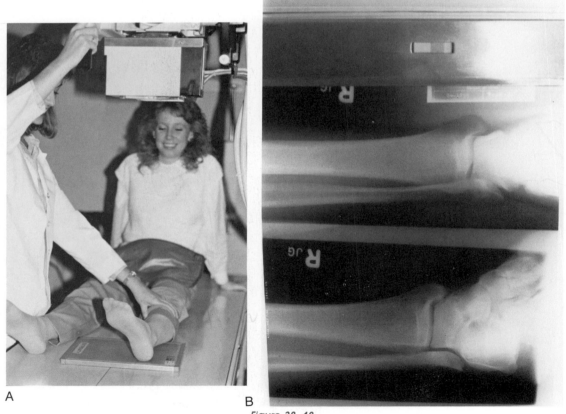

Figure 38–18
A, *Oblique view. The body part is usually inclined at a 45-degree angle to the x-ray beam.* **B,** *Resulting x-ray.*

Exposing X-Ray Film

X-rays, which can be produced by high-velocity electrons in a vacuum tube, expose (turn black) a sheet of x-ray film. X-rays can also be absorbed by substances, to a degree relative to the density of that substance. Thus, if part of the body is positioned on a *cassette* (film holder) and x-rays are directed through it, the rays will be absorbed or scattered by the various substances in the body and will expose the film to varying degrees. The resulting image will show the pattern of substances inside the body. Air, for instance, is least dense and appears as black areas, whereas water, fat, and metal appear increasingly white. Since the human body is made of different materials and is of varying thicknesses, the final image is composed of various degrees of black and white, as in Figure 38–19.

Processing X-Ray Film

Film development takes place in a darkroom. No natural light is permitted in this area. The only artificial light used is a specially designed low-wattage bulb that will not expose the film. For x-ray film processing, most modern medical offices use automatic developers, which produce images quickly and automatically. Some offices use the manual method, which is pictured in Figure 38–20.

Filing X-Ray Films and Reports

X-ray films are permanent records that must be preserved many years for both medical and legal reasons. Medical assistants are often responsible for storing the patient's films after processing is completed and after the physician has read them. The films are placed in large envelopes, with the patient's name, the patient's number (if used), and the date clearly marked on the outside. These films should be stored in a dry, cool place. In a general practice office, the films are usually kept in a readily accessible area for viewing.

X-ray films are the property of the medical office where the films are taken. They do not belong to the patient. Written x-ray reports may be sent out, but the actual films must remain as part of the patient's file.

38

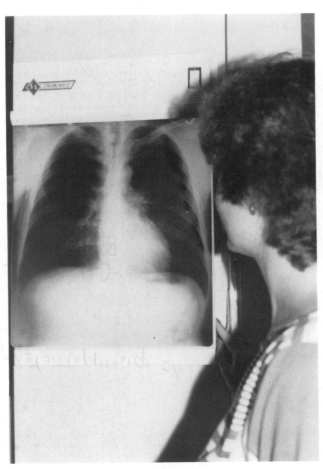

Figure 38–19
Chest x-ray showing varying degrees of black and white.

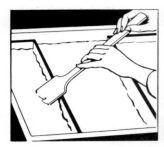

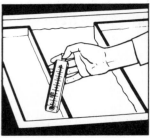

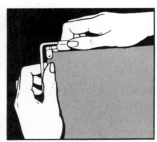

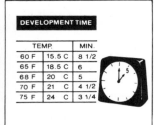

DEVELOPMENT TIME		
TEMP.		MIN.
60 F	15.5 C	8 1/2
65 F	18.5 C	6
68 F	20 C	5
70 F	21 C	4 1/2
75 F	24 C	3 1/4

1 Stir Solutions Stir developer and fixer solutions to equalize their temperature. (Use separate paddle for each to avoid possible contamination.)

2 Check Temperature Check temperature of solutions with accurate thermometer. Rinse thermometer after each measurement to avoid contaminating next solution. Adjust to recommended temperature.

3 Load Film on Hanger Attach film carefully to hanger of proper size. (Attach at lower corners first.) Avoid finger marks, scratches, or bending.

4 Set Timer Set timer for recommended period of development based on temperature of developer solution.

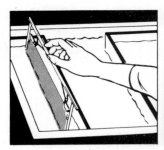

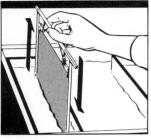

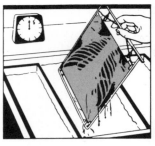

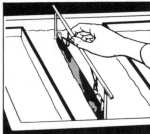

5 Immerse Film in Developer Completely immerse film. Do it smoothly and without pause to avoid streaking. Start timer. Rap film against side of tank to remove film surface air bubbles.

6 Agitate Film—If Recommended Follow manufacturer's instructions as to vigor and frequency and whether the film should be agitated within the tank or raised and lowered.

7 Drain Outside Developer Tank When alarm rings, lift hanger out quickly. Then drain film for a moment into space between tanks. For fast drainage, tilt hanger.

8 Rinse Thoroughly Place film in acid rinse bath or running water. Agitate hanger continuously. Rinse film about 30 seconds. Lift from rinse bath. Drain well.

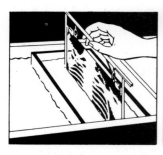

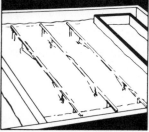

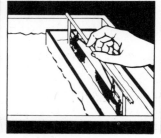

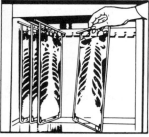

9 Fix Adequately Immerse film. Agitate hanger vigorously at start. Follow manufacturer's recommendations for time and temperature— at least twice time required to "clear" film (when its milky look has disappeared).

10 Wash Completely Remove film to tank of running water (flow rate of about 8 complete changes per hour). Keep ample space between hangers (water must flow over their tops). Allow adequate time for thorough washing— usually from 5 to 30 minutes, depending on film.

11 Use Final Rinse If facilities permit, use a final rinse in a solution containing a wetting agent to speed drying and prevent water marks. Immerse film for 30 seconds, and drain for several seconds.

12 Dry Dry in dust-free area at room temperature or in suitable drying cabinet. Keep films well separated. When dry, remove films from hangers and trim corners to remove clip marks. Insert in identified envelopes.

Figure 38–20
The basic steps involved in processing x-ray film. (Reprinted courtesy of Eastman-Kodak Company, Rochester, NY. ©Eastman-Kodak Company.)

Procedure 38–1

PROCEDURAL GOAL

To assist with an x-ray examination under the supervision of a physician.

EQUIPMENT AND SUPPLIES

Physician's order for an x-ray examination
X-ray machine
X-ray film and holder
X-ray darkroom
X-ray automatic developer or manual processing solutions

PROCEDURE

1. Introduce yourself, and confirm the identity of the patient. Ascertain if any special preparations were followed.
   Purpose: If special preparations were not followed, the examination may need to be rescheduled.
2. Explain the procedure.
   Purpose: Helps to reassure the patient and alleviates fear and anxiety.
3. Check to make certain that the patient has removed all metal objects from the area to be examined.
   Purpose: Metal objects appear on the film and may obscure the final image.
4. Drape the patient as necessary, and shield the abdominal area.
   Purpose: Drapes provide warmth, and shields protect the reproductive areas.
5. Position the patient properly, and immobilize the part, if necessary.
   Purpose: Proper positioning and complete stillness are necessary to achieve a clear, readable radiograph.
6. Stand behind a lead shield during the exposure.
   Purpose: Lead shields provide protection from scattered radiation.
7. Ask the patient to assume a comfortable position after the examination is completed, and wait until the films are processed.
   Purpose: In the event that it is necessary to retake an x-ray film, the patient will be readily accessible.
8. Develop the film, using automatic or manual film processing.
9. Dismiss the patient if all films are satisfactory.
10. Place the dry, finished x-ray film in a properly labeled envelope, and file it according to the policies of the office.
11. Record the x-ray examination on the patient's chart, along with the final written x-ray findings.

TERMINAL PERFORMANCE OBJECTIVE

Under proper supervision, and given the necessary patient, equipment and supplies, assist with the preparation and positioning of the patient, and with exposing and development of the film to achieve a clear crisp image, while adhering to the principles of radiation safety, and correctly complete each step of the procedure in the proper order as determined by your evaluator.

38

REFERENCES AND READINGS

Bartrum, R. J., and Crow, H. C.: *Real-time Ultrasound*, 2nd ed. Philadelphia, W. B. Saunders Co., 1983.
Fundamentals of Radiography, 12th ed. Rochester, NY, Eastman Kodak, 1980.

Klein, E.: *Medical Tests and You.* New York, Grosset & Dunlap, 1978.
Meschan, I.: *Radiographic Positioning and Related Anatomy*, 2nd ed. Philadelphia, W. B. Saunders Co., 1978.
Meschan, I., and Ott, D. J.: *Introduction to Diagnostic Imaging*, Philadelphia, W. B. Saunders Co., 1984.
Snopek, A.: *Fundamentals of Special Radiographic Procedures*, 2nd ed. Philadelphia, W. B. Saunders Co., 1984.

CHAPTER OUTLINE

VOCABULARY

See Glossary at end of book for definitions.

anaphylactic shock	insulin shock	paroxysm
anaphylaxis	lethargic	traumatic
convulsion		

Breathing
Circulation

Airways breathing—N Circulation

First Aid and Medical Emergencies

OBJECTIVES

Upon successful completion of this chapter you should be able to

1. Define and spell the words in the Vocabulary for this chapter.
2. Describe the medical assistant's legal responsibility in emergencies.
3. Recall two resources that can help you to make your medical office accident-proof.
4. List the basic items necessary for a crash tray.
5. Explain how and why a defibrillator is used in an emergency.
6. Recognize the actions of a choking victim.
7. Recall the conditions that necessitate the implementation of CPR.
8. Identify the major symptoms associated with heart attack.
9. List four medications that are indicated for a victim experiencing a severe cardiac disorder.
10. Describe the emergency medical care that is usually given to victims of asthma, anaphylactic shock, convulsions, and hemorrhagic shock.
11. State the functions of a Poison Control Center.

Upon successful completion of this chapter you should be able to perform the following activity:

1. Demonstrate CPR on an American Heart Association–approved manikin.

First aid is defined as the immediate care given to a person who has been injured or has been suddenly taken ill. It includes well-chosen words of encouragement, a willingness to help, a promotion of confidence by the demonstration of competence, and the performance of temporary physical care to alleviate pain or a life-threatening situation. First-aid knowledge and skill can often mean the difference between life and death, temporary and permanent disability, and rapid recovery and long-term hospitalization.

It is frequently the medical assistant who is responsible for initiating first aid in the office and continuing to administer first aid until the physician or other trained medical teams arrive. Each medical assistant should enroll in an American Red Cross Advanced First-Aid Course and American Heart Association Cardiopulmonary Resuscitation (CPR) Course. Basic knowledge of CPR and life-support skills need to be updated periodically because of recommended changes for procedures as new techniques are developed. It is strongly recommended that medical assistants encourage their local chapters of the American Association of Medical Assistants (AAMA) to offer workshops conducted by physicians and emergency personnel from the community.

There are many acceptable approaches to emergency care. All offices should establish written policies concerning the handling of medical emergencies. The medical assistant should consult with the physician-employer for the preferences in handling emergencies in that particular practice. Medical assistants should perform only emergency procedures that they have been trained to handle, and while in the office, only those designated by the physician. If an emergency occurs in the office, the medical assistant should notify the physician or any other available physician. If a physician is not located, then the assistant should contact the local emergency medical services team.

Medical assistants do not assume the responsibility of diagnosing but are expected to make decisions based on their medical knowledge. A major goal in emergency care of the injured is to cause no further harm.

In a true emergency, the law permits anyone to do whatever is reasonably necessary, provided that the care given is within the scope of competence of the person administering first aid. The law holds persons giving emergency care to be responsible for any injury that they cause as a result of their negligence or failure to exercise reasonable care. You, the medical assistant, are limited to the standards of your state laws, and your physician-employer is legally responsible for your mistakes.

MAKING THE OFFICE ACCIDENT-PROOF

Usually, it is the medical assistant's responsibility to make the office as accident-proof as possible. Do not use scatter rugs or delicate chairs, and be sure that floors are not slippery. Keep cupboard doors and drawers closed. Wipe up spills immediately, and pick up dropped objects. All medications should be kept out of sight; dangerous drugs should be kept in locked cupboards. If there are children in the office, keep all sharp objects out of reach. Never leave a seriously ill patient or a restless, depressed, or unconscious patient unattended.

PLANNING AHEAD

The office staff should discuss possible emergencies that may occur in that office or area. For instance, local industries may present unique problems that call for very specialized care. Plan for these, and ask the physician's advice on what procedures to follow. If there are several employees, each should be assigned specific duties. Organization and planning make the difference between organized care for the patient and complete chaos. Some offices have set up the "buddy system." This system allows one person to take immediate charge of the patient while another obtains needed materials and calls for assistance. They can also relieve each other in more strenuous work such as resuscitation and external heart massage.

Using Community Emergency Services. Many communities have established an Emergency Medical Services (EMS) system. This system includes an efficient communications network, such as the emergency telephone number 911; well-trained rescue personnel; properly equipped vehicles; an emergency facility that is open 24 hours a day to provide advanced life-support; and hospital intensive care for the victims.

There are over 300 Poison Control Centers in the United States ready to provide emergency information for treating victims of poisonings. Many of the centers have toll-free lines. Some have systems for communicating with deaf persons.

Every office should post a list of local emergency numbers. This list should be in plain sight and should be known to all office personnel. Include on the list the local emergency medical service system, poison control center, ambulance, fire, rescue squad, and police department numbers.

Preventing Children's Accidents. Accidents are the leading cause of death among children under 15 years of age. Even more common are home accidents that cause injuries that do not kill but require hospitalization. Such accidents exceed half a million each year. The Children's Bureau of the Department of Health, Education, and Welfare has published pamphlets containing helpful tips on preventing accidents. Child-resistant bottle caps, safer toys, better-educated parents, more responsible toy manufacturers, and government regulations have helped to cut dramatically the number of childhood deaths and injuries. Parents should be encouraged to use car safety seats, make their homes accident-proof, purchase safe toys, become familiar with basic first-aid procedures, and know the local emergency numbers. Medical assistants in both pediatrics and family practice specialties may be called upon to educate families in these matters.

SUPPLIES AND EQUIPMENT FOR EMERGENCIES

Crash Tray. The emergency, or crash, tray is a properly equipped tray of first aid items needed for a variety of emergencies. Contents of the tray vary to some degree, according to the type of emergencies each office encounters. The tray should be kept in an easily accessible place known to all personnel in the office. A firm rule must be made that no one borrows any items from the tray. Medication expiration dates should be checked and the tray replenished with fresh supplies after use.

BASIC CRASH TRAY ITEMS

Activated charcoal, bottle of 30 to 50 gm
Adhesive tape
Airways in assorted sizes
Amobarbital sodium (Amytal Sodium)
Antihistamine, injectable and oral
Apomorphine hydrochloride
Atropine
Dextrose
Diazepam (Valium)
Digoxin (Lanoxin)
Disposable syringe and needle units
Epinephrine (Adrenalin), injectable
Furosemide (Lasix)
Glucagon
Hot and cold packs (instant type)
Ipecac syrup
Isoproterenol hydrochloride aerosol spray (Isuprel)
Lidocaine (Xylocaine)
Metaraminol (Aramine)
Muslin sling or cravat bandage to be used as a tourniquet
Orange juice
Sterile dressings (miscellaneous sizes, including two abdominal pads)

Epinephrine is a vasoconstrictor used to check hemorrhage. It relaxes the bronchioles, is used to relieve asthmatic **paroxysm**, and is an emergency heart stimulant used to treat shock. Epinephrine should be in a ready-to-use cartridge syringe and needle unit. These are supplied in 1.0-cc cartridges.

Other drugs used are atropine, digoxin (Lanoxin), and lidocaine (Xylocaine). Atropine decreases secretions, increases respiration and heart rates, and is a smooth muscle relaxant. It dilates the pupil of the eye and is a general cerebral stimulant. Atropine relieves gastrointestinal cramps and hypermotility and may also be used to relieve pain locally. Digoxin is a cardiotonic. It is used to treat congestive heart failure and is good for emergency use because it has a relatively rapid action. Lidocaine is used as both a local and a topical anesthetic.

Apomorphine hydrochloride is a prompt and effective emetic and is used in cases of poisoning when a stomach pump cannot be employed. Syrup of ipecac is also an emetic and one that many physicians are recommending be kept on hand in the home for use in emergencies.

Antihistamines are used to counteract the effect of histamine and are used in the treatment of allergic reactions and **anaphylaxis**.

Isoproterenol, an antispasmodic, is used in bronchial spasm and is also a cardiac stimulant. Some trademarks for this product are Isuprel (Winthrop-Breon), Medihaler-Iso (Riker), and Norisodrine (Abbott).

Other medications that may be found on a crash tray are metaraminol (Aramine) (50 percent, in a prefilled syringe), for severe shock; amobarbital sodium (Amytal) and diazepam (Valium), for convulsions and as sedatives; dextrose and insulin, to treat diabetic patients; and furosemide (Lasix), for congestive heart failure. Glucagon is primarily used to counteract severe hypoglycemic reactions in diabetic patients taking insulin.

Small cans, with pull-tab openers, of orange juice are handy for quick sugar administration in cases of diabetic patients experiencing **insulin shock.**

Most physicians and others involved in emergency care do not recommend a tourniquet because of the danger from incorrect usage. A tourniquet that completely stops blood flow to the point of no measurable pulse is potentially hazardous and should be used very cautiously. It is much better to apply pressure directly over the bleeding area. Today, rather than a tourniquet, a constricting band is employed for the purpose of decreasing lymphatic and superficial venous blood flow for insect and snakebites. In these cases, the constricting band is applied just above the bite area.

Crash Cart. As more patients come to clinics and physicians' offices to seek emergency care, the medical assistant will need to become even more familiar with specialized equipment on the emergency, or "crash," cart to help save lives. This cart contains many more items than the smaller crash tray commonly found in most physicians' offices. Figure 39–1 shows the outside and the inside of a typical crash cart. The cart contains numerous locking drawers in which supplies and medicines are kept.

Defibrillators. The medical assistant who works in a large clinic or in an urgent-care center may be required to assist the team with defibrillation of

39

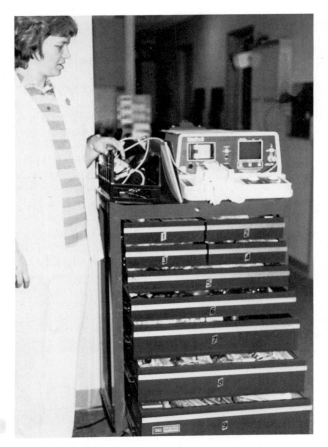

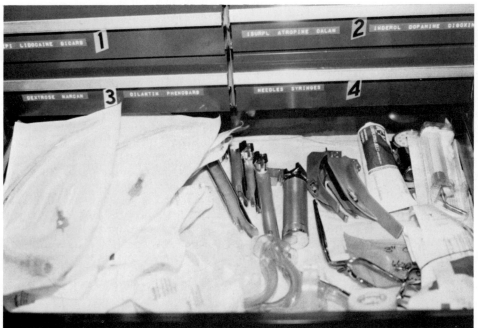

Figure 39–1

A, A typical crash cart used in clinics and urgent care centers. It is on wheels, and the top is large enough to hold a defibrillator. **B,** The interior of the crash cart drawer reveals a good supply of airways, a laryngoscope with extra batteries, and some sterile wrapped supplies that are readily available in an emergency situation. (**A** and **B** courtesy of Dean West Urgent Care, Madison, WI.)

emergency patients. Defibrillators are instruments that send a massive jolt of electricity into the heart muscle by means of plates or paddles applied to the chest in order to re-establish the proper rhythm of the heartbeat. One paddle is placed to the right of the upper sternum and the other is placed just to the left of the nipple, at the apex of the heart.

The office defibrillator is portable and is powered by batteries. The monitor has a nonfading display, and it is possible to freeze the monitor for prolonged viewing. If a permanent record of the victim's heart rate is desired, the machine can make a copy.

GENERAL RULES FOR EMERGENCIES

The general rules to follow in an emergency are few but very important.

- The first and most important rule is to keep calm. Reassure the patient and make him or her as comfortable as possible.
- Survey the situation to determine the nature of the emergency. A decision must be made as to whether the need is immediate. This decision requires calm judgment and may call for some medical knowledge.
- Take immediate steps to remedy the situation. Calmly but firmly give specific instructions to the patient and to other office personnel. Never say, "Will someone call the doctor?" Say, "YOU call the doctor," "YOU get a blanket," and "YOU get the emergency tray."
- After the emergency is under control, make certain that all the events and the medications used are recorded accurately. Be precise when recording. Have statements of how the accident happened or what events just preceded the emergency.
- Follow the universal blood and body-fluid precautions (see Appendix C, Recommendations for Prevention of AIDS Transmission).

COMMON EMERGENCIES

The basic principles and procedures for the following emergencies are covered thoroughly in the manuals published by the American Red Cross, which are listed at the end of this chapter. Wound care, dressings and bandages, burns, and poisonings are among the topics included in the American Red Cross Basic First-Aid course, which is the minimum requirement for accredited programs of medical assisting as defined by the Committee on Allied Health Education of the American Medical Association. These manuals are readily available at modest cost everywhere in the United States. The following sections of this chapter serve as a review and reference source for administering first aid in common emergencies.

Fainting (Syncope)

One of the most common emergency problems to confront the medical assistant is fainting. Fainting is usually caused by lack of oxygen in the blood, with a consequent lack of oxygen to the brain. Prior to fainting, a person may appear pale, may feel cold, weak, dizzy, or nauseated, and may have numbness of the extremities. Immediately lay the patient flat, with the head lower than the heart. Loosen all tight clothing. Maintain an open airway. Apply a cold washcloth to the forehead. Pass aromatic spirits of ammonia back and forth under the patient's nostrils. Be careful not to hold the ammonia too close to the nose. Obtain the patient's pulse, respiration rate, and blood pressure; and then report the findings to the physician. Keep the patient in a supine position for at least ten minutes after consciousness has been regained.

If recovery is not prompt, summon the physician or emergency medical rescue team for transportation to the hospital. This might be a brief episode in the development of a serious underlying illness.

Emergency Respiratory Resuscitation

Breathing may suddenly cease for a variety of reasons, including shock, disease, and trauma. The most obvious sign that breathing has stopped is when the chest is no longer moving. Artificial respiration must be begun immediately, since death may follow within four to six minutes.

Resuscitation techniques should be studied and practiced in courses directed toward this purpose. The basics are presented here as an introduction or a reference. First, the airway must be opened by positioning the patient on the back and relieving possible obstruction of the air passage by the tongue. Extreme caution must be used if there is any chance that the patient has suffered a cervical neck injury, as should be assumed in any accident. If neck injury is not suspected, the head is tilted by downward pressure on the forehead and upward pressure under the chin. If neck injury may be present, grasp the angle of the victim's lower jaw without extending the neck.

Mouth-to-mouth resuscitation is begun if breathing does not follow opening of the airway. Position yourself on the side of the patient's head. One hand should continue pressing on the forehead and should also be turned so that the fingers can hold the nose shut. The other hand should continue lifting the chin upward. Place your mouth over the mouth of the victim and give two full breaths. Check for the carotid pulse. If the pulse is present, continue ventilating the lungs every five seconds. If the pulse is absent, you must provide artificial circulation in addition to artificial respiration (see the section on cardiopulmonary resuscitation).

39

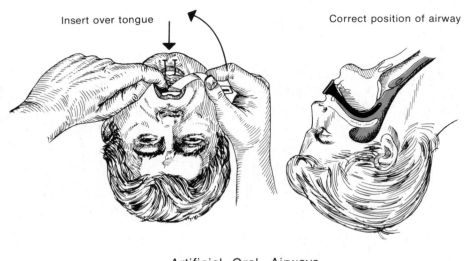

Insert over tongue   Correct position of airway

Artificial Oral Airways

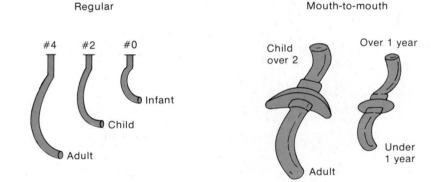

Regular   Mouth-to-mouth

#4 #2 #0

Infant

Child

Adult

Child over 2   Over 1 year

Adult

Under 1 year

Figure 39–2
Recommended placement of an artificial airway device. The mouth-to-mouth devices are recommended for use by the rescuer when diseases that can be transferred (such as AIDS) are present in the victim.

There is a mouth-to-nose and a mouth-to-stoma method for resuscitation of victims with tracheotomies. Please refer to the American Red Cross *Standard First Aid Manual* for specific procedures and precautions.

Artificial airways may be inserted by trained personnel to establish or maintain breathing. Airways of various types and sizes should be kept ready on the emergency tray and cart (Fig. 39–2).

Cardiopulmonary Resuscitation

Cessation of breathing may be accompanied by a cessation of the heartbeat (cardiac arrest), which is identified by the lack of a pulse. Artificial respiration must then be accompanied by external (closed) cardiac massage. This is called cardiopulmonary resuscitation (CPR), which is the combination of artificial circulation and artificial breathing.

The basic ABC steps of CPR include

A—airway
B—breathing
C—circulation

When both breathing and pulse stop, the victim has suffered sudden death. There are many causes of sudden death, including choking, drowning, poisoning, suffocation, electrocution, and smoke inhalation. CPR must be started immediately in an attempt to prevent death or permanent damage to body organs, especially the brain.

Since CPR may cause injuries to the ribs, heart, liver, lungs, and blood vessels, it should be performed only by individuals properly trained in the techniques and only if cardiac arrest has occurred.

In CPR, the heart is compressed by downward pressure on the sternum, which should cause the blood to circulate. The proper position is for the heel of the one hand to be placed on the sternum, two finger widths above the lower notch where the ribs join. The other hand is placed on top, and the rescuer presses straight down. The sternum will be depressed one and one-half to two inches with sufficient pressure.

If there is only *one rescuer*, compressions should be given at a rate of 80 to 100 times per minute. After every 15 compressions, move back to the mouth to give two full breaths. With *two rescuers*,

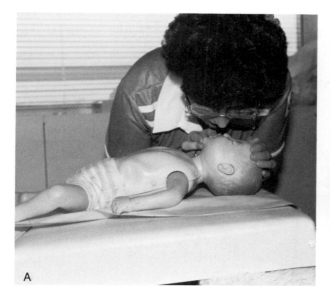

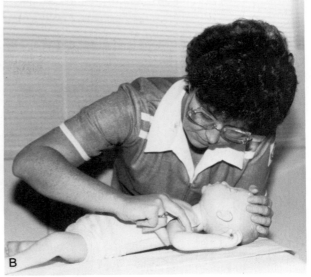

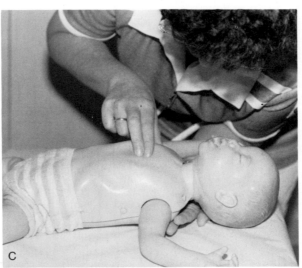

Figure 39–3

Modifications necessary for the CPR procedure when the victim is an unresponsive infant. **A,** *Gently tilt the head backward but do not hyperextend it.* **B,** *Locate the brachial pulse, between the elbow and the shoulder.* **C,** *Place the fingers one finger width below the nipple line. Remember to support the upper back with the other hand.*

ventilation and compression can be performed simultaneously. Compressions should be given at a rate of 60 to 80 times per minute, with a pause for a ventilation by the second rescuer after every fifth compression. Continue cardiopulmonary resuscitation until advanced life support is available.

Cardiopulmonary resuscitation for infants and small children is similar to that for adults. The few important differences must be remembered. When handling an infant be careful that you do not overextend the head when tilting it back (Fig. 39–3A). The infant's neck is so pliable that forceful backward tilting might block breathing passages instead of opening them. With an infant who is not breathing, be certain to cover both the mouth and

the nose with your mouth and deliver two slow "puffs" that are just strong enough to make the chest rise. With a small child, pinch the nose, cover the mouth, and breathe as for an infant. In an infant. check the brachial pulse (Fig. 39–3B) between the elbow and the shoulder. Use only the finger tips at the center of the sternum for compressions on the infant (Fig. 39–3C). Compress the sternum between one-half and one inch, at a rate of at least 100 times per minute. Only the heel of one hand is used for compressions on a small child. Depress the sternum one to one and one-half inches, at a rate of 80 to 100 times per minute. CPR for children over eight years is the same as that for adults.

Procedure 39–1

PERFORMING CARDIOPULMONARY RESUSCITATION

PROCEDURAL GOAL

To restore breathing and blood circulation when a victim's respiration and pulse stop.

EQUIPMENT AND SUPPLIES

Blood and body-fluid protection barriers (goggles, masks, and aprons or gowns), as necessary (see Appendix C, Recommendations for Prevention of AIDS Transmission)

Nonsterile gloves (sterile gloves may be preferred)

An American Heart Association–approved manikin equipped with a printout for demonstration of the proper technique for your instructor.

PROCEDURE

(Performed on a manikin only)

1. Wash and dry your hands. Follow universal blood and body-fluid precautions (see Appendix C). Glove yourself with nonsterile or sterile gloves.
2. Shake the "victim's" shoulder gently and shout, "Are you all right?" If there is no response, shout for help.
   Purpose: To determine whether the victim is conscious. The call for help will alert other rescue personnel to the problem.
3. Tilt the head, and lift the chin. Look, listen, and feel for signs of breathing. Place your ear over the mouth, and listen for breathing. Look for evidence that the chest is rising and falling.
   Purpose: To determine whether the victim is breathing and to open the airway.

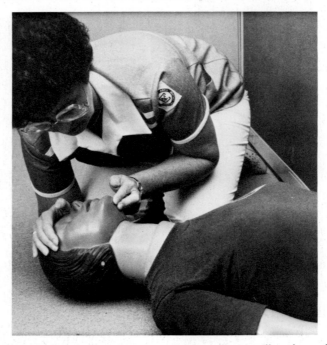

4. Begin rescue breathing by pinching the nose tightly with your thumb and forefinger if none of the signs are present (facing page, top left).
   Purpose: There must be an airtight seal so that air cannot escape through the nose when you perform mouth-to-mouth resuscitation.
5. Maintain an airtight seal with your mouth on the victim's mouth (facing page, top right).
6. Give two full breaths.
   Purpose: May be sufficient stimulus to initiate breathing by the victim.
7. Check the carotid pulse (facing page, bottom left).
   Purpose: The pulse is easier to feel in this area.

Procedure continued on opposite page

8. Continue mouth-to-mouth resuscitation at the rate of approximately one full breath every five seconds, *if the pulse is present.*
9. Initiate CPR, *if there is no pulse.*
10. Kneel at the victim's side near the chest. Move your fingers up the ribs to the point where the sternum and ribs join. Your middle fingers should fit into this area, and your index finger should be next to it across the sternum.
11. Place the heel of your hand on the chest midline, over the sternum, just above your index finger (bottom right).

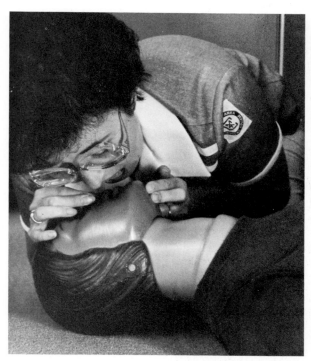

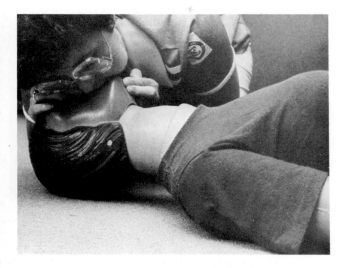

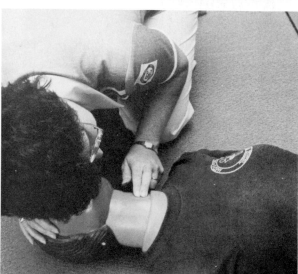

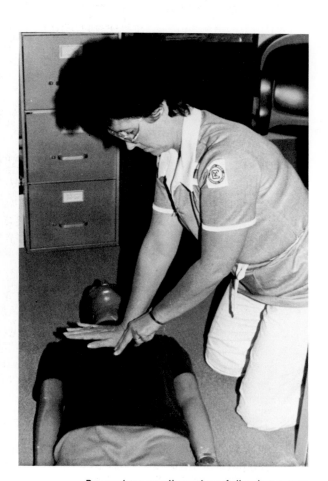

Procedure continued on following page

39

12. Place your second hand on top of your first hand, and lift your fingers upward and off the chest (below, left).
    Purpose: This position gives you the most control, allowing you to avoid cracking the victim's rib when you compress the chest.
13. Bring your shoulders directly over the victim's sternum as you compress downward, and keep your arms straight.
14. Depress the sternum one and one-half to two inches for an adult victim. Relax the pressure on the sternum after each compression but do not remove your hands from the victim's sternum.
    Purpose: The depth of depression needed to circulate blood through the heart. Movement of the hand from the original site could cause injury to the victim.
15. Perform 15 compressions. After performing the 15 compressions, open the airway, pinch the nose, take a deep breath, cover the mouth completely with your lips, and blow 2 full breaths (below, right).

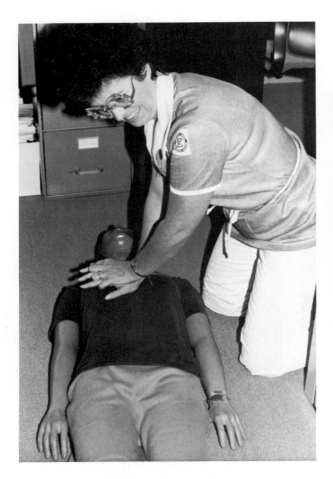
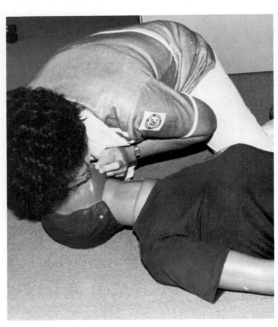

16. Continue CPR at the rate of 15 compressions and 2 ventilations, at a compression rate of 80 to 100 times per minute.

TERMINAL PERFORMANCE OBJECTIVE

Given a simulated emergency situation with an unconscious victim (manikin) who is not breathing and has no pulse, assess the situation, open the airway, initiate mouth-to-mouth resuscitation, and provide artificial circulation, maintaining 15 compressions to 2 full breaths at a compression rate of 80 to 100 times per minute until emergency help is available. The CPR procedure should be observed by a certified instructor and should be performed according to accepted standards as approved by the American Heart Association. Correctly complete each step of the procedure in the proper order as determined by your instructor.

Choking

Choking is caused by a foreign object, usually food, lodged in the upper airway. Often, exhalation can take place, but inhalation is blocked. Thus, the lungs quickly empty. The choking victim who has food or a foreign object lodged in the throat cannot speak, breathe, or cough. The victim may clutch the neck between the thumb and index finger. This universal distress signal should be viewed as a sign that the victim needs help (Fig. 39–4). The face pales and turns blue. Eventually, there is loss of consciousness and cardiopulmonary arrest. If the object is not removed, the victim may die within four to six minutes.

If the victim has good air exchange, or only partial obstruction, and can speak, cough, or breathe, do not interfere. If the victim cannot speak, cough, or breathe, use the Heimlich maneuver. Give subdiaphragmatic abdominal thrusts until the foreign body is expelled or the victim becomes unconscious (Fig. 39–5). If the victim becomes unconscious, position the victim on his or her back, and call out for help. Sweep your finger in the victim's throat in an attempt to remove the foreign body. Open the airway, and attempt rescue breathing. If you are still unsuccessful in removing the foreign body, use the Heimlich maneuver and give six to ten subdiaphragmatic abdominal thrusts. Repeat the sequence until you are successful. After the obstruction is removed, begin the ABC's of CPR, if necessary.

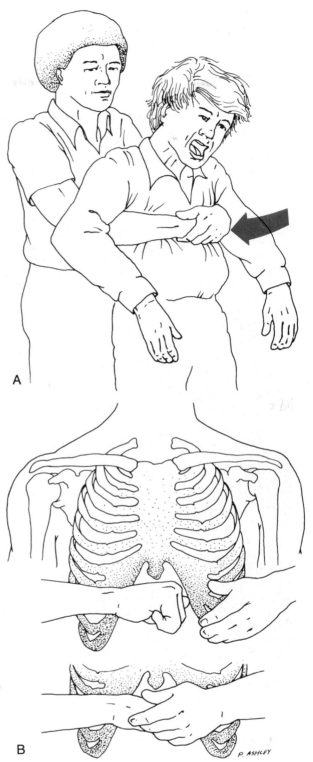

A

B

Figure 39–5

The Heimlich maneuver. **A,** *If the victim is standing, get behind him and put both of your arms around his waist. Put your fist on the victim's abdominal area just above the umbilicus, and pound your fist with your other hand to give a quick, sharp upward thrust like a "bear hug."* **B,** *Hand placement for abdominal thrust. Rescuer makes a fist with one hand and covers it with the other hand. Flat side of the fist is placed against the upper abdomen.*

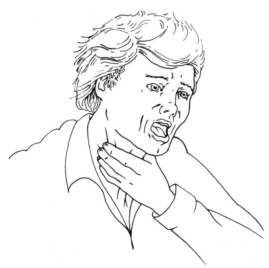

Figure 39–4

The choking sign. The distress of the choking victim must be distinguished from that of the coronary victim. The face develops a blue color, owing to the lack of oxygen in both cases. The choking sign consists of the victim grasping at the throat. The immediate use of the Heimlich maneuver is indicated.

39

To dislodge a foreign object from an infant, place the victim face down, over your forearm and across your thigh. The head should be lower than the trunk. Next, support the head and neck of the victim with one hand. Using the heel of the other hand, deliver four blows to the back, between the infant's shoulder blades. Place the infant on his or her back, with the head lower than the trunk. Using two or three fingers, deliver four thrusts in the sternum area. Repeat the sequence until the foreign body is expelled or the infant becomes unconscious.

If the infant becomes unconscious, position the infant on his or her back and call out for help. Sweep your finger in the throat in an attempt to remove the foreign body. Open the airway, and attempt rescue breathing. If you are still unsuccessful in removing the foreign body, perform the sequence of back blows and chest thrusts until you are successful. After the obstruction is removed, begin the ABC's of CPR, if necessary.

Chest Pain

Chest pain can be associated with both heart and lung disease as well as a few other conditions. It can be quite serious, and all patients with chest pain are treated as cardiac emergencies until a physician has ruled out this diagnosis. The patient is usually sweating and has a gray, ashen appearance. The lips and fingernails may be blue (cyanotic). Frequently, the patient is clutching the chest in pain. This pain may radiate out the left arm and up the left side of the neck. The pulse may be rapid and weak. Frequently, there is nausea.

Do not have the patient walk any distance. A wheelchair or a chair with rollers is an excellent method of moving this patient to a quiet room. The patient will probably prefer to have his or her head slightly elevated or even to be in a semisitting position. Keep the patient quiet and warm. Loosen all tight clothing. Administer oxygen if the physician has previously given these instructions. *Absolutely no smoking should be allowed by the patient or by anyone within the vicinity.* Prepare the medication that the physician is most likely to use. This may be epinephrine (Adrenalin), atropine, digitalis, calcium chloride 10 percent, or morphine. Determine whether the conscious patient is carrying any medication. Ask about the medication. Usually, this medication is nitroglycerin tablets that are administered sublingually. You may give them to the patient with the patient's consent. Do not give the patient alcohol, food, or water by mouth without the physician's permission. Do not give spirits of ammonia.

If the physician is in the office or is on the way, connect the patient to the electrocardiograph, and record a few tracings. Lead II is usually considered to be the monitoring lead. If the physician cannot be reached, call the emergency rescue team. It may be necessary to start mouth-to-mouth resuscitation if the patient is unconscious and there is no evidence of breathing. If chest pain progresses to cardiac arrest, CPR must be performed.

The office staff must remain calm and offer emotional support and reassurance, since all heart patients are extremely frightened and anxious.

Signals of Heart Attack

A heart attack is caused by a blockage of the coronary arteries, so that the blood supply to the heart muscles is stopped. The most common signal of heart attack is an uncomfortable pressure, squeezing, fullness, or pain in the center of the chest, behind the breastbone. This may spread to the shoulder, neck, jaw, or arms. The pain may not be severe. Other symptoms include sweating, nausea, indigestion, shortness of breath, cold and clammy skin, a feeling of weakness, and extreme apprehension.

Cerebrovascular Accident (Stroke) [permanent]

A cerebrovascular accident (CVA) is a disorder of the blood vessels serving the cerebrum, resulting in an impairment of the blood supply to a part of the brain. The term "stroke" is often applied to this problem. This interruption in the normal circulation of blood through the brain leads to a sudden loss of consciousness and some degree of paralysis, which may be temporary or permanent depending on the severity of the oxygen deprivation of the brain cells.

Usually, minor strokes do not produce unconsciousness, and the symptoms depend upon the location of the hemorrhage and the amount of brain damage. Symptoms include headache, confusion, slight dizziness, and ringing in the ears. This may be followed by minor difficulties in speech, memory changes, weakness of the extremities, and some disturbance of personality.

Symptoms of a major stroke include unconsciousness, paralysis on one side of the body, difficulty in breathing and swallowing, loss of bladder and bowel control, unequal pupil size, and slurring of speech.

The patient should be protected against any further injury or physical exertion. Keep the patient lying down and covered lightly. Maintain an open airway. Position the head so that any secretions will drain from the side of the mouth, to prevent choking. Do not give the patient anything to eat or drink. Vital signs should be taken at regular intervals and recorded for the physician. Have an ambulance take the patient to the hospital as soon as possible.

TIA Trans inchemic Attack = A Temporary Loss of Blood to the Brain

Poisonings

All poisonings are considered medical emergencies. Poisoning can occur by mouth, absorption, inhalation, and injection. Aspirin is by far the most common poison seen in young children. Other typical household poisons include medicines, detergents, cleaners, disinfectants, bleaches, insecticides, ammonia, glues, cosmetics, and poisonous plants. Symptoms of poisoning vary greatly. Important signs of poisoning include open bottles of medicines or chemicals, stains on clothing, burns on hands and mouth, changes in skin color, nausea, shallow breathing, *convulsions*, stomach cramps, heavy perspiration, dizziness, drowsiness, and unconsciousness.

When a person calls to report a poisoning, ask for

- The location and the phone number
- The name of the poison taken
- How much was taken
- How long ago the poison was taken
- Whether or not vomiting has occurred
- The name, weight, and age of the victim
- Any first aid being given

Instruct the caller not to hang up and not to leave the victim unattended, and then you call the local poison control center. Quickly forward all directions to the caller. Tell the caller to bring the container of poison or of vomitus to the office or hospital.

Speed is essential in administering first aid in poisonings. In all cases, it is most important to dilute the poison, to induce vomiting (except when the person has swallowed a corrosive poison), and to seek medical attention. Generally, it is safe to try to dilute the poison with one or two cups of water or milk. It is important to dilute the poison before vomiting is induced. Do not induce vomiting if the victim is unconscious or having a **convulsion.** Do not attempt to induce vomiting when the victim has swallowed a strong corrosive or petroleum product. Give one tablespoon of syrup of ipecac and one cup of water. If vomiting does not occur after 20 minutes, repeat the procedure. It may be necessary to make the victim gag to start vomiting. The gag reflex is started by touching the back of the tongue lightly. Encourage the victim to drink fluids until the emesis is reasonably clear. When vomiting has stopped, administer 30–50 gm of activated charcoal, which will absorb any residual toxic substance and inhibits the absorption of poisons.

Insect Stings

Remove the stinger, if there is one, by gently brushing it off or by using forceps or tweezers. Be careful not to squeeze the stinger. This further injects more venom into the skin. Place the forceps as close to the skin as possible, not over the stinger sac, and gently remove the stinger. Apply ice in a towel or a plastic bag around the area, to relieve the pain and slow the absorption of the venom. Calamine lotion or a paste of baking soda may be applied to relieve itching. Keep the patient's activities to a minimum, in order to slow down circulation and, thus, the spread of the venom.

If the patient gives a history of allergies, especially to insect venom, the patient should be transported to the nearest hospital for immediate care. This patient may experience dyspnea and a decrease in blood pressure. A wet, itchy, swollen rash may occur. The victim may complain of shortness of breath or difficulty in breathing. Sometimes, there is edema of the lips and the face. Difficulty in talking is a sign of edema in the throat. In this situation, there is the possibility of complete airway obstruction. These are signs of a true emergency. Epinephrine and oxygen should be ready for immediate administration on the physician's orders. Antihistamines may be used, as well as cortisone, but the action of these are considerably slower than that of epinephrine. If the patient experiences acute **anaphylactic shock**, death may occur within one hour without the intervention of a physician.

Shock

Shock is a condition that produces a depressed state of many vital body functions. It is a physiologic reaction resulting from a **traumatic** condition to the body. Shock is often caused by an injury, accident, hemorrhage, illness, surgical operation, or overdose of drugs or by burns, pain, fear, or emotional stress. Shock may be immediate or delayed, mild or severe, and even fatal.

The patient may be pale and clammy and often has dilated pupils, a weak and rapid pulse, and low blood pressure. The patient may complain of thirst and feel **lethargic** and faint. There may be labored breathing.

Ensure an open airway, and check for breathing and circulation. Place the patient on his or her back, with the legs elevated, loosen all tight clothing. Cover the patient with a blanket for warmth. Do not move the patient unnecessarily. Fluids may be given by mouth if not contraindicated or if medical care will be delayed for more than 60 minutes. Because there are so many different causes of shock, it is advisable to administer only basic first-aid care and to have the patient transported to the hospital.

Asthmatic Attack

Asthma is a condition characterized by wheezing, coughing, choking, and shortness of breath resulting from spasmodic constriction of the bronchi in the lungs. Attacks vary greatly. Severe attacks rarely

39

last for more than a few hours, but milder symptoms may persist much longer.

Some asthmatic patients carry respiratory inhalators with them. You may assist them with using this inhalator. A bronchodilator such as epinephrine or aminophylline may be ordered by the physician. Other medications are used to thin the mucus in the air passages so that the patient can clear the lungs more easily.

The patient should be warned of the hazards of overstimulation of the body, such as exercise and emotional upsets causing laughing or crying. Explain the importance of relaxation to the patient with asthma.

Seizures

Seizures are frightening to witness, but usually the patient is not suffering, nor is there great danger. Establishing a tranquil environment is usually an essential component of caring for patients experiencing seizures. Loosen clothing, but do not attempt to restrain the patient's movements, except to prevent injury. Remove anything that might be in the way that could cause harm. Always protect the head. Give neither fluids nor medication by mouth. If the patient remains unconscious after the jerking has subsided, position the patient in a semiprone position in order to maintain an open airway and to allow drainage of excess saliva. Do not attempt to place anything between the teeth during the convulsion because forcing an object through a tightly clenched mouth may damage the teeth. After the seizure is over, let the patient rest or sleep in a quiet room. If the patient has not regained consciousness within 10 to 15 minutes, it may be advisable to contact the physician.

Abdominal Pain

Abdominal pain is any pain or discomfort in the abdomen. The pain can be caused by stress, inflammation, hemorrhage, obstruction, ulcers, tumors, or excessive eating, drinking, or smoking. All abdominal pain should be investigated. Severe and persistent abdominal pain, especially when accompanied by fever, should have medical attention as soon as possible.

Treatment varies with the cause of the pain. Keep the patient warm and quiet. Have an emesis basin available. Administer nothing by mouth. Do not apply heat to the abdomen unless so instructed by the physician. Check and record the patient's vital signs.

Obstetric Emergencies

The types of problems found in an obstetric office are unique to this specialty. Every medical assistant employed in an office where the physician delivers babies should be trained to handle emergencies. The majority of these problems will be presented to you over the telephone. If there are physicians in the office, those calls should be transferred to them immediately.

If a pregnant patient calls in to report vaginal bleeding, you must ask some specific questions. Is the bleeding like a menstrual flow or is it a gushing type of hemorrhage? Is it painful or without any pain? If the bleeding is gushing, the patient must be told to lie down immediately while you send for an ambulance. In such a situation, the mother and baby could bleed to death in a matter of a few minutes as the result of a ruptured uterus. If the bleeding is like a normal menstrual flow, have the patient go to bed, with the foot of the bed elevated. Tell her that you will report this to the physician immediately. If the tissue passed is liver-like, it may be a blood clot; white tissue may be fetus. No matter what the appearance of the tissue, have the patient take it with her to the hospital.

Sprains

A sprain is an injury to a ligamentous structure surrounding a joint and is frequently due to twisting or wrenching of that part. Today, the most accepted first aid is elevation, mild compression, and immediate application of ice. There is considerable advantage if the ice is applied within 20 to 30 minutes after the injury has occurred. The ice should remain on the part for 24 hours, with the injured area elevated. After 24 to 36 hours, application of mild heat is usually indicated. The patient may be advised to immobilize the part.

Fractures

A fracture is a break or crack in a bone and can result from trauma or disease (Fig. 39–6). Fractures in which the bone penetrates the skin, causing an open wound, are called open, or compound, fractures. Fractures in which there is no break in the skin are called closed, or simple, fractures.

When a patient with a fracture is brought into the office, the medical assistant should make the patient as comfortable as possible. Have the patient lie down in a position that does not place strain on the area. First aid includes preventing movement of the injured part; elevation of the affected extremity; application of ice; and control of bleeding, if present. Do not apply too much pressure on the bleeding area if there is a fracture beneath. Be gentle. Do not attempt to straighten the fracture or move it in any way . If the patient must be moved, give support to the fractured area before moving. If possible, an x-ray film of the area should be ready when the physician arrives.

Simple (closed) fracture — No open wound

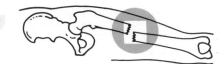

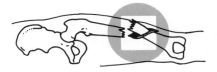

Compound (open) fracture—Wound in skin communicates with fracture

Extracapsular fracture—Bone broken outside joint

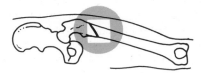

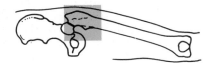

Intracapsular fracture—Bone broken inside joint

Comminuted fracture—Bone splintered into fragments

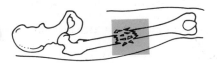

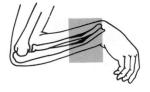

Greenstick fracture—Bone broken, bent but still securely hinged at one side

Longitudinal fracture—Break runs parallel with bone

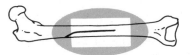

Figure 39–6
Various types of fractures encountered in emergency care. (From Ethicon, Inc.: Nursing Care of the Patient in the O.R.)

Illustration continued on following page

39

Transverse fracture—Break runs across bone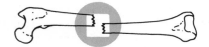

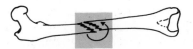 Oblique fracture—Break runs in slanting direction on bone

Spiral fracture—Break coils around bone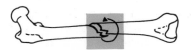

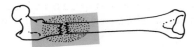 Pathologic fracture—Break is at site of bone disease

Impacted fracture—Bone broken and wedged into other break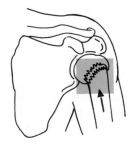

Fracture dislocation—Break complicated by bone out of joint

Depressed fracture—Broken skull bone driven inward

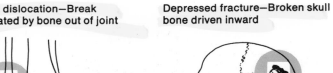

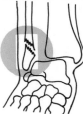

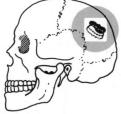

Figure 39–6 Continued

Burns

Burns are the most frequent cause of all injuries and the leading cause of accidental death in the United States. Burn injuries can result from heat, chemicals, or radiation. Burns are classified as first-degree, second-degree, or third-degree, depending on the depth of the wound (Fig. 39–7). A first degree burn shows erythema of the epidermis only. The tissue destruction is superficial, without blistering. The use of cold packs on a first-degree burn until the pain stops may prevent it from becoming a second-degree burn. A second-degree burn includes the entire epidermal layer and varying depths of the dermis. Blisters are usually formed, and there is some pain. There is also danger of infection in the blistered area. If the burn is deep enough, there may be some destruction of the hair follicles and the sebaceous glands. A third-degree burn is the destruction of all the epithelium and may involve underlying muscle tissue. Destroyed skin sloughs leaving a raw area. There is danger of infection. Third-degree burns themselves do not cause pain, as the nerve endings are destroyed.

Burns are also classified according to the percentage of body surface involved (Fig. 39–8). A method called the Rule of Nines has been developed to determine burn surface involvement. The front and back of the trunk constitute 36 percent of the total body surface; with the head and neck, 9 percent; each arm, 9 percent; and each leg, 18 percent. In general, an adult who has suffered burns over 15 percent of the body surface or a child who has burns over 10 percent requires hospitalization.

First aid for burns includes relief of the pain, prevention of infection, and treatment of shock. Burns are extremely painful and dangerous. Recommended first aid for a first-degree burn is to immerse it immediately in cool water. This gives fast relief from the pain. If immersion in water is not possible, then apply sterile, wet compresses to the area. There is always the danger of infection from contamination because the burned tissue acts as a culture medium for bacteria and there is poor circulation through this tissue to carry medications such as antibiotics. Apply a sterile, dry dressing over the wet compress. If the burn is over a large area, wrap a sterile towel over the area, and get the patient to the hospital as soon as possible.

Second-degree burns are immersed in cold water for one to two hours. Do not open blisters. Do not apply any medications or ointments unless instructed to do so by the physician. Apply a dry, sterile protective bandage.

For third-degree burns, do not remove adhered particles or charred clothing. Cover the burns with thick, sterile dressings. Keep the patient warm and quiet, and provide him or her with emotional support. Chemical burns should be thoroughly rinsed with plenty of running water and should be covered with a sterile dressing.

The most serious effect of extensive burns is shock. Observe the patient for any signs and symptoms of shock, and begin first aid immediately.

Lacerations

Lacerations are a common presentation in general practice and pediatrics. A lacerated wound displays a jagged or irregular tearing of the tissues. Bleeding may be profuse. Since there is much tissue destruction, the possibility of contamination exists.

Have the patient lie down. The patient should be

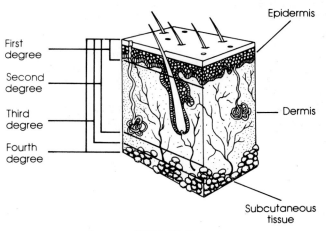

Figure 39–7
Depths of burns.

First degree
Second degree
Third degree
Fourth degree

Epidermis
Dermis
Subcutaneous tissue

39

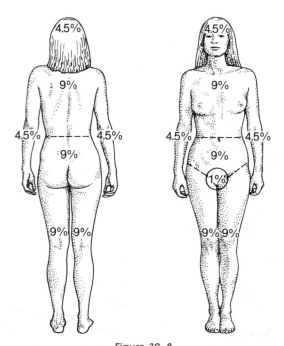

Figure 39–8
The extent of burn to the entire body surface is the usual method for determining the severity of burns. For example, a burn that involves the back, chest, and one arm would be calculated to be approximately 22 percent of the total body surface. Such a burn is considered severe enough to demand medical care. The figure shows how the percentages are determined. This is called the "Rule of Nines."

kept quiet. Cover the injured area with a sterile dressing. Use a dressing that is thick enough to absorb the bleeding. If bleeding persists or is profuse, apply direct pressure to the dressing and also to the area just above the wound. The injured part of the body should be elevated above the level of the victim's heart.

Wounds that are not bleeding severely and that do not involve deep tissues should be cleansed. Wash in and around the wound with soap and water to remove bacteria and other foreign matter. If the laceration is extremely dirty, it may be irrigated with sterile normal saline solution. Hydrogen peroxide is not generally recommended for fresh wounds as it may damage tissue. Rinse the wound thoroughly with clean water, and blot dry. Then cover the injured area with a sterile dressing.

A butterfly closure strip may be used over small lacerations, to hold the edges together. If the wound is superficial and has straight edges, it may be closed with a microporous tape, which eliminates the discomfort of suturing and suture removal as well as some of the potential risks of infected sutures. The tape (available in 1/4- or 1/2-inch widths) is placed at approximately 1/4-inch intervals until the wound is closed. Generally, closure is started near one end. However, a longer wound could be brought together in quarters, and then the intervening spaces closed next. Figure 39–9 shows an excellent method of informing patients as to the nature of their injury and of both the office and the home treatment required.

Animal Bites

Any animal bite that breaks the skin should be seen by a physician and reported to the authorities. The animal must be identified and confined for quarantine. The animal should not be killed because a positive rabies identification is almost impossible to make if the animal has been dead for a while. Many pet owners will not admit that their pet has bitten a person because they fear that the animal will be killed. Assure them that the Health Department authorities only want to confine the animal for observation. The bite should be washed thoroughly with soap and water and should be treated as any other wound would be. The victim should be seen by a physician.

Nosebleeds (Epistaxis)

Nosebleed, or epistaxis, is a hemorrhage from the nose usually resulting from the rupture of small vessels within the nose. Nosebleeds can result from injury, disease, strenuous activity, high altitudes, and exposure to cold. Keep the patient quiet and in a sitting position. Apply external pressure to the affected nostril. Cold compresses to the nose and

Medic East

David A. Goodman, M.D.
Medical Director

2810 East Washington Ave.
Madison, WI 53704
(608) 244–1213

Member of National Association
For Ambulatory Care

Injury: Abrasions, Cuts, Lacerations

Description: An abrasion occurs when a wide area of skin is
scraped off. Although there may not be much
bleeding, there is often much pain and the possibility of infection.
When the skin is cut, it requires rapid repair
to prevent infection and scarring. If the cut
is more than 8 hours old, significant healing
has already started, preventing the physician
from suturing it closed. (If an old wound is
sutured, there is a greater possibility of
infection).

Treatment: Abrasions must be carefully cleansed, especially
if much dirt is in the wound. After cleansing,
a thin layer of ointment is applied to promote
healing and comfort. This may or may not be covered with a dressing depending on the location of
the wound. Lacerations that are clean and recent
are often closed with suture. Sutures under the
skin dissolve and do not have to be removed.
Sutures on top of the skin need to be removed
according to doctor's instructions (generally
4–7 days in the face and up to 2 weeks in legs
and arms). Dressings are applied to keep the
wound clean and dry. These dressings should be
changed every 1–2 days, and the wound cleansed
with mild soap and water. After about 4 days,
the wound should be covered only to protect it
from getting dirty or wet.

The main complication of abrasions and lacerations
is infection, which if left unchecked, may cause
significant problems. Return to MedicEast if any
of the following signs are noted:
        *Fever
        *Pus type drainage
        *Swelling or redness
        *Red streaks near wound
        *Severe pain

39

Figure 39–9
Typical educational and informational literature given to the patient to help the home care of a wound. (Courtesy of Medic East, Madison, WI.)

face may also be of value. If bleeding cannot be controlled, insert a clean pad of gauze into the nostril.

Hemorrhages

Bleeding may be external or internal. Those administering first aid can do little about internal bleeding, except to keep the patient quiet and warm to minimize shock. Get medical help immediately.

External bleeding is not as complex as internal bleeding in that you can frequently see the source of the bleeding. Shock and loss of consciousness may occur from a rapid loss of blood in a short period of time. There are four practical ways of controlling severe bleeding.

The first technique is to use direct pressure over the area, by applying a sterile dressing. If blood soaks through the entire pad, do not remove the pad, but add additional pads of thick cloth and continue direct pressure. The second method is elevation of the injured part. Elevation uses the forces of gravity to control blood flow. The third method is to apply pressure over the nearest pressure point between the bleeding area and the heart. This compresses the main artery supplying the affected limb. The last resort is the application of a tourniquet. The use of a tourniquet is dangerous and should be used only for a life-threatening hemorrhage. By deciding to use a tourniquet, you have made a decision that the patient will bleed to death without it.

The types of wounds that would most probably require a tourniquet involve deep lacerations into an artery of the midupper arm, or amputation of the arm at the same level, and deep lacerations into an artery of the thigh, or amputation of the leg at the thigh level.

A tourniquet must be at least 2 inches wide. Less width may cause tissue damage under the tourniquet and, then, the possibility of amputation at a higher level on the extremity. A broad, flat tourniquet is best, and a pad should be used under the area of the tie. Wrap it twice around the extremity, about 1 to 2 inches above the wound. Tie a half-knot, and place a short stick on this knot. Tie a full knot over this stick. Twist the stick to tighten the tourniquet until you can no longer feel a pulse. Gently tighten the tourniquet until the bleeding is stopped. Do not make it any tighter, since the tissues beyond the tourniquet can die without blood circulation. Do not release the tourniquet but seek medical help immediately. If possible, avoid covering the tourniquet, so that emergency medical personnel will see it immediately. Also, write the time of the application on the victim's forehead, or pin a note on their clothing.

Because a tourniquet completely obstructs the flow of blood to an extremity, the victim may lose the injured extremity. In other words, the extremity may be sacrificed in order to save the victim's life.

Head Injuries

The severity of a head injury can vary greatly. With a head injury, the patient may appear normal, may experience dizziness, severe headache, or memory loss, or may even be unconscious. The loss of consciousness may be brief or prolonged; it may appear immediately or may be delayed. The victim may experience vomiting, loss of bladder and bowel control, and bleeding from the nose, mouth, or ears. The pupils of the eyes may be of unequal diameters.

All head injuries must be considered serious. Seek medical attention immediately. Have the victim lie flat unless there is difficulty in breathing. In such case, raise the head and shoulders slightly unless there is evidence of neck injury. Control any hemorrhage. Do not administer anything by mouth. Keep the patient warm and quiet. Watch the pupils of the eyes, and record any changes. Obtain the vital signs. Record the extent and duration of any unconsciousness.

Foreign Bodies in the Eye

This kind of emergency is most uncomfortable, and it is often extremely difficult to keep the patient from rubbing the eye. Tell the patient not to touch the eye in any way. If the doctor has given you prior permission, you may put a few drops of ophthalmic topical anesthetic in the eye. The patient will greatly appreciate this and will experience almost immediate relief. The eye may be rinsed with tepid tap water in an attempt to remove the object. Unless the foreign object is clearly visible, do not attempt to search for it or to remove it.

The medical assistant should never attempt to remove a foreign body from the cornea. The patient should be placed in a darkened room to wait. Have plenty of tissues available. If there is a contusion and swelling, cold wet compresses will help. If you have been trained to turn an upper eyelid out, then do so gently and search for the foreign body. Be very careful not to place any pressure on the eye. If the foreign body cannot be found, then ask the patient to close the eyes. Cover both eyes with eye pads and hold them in place with a strip of tape until the physician arrives.

Remember, emergencies can occur in the home, while you are vacationing, or in the physician's office. The medical assistant must remain calm, take charge of the situation, call for help, and be prepared to administer appropriate first-aid measures. Keep your Red Cross and American Heart Association cards current. Attend community workshops to maintain and extend your skills. Your participation in emergency care may help to save lives!

REFERENCES AND READINGS

American National Red Cross: *Cardiopulmonary Resuscitation, USA.* 1981
————:*Advanced First Aid and Emergency Care,* 2nd ed. 1981.
————:*Child Saver CPR.* 1985.
————:*Infant Saver.* 1984.
————:*Standard First Aid and Personal Safety,* 2nd ed. 1981.
Dugas, B. W.: *Introduction To Patient Care: A Comprehensive Approach to Nursing,* 4th ed. Philadelphia, W. B. Saunders Co., 1983.

Efferon, D. M.: *Cardiopulmonary Resuscitation,* 2nd ed. Tulsa, OK, CPR Publisher, Inc., 1984.
Marsh, J. D.: *Emergency! Basic Emergency Care.* Madison, WI, Madison General Hospital, 1984.
Reilly, B.: *Practical Strategies In Outpatient Medicine.* Philadelphia, W. B. Saunders Co., 1984.
Roberts, J. R., and Hedges, J. R.: *Clinical Procedures in Emergency Medicine.* Philadelphia, W. B. Saunders Co., 1985.
Wood, L. A.: *Nursing Skills for Allied Health Services.* Philadelphia, W. B. Saunders Co., 1984.

39

Combining Forms in Medical Terminology*

The following is a list of combining forms encountered frequently in the vocabulary of medicine. A dash or dashes are appended to indicate whether the form usually precedes (as *ante-*) or follows (as *-agra*) the other elements of the compound or usually appears between the other elements (as *-em-*). Following each combining form, the first item of information is the Greek or Latin word, or both a Greek and a Latin word, from which it is derived. Those words that are not printed in Greek characters are Latin. Information necessary to an understanding of the form appears next in parentheses. Then the meaning or meanings of the word are given, followed where appropriate by reference to a synonymous combining form. Finally, an example is given to illustrate the use of the combining form in a compound English derivative.

a-	*a-* (*n* is added before words beginning with a vowel) negative prefix. Cf. in-³. a*metria*
ab-	*ab* away from. Cf. apo-. *ab*ducent
abdomin-	*abdomen, abdominis.* *abdomi*noscopy
ac-	See ad-. *ac*cretion
acet-	*acetum* vinegar. *acet*ometer
acid-	*acidus* sour. *acid*uric
acou-	ἀκούω hear. *acou*esthesia. (Also spelled acu-)
acr-	ἄκρον extremity, peak. *acr*omegaly
act-	*ago, actus* do, drive, act. *act*reaction
actin-	ἀκτίς, ἀκτῖνος ray, radius. Cf. radi-. *actin*ogenesis
acu-	See acou-. osteo*acu*sis
ad-	*ad* (*d* changes to *c, f, g, p, s,* or *t* before words beginning with those consonants) to. *ad*renal
aden-	ἀδήν gland. Cf. gland-. *aden*oma
adip-	*adeps, adipis* fat. Cf. lip- and stear-. *adip*ocellular
aer-	ἀήρ air. an*aer*obiosis
aesthe-	See esthe-. *aesthe*sioneurosis
af-	See ad-. *af*ferent
ag-	See ad-. *ag*glutinant
-agogue	ἀγωγός leading, inducing. galact*agogue*
-agra	ἄγρα catching, seizure. pod*agra*
alb-	*albus* white. Cf. leuk-. *alb*ocinereous
alg-	ἄλγος pain. neur*alg*ia
all-	ἄλλος other, different. *all*ergy
alve-	*alveus* trough, channel, cavity. *alve*olar
amph-	See amphi-. *amph*eclexis
amphi-	ἀμφί (*i* is dropped before words beginning with a vowel) both, doubly. *amphi*celous
amyl-	ἄμυλον starch. *amyl*osynthesis
an-¹	See ana-. *an*agogic
an-²	See a-. *an*omalous
ana-	ἀνά (final *a* is dropped before words beginning with a vowel) up, positive. *ana*phoresis
ancyl-	See ankyl-. *ancyl*ostomiasis
andr-	ἀνήρ, ἀνδρός man. gyn*andr*oid
angi-	ἀγγεῖον vessel. Cf. vas-. *angi*emphraxis
ankyl-	ἀγκύλος crooked, looped. *anky*lodactylia. (Also spelled ancyl-)
ant-	See anti-. *ant*ophthalmic
ante-	*ante* before. *ante*flexion
anti-	ἀντί (*i* is dropped before words beginning with a vowel) against, counter. Cf. contra-. *anti*pyogenic
antr-	ἄντρον cavern. *antr*odynia
ap-¹	See apo-. *ap*heter
ap-²	See ad-. *ap*pend
-aph-	ἅπτω, ἀφ- touch. dys*aph*ia. (See also hapt-)
apo-	ἀπό (*o* is dropped before words beginning with a vowel) away from, detached. Cf. ab-. *apo*physis
arachn-	ἀράχνη spider. *arachn*odactyly
arch-	ἀρχή beginning, origin. *arch*enteron
arter(i)-	ἀρτηρία elevator (?), artery. *arterio*sclerosis, peri*arter*itis
arthr-	ἄρθρον joint. Cf. articul-. syn*arthr*osis
articul-	*articulus* joint. Cf. arthr-. dis*articul*ation

*Compiled by Lloyd W. Daly, A.M., Ph.D., Litt.D., Allen Memorial Professor of Greek, University of Pennsylvania. *In* Dorland's Pocket Medical Dictionary, 21st ed. Philadelphia, W. B. Saunders Co., 1968.

as-   See ad-. *assimilation*

at-   See ad-. *attrition*

aur-   *auris* ear. Cf. ot-. *aur*inasal

aux-   αὔξω increase. enter*auxe*

ax-   ἄξων or *axis* axis. *ax*ofugal

axon-   ἄξων axis. *axon*ometer

ba-   βαίνω, βα- go, walk, stand. hypno*batia*

bacill-   *bacillus* small staff, rod. Cf. bacter-. actino*bacill*osis

bacter-   βακτήριον small staff, rod. Cf. bacill-. *bacter*iophage

ball-   βάλλω, βολ- throw. *ball*istics. (See also bol-)

bar-   βάρος weight. pedo*bar*ometer

bi-¹   βίος life. Cf. vit-. aero*bic*

bi-²   *bi*- two (see also di-¹). *bi*lobate

bil-   *bilis* bile. Cf. chol-. *bil*iary

blast-   βλαστός bud, child, a growing thing in its early stages. Cf. germ-. *blast*oma, zygoto*blast*.

blep-   βλέπω look, see. hemia*blep*sia

blephar-   βλέφαρον (from βλέπω; see blep-) eyelid. Cf. cili-. *blephar*oncus

bol-   See ball-. em*bol*ism

brachi-   βραχίων arm. *brachi*ocephalic

brachy-   βραχύς short. *brachy*cephalic

brady-   βραδύς slow. *brady*cardia

brom-   βρῶμος stench. podo*brom*idrosis

bronch-   βρόγχος windpipe. *bronch*oscopy

bry-   βρύω be full of life. em*bry*onic

bucc-   *bucca* cheek. disto*bucc*al

cac-   κακός bad, abnormal. Cf. mal-. *cac*odontia, arthro*cac*e. (See also dys-)

calc-¹   *calx, calcis* stone (cf. lith-), limestone, lime. *calc*ipexy

calc-²   *calx, calcis* heel. *calc*aneotibial

calor-   *calor* heat. Cf. therm-. *calor*imeter

cancr-   *cancer, cancri* crab, cancer. Cf. carcin-. *cancr*ology. (Also spelled chancr-)

capit-   *caput, capitis* head. Cf. cephal-. de*capit*ator

caps-   *capsa* (from *capio;* see cept-) container. en*caps*ulation

carbo(n)-   *carbo, carbonis* coal, charcoal. *carbo*hydrate, *carbon*uria

carcin-   καρκίνος crab, cancer. Cf. cancr-. *carcin*oma

cardi-   καρδία heart. lipo*cardi*ac

cary-   See kary-. *cary*okinesis

cat-   See cata-. *cat*hode

cata-   κατά (final *a* is dropped before words beginning with a vowel) down, negative. *cata*batic

caud-   *cauda* tail. *caud*ad

cav-   *cavus* hollow. Cf. coel-. con*cav*e

cec-   *caecus* blind. Cf. typhl-. *cec*opexy

cel-¹   See coel-. amphi*cel*ous

cel-²   See -cele. *cel*ectome

-cele   κήλη tumor, hernia. gastro*cele*

cell-   *cella* room, cell. Cf. cyt-. *cell*iferous

cen-   κοινός common. *cen*esthesia

cent-   *centum* hundred. Cf. hect-. Indicates fraction in metric system. [This exemplifies the custom in the metric system of identifying fractions of units by stems from the Latin, as *cent*imeter, *deci*meter, *milli*meter, and multiples of units by the similar stems from the Greek, as *hecto*meter, *deca*meter, and *kilo*meter.] *cent*imeter, *centi*pede

cente-   κεντέω puncture. Cf. punct-. entero*cente*sis

centr-   κέντρον or *centrum* point, center. neuro*centr*al

cephal-   κεφαλή head. Cf. capit-. en*cephal*itis

cept-   *capio, -cipientis, -ceptus* take, receive. re*cept*or

cer-   κηρός or *cera* wax. *cer*oplasty, *cer*omel

cerat-   See kerat-. a*cerat*osis

cerebr-   *cerebrum.* *cerebr*ospinal

cervic-   *cervix, cervicis* neck. Cf. trachel-. *cervic*itis

chancr-   See cancr-. *chancr*iform

cheil-   χεῖλος lip. Cf. labi-. *cheil*oschisis

cheir-   χείρ hand. Cf. man-. macro*cheir*ia. (Also spelled chir-)

chir-   See cheir-. *chir*omegaly

chlor-   χλωρός green. a*chlor*opsia

chol-   χολή bile. Cf. bil-. hepato*chol*angeitis

chondr-   χόνδρος cartilage. *chondr*omalacia

chord-   χορδή string, cord. peri*chord*al

chori-   χόριον protective fetal membrane. endo*chori*on

chro-   χρώς color. poly*chro*matic

chron-   χρόνος time. syn*chron*ous

chy-   χέω, χυ- pour. ec*chy*mosis

-cid(e)   *caedo, -cisus* cut, kill. infanti*cide,* germi*cid*al

cili-   *cilium* eyelid. Cf. blephar-. super*cili*ary

cine-   See kine-. auto*cine*sis

-cipient-   See cept-. in*cipient*

circum-   *circum* around. Cf. peri-. *circum*ferential

-cis-   *caedo, -cisus* cut, kill. ex*cis*ion

clas-   κλάω, κλασ- break. cranio*clast*

clin-   κλίνω bend, incline, make lie down. *clin*ometer

clus-   *claudo, -clusus* shut. Maloc*clus*ion

co-   See con-. *co*hesion

cocc-   κόκκος seed, pill. gono*cocc*us

coel-   κοῖλος hollow. Cf. cav-. *coel*enteron. (Also spelled cel-)

col-¹   See colon-. *col*ic

col-²   See con-. *col*lapse

colon-   κόλον lower intestine. *colon*ic

colp-   κόλπος hollow, vagina. Cf. sin-. endo*colp*itis

com-   See con-. *com*masculation

con-   *con*- (becomes *co*- before vowels or *h; col*- before *l; com*- before *b, m,* or *p; cor*- before *r*) with, together. Cf. syn-. *con*traction

contra-   *contra* against, counter. Cf. anti-. *contra*indication

copr-   κόπρος dung. Cf. sterco-. *copr*oma

cor-¹   κόρη doll, little image, pupil. iso*cor*ia

cor-²   See con-. *cor*rugator

corpor-   *corpus, corporis* body. Cf. somat-. intra*corpor*al

cortic-   *cortex, corticis* bark, rind. *cortic*osterone

cost-   *costa* rib. Cf. pleur-. inter*cost*al

crani-   κρανίον or *cranium* skull. peri*crani*um

creat-   κρέας, κρεατ- meat, flesh. *creat*orrhea

-crescent   *cresco, crescentis, cretus* grow. ex*crescent*

cret-¹   *cerno, cretus* distinguish, separate off. Cf. crin-. dis*cret*e

cret-²   See -crescent. ac*cret*ion

crin-   κρίνω distinguish, separate off. Cf. cret-¹. endo*crin*ology

crur-   *crus, cruris* shin, leg. brachio*crur*al

cry-   κρύος cold. *cry*esthesia

crypt-   κρύπτω hide, conceal. *crypt*orchism

cult-   *colo, cultus* tend, cultivate. *cult*ure

cune-   *cuneus* wedge. Cf. sphen-. *cune*iform

cut-   *cutis* skin. Cf. derm(at)-. sub*cut*aneous

cyan-   κύανος blue. antho*cyan*in

cycl-   κύκλος circle, cycle. *cycl*ophoria

cyst-   κύστις bladder. Cf. vesic-. nephro*cyst*itis

cyt-   κύτος cell. Cf. cell-. plasmo*cyt*oma

dacry-   δάκρυ tear. *dacry*ocyst

dactyl-   δάκτυλος finger, toe. Cf. digit-. hexa*dactyl*ism

de-   *de* down from. *de*composition

dec-¹   δέκα ten. Indicates multiple in metric system. Cf. dec-². *deca*gram

dec-²   *decem* ten. Indicates fraction in metric system. Cf. dec-¹. *deci*para, *deci*meter

dendr-   δένδρον tree. neuro*dendr*ite

dent-   *dens, dentis* tooth. Cf. odont-. inter*dent*al

derm(at)-   δέρμα, δέρματος skin. Cf. cut-. endo*derm,* *dermat*itis

desm-   δεσμός band, ligament. syn*desm*opexy

dextr- — *dexter, dextr-* right-hand. ambi*dextr*ous

di-¹ — *di-* two. *di*morphic. (See also bi-²)

di-² — See dia-. *di*uresis.

di-³ — See dis-. *di*vergent.

dia- — διά (a is dropped before words beginning with a vowel) through, apart. Cf. per-. *dia*gnosis

didym- — δίδυμος twin. Cf. gemin-. epi*didym*al

digit- — *digitus* finger, toe. Cf. dactyl-. *digit*igrade

diplo- — διπλόος double. *diplo*myelia

dis- — *dis-* (s may be dropped before a word beginning with a consonant) apart, away from. *dis*location

disc- — δίσκος or *discus* disk. *disco*placenta

dors- — *dorsum* back. ventro*dors*al

drom- — δρόμος course. hemo*drom*ometer

-ducent — See duct-. ad*ducent*

duct- — *duco, ducentis, ductus* lead, conduct. ovi*duct*

dur- — *durus* hard. Cf. scler-. in*dura*tion

dynam(i)- — δύναμις power. *dynam*oneure, neuro*dynam*ic

dys- — δυσ- bad, improper. Cf. mal-. *dys*trophic. (See also cac-)

e- — *e* out from. Cf. ec- and ex-. *e*mission

ec- — ἐκ out of. Cf. e- *ec*centric

-ech- — ἔχω have, hold, be. syn*ech*otomy

ect- — ἐκτός outside. Cf. extra-. *ecto*plasm

ede- — οἰδέω swell. *ede*matous

ef- — See ex-. *ef*florescent

-elc- — ἕλκος sore, ulcer. enter*elc*osis. (See also helc-)

electr- — ἤλεκτρον amber. *electr*otherapy

em- — See en-. *em*bolism, *em*pathy, *em*phlysis

-em- — αἷμα blood. an*em*ia. (See also hem(at)-)

en- — ἐν (n changes to m before b, p, or ph) in, on. Cf. in-². *en*cellitis

end- — ἔνδον inside. Cf. intra-. *end*angium.

enter- — ἔντερον intestine. dys*enter*y

ep- — See epi-. *ep*axial

epi- — ἐπί (i is dropped before words beginning with a vowel) upon, after, in addition. *epi*glottis

erg- — ἔργον work, deed. *erg*y

erythr- — ἐρυθρός red. Cf. rub(r)-. *erythr*ochromia

eso- — ἔσω inside. Cf. intra-. *eso*phylactic

esthe- — αἰσθάνομαι, αἰσθη- perceive, feel. Cf. sens-. an*esthe*sia

eu- — εὖ good, normal. *eu*pepsia

ex- — ἐξ or *ex* out of. Cf. e-. *ex*cretion

exo- — ἔξω outside. Cf. extra-. *exo*pathic

extra- — *extra* outside of, beyond. Cf. ect- and exo-. *extra*cellular

faci- — *facies* face. Cf. prosop-. brachio*faci*olingual

-facient — *facio, facientis, factus, -fectus* make. Cf. poie-. cale*facient*

-fact- — See facient-. arte*fact*

fasci- — *fascia* band. *fasci*orrhaphy

febr- — *febris* fever. Cf. pyr-. *febr*icide

-fect- — See -facient. de*fect*ive

-ferent — *fero, ferentis, latus* bear, carry. Cf. phor-. ef*ferent*

ferr- — *ferrum* iron. *ferr*oprotein

fibr- — *fibra* fibre. Cf. in-¹. chondro*fibr*oma

fil- — *filum* thread. *fil*iform

fiss- — *findo, fissus* split. Cf. schis-. *fiss*ion

flagell- — *flagellum* whip. *flagell*ation

flav- — *flavus* yellow. Cf. xanth-. ribo*flav*in

-flect- — *flecto, flexus* bend, divert. de*flect*ion

-flex- — See -flect-. re*flex*ometer

flu- — *fluo, fluxus* flow. Cf. rhe-. *flu*id

flux- — See flu-. af*flux*ion

for- — *foris* door, opening. *for*ated

-form — *forma* shape. Cf. -oid. ossi*form*

fract- — *frango, fractus* break. re*fract*ive

front- — *frons, frontis* forehead, front. naso*front*al

-fug(e) — *fugio* flee, avoid. vermi*fuge*, centri*fug*al

funct- — *fungor, functus* perform, serve, function. mal*function*

fund- — *fundo, fusus* pour. in*fund*ibulum

fus- — See fund-. dif*fus*ible

galact- — γάλα, γάλακτος milk. Cf. lact-. dys*galact*ia

gam- — γάμος marriage, reproductive union. a*gam*ont

gangli- — γάγγλιον swelling, plexus. neuro*gangli*itis

gastr- — γαστήρ, γαστρός stomach. cholangio*gastr*ostomy

gelat- — *gelo, gelatus* freeze, congeal. *gelat*in

gemin- — *geminus* twin, double. Cf. didym-. quadri*gemin*al

gen- — γίγνομαι, γεν-, γον- become, be produced, originate, or γεννάω produce, originate. cyto*gen*ic

germ- — *germen, germinis* bud, a growing thing in its early stages. Cf. blast-. *germ*inal, ovi*germ*

gest- — *gero, gerentis, gestus* bear, carry. con*gest*ion

gland- — *glans, glandis* acorn. Cf. aden-. intra*gland*ular

-glia — γλία glue. neuro*glia*

gloss- — γλῶσσα tongue. Cf. lingu-. tricho*gloss*ia

glott- — γλῶττα tongue, language. *glott*ic

gluc- — See glyc(y)-. *gluc*ophenetidin

glutin- — *gluten, glutinis* glue. ag*glutin*ation

glyc(y)- — γλυκύς sweet. *glyc*emia, *glycy*rrhizin. (Also spelled gluc-)

gnath- — γνάθος jaw. ortho*gnath*ous

gno- — γιγνώσκω, γνω- know, discern. dia*gno*sis

gon- — See gen-. amphi*gon*y

grad- — *gradior* walk, take steps. retro*grad*e

-gram — γράφω, γραφ- + -μα scratch, write, record. cardio*gram*

gran- — *granum* grain, particle. lipo*gran*uloma

graph- — γράφω scratch, write, record. histo*graph*y

grav- — *gravis* heavy. multi*grav*ida

gyn(ec)- — γυνή, γυναικός woman, wife. andro*gyn*y, *gynec*ologic

gyr- — γῦρος ring, circle. *gyr*ospasm

haem(at)- — See hem(at)-. *haem*orrhagia, *haemat*oxylon

hapt- — ἅπτω touch. *hapt*ometer

hect- — ἑκτ- hundred. Cf. cent-. Indicates multiple in metric system. *hect*ometer

helc- — ἕλκος sore, ulcer. *helc*osis

hem(at)- — αἷμα, αἵματος blood. Cf. sanguin-. *hem*angioma, *hemat*ocyturia. (See also -em-)

hemi- — ἡμι- half. Cf. semi-. *hemi*ageusia

hen- — εἷς, ἑνός one. Cf. un-. *hen*ogenesis

hepat- — ἧπαρ, ἥπατος liver. gastro*hepat*ic

hept(a)- — ἑπτά seven. Cf. sept-². *hept*atomic, *hepta*valent

hered- — *heres, heredis* heir. *hered*oimmunity

hex-¹ — ἕξ six. Cf. sex-. *hex*yl-. An a is added in some combinations.

hex-² — ἔχω, ἑχ- (added to σ becomes ἑξ-) have, hold, be. ca*hex*y

hexa- — See hex-¹. *hexa*chromic

hidr- — ἱδρώς sweat. hyper*hidr*osis

hist- — ἱστός web, tissue. *hist*odialysis

hod- — ὁδός road, path. *hod*oneuromere. (See also od- and -ode¹)

hom- — ὁμός common, same. *hom*omorphic

horm- — ὁρμή impetus, impulse. *horm*one

hydat- — ὕδωρ, ὕδατος water. *hydat*ism

hydr- — ὕδωρ, ὑδρ- water. Cf. lymph-. achlor*hydr*ia

hyp- — See hypo-. *hyp*axial

hyper- — ὑπέρ above, beyond, extreme. Cf. super-. *hyper*trophy

hypn- — ὕπνος sleep. *hypn*otic

hypo- — ὑπό (o is dropped before words beginning with a vowel) under, below. Cf. sub-. *hypo*metabolism

hyster- — ὑστέρα womb. colpo*hyster*opexy

iatr- — ἰατρός physician. ped*iatr*ics

idi-	ἴδιος peculiar, separate, distinct. *idi*osyncrasy
il-	See in-². ³. *il*linition (in, on), *il*legible (negative prefix)
ile-	See ili- [ile- is commonly used to refer to the portion of the intestines known as the ileum]. *ile*ostomy
ili-	*ilium (ileum)* lower abdomen, intestines [ili- is commonly used to refer to the flaring part of the hip bone known as the ilium]. *ili*osacral
im-	See in-². ³. *im*mersion (in, on), *im*perforation (negative prefix)
in-¹	ἴς, ἰνός fiber. Cf. fibr-. *in*osteatoma
in-²	*in (n* changes to *l, m,* or *r* before words beginning with those consonants) in, on. Cf. en-. *in*sertion
in-³	*in- (n* changes to *l, m,* or *r* before words beginning with those consonants) negative prefix. Cf. a-. *in*valid
infra-	*infra* beneath. *infra*orbital
insul-	*insula* island. *insul*in
inter-	*inter* among, between. *inter*carpal
intra-	*intra* inside. Cf. end- and eso-. *intra*venous
ir-	See in-². ³. *ir*radiation (in, on), *ir*reducible (negative prefix)
irid-	ἴρις, ἴριδος rainbow, colored circle. kerato*irid*ocyclitis
is-	ἴσος equal. *is*otope
ischi-	ἴσχιον hip, haunch. *ischi*opubic
jact-	*iacio, iactus* throw. *jact*itation
ject-	*iacio, -iectus* throw. in*ject*ion
jejun-	*ieiunus* hungry, not partaking of food. gastro*jejun*ostomy
jug-	*iugum* yoke. con*jug*ation
junct-	*iungo, iunctus* yoke, join. con*junct*iva
kary-	κάρυον nut, kernel, nucleus. Cf. nucle-. mega*kary*ocyte. (Also spelled cary-)
kerat-	κέρας, κέρατος horn. *kerat*olysis. (Also spelled cerat-)
kil-	χίλιοι one thousand. Cf. mill-. Indicates multiple in metric system. *kil*ogram
kine-	κινέω move. *kine*matograph. (Also spelled cine-)
labi-	*labium* lip. Cf. cheil-. gingivo*labi*al
lact-	*lac, lactis* milk. Cf. galact-. gluco*lact*one
lal-	λαλέω talk, babble. glosso*lal*ia
lapar-	λαπάρα flank. *lapar*otomy
laryng-	λάρυγξ, λάρυγγος windpipe. *laryng*endoscope
lat-	*fero, latus* bear, carry. See -ferent. trans*lat*ion
later-	*latus, lateris* side. ventro*later*al
lent-	*lens, lentis* lentil. Cf. phac-. *lent*iconus
lep-	λαμβάνω, ληπ- take, seize. cata*lep*tic
leuc-	See leuk-. *leuc*inuria
leuk-	λευκός white. Cf. alb-. *leuk*orrhea. (Also spelled leuc-)
lien-	*lien* spleen. Cf. splen-. *lien*ocele
lig-	*ligo* tie, bind. *lig*ate
lingu-	*lingua* tongue. Cf. gloss-. sub*lingu*al
lip-	λίπος fat. Cf. adip-. glyco*lip*in
lith-	λίθος stone. Cf. calc-¹. nephro*lith*otomy
loc-	*locus* place. Cf. top-. *loc*omotion
log-	λέγω, λογ- speak, give an account. *log*orrhea, embry*olog*y
lumb-	*lumbus* loin. dorso*lumb*ar
lute-	*luteus* yellow. Cf. xanth-. *lute*oma
ly-	λύω loose, dissolve. Cf. solut-. kerato*ly*sis
lymph-	*lympha* water. Cf. hydr-. *lymph*adenosis
macr-	μακρός long, large. *macr*omyeloblast
mal-	*malus* bad, abnormal. Cf. cac- and dys-. *mal*function
malac-	μαλακός soft. osteo*malac*ia
mamm-	*mamma* breast. Cf. mast-. sub*mamm*ary
man-	*manus* hand. Cf. cheir-. *man*iphalanx
mani-	μανία mental aberration. *mani*graphy, klepto*mani*a
mast-	μαστός breast. Cf. mamm-. hyper*mast*ia
medi-	*medius* middle. Cf. mes-. *medi*frontal
mega-	μέγας great, large. Also indicates multiple (1,000,000) in metric system. *mega*colon, *mega*dyne. (See also megal-)
megal-	μέγας, μεγάλου great, large. acro*megal*y
mel-	μέλος limb, member. sym*mel*ia
melan-	μέλας, μέλανος black. hippo*melan*in
men-	μήν month. dys*men*orrhea
mening-	μῆνιγξ, μήνιγγος membrane. encephalo*mening*itis
ment-	*mens, mentis* mind. Cf. phren-, psych- and thym-. de*ment*ia
mer-	μέρος part. poly*mer*ic
mes-	μέσος middle. Cf. medi-. *mes*oderm
met-	See meta-. *met*allergy
meta-	μετά (*a* is dropped before words beginning with a vowel) after, beyond, accompanying. *meta*carpal
metr-¹	μέτρον measure. stereo*metr*y
metr-²	μήτρα womb. endo*metr*itis
micr-	μικρός small. photo*micr*ograph
mill-	*mille* one thousand. Cf. kil-. Indicates fraction in metric system. *mill*igram, *mill*ipede
miss-	See -mittent. intro*miss*ion
-mittent	*mitto, mittentis, missus* send. inter*mittent*
mne-	μιμνήσκω, μνη- remember. pseudo*mne*sia
mon-	μόνος only, sole. *mon*oplegia
morph-	μορφή form, shape. poly*morph*onuclear
mot-	*moveo, motus* move. vaso*mot*or
my-	μῦς, μυός muscle. inoleio*my*oma
-myces	μύκης, μύκητος fungus. myelo*myces*
myc(et)-	See -myces. asco*myc*etes, strepto*myc*in
myel-	μυελός marrow. polio*myel*itis
myx-	μύξα mucus. *myx*edema
narc-	νάρκη numbness. topo*narc*osis
nas-	*nasus* nose. Cf. rhin-. palato*nas*al
ne-	νέος new, young. *ne*ocyte
necr-	νεκρός corpse. *necr*ocytosis
nephr-	νεφρός kidney. Cf. ren-. para*nephr*ic
neur-	νεῦρον nerve. esthesio*neur*e
nod-	*nodus* knot. *nod*osity
nom-	νόμος (from νέμω deal out, distribute) law, custom. tax*onom*y
non-	*nona* nine. *non*acosane
nos-	νόσος disease. *nos*ology
nucle-	*nucleus* (from *nux, nucis* nut) kernel. Cf. kary-. *nucle*ide
nutri-	*nutrio* nourish. mal*nutri*tion
ob-	*ob (b* changes to *c* before words beginning with that consonant) against, toward, etc. *ob*tuse
oc-	See ob-. *oc*clude.
ocul-	*oculus* eye. Cf. ophthalm-. *ocul*omotor
-od-	See -ode¹. peri*od*ic
-ode¹	ὁδός road, path. cath*ode*. (See also hod-)
-ode²	See -oid. nemat*ode*
odont-	ὀδούς, ὀδόντος tooth. Cf. dent-. orth*odont*ia
-odyn-	ὀδύνη pain, distress. gastr*odyn*ia
-oid	εἶδος form. Cf. -form. hy*oid*
-ol	See ole-. cholester*ol*
ole-	*oleum* oil. *ole*oresin
olig-	ὀλίγος few, small. *olig*ospermia
omphal-	ὀμφαλός navel. peri*omphal*ic
onc-	ὄγκος bulk, mass. hemat*onc*ometry
onych-	ὄνυξ, ὄνυχος claw, nail. an*onych*ia
oo-	ὠόν egg. Cf. ov-. peri*oo*thecitis
op-	ὁράω, ὀπ- see. erythr*op*sia
ophthalm-	ὀφθαλμός eye. Cf. ocul-. ex*ophthalm*ic

or-   *os, oris* mouth. Cf. stom(at)-. intra*or*al

orb-   *orbis* circle. sub*orb*ital

orchi-   ὄρχις testicle. Cf. test-. *orchi*opathy

organ-   ὄργανον implement, instrument. *organ*oleptic

orth-   ὀρθός straight, right, normal. *orth*opedics

oss-   *os, ossis* bone. Cf. ost(e)-. *oss*iphone

ost(e)-   ὀστέον bone. Cf. oss-. en*ost*osis, *oste*anaphysis

ot-   οὖς, ὠτός ear. Cf. aur-. par*ot*id

ov-   *ovum* egg. Cf. oo-. syn*ov*ia

oxy-   ὀξύς sharp. *oxy*cephalic

pachy(n)-   παχύνω thicken. *pachy*derma, myo*pachy*nsis

pag-   πήγνυμι, παγ- fix, make fast. thoraco*pag*us

par-¹   *pario* bear, give birth to. primi*par*ous

par-²   See para-. *par*epigastric

para-   παρά (final *a* is dropped before words beginning with a vowel) beside, beyond. *para*mastoid

part-   *pario, partus* bear, give birth to. *part*urition

path-   πάθος that which one undergoes, sickness. psycho*path*ic

pec-   πήγνυμι, πηγ- (πηκ- before τ) fix, make fast. sym*pec*tothiene. (See also pex-)

ped-   παῖς, παιδός child. ortho*ped*ic

pell-   *pellis* skin, hide. *pell*agra

-pellent   *pello, pellentis, pulsus* drive. re*pellent*

pen-   πένομαι need, lack. erythrocyto*pen*ia

pend-   *pendeo* hang down. ap*pend*ix

pent(a)-   πέντε five. Cf. quinque-. *pent*ose, *penta*ploid

peps-   πέπτω, πεψ- (before σ) digest brady*peps*ia

pept-   πέπτω digest. dys*pept*ic

per-   *per* through. Cf. dia-. *per*nasal

peri-   περί around. Cf. circum-. *peri*phery

pet-   *peto* seek, tend toward. centri*pet*al

pex-   πήγνυμι, πηγ- (added to σ becomes πηξ-) fix, make fast. hepato*pex*y

pha-   φημί, φα- say, speak. dys*pha*sia

phac-   φακός lentil, lens. Cf. lent-. *phac*osclerosis. (Also spelled phak-)

phag-   φαγεῖν eat. lipo*phag*ic

phak-   See phac-. *phak*itis

phan-   See phen-. dia*phan*oscopy

pharmac-   φάρμακον drug. *pharmac*ognosy

pharyng-   φάρυγξ, φαρυγγ- throat. glosso*pharyng*eal

phen-   φαίνω, φαν- show, be seen. phos*phen*e

pher-   φέρω, φορ- bear, support. peri*pher*y

phil-   φιλέω like, have affinity for. eosino*phil*ia

phleb-   φλέψ, φλεβός vein. peri*phleb*itis

phleg-   φλέγω, φλογ- burn, inflame. adeno*phleg*mon

phlog-   See phleg-. anti*phlog*istic

phob-   φόβος fear, dread. claustro*phob*ia

phon-   φωνή sound. echo*phon*y

phor-   See pher-. Cf. -ferent. exo*phor*ia

phos-   See phot-. *phos*phorus

phot-   φῶς, φωτός light. *phot*erythrous

phrag-   φράσσω, φραγ- fence, wall off, stop up. Cf. sept-¹. dia*phrag*m

phrax-   φράσσω, φραγ- (added to σ becomes φραξ-) fence, wall off, stop up. em*phrax*is

phren-   φρήν mind, midriff. Cf. ment-. meta*phren*ia, meta*phren*on

phthi-   φθίνω decay, waste away. ophthalmo*phthi*sis

phy-   φύω beget, bring forth, produce, be by nature. noso*phy*te

phyl-   φῦλον tribe, kind. *phyl*ogeny

-phyll   φύλλον leaf. xantho*phyll*

phylac-   φύλαξ guard. pro*phylac*tic

phys(a)-   φυσάω blow, inflate. *phys*ocele, *phys*alis

physe-   φυσάω, φυση- blow, inflate. em*physe*ma

pil-   *pilus* hair. e*pil*ation

pituit-   *pituita* phlegm, rheum. *pituit*ous

placent-   *placenta* (from πλακοῦς) cake. extra*placent*al

plas-   πλάσσω mold, shape. cine*plas*ty

platy-   πλατύς broad, flat. *platy*rrhine

pleg-   πλήσσω, πληγ- strike. di*pleg*ia

plet-   *pleo, -pletus* fill. de*plet*ion

pleur-   πλευρά rib, side. Cf. cost-. peri*pleur*al

plex-   πλήσσω, πληγ- (added to σ becomes πληξ-) strike. apo*plex*y

plic-   *plico* fold. com*plic*ation

pne-   πνοιά breathing. traumato*pne*a

pneum(at)-   πνεῦμα, πνεύματος breath, air. *pneum*odynamics, *pneumat*othorax

pneumo(n)-   πνεύμων lung. Cf. pulmo(n)-. *pneumo*centesis, *pneumon*otomy

pod-   πούς, ποδός foot. *pod*iatry

poie-   ποιέω make, produce. Cf. -facient. sarco*poie*tic

pol-   πόλος axis of a sphere. peri*pol*ar

poly-   πολύς much, many. *poly*spermia

pont-   *pons, pontis* bridge. *pont*ocerebellar

por-¹   πόρος passage. myelo*por*e

por-²   πῶρος callus. *por*ocele

posit-   *pono, positus* put, place. re*posit*or

post-   *post* after, behind in time or place. *post*natal, *post*oral

pre-   *prae* before in time or place. *pre*natal, *pre*vesical

press-   *premo, pressus* press. *press*oreceptive

pro-   πρό or *pro* before in time or place. *pro*gamous, *pro*cheilon, *pro*lapse

proct-   πρωκτός anus. entero*proct*ia

prosop-   πρόσωπον face. Cf. faci-. di*prosop*us

pseud-   ψευδής false. *pseud*oparaplegia

psych-   ψυχή soul, mind. Cf. ment-. *psych*osomatic

pto-   πίπτω, πτω- fall. nephro*pto*sis

pub-   *pubes & puber, puberis* adult. ischio*pub*ic. (See also puber-)

puber-   *puber* adult. *puber*ty

pulmo(n)-   *pulmo, pulmonis* lung. Cf. pneumo(n)-. *pulmo*lith, cardio*pulmon*ary

puls-   *pello, pellentis, pulsus* drive. pro*puls*ion

punct-   *pungo, punctus* prick, pierce. Cf. cente-. *punct*iform

pur-   *pus, puris* pus. Cf. py-. sup*pur*ation

py-   πύον pus. Cf. pur-. nephro*py*osis

pyel-   πύελος trough, basin, pelvis. nephro*pyel*itis

pyl-   πύλη door, orifice. *pyl*ephlebitis

pyr-   πῦρ fire. Cf. febr-. galacto*pyr*a

quadr-   *quadr-* four. Cf. tetra-. *quadr*igeminal

quinque-   *quinque* five. Cf. pent(a)-. *quinque*cuspid

rachi-   ῥαχίς spine. Cf. spin-. encephalo*rachi*dian

radi-   *radius* ray. Cf. actin-. ir*radi*ation

re-   *re-* back, again. *re*traction

ren-   *renes* kidneys. Cf. nephr-. ad*ren*al

ret-   *rete* net. *ret*othelium

retro-   *retro* backwards. *retro*deviation

rhag-   ῥήγνυμι, ῥαγ- break, burst. hemor*rhag*ic

rhaph-   ῥαφή suture. gastror*rhaph*y

rhe-   ῥέω flow. Cf. flu-. diar*rhe*al

rhex-   ῥήγνυμι, ῥηγ- (added to σ becomes ῥηξ-) break, burst. metror*rhex*is

rhin-   ῥίς, ῥινός nose. Cf. nas-. basi*rhin*al

rot-   *rota* wheel. *rot*ator

rub(r)-   *ruber, rubri* red. Cf. erythr-. bili*rub*in, *rubr*ospinal

salping-   σάλπιγξ, σάλπιγγος tube, trumpet. *salping*itis

sanguin-   *sanguis, sanguinis* blood. Cf. hem(at)-. *sanguin*eous

sarc-   σάρξ, σαρκός flesh. *sarc*oma

schis-   σχίζω, σχιδ- (before τ or added to σ becomes σχισ-) split.

	Cf. fiss-. *schistorachis, rachischisis*
scler-	σκληρός hard. Cf. dur-. *sclerosis*
scop-	σκοπέω look at, observe. *endoscope*
sect-	*seco, sectus* cut. Cf. tom-. *sectile*
semi-	*semi-* half. Cf. hemi-. *semiflexion*
sens-	*sentio, sensus* perceive, feel. Cf. esthe-. *sensory*
sep-	σήπω rot, decay. *sepsis*
sept-¹	*saepio, saeptus* fence, wall off, stop up. Cf. phrag-. *naseptal*
sept-²	*septem* seven. Cf. hept(a)-. *septan*
ser-	*serum* whey, watery substance. *serosynovitis*
sex-	*sex* six. Cf. hex-¹. *sexdigitate*
sial-	σίαλον saliva. *polysialia*
sin-	*sinus* hollow, fold. Cf. colp-. *sinobronchitis*
sit-	σῖτος food. *parasitic*
solut-	*solvo, solventis, solutus* loose, dissolve, set free. Cf. ly-. *dissolution*
-solvent	See solut-. *dissolvent*
somat-	σῶμα, σώματος body. Cf. corpor-. *psychosomatic*
-some	See somat-. *dictyosome*
spas-	σπάω, σπασ- draw, pull. *spasm, spastic*
spectr-	*spectrum* appearance, what is seen. *microspectroscope*
sperm(at)-	σπέρμα, σπέρματος seed. *spermacrasia, spermatozoon*
spers-	*spargo, -spersus* scatter. *dispersion*
sphen-	σφήν wedge. Cf. cune-. *sphenoid*
spher-	σφαῖρα ball. *hemisphere*
sphygm-	σφυγμός pulsation. *sphygmomanometer*
spin-	*spina* spine. Cf. rachi-. *cerebrospinal*
spirat-	*spiro, spiratus* breathe. *inspiratory*
splanchn-	σπλάγχνα entrails, viscera. *neurosplanchnic*
splen-	σπλήν spleen. Cf. lien-. *splenomegaly*
spor-	σπόρος seed. *sporophyte, zygospore*
squam-	*squama* scale. *desquamation*
sta-	ἵστημι, στα- make stand, stop. *genesistasis*
stal-	στέλλω, σταλ- send. *peristalsis*. (See also stol-)
staphyl-	σταφυλή bunch of grapes, uvula. *staphylococcus, staphylectomy*
stear-	στέαρ, στέατος fat. Cf. adip-. *stearodermia*
steat-	See stear-. *steatopygous*
sten-	στενός narrow, compressed. *stenocardia*
ster-	στερεός solid. *cholesterol*
sterc-	*stercus* dung. Cf. copr-. *stercoporphyrin*
sthen-	σθένος strength. *asthenia*
stol-	στέλλω, στολ- send. *diastole*
stom(at)-	στόμα, στόματος mouth, orifice. Cf. or-. *anastomosis, stomatogastric*
strep(h)-	στρέφω, στρεπ- (before τ) twist. Cf. tors-. *strephosymbolia, streptomycin*. (See also stroph-)
strict-	*stringo, stringentis, strictus* draw tight, compress, cause pain. *constriction*
-stringent	See strict-. *astringent*
stroph-	στρέφω, στροφ- twist. *anastrophic*. (See also strep(h)-)
struct-	*struo, structus* pile up (against). *obstruction*
sub-	*sub* (*b* changes to *f* or *p* before words beginning with those consonants) under, below. Cf. hypo-. *sublumbar*
suf-	See sub-. *suffusion*
sup-	See sub-. *suppository*
super-	*super* above, beyond, extreme. Cf. hyper-. *supermotility*
sy-	See syn-. *systole*
syl-	See syn-. *syllepsiology*
sym-	See syn-. *symbiosis, symmetry, sympathetic, symphysis*
syn-	σύν (*n* disappears before *s*, changes to *l* before *l*, and changes to *m* before *b, m, p,* and *ph*) with, together. Cf. con-. *myosynizesis*
ta-	See ton-. *ectasis*
tac-	τάσσω, ταγ- (τακ- before τ) order, arrange. *atactic*
tact-	*tango, tactus* touch. *contact*
tax-	τάσσω, ταγ- (added to σ becomes ταξ-) order, arrange. *ataxia*
tect-	See teg-. *protective*
teg-	*tego, tectus* cover. *integument*
tel-	τέλος end. *telosynapsis*
tele-	τῆλε at a distance. *teleceptor*
tempor-	*tempus, temporis* time, timely or fatal spot, temple. *temporomalar*
ten(ont)-	τένων, τένοντος (from τείνω stretch) tight stretched band. *tenodynia, tenonitis, tenontagra*
tens-	*tendo, tensus* stretch. Cf. ton-. *extensor*
test-	*testis* testicle. Cf. orchi-. *testitis*
tetra-	τετρα- four. Cf. quadr-. *tetragenous*
the-	τίθημι, θη- put, place. *synthesis*
thec-	θήκη repository, case. *thecostegnosis*
thel-	θηλή teat, nipple. *thelerethism*
therap-	θεραπεία treatment. *hydrotherapy*
therm-	θέρμη heat. Cf. calor-. *diathermy*
thi-	θεῖον sulfur. *thiogenic*
thorac-	θώραξ, θώρακος chest. *thoracoplasty*
thromb-	θρόμβος lump, clot. *thrombopenia*
thym-	θυμός spirit. Cf. ment-. *dysthymia*
thyr-	θυρεός shield (shaped like a door θύρα). *thyroid*
tme-	τέμνω, τμη- cut. *axonotmesis*
toc-	τόκος childbirth. *dystocia*
tom-	τέμνω, τομ- cut. Cf. sect-. *appendectomy*
ton-	τείνω, τον- stretch, put under tension. Cf. tens-. *peritoneum*
top-	τόπος place. Cf. loc-. *topesthesia*
tors-	*torqueo, torsus* twist. Cf. strep-. *extorsion*
tox-	τοξικόν (from τόξον bow) arrow poison, poison. *toxemia*
trache-	τραχεῖα windpipe. *tracheotomy*
trachel-	τράχηλος neck. Cf. cervic-. *trachelopexy*
tract-	*traho, tractus* draw, drag. *protraction*
traumat-	τραῦμα, τραύματος wound. *traumatic*
tri-	τρεῖς, τρία or *tri-* three. *trigonid*
trich-	θρίξ, τριχός hair. *trichoid*
trip-	τρίβω rub. *entripsis*
trop-	τρέπω, τροπ- turn, react. *sitotropism*
troph-	τρέφω, τροφ- nurture. *atrophy*
tuber-	*tuber* swelling, node. *tubercle*
typ-	τύπος (from τύπτω strike) type. *atypical*
typh-	τῦφος fog, stupor. *adenotyphus*
typhl-	τυφλός blind. Cf. cec-. *typhlectasis*
un-	*unus* one. Cf. hen-. *unioval*
ur-	οὖρον urine. *polyuria*
vacc-	*vacca* cow. *vaccine*
vagin-	*vagina* sheath. *invaginated*
vas-	*vas* vessel. Cf. angi-. *vascular*
vers-	See vert-. *inversion*
vert-	*verto, versus* turn. *diverticulum*
vesic-	*vesica* bladder. Cf. cyst-. *vesicovaginal*
vit-	*vita* life. Cf. bi-¹. *devitalize*
vuls-	*vello, vulsus* pull, twitch. *convulsion*
xanth-	ξανθός yellow, blond. Cf. flav- and lute-. *xanthophyll*
-yl-	ὕλη substance. *cacodyl*
zo-	ζωή life, ζῷον animal. *microzoaria*
zyg-	ζυγόν yoke, union. *zygodactyly*
zym-	ζύμη ferment. *enzyme*

Common Abbreviations, Acronyms, and Symbols

abd	abdomen	CO_2	carbon dioxide
a.c.	before meals	COPD	chronic obstructive pulmonary disease
ad lib	as desired		
$AgNO_3$	silver nitrate	CPR	cardiopulmonary resuscitation
A/KA	above knee amputation		
Anesth	anesthesia	C/S	cesarean section
A & P	anterior and posterior, auscultation and percussion	CSF	cerebrospinal fluid
		CVA	cerebrovascular accident
		cysto	cystoscopy
ASCVD	arteriosclerotic cardio-vascular disease		
		D & C	dilatation and curettage
ASHD	arteriosclerotic heart disease	disch	discharge
		DJD	degenerative joint disease
A & W	alive and well	DM	diabetes mellitus
		DNA	deoxyribonucleic acid
BE	barium enema	DOA	dead on arrival
BID	twice a day	DOB	date of birth
B/KA	below knee amputation	DPT	diphtheria, pertussis, tetanus
BM	bowel movement	DR	delivery room
BMR	basal metabolic rate		
BP	blood pressure	Dx	diagnosis
BPH	benign prostatic hypertrophy		
BUN	blood urea nitrogen	EDC	estimated date of confinement
Bx	biopsy		
		EEG	electroencephalogram
C	centigrade	EENT	eye, ear, nose, and throat
Ca	calcium	EKG	electrocardiogram
CA	carcinoma	ENT	ear, nose, and throat
cal	calorie	EOM	extraocular movements
CBC	complete blood count	ER	emergency room
cc	cubic centimeter	EUA	examination under anesthesia
CCU	Coronary Care Unit	expl lap	exploratory laparotomy
CHF	congestive heart failure		
cm	centimeter	F	female
CNS	central nervous system	Fa or F	Fahrenheit

FB	foreign body	NB	newborn
FBS	fasting blood sugar	NP	neuropsychiatric
FH	family history	NPN	nonprotein nitrogen
FHT	fetal heart tones	N.P.O.	nothing by mouth
FS	frozen section	N & V	nausea and vomiting
FTG	full thickness graft		
FU	follow up	OB	obstetrics
FUO	fever of unknown origin	O.C.	oral contraceptive
Fx	fracture	OD	overdose
		O.D.	right eye
GB	gallbladder	OP	outpatient
GE	gastroenterology	O.R.	operating room
GI	gastrointestinal	O.S.	left eye
gm	gram	O.U.	both eyes
GP	general practitioner		
GTT	glucose tolerance test	Path	pathology
gtt	drops	PBI	protein bound iodine
GU	genitourinary	p.c.	after meals
GYN	gynecology	PCCU	Postcoronary Care Unit
		Peds	pediatrics
HCl	hydrochloric acid	PERRLA	pupils equal, round, regular,
HCVD	hypertensive cardiovascular		react to light and
	disease		accommodation
Hgb	hemoglobin	PFT	pulmonary function test
hs	at bedtime	PH	past history
Hx	history	PID	pelvic inflammatory disease
		PKU	phenylketonuria
ICU	Intensive Care Unit	PMR	Paramedic run
I & D	incision and drainage	PND	paroxysmal nocturnal
IM	intramuscular		dyspnea
inj	injection	PO	by mouth (per os)
int & ext	internal and external	PROM	premature rupture of
I & O	intake and output		membranes
IP	inpatient	pro time	prothrombin time
IPPB	intermittent positive	prn	when needed
	pressure breathing	Psych	psychiatry
IT	inhalation therapy	pt	patient
IUD	intrauterine device	PT	physical therapy
IV	intravenous	PU	peptic ulcer
IVP	intravenous pyelogram	Px	physical examination
K	potassium	q	every
KJ	knee jerk	qd	every day
KUB	kidney, ureter, and bladder	qh	every hour
		QID	four times a day
L	left	qn	every night
L & A	light and accommodation	qns	quantity not sufficient
lat	lateral		
LLQ	left lower quadrant	R	right
LMP	last menstrual period	Ra	radium
LOM	limitation of motion	R.A.	rheumatoid arthritis
LUQ	left upper quadrant	RBC	red blood cell
		REM	rapid eye movement
M	male	RHD	rheumatic heart disease
MH	marital history	R/O	rule out
MS	multiple sclerosis	ROS	review of systems

R.R.	recovery room		VDRL	Venereal Disease Research Laboratory
Rx	prescription		VS	vital signs
SH	social history		Wass	Wassermann
sig	directions		WBC	white blood cell
SMR	submucous resection		WDWN	well developed and well nourished
SOB	shortness of breath		WF	white female
stat	immediately		WM	white male
STG	split thickness graft		WNL	within normal limits
subq	subcutaneous			
SWD	short wave diathermy			

Symbols

T	temperature		$\bar{a}$	before
T & A	tonsillectomy & adenoidectomy		$\bar{aa}$	of each
tab	tablet		$\bar{c}$	with
TB	tuberculosis		$\bar{p}$	after
TIA	transient ischemic attack		$\bar{s}$	without
TID	three times a day		↓	decreased
TPR	temperature, pulse, respiration		↑	increased
TUR	transurethral resection		>	greater than
			<	less than
UA	urinalysis		✿	birth
UCHD	usual childhood diseases		—	negative
UR	utilization review		+	positive
URI	upper respiratory infection		±	negative or positive (indefinite)
UTI	urinary tract infection		♂	male
			♀	female
VA	visual acuity		μ	micron
VD	venereal disease		†	death

Recommendations for Prevention of AIDS Transmission

There is no evidence of person-to-person transmission of AIDS through ordinary daily or occupational contact, nor is there evidence that AIDS can be communicated through airborne transmission or contact with food or beverages. The epidemiologic pattern of AIDS appears to resemble closely that of hepatitis B virus infection, that is, it is a bloodborne, sexually transmitted disease. However, the number of AIDS cases continues to increase, and that increases the risk that medical assistants will be exposed to the blood of patients infected with the AIDS virus, especially if the precautions for blood and body fluids are not followed for *all* patients. This appendix of infection-control precautions should be adhered to rigorously to minimize your risk of exposure to the blood and body fluids of *all* patients.

DEFINITIONS

Acquired Immunodeficiency Syndrome (AIDS). Disease involving the total collapse of the human immune system. The body becomes defenseless and eventually succumbs to certain cancers, pneumonia, and other infections. There is strong evidence that the cause is the human immunodeficiency virus (HIV; formerly, HTLV III), although other factors, as yet unknown, may contribute. The H Group

Body Fluids. External and internal fluids, secretions, and excretions of the human body, including blood, semen, vaginal secretions, saliva, tears, breast milk, cerebrospinal fluid, amniotic fluid, and urine.

High-Level Disinfection. A chemical procedure that kills vegetative organisms and viruses but not large numbers of bacterial spores. The chemicals are termed "sterilants" and may be used for sterilization or high-level disinfection, provided that the contact time is correct. Chemical germicides are registered with the U.S. Environmental Protection Agency (EPA). Information on chemical germicides can be obtained by writing to the Disinfectants Branch, Office of Pesticides, Environmental Protection Agency, 401 M Street, SW, Washington, D.C. 20460.

Human Immunodeficiency Virus (HIV). A virus that causes acquired immunodeficiency syndrome (AIDS), transmitted through sexual contact and exposure to infected blood or blood components, and through mother to newborn. Although HIV has been isolated from other body fluids, secretions, and excretions, epidemiologic evidence suggests that transmission of HIV has implicated only blood, semen, vaginal secretions, and possibly breast milk.

Invasive Procedure. Surgical entry into tissues, cavities, or organs; repair of traumatic injuries in which skin is not intact; catheterization and angiographic procedures; vaginal or cesarean delivery or other gynecologic or obstetric procedures; or any procedure in the oral cavity during which bleeding occurs or the potential for bleeding exists.

UNIVERSAL PRECAUTIONS

The recommendations for preventing the transmission of HIV in health-care settings emphasize that *universal blood and body-fluid precautions* be consistently used for *all* patients in all situations, including emergency care, when there is an increased risk of exposure to blood, and when the infectious status of the patient is unknown.

The universal precaution system differs from the traditional isolation precaution system. The traditional isolation precaution system is based on a specific isolation technique that is used for a specific diagnosis or in the known presence of a specific disease category. Some isolation techniques include signs placed on doors and warning labels on specimens.

The universal precaution system is a body-substance isolation system and is not dependent on knowing whether or not a patient is infected with AIDS or any other blood-borne pathogen, such as hepatitis B. Since we cannot reliably identify all patients infected with HIV or other blood-borne pathogens, these recommendations emphasize the need to treat the blood and body fluids of *all* patients as potentially infectious.

This very simple strategy is based on the consistent application of procedures for contact with body substances of *all* patients. Implementation of the universal precaution system eliminates the need for warnings. No additional precautions are necessary, even if the patient is known to be infectious. The only exception is for airborne infections. Diagnosed or suspected airborne infections still require the use of traditional isolation techniques with regard to the patient, including the segregation of the patient from other patients and the use of masks (although the effectiveness of masks in preventing the inhalation of airborne pathogens has not been proved).

The universal precaution system is designed to reduce the risk of cross-infection of *any* infective agent in *any* body substance in *any* patient. The result is greater protection for health care workers and patients.

Barrier Protection

Medical assistants should routinely use appropriate barrier precautions when contact with blood or other body fluids is anticipated.

Gloves. Gloves should be changed after contact with each patient and after the handling of each specimen. Gloves should be worn for

- Touching a patient's blood and body fluids, mucous membranes, or skin that is not intact.
- Handling items and surfaces contaminated with blood and body fluids.
- Performing venipuncture and other vascular access procedures.
- Any invasive procedure. If a glove is torn or an injury occurs, the glove should be removed and replaced with a new glove as soon as safety permits. The instrument involved in the incident should be removed from the sterile field to a safe container.
- Dressing changes. Enclose small dressings inside the glove as you remove it, by grasping the dressing as you pull the glove off inside out.
- Handling and processing all specimens of blood and body fluids.
- Cleaning and decontaminating spills of blood or other body fluids.
- Disposing bulk blood, suctioned fluids, excretions, and secretions down a drain connected to a sanitary sewer.

Gowns and Aprons. Cover gowns or disposable plastic aprons should be worn

- If it is probable that your clothing will be soiled with body substances.
- When procedures are likely to generate splashes of blood or other body fluids.
- During invasive procedures that are likely to splash blood or other body fluids.
- When cleaning and decontaminating spills of blood or other body fluids.

Masks, Glasses, and Goggles. Protect your eyes and oral and nasal mucous membranes from contamination by shielding your face. Use disposable masks. Reusable goggles should be on hand for each physician and assistant and should be washed after each use. Eyeglasses are considered an effective barrier. Use masks and protective eyewear when

- Procedures are likely to generate droplets of blood or body fluids.
- Mucous-membrane contact with blood or body fluids is anticipated during the handling of blood or body fluid specimens.
- High-speed suctioning or evacuation equipment is likely to generate aerosol contamination.
- Laboratory procedures have a high potential for generating droplets (for example, blending, ultrasonic procedures, centrifugation, and vigorous mixing).

Hands and Skin Surfaces

If you have exudative lesions or weeping dermatitis, you should not perform any duties involving direct patient care. In addition, you should not handle any equipment used in patient care, until the condition resolves. Hands and skin surfaces should be washed

- Immediately after gloves are removed.
- Immediately and thoroughly after any accidental contact with blood or other body fluids.
- Immediately after the completion of any specimen processing.
- After completing daily clinical or laboratory activities, before leaving the office.

Needles and Sharp Instruments

Special care must be taken to prevent injuries caused by needles and sharp instruments during procedures, when cleaning used instruments, and during the disposal of instruments. These precautions should be followed:

- Do not recap used needles and scalpel blades.
- Do not bend or break needles and scalpel blades.
- Do not remove used needles from syringes.
- Do not otherwise manipulate used needles by hand.
- Do not remove used scalpel blades from handles by hand. Use a hemostat to remove the blade.
- Immediately after use, dispose of syringes and needles, scalpel blades, and other sharp items in puncture-resistant containers. The containers must be located as close as possible to the area where the instruments are used.
- Immediately after use, place reusable sharp materials in a puncture-resistant container for transport to the reprocessing room.
- If a needle cap must be replaced during work with specimens, recap with only one hand. Place the cap on a clean surface, and insert the needle into it.

Laboratory Specimens

All blood and other body fluids from every patient should be considered infective. The following precautions should be followed when handling specimens:

- Place all specimens in well-constructed containers with secure lids. Place this in a second container, such as an impervious bag, for transport. Check the bag for cracks or leaks.
- Avoid contaminating the outside of the container or the label with the specimen substance. If the outside is contaminated, the container should be disinfected, for example with 1:10 dilution of 5.25 percent sodium hypochlorite (household chlorine bleach and water), and placed in an impervious bag for transport.

- Biologic safety cabinets should be used if procedures are performed that generate droplets or spattering.
- Mouth pipetting must not be done.
- Laboratory work surfaces must be immediately decontaminated with a disinfectant (such as sodium hypochlorite) after accidental spills of blood or body fluids, and at the end of each procedure.
- Contaminated test materials should be decontaminated before reprocessing or should be placed in impervious bags and disposed of according to policy.
- Equipment that has been contaminated with blood or body fluid should be decontaminated before being repaired in the office or transported to the manufacturer.

ENVIRONMENTAL CONSIDERATIONS

There is no documentation of the transmission of HIV through the environment mode. However, certain precautions should be consistently practiced on *all* patients.

Sterilization and Disinfection

Current standards for sterilization and disinfection techniques are considered satisfactory for sterilizing and disinfecting items contaminated with blood and body fluids from patients infected with blood-borne pathogens, including HIV.

- Instruments that invade the tissues or the vascular system should be sterilized before reuse.
- Instruments and equipment that come into contact with the mucous membranes should be sterilized or receive high-level disinfection.
- HIV is rapidly inactivated after being exposed to common household bleach (sodium hypochlorite), prepared daily, in dilutions ranging from 1:100 to 1:10, depending on the amount of blood or body fluid present on the surface to be cleaned and disinfected. This method is inexpensive and effective.
- Many commercial germicides are effective and may be more compatible with certain medical devices and equipment that might be corroded by exposure to household bleach. Read the manufacturers' recommendations.

Housekeeping

Walls, floors, and other surfaces that are not in direct contact with treatment routines are not considered a source of infection. The strategies for cleaning and disinfecting these areas do not need to be changed.

- Cleaning and removing soil should be routine.
- Horizontal surfaces in the patient treatment areas should be cleaned on a regular basis, after spills, and after each patient.
- Scrubbing is as important as the disinfectant or detergent used.

Blood or Other Body Fluid Spills

The following procedure should be used for all spills involving blood or body fluids:

1. Do not proceed without the proper barrier protections (gloves, apron, goggles, and mask).
2. First, remove the visible material with disposable towels.
3. Place the spilled material and the towels immediately into an impervious bag, at the spill site.
4. Decontaminate the area with chemical germicides that are approved for use as "hospital disinfectants." The label should state that the disinfectant is tuberculocidal when used at room temperature. Household bleach (1:10 dilution of 5.25 percent sodium hypochlorite with water) may be used.
5. If the spill is large, the contaminated area should be flooded with a liquid germicide and then cleaned and decontaminated with fresh germicidal chemical.
6. Dispose of all materials, including your gloves, apron, and mask, in a second impervious bag.
7. Clean your goggles, and wash your hands thoroughly.

Laundry

The risk of HIV transmission from soiled linen is negligible. Good hygienic procedures are adequate.

- Handle soiled linen as little as possible.
- Handle linens with minimum agitation to prevent airborne transmission of microorganisms.
- Bag linens where they are used. Do not sort them.
- Linens soiled with blood or body fluids should be bagged and transported in bags that will not leak. Wear gloves and other protective clothing, as necessary.

Infective Waste

Every office should develop written policies for the removal of infective materials from the facility.

- Contaminated materials should be decontaminated before being placed in bags and disposed of.

- Infective waste should be autoclaved before disposal in a sanitary landfill or by incineration.
- Bulk blood and body fluids may be carefully poured down a drain connected to a sanitary sewer.

Special Ophthalmic Considerations

- Contact lenses used for trial fittings should be disinfected with a hydrogen peroxide contact lens disinfecting system or heat (172.4 to 176.0°F, 78 to 80°C) for ten minutes.
- Gloves should be worn during eye examinations and procedures involving contact with tears, or hands should be washed immediately after such examinations and procedures.

Miscellaneous Considerations

- Because the infant is at risk of infection during a pregnancy, pregnant health-care workers should be extremely familiar with and should strictly adhere to the precautions associated with HIV transmission.
- Although saliva has not been implicated in HIV transmission, mouthpieces, resuscitation bags, and other ventilation devices should be available for use in cardiopulmonary resuscitation (CPR).

MANAGEMENT AND RESPONSIBILITIES

All medical personnel should be charged with the following responsibilities:

- Establishing policies and procedures for the education of all personnel in the need for the routine use of universal blood and body fluid precautions for *all* patients.
- Providing the equipment and supplies necessary to minimize the risk of HIV transmission.
- Monitoring, with discipline, adherence to the universal blood and body-fluid precautions, and following this with counseling and retraining, when necessary.

REFERENCES AND READINGS

Acquired Immunodeficiency Syndrome Recommendations and Guidelines, November 1982 to November 1986. Atlanta, GA, Centers for Disease Control, 1986.

Centers for Disease Control: Recommendations for prevention of HIV transmission in health-care settings. MMWR 36 (Suppl. 2S), 1987.

Centers for Disease Control: Revision of the CDC surveillance case definition for acquired immunodeficiency syndrome. MMWR 36 (Suppl. 1S), 1987.

Jackson, M. M., Lynch, P., et al.: Why not treat all body substances as infectious? *American Journal of Nursing*, September 1987, pp. 1137–1139.

Model Hospital Protocol for Management of Patients with AIDS. Prepared by The AIDS Sub-Committee of the Personnel Resources Committee of the Hospital Council of Southern California. Los Angeles, 1985.

THE HUMAN BODY
HIGHLIGHTS of STRUCTURE and FUNCTION
SKELETAL SYSTEM

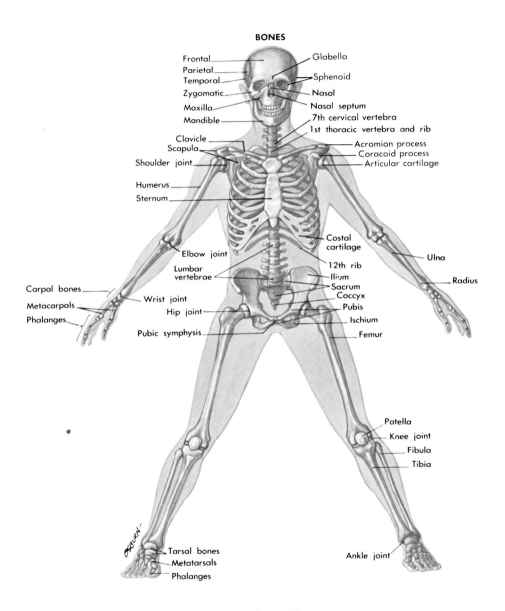

BONES

Frontal
Parietal
Temporal
Zygomatic
Maxilla
Mandible
Clavicle
Scapula
Shoulder joint
Humerus
Sternum
Elbow joint
Lumbar vertebrae
Carpal bones
Metacarpals
Phalanges
Wrist joint
Hip joint
Pubic symphysis

Glabella
Sphenoid
Nasal
Nasal septum
7th cervical vertebra
1st thoracic vertebra and rib
Acromion process
Coracoid process
Articular cartilage
Costal cartilage
12th rib
Ilium
Sacrum
Coccyx
Pubis
Ischium
Femur
Ulna
Radius

Patella
Knee joint
Fibula
Tibia

Tarsal bones
Metatarsals
Phalanges

Ankle joint

Designed by
WILLIAM A. OSBURN, M.M.A.
Artwork by
ELLEN COLE
ROBERT DEMAREST
GRANT LASHBROOK
WILLIAM OSBURN
W. B. SAUNDERS COMPANY
Philadelphia — London — Toronto

Plate 1

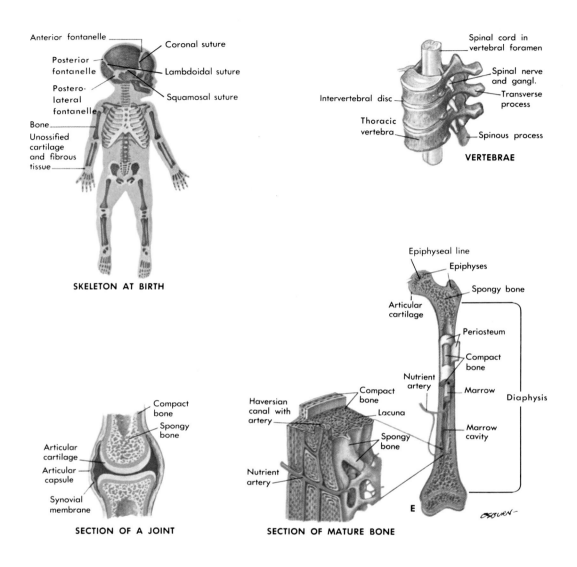

SKELETON AT BIRTH

Anterior fontanelle
Coronal suture
Posterior fontanelle
Lambdoidal suture
Postero-lateral fontanelle
Squamosal suture
Bone
Unossified cartilage and fibrous tissue

VERTEBRAE

Spinal cord in vertebral foramen
Spinal nerve and gangl.
Intervertebral disc
Transverse process
Thoracic vertebra
Spinous process

SECTION OF A JOINT

Compact bone
Spongy bone
Articular cartilage
Articular capsule
Synovial membrane

SECTION OF MATURE BONE

Haversian canal with artery
Compact bone
Lacuna
Nutrient artery
Spongy bone

Epiphyseal line
Epiphyses
Spongy bone
Articular cartilage
Periosteum
Compact bone
Nutrient artery
Marrow
Marrow cavity
Diaphysis
E

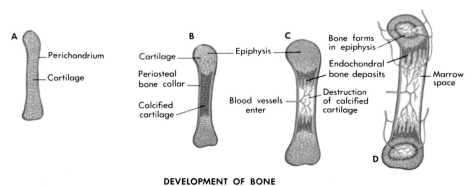

DEVELOPMENT OF BONE

A
Perichondrium
Cartilage

B
Cartilage
Epiphysis
Periosteal bone collar
Calcified cartilage

C
Bone forms in epiphysis
Endochondral bone deposits
Blood vessels enter
Destruction of calcified cartilage

D
Marrow space

Plate 2

SKELETAL MUSCLES

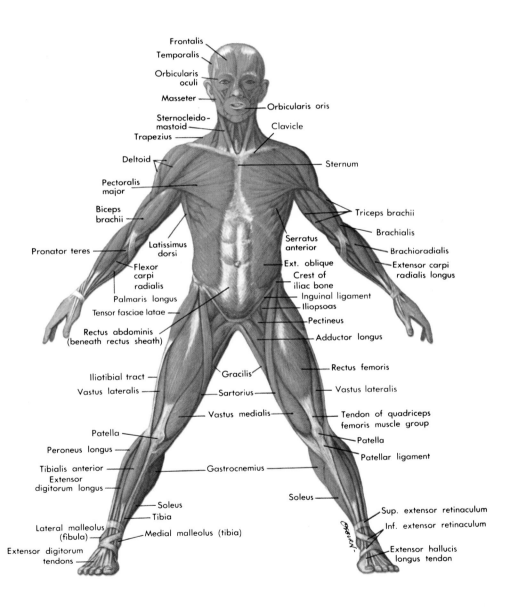

Frontalis
Temporalis
Orbicularis oculi
Masseter
Orbicularis oris
Sternocleido-mastoid
Clavicle
Trapezius
Deltoid
Sternum
Pectoralis major
Biceps brachii
Triceps brachii
Brachialis
Pronator teres
Latissimus dorsi
Serratus anterior
Brachioradialis
Flexor carpi radialis
Ext. oblique
Extensor carpi radialis longus
Crest of iliac bone
Palmaris longus
Inguinal ligament
Iliopsoas
Tensor fasciae latae
Pectineus
Rectus abdominis (beneath rectus sheath)
Adductor longus
Iliotibial tract
Gracilis
Rectus femoris
Vastus lateralis
Sartorius
Vastus lateralis
Vastus medialis
Tendon of quadriceps femoris muscle group
Patella
Patella
Peroneus longus
Patellar ligament
Tibialis anterior
Gastrocnemius
Extensor digitorum longus
Soleus
Soleus
Sup. extensor retinaculum
Tibia
Inf. extensor retinaculum
Lateral malleolus (fibula)
Medial malleolus (tibia)
Extensor digitorum tendons
Extensor hallucis longus tendon

Plate 3

HOW A MUSCLE CONTRACTS

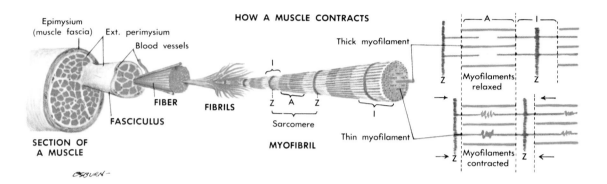

Epimysium (muscle fascia)
Ext. perimysium
Blood vessels
FIBER
FASCICULUS
SECTION OF A MUSCLE
OSBURN

FIBRILS

I
Z A Z
Sarcomere
MYOFIBRIL

Thick myofilament
Thin myofilament
I

A I
Z
Myofilaments relaxed
Z
Z
Myofilaments contracted
Z

HOW A MUSCLE ATTACHES TO BONE

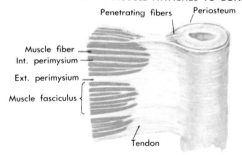

Penetrating fibers
Periosteum
Muscle fiber
Int. perimysium
Ext. perimysium
Muscle fasciculus
Tendon

The connective tissue which surrounds the muscle fibers and bundles may (1) form a tendon which fuses with the periosteum, or (2) may fuse directly with the periosteum without forming a tendon.

HOW A MUSCLE PRODUCES MOVEMENT

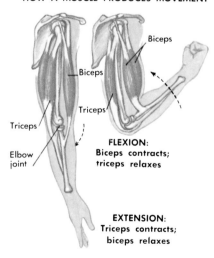

Biceps
Biceps
Triceps
Triceps
Elbow joint

FLEXION:
Biceps contracts; triceps relaxes

EXTENSION:
Triceps contracts; biceps relaxes

Plate 4

RESPIRATION AND THE HEART

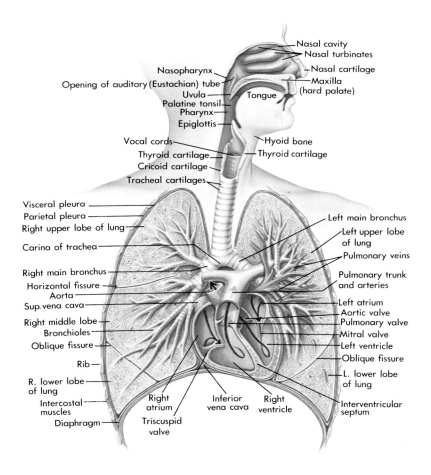

Nasal cavity
Nasal turbinates
Nasopharynx
Nasal cartilage
Opening of auditory (Eustachian) tube
Maxilla
(hard palate)
Uvula
Tongue
Palatine tonsil
Pharynx
Epiglottis
Vocal cords
Hyoid bone
Thyroid cartilage
Thyroid cartilage
Cricoid cartilage
Tracheal cartilages
Visceral pleura
Parietal pleura
Left main bronchus
Right upper lobe of lung
Left upper lobe
of lung
Carina of trachea
Pulmonary veins
Right main bronchus
Pulmonary trunk
and arteries
Horizontal fissure
Aorta
Sup. vena cava
Left atrium
Aortic valve
Right middle lobe
Pulmonary valve
Bronchioles
Mitral valve
Oblique fissure
Left ventricle
Rib
Oblique fissure
R. lower lobe
of lung
L. lower lobe
of lung
Intercostal
muscles
Right
atrium
Inferior
vena cava
Right
ventricle
Interventricular
septum
Diaphragm
Triscuspid
valve

Plate 5

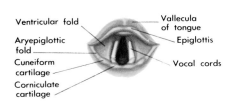

Ventricular fold

Vallecula
of tongue

Aryepiglottic
fold

Epiglottis

Cuneiform
cartilage

Vocal cords

Corniculate
cartilage

SUPERIOR VIEW OF LARYNX

Epiglottis

Hyoid
bone

Thyrohyoid
membrane

Cricothyroid
membrane

Thyroid
cartilage

Cricoid
cartilage

LATERAL VIEW OF THE LARYNX

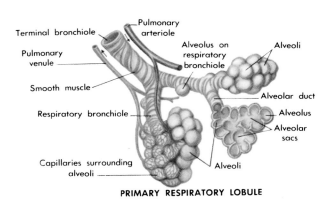

Terminal bronchiole

Pulmonary
arteriole

Pulmonary
venule

Alveolus on
respiratory
bronchiole

Alveoli

Smooth muscle

Alveolar duct

Respiratory bronchiole

Alveolus

Alveolar
sacs

Capillaries surrounding
alveoli

Alveoli

PRIMARY RESPIRATORY LOBULE

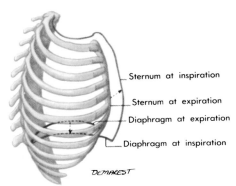

Sternum at inspiration

Sternum at expiration

Diaphragm at expiration

Diaphragm at inspiration

DEMAREST

THORACIC RESPIRATORY MOVEMENTS

Plate 6

BLOOD VASCULAR SYSTEM
VEINS

STRUCTURE

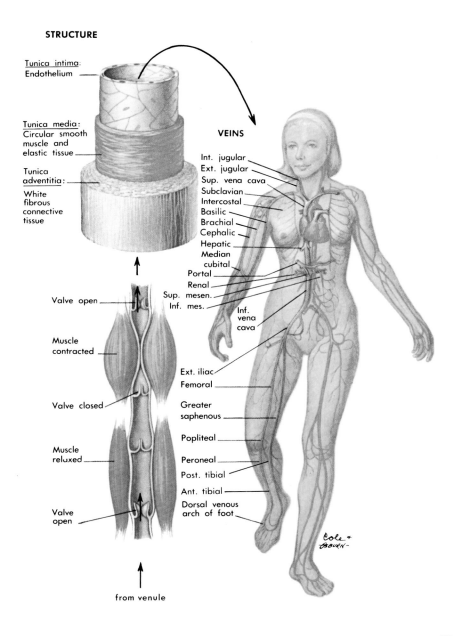

Tunica intima:
Endothelium

Tunica media:
Circular smooth
muscle and
elastic tissue

Tunica
adventitia:

White
fibrous
connective
tissue

Valve open

Muscle
contracted

Valve closed

Muscle
reluxed

Valve
open

from venule

VEINS

Int. jugular
Ext. jugular
Sup. vena cava
Subclavian
Intercostal
Basilic
Brachial
Cephalic
Hepatic
Median
cubital
Portal
Renal
Sup. mesen.
Inf. mes.
Inf.
vena
cava

Ext. iliac
Femoral

Greater
saphenous

Popliteal

Peroneal
Post. tibial

Ant. tibial

Dorsal venous
arch of foot

Cole +
Osburn

Plate 7

ARTERIES

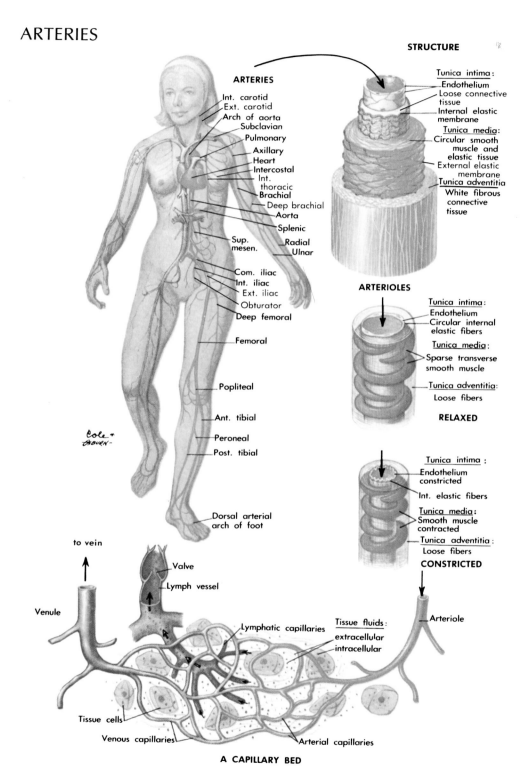

STRUCTURE

Tunica intima:
Endothelium
Loose connective tissue
Internal elastic membrane
Tunica media:
Circular smooth muscle and elastic tissue
External elastic membrane
Tunica adventitia
White fibrous connective tissue

ARTERIES

Int. carotid
Ext. carotid
Arch of aorta
Subclavian
Pulmonary
Axillary
Heart
Intercostal
Int. thoracic
Brachial
Deep brachial
Aorta
Splenic
Sup. mesen.
Radial
Ulnar
Com. iliac
Int. iliac
Ext. iliac
Obturator
Deep femoral
Femoral
Popliteal
Ant. tibial
Peroneal
Post. tibial
Dorsal arterial arch of foot

ARTERIOLES

Tunica intima:
Endothelium
Circular internal elastic fibers
Tunica media:
Sparse transverse smooth muscle
Tunica adventitia:
Loose fibers

RELAXED

Tunica intima:
Endothelium constricted
Int. elastic fibers
Tunica media:
Smooth muscle contracted
Tunica adventitia:
Loose fibers

CONSTRICTED

to vein
Valve
Lymph vessel
Venule
Lymphatic capillaries
Tissue fluids:
extracellular
intracellular
Arteriole
Tissue cells
Venous capillaries
Arterial capillaries

A CAPILLARY BED

Plate 8

DIGESTIVE SYSTEM

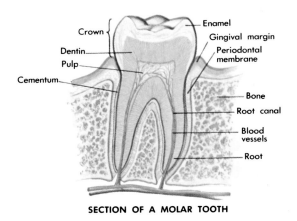

SECTION OF A MOLAR TOOTH

Crown
Dentin
Pulp
Cementum

Enamel
Gingival margin
Periodontal membrane
Bone
Root canal
Blood vessels
Root

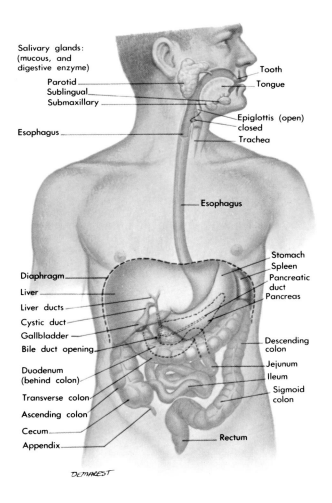

Salivary glands:
(mucous, and digestive enzyme)
Parotid
Sublingual
Submaxillary
Esophagus

Tooth
Tongue
Epiglottis (open)
closed
Trachea

Esophagus

Diaphragm
Liver
Liver ducts
Cystic duct
Gallbladder
Bile duct opening
Duodenum (behind colon)
Transverse colon
Ascending colon
Cecum
Appendix

Stomach
Spleen
Pancreatic duct
Pancreas
Descending colon
Jejunum
Ileum
Sigmoid colon
Rectum

DEMAREST

Plate 9

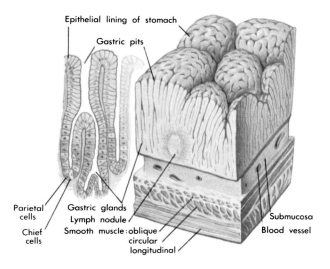

Epithelial lining of stomach

Gastric pits

Parietal cells

Chief cells

Gastric glands

Lymph nodule

Smooth muscle: oblique
circular
longitudinal

Submucosa

Blood vessel

SECTION OF STOMACH WALL

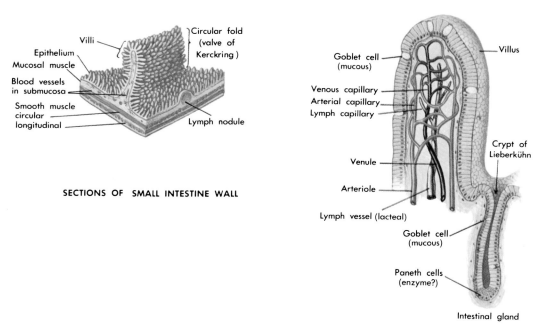

Villi

Epithelium

Mucosal muscle

Blood vessels in submucosa

Smooth muscle
circular
longitudinal

Circular fold (valve of Kerckring)

Lymph nodule

SECTIONS OF SMALL INTESTINE WALL

Goblet cell (mucous)

Venous capillary

Arterial capillary

Lymph capillary

Venule

Arteriole

Lymph vessel (lacteal)

Villus

Crypt of Lieberkühn

Goblet cell (mucous)

Paneth cells (enzyme?)

Intestinal gland

Epithelial lining

Openings of glands

Intestinal gland

Submucosal blood vessels

Smooth muscle (circular)

Longitudinal muscle band

DEMAREST

SECTION OF LARGE INTESTINE (COLON)

Plate 10

GENITOURINARY SYSTEM

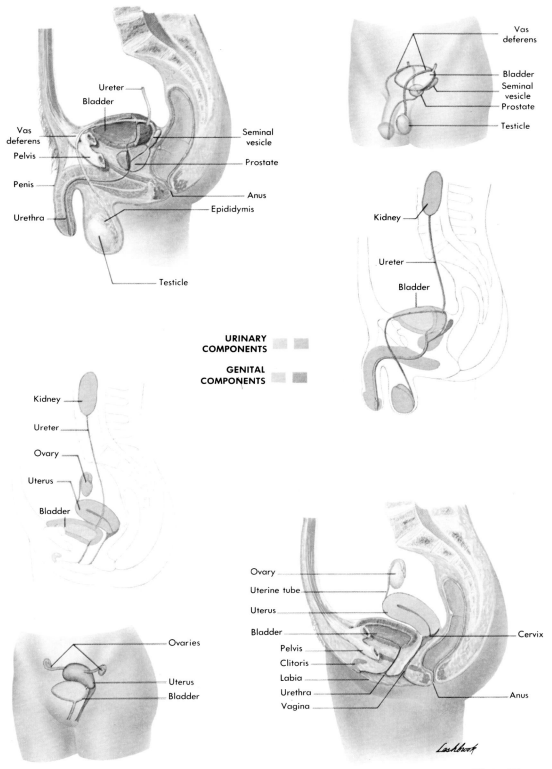

Ureter

Bladder

Vas deferens

Pelvis

Penis

Urethra

Seminal vesicle

Prostate

Anus

Epididymis

Testicle

Vas deferens

Bladder
Seminal vesicle
Prostate

Testicle

Kidney

Ureter

Bladder

URINARY COMPONENTS

GENITAL COMPONENTS

Kidney

Ureter

Ovary

Uterus

Bladder

Ovaries

Uterus

Bladder

Ovary

Uterine tube

Uterus

Bladder

Pelvis

Clitoris

Labia

Urethra

Vagina

Cervix

Anus

Plate 11

STRUCTURAL HIGHLIGHTS OF THE NERVOUS SYSTEM

GENERAL ARCHITECTURE AND PHYSIOLOGY

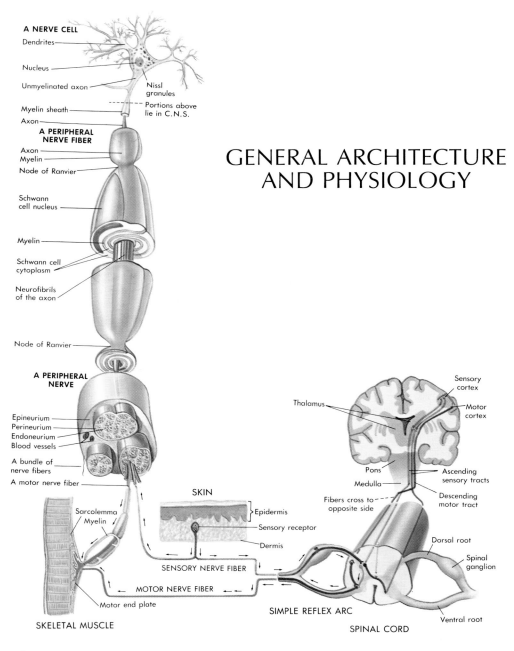

A NERVE CELL
- Dendrites
- Nucleus
- Unmyelinated axon
- Nissl granules
- Myelin sheath
- Axon
- Portions above lie in C.N.S.

A PERIPHERAL NERVE FIBER
- Axon
- Myelin
- Node of Ranvier
- Schwann cell nucleus
- Myelin
- Schwann cell cytoplasm
- Neurofibrils of the axon
- Node of Ranvier

A PERIPHERAL NERVE
- Epineurium
- Perineurium
- Endoneurium
- Blood vessels
- A bundle of nerve fibers
- A motor nerve fiber

- Sarcolemma
- Myelin
- Motor end plate

SKELETAL MUSCLE

SKIN
- Epidermis
- Sensory receptor
- Dermis

SENSORY NERVE FIBER

MOTOR NERVE FIBER

- Sensory cortex
- Thalamus
- Motor cortex
- Pons
- Medulla
- Fibers cross to opposite side
- Ascending sensory tracts
- Descending motor tract
- Dorsal root
- Spinal ganglion
- Ventral root

SIMPLE REFLEX ARC

SPINAL CORD

Plate 12

BRAIN AND SPINAL NERVES

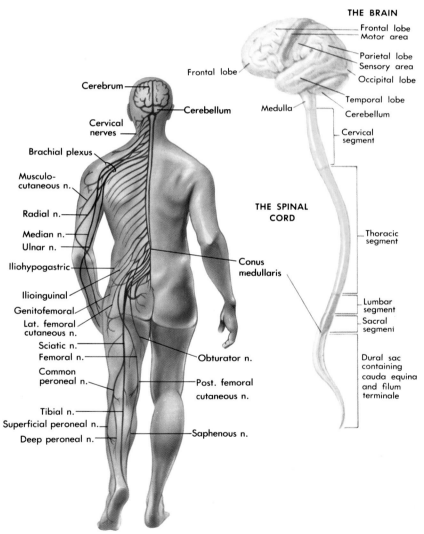

THE BRAIN

Frontal lobe
Motor area
Parietal lobe
Sensory area
Occipital lobe
Temporal lobe
Cerebellum

Frontal lobe

Medulla

Cervical
segment

**THE SPINAL
CORD**

Thoracic
segment

Lumbar
segment

Sacral
segmeni

Dural sac
containing
cauda equina
and filum
terminale

Cerebrum
Cerebellum

Cervical
nerves

Brachial plexus

Musculo-
cutaneous n.

Radial n.

Median n.
Ulnar n.

Iliohypogastric

Ilioinguinal

Genitofemoral

Lat. femoral
cutaneous n.

Sciatic n.
Femoral n.

Common
peroneal n.

Tibial n.

Superficial peroneal n.

Deep peroneal n.

Conus
medullaris

Obturator n.

Post. femoral
cutaneous n.

Saphenous n.

THE MAJOR SPINAL NERVES

Plate 13

AUTONOMIC NERVES

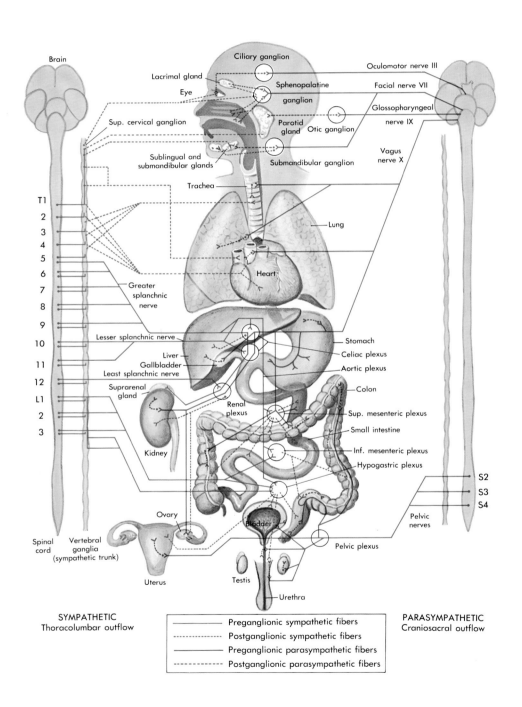

Brain

Ciliary ganglion

Oculomotor nerve III

Lacrimal gland

Sphenopalatine
ganglion

Facial nerve VII

Eye

Glossopharyngeal
nerve IX

Sup. cervical ganglion

Parotid
gland

Otic ganglion

Submandibular ganglion

Vagus
nerve X

Sublingual and
submandibular glands

Trachea

T1

2

3

4

Lung

5

6

Heart

7

Greater
splanchnic
nerve

8

9

Lesser splanchnic nerve

Stomach

10

Liver

Celiac plexus

Gallbladder

Aortic plexus

11

Least splanchnic nerve

12

Colon

Suprarenal
gland

L1

Renal
plexus

Sup. mesenteric plexus

2

Small intestine

3

Inf. mesenteric plexus

Kidney

Hypogastric plexus

S2

S3

S4

Ovary

Bladder

Pelvic
nerves

Spinal
cord

Vertebral
ganglia
(sympathetic trunk)

Pelvic plexus

Uterus

Testis

Urethra

SYMPATHETIC
Thoracolumbar outflow

———————— Preganglionic sympathetic fibers
- - - - - - - - Postganglionic sympathetic fibers
———————— Preganglionic parasympathetic fibers
- - - - - - - - Postganglionic parasympathetic fibers

PARASYMPATHETIC
Craniosacral outflow

Plate 14

ORGANS OF SPECIAL SENSE

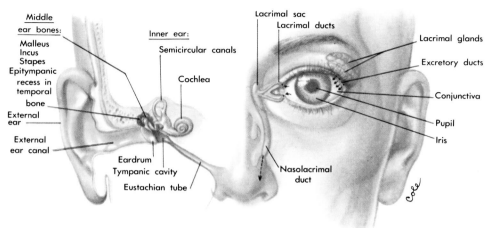

Middle ear bones:
Malleus
Incus
Stapes
Epitympanic recess in temporal bone
External ear
External ear canal

Inner ear:
Semicircular canals
Cochlea

Eardrum
Tympanic cavity
Eustachian tube

Lacrimal sac
Lacrimal ducts
Lacrimal glands
Excretory ducts
Conjunctiva
Pupil
Iris
Nasolacrimal duct

THE ORGAN OF HEARING

THE LACRIMAL APPARATUS AND THE EYE

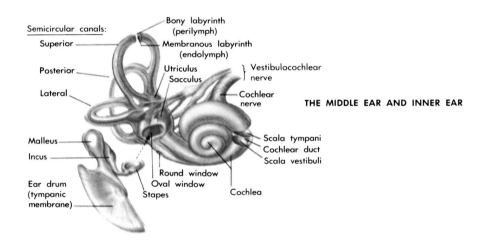

Semicircular canals:
Superior
Posterior
Lateral

Bony labyrinth (perilymph)
Membranous labyrinth (endolymph)
Utriculus
Sacculus
Vestibulocochlear nerve
Cochlear nerve

Malleus
Incus

Ear drum (tympanic membrane)

Round window
Oval window
Stapes

Scala tympani
Cochlear duct
Scala vestibuli

Cochlea

THE MIDDLE EAR AND INNER EAR

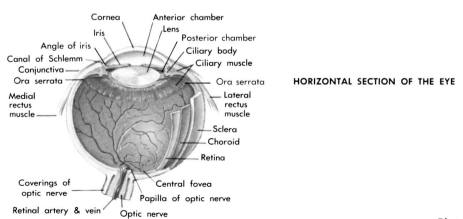

Cornea
Iris
Angle of iris
Canal of Schlemm
Conjunctiva
Ora serrata
Medial rectus muscle

Anterior chamber
Lens
Posterior chamber
Ciliary body
Ciliary muscle
Ora serrata
Lateral rectus muscle
Sclera
Choroid
Retina

Coverings of optic nerve
Retinal artery & vein
Central fovea
Papilla of optic nerve
Optic nerve

HORIZONTAL SECTION OF THE EYE

Plate 15

PARANASAL
SINUSES

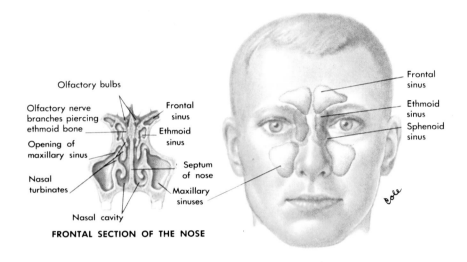

Olfactory bulbs

Olfactory nerve
branches piercing
ethmoid bone

Frontal
sinus

Ethmoid
sinus

Opening of
maxillary sinus

Septum
of nose

Nasal
turbinates

Maxillary
sinuses

Nasal cavity

FRONTAL SECTION OF THE NOSE

Frontal
sinus

Ethmoid
sinus

Sphenoid
sinus

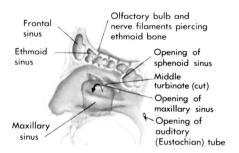

Frontal
sinus

Olfactory bulb and
nerve filaments piercing
ethmoid bone

Ethmoid
sinus

Opening of
sphenoid sinus

Middle
turbinate (cut)

Opening of
maxillary sinus

Maxillary
sinus

Opening of
auditory
(Eustachian) tube

SAGITTAL SECTION OF THE NOSE

Plate 16

abet Encourage or support. (4)*

abrasion Rubbing or scraping of the skin or mucous membrane, such as a "skinned knee." (30)

abscess A localized collection of pus located directly under the skin or deep within the body that may result in tissue destruction. (24)

accelerating Causing to act or move faster. (3)

account balance The difference between the total debits (charges) and the total credits (payments). (13)

accounting equation Assets = Liabilities + Proprietorship. (13)

accounts payable Amounts charged and not paid. (13)

accounts receivable ledger A record of the amounts owed by all the physician's patients. (13)

accounts receivable ratio A formula for measuring how fast outstanding accounts are being paid. (15)

accuracy How close a determination is to the actual value. (33)

acidosis Chemical imbalance caused by a decrease in the alkaline content of body fluids. (28)

administrative Having to do with management duties. In medical assisting, refers to all "front office" activities. (1)

agar A substance extracted from algae that is used in the laboratory to grow cultures of bacteria and other microorganisms. (22)

age analysis A procedure for classifying accounts receivable by age from the first date of billing. (15)

agenda A list of the specific items under each division of the order of business to be presented at a business meeting. (17)

agglutination The clumping together of particles (antigens or antibodies) resulting from their interaction with specific antibodies (or antigens), with a visible aggregate being formed; used in laboratory tests for blood typing and many tests for disease. (34)

aliquot A portion of well-mixed sample that is removed for testing. (33)

allergic reaction Bodily response brought about by a hypersensitivity to certain irritating substances. (7)

allied health professionals Health-related personnel who fulfill necessary functions, including those of assisting, facilitating, and complementing the work of physicians and other specialists in health care systems. (1)

alphabetic filing Any system that arranges names or topics according to the sequence of letters in the alphabet. (11)

alpha-numeric Systems made up of combinations of letters and numbers. (11)

amenorrhea Absence of menstruation. (29)

amino acid One of 20 organic compounds that form the chief constituents of proteins. (21)

ampule A small (usually one dose) glass container of medication prepared for parenteral administration. (30)

anaphylactic shock A serious and profound state of shock brought about by anaphylaxis to an allergen. (39)

anaphylaxis An exaggerated reaction to a foreign protein; hypersensitivity. (39)

ancillary Subordinate, auxiliary. (19)

anemia An abnormal decrease in the red blood cell count, hemoglobin, or hematocrit caused by increased red blood cell destruction or inability to produce sufficient amounts of normal red blood cells. (36)

angina pectoris Acute pain in the chest, resulting from a decreased blood supply to the heart muscles. (26)

anhydrosis Reduced or suppressed sweating. (23)

ankylosis Stiffening or immobility of a joint resulting from disease, trauma, heredity, or surgery. (29)

annotate To furnish with notes, which are usually critical or explanatory. (10)

anorexia nervosa An emotional condition characterized by a refusal to eat and an altered physical image. (21)

antibody An immunoglobulin produced by lymphoid tissue in response to stimulus by bacterial, viral, or other antigens that protects the body from infection by that organism. (33)

anticoagulant A substance added to a blood sample that prevents coagulation. (33)

appraisal Setting a value on, or judging as to quality. (19)

approximate To bring wound or skin edges together. (31)

approximation The act or process of drawing together skin or wound edges. (30)

arbitration The hearing and determination of a cause in controversy by a person or persons either chosen by the parties involved or appointed under statutory authority. (5)

arbitrator A neutral person chosen to settle differences between two parties in controversy. (5)

---

*Number(s) in parentheses refers to chapter(s) in which term is primarily used.

arrhythmia Irregular heartbeat. (25, 29, 37)

arteriosclerosis A condition caused by diseases that thicken, and thus decrease the elasticity of, artery walls. (25)

arthritis Inflammation of a joint or many joints. (32)

artificial insemination The introduction of semen into the vagina or cervix by artificial means. (4)

assault An intentional, unlawful attempt of bodily injury to another by force. (5)

assignment of insurance benefits A statement authorizing the insurance company to pay benefits directly to the physician. (12, 16)

asthma Panting and wheezing caused by bronchial tube swelling or spasm. (29)

atherosclerosis A specific type of arteriosclerosis in which the artery walls become thick and, thus, less elastic. (25)

atrophy Wasting away, decrease in size from normal. (32)

auscultation The act of listening for sounds within the body. (2)

avocational Pertaining to a subordinate occupation or a hobby. (20)

bacteria One-celled microscopic organisms. (2)

bariatrics Medical specialty for the prevention, control, and treatment of obesity. (29)

battery A willful and unlawful use of force or violence upon the person of another. (5)

beneficiary The person receiving the benefits of an insurance policy. (16)

bilirubin The orange-yellow pigment that is formed from the breakdown of hemoglobin in old red blood cells. (28)

biopsy The excision of a small sample of living tissue from the human body for diagnostic or therapeutic purposes. (24)

biotin A type of B-complex vitamin. (21)

bruit An abnormal sound or murmur heard on auscultation of an organ or gland. (28)

buffy coat The white layer separating the plasma and the red blood cell layers in a centrifuged hematocrit; it contains the white cells and the platelets. An increase in the size of the buffy layer, or buffy coat, should be investigated. (36)

bulimia An abnormal increase in hunger characterized by binge eating and self-induced vomiting. (21)

bursitis Inflammation of a bursa, especially in the shoulder or knee. (32)

calorie The amount of heat necessary to raise the temperature of 1 kilogram of water 1 degree Celsius, or a pint of water 4 degrees Fahrenheit. (21)

candid Frank, straightforward. (19)

cannula A flexible tube that surrounds a sharp pointed trocar for insertion. The trocar is withdrawn and fluid escapes from the body through the cannula. (24)

capital purchase Purchase of a major item of furniture or equipment. (18)

caption A heading, title, or subtitle under which records are filed. (11)

cardiac arrest Sudden stopping of the heart and circulatory system. (37)

cardiotonic Increasing tonicity of the heart. (26)

carotene The yellow or red pigment from, for example, carrots, sweet potatoes, milk fat, and egg yolk that the body converts to vitamin A. (21)

categorically Pertaining to a division in any classification system. (18)

causative The organism or substance that is responsible for an effect or condition. (23)

caustics Substances that burn or destroy organic tissue by chemical action. (18, 30)

cauterization Destruction of tissue by chemicals, heat, electricity, or freezing. (29)

cellulose A carbohydrate that forms the structure of most plants. (21)

censure Act of blaming or condemning sternly. (4)

centrifuge An instrument that separates portions of samples by rapidly spinning them in a container. (36)

cerebrospinal fluid (CSF) The fluid that flows through and protects the ventricles of the brain and that can be removed by lumbar puncture for the purpose of analysis. (33)

cerumen The soft, brown wax-like secretion of the sebaceous glands found in the external ear canal. (24)

chancre A hard ulcer appearing in primary syphilis that is filled with spirochetes and is highly contagious. (29)

chemotherapy The treatment of disease by chemical agents. (2)

cholesterol A substance found in plant and animal fats, such as saturated oils, egg yolk, and milk, that is currently thought to produce fatty deposits in blood vessels. (21)

choline An essential part of the diet of mammals that helps to prevent the deposition of fat in the liver. (21)

chronologic In the order of time. (20)

chronologic file A file in which items are filed by date. (11)

circumvention Going around, or avoidance. (19)

claim A demand to the insurer by the insured person for the payment of benefits under a policy. (16)

clarity The state of being clear; lucidity. (9)

clinical Pertaining to actual observation and treatment of patients. (1)

coagulable Capable of being formed into clots. (23)

coagulative Capable of forming clots.

coagulum A blood clot. (31)

coinsurance/copayment A policy provision by

which both the insured person and the insurer share in a specified ratio the expenses resulting from an illness or injury. (16)

collection ratio A formula for measuring the effectiveness of the billing system. (15)

colloquialism An expression acceptable and correct in ordinary conversation, or informal speech, but unsuited to formal speech or writing. (17)

colony The visible growth on a culture plate, usually resulting from a single bacterium. (34)

colony count The number of colonies on a culture plate that directly indicates the number of bacteria (colony-forming units) in a volume of urine, usually 1 milliliter. (34)

communicable Capable of being transmitted from one person to another. (5)

compulsory Obligatory; enforced. (4)

concise Expressing much in brief form. (10)

condylomata Soft, moist, pink or red swellings that grow rapidly and have a cauliflower appearance. Sexually transmitted, they are known as "genital warts." (31)

congenital Diseases or deformities that are present at birth or transmitted directly from the parent(s). Syphilis, German measles, and AIDS are examples. (29)

congestive heart failure A condition in which the heart is unable to pump the body's required amount of blood, resulting in accumulation of fluid in the abdomen, legs, or lungs. (25)

contagious Transmitted readily from one person to another by direct or indirect contact. (5)

contamination The act of soiling, staining, or polluting, especially the introduction of infectious materials or germs that produce disease. (2)

continuation page The second and following pages of a letter. (10)

continuing education units (CEUs) Units granted for attending approved seminars, lectures, and scientific meetings as well as formal courses in accredited colleges and universities. (5)

continuity Quality or state of being continuous. (11)

contraindication The presence of a disease or condition that renders a specific type of treatment improper or undesirable. (29)

controversial Disputable; leading to conflict. (7)

convulsion An involuntary contraction or a series of contractions of voluntary muscles. (39)

corporeal Pertaining to the human body. (23)

correlation The act or process of correlating; mutual relation. (11)

cretinism Congenital condition characterized by diminished development and dystrophy of bones and soft tissues as well as some mental retardation resulting from hypofunctioning of the thyroid gland. (21)

cross-reference A notation in a file indicating that a record is stored elsewhere and giving the reference. (11)

curettage The act of scraping a body cavity with a surgical instrument such as a curette. (24)

cyanosis A state of bluish coloration of the skin and mucous membranes caused by a lowered level of oxygen in the blood. (28)

cyst A sac of fluid or semisolid material located in or under the skin. (24)

daisy wheel A printing element of an electric typewriter or printer that consists of a disc with spokes bearing type. (10)

débridement The surgical removal of damaged, diseased, or contaminated tissue until healthy tissue is exposed. (30, 31)

deductible A statement in an insurance policy that the insuring company will pay the expenses incurred after the insured person has paid a specified amount. (16)

defibrillator A machine that stops atrial or ventricular fibrillation by electric shock. (37)

deficiencies Conditions characterized by a less than normal intake of a particular substance. (21)

demographic Relating to the statistical characteristics of populations, such as births, marriages, mortality, health, and so forth. (11)

denervation A condition in which the nerve supply has been blocked. (32)

desiccation Drying. (23)

desquamation The shedding, in scales or sheets, of epithelial cells of the skin. (30)

deviation A noticeable or marked departure from accepted norms of behavior. (8)

diabetes mellitus A disorder of carbohydrate metabolism caused by underproduction of insulin and characterized by excessive urinary output. (21)

dialysis The process of separating out from the blood the harmful waste products of the body that are normally removed by the kidney. (2)

diction Choice of words to express ideas, especially with regard to correctness, clearness, or effectiveness. (9)

dietitian A member of the health care team holding a bachelor's degree in foods and nutrition who is concerned with the maintenance and promotion of health and the treatment of disease via use of the diet. (21)

digestion The process of converting food into chemical substances that can be used by the body. (21)

dilatation Opening or widening the circumference of a body orifice with a dilating instrument. (24)

dilemma A situation involving choice between equally unsatisfactory alternatives. (4)

diluent A substance, such as water, that renders a drug or a solution less potent. (30)

diplopia Double vision resulting from muscle irregularity, which places the eyes so that light rays fall upon different parts of the retinas and produce two images. (29)

direct filing system A filing plan whereby materials can be located without consulting an intermediary source of reference. (11)

disability The condition resulting from illness or injury that makes an individual unable to be employed. (16)

disbursements Funds paid out. (13, 14)

discrepancy A state of disagreement. (4)

discretion Quality of being discreet, tactful, or prudent. (1)

discrimination A distinction based on race, religion, sex, or some other factor, especially one resulting in unfair or injurious treatment of an individual belonging to a particular group. (19)

disruption A breaking down or an upset. (8)

dissect To cut or separate tissues with a cutting instrument or surgical scissors. (24)

dissemination The act of broadcasting or spreading over a considerable area. (3, 19)

diuretic An agent or drug that causes the body to produce and excrete an increased amount of urine. (21)

dual pitch Capability of a typewriter or printer to produce either elite or pica spacing. (10)

dyspnea Labored or difficult breathing. (37)

eczema A skin reaction to stimulants or irritants that causes redness, blistering, itching, and, later, scaling. This allergic reaction occurs most frequently in childhood. (29)

edit To correct and prepare for publication. (10)

effective date The date on which an insurance policy starts to take effect. (16)

elite type Type that produces 12 characters to the inch. (10)

emancipated minor A person under legal age who is self-supporting and living apart from parents or guardian. (5, 15)

embryology The science of the development of the individual during the embryonic stage. (2)

empathy Projection of one's own consciousness into the state of mind of another being, and understanding that person's feelings, wishes, ideas, and so on. (1)

emphysema A pathologic accumulation of air in the tissues or organs such as in pulmonary emphysema, in which the bronchioles become plugged with mucus and lose elasticity. (28)

endogenous Produced within, or caused by factors within, the organism. (21, 28)

endorsement Sanction or approval. (5)

endorser Person who signs his or her name on the back of a check for the purpose of transferring title to another person. (14)

endotoxin A poisonous substance found in the walls of certain bacteria (usually Gram-negative rods) that is released after the death of the bacterium, causing fever, chills, and other symptoms. (34)

enunciation Act of pronouncing words distinctly. (9)

enzymatic reaction A chemical reaction that is controlled by an enzyme. (35)

erythema A red color of the skin due to capillary congestion resulting from injury, infection, or inflammation. (29, 32)

exclusions Specific hazards or conditions listed in an insurance policy for which the policy will not provide benefit payments. (16)

excoriation Any injury to the skin caused by an abrasion or by scratching. (28)

exogenous Produced outside or caused by factors outside the organism. (21, 28)

exophthalmos An abnormal protrusion of the eye. (28)

expeditiously Efficiently and quickly. (19)

expendable Supplies or equipment that are normally used up or consumed in service. (18)

expulsion Act of expelling or forcing out. (4)

externship The practice of receiving employment experience in qualified health care facilities under the cooperative supervision of the medical staff and the program instructor as part of the education curriculum. (1, 20)

extracurricular Relating to those activities that form part of the life of students but are not part of the courses of study. (20)

extravasation Bleeding into the tissues. (32)

facilitate Make easier or more convenient. (18)

fascia A sheet or band of fibrous tissue, deep in the skin, that covers muscles and body organs. (30)

fast(ing) To go without food for a specified period of time (usually 12 to 14 hours) prior to the collection of samples for analysis. (33)

fee profile A compilation of a physician's fees over a given period of time. (12)

fee schedule A list of services or procedures indemnified by the insurance company and the specific dollars that will be paid for each service. (16)

fee splitting Sharing a fee with another physician, laboratory, or drug company, not based on services performed. (4)

fiber Component of food resistant to chemical digestion. (21)

filing system A plan for organizing records so that they can be found when needed. (11)

fiscal agent A financial representative. (12)

fistula An abnormal, tube-like passage within the body tissues. (24)

format Shape, size, and general makeup of a publication. (20)

freestanding emergency center An emergency facility not associated with a hospital. (1)

galley proof A proof from type on a galley before it is made up into pages. (17)

galvanometer An instrument that measures current by electromagnetic action. (37)

general journal A book of original entry in accounting. (13)

genetics The branch of biology dealing with heredity and variation among related organisms. (4)

ghost surgery A situation in which a patient has consented to have surgery done by surgeon A, but without the patient's knowledge or consent the surgery is actually performed by surgeon B. (4)

glaucoma A disease of the eye in which an increase in intraocular pressure may cause blindness as a result of shrinking of the optic nerve. (24)

gliadin A protein, from wheat, that is soluble in alcohols. (21)

glycogen A polysaccharide that is the principal form in which carbohydrate is stored in animal tissues. (21)

goiter An enlargement of the thyroid gland. (21)

gonadal Pertaining to the sex glands, the ovary in the female, and the testis in the male. (21)

group practice The provision of services by a group of at least three practitioners. (1)

haughty Arrogant; disdainfully or contemptuously proud. (7)

health maintenance organization (HMO) An organization that provides for comprehensive health care to an enrolled group for a fixed periodic payment. (1)

hemangioma A benign tumor of dilated blood vessels. (31)

hematoma A localized collection of clotted blood caused by a broken blood vessel. (31)

hemiplegia Paralysis of one side of the body. (2)

hemolysis The destruction of red blood cells. (34)

hemolyzed A blood sample in which the red cells have ruptured. (33)

hermetically sealed Sealed so that no air is allowed to enter. (27)

histologist One who specializes in the study of the minute structure, composition, and function of the tissues. (2)

hydrocele A painless swelling of the scrotum caused by a collection of fluid in the testis. (28)

hydrocephaly An abnormal accumulation of cerebral spinal fluid (CSF) within the skull resulting from defective absorption of CSF, excessive production of CSF, or circulatory blockage of CSF (also referred to as "water on the brain"). (29)

hydrogenated Combined with, treated with, or exposed to hydrogen. (21)

hyperventilation A condition caused by excessively prolonged deep breathing that results in an abnormally high level of air in the lungs. It is usually associated with anxiety and emotional tension. (25)

immunology A science that deals with the phenomena and the causes of immunity and immune responses. (2)

in situ Localized. (31)

in vitro In glass; in a test tube or other artificial environment. (4)

incontinence The inability to control the excretion of urine or feces. (29)

indemnity A benefit paid by an insurer for a loss insured under a policy. (16)

induration The process of hardening or an abnormally hard spot or place in the tissues. (29)

informed consent A consent in which there is understanding of what is to be done and the risks involved, why it should be done, and alternative methods of treatment available and their attendant risks. The alternatives include the failure to treat and the attendant risk. (5)

innovation Act of introducing something new or novel. (2)

inoculate To place a specimen in a culture medium to allow it to grow so that it can be identified. (34)

insubordination Refusing to submit to authority. (19)

insulin shock Shock brought about by too much insulin, too little food, or excessive exercise. When untreated, can result in death. (39)

integral Essential; being an indispensable part of a whole. (8)

intercom An intercommunication system; a direct telephone line from one station to another. (7)

intermittent Coming and going at intervals; not continuous. (8)

invasion of privacy Unauthorized disclosure of a person's private affairs. (15)

inventory A list of articles with the description and quantity of each. (18)

invoice A paper describing a purchase and the amount due. (13)

ion An electrically charged particle. (26)

ionizing Process in which a neutral atom or molecule gains or loses electrons and then acquires a negative or positive electric charge. (38)

irrigation The flushing out of a cavity or wound with a solution. (31)

ischemia Decreased blood flow to a body part or organ that is caused by constriction or plugging of the supplying artery. (35)

isolation The act of placing alone, apart from others. (3)

jargon The technical vocabulary of a special group. (1)

jaundice Yellow color of the skin, sclera, and secretions resulting from increased levels of bilirubin in the blood and deposition of bile pigments (also called icterus). (28)

keratosis Any horny growth, such as warts. (31)

lesion A wound, sore, ulcer, tumor, or any traumatic tissue damage that causes a lack of tissue continuity or a loss of function. (30)

lethargic Pertaining to a condition of drowsiness or indifference. (39)

leukemia A cancerous condition of the white blood cells usually resulting in the overproduction of one type of white blood cell. (36)

leukoderma A localized loss of skin pigmentation, such as the ring around a nevus. (29)

lexicographic Pertaining to an alphabetic arrangement of the words in a language. (17)

liability State or quality of being liable; that for which one is liable, such as debts. (5)

litigation Contest in a court of justice for the purpose of enforcing a right. (5, 11)

lumen An open space such as that within a blood vessel, the intestine, or an examining instrument. (24)

maker (of a check) Any individual, corporation, or legal party who signs a check or any type of negotiable instrument. (14)

malfeasance The doing of an act that is wholly wrongful and unlawful. (5)

malpractice Professional misconduct, improper discharge of professional duties, or a failure to meet the standard of care by a professional, resulting in harm to another. (5)

mandatory In the nature of a mandate or command; obligatory. (1)

matrix Something in which something else originates, develops, takes shape, or is contained. (8)

medical indigent One who is able to take care of ordinary living expenses but who cannot afford medical care. (12, 16)

member physician A physician who has agreed to accept the contracts of an insurer, which usually include accepting the insurance benefits as payment in full. (16)

meniscus The concave or convex surface of a column of liquid, such as the mercury in a sphygmomanometer. (25)

meticulous Excessively careful of small details. (19)

microcephaly Abnormal smallness of the skull. (29)

microfilming Photographing records in reduced size on film. (11)

microorganism An organism of microscopic or ultramicroscopic size. (2)

microsurgery Surgery performed under a microscope with very small instruments. (30)

misfeasance The improper performance of a lawful act. (5)

monitor To listen to the matter transmitted by telephone. (9)

monograph A learned treatise on a small area of learning; a written account of a single thing or class. (17)

mordant A chemical (Gram's iodine) used to make the primary stain (crystal violet) adhere to the cells it stains. (34)

morphology The study of the size, shape, and staining characteristics of a cell. (36)

motivation Process of inciting a person to some action or behavior. (19)

multiparous Referring to a woman who has had two or more live births. (29)

multiple-dose vial A small bottle that contains more than one dose of a medication. (30)

myoglobinuria The abnormal presence of myoglobin (a hemoglobin-like chemical of muscle tissue) in urine, as a result of muscle deterioration. (35)

myringotomy An incision into the tympanic membrane. (29)

negotiable Legally transferable to another party. (14)

neophyte A beginner. (2)

nevi Moles or birthmarks characterized by round, pigmented, flat, or raised areas varying in color from yellow-brown to black. May be present at birth or may develop later. (28)

nomogram A representation by graphs, diagrams, or charts of the relationships between numeric variables. (26)

nonfeasance The failure to do something that should have been done. (5)

numeric filing Filing records, correspondence, or cards by number. (11)

obesity An excess accumulation of body fat, usually defined as more than 20 percent above the recommended body weight. (21)

objective Something toward which effort is directed; an aim or end of action. (20)

obturator A metal rod with a smooth rounded tip, placed in hollow instruments to decrease destruction of the mucous membrane during insertion. (24)

occult Hidden, as occult disease. (33)

oral hygiene The proper care of the mouth and teeth for the maintenance of health and the prevention of disease. (7)

order of business A list of the different divisions of business in the order in which each will be called for at business meetings. (17)

orientation The determination or adjustment of one's intellectual or emotional position with reference to circumstances. (19)

osteoarthritis The most common type of arthritis, which causes the joints to degenerate. (32)

osteoporosis A disorder characterized by loss of bone tissue, occurring most frequently in small-boned, postmenopausal, sedentary women. (32)

oviducts The pair of tubes in the female that carry the egg from the ovary to the uterus; fallopian tubes. (2)

packing slip An itemized list of items in a package. (13)

pallor The absence of color of the skin, which causes unnatural paleness. (28)

pandemic Affecting the majority of the people in a country or a number of countries. (2)

pantothenic acid B complex vitamin present in all living tissues. (21)

paraplegia Paralysis of the legs and, sometimes, the lower body below the site of injury or infection of the spinal cord. (29)

parenteral Referring to administration of medication routes other than the alimentary canal, such as subcutaneous, intramuscular, or intravenous. (30)

paroxysm The sudden return or amplification of symptoms, such as a spasm or a seizure. (30, 39)

passive Referring to the movement or exercising of a part of the body by an externally applied force. (28)

patency The open condition of a body cavity or canal. (24)

pathologic Altered or caused by disease. (2)

payables Amounts owed to others. (13)

payee Person named on a draft or check as the recipient of the amount shown. (14)

payer Person who writes a check in favor of the payee. (14)

pedunculated Having a stem-like connected part. (31)

pejorative Having a negative connotation; a depreciatory word. (11)

percussion The act of striking a part with short, sharp blows, as an aid in diagnosing the condition of the underlying parts by the sound obtained. (2)

periodical A journal published with a fixed interval (more than one day) between the issues or numbers. (17)

perjured testimony Telling what is false when sworn to tell the truth. (5)

permeability The ability to allow solutions to pass through. (26)

permeable Capable of allowing a substance to pass through, such as salt through a membrane. (23)

personal inventory A complete summary of pertinent information about oneself. (20)

phagocytosis The engulfing of microorganisms, other cells, and foreign particles by phagocytes. (2)

phenylalanine An essential amino acid found in milk, eggs, and other common foods that is necessary for normal growth and development. (35)

phenylketonuria (PKU) A congenital disease resulting from a defect in protein metabolism that, when untreated, causes severe mental retardation. (21)

philosophy The general laws that furnish the rational explanation of anything. (19)

phonetic Of or pertaining to the voice or its use. (7)

photocoagulation Clotting of blood with light. (31)

photometer An instrument that measures the intensity of a beam of light passing through it; the intensity of the light beam is directly related to the concentration of the substance the beam passes through. (33)

physiologic saline A salt and water solution of 0.9 percent that is the same osmotic pressure as blood serum. (30)

pica type Type that produces ten characters to the inch. (10)

pitch The vibration frequency of a tone or sound. (9)

planing The rubbing away of a layer of tissue. (31)

polycythemia vera A condition that causes an overproduction of all formed elements of the blood, including red blood cells, white blood cells, and platelets. (36)

polyp A tumor on a stem, frequently found on the mucous membrane. (24)

posting The transfer of information from one record to another. (13)

postpartum The period of time after giving birth. (28)

power of attorney A legal statement in which a person authorizes another person to act as his or her attorney or agent; may be limited to the handling of certain procedures. The person authorized to act as agent is known as an attorney in fact. (14)

preamble An introductory portion; a preface. (4)

precept A practical rule guiding behavior or technique. (4)

precordial Pertaining to the region over the heart and lower thorax. (37)

pre-existing condition A physical condition of an insured person that existed prior to the issuance of the insurance policy. (16)

premium The periodic payment required to keep a policy in force. (16)

prerogative An exclusive and unquestionable right belonging to a person or body of persons. (8)

presbyopia Loss of elasticity of the lens of the eye, causing the near point of distinct vision to be removed farther from the eye; generally occurs after age 40. (29)

preservative A substance added to a specimen that prevents deterioration of cells or chemicals in the specimen. (33)

prevail To be common, or usual. (7)

probate Official proof, especially of an instrument offered as the last will and testament of a person deceased. (5)

probationary Pertaining to a trial or a period of trial to ascertain fitness for a job. (19)

professional courtesy Reduction or absence of fees to professional associates. (12)

Professional Standards Review Organization (PSRO) A group of physicians working with the government to review cases for hospital admission and discharge under government guidelines; sometimes referred to as Peer Review. (16)

prognosis Forecast of the course of a disease. (17)

pronunciation Act or manner of pronouncing words. (9)

proofread To check written copy for errors. (10)

propriety Quality of being proper or fitting. (7)

protein A group of organic compounds occurring in plants and animals and containing the major elements nitrogen and the amino acids, which are essential for the maintenance of life. (21)

prothrombin A substance present in blood plasma

that is converted into thrombin during the process of clotting. (21)

protocols Rules of performance. (1)

protozoa Primitive animal organisms consisting of a single cell. (2)

prudent Capable of directing or conducting oneself wisely and judiciously. (3, 5)

pruritus Itching of the skin or mucous membrane. (29)

psychologic Directed toward the mind or will. (7)

ptosis Prolapse (drooping) of an organ or body part. (29)

public domain The realm embracing property rights that belong to the community at large and are subject to appropriation by anyone. (4)

pulses The expansion and contraction of arteries that may be felt with the finger. (25)

  bounding A pulse that is faster than normal and then disappears.

  elastic A pulse that gives an elastic sensation to the finger.

  intermittent Characterized by skipped or missing pulse beats.

  irregular The pulse rate varies in strength and recurrence.

  thready A pulse that is scarcely perceptible.

  unequal Uneven, dissimilar pulse beats.

purulent Consisting of or containing pus. (2)

pyogenic Producing pus. (23)

quackery Pretense of medical skill. (5)

quality control A program required by law that monitors all phases of specimen collection, processing, testing, and reporting to ensure the accuracy of the results. (33)

rad A measurement of the actual absorbed dose of radiation (see *rem*). (38)

radiation The transfer through space of any form of energy, such as light, heat, or x-rays. (38)

radical mastectomy The complete surgical removal of a breast, the surrounding muscles, and lymphatic glands. (27)

reciprocity An obligation under which something is done or given by each of two to the other. (5)

recruitment The supplying of new members or help. (19)

reference laboratory A large laboratory that accepts specimens from smaller laboratories to perform tests not done by the smaller laboratories. (33)

regional Pertaining to a region or territory; local. (1)

rem A newer method for measuring the amount of radiation absorbed by a patient while exposed to x-rays. Similar to a *rad*. (38)

reputable Honorable; having a good reputation. (18)

requisition A multiple copy form containing patient identification, filled out when a laboratory test is requested. Copies go to the patient's chart and the business office for billing. The laboratory copy stays in the laboratory. (33)

resident A graduate and licensed physician receiving training in a specialty in a hospital. (4)

resonance Sound or echo produced by percussion of a body organ or cavity. (28)

resumé A selective summary of one's education and employment record tailored to the position being sought. (20)

retention schedule A listing of dates until which records are to be kept, based on statutes of limitations, tax regulations, and other factors. (11)

revocation The act of annulling by recalling or taking back. (4, 5)

rhinitis Acute or chronic inflammation of the mucous membrane of the nose. (29)

rider A legal document that modifies the protection of a policy. (16)

roentgen Unit used as x-ray dosage. (38)

rural Pertaining to the country, as distinguished from a city or town. (1)

screening test A laboratory test done on large numbers of people for the purpose of detecting occult disease. (34)

scurvy A condition resulting from an ascorbic acid (vitamin C) deficiency, characterized by bleeding gums and black and blue spots on the skin. (21)

seminar A group of students meeting regularly and informally with a professor for discussion of ideas and problems. (20)

senile Pertaining to old age. (31)

sensitivity disk An antibiotic-impregnated paper disc that is placed on a specially inoculated culture plate to determine whether an organism is sensitive or resistant to that antibiotic. (34)

sequential Succeeding or following in order or as a result. (11)

serum The clear, straw-colored liquid part of the blood that remains after the blood cells and fibrinogen have been filtered out. (22)

shelf filing System that uses open shelves (rather than cabinets) for storing records. (11)

slough The shedding away of dead tissue cells. (31)

solo private practice One physician practicing alone. (1)

specimen A sample of body fluid, waste product, or tissue that is collected for analysis. (33)

spermatozoa Mature male germ cells. (2)

spore The reproductive stage of certain bacteria, enabling the organism to resist unfavorable conditions, such as in the diseases tetanus, gas gangrene, and botulism. Also, the reproductive stage of fungi. (22)

sprain A traumatic injury without separation to the muscles, tendons, and ligament surrounding a joint. (32)

Stat. Do immediately (from the Latin *statim*, meaning "at once"). (33)

stat. report An immediate report. (8)

statement A request for payment. (13)

statute of limitations The time limit within which

an action may legally be brought upon a contract. (11, 15)

statutory body A part of the legislative branch of a government. (3)

stethoscope An instrument for listening to sounds within the body. (2)

strain A muscular injury resulting from excessive physical exertion. (32)

stylus A metal probe that is inserted or passed through a catheter, needle, or tube for cleaning purposes or to facilitate passage into the body orifice. (24)

subject filing Arranging records alphabetically by names of topics or things rather than by names of individuals. (11)

subscriber One named as principal in an insurance contract. (16)

subsidize To aid or promote, as a private enterprise, with public money. (15)

substantiated Having been established as true by proof or competent evidence; verified. (3)

substantive law Pertaining to or constituting the essential part or principles of the law; substantive law creates rights and obligations. (5)

superbill A combination charge slip, statement, and insurance reporting form. (15)

suppuration The production of purulent material (pus) from a wound. (24)

suspension The act of interrupting or discontinuing temporarily, but with an expectation or purpose of resumption. (4, 5)

symmetry Relative proportion of opposite sides of the body and its parts to each other. (28)

syphilitic chancre The primary sore of syphilis. (2)

tab The projection on a file folder or guide on which the caption is written. (11)

tabulation Arranging into a table or list. (10)

technical Pertaining to the practical or procedural details of a trade or profession. (1)

technologic Relating to the application of scientific knowledge or methods. (4)

teller A bank employee who is assigned the duty of waiting on the bank's customers. (14)

termination conversion An agreement by an insurance company to continue coverage of an employee after retirement or termination of employment, upon request of the insured person. (16)

tetany A continuous contraction or muscle spasm, without noticeable twitching, caused by an inadequate blood calcium level or by accidental surgical removal of the parathyroid gland. (21)

therapeutic Pertaining to the art of healing; curative. (1)

third-party check A check written to the order of the person offering payment and unknown to the payee, who is a third party in the process. (14)

third-party payer Someone other than the patient, spouse, or parent who is responsible for paying all or part of the patient's medical costs. (12)

thrombosed Enlarged because filled with clotted blood. (28)

tickler (file) A chronologic file used as a reminder that something must be taken care of on a certain date. (8, 11)

tinnitus Ringing in the ears. (28)

tone A normal state of balanced tension in muscle tissue when the muscles are at rest. (32)

tort An act that brings harm to a person or damage to property, caused negligently or intentionally. (5)

toxin A poisonous protein substance produced by some plants, animals, and pathogenic bacteria that builds up in the body as the microorganisms multiply. Toxins ingested from foods are responsible for some forms of food poisoning. (22, 34)

transcription The process of taking input in person or by machine dictation and keyboarding it by typewriter or word processor into mailable form. (10)

transfer Removing inactive records from the active files. (11)

transmitter The part of a telephone into which one speaks. (9)

traumatic Pertaining to, resulting from, or causing physical injury or emotional shock. (39)

treatise A systematic exposition or argument in writing. (17)

trespass To exceed the bounds of what is lawful, right, or just. (5)

tryptophan Essential amino acid present in high concentration in animal and fish protein. (21)

UCR (usual, customary, and reasonable) A formula for determining medical insurance benefits payable. (12)

unit Each part of a name that is used in indexing. (11)

untoward Hard to manage. (31)

urban Characteristic of or pertaining to a city or town. (1)

uremia A toxic condition in renal insufficiency that is characterized by the lack of excretion of waste nitrogenous substances in the blood. (28)

venereal Due to or propagated by sexual intercourse. (5)

vertigo Sensation of moving around in space; dizziness. (28)

vesiculation The formation of blister-like elevations on the skin. (29)

viable Able to maintain an independent state of life, such as life after birth. (23)

virulent Exceedingly pathogenic, noxious, or deadly. (2)

viscosity The quality of being a gluey substance lacking easy movement. (27)

vitiligo The loss of melanin in the skin, characterized by white patches. (28)

volatile Referring to an explosive substance's capacity to vaporize at a low temperature. (27)

Page numbers referring to illustrations and procedures are italicized; those referring to tables are followed by *t*.